INTENSIVE CAR

DEDICATION

To our wives and families without whose support this book could never have been completed. Also to the nurses, medical students and doctors in training who stimulated us to undertake this task and, through their encouragement, persuaded us to persevere to its completion.

CJH
DW

To Michael White, Professor of Medicine, University of Hull, a dear friend who died on Sunday 13th August 1995.

CJH

Commissioning Editors: Michael Parkinson, Alison Taylor
Development Editor: Hannah Kenner
Project Manager: Nancy Arnott
Design Direction: George Ajayi
Illustration Manager: Bruce Hogarth
Illustrator: Richard Prime

INTENSIVE CARE

A concise textbook

THIRD EDITION

Charles Hinds FRCP FRCA

Professor of Intensive Care Medicine
William Harvey Research Institute, Barts and The London School of Medicine and Dentistry and Barts and the London NHS Trust, London, UK

David Watson BSc (Hons) FRCA

Consultant and Senior Lecturer in Intensive Care Medicine
William Harvey Research Institute, Barts and The London School of Medicine and Dentistry and Homerton University Hospital NHS Trust, London, UK

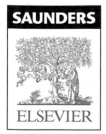

SAUNDERS

ELSEVIER

Edinburgh   London   New York   Oxford   Philadelphia   St Louis   Sydney   Toronto   2008

SAUNDERS
ELSEVIER

An imprint of Elsevier Limited

First edition 1987
Second edition 1996
Third edition 2008

ISBN: 978-0-702-02596-9

British Library Cataloguing in Publication Data
A catalogue record for this book is available from the British Library

Library of Congress Cataloging in Publication Data
A catalog record for this book is available from the Library of Congress

Note
Knowledge and best practice in this field are constantly changing. As new research and experience broaden our knowledge, changes in practice, treatment and drug therapy may become necessary or appropriate. Readers are advised to check the most current information provided (i) on procedures featured or (ii) by the manufacturer of each product to be administered, to verify the recommended dose or formula, the method and duration of administration, and contraindications. It is the responsibility of the practitioner, relying on their own experience and knowledge of the patient, to make diagnoses, to determine dosages and the best treatment for each individual patient, and to take all appropriate safety precautions. To the fullest extent of the law, neither the Publisher nor the Authors assume any liability for any injury and/or damage to persons or property arising out of or related to any use of the material contained in this book.

The Publisher

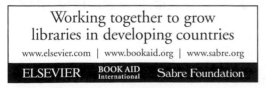

Printed in China

Contents

Preface

The last decade has witnessed tremendous advances in the theory and practice of intensive care medicine, most obviously in the number and quality of clinical trials affecting the care of our patients. To incorporate this vast amount of new knowledge succinctly has been a major challenge in preparing a new edition of our concise textbook.

This third edition has been further expanded, extensively revised and updated. In particular new, evidence-based approaches to management have been included. Additional topics, such as relative adrenal suppression, tight glycaemic control, acute coronary syndromes, ventilator-associated and community-acquired pneumonia, non-invasive and 'protective' ventilation, meningoencephalitis and intracranial haemorrhage have been introduced. Antibiotic guidelines have been updated and the latest Advanced Life Support/Advanced Trauma Life Support and surviving sepsis guidelines have been included, whilst a number of topics such as fluid and electrolyte balance, nutrition and alternatives to the pulmonary artery catheter for haemodynamic monitoring are considered in more detail. The large number of new references focus on key prospective, randomized, controlled trials, meta-analyses and systematic reviews; throughout there is an emphasis on the practice of evidence based medicine, with clear guidelines for the management of specific conditions. Where there are controversies we attempt to provide a balanced view and we cite the most relevant publications. Important physiological and scientific concepts and principles that underpin the management of critically ill patients are emphasized. Despite the inclusion of so much new material we have tried to ensure that the book remains concise and that the information continues to be readily accessible.

As before, the book is intended primarily as an introductory text for trainees in intensive care medicine. This latest edition has also been written bearing in mind the needs of those preparing for the increasingly important examinations in the specialty (e.g. the European, UK and Irish Diplomas of Intensive Care). The book is aimed not only at those embarking on specialist training in intensive care but also at trainees in other acute specialities who are increasingly becoming involved in the management of critically ill patients and those who may be sitting other postgraduate exams that include aspects of intensive care and acute medicine in the syllabus (e.g. FRCA, FRCS, MRCP). We hope the book will also prove useful for nurses and other allied health care professionals specializing in intensive care, as well as for undergraduate medical students. It may also serve as a reference text for both trainees and qualified specialists.

Once again the book has been written entirely by the two of us in an effort to ensure consistency of style and content, avoid repetition and facilitate extensive cross-referencing. For this third edition, however, every chapter has also been reviewed by an expert colleague to ensure that the content is accurate and up-to-date and that there are no serious omissions. We are deeply indebted to the following friends and colleagues who so willingly gave of their time and expertise:

Chapters 1 and 2	Dr Saxon Ridley, Glan Clwyd Hospital, Wales
Chapter 4	Dr Neil Soni, Chelsea and Westminster Hospital, London
Chapter 5	Prof. Mervyn Singer, University College Hospital, London
Chapters 6 and 7	Dr Brian Keogh, Royal Brompton Hospital, London
Chapter 8	Prof. Tim Evans, Royal Brompton Hospital, London
Chapter 9	Dr David Lipkin, Royal Free Hospital, London
Chapter 10	Mr David Skinner, John Radcliffe Hospital, Oxford
Chapter 11	Prof. Richard Griffiths, University of Liverpool, Liverpool
Chapter 12	Dr David Wareham, Barts and The London NHS Trust, London
Chapter 13	Dr Alasdair Short, Broomfield Hospital, Chelmsford, Essex
Chapter 14	Dr Julia Wendon, King's College Hospital, London
Chapter 15	Dr Peter Andrews, Western General Hospital, Edinburgh, Scotland
Chapter 16	Dr Anne Ballinger, Homerton University Hospital, London
Chapter 17	Prof. John Monson, Barts and The London NHS Trust, London
Chapter 18	Dr Catherine Nelson-Piercy, St Thomas' Hospital, London
Chapter 19	Prof. John Henry, Imperial College, London

Chapter 20	Dr Colin Ferguson, Derriford Hospital, Plymouth, Devon
Chapter 21	Dr Peter Shirley, Barts and The London NHS Trust, London

Lastly, we would like to thank the publishers for their help and forebearance. We are indebted once again to Miss Sandra Sims, our Academic Secretary, for typing the manuscript, incorporating numerous corrections and revisions with unstinting patience, and for her continued support and enthusiasm for the project. We are also grateful to Philip Salter and St Bartholomew's Hospital for providing several of the images for this book.

CJ Hinds
D Watson

List of physiological abbreviations

C_aO_2	Arterial oxygen content
$C_{a-v}O_2$	Arteriovenous oxygen content difference
$C_{a-j}O_2$	Cerebral arteriovenous (arterio-jugular bulb) oxygen content difference (also commonly abbreviated $AJDO_2$)
$C_{\bar{v}}O_2$	Mixed venous oxygen content
DO_2	Oxygen delivery
F_AO_2	Fractional concentration of oxygen in alveolar gas
F_IO_2	Fractional concentration of oxygen in inspired gas
$M\dot{V}O_2$	Myocardial oxygen consumption
PO_2	Partial pressure of oxygen
P_aO_2	Arterial oxygen tension
P_AO_2	Alveolar oxygen tension
P_aCO_2	Arterial carbon dioxide tension
P_ACO_2	Alveolar carbon dioxide tension
$P_{A-a}O_2$	Alveolar–arterial oxygen difference
P_ECO_2	End-tidal carbon dioxide tension
$P_{\bar{v}}CO_2$	Mixed venous carbon dioxide tension
$P_{\bar{v}}O_2$	Mixed venous oxygen tension
$\dot{Q}$	Perfusion per unit time
$\dot{Q}_t$	Cardiac output
SO_2	Oxygen saturation
S_aO_2	Arterial oxygen saturation
S_jO_2	Jugular bulb oxygen saturation
S_pO_2	Oxygen saturation determined by pulse oximetry
$S_{\bar{v}}O_2$	Mixed venous oxygen saturation
$\dot{V}$	Ventilation per unit time
$\dot{V}_A$	Effective alveolar ventilation per unit time
$\dot{V}CO_2$	Amount of carbon dioxide excreted per unit time
V_D	Dead space
$\dot{V}_E$	Expired minute volume
$\dot{V}O_2$	Oxygen consumption
V_T	Tidal volume

1 Planning, organization and management

INTRODUCTION

Intensive care medicine (or critical care medicine) is predominantly concerned with the management of patients with acute life-threatening conditions (the critically ill) in specialized units, but also encompasses the resuscitation and transport of those who become acutely ill or are injured, either elsewhere in the hospital (e.g. in coronary care units, acute admission wards, postoperative recovery areas or accident and emergency units) or in the community. Intensive care has been defined as 'a service for patients with potentially recoverable diseases who can benefit from more detailed observation and treatment than is generally available in the standard wards and departments' (Spiby, 1989).

The creation of intensive care units (ICUs) and the subsequent development of intensive care medicine owe much to the introduction of intermittent positive-pressure ventilation (IPPV) for the treatment of patients with respiratory failure. The therapeutic potential of this technique was first recognized during the 1950s when positive-pressure ventilation via a tracheostomy was used to support patients with respiratory failure due to neuromuscular disorders such as poliomyelitis or acute exacerbations of chronic obstructive pulmonary disease (see Chapter 7), and occasionally those with postoperative respiratory insufficiency. The more widespread adoption of therapeutic IPPV (as opposed to its established role in anaesthesia) during the early 1960s prompted many institutions to create respiratory care units to facilitate the management of patients requiring mechanical ventilation. At the same time, it was appreciated that patients who had undergone cardiac surgery, which was then associated with an appreciable mortality, could benefit from intensive postoperative care, and that the complications of myocardial infarction could be detected and treated more effectively within specialized coronary care units. It soon became apparent that other critically ill patients could be better managed within purpose-built units fully equipped with monitoring and technical facilities in which they could receive continuous expert nursing care and the constant attention of appropriately trained medical staff. It also seemed likely that this concentration of special facilities and expertise would improve patient outcomes and reduce costs.

The scope of intensive care medicine has since developed and expanded to include the management of patients with a wide variety of underlying medical and surgical disorders (Table 1.1). In addition, patients with acute cardiorespiratory disturbances frequently develop failure of other organs or systems and, once the initial objective of sustaining life has been achieved, the primary disease must be diagnosed and appropriately treated. Teamwork and a multidisciplinary approach are central to the provision of optimal intensive care and are most effective when directed and coordinated by committed specialists. Apart from their clinical expertise, such specialists can facilitate communication and coordination, provide effective and informed management of admissions and discharges and offer valuable insights into difficult ethical decisions (Vincent, 2000). More recently the value of extending the responsibilities of the intensive care team to encompass the recognition and management of seriously ill patients throughout the hospital, including critically ill patients who have been discharged to the ward (outreach care: see below) has been generally accepted, although some remain concerned by the lack of convincing evidence that this approach leads to tangible benefits.

A high-quality intensive care service should provide equitable, humane and effective care as cost-effectively as possible.

LEVELS OF CARE AND FACILITIES REQUIRED TO DELIVER A CRITICAL CARE SERVICE (Intensive Care Society Standards for Intensive Care Units, 1997)

ICUs are usually reserved for patients with potential or established organ failure and must therefore provide the facilities for the diagnosis, prevention and treatment of multiple organ failure.

High-dependency units (HDUs) (Ridley, 1998) offer a standard of care intermediate between that available on the general ward and that in the ICU. These units, also sometimes called *intermediate care units* or *progressive care units,* provide monitoring and support for patients with acute (or acute on chronic) single-organ failure and for those who are

Table 1.1 Some common indications for admission to intensive care

Surgical emergencies	Medical emergencies
Acute intra-abdominal catastrophe	**Respiratory failure**
Ruptured/leaking abdominal aortic aneurysm	Exacerbation of chronic obstructive pulmonary disease
Perforated viscus, especially with faecal soiling of peritoneum (often complicated by sepsis/septic shock)	Acute severe asthma
	Severe pneumonia (may be complicated by septic shock)
Trauma (often complicated by hypovolaemic and later septic shock)	
Multiple injuries	**Meningococcal infection**
Massive blood loss	**Status epilepticus**
Severe head injury	**Severe diabetic ketoacidosis**
	Coma
Elective surgery	**Obstetric emergencies**
Extensive/prolonged procedures (e.g. oesphagogastrectomy)	Severe pre-eclampsia/eclampsia
Cardiothoracic surgery	Amniotic fluid embolism
Major head and neck surgery	
Coexisting cardiovascular or respiratory disease	

at risk of developing organ failure, including facilities for short-term respiratory support and immediate resuscitation. They can also provide a 'step-down' facility for patients being discharged from intensive care, thereby avoiding the abrupt change in the level of support that occurs when patients are discharged to a general ward and perhaps allowing earlier discharge of patients from the ICU. These units also provide a more comfortable environment for less severely ill patients, who are often conscious and alert. Intermediate care units should not be used for patients requiring multiple-organ support or prolonged, sophisticated mechanical ventilation. Guidelines to promote safe triage of patients to intermediate care units have been published (Nasraway et al., 1998).

It is suggested that HDUs can reduce the pressure on the general wards or overloaded ICUs, improve efficiency and reduce costs without compromising patient care. It has been estimated that the total cost per patient-day on an HDU running at 70% occupancy is around £250 – much less than the total daily cost of intensive care, which is in excess of £500 (Edbrooke et al., 1997) and is probably more than £1000 (Singer et al., 1994). These costs have of course increased significantly since these figures were published. Certainly it seems that there are a large number of patients who require intermediate care (mainly concentrated nursing care with a nurse/patient ratio of 1:3 or 1:4 and simple monitoring) (Zimmerman et al., 1996), and an impressive reduction in cardiac arrest calls from the general ward has been reported following the introduction of an intermediate care unit (Franklin et al., 1988). It has also been reported

that the introduction of an HDU reduced the number of ICU readmissions (Fox et al., 1999). In one centre the opening of a six-bedded HDU, adjacent to an eight-bedded ICU, was followed by a 49% increase in the total number of patients admitted to the critical care facility. Most of this increase was accounted for by patients admitted to the new HDU, with the number of patients referred for postoperative high-dependency care increasing dramatically. Only a few patients admitted to the HDU subsequently deteriorated and 'stepped up' to the ICU (Dhond et al., 1998). Importantly, there was a suggestion in this study that the opening of an HDU was associated with a reduction in the severity of illness of patients throughout the hospital, perhaps because of earlier referral to the ICU or stabilization of patients on HDU prior to discharge to the ward (Dhond et al., 1998). It seems, therefore that the opening of HDU facilities is likely to generate new, previously unmet, demand for critical care services and is unlikely to relieve the pressure on ICU beds or reduce the overall cost of critical care. Nevertheless this should be offset by improvements in the quality of care (Ridley, 1998), although there is a paucity of objective evidence to support the efficacy of intermediate care (Vincent and Burchadi, 1999). It is also important to be aware of the dangers of deskilling ward staff, as well as compromising recruitment and retention on the general wards.

Although it is important that the provision of staff and the level of technical support match the needs of the individual patient, many now believe that resources are used more efficiently when combined in a single critical care facility rather than being divided between physically and managerially separate units, staffed independently (Vincent and Burchadi, 1999). A frequently adopted, and successful, compromise is to create physically adjacent ICUs and HDUs, clearly separated by, for example, doors or an archway but covered by the same team of medical and nursing staff. Administrative control of both units, and supervision of clinical management should reside with senior ICU staff in order to avoid conflicts in bed management and triage of patients and to ensure that quality of care is maintained (see below) (Ridley, 1998).

In Australia three levels of intensive care provision have been defined:

- *Level 1 (small district hospital)* provides close nursing observation, basic monitoring, immediate resuscitation and short-term (24 hours or less) ventilation. These units are equivalent to HDUs.
- *Level 2 (larger general hospital)* provides more prolonged ventilation, a resident doctor, and access to pathology, radiology and physiotherapy at all times. These units are equivalent to the ICUs sometimes found in smaller district general hospitals in the UK. They do not provide more advanced organ support (e.g. haemofiltration) and more complex invasive monitoring (e.g. intracranial pressure monitoring, pulmonary artery catheterization).
- *Level 3 (tertiary referral hospital)* provides all aspects of intensive care and is staffed by specialists in intensive care with trainees, specialist nurses and allied health professionals. These units have access to complex investigations, advanced imaging techniques and specialists from all disciplines. In the UK such units have sometimes been referred to as regional ICUs.

Stratification of ICUs in this way may have the advantage of avoiding unnecessary duplication of expensive intensive care facilities, and more flexible utilization of personnel and beds. It does mean, however, that the transfer of critically ill patients between hospitals becomes increasingly common, often displacing them from their local support environment. Another disadvantage of regionalization may be a loss of skills and knowledge in the smaller hospitals. It has been suggested that early referral to a regional (level 3) unit may decrease mortality in patients with complex critical illness and that sicker patients benefit from early referral. Mortality is, however, likely to be extremely high in those patients transferred after more than 10 days of intensive care (Purdie et al., 1990).

Following a review of adult critical care services in the UK by a National Expert Group, the Department of Health (2000) published a document entitled *Comprehensive Critical Care* in which a new classification of critically ill patients according to clinical need was proposed:

- *Level 0*: patients whose needs can be met through normal ward care in an acute hospital;
- *Level 1*: patients at risk of their condition deteriorating, or those recently relocated from higher levels of care whose needs can be met on an acute ward with additional advice and support from the critical care team;
- *Level 2*: patients requiring more detailed observation or interventions, including support for a single failing organ system or postoperative care, and those stepping down from higher levels of care;
- *Level 3*: patients requiring advanced respiratory support alone or basic respiratory support together with support of at least two organ systems. This level includes all complex patients requiring support for multiorgan failure.

More recently the UK Intensive Care Society has expanded on this guidance (Intensive Care Society, 2002).

Clearly the precise number of critical care beds required to meet fluctuating demand in an individual hospital will depend on a variety of local factors, including the number of acute beds, the number and size of different units in that hospital, the acceptability of transferring patients to another hospital and local case mix. The need for flexibility and for local, rather than national, planning has been emphasized (Association of Anaesthetists of Great Britain and Ireland, 1988), although adherence to national and international standards and guidelines is clearly essential. Many years ago the Department of Health and Social Security recommended that approximately 1–2% of the acute beds of a general hospital should be allocated to intensive care, and suggested that bed numbers should be increased if there are special units within the hospital for cardiac, major vascular and neurosurgery (Department of Health and Social Security, 1970, revised 1992). Since then, however, there has been a progressive and substantial increase in the demand for intensive care, largely because, despite the recent decrease in the number of long-stay acute hospital beds (a trend that is likely to continue), the proportion of seriously ill patients has steadily increased. As a result it is now generally accepted that the proportion of hospital beds that should be allocated to intensive care is considerably greater than originally suggested, although there is still wide variation in the provision of critical care facilities. In one study involving 40 ICUs in North America, the average number of beds in each hospital was 359 and the average number of intensive care beds in each institution was 21 (Knaus et al., 1991). Overall in the USA, intensive care accounts for about 6–11% of all hospital beds and an expenditure of as much as 1% of gross national product (Osborne and Evans, 1994). By contrast, the UK has spent only about 0.05% of gross national product on intensive care and only around 2.6% of hospital beds have been designated for intensive care. Similarly, the provision of intermediate-care beds in the UK has been inadequate (Edbrooke et al., 1997; Ridley, 1998), although more recently expenditure on critical care facilities has increased.

It has been estimated that to meet the needs of a population of 500 000 individuals for 95% of the time requires 30 intensive care and 55 high-dependency beds in a single critical care area. These numbers increase to 48 and 81 respectively if resources are divided among three separate critical care areas (Lyons *et al.,* 2000). Two years prior to the publication of this study, it was estimated that there were around 70 adult critical care beds per million of the population in Wales and 55 per million in England. In terms of demand for HDU facilities it has been estimated that for a hospital of around 1200 beds an eight-bed unit would be full 50% of the time whilst seven beds would be full 63% of the time (Leeson-Payne and Aitkenhead, 1995). Recent developments, such as the improvements in outcome which can be achieved by intensive management of high-risk surgical patients (see Chapter 5) are likely to increase the demand on critical care facilities and may negate the recent modest increases (about 22%) in intensive care beds in England.

DESIGNING CRITICAL CARE AREAS

The size of a critical care unit should be governed by the fact that those with fewer than four beds and less than 200 admissions a year, or a bed occupancy less than 60%, are unlikely to acquire and retain the necessary expertise, and are probably uneconomic (Association of Anaesthetists of Great Britain and Ireland, 1988), whereas units with more than 15–20 beds become increasingly difficult for one team to manage. Although the average district general hospital is likely to have around 6–10 beds, units with 20–30 beds, or even more, may be appropriate in larger institutions, and can operate effectively, provided they are adequately staffed and working practices are adapted to cope with the increased workload.

In the UK and Australasia there has been a preference for developing general ICUs, managed wherever possible by intensive care specialists, and for providing separate units only for neonatal, paediatric, post cardiac surgery and, sometimes, neurosurgical intensive care. In some hospitals intermediate care units are also established for specific patient groups such as cardiac, neurosurgical or respiratory patients. Coronary care units are usually separated from the other intensive care areas. In some large North American hospitals units may be further subdivided (e.g. into medical, respiratory, surgical and trauma). Whatever the arrangements, the various units, including intermediate care facilities, should be close to each other, in order to make optimal use of pooled medical, nursing and technical staff, as well as equipment. They should also be adjacent, horizontally or vertically, to other acute areas such as the accident and emergency department, the operating theatres and the labour ward, and to imaging facilities. The intensive care areas must also be easily accessible via capacious, reliable lifts, wide corridors (≥ 2 m) and large doors. Provision must be made for escape from fire.

ICUs must be spacious and allow easy access to the patient (**Fig. 1.1**); 20–21 m² per bed space, with an unobstructed corridor space of 2.5 m beyond the working area is recommended. Single-bed areas should be provided with a

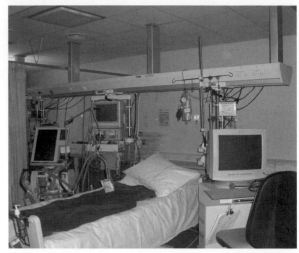

(a)

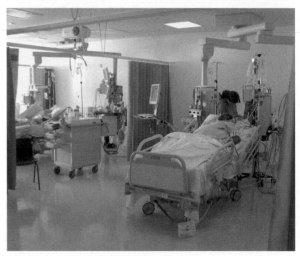

(b)

Fig. 1.1 Access to intensive care patients must be unrestricted. This is achieved by allowing adequate floor space for each bed area. The available space and access to the patient can be optimized by using (a) an overhead rail or (b) a pendant system.

gowning lobby of 6 m² (Facilities for Critical Care, 2003; Intensive Care Society Standards for Intensive Care Units 1997; Society of Critical Care Medicine, 1995). Isolation rooms require an additional anteroom of 1.9–2.5 m² for hand-washing and gowning. The overall floor plan should minimize unnecessary through traffic (Aitkenhead *et al.,* 1993). The patient areas should consist of a large open-plan area containing several beds, with some adjacent single-bedded cubicles, the exact proportion being determined by the types of patient being treated. Open-plan areas make the most efficient use of nursing staff, while single cubicles may be used to minimize the risks of cross-infection by isolating patients with impaired immune responses or those harbouring dangerous microorganisms, as well as to provide privacy for mentally alert, long-stay patients. It is generally recommended that not more than two or possibly three single rooms should be provided for every 10 beds, but this may have to be reviewed in light of the increased incidence of infection with multiresistant organisms (see Chapter 12), more frequent patient transfers and the hazards associated with highly infectious viral illnesses such as severe acute respiratory syndrome (SARS).

Positive/negative-pressure air-conditioning systems for single isolation rooms are expensive and of unproven efficacy. Air conditioning is, however, essential to ensure a reasonable working environment.

Each bed space must be equipped with monitors, suction apparatus, piped oxygen and air, and a vacuum supply. Three oxygen, two air and four suction outlets have been recommended. Low-pressure suction should be available. Some recommend installation of a scavenging system. There should also be a bedside light. A plentiful supply of mains sockets (e.g. 20–24 per bed) is essential, as are power points for mobile X-ray equipment. Outlets for radio, television and telephone can be included, even though they may not often be used, and a computer terminal may be provided at each bedside. There must be emergency back-up supplies of air, oxygen, suction and power that are immediately available in the event of failure (Aitkenhead et al., 1993). Facilities for haemodialysis, such as filtered water, are sometimes provided at selected bed areas. To avoid restricting access to the patient, services are normally delivered via trunking and equipment is traditionally mounted on a rail system, both being located behind the bed. Currently, services and some equipment are more often ceiling-mounted or delivered via an overhead rail (see **Fig. 1.1**) or through a floor column. Space for additional monitoring equipment may, however, be limited with these alternative designs.

Bed dividers can be used not only to provide a degree of privacy for the patients, but also as storage space. By keeping all essential equipment at the bedside, staff movement can be reduced. Lining the bed divider with lead will help to minimize the risks of radiation exposure to patients and staff. A chart table and writing surface are also required at the bedside. There should be a central nursing station from where it is possible to access local and remote computing facilities and to see all patients and their bedside monitors. It is important to provide adequate radiograph viewing facilities. Digital technology can now be used to retrieve radiographs from the radiology department to be viewed and manipulated on screens in the unit or at the bedside. A good communication network using telephones and an intercom system is essential.

There should be separate 'clean' and 'dirty' utility rooms, with adequate facilities for the disposal of soiled linen and waste. Surfaces should be easily cleaned and there should be a good supply of non-splash washbasins, with one in each single room (Aitkenhead et al., 1993). Elbow-, knee-, foot- or infrared-operated taps are recommended to minimize contamination.

As well as plenty of storage space (25–30% of the patient and central nursing station areas is recommended), it is important to provide a doctor's on-call room, adequate office accommodation, a staff rest room, changing rooms, a waiting area, overnight accommodation for relatives and an interview room. Other facilities may include a reception area, a library and a tutorial room.

In most units there will be an onsite 'stat' laboratory allowing immediate blood gas analysis and determination of plasma electrolytes, blood sugar levels, haemoglobin concentration and packed cell volume. In some units this laboratory will also be equipped with devices for measuring haemoglobin saturation with oxygen, blood lactate levels and plasma osmolality. Overall, more than 50% of the total floor space of the unit should be for non-patient areas.

Finally, it is important for the psychological well-being of both patients and staff that all bed areas are well illuminated with natural daylight (Wilson, 1972) (see Chapter 11). Ideally patients should be positioned facing a window with a view of the outside world.

EQUIPMENT

Clearly the quantity and level of sophistication of the equipment and monitoring required will be influenced by the size and role of the ICU (**Table 1.2**). Monitoring equipment should preferably have the capacity for data storage and retrieval. The equipment for the following therapeutic interventions should be immediately available (Aitkenhead et al., 1993):

- tracheal intubation;
- direct current (dc) cardioversion;
- bronchoscopy;
- insertion of chest drains;
- cardiac pacing;
- intra-aortic balloon pumping (cardiothoracic and some level 3 units);
- invasive haemodynamic monitoring;
- establishing extracorporeal renal support (level 3 units).

MANAGEMENT OF THE CRITICAL CARE SERVICE

MEDICAL STAFF

It is essential that a suitably trained resident doctor is immediately available throughout the day and night to deal with emergencies occurring on the unit. Often this doctor is an anaesthetist, but if not must be capable of emergency intubation and have a thorough knowledge of the techniques of respiratory support and cardiopulmonary resuscitation and their complications. Resident doctors must be closely supervised at all times by a senior member of the medical staff and an experienced intensive care specialist should always be immediately available for advice and be ready to attend the unit at short notice. In many larger units trainees

Table 1.2 Some of the equipment required in a regional (level 3) intensive care unit

Monitoring and investigations	Equipment for:
Bedside monitors Central monitors Portable monitors	Blood gas/acid–base analysis Determination of electrolytes Measurement of haemoglobin/packed cell volume Measurement of blood lactate Measurement of oxygen content Bedside blood sugar measurements Assessment of coagulation 12-lead electrocardiogram Monitoring lung function Weighing patients
Facilities for monitoring:	
Intravascular pressures Intracranial pressure Cerebral function (Jugular venous bulb oxygen) (Cerebral blood flow) Cardiac output Echocardiography Pulse oximetry Capnography Temperature monitoring	
Respiratory therapy	**Renal support**
Ventilators (bedside and portable, non-invasive) Humidifiers Oxygen masks Masks/hoods for applying CPAP and non-invasive ventilation Circuits Self-inflating bags for manual ventilation Fibreoptic bronchoscope Anaesthetic machine	(Equipment for peritoneal dialysis) Equipment for continuous venovenous haemo(dia)filtration Access to haemodialysis machine
Cardiovascular therapy	**Other**
Defibrillators (including portable devices) Intra-aortic balloon pump Infusion pumps and syringe pumps Pacemakers	Pressure-relieving beds and mattresses Heating/cooling blankets/devices Drip stands Dressing trolleys Mobile curtains
Radiology	
Portable X-ray machine Image intensifier Portable ultrasound device	

CPAP, continuous positive-airway pressure.

specializing in intensive care and research fellows will be important members of the medical team.

Each ICU must have a nominated director who should be an intensive care specialist. There is now general agreement among those closely involved in intensive care that the base specialty (anaesthesia, medicine, surgery or emergency medicine) of the director is largely irrelevant, provided that he or she is motivated and appropriately trained. The proportion of the senior specialists' time allocated to intensive care will depend largely on the size and type of hospital. In a large university hospital, most or all of their sessions may be devoted to intensive care so that additional administra-tive, teaching, training and research commitments can be fulfilled, while in some smaller general hospitals it may be appropriate to appoint senior specialists 'with an interest in intensive care' who will also have a significant number of sessions in their base specialty.

The on-call commitment will necessarily be shared between several suitably trained senior doctors. In many hospitals in the UK, the ICU is run by a group of anaesthetists specializing in intensive care, while in others the team consists of both anaesthetists and physicians. Only a few units are managed exclusively by physicians. In North America, surgeons also specialize in intensive care and are particularly involved in the management of critically ill trauma patients. These intensive care specialists should control and coordinate patient care in conjunction with the primary clinician; they should also, when appropriate, be guided by advice obtained from other specialists. Clear lines of responsibility must be established between the medical staff. All those involved in the patients' care, including nurses and physiotherapists, must communicate effectively.

NURSING STAFF

An adequate complement of suitably trained nurses is crucial to the success of an ICU. In level 3 units in the UK, nurse-to-patient ratios of 1:1, with an additional nurse in charge and sometimes a 'runner', are conventionally considered to be ideal. Allowing for holidays, off-duty and sickness, this requires a total of approximately 6.5 nurses per bed, as well as a nurse manager, who assumes overall administrative responsibility. A clinical teacher who can develop the skills of the less experienced staff is an invaluable addition to the team.

High-dependency beds are usually staffed at a lower nurse-to-patient ratio, typically 1:2. Nurse-to-patient ratios vary widely across Europe, however, and in one study it appeared that the UK was the least efficient in terms of work delivered per nurse (Moreno and Reis Miranda, 1998), whereas in the USA the nurse-to-patient ratio is commonly 1:2 or 1:3 (although this may partly reflect differences in case mix and the provision of additional non-nursing support staff). Although there is some evidence to suggest that lower nurse-to-patient ratios and in particular excessive workload can be associated with worse outcomes (Amaravadi et al., 2000; Tarnow-Mordi et al., 2000), global outcome measures do not appear to be demonstrably worse in systems with fewer nurses per patient. Moreover, because of economic constraints and a shortage of suitably qualified personnel, it can be difficult consistently to achieve one-to-one nursing without closing beds. Further problems are posed by the inevitable fluctuations in both patient numbers and the level of nursing care that each requires. Although the optimum bed occupancy is said to be approximately 80%, in some units this figure is closer to 60%, while in others occupancy approaches 100%. Furthermore, some units deal almost exclusively with seriously ill, ventilated, long-stay patients, while others admit a larger proportion of relatively stable cases, mainly for short-term observation. Units that are adequately staffed when full of highly dependent patients will therefore have an excess of nurses at other times. The alternative is a relatively understaffed unit, unable to cope during periods of peak demand. In an attempt to solve this problem and to achieve a balance between these two extremes, more exact methods of assessing the overall nursing requirements of a particular unit have been developed (Intensive Care Society Standards for Intensive Care Units, 1997). In general a flexible and innovative approach to nurse staffing (including, for example, adjusting the skill mix to match local demands and the employment of support staff) is the best means of achieving efficiency without compromising standards of care or job satisfaction.

Recruitment, retention and the commitment of nursing staff to the organization can be improved by attention to the design and planning of units, as well as to the organizational, administrative and stress management aspects of intensive care discussed elsewhere in this chapter. Attention to education, training and career development is also essential.

ADMINISTRATIVE AND ANCILLARY STAFF

A *receptionist/ward clerk* who can answer the telephone, attend to relatives and perform clerical duties is a valuable addition to the team and can relieve the nurses' workload. *Secretarial assistance* will also be required. *Cleaners* fulfil a vital role in minimizing the risk of cross-infection.

OTHER HEALTH CARE PROFESSIONALS

Physiotherapists who are experienced in dealing with critically ill, ventilated patients have a vital role in successful intensive care (see later chapters) and must be integrated into the team.

Adequate *technical support* for repair and maintenance of equipment is also essential. It is particularly important that on-site laboratory equipment such as automated blood gas analysers is subjected to a strict quality control programme performed by experienced laboratory staff (see Chapter 6). These members of the team should also be involved in selecting and buying equipment.

Expert imaging (e.g. chest radiography, ultrasound, computed tomographic (CT) scanning) is an important aspect of intensive care and requires the services of skilled radiographers and close liaison with radiologists.

A *pharmacist* should be identified as having responsibility for the ICU and should be available for advice. Importantly, the participation of a pharmacist in daily, multidisciplinary ward rounds has been shown to reduce costs and the incidence of adverse drug events (Leape et al., 1999). It is also important to be able to consult suitably experienced *dietitians*. Specialized *respiratory therapists* are important members of the team in North America, but have not established a role in the UK, Europe or Australasia.

Finally access to social workers, counselling services and ministers of religion is essential.

EDUCATION AND RESEARCH

Staff morale and job satisfaction and the quality of patient care can be substantially enhanced by providing structured introductory training, offering specific opportunities for career development and encouraging participation in continuing education, including attendance at national and international meetings. Larger units may also offer approved courses in intensive care nursing and more specialist training in intensive care medicine. An active research programme can also have a beneficial influence on *esprit de corps* by stimulating enquiry, discussion and enthusiasm for the specialty.

AUDIT

A system of continuing audit is essential to document activity, identify deficiencies and suggest ways of improving patient care. It is recommended that audit should involve regular objective assessments of structure, processes and outcome (Aitkenhead *et al.*, 1993). It is important to 'close the loop' by auditing the impact of any changes that are made on the chosen outcome measures. Data managers may be employed to collect and collate the information required.

Incidents that either could, or did, reduce the margin of safety for a patient or staff member should be documented in a structured report so that measures can be taken to minimize the risk of a similar event in the future.

Diagnostic discrepancies have been found in almost 20% of non-surviving ICU patients who undergo postmortem, and in a fifth of these their chances of survival may have been adversely affected (Twigg *et al.*, 2001). Many therefore believe that the postmortem examination continues to have an important role in auditing clinical practice and diagnostic performance.

POLICIES AND CLINICAL PROTOCOLS

Policies facilitate the delivery of high-quality patient care. ICUs and HDUs should, for example, have agreed written policies for the admission and discharge of patients and for dealing with patient referrals. Management responsibilities and the clinical chains of command should also be clearly defined.

Written, evidence-based clinical protocols or guidelines for all the common intensive care activities and procedures should be produced and adhered to, and should be regularly reviewed. Safe practice demands that protocols for all procedures should stipulate that (Aitkenhead *et al.*, 1993):

- the availability, correct functioning and calibration of all equipment should be checked in advance;
- the operator should be appropriately experienced or must be supervised;
- competent assistance should be available;
- the expected benefits should outweigh the anticipated risks.

Examples of activities for which protocols should normally be established include:

- vascular cannulation, including pulmonary artery catheterization;
- tracheal intubation and extubation, percutaneous tracheostomy;
- mechanical ventilation;
- antimicrobial policies and prevention of infection.

Written guidelines for the management of specific conditions, especially those that are encountered less frequently, are also valuable.

DOCUMENTATION

Regular systematic clinical assessments of the patient should be recorded in the progress notes, including comments on vital signs, the function of each organ or system and the results of haematological, biochemical and microbiological investigations. The treatment plan for the day and any alterations or additions to the drug regimen, including microbiological findings and alterations to the antibiotic regimes, must be recorded. Interviews with relatives should also be documented, as should decisions to limit or withdraw treatment. Physiological measurements, clinical signs and blood results should be recorded on flow charts or in a computerized patient data management system. Accurate fluid balance charts are essential.

EMERGENCY TEAMS, EARLY-WARNING SYSTEMS AND OUTREACH CARE

The National Confidential Enquiries into Perioperative Deaths (NCEPOD) (Callum *et al.*, 2002) have shown that about two-thirds of deaths occur more than 3 days after surgery, mostly on the ward. It is also well recognized that patients admitted to ICUs from the general wards have a higher mortality than those admitted from other areas of the hospital (Goldhill and Sumner, 1998). A considerable proportion of such patients have received cardiopulmonary resuscitation before admission to intensive care (Goldhill *et al.*, 1999a) and many of these unexpected cardiac arrests are preceded by marked physiological deterioration, which is often unrecognized or inappropriately treated (Franklin and Mathew, 1994; Schein *et al.*, 1990). Similarly, Goldhill and his colleagues (1999a) found that physiological variables are frequently abnormal in the 24-hour period before admission to intensive care from the ward: the most important indicators of risk are respiratory rate, heart rate and the adequacy of oxygenation. Moreover there is now good evidence to indicate that the care received by emergency patients before their admission to ICUs is frequently suboptimal, that this poor management adversely influences outcome and that a proportion of deaths may be avoidable (Goldhill *et al.*, 1999a; McGloin *et al.*, 1999; McQuillan *et al.*, 1998). In one study the principal causes of suboptimal care were identified as failure of organization, lack of knowledge, failure to appreciate clinical urgency, lack of experience, lack of supervision and failure to seek advice from senior colleagues (McQuillan *et al.*, 1998).

It seems clear, therefore, that the care of seriously ill patients on the general wards is often less than adequate and it is likely that in some cases intensive care admission could be avoided by the early institution of appropriate management. It has been suggested, therefore, that the skills of the critical care team should be exported beyond the confines of their specialized units to encompass the rest of the hospital (a concept sometimes termed *critical care without walls*). The development of such *outreach services* was advocated in *Comprehensive Critical Care* (Department of Health, 2000), in which it was envisaged that the outreach service would:

- provide education and support for ward staff in the management of the severely ill;
- avert intensive care admissions by early identification and timely, appropriate resuscitation;
- facilitate early admission of appropriate cases to an ICU/HDU;
- facilitate safe discharge of patients from critical care units to the ward, and home, by providing continuing support and advice;
- promote continuity of care;
- ensure thorough audit and evaluation of performance.

In some cases the outreach team may facilitate decisions to withhold or withdraw life-sustaining treatment (see below).

The exact composition of the outreach team varies depending on local priorities and perceived needs, but membership should reflect the multidisciplinary approach required for optimal management of the acutely ill patient. The number of staff involved will be influenced by the size and geography of the hospital and whether the team is to be available 24 hours a day, 7 days a week or only during normal working hours. The team requires the involvement of senior medical intensive care specialists and resident doctors, as well as nursing input from senior nurses trained in critical care, and can benefit from the advice and support of physiotherapists, as well as dietitians, pharmacists and rehabilitation staff. The critical care technicians have a role in providing monitoring facilities, both on the wards and for transfer, and the resuscitation officer should be involved in developing an integrated training programme. The team leader may be a medical intensive care specialist or a senior critical care nurse, who in the UK may be a nurse consultant or clinical nurse specialist. Team members must be good teachers and communicators who are capable of independent practice and are committed to the concept of outreach care. They must continue to be exposed to critical care practice in order to ensure retention of skills.

The success of the outreach service will depend on the level of support received from senior medical and nursing staff on the wards. It is important, therefore, that the outreach team functions in a cooperative and supportive manner, and that confrontation is avoided. Ideally a collaborative partnership should be developed between the critical care team and other departments in the hospital to provide a continuum of care, regardless of the patient's location. Deskilling of ward staff must be avoided. It is worth emphasizing that outreach care should not be viewed as a remedy for inadequate resource provision; indeed, there is a danger that the additional workload generated by an outreach team could overwhelm a poorly resourced critical care department (Intensive Care Society Standards and Guidelines, 2000).

In order to facilitate recognition of 'at-risk' patients on the wards and subsequent early referral to the critical care emergency or outreach team, a number of *early-warning systems* have been devised (Goldhill et al., 1999a; Lee et al., 1995). These are based primarily on bedside recognition of

deteriorating physiological variables and can be used to supplement clinical intuition. Early-warning systems should be used in conjunction with the prior identification of patients in high-risk groups, such as those recently discharged from ICU/HDU, those who have recently undergone high-risk surgery, victims of major trauma, patients with pancreatitis and those with a decreased conscious level. The first such system to be described was the *medical emergency team* (MET) (Lee et al., 1995), which was originally conceived in an attempt to reduce the incidence and improve the outcome of cardiopulmonary arrest on the ward. In this system doctors and nurses use specified calling criteria to assist in the recognition of patients at risk and to trigger urgent intervention. Other similar systems have since been developed, including the *patient-at-risk team* (PART) (Goldhill et al., 1999b), and the *(modified) early-warning score* (Subbe et al., 2001) as well as updated MET calling criteria (Hillman et al., 2005) (**Table 1.3**). It has also been suggested that the outcome of high-risk surgical patients could be improved by widening the remit of the acute pain service to form a postoperative care team (Goldhill, 1997).

To date, however, the introduction of outreach services has been haphazard and inconsistent. In 2001 only 50% of hospitals surveyed in England had established such a service. In more than half of these there was no medical input; the majority ceased to function outside normal working hours and eight different alerting systems were used. Moreover, although the concept of outreach care has many enthusiastic supporters and is intuitively attractive, there is only limited evidence to show that this approach is effective (Ball et al., 2003; Priestley et al., 2004). Two cohort studies have indicated that the MET system can reduce unexpected intensive care admission (Bristow et al., 2000) and the incidence of, and mortality from, unexpected cardiac arrest and adverse postoperative outcomes (Bellomo et al., 2004). Hospital mortality may also be reduced (Bellomo et al., 2003; Buist et

Table 1.3 Medical emergency team-calling criteria (from Hillman et al., 2005)

Airway	If threatened
Breathing	All respiratory arrests Respiratory rate < 5 breaths/minute Respiratory rate > 36 breaths/minute
Circulation	All cardiac arrests Pulse rate < 40 beats/minute Pulse rate > 140 beats/minute Systolic blood pressure < 90 mm Hg
Neurology	Sudden fall in level of consciousness (fall in Glasgow Coma Scale of > 2 points) Repeated or prolonged seizures
Other	Any patient who does not fit the criteria above, but about whom you are seriously worried

al., 2002). On the other hand, in one hospital the introduction of the modified early-warning score failed to influence mortality or the rates of cardiopulmonary arrest or ICU/HDU admissions (Subbe *et al.*, 2003), and in a recent cluster-randomized controlled trial in 23 hospitals the MET system did not substantially affect the incidence of cardiac arrest, unplanned ICU admission or unexpected death (Hillman *et al.*, 2005). Overall the evidence to support the introduction of such rapid-response teams is weak and it is unclear whether any possible benefit derives from the delivery of specialized treatment to a deteriorating patient or from educating ward staff in the early recognition of deterioration (Winters *et al.*, 2006). Hopefully, over the next few years the role and value of outreach care, as well as the most effective team composition, organization and call-out criteria, will be established.

THE INFLUENCE OF ORGANIZATION AND RESOURCES ON OUTCOMES

Accumulating evidence indicates that the organizational characteristics of ICUs, including the extent of involvement of specialist intensive care clinicians and nurse staffing levels, can significantly affect patient outcome (Vincent, 2000).

Several studies have suggested that morbidity and mortality rates are lower in so-called 'closed units' (in which patient care is directed and coordinated by appointed intensive care specialists) than in 'open units' (in which patients are managed by their admitting clinicians) (Baldock *et al.*, 2001). Also, in high-risk surgical patients the absence of regular bedside rounds by intensive care specialists has been associated with an increased length of stay in ICU and hospital, increased hospital costs, a higher incidence of postoperative complications (Dimick *et al.*, 2001; Pronovost *et al.*, 1999) and a threefold increase in mortality (Pronovost *et al.*, 1999), whilst a recent systematic review confirmed that 'high-intensity' staffing by intensive care physicians is associated with reduced hospital and ICU mortality and length of stay (Pronovost *et al.*, 2002). Moreover there is evidence to indicate that providing out-of-hours cover by intensive care specialists, as opposed to weekday cover only, can significantly reduce mortality rates (Blunt and Burchett, 2000).

It has recently been suggested that 'telemedicine' may enable ICUs to achieve improvements in quality of care when there is a shortage of specialist intensive care clinicians (Breslow *et al.*, 2004). There is also some evidence to suggest that better outcomes are achieved by units with greater availability of technological support (Bastos *et al.*, 1996) and higher case volumes (Kahn *et al.*, 2006).

Lastly a low night time nurse-to-patient ratio (one nurse caring for more than two patients) has been associated with an increased risk of complications and resource use after oesophagectomy (Amaravadi *et al.*, 2000) and excessive unit workload appears to increase mortality (Tarnow-Mordi *et al.*, 2000). Similarly, eliminating extended work shifts and reducing the hours worked by resident medical staff in the ICU decreases failures due to lack of attention during the night and reduces serious medical errors (Landrigan *et al.*, 2004; Lockley *et al.*, 2004).

The consequences of a shortage of intensive care beds include high occupancy rates, cancelled elective surgery, frequent refused admissions and premature discharge of patients from intensive care. Disturbingly, the frequency of night time discharges (a surrogate measure of pressure on intensive care beds) appears to be increasing in the UK; moreover, many of these discharges are premature and are associated with a worse outcome (Goldfrad and Rowan, 2000). Similarly, it has been shown that patients discharged during the night to a general ward rather than an HDU are more likely to die in hospital (Beck *et al.*, 2002). Partly as a response to these findings, as well as to the unacceptably high mortality and readmission rates following discharge from intensive care areas to the ward, it has been suggested that the Therapeutic Intervention Scoring System (TISS: see Chapter 2) might be a useful aid to discharge decision making (Beck *et al.*, 2002; Smith *et al.*, 1999). Others have developed a logistic regression triage model to identify patients at risk from early discharge (Daly *et al.*, 2001). These latter authors concluded that up to 34% of intensive care patients could be at risk and that an increase in intensive care bed numbers of around 16% would be required to avoid deaths caused by inappropriate early discharge (Daly *et al.*, 2001). Importantly, but perhaps not surprisingly, there is also objective evidence to indicate that appropriately referred cases who are refused admission to intensive care have an increased rate of attributable mortality and it has been suggested that the number of potentially avoidable deaths in England caused by such refusals could amount to as many as 2500 cases every year (Metcalfe *et al.*, 1997).

WORK-RELATED STRESS

It is widely acknowledged that the medical and nursing professions are exposed to considerable occupational stress. Many believe that this stress accounts, at least in part, for the observation that doctors have twice as many road accidents, three times the incidence of cirrhosis and suicide and 30 times the incidence of drug addiction compared to the general population. Similarly, nurses have the highest suicide rate amongst professional groups and constitute the greatest number of psychiatric outpatient referrals. The psychological pressures on those who work in ICUs are particularly intense (Table 1.4). Although moderate stress or pressure may improve health and performance, high levels of stress, if prolonged, can, depending on the individual, lead to ill health. As well as the usual signs and symptoms of stress (Table 1.5), the syndrome of 'burn-out' (Table 1.6) has been well described in intensive care staff (Roberts, 1986). This is a process in which high and sustained levels of job stress produce feelings of tension, irritability and fatigue, ending with a defensive reaction of detachment, apathy, cynicism or rigidity. Such work-related stress disorders are more likely to occur in the most dedicated, enthusiastic and idealistic members of staff.

Because of the sustained intimate contact between intensive care nurses and their patients, a close relationship is inevitably established, particularly with those whose stay in

Table 1.4 Causes of stress in the intensive care unit

Death and dying

Staff shortages/high turnover

Workload/shift work/fatigue

Job insecurity

Inadequate teaching, training and support

Lack of job satisfaction

Lack of recognition of expertise and contribution/feeling undervalued

Bureaucracy/administrative workload

Accountability/responsibility

Lack of resources/poor equipment

Increasingly sophisticated technology

Interpersonal communication difficulties and conflict (between staff/between staff and relatives)

Difficulty communicating with patients

Table 1.5 Some effects of stress

Physiological

Fatigue
Muscle tension
Headache, neck ache, backache
Eating disturbances
Sexual difficulties
? Hypertension
? Peptic ulceration
? Coronary artery disease
? Recurrence of previous diseases

Psychological

Anxiety
Depression
Indecision
Obsessional behaviour
Reduced self-esteem
Reduced enthusiasm
Irritability

Behavioural

Drug or alcohol abuse
Prone to accidents
Poor work performance
Aggressiveness
Relationship problems
Insomnia
Withdrawal

Table 1.6 Signs and symptoms of 'burn-out' (Roberts, 1986)

Emotional

Loss of humour: 'gallows humour'
Persistent sense of failure, guilt, blame
Cynical, blaming attitude towards patients
Frequent anger, resentment and bitterness
Increasing irritability, family and marital conflict
Feelings of discouragement and indifference
Eventual resignation to lack of power
Preoccupation with own needs and personal survival

Behavioural

Frequent clock-watching
Increasing resistance to go to work each day
Postpone patient contacts, resist calls and visits
Increasingly go by the book, loss of creative problem solving
Work harder to achieve less
Avoid discussing work with colleagues
Increasing social isolation
Increasing use of mood-altering drugs

Physical

Feel tired and exhausted all day
Sleep disorders
Frequent and long-lasting minor ailments
Increasing use of sick leave, high absenteeism
Prone to accidents

Cognitive

Increasing thoughts of leaving job
Inability to concentrate on or listen to what patient is saying
Rigid thinking, resist all change
Increasing suspiciousness and distrust
See patients as objects rather than people
Stereotype patients

the unit is prolonged. This exposes the nurse to considerable emotional pressures, which are often exacerbated by frequent close contact with the patient's anxious and distressed relatives. The work of an intensive care nurse is both physically and mentally demanding, involving the ability to use complex equipment and to diagnose acute life-threatening events and administer appropriate emergency treatment. Moreover, although nurses are usually well supported by their colleagues, many are reluctant to seek advice, fearing that this might be interpreted as incompetence.

Medical staff on the ICU are also subjected to stress (Lask, 1987), often exacerbated by poor support from colleagues, distractions (examinations, research, work in other areas) and taking ultimate responsibility for key decisions. It has also been suggested that doctors' frustration at being unable to help an individual patient may precipitate excessive criticism of colleagues, overzealous treatment or even avoidance of the unit altogether.

Finally, both medical and nursing staff are occasionally exposed to abuse and violence by patients and relatives (Lynch et al., 2003), experiences that are likely to exacerbate work-related stress.

Maintenance of staff morale is therefore crucial. Important aspects to be considered include the provision of adequate numbers of appropriately qualified personnel, close cooperation and discussion of management decisions among all members of staff, consistent unit policies and comprehensive teaching in all aspects of intensive care. Unit design may also be important; for example, it has long been recognized that working in an environment devoid of natural light increases stress (Wilson, 1972).

Finally, faulty job design is an important cause of burnout. Confusion about the exact nature and extent of one's responsibilities can lead to exhaustion, while overlapping responsibilities may precipitate competition and conflict with colleagues. These factors will be exacerbated by lack of meaningful support, negative feedback and teaching that creates false expectations.

Measures that may reduce the incidence of stress-related ill health include:

- teaching stress awareness and personal stress management;
- improving interpersonal communication skills;
- encouraging effective communication between all members of the multidisciplinary team;
- improved management and organizational changes;
- adequate leave of absence;
- access to further education and opportunities for professional advancement;
- adequate support;
- team approach;
- personal changes (e.g. exercise, relaxation).

REFERENCES

Aitkenhead AR, Booij LH, Dhainaut JF et al. (1993) International standards for safety in the intensive care unit. Intensive Care Medicine 19: 178–181.

Amaravadi RK, Dimick JB, Pronovost PJ, et al. (2000) ICU nurse-to-patient ratio is associated with complications and resource use after esophagectomy. Intensive Care Medicine 26: 1857–1862.

Association of Anaesthetists of Great Britain and Ireland (1988) Intensive Care Services – Provision for the Future. Available from the Association of Anaesthetists.

Baldock G, Foley P, Brett S (2001) The impact of organisational change on outcome in an intensive care unit in the United Kingdom. Intensive Care Medicine 27: 865–872.

Ball C, Kirkby M, Williams S (2003) Effect of the critical care outreach team on patient survival to discharge from hospital and readmission to critical care: non-randomised population based study. British Medical Journal 327: 1014.

Bastos PG, Knaus WA, Zimmerman JE, et al. (1996) The importance of technology for achieving superior outcomes from intensive care. Intensive Care Medicine 22: 664–669.

Beck DH, McQuillan P, Smith GB (2002) Waiting for the break of dawn? The effects of discharge time, discharge TISS scores and discharge facility on hospital mortality after intensive care. Intensive Care Medicine 28: 1287–1293.

Bellomo R, Goldsmith D, Uchino S, et al. (2003) A prospective before-and-after trial of a medical emergency team. Medical Journal of Australia 179: 283–287.

Bellomo R, Goldsmith D, Uchino S, et al. (2004) Prospective controlled trial of effect of medical emergency team on postoperative morbidity and mortality rates. Critical Care Medicine 32: 916–921.

Blunt MC, Burchett KR (2000) Out-of-hours consultant cover and case-mix adjusted mortality in intensive care. Lancet 356: 735–736.

Breslow MJ, Rosenfeld BA, Doerfler M, et al. (2004) Effect of a multiple-site intensive care unit telemedicine program on clinical and economic outcomes: an alternative paradigm for intensivist staffing. Critical Care Medicine 32: 31–38.

Bristow PJ, Hillman KM, Chey T, et al. (2000) Rate of in-hospital arrests, deaths and intensive care admissions: the effect of a medical emergency team. Medical Journal of Australia 173: 236–240.

Buist MD, Moore GE, Bernard SA, et al. (2002) Effects of a medical emergency team on reduction of incidence of and mortality from unexpected cardiac arrests in hospital: preliminary study. British Medical Journal 324: 387–390.

Callum KG, Carr MJ, Gray AJC, et al. (2002) The 2002 Report of the National Confidential Enquiry into Perioperative Deaths. NCEPOD: London.

Daly K, Beale R, Chang RW (2001) Reduction in mortality after inappropriate early discharge from intensive care unit: logistic regression triage model. British Medical Journal 322: 1274–1276.

Department of Health (2000) Comprehensive Critical Care: A Review of Adult Critical Care Services. Department of Health: London.

Department of Health and Social Security (1970) Intensive Therapy Unit. Hospital Building Note (HBN) 27. Revised 1992. Department of Health and Social Security: London.

Dhond G, Ridley S, Palmer M (1998) The impact of a high-dependency unit on the workload of an intensive care unit. Anaesthesia 53: 841–847.

Dimick JB, Pronovost PJ, Heitmiller RF, et al. (2001) Intensive care unit physician staffing is associated with decreased length of stay, hospital cost, and complications after esophageal resection. Critical Care Medicine 29: 753–758.

Edbrooke DL, Stevens VG, Hibbert CL, et al. (1997) High dependency units in England – the lack of provision and the cost of the shortfall. Care of the Critically Ill 13: 112–115.

Facilities for Critical Care (2003) Health Building Note 57. NHS Estates, The Stationery Office: London.

Fox AJ, Owen-Smith O, Spiers P (1999) The immediate impact of opening an adult high dependency unit on intensive care unit occupancy. Anaesthesia 54: 280–283.

Franklin C, Mathew J (1994) Developing strategies to prevent in-hospital cardiac arrest: analyzing responses of physicians and nurses in the hours before the event. Critical Care Medicine 22: 244–247.

Franklin CM, Rackow EG, Mamdani B, et al. (1988) Decreases in mortality on a large urban medical service by facilitating access to critical care. Archives of Internal Medicine 148: 1403–1405.

Goldfrad C, Rowan K (2000) Consequences of discharges from intensive care at night. Lancet 355: 1138–1142.

Goldhill DR (1997) Introducing the postoperative care team. British Medical Journal 314: 389.

Goldhill DR, Sumner A (1998) Outcome of intensive care patients in a group of British intensive care units. Critical Care Medicine 26: 1337–1345.

Goldhill DR, White SA, Sumner A (1999a) Physiological values and procedures in the 24 h before ICU admission from the ward. Anaesthesia 54: 529–534.

Goldhill DR, Worthington L, Mulcahy A, et al. (1999b) The patient-at-risk team: identifying and managing seriously ill ward patients. Anaesthesia 54: 853–860.

Hillman K, Chen J, Cretikos M, et al. (2005) Introduction of the medical emergency team (MET) system: a cluster-randomised controlled trial. Lancet 365: 2091–2097.

Intensive Care Society (2002) Levels of Critical Care for Adult Patients. Intensive Care Society: London, UK.

Intensive Care Society Standards and Guidelines (2000) Guidelines for the Introduction of Outreach Services. Intensive Care Society: London, UK. Available online at: www.ics.ac.uk.

Intensive Care Society Standards for Intensive Care Units (1997) Biomedica. Intensive Care Society: London, UK. Available online at: www.ics.ac.uk.

Kahn JM, Goss CH, Heagerty PJ, et al. (2006) Hospital volume and the outcomes of mechanical ventilation. New England Journal of Medicine 355: 41–50.

Knaus WA, Wagner DP, Draper EA, et al. (1991) The APACHE III prognostic system: risk prediction of hospital mortality for critically ill hospitalized adults. Chest 100: 1619–1636.

Landrigan CP, Rothschild JM, Cronin JW, et al. (2004) Effect of reducing interns' work hours on serious medical errors in intensive care units. *New England Journal of Medicine* **351**: 1838–1848.

Lask B (1987) Forget the stiff upper lip. *British Medical Journal* **295**: 1584–1585.

Leape LL, Cullen DJ, Clapp MD, *et al.* (1999) Pharmacist participation on physician rounds and adverse drug events in the intensive care unit. *Journal of the American Medical Association* **282**: 267–270.

Lee A, Bishop G, Hillman KM, *et al.* (1995) The medical emergency team. *Anaesthesia and Intensive Care* **23**: 183–186.

Leeson-Payne CG, Aitkenhead AR (1995) A prospective study to assess the demand for a high dependency unit. *Anaesthesia* **50**: 383–387.

Lockley SW, Cronin JW, Evans EE, *et al.* (2004) Effect of reducing interns' weekly work hours on sleep and attentional failures. *New England Journal of Medicine* **351**: 1829–1837.

Lynch J, Appelboam R, McQuillan PJ (2003) Survey of abuse and violence by patients and relatives towards intensive care staff. *Anaesthesia* **58**: 893–899.

Lyons RA, Wareham K, Hutchings HA, *et al.* (2000) Population requirement for adult critical-care beds: a prospective quantitative and qualitative study. *Lancet* **355**: 595–598.

McGloin H, Adam SK, Singer M (1999) Unexpected deaths and referrals to intensive care of patients on general wards. Are some cases potentially avoidable? *Journal of the Royal College of Physicians of London* **33**: 255–259.

McQuillan P, Pilkington S, Allan A, *et al.* (1998) Confidential inquiry into quality of care before admission to intensive care. *British Medical Journal* **316**: 1853–1858.

Metcalfe MA, Sloggett A, McPherson K (1997) Mortality among appropriately referred patients refused admission to intensive-care units. *Lancet* **350**: 7–11.

Moreno R, Reis Miranda D (1998) Nursing staff in intensive care in Europe: the mismatch between planning and practice. *Chest* **113**: 752–758.

Nasraway SA, Cohen IL, Dennis RC, *et al.* (1998) Guidelines on admission and discharge for adult intermediate care units. *Critical Care Medicine* **26**: 607–610.

Osborne M, Evans TW (1994) Allocation of resources in intensive care: a transatlantic perspective. *Lancet* **343**: 778–780.

Priestley G, Watson W, Rashidian A, *et al.* (2004) Introducing Critical Care Outreach: a ward-randomised trial of phased introduction in a general hospital. *Intensive Care Medicine* **30**: 1398–1404.

Pronovost PJ, Jenckes MW, Dorman T, *et al.* (1999) Organizational characteristics of intensive care units related to outcomes of abdominal aortic surgery. *Journal of the American Medical Association* **281**: 1310–1317.

Pronovost PJ, Angus DC, Dorman T, *et al.* (2002) Physician staffing patterns and clinical outcomes in critically ill patients. *Journal of the American Medical Association* **288**: 2151–2162.

Purdie JA, Ridley SA, Wallace PG (1990) Effective use of regional intensive therapy units. *British Medical Journal* **300**: 79–81.

Ridley SA (1998) Intermediate care, possibilities, requirements and solutions. *Anaesthesia* **53**: 654–664.

Roberts GA (1986) Burnout: psychobabble or valuable concept? *British Journal of Hospital Medicine* **36**: 194–197.

Schein RM, Hazday N, Pena M, *et al.* (1990) Clinical antecedents to in-hospital cardiopulmonary arrest. *Chest* **98**: 1388–1392.

Singer M, Myers S, Hall G, *et al.* (1994) The cost of intensive care: a comparison on one unit between 1988 and 1991. *Intensive Care Medicine* **20**: 542–549.

Smith L, Orts CM, O'Neil I, *et al.* (1999) TISS and mortality after discharge from intensive care. *Intensive Care Medicine* **25**: 1061–1065.

Society of Critical Care Medicine (Guidelines/ Practices Parameters Committee of the American College of Critical Care Medicine,

Society of Critical Care Medicine) (1995) Guidelines for intensive care unit design. *Critical Care Medicine* **23**: 582–588.

Spiby J (1989) Intensive care in the United Kingdom: report from the King's Fund Panel. *Anaesthesia* **44**: 428–431.

Subbe CP, Kruger M, Rutherford P, *et al.* (2001) Validation of a modified early warning score in medical admissions. *Quarterly Journal of Medicine* **94**: 521–526.

Subbe CP, Davies RG, Williams E, *et al.* (2003) Effect of introducing the modified early warning score on clinical outcomes, cardio-pulmonary arrests and intensive care utilisation in acute medical admissions. *Anaesthesia* **58**: 797–802.

Tarnow-Mordi WO, Hau C, Warden A, *et al.* (2000) Hospital mortality in relation to staff workload: a 4-year study in an adult intensive care unit. *Lancet* **356**: 185–189.

Twigg SJ, McCrirrick A, Sanderson PM (2001) A comparison of post mortem findings with post hoc estimated clinical diagnoses of patients who die in a United Kingdom intensive care unit. *Intensive Care Medicine* **27**: 706–710.

Vincent J-L (2000) Need for intensivists in intensive care units. *Lancet* **356**: 695–696.

Vincent J-L, Burchadi H (1999) Do we need intermediate care units? *Intensive Care Medicine* **25**: 1345–1349.

Wilson LM (1972) Intensive care delirium. The effect of outside deprivation in a windowless unit. *Archives of Internal Medicine* **130**: 225–226.

Winters BD, Pham J, Pronovost PJ (2006) Rapid response teams – walk, don't run. *Journal of the American Medical Association* **296**: 1645–1647.

Zimmerman JE, Wagner DP, Sun X, *et al.* (1996) Planning patient services for intermediate care units: insights based on care for intensive care unit low-risk monitor admissions. *Critical Care Medicine* **24**: 1626–1632.

2 Outcome and costs

MORTALITY, LONG-TERM SURVIVAL AND QUALITY OF LIFE

Intensive care outcomes can be assessed in terms of mortality, morbidity, disability, functional health status and quality of life.

For many critically ill patients, intensive care is undoubtedly life-saving and resumption of a normal lifestyle is to be expected. In certain patients (e.g. trauma victims or drug overdose patients and those recovering from cardiac surgery), mortality rates should be very low and the majority will make a good recovery. It is also widely accepted that the elective admission of selected high-risk patients into an intensive care or high-dependency unit, particularly in the immediate perioperative period, can minimize morbidity and mortality and reduce costs (see Chapter 5), as well as reducing the demands on medical and nursing personnel on the general wards.

In the more seriously ill patients, however, immediate mortality rates are high, while a significant number succumb soon after discharge from the intensive care unit (ICU) and the quality of life for some of those who do survive may be poor. In one study of outcome in a heterogeneous group of critically ill patients admitted to a typical general ICU in the UK, 24% died in the unit and a further 24% died within 2 years of discharge (Ridley et al., 1990). Long-term survival was related to age and severity of illness, but unsurprisingly, mortality was also influenced by the diagnosis: 71% of trauma patients survived to 1 year compared with only 41% of those admitted with gastrointestinal pathology (Ridley et al., 1990). Morbidity and mortality are also higher in morbidly obese patients (El-Solh et al. 2001) and patients readmitted to the ICU have a particularly poor outcome (Rosenberg et al., 2001). Patients referred to intensive care from medical specialties tend to be younger, more severely ill and have a worse short-term outcome than other categories of critically ill patients. Long-term outcome is better, however, and is almost equivalent to the general population (Lam and Ridley, 1999). In another study from the UK the ICU mortality rate was 29%, rising to a cumulative mortality rate of 39% at 3 months, 41% at 6 months and 43% at 1 year

after discharge from ICU (Eddleston et al., 2000). It is not clear how long it takes for the survival curves of intensive care survivors to become equivalent to those of the general population; some have suggested that it may take at least 3 years (Ridley and Plenderleith, 1994) and that after 4 years survival matches that of the normal population (Wright et al., 2003). When compared to patients who have been admitted to hospital, rather than to the general population, however, it seems that admission to intensive care has minimal independent effect on mortality after discharge (Keenan et al., 2002).

Quality of life following intensive care is influenced by both the extent of any persisting physical disability and the degree of cognitive and/or psychological impairment. Physical disabilities in intensive care survivors may include residual pulmonary dysfunction, neuromuscular weakness, entrapment neuropathies and altered sensation. Heterotopic calcification (the deposition of para-articular ectopic bone) is an unusual complication of critical illness but can cause complete immobilization of large joints. Neuropsychological disability may be related to memory loss, impaired attention/concentration, depression or posttraumatic stress disorder (Herridge, 2002). Prolonged cognitive dysfunction is also common (Sukantarat et al., 2005). Fatigue and a disturbed sleep pattern are common, while women may suffer significant hair loss (Eddleston et al., 2000).

Although some investigators have concluded that quality of life after intensive care is good, and is generally determined by premorbid health (Sage et al., 1986), others have detected significant decreases in quality of life in some subgroups, including younger patients, trauma victims, patients admitted with respiratory problems and those who previously had a good quality of life (Ridley and Wallace, 1990; Ridley et al., 1994). It has been shown that the patients' perceived quality of life may be reduced by a decreased ability to think and remember, limitations on their contact with other family members, a perceived decrease in their contribution to society, a reduction in activities outside work and a fall in income (Ridley et al., 1994). In young trauma patients the reduction in quality of life after intensive care is associated with significant psychological difficulties as well as concerns about employment and leisure activities, and it has been suggested that rehabilitation programmes should concentrate on these areas (Thiagarajan *et al.*, 1994).

More recently other investigators have suggested that, although quality of life scores are lower than in the general population at 3 months after intensive care discharge, the majority of patients are satisfied with their recovery. The incidence of psychological disturbance seems to be low, although fatigue, poor concentration and sleep disturbance are common (Eddleston *et al.*, 2000). Similarly, long-term survivors of acute respiratory distress syndrome (ARDS) describe a good overall health-related quality of life, although in a subgroup of patients traumatic experiences seemed to be related to the development of posttraumatic stress disorder and a reduction in quality of life (Schelling *et al.*, 1998). Even in a group of elderly patients (> 70 years old) who remained in intensive care for more than 30 days, most of the 47% of patients who survived to leave hospital remained independent with a good quality of life, despite moderate disability (Montuclard *et al.*, 2000). Moreover measures of quality of life tend to improve with time and significant improvements in mental health, vitality and social functioning, together with a reduction in pain scores, have been described after 6 months' convalescence (Ridley *et al.*, 1997).

COSTS

Intensive care is thought to be around 3–4 times more expensive than routine ward care (£1000–£1800 per bed-day) and costs continue to increase. In the UK, it has been estimated that the incremental cost per quality-adjusted life-year gained of treatment in intensive care is £7010. Cost-effectiveness can therefore be considered to be excellent and to compare favorably with other commonly used health care interventions (Ridley & Morris, 2007). This does, however, place intensive care at the higher end of health care expenditure, equivalent to heart transplantation, but cheaper than haemodialysis, and the costs increase considerably if expenditure on non-survivors, who frequently cost more than the survivors, is included in the calculation. In another study from the UK the median daily cost of treating a patient without sepsis was $750 (range $644–$909), whilst the median total cost was $1666 (range $980–$2772). Total expenditure on patients with sepsis was much higher than for those without sepsis, rising to a median cost of $17 962 (range $13 031–$28 547) for those who developed sepsis more than 2 days after ICU admission. This increased total cost was largely explained by a more prolonged stay in the ICU and an increased number of therapeutic interventions (Edbrooke *et al.*, 1999). In a group of elderly, long-stay, mechanically ventilated patients in a Parisian ICU, the estimated cost per hospital survivor was €55 272 ($60 246) (Montuclard *et al.*, 2000). Unusually in this study, resource utilization was similar in survivors and non-survivors.

END-OF-LIFE DECISION MAKING, WITHHOLDING AND WITHDRAWING TREATMENT (Carlet *et al.*, 2004; Intensive Care Society, 1998)

Apart from considerations of cost, inappropriate use of intensive care facilities has other implications (Jennett, 1984). The patient may experience unnecessary suffering and loss of dignity, while relatives may also have to endure extreme stress and emotional pressures. In some cases, treatment may simply prolong the process of dying or sustain life of dubious quality, and in others the risks of interventions may outweigh the potential benefits. Some time ago Jennett (1984) summarized the circumstances in which intensive care might be considered to be inappropriate as:

- unnecessary, because routine care would have achieved the same result;
- unsuccessful, because the patient is too ill to recover;
- unsafe, because the risks of complications exceed the potential benefits;
- unkind, because the subsequent quality of life is unacceptable;
- unwise, because of the diversion of limited resources.

To ensure a humane approach to the management of the critically ill and that limited resources are used appropriately, it is important to identify those patients who are most likely to benefit from intensive care (who ideally should never be denied admission), and to withhold, limit or withdraw intensive treatment when there is no prospect of recovery. The challenge is to avoid the futile prolongation of suffering, whilst at the same time avoiding precipitous decisions to withdraw treatment which could potentially result in avoidable deaths. It is also important to avoid admitting those who will make a good recovery even without admission to intensive care.

Because high mortality rates in the ICU and soon after discharge contribute significantly to the costs of intensive care, it has been suggested that efforts to contain costs should concentrate on prior selection of patients with a 'reasonable' prospect of survival (Ridley *et al.*, 1994). In practice, however, it is not usually acceptable to deny critically ill patients admission to intensive care, even when the chances of recovery from the acute illness seem to be remote. The long-term prognosis is usually uncertain, except perhaps in patients with disseminated, incurable malignancy or terminal chronic respiratory failure and those with severe permanent brain damage, and it is often difficult to make a precise diagnosis on initial referral. In addition, the patient's response to treatment can rarely be anticipated with any degree of certainty. Decisions to deny patients access to intensive care may also be tempered by the knowledge that the prognosis of individual disorders may change as standards of care improve or new treatments are introduced.

In the very early days of intensive care some considered it reasonable to deny admission simply on the grounds of old age, but it was soon recognized that this approach could not be justified. Although it is clear that some elderly patients may have little or no chance of returning to an independent existence and there is evidence that age can affect long-term survival (Ridley *et al.*, 1990), it has been shown that old age alone does not influence either the cost or the outcome of intensive care (Fedullo and Swinburne, 1983), neither does it preclude a good quality of life for survivors (Montuclard *et al.*, 2000). There is also evidence to suggest that age should not be a consideration when allocating intensive care beds to patients with malignancy (Chalfin and Carlon, 1990). It would seem that physiological age is more important than chronological age in determining survival and that a careful assessment of the patient's previous health, physical independence and social circumstances provides a better indication of the likely benefits of intensive care (Editorial, 1991).

Because it is rarely possible or acceptable to discriminate between critically ill patients before admission, the humanitarian and cost-effective practice of intensive care largely depends on a willingness to make decisions about withholding, withdrawing or limiting treatment once it becomes clear that the prognosis is hopeless. To persist with futile treatment is undignified and sometimes distressing for the patient, as well as upsetting and disruptive for the relatives, demoralizing for the staff and wasteful of limited resources. It is also now generally accepted that physicians are not obliged to administer *extraordinary care*. This has been defined (Schneiderman and Spragg, 1988) as care that is not morally obligatory because:

- it is medically impossible or futile;
- it provides no benefits in terms of prolonging life or alleviating suffering;
- the resulting burdens on the patient are excessive in relation to the benefits.

Increasingly, therefore, it is accepted that prolonged, aggressive treatment may not always be in the patients' best interests; consequently death in North American and European ICUs now frequently follows limitation of life-sustaining treatments (Esteban *et al.*, 2001; Ferrand *et al.*, 2001; Pochard *et al.*, 2001a; Prendergast and Luce, 1997, Prendergast *et al.*, 1998; Smedira *et al.*, 1990; Sprung *et al.*, 2003; Vincent, 1990, 1999). There are, however, substantial differences in the rates of withdrawing and withholding treatment between and within countries, as well as between individual units (McClean *et al.*, 2000) and clinicians. In one European survey, for example, the incidence of withdrawing life-sustaining treatments ranged from 48% in the north to 18% in the south of Europe (Sprung *et al.*, 2003).

DECISION MAKING

When making decisions to forgo life-sustaining treatment, clinicians may be helped by some of the statements that have appeared in landmark court decisions in the USA relating to patients in a persistent vegetative state (Schneiderman and Spragg, 1988). These have included the contention that 'prolongation of life does not mean a mere suspension of the act of dying, but contemplates at the very least a remission of symptoms enabling return towards a normal, functioning, integrated existence' and the recommendation that 'the focal point of decision should be the prognosis as to the reasonable possibility of return to cognitive and sapient life, as distinguished from the forced continuance of that biological vegetative existence'. In another case it was stated that life-sustaining treatment can be withdrawn when it is clear that the patient will never 'regain cognitive behaviour, the ability to communicate, or the capability of interacting purposefully with their environment' (Ruark and Raffin, 1988). Most would agree that these decisions should not be influenced by 'assessments of the personal worth, or social utility of another's life, or of that life to others' (Schneiderman and Spragg, 1988). Finally, as in all branches of medicine, decision making in intensive care should be based on the overriding priority to act in the patients' best interests and on generally accepted ethical principles (Ruark and Raffin, 1988), including:

- beneficence (health care should benefit the patient) – the primary objective is to preserve life, but this should be tempered by the need to alleviate suffering;
- non-maleficence – first do no harm (*primum non nocere*);
- respect the autonomy of the patient;
- distributive justice – allocate medical resources fairly;
- tell the truth.

These judgements can be difficult and onerous, not least because it is usually difficult to identify at an early stage and without reasonable doubt those patients who will inevitably die, and typically the prognosis only becomes obvious relatively late in the evolution of the acute illness. Unfortunately the available severity-scoring systems do not predict outcome in individual patients with sufficient accuracy to be useful in end of life decision making (see below) and even experienced clinicians find it difficult to assess prognosis with confidence. Although the concept of *futility* is often evoked as a justification for limiting treatment, there is no universally accepted definition of this term and the likelihood of benefit must be extremely small before an intervention can be considered 'futile' (some ethicists have suggested < 1%). Decision making is further complicated by the need to consider not only the chances of survival but also the anticipated quality of life if the patient were to survive, bearing in mind that there must always be a presumption in favour of preserving life.

Decisions to withhold or withdraw treatment should therefore always be taken by senior staff who are regularly present on the unit and continuously involved in patient care. These decisions should be reached in consultation with other intensive care clinicians and the primary physician or surgeon, sometimes with the assistance of clinicians with expertise in the prognosis of particular diseases. Nurses should also be involved in decisions to limit care, since they often have closer, more prolonged contact with patients and their families and may provide valuable insights into their feelings and opinions. Other health team members, for example physiotherapists, may also be valuable participants in the decision-making process, whilst clergy, social workers or psychologists can play a vital role in assisting patients, their friends and relatives to cope with the stress and depression that often accompany such decisions. Again, however, there appear to be differences between southern European countries, where decisions are more often made by the doctors acting alone, and the UK and Switzerland, where normally all the ICU staff are consulted (Vincent, 1999). Indeed, in one Spanish study, nurses were never involved in decisions to withhold or withdraw life support, although they were always informed of the decision (Esteban *et al.*, 2001).

It is important to appreciate that patients have the right to control what happens to them – *patient autonomy.* Informed, rational and competent patients therefore have the unambiguous right to refuse life-sustaining treatment. Not only do clinicians not have the right to force treatment on competent, unwilling patients, but if a competent patient requests that an intervention such as mechanical ventilation be discontinued, his or her wish should normally be honoured. Patients do not, however, have the right to demand life-sustaining treatment when the clinician considers it is inappropriate (Ruark and Raffin, 1988; Schneiderman and Spragg, 1988); neither is there any legal or moral obligation to provide treatment on request when there appears to be no possibility of benefit. Clinicians should not, therefore, feel obligated to intervene with mechanical ventilation if respiratory support will not contribute to preserving life or alleviating suffering. Finally, the patient's refusal, request or consent can only be truly informed when the clinician has communicated *all* the information the patient needs to make a knowledgeable decision, including any uncertainties.

The concept of patient autonomy is not usually directly applicable to intensive care patients, however, since fewer than 5% retain their decision-making capacity. Moreover it is difficult for medical and nursing staff to predict or understand the end-of-life preferences of individual patients and misunderstandings may be compounded by a failure to appreciate the varied cultural, spiritual and religious needs of patients and their families. Because respect for the autonomy of the patient is now paramount in medical practice in the USA, and since US law is determined to support this principle under all circumstances, *advance health care directives, health care proxies* (surrogates) and the choice of proxy based on a hierarchical list have all received legal recognition. Also *durable power of attorney* can be used to allow the patient to select surrogate decision-makers in advance, and this may help to minimize subsequent family conflicts during the decision-making process.

Advance directives or *living wills* enable patients to anticipate some end-of-life decisions while still capable and ratio-

nal and to make a formal statement about how they would want to be treated should they become incompetent. Unfortunately, advance directives have not proved to be particularly useful in the management of mentally incompetent critically ill patients and they are not, of course, a substitute for effective communication between staff, patients and relatives. In practice they are often ignored by caregivers, they have been completed by fewer than 10% of patients admitted to ICUs and they do not seem to affect patients' outcomes, including quality of life, hospital length of stay or use of cardiopulmonary resuscitation (Schneiderman *et al.*, 1992). Some have also expressed concern that patients might be (or feel themselves to be) under pressure from friends, relatives or health workers to indicate their willingness to have treatment discontinued because they think of themselves as a burden that nobody wishes (or can afford) to support. Occasionally the likely progression of an illness may have been explained to the patient who may then have indicated the choices he or she would wish to make at each stage.

Although the *views of the family* concerning the patient's best interests are often invaluable, the use of surrogates also has limitations, not least because most patients have not discussed their end-of-life preferences in advance. Some studies have found that *surrogates* often fail to represent the patient's wishes accurately (Seckler *et al.,* 1991) and others have shown that relatives of dying patients have high rates of anxiety and depression (Pochard *et al.,* 2001b), perhaps compromising their decision-making capability. Surrogates may also have limited ability to comprehend medical aspects of care and they may have conflicts of interest, believing, for example, that they will benefit financially from their relative's demise. Some clinicians have suggested that family/ surrogates should not be burdened with making end-of-life decisions, although anxious and depressed family members rarely express a desire to be excluded from decision making and there is a possibility that exclusion could increase, rather than decrease, stress and anxiety. Although most would advocate that family members should be involved in end-of-life decisions, in practice this is not always the case (Ferrand *et al.,* 2001; Pochard *et al.,* 2001a) and it seems that the family is less likely to be involved in southern European than in northern European countries (Vincent, 1999).

It must be recognized that most societies are increasingly multicultural and multiracial, with a diversity of religious beliefs, and that deficiencies in end-of-life care tend to be more frequent in ethnic-minority populations. There is also evidence to suggest that the religious background of the clinician can influence the provision of end-of-life care (Vincent, 1999). Not only may the religion, ethnicity and culture of clinicians shape their attitudes and approaches to end-of-life care, but these factors can also fundamentally influence the hopes and aspirations of their families.

Importantly, medical and nursing staff involved in making end-of-life decisions should be aware that their assessment of the usefulness of intensive care for an individual patient may differ substantially from that of patients or their relatives. In one study, for example, nurses significantly underestimated the usefulness of intensive care in comparison to the evaluation of patients or their families, and patients believed that quality of life was a less important consideration than did their nurses (Danis *et al.*, 1987). Moreover, the demand and expectations of patients and their families may conflict with efforts to ration intensive care on the basis of age, function or quality of life. Danis *et al.* (1988) found that 70% of a group of medical intensive care patients or their families were 100% willing to undergo intensive care again to achieve even just 1 month of survival, while only 8% were completely unwilling to undergo intensive care to achieve any prolongation of life. In the majority of cases, preferences did not seem to be closely related to functional status or quality of life and were not altered by life expectancy. The willingness to undergo intensive care again was not influenced by age, severity of the acute illness, length of stay or the cost of intensive care (Danis *et al.*, 1988).

To date the role of ethics committees and ethics consultants has largely been limited to exceptional cases and their impact on day-to-day end-of-life decision making has been minimal. Some recent evidence suggests, however, that the more routine use of a readily available and responsive ethics consultant may result in a measurable improvement in end-of-life care (Schneiderman *et al.*, 2000) and ethics committees can be helpful when establishing institutional policies and guidelines.

WITHDRAWING LIFE-SUSTAINING TREATMENT AND END-OF-LIFE CARE

Once the decision to withdraw life-sustaining treatment has been made, the responsible clinicians, in consultation with the nurses and sometimes the patient's family, must decide which interventions should be discontinued. Such choices are important because they can influence the rapidity, the degree of discomfort and the dignity of the patient's death. It is worth bearing in mind that ethically, withdrawing life support, including mechanical ventilation, is considered to be no different from discontinuing any other inappropriate medical intervention (Schneiderman and Spragg, 1988) and that there is no ethical difference between withholding or withdrawing a life-sustaining treatment. Discussions with family and friends should stress the alleviation of suffering and emphasize that priority will be given to the comfort and dignity of the patient. Such *comfort care* has physical, social and spiritual dimensions. First and foremost, the patient must be assured of a painfree death. Moral principles and legislation prohibit administering treatments specifically designed to hasten death (except under certain special circumstances in a few countries), but the patient must be given sufficient analgesia to alleviate pain and distress; if such analgesia hastens death this *double effect* should not inhibit the primary aim of assuring comfort. When mechanical ventilation is to be discontinued, the patient must be given narcotics and sedatives to eliminate the discomfort of agonal efforts to breathe. Unfortunately, it seems that in practice major problems such as pain, discomfort, anxiety, sleep disturbance, unsatisfied hunger, thirst and depression are often not adequately addressed (Nelson *et al.*, 2001).

Importantly, the provision of comfort should involve the family as well as the patient. In this respect the importance of the nurses' rapport with the family must be understood and encouraged, since the comfort and satisfaction of the family during and after the dying process often depend on this relationship. Providing relatives of patients who are dying on the ICU with a bereavement brochure, using a proactive communication strategy that includes longer conferences, and allowing family members more time to talk seem to lessen the burden of bereavement (Lautrette *et al.*, 2007). The feelings of family and friends may also influence the manner in which treatment is withdrawn. Thus in some cases it may be appropriate to delay withdrawing treatment to allow them to cope with grief or to assimilate and come to terms with their loss.

It also seems that organizational factors may influence the approach to end-of-life care. For example, patients dying in a medical ICU under the care of staff intensivists were more likely to undergo the active withdrawal of life-sustaining therapies than those with a private attending physician (Kollef and Ward, 1999), perhaps because, usually, intensive care specialists have more relevant experience, are more available, provide more appropriate care for dying patients and are more comfortable with treatment limitation. It has also been suggested that patient reimbursement status (Rapoport *et al.*, 1992), case mix and hospital type (university versus community) (Bach *et al.*, 1998) may influence the frequency with which life-sustaining treatments are withdrawn, although such factors are certainly not the most important influences on decisions to withhold or withdraw care. The influence of the availability of intensive care facilities on end-of-life care is unclear. In one survey, ICU admissions were frequently limited by lack of beds (especially in Greece, Italy, Portugal and the UK) and yet three-quarters of clinicians stated that they would admit patients with no hope of surviving for more than a few weeks (Vincent, 1999).

CONSENSUS IN END-OF-LIFE CARE?

There can be no doubt that there are significant differences between end-of-life care in Europe and North America, as well as wide variations between and within countries and between individual units. The attitudes of individual clinicians to end-of-life care also differ and doctors will often admit to discrepancies between their clinical practice and their personal philosophy and beliefs. As well as differences in the rates of withholding and withdrawing treatments, the frequency with which intensive care admission is refused and the proportion of intensive care deaths preceded by a 'do not resuscitate' (DNR) order, there are other differences including the use of advance directives, the designation of

Table 2.1 Similarities between the views of European professional societies on end-of-life care

Refer to the basic ethical principles of: autonomy; beneficence; non-malificence; proportionate treatment and distributive justice. Several state explicitly that the need for an intensive care unit bed for another patient should not be a reason for withdrawing treatment

Recognize the necessity for the limitation of life-prolonging treatments when the clinical situation is hopeless and a treatment appears either futile or inadvisable. Several societies state that there is no ethical difference between withholding and withdrawing life-prolonging treatments. Although many clinicians are reluctant to withdraw treatments once they have been introduced, it is suggested that a treatment may be withdrawn if it has proved to be ineffective

Underline the importance of the decision-making process which must be based on a thorough evaluation of the situation made by the attending intensive care unit physician over a sufficient time course to ascertain the hopelessness of the situation

Advocate taking into account the patient's will when he/she is capable of expressing it

Recommend keeping the family totally informed and taking their opinion into account. Some underline the desirability of consensus amongst the family. All recommend that the burden of the decision should not be put upon the family. Most recommend more or less explicitly the need to provide psychological support to the family

Stress the need for a general consensus between all the medical staff and the nurses taking care of the patient. In all countries, the final decision is the personal responsibility of the clinician alone

Strongly recommend that all decisions, and discussions for some, be recorded in the patient's notes

Recommend that it is the physician's duty to initiate the withdrawing of life-sustaining techniques but indicate that the nurse may be involved depending on the procedure to be withdrawn

Recommend implementing a thorough palliative care strategy once the decision to withhold or withdraw life-sustaining treatments has been made. Recommendations include analgesic and sedative agents in adequate doses, compassionate care, maximal possible access for relatives and friends, and privacy

Religious rites must be allowed and respected

Take a strong position against euthanasia, which is illegal or forbidden by national medical associations in most countries

surrogates and the involvement of families in end-of-life decision making. There also appears to be considerable variation in the extent to which nurses and other professionals are involved in these decisions, the type of therapeutic interventions most frequently withdrawn and the role played by ethics consultants or committees. Some of these differences may be more apparent than real, however, and recent evidence suggests that there has been some convergence in opinion about good practice at the end of life among professional societies in the UK and Europe (**Table 2.1**) as well as in the USA.

Nevertheless, some continue to remark on the apparent differences between the approach to end-of-life decisions in North America (favouring *patient autonomy*, i.e. a patient/surrogate-directed approach) and certain European countries, particularly those in the south, which favour a *paternalistic* (i.e. doctor-directed) approach. Certainly guidelines from the UK (e.g. those published by the General Medical Council and the British Medical Association) and other professional societies in Europe clearly indicate that if the patient is incompetent the final decision is the sole responsibility of the doctor in charge of the patient's care. In the USA, on the other hand, none of the professional societies advocates that the ultimate or primary decision should rest with clinicians. More recently North America and many European countries have been moving towards the adoption

of the *shared decision-making* model, an approach which seems to be favoured by the majority of patients, family members and the general public. The objective is to achieve consensus with the family on a course of action which is in accordance with the patient's values.

Clearly, sensitive, inclusive and effective communication with the family or patient's representative(s) is a prerequisite. Such discussions are easier when the family has been kept fully informed during all stages of the patient's illness, with regular updates on progress, and when they have been prepared for the possibility that the patient may not survive and that it may be appropriate to limit treatment in the event of failure to improve or further deterioration. The shared decision-making process involves the intensive care team providing information concerning the patient's medical condition and prognosis, as well as recommendations and guidance as to the best course of management, whilst the family provides insight into the patient's premorbid health status and wishes. These meetings are also an opportunity to gain a better understanding of the patient's background, including religion and culture, and to build a collaborative relationship with the family. Ultimately the doctor leading the health care team takes responsibility for the proposed course of action. With this approach conflicts are rare, except when there has been a failure of communication, but may arise, for example, when the family insists on continuation of life-sustaining therapy against the advice of the intensive care team. Under these circumstances it may be reasonable to continue support for a predetermined period, following which the situation is reassessed with the family. On the rare occasions when conflict cannot be resolved, a second opinion, perhaps from a clinician from another institution, or an ethics consultation may be helpful. Occasionally it may be advisable to obtain legal advice.

Finally the importance of adequate documentation of the decision-making process, of audit and of training for medical and nursing staff in end-of-life care must be emphasized.

■ SEVERITY-SCORING SYSTEMS

The outcome of critical illness is determined by:

- the severity of the acute illness;
- the patient's previous state of health;
- the nature of the underlying disease;
- the treatment given;
- the patient's response to treatment.

Early attempts to quantify the relationship between severity of illness and outcome were based on disease-specific indices such as the Glasgow Coma Scale (GCS) for patients with acute brain injury (see Chapter 15) and the Ranson criteria for acute pancreatitis (see Chapter 16). Although these systems do accurately stratify patients according to risk, they are limited by their disease specificity. A variety of more generally applicable methods for assessing illness severity, and thereby estimating probabilities of death, have therefore been developed. These 'generic' scoring systems have included:

- assessments of the severity of the acute disturbance of physiological function: Acute Physiology and Chronic Health Evaluation (APACHE) and the Simplified Acute Physiology Score (SAPS) (Knaus et al., 1981, 1985, 1991; Le Gall et al., 1984, 1993);
- a measure of the therapeutic effort expended on a patient: Therapeutic Intervention Scoring System (TISS) (Cullen et al., 1974; Keene and Cullen, 1983);
- Mortality Prediction Model (MPM) (Lemeshow et al., 1988) later updated to a Mortality Probability Model (MPMII) (Lemeshow et al., 1993);
- an assessment of organ dysfunction: Sepsis-related Organ Failure Assessment (SOFA) score (Vincent et al., 1996), Multiple Organ Dysfunction (MOD) score (Marshall et al., 1995).

Other systems have been devised for particular categories of patients, such as the combined Trauma and Injury Severity Scoring System (TRISS) (Boyd et al., 1987), which consists of calculations based on the Injury Severity Score (ISS) and the Revised Trauma Score (RTS).

These scoring systems have been used for comparative audit of clinical effectiveness, for research and to inform the clinical management of individual patients.

THE ACUTE PHYSIOLOGY AND CHRONIC HEALTH EVALUATION SYSTEM

The APACHE scoring system is a widely applicable method for assessing severity of illness in the critically ill and has been extensively validated. It was originally designed as a classification system (Knaus et al., 1981), which would:

- control for case mix (that is, the characteristics of the patient population in terms of diagnosis, comorbidities, presentation, age, sex, severity of illness and available treatment) – case mix adjustment;
- allow meaningful comparisons of outcomes;
- assist in the evaluation of new therapies;
- be used to study the use of intensive care.

The original score consisted of two parts: the Acute Physiology Score (APS) based on 34 physiological variables, and an assessment of the patient's previous state of health. Scores were assigned to each physiological variable depending on the extent to which they deviated from normal and their relative importance in determining outcome. There was a direct relationship between the calculated APS and the relative risk of death, although the chronic health indicators were associated with an increased risk of death only in patients with very poor and failing health before admission.

APACHE II

Largely because a number of the 34 physiological variables are not routinely measured in all patients, the relatively complex APACHE system was simplified, refined and improved to produce the clinically more practical and now extensively used APACHE II score (Knaus et al., 1985) (Table 2.2). The number of physiological variables was reduced to 12 easily measured values, the assessment of chronic health was changed to a system in which points were assigned for long-standing organ dysfunction, and increasing age attracted additional risk points. The impact of emergency surgery on outcome was also incorporated into the risk assessment. The final APACHE II score is the sum of the acute physiology, age and chronic health points, calculated from the worst values during the first 24 hours of intensive care.

It is important to appreciate that the relationship between this score and outcome is crucially dependent on the underlying disease. For example, for a given score the prognosis for a patient with septic shock is considerably worse than that for a patient with asthma or diabetic ketoacidosis. To provide an accurate assessment of illness severity and risk of death it is therefore essential to weight the score using coefficients assigned to specific diagnoses (Table 2.3). When this is done there is a consistent relationship between APACHE II mortality predictions and observed hospital death rates throughout the spectrum from low to high risk of death.

Since APACHE II can accurately quantify the severity of illness and predict overall mortality for large groups of acutely ill patients, it may be useful for auditing a unit's

Table 2.2 Assignment of points to derive Acute Physiology and Chronic Health Evaluation (APACHE) II score

Table 2.2A Assignment of points in acute physiology score

	4	3	2	1	0	1	2	3	4
Rectal temperature (°C)	≥ 41.0	39.0–40.9		38.5–38.9	36.0–38.4	34.0–35.9	32.0–33.9	30.0–31.9	≤ 29.9
Mean blood pressure (mmHg)	≥ 160	130–159	110–129		70–109		50–69		≤ 49
Heart rate (ventricular response/min)	≥ 180	140–179	110–139		70–109		55–69	40–54	≤ 39
Respiratory rate (breaths/min, spontaneous or mechanical)	≥ 50	35–49		25–34	12–24	10–11	6–9		≤ 5
Oxygenation (mmHg)									
$F_IO_2 \geq 0.5$ (record A-adO$_2$)	≥ 500	350–499	200–349		< 200				
$F_IO_2 < 0.5$ (record only PaO$_2$)					> 70	61–70		55–60	< 55
Arterial pH	≥ 7.70	7.60–7.69		7.50–7.59	7.33–7.49		7.25–7.32	7.15–7.24	< 7.15
Serum sodium (mmol/L)	≥ 180	160–179	155–159	150–154	130–149		120–129	111–119	≤ 110
Serum potassium (mmol/L)	≥ 7.0	6.0–6.9		5.5–5.9	3.5–5.4	3.0–3.4	2.5–2.9		< 2.5
Serum creatinine (mg/100 mL)	≥ 3.5	2.0–3.4	1.5–1.9		0.6–1.4		< 0.6		
Haematocrit	≥ 60		50–59.9	46–49.9	30–45.9		20–29.9		< 20
White blood cell count ($\times 10^3$/mL^3)	≥ 40		20–39.9	15–19.9	3–14.9		1–2.9		< 1

Glasgow Coma Scale (GCS): subtract GCS from 15 to obtain points assigned

Table 2.2B Points assigned to age and chronic disease as part of the APACHE II score

Age (years)	Score
< 45	0
45–54	2
55–64	3
65–74	5
≥ 75	6
History of chronic conditions	
None	0
Present:	
Elective surgical patient:	2
Emergency surgical or non-surgical patient	5

Table 2.3 Diagnostic categories used to provide an accurate assessment of illness severity and risk of death from the Acute Physiology and Chronic Health Evaluation (APACHE) II score

Primary system

R, respiratory; C, cardiovascular; N, neurological; G, gastrointestinal; K, renal; M, metabolic; H, haematological

Precipitating factor

01 Infection
02 Neoplasm
03 Trauma
04 Self-intoxication (overdose)
05 Intracerebral haemorrhage
06 Cranial haemorrhage
07 Seizures
08 Neuromuscular failure
09 Coronary artery disease
10 Myocardial infarction
11 Valvar heart disease
12 Peripheral vascular disease
13 Embolus
14 Congenital anomaly/anatomical defect
15 Congestive heart failure/pulmonary oedema
16 Hypertension
17 Rhythm disturbance
18 Pericardial disease
19 Cardiogenic shock/cardiomyopathy
20 Septic shock/sepsis
21 Anaphylactic/drug-induced shock
22 Haemorrhagic shock/hypovolaemic shock
23 Bleeding (significant but not shock)
24 Cardiac/respiratory arrest
25 Allergic reaction
26 Obstruction/perforation
27 Coma/mental derangement
28 Electrolyte imbalance/acid–base disturbance
29 Diabetic ketoacidosis
30 Endocrine emergency
31 Hypothermia/hyperthermia
32 Haematological insufficiency/crisis
33 Transplant surgery
34 Postoperative ventilation or respiratory support (unplanned)
35 Acute exacerbation of chronic end-stage disease
36 Toxic/chemical poisoning

clinical activity, for evaluating the use of resources and for characterizing groups of patients in clinical studies. Severity scores such as APACHE II may also be useful as a means of adjusting for case-mix differences between groups of patients in non-randomized or observational studies and to aid stratification in randomized controlled trials. Many believe that despite its limitations (see below), APACHE II mortality predictions can also be used to compare the efficacy of intensive care between different units and over time in the same unit. This involves calculating the expected mortality rate by dividing the sum of the predicted risks of death for all patients by the total number of patients. It is suggested that by relating the actual to the predicted mortality – the *standardized mortality ratio* (SMR) – the performance of individual units is adjusted for case mix and can be assessed and compared with other units. When this technique was used to compare outcome in 13 major medical centres in the USA, results were significantly better than average in one hospital, while in another, outcome was significantly worse than predicted. These differences were thought to be related more to the interaction and coordination of each ICU's staff than the administrative structure, amount of specialized treatment used or the hospital's teaching status (Knaus *et al.*, 1986). The calculation of SMRs is, however, a fairly blunt instrument for between-unit comparisons. Only extreme differences in SMR (0.59 and 1.58 respectively in the study just mentioned) can be considered to be significant, and then only when based on large numbers. In addition, serious errors can be introduced, for example by overscoring on the GCS or the chronic health evaluation, or by misclassifying the diagnostic category. When using the APACHE II methodology it is important to appreciate that:

- it must not be used without taking into account the underlying disease;
- it cannot be used on samples of patients selected according to different criteria;
- it cannot be applied at times other than the first 24 hours of intensive care;
- the risk of death may not be accurately assessed in patients with rare conditions or in those with unusual presentations of common conditions;
- the accuracy of predictions will be reduced when data collection is incomplete;
- mortality predictions are of limited value because they are based on treatment outcomes.

The international applicability of the American-derived APACHE II equation has been assessed in a number of studies (Rowan *et al.*, 1993; Sirio *et al.*, 1992; Zimmerman *et al.*, 1988). When APACHE II was used in two hospitals in New Zealand (Zimmerman *et al.*, 1988) and in ICUs in six hospitals in Japan (Sirio *et al.*, 1992), the observed mortality did not differ significantly from that predicted by the American equation. In the UK and Ireland, however, it was found that, although the overall predictive ability was good, the

Table 2.4A Simplified Acute Physiology Score (SAPS II) score sheet

Variable/points	26	13	12	11	9	7	6	5	4	3	2	0
Age (years)												< 40
Heart rate (beats/min)				< 40							40–69	70–119
Systolic BP (mmHg)		< 70						70–99				100–199
Body temperature (°C)												< 39
(°F)												< 102.2
Only if VENT or CPAP:												
$Pa0_2$ (mmHg)/F_10_2 (0.xx)				< 100	100–199		≥ 200					
$Pa0_2$ (kPa)/F_10_2 (0.xx)				< 13.3	13.3–26.5		≥ 26.6					
Urinary output (L/day)				< 0.500					0.500–0.999			≥ 1.000
Blood urea (mmol/L)												< 10.0
(g/L)												< 0.60
WBC (10^3/mm^3)			< 1.0									1.0–19.9
Serum K$^+$ (mmol/L)										< 3.0		3.0–4.9
Serum Na$^+$ (mmol/L)								< 125				125–144
Serum HCO$_3^-$ (mmol/L)							< 15			15–19		≥ 20
Bilirubin (μmol/L)												< 68.4
(mg/L)												< 4.0
GCS	< 6	6–8				9–10		11–13				14–15
Chronic diseases												
Type of admission												
Sum of points												
Total SAPS II												
Risk of hospital death												

AIDS, acquired immune deficiency syndrome; BP, blood pressure; CPAP, continuous positive airways pressure; GCS, Glasgow Coma Scale; Haem. mal., haematological malignancy; Met. can., metastatic cancer; VENT, ventilated; WBC, white blood cells.

observed mortality was rather higher than predicted in two of the lower-risk groups and lower than expected in some of the highest-risk patients. Moreover, the equation did not adjust uniformly across some of the subgroups defined according to factors such as age and diagnosis. There are a number of possible explanations for these disparities, including systematic differences in medical definitions and diagnostic labelling between the two countries, systematic variations in the effectiveness of treatment and the possibility that there are age-specific differences in health status between countries. These findings highlight some of the complexities of severity scoring (Rowan et al., 1993).

APACHE III

Knaus et al. (1991) later attempted to improve on the prognostic estimates derived from APACHE II by re-evaluating the selection and weighting of physiological variables, as well as examining the influence of differences in patient selection

and timing of intensive care admission on outcome. The improved explanatory power of this APACHE III score can be combined with major disease category and previous patient location to produce an estimated risk of death for each patient. As with APACHE II, the difference between predicted and actual death rates can be used to compare mortalities between units and to provide a quantitative assessment of quality of care. APACHE III could also be used to improve ICU discharge decisions (Zimmerman et al., 1994). Finally, further development of the APACHE III score provides equations to estimate the length of stay in ICU, the amount and type of therapy required and the intensity of nursing care. When used in Scottish ICUs, however, the predicted length of stay, which is based on practice in the USA, was consistently longer than the actual length of stay (Woods et al., 2000).

The improvements in predictive power achieved with APACHE III are, however, relatively modest and the coeffi-

Table 2.4A *continued*

1	2	3	4	6	7	8	9	10	12	15	16	17	18
					40–59				60–69	70–74	75–79		≥ 80
			120–159		≥ 160								
	≥ 200												
		≥ 39											
		≥ 102.2											
				10.0–29.9				≥ 30.0					
				0.60–1.79				≥ 1.80					
		≥ 20.0											
		≥ 5.0											
≥ 145													
			68.4–102.5					> 102.6					
			40.0–59.9					≥ 60.0					
							Met. can.	Haem. mal.				AIDS	
Scheduled surgical				Medical	Unscheduled surgical								

cients and equation for calculation of risk are not in the public domain (Bion, 1993); most units therefore continue to use the APACHE II methodology for clinical audit and research.

OTHER SCORING SYSTEMS
Simplified Acute Physiology Score
This arose from an independent attempt to simplify the APACHE system by reducing the original 34 variables to 13. The weights assigned to each physiological variable were nearly equivalent to those used in APACHE and the accuracy of predictions was comparable to that obtained using the original APACHE system.

SAPSII (Le Gall *et al.*, 1993) was developed by logistic regression analysis of data from a joint European/North American study. Seventeen readily available variables are used to derive a score (**Table 2.4**) from which the probability of death is calculated directly without correcting for the acute disease.

Sepsis-related Organ Failure Assessment (SOFA) score
Because organ dysfunction develops and resolves over a variable time course, meaningful assessment requires repeated evaluation, usually on a daily basis. Effective organ failure assessment systems need to be simple to apply and should be based on reliable, repeatable and readily available variables. The SOFA system (also known as the sequential organ failure score) was developed by the European Society of Intensive Care Medicine as a means of assessing the degree of individual organ dysfunction in critically ill patients easily and repeatedly (Vincent *et al.*, 1996) (**Table 2.5**). This score is intended to quantify morbidity and therefore complements other systems which focus on mortality. The score is limited to six organs, each being awarded a score between zero (normal) and 4,

Table 2.4B Variables and definitions for Simplified Acute Physiology Score (SAPS II)

Variable	Definition
Age	Use the patient's age at last birthday in years
Heart rate	Use the worst value in 24 hours, either low or high heart rate (e.g. if it varies from cardiac arrest (11 points) to extreme tachycardia (3 points), assign 4 points)
Systolic BP	Use the same method as for heart rate (e.g. if it varies from 60 mmHg to 195 mmHg, assign 13 points)
Body temperature	Use the highest temperature in Celsius or Fahrenheit
Pao_2/F_iO_2 ratio	If ventilated or CPAP, use the lowest value of the ratio
Urinary output	If the patient is in the ICU for less than 24 hours, make the calculation for 24 hours (e.g. 1 litre in 8 hours = 3 litres in 24 hours)
Blood urea	Use the highest value in mmol/L or g/L
WBC	Use the worst (high or low) WBC count according to the score sheet
Serum K^+	Use the worst (high or low) value in mmol/L according to the score sheet
Serum Na^+	Use the worst (high or low) value in mmol/L according to the score sheet
Serum HCO_3^-	Use the lowest value in mmol/L
Bilirubin	Use the highest value in µmol/L or mg/L
GCS	Use the lowest value: if the patient is sedated, record the estimated GCS before sedation
Type of admission	Unscheduled surgical*, scheduled surgical† or medical‡
AIDS	Yes, if positive HIV with clinical complications such as *Pneumocystis jirovecii* pneumonia, Kaposi's sarcoma, lymphoma, tuberculosis, *Toxoplasma* infection
Haematological malignancy	Yes, if lymphoma, acute leukaemia, multiple myeloma
Metastatic cancer	Yes, if proven metastasis by surgery, CT scan or any other method

AIDS, acquired immunodeficiency syndrome; BP, blood pressure; CPAP, continuous positive airways pressure; GCS, Glagow Coma Score; ICU, intensive care unit; WBC, white blood cells.
*Patients added to operating room schedule within 24 hours of the operation.
†Patients whose surgery was scheduled at least 24 hours in advance.
‡Patients having no surgery within 1 week of ICU admission.

based on the worst values on each day. Because mortality is directly related to the degree of organ failure, it is not surprising that retrospective studies have confirmed that increasing SOFA scores are associated with increased mortality.

Multiple Organ Dysfunction (MOD) score (Table 2.6) (Marshall et al., 1995)

This score uses variables which reflect physiological derangement, rather than therapeutic interventions used to support failing organs. Only postresuscitation values are used in the calculation of the MOD score, values are recorded at the same time each day and missing or unobtainable values are presumed to be normal. Incremental increases in aggregate MOD scores are associated with increased ICU mortality and daily MOD component scores provide additional prognostic information when compared to baseline scores (Cook et al., 2001). The MOD score may provide a measure of

admission severity of illness, intensity of therapeutic intervention and global ICU morbidity, and may be useful as an outcome measure in clinical trials.

Mortality Prediction Models (MPMs)

Lemeshow et al. (1988) devised MPMs based on stepwise linear discriminant function and multiple logistic regression analysis of data from a large cohort of adult general intensive care patients in a single hospital. A series of questions with predominantly yes or no answers relating to 11 admission variables are answered and these are weighted according to their individual contribution to mortality. Serial observations of the changing probability of mortality are then used to anticipate the likely outcome. Later it was shown that APACHE II is superior to the MPM as a means of predicting outcome in groups of adult intensive care patients from the UK and Ireland (Rowan et al., 1994), although later develop-

Table 2.5 The Sepsis related Organ Failure Assessment (SOFA) score

SOFA score	1	2	3	4
Respiration				
PaO_2/F_iO_2 (mmHg)	< 400	< 300	< 200	< 100
(kPa)	(< 53.3)	(< 40)	(< 26.7)	(< 13.3)
			⟵ with respiratory support ⟶	
Coagulation				
Platelets ($\times 10^9$/L)	< 150	< 100	< 50	< 20
Liver				
Bilirubin (mg/dL)	1.2–1.9	2.0–5.9	6.0–11.9	> 12.0
(μmol/L)	(20–32)	(33–101)	(102–204)	(> 204)
Cardiovascular				
Hypotension [a]	MAP < 70 mmHg	Dopamine ≤ 5 or dobutamine (any dose)	Dopamine > 5 or adrenaline ≤ 0.1 or noradrenaline ≤ 0.1	Dopamine > 15 or adrenaline > 0.1 or noradrenaline > 0.1
Central nervous system				
Glasgow Coma Scale	13–14	10–12	6–9	< 6
Renal				
Creatinine (mg/dl)	1.2–1.9	2.0–3.4	3.5–4.9	> 5.0
(μmol/L)	(110–170)	(171–299)	(300–440)	(> 440)
or				
Urine output (mL/day)			< 500	< 200

MAP, mean arterial pressure.
*Adrenergic agents administered for at least 1 hour (doses are in μg/kg per min).

ments of the MPM (MPM II at 24, 48 and 72 hours) may provide more accurate estimates of the probability of hospital mortality (Lemeshow et al., 1994).

Therapeutic Intervention Scoring System (Table 2.7)

The TISS was originally designed to measure the severity of illness by quantifying the type and intensity of the treatment provided (Cullen et al., 1974). Because TISS points are dependent on local, or even individual, treatment strategies, and the therapeutic capability of the unit, as well as the appropriateness of an intervention, the score cannot be used to compare the efficacy of intensive care in different units. Also TISS is not an ideal method for assessing the relationship between severity of illness and outcome. It does, however, provide an accurate assessment of the level of care and monitoring and can be performed daily. It is therefore a valuable administrative tool. TISS can, for example, be used to assess the workload required by each patient, to establish nurse-to-patient ratios, to determine a hospital's requirement for ICU beds and to calculate costs. More recently, an intermediate TISS has been developed for use in patients who do not require intensive care (Cullen et al., 1994).

Injury Severity Score and Combined Trauma and Injury Severity Score

The ISS and TRISS system was developed to provide a standard approach for the evaluation of trauma care (Boyd et al., 1987). Mortality following traumatic injury depends on the degree of physiological derangement, the extent of the anatomical injury, the age of the patient and whether the trauma was blunt or penetrating. The TRISS methodology combines these factors – the RTS, the ISS, age, blunt or penetrating injury – to provide a measure of the probability of survival.

PREDICTING DEATH IN INDIVIDUAL PATIENTS

Although the APACHE methodology and other severity-scoring systems can be used to estimate individual probabilities of death, they clearly cannot predict with certainty the outcome in an individual patient, and were not designed to do so. Objective probabilities should not therefore be used in isolation as a basis for limiting or discontinuing treatment and should not be used as a substitute for clinical decision making, as outlined earlier in this chapter. It is, however, possible that reliable, well-calibrated prognostic scoring systems may be useful aids to such subjective assessments.

Table 2.6A The Multiple Organ Dysfunction (MOD) score

Organ system	0	1	2	3	4
Respiratory*					
PO_2/F_iO_2	> 300	226–300	151–225	76–150	≤ 75
Renal†					
Serum creatinine (μmol/L)	≤ 100	101–200	201–350	351–500	> 500
Hepatic					
Serum bilirubin (μmol/L)	≤ 20	21–60	61–120	121–240	> 240
Cardiovascular‡					
PAR	≤ 10.0	10.1–15.0	15.1–20.0	20.1–30.0	> 30.0
Haematological					
Platelet count (platelets/mL)	> 120	81–120	51–80	21–50	≤ 20
Neurological§					
GCS	15	13–14	10–12	7–9	≤ 6

Selected values are those obtained at a standard time of day (preferably morning) rather than the worst values during the day; missing data receive a score of zero. *The PO_2/F_iO_2 ratio is calculated without reference to the use or mode of mechanical ventilation, and without reference to the use or level of positive end-expiratory pressure. †The serum creatinine level is measured without reference to the use of dialysis. ‡The pressure-adjusted heart rate (PAR). §The Glasgow Coma Scale (GCS) is preferably calculated by the patient's nurse, and is scored conservatively (for the patient receiving sedation or muscle relaxants, normal function is assumed unless there is evidence of intrinsically altered mentation). Reproduced with permission from Marshall *et al.* (1995).

Table 2.6B Calculation of Multiple Organ Dysfunction (MOD) scores*

Admission MOD score

The sum of the values for the six MOD score variables obtained on the first ICU day

Daily MOD score

The sum of the values for the six MOD score variables calculated separately for each ICU day

Cumulative MOD score

The sum of the worst daily values for each variable up to the current day. The baseline score is the admission MOD score. Further deterioration in any given variable is reflected by increasing the score for that system, while improvement is not recorded. In contrast with the daily score, the cumulative score reflects only worsening of function, and provides a measure of the time course and severity of clinical deterioration following ICU admission

Aggregate MOD score

The sum of the worst day's value for each of the six variables over the entire ICU stay. Thus the value for the respiratory component may be obtained on day 2 and that for the renal component on day 11. This has been the standard approach used to quantify organ failure or dysfunction; it can be appreciated that the aggregate MOD score will be identical with the cumulative score on the last ICU day

ΔMOD score

The difference between the aggregate score, or the cumulative score over a defined period, and the admission MOD score. As a measure of the deterioration in organ function occurring over a set time interval, it provides a measure of morbidity attributable to events occurring following admission to the ICU and therefore potentially amenable to therapeutic intervention

Mortality-adjusted score

The aggregate score, adjusted so that a maximal score of 24 is given to any patient who dies during the ICU stay, regardless of the score at the time of death. The mortality-adjusted score is a combined measure of clinically significant morbidity and mortality during the ICU stay

ICU, intensive care unit. *Raw data for each of the six systems are recorded daily. For each variable, the value selected is representative, usually the first recorded value of the day. Pre-resuscitation values or obvious laboratory errors are omitted; missing data are assigned the value recorded for the previous day or, if none are available, are scored zero.

Table 2.7 Therapeutic Intervention Scoring System

Four points

(a) Cardiac arrest and/or countershock within past 48 hours
Point score for 2 days after most recent cardiac arrest

(b) Controlled ventilation with or without positive end-expiratory pressure
Does not mean intermittent mandatory ventilation, which is a 3-point intervention. If the patient's full ventilatory needs are being supplied by the machine, score 4 points

(c) Controlled ventilation with intermittent or continuous muscle relaxants

(d) Balloon tamponade of varices

(e) Continuous arterial infusion
e.g. intra-arterial pitressin infusion. Does not include standard 3-mL/h heparin flush to maintain cardiac patency

(f) Pulmonary artery catheter

(g) Atrial and/or ventricular pacing
Active pacing even if a chronic pacemaker

(h) Haemodialysis in unstable patient
Include first two rounds of an acute dialysis. Include chronic dialysis in patient whose medical situation now renders dialysis unstable

(i) Peritoneal dialysis

(j) Induced hypothermia
Continuous or intermittent cooling to achieve body temperature less than 33°C

(k) Pressure-active blood infusion
Use of a blood pump or manual pumping of blood in the patient who requires rapid blood replacement

(l) G-suit

(m) Intracranial pressure monitoring

(n) Platelet transfusion

(o) Intra-aortic balloon assist

(p) Emergency operative procedures (within past 24 hours)
Can include the initial emergency operative procedure, not including diagnostic tests (i.e. angiography, computed tomography scan)

(q) Lavage of acute gastrointestinal bleeding

(r) Emergency endoscopy or bronchoscopy

(s) Vasoactive drug infusion (> one drug)

Three points

(a) Central intravenous hyperalimentation (includes renal, cardiac, hepatic failure fluid)

(b) Pacemaker on standby

(c) Chest tubes

(d) Intermittent mandatory ventilation or assisted ventilation

(e) Continuous positive airways pressure

(f) Concentrated K^+ infusion via central catheter

(g) Nasotracheal or orotracheal intubation

(h) Blind intratracheal suctioning

(i) Complex metabolic balance (frequent intake and output)
Measurement of intake/output above and beyond the normal 24-hour routine. Frequent adjustment of intake according to total output

(j) Multiple blood gas, bleeding and/or stat studies (> four per shift)

(k) Frequent infusions of blood products (> 5 units/24 hours)

(l) Bolus intravenous medication (non-scheduled)

(m) Vasoactive drug infusion (one drug)

(n) Continuous antiarrhythmia infusions

(o) Cardioversion for arrhythmia (not defibrillation)

(p) Hypothermia blanket

(q) Arterial line

(r) Acute digitalization (within 48 hours)

(s) Measurement of cardiac output by any method

(t) Active diuresis for fluid overload or cerebral oedema

(u) Active therapy for metabolic alkalosis

(v) Active therapy for metabolic acidosis

(w) Emergency thora-, para- and pericardiocentesis

(x) Acute anticoagulation (initial 48 hours)
Includes Rheomacrodex

(y) Phlebotomy for volume overload

(z) Coverage with more than two intravenous antibiotics

(aa) Therapy of seizures or metabolic encephalopathy (within 48 hours of onset)

(bb) Complicated orthopaedic traction (e.g. Stryker frame, CircOlectric bed)

Two points

(a) Central venous pressure

(b) Two peripheral intravenous catheters

(c) Haemodialysis (stable patient)

(d) Fresh tracheostomy (less than 48 hours)

Table 2.7 *Continued*

(e)	Spontaneous respiration via endotracheal tube or tracheostomy (T-piece or tracheostomy mask)	(f)	Stat blood tests
(f)	Gastrointestinal feedings	(g)	Intermittent scheduled intravenous medications
(g)	Replacement of excess fluid loss (over and above the ordered maintenance level)	(h)	Routine dressing changes
		(j)	Standard orthopaedic traction
(h)	Parenteral chemotherapy	(j)	Tracheostomy care
(i)	Hourly neurological vital signs	(k)	Decubitus ulcer (preventive therapy)
(j)	Multiple dressing changes	(l)	Urinary catheter
(k)	Pitressin infusion	(m)	Supplemental oxygen (nasal or mask)

One point

(a)	Electrocardiogram monitoring	(n)	Intravenous antibiotics (two or fewer)
(b)	Hourly vital signs	(o)	Chest physiotherapy
(c)	One peripheral intravenous catheter	(p)	Extensive irrigations, packings or debridement of wounds, fistulas or colostomy
(d)	Chronic anticoagulation	(q)	Gastrointestinal decompression
(e)	Standard intake and output (every 24 hours)	(r)	Peripheral hyperalimentation/intralipid therapy

Reproduced from Cullen and Nemeskal (1989). Therapeutic Intervention Scoring System (TISS). In: Farmer JC (ed.) *Problems in Critical Care*, vol. 3. JP Lippincott: Philadelphia, PA.

Certainly objective outcome predictions do have a number of potential advantages compared with clinical judgement (Knaus *et al.*, 1991), including the following:

- Past experiences are taken into account in an unbiased manner, whereas, with human decisions, recent experience has a disproportionate influence.
- Objective outcome predictions should be more reliable because they are based on reproducible data.
- The database supporting the risk estimate is substantially larger than any one clinician's experience.
- The risk estimates are based solely on the patient's response to treatment.

In practice APACHE III outcome predictions compare favourably with clinicians' assessments; indeed, the objective system is better calibrated, and there is evidence that daily prognostic estimates are sufficiently accurate to be used to assist clinical decision making (Wagner *et al.*, 1994). Usually, however, daily risk assessments only serve to confirm prognostic uncertainty, albeit with a reduced chance of error, and most difficult clinical problems are unlikely to be resolved solely by objective probability estimates.

CRITICISMS OF SEVERITY SCORING

The introduction of prognostic scoring systems has been accompanied by considerable debate and controversy. Whereas some have been concerned with practical difficulties related to data collection and consistency of scoring methods, others have questioned their accuracy, as well as their use for audit, evaluating a unit's performance, between-unit comparisons and patient selection (Boyd and Grounds,

1993; Civetta, 1990). Some have gone so far as to suggest that it is virtually impossible to develop a useful scoring system (Civetta, 1990). Certain limitations of prognostic scoring systems, such as their inability to predict either the sudden unexpected complications that often affect outcome or the subsequent development of multiple organ dysfunction, are intuitively obvious. Also the fact that different scoring systems yield different probabilities for the same patient seems to indicate that other factors, not incorporated into current scoring systems, are important determinates of outcome.

Of more concern is the suggestion that scores based on physiological data that can be influenced by medical and nursing interventions, such as APACHE, cannot be used to compare unit performances and are not suitable for audit (Boyd and Grounds, 1993). It is claimed that the accuracy of such systems is compromised by *lead time bias*; that is, they fail to take into account the effect that management before the initiation of intensive care (e.g. stabilization in the operating theatre or prompt retrieval and resuscitation of trauma patients) may have on physiological variables. This issue was, however, addressed in the development of APACHE III (see earlier in this chapter). Conversely, the use of intentional hypotension, hypothermia, muscle relaxation and mechanical ventilation can result in a high APACHE score, despite a low risk of death (Civetta, 1990). It is probably for this reason that APACHE II predictions cannot be applied to post cardiac surgery patients.

There is also concern that interobserver variations may have a profound effect on calculated probabilities of survival. Assessment of APACHE II scores, for example, varies widely between both less experienced trainees and experienced intensivists (Polderman *et al.*, 1999) and can be unreliable, with numerous errors. It has been shown that in everyday practice scores are usually overestimated (Polderman *et al.*, 2001). With the TRISS system it has been shown that individual predictions of survival are also potentially inaccurate, except at the extremes of probabilities (Zoltie and de Dombal, 1993).

Finally, some have contended that exclusion of patients from intensive care on the basis of APACHE II scores will not result in significant savings, but will instead create risks of increased morbidity, mortality and costs (Civetta, 1990).

REFERENCES

Bach PB, Carson SS, Leff A (1998) Outcomes and resource utilisation for patients with prolonged critical illness managed by university-based or community-based subspecialists. *American Journal of Respiratory and Critical Care Medicine* **158**: 1410–1415.

Bion J (1993) Outcomes in intensive care. *British Medical Journal* **307**: 953–954.

Boyd O, Grounds RM (1993) Physiological scoring systems and audit. *Lancet* **341**: 1573–1574.

Boyd CR, Tolson MA, Copes WS (1987) Evaluating trauma care: the TRISS method. *Journal of Trauma* **27**: 370–378.

Carlet J, Thijs LG, Antonelli M, *et al.* (2004) Challenges in end-of-life care in the ICU. Statement of the 5th International Consensus Conference in Critical Care: Brussels, Belgium, April 2003. *Intensive Care Medicine* **30**: 770–784.

Chalfin DB, Carlon GC (1990) Age and utilization of intensive care unit resources of critically ill cancer patients. *Critical Care Medicine* **18**: 694–698.

Civetta JM (1990) 'New and improved' scoring systems. *Critical Care Medicine* **18**: 1487–1490.

Cook R, Cook D, Tilley J, *et al.* (2001) Multiple organ dysfunction: baseline and serial component scores. *Critical Care Medicine* **29**: 2046–2050.

Cullen DJ, Nemeskal AR (1989) Therapeutic Intervention Scoring System (TISS). In: Farmer JC (ed.) *Problems in Critical Care*, vol. 3. JP Lippincott: Philadelphia, PA.

Cullen DJ, Civetta JM, Briggs BA, *et al.* (1974) Therapeutic intervention scoring system: a method for quantitative comparison of patient care. *Critical Care Medicine* **2**: 57–60.

Cullen DJ, Nemeskal AR, Zaslavsky AM (1994) Intermediate TISS: a new therapeutic intervention scoring system for non-ICU patients. *Critical Care Medicine* **22**: 1406–1411.

Danis M, Jarr SL, Southerland LI, *et al.* (1987) A comparison of patient, family, and nurse evaluations of the usefulness of intensive care. *Critical Care Medicine* **15**: 138–143.

Danis M, Patrick DL, Southerland LI, *et al.* (1988) Patients' and families' preferences for medical intensive care. *Journal of the American Medical Association* **260**: 797–802.

Edbrooke DL, Hibbert CL, Kingsley JM, *et al.* (1999) The patient-related costs of care for sepsis patients in a United Kingdom adult general intensive care unit. *Critical Care Medicine* **27**: 1760–1767.

Eddleston J, White P, Guthrie E (2000) Survival, morbidity, and quality of life after discharge from intensive care. *Critical Care Medicine* **28**: 2293–2299.

Editorial (1991) Intensive care for the elderly. *Lancet* **337**: 209–210.

El-Solh A, Sikka P, Bozkanat E, *et al.* (2001) Morbid obesity in the medical ICU. *Chest* **120**: 1989–1997.

Esteban A, Gordo F, Solsona JF, *et al.* (2001) Withdrawing and withholding life support in the intensive care unit: a Spanish prospective multi-center observational study. *Intensive Care Medicine* **27**: 1744–1749.

Fedullo AJ, Swinburne AJ (1983) Relationship of patient age to cost and survival in a medical ICU. *Critical Care Medicine* **11**: 155–159.

Ferrand E, Robert R, Ingrand P, *et al.* (2001) Withholding and withdrawal of life support in intensive care units in France: a prospective survey. *Lancet* **357**: 9–14.

Herridge MS (2002) Long-term outcomes after critical illness. *Current Opinion in Critical Care* **8**: 331–336.

Intensive Care Society (1998) *Guidelines for Bereavement Care in Intensive Care Units.* Intensive Care Society: London, UK. Available online at: www.ics.ac.uk

Jennett B (1984) Inappropriate use of intensive care. *British Medical Journal* **289**: 1709–1711.

Keenan SP, Dodek P, Chan K, *et al.* (2002) Intensive care unit admission has minimal impact on long term mortality. *Critical Care Medicine* **30**: 501–507.

Keene AR, Cullen DJ (1983) Therapeutic intervention scoring system: update 1983. *Critical Care Medicine* **11**: 1–3.

Knaus WA, Zimmerman JE, Wagner DP, *et al.* (1981) APACHE – acute physiology and chronic health evaluation: a physiologically based classification system. *Critical Care Medicine* **9**: 591–597.

Knaus WA, Draper EA, Wagner DP, *et al.* (1985) APACHE II: a severity of disease classification system. *Critical Care Medicine* **13**: 818–829.

Knaus WA, Draper EA, Wagner DP, *et al.* (1986) An evaluation of outcome from intensive care in major medical centers. *Annals of Internal Medicine* **104**: 410–418.

Knaus WA, Wagner DP, Draper EA, *et al.* (1991) The APACHE III prognostic system: risk prediction of hospital mortality for critically ill hospitalized adults. *Chest* **100**: 1619–1636.

Kollef MH, Ward S (1999) The influence of access to a private attending physician on the withdrawal of life-sustaining therapies in the intensive care unit. *Critical Care Medicine* **27**: 2125–2132.

Lam S, Ridley S (1999) Critically ill medical patients, their demographics and outcome. *Anaesthesia* **54**: 845–852.

Lautrette A, Darmen M, Megarlane B, et al. (2007) A communication strategy and brochure for relatives of patients dying in the ICU. *New England Journal of Medicine* **356**: 469–478.

Le Gall JR, Loirat P, Alperovich A, *et al.* (1984) A simplified acute physiology score for ICU patients. *Critical Care Medicine* **12**: 975–977.

Le Gall J-R, Lemeshow S, Saulnier F (1993) A new simplified acute physiology score (SAPS II) based on a European/North American multicenter study. *Journal of the American Medical Association* **270**: 2957–2963.

Lemeshow S, Teres D, Avrunin JS, *et al.* (1988) Refining intensive care unit outcome prediction by using changing probabilities of mortality. *Critical Care Medicine* **16**: 470–477.

Lemeshow S, Teres D, Klar J, *et al.* (1993) Mortality probability models (MPM II) based on an international cohort of intensive care unit patients. *Journal of the American Medical Association* **270**: 2478–2486.

Lemeshow S, Klar J, Teres D, *et al.* (1994) Mortality probability models for patients in the intensive care unit for 48 or 72 hours: a prospective, multicenter study. *Critical Care Medicine* **22**: 1351–1358.

McLean RF, Tarshis J, Mazer CD, *et al.* (2000) Death in two Canadian intensive care units: institutional difference and changes over time. *Critical Care Medicine* **28**: 100–103.

Marshall JC, Cook DJ, Christou NV, *et al.* (1995) Multiple organ dysfunction score: a reliable descriptor of a complex clinical outcome. *Critical Care Medicine* **23**: 1638–1652.

Montuclard L, Garrouste-Orgeas M, Timsit J-F, *et al.* (2000) Outcome, functional autonomy, and quality of life of elderly patients. *Critical Care Medicine* **28**: 3389–3395.

Nelson JE, Meier DE, Oei FJ, *et al.* (2001) Self-reported symptom experience of critically ill cancer patients receiving intensive care. *Critical Care Medicine* **29**: 277–282.

Pochard F, Azoulay E, Chevret S, *et al.* (2001a) French intensivists do not apply American recommendations regarding decisions to forgo life-sustaining therapy. *Critical Care Medicine* **29**: 1887–1892.

Pochard F, Azoulay E, Chevret S, *et al.* (2001b) Symptoms of anxiety and depression in family members of intensive care unit patients: ethical hypothesis regarding decision-making capacity. *Critical Care Medicine* **29**: 1893–1897.

Polderman KH, Thijs LG, Girbes AR (1999) Interobserver variability in the use of APACHE II scores. *Lancet* **353**: 380.

Polderman KH, Girbes AR, Thijs LG, *et al.* (2001) Accuracy and reliability of APACHE II scoring in two intensive care units. *Anaesthesia* **56**: 47–50.

Prendergast TJ, Luce JM (1997) Increasing incidence of withholding and withdrawal of life support from the critically ill. *American Journal of Respiratory and Critical Care Medicine* **155**: 15–20.

Prendergast TJ, Claessens MT, Luce JM (1998) A national survey of end-of-life care for critically ill patients. *American Journal of Respiratory and Critical Care Medicine* **158**: 1163–1167.

Rapoport J, Gehlbach S, Lemeshaw S, *et al.* (1992) Resource utilization among intensive care patients. Managed care vs traditional insurance. *Archives of Internal Medicine* **152**: 2207–2212.

Ridley S, Morris S (2007) Cost effectiveness of adult intensive care in the UK. *Anaesthesia* **62**: 547–554.

Ridley S, Plenderleith L (1994) Survival after intensive care comparison with a matched normal population as an indicator of effectiveness. *Anaesthesia* **49**: 933–935.

Ridley SA, Wallace PG (1990) Quality of life after intensive care. *Anaesthesia* **45**: 808–813.

Ridley S, Jackson R, Findlay J, *et al.* (1990) Long term survival after intensive care. *British Medical Journal* **301**: 1127–1130.

Ridley S, Biggam M, Stone P (1994) A cost–utility analysis of intensive therapy. II. Quality of life in survivors. *Anaesthesia* **49**: 192–196.

Ridley SA, Chrispin PS, Scotton H, *et al.* (1997) Changes in quality of life after intensive care: comparison with normal data. *Anaesthesia* **52**: 195–202.

Rosenberg AL, Hofer TP, Hayward RA, *et al.* (2001) Who bounces back? Physiologic and other predictors of intensive care unit readmission. *Critical Care Medicine* **29**: 511–518.

Rowan KM, Kerr JH, Major E, *et al.* (1993) Intensive Care Society's APACHE II study in Britain and Ireland. II. Outcome comparisons of intensive care units after adjustment for case mix by the American APACHE II method. *British Medical Journal* **307**: 977–981.

Rowan KM, Kerr JH, Major E, *et al.* (1994) Intensive Care Society's acute physiology and chronic health evaluation (APACHE II) study in Britain and Ireland: a prospective, multicenter, cohort study comparing two methods for predicting outcome for adult intensive care patients. *Critical Care Medicine* **22**: 1392–1401.

Ruark JE, Raffin TA (1988) Initiating and withdrawing life support. Principles and practice in adult medicine. *New England Journal of Medicine* **318**: 25–30.

Sage WM, Rosenthal MH, Silverman JF (1986) Is intensive care worth it? An assessment of input and outcome for the critically ill. *Critical Care Medicine* **14**: 777–782.

Schelling G, Stoll C, Haller M, *et al.* (1998) Health-related quality of life and posttraumatic stress disorder in survivors of the acute respiratory distress syndrome. *Critical Care Medicine* **26**: 651–659.

Schneiderman LJ, Spragg RG (1988) Ethical decisions in discontinuing mechanical ventilation. *New England Journal of Medicine* **318**: 984–988.

Schneiderman LJ, Pearlman RA, Kaplan RM, *et al.* (1992) Relationship of general advance directive instructions to specific life-sustaining treatment preferences in patients with serious illness. *Archives of Internal Medicine* **152**: 2114–2122.

Schneiderman LJ, Gilmer T, Teetzel HD (2000) Impact of ethics consultations in the intensive care setting: a randomized, controlled trial. *Critical Care Medicine* **28**: 3920–3924.

Seckler AB, Meier DE, Mulvihill M, *et al.* (1991) Substituted judgement: how accurate are proxy predictions? *Annals of Internal Medicine* **115**: 92–98.

Sirio CA, Tajimi K, Tase C, *et al.* (1992) An initial comparison of intensive care in Japan and the United States. *Critical Care Medicine* **20**: 1207–1215.

Smedira NG, Evans BH, Grais LS, *et al.* (1990) Withholding and withdrawal of life support from the critically ill. *New England Journal of Medicine* **322**: 309–315.

Sprung CL, Cohen SL, Sjokvist P, *et al.* (2003) End of life practices in European intensive care units – the Ethicus study. *Journal of the American Medical Association* **290**: 790–797.

Sukantarat KT, Burgess PW, Williamson RC, *et al.* (2005) Prolonged cognitive dysfunction in survivors of critical illness. *Anaesthesia* **60**: 847–853.

Thiagarajan J, Taylor P, Hogbin E, *et al.* (1994) Quality of life after multiple trauma requiring intensive care. *Anaesthesia* **49**: 211–218.

Vincent J-L (1990) European attitudes towards ethical problems in intensive care medicine: results of an ethical questionnaire. *Intensive Care Medicine* **16**: 256–264.

Vincent J-L (1999) Forgoing life-support in western European intensive care units: the results of an ethical questionnaire. *Critical Care Medicine* **27**: 1626–1633.

Vincent J-L, Moreno R, Takala J, *et al.* (1996) The Sepsis-related Organ Failure Assessment (SOFA) score to describe organ dysfunction/failure. *Intensive Care Medicine* **22**: 707–710.

Wagner DP, Knaus WA, Harrell FE, *et al.* (1994) Daily prognostic estimates for critically ill adults in intensive care units: results from a prospective, multicenter, inception cohort analysis. *Critical Care Medicine* **22**: 1359–1372.

Woods AW, MacKirdy FN, Livingston BM, *et al.* (2000) Evaluation of predicted and actual length of stay in 22 Scottish intensive care units using the APACHE III system. *Anaesthesia* **55**: 1058–1065.

Wright JC, Plenderleith L, Ridley SA (2003) Long-term survival following intensive care: subgroup analysis and comparison with the general population. *Anaesthesia* **58**: 637–642.

Zimmerman JE, Knaus WA, Judson JA, *et al.* (1988) Patient selection for intensive care: a comparison of New Zealand and United States hospitals. *Critical Care Medicine* **16**: 318–326.

Zimmerman JE, Wagner DP, Draper EA, *et al.* (1994) Improving intensive care unit discharge decisions: supplementing physician judgment with predictions of next day risk for life support. *Critical Care Medicine* **22**: 1373–1384.

Zoltie N, de Dombal FT on behalf of the Yorkshire Trauma Audit Group (1993) The hit and miss of ISS and TRISS. *British Medical Journal* **307**: 906–909.

3 Applied cardiovascular and respiratory physiology

In all critically ill patients the immediate priority must be to preserve life and prevent, reverse or minimize damage to vital organs such as the brain, gut and kidneys. This is achieved by optimizing cardiovascular and respiratory function in order to *maintain perfusion pressure* and *deliver sufficient oxygen* to the tissues. Subsequently, it is hoped that the underlying abnormality will resolve either spontaneously (e.g. postoperatively and in some viral illnesses such as Guillain–Barré syndrome) or as a result of specific treatment aimed at the underlying disease, such as the administration of antibiotics to a patient with pneumonia or surgery to control a source of infection. Occasionally, when the aetiology of the acute illness is unknown, successful resuscitation and stabilization provide a 'breathing space' during which the diagnosis can be made and specific therapy started.

OXYGEN DELIVERY

Oxygen delivery (DO_2) or *oxygen despatch* is defined as the total amount of oxygen delivered to the tissues per unit time. It is dependent on:

- the volume of blood flowing through the microcirculation per unit time (i.e. the cardiac output, $\dot{Q}_t$)
- the amount of oxygen contained in that blood (i.e. the arterial oxygen content, C_aO_2) (**Table 3.1**).

Oxygen is transported in combination with haemoglobin (Hb) and dissolved in plasma, the amount combined with Hb being determined by its oxygen capacity (usually taken as being 1.34 mL O_2/g Hb) and its percentage saturation with oxygen (SO_2), while the volume dissolved in plasma depends on the partial pressure of oxygen (PO_2) (see **Table 3.1**). For most practical purposes, except when hyperbaric oxygen is administered, the amount of dissolved oxygen is sufficiently small to be ignored.

In the normal, healthy adult approximately 1000 mL (550 mL/min per m²) of oxygen is delivered to the tissues each minute (see **Table 3.1**) and, since the normal oxygen consumption ($\dot{V}O_2$) is 250 mL/min (140 mL/min per m²), only about 25% of the available oxygen is used. Normal arterial blood, in which the Hb is fully saturated, contains 20 vol% of oxygen, and since 25% (or 5 vol%) is extracted by the tissues, this leaves 15 vol% in mixed venous blood, which is, therefore, 75% saturated with oxygen. The normal arteriovenous oxygen content difference is therefore 5 mL/100 mL of blood (**Fig. 3.1**; Appendices 1 and 2).

Clinically, however, the utility of this global concept of oxygen despatch is limited because:

- Some organs, notably the heart, have a very high oxygen requirement relative to their blood flow and may, therefore, receive insufficient supplies of oxygen even when overall oxygen delivery (DO_2) is apparently adequate.
- It does not take into account changes in the relative blood flow to individual organs or its distribution in the microcirculation (i.e. the efficiency with which oxygen delivery is matched to the metabolic requirements of individual tissues or cells).
- Microcirculatory flow is influenced by viscosity.

CARDIAC OUTPUT

The factors that determine the volume of blood delivered to the tissues (i.e. the cardiac output) will be considered first. It is useful to index the cardiac output and other haemodynamic and oxygen transport variables to the body surface area (in square metres). In this way, comparisons can be made between patients, and the normal limits can be more closely defined (see Appendices 1 and 2).

Maintenance of an adequate cardiac output is obviously crucial to survival; both the heart rate and the determinants of the stroke volume need to be considered (**Fig. 3.2**).

HEART RATE AND RHYTHM

The heart rate is largely dependent on the balance of sympathetic and parasympathetic nervous activity and, in health, is directly related to the metabolic rate. At rest, vagal tone predominates and maintains the heart rate at about 70 beats/min. If both the sympathetic and parasympathetic supply to the heart are interrupted, a rate of approximately 100 beats/min results.

Table 3.1 Determinants of oxygen delivery

Oxygen delivery = cardiac output × arterial oxygen content

Oxygen delivery = cardiac output × [(Hb × S_aO_2 × 1.34) + (P_aO_2 × 0.003)]

For representative values in a normal adult, and ignoring the small amount of dissolved oxygen:
1000 mL/min ≈ 5000 mL × 15/100 g/mL × 99/100 × 1.34

Since oxygen consumption is normally approximately 250 mL/min, there is an excess of supply over demand, which provides a margin of safety if oxygen consumption increases or oxygen delivery falls

Hb, haemoglobin; P_aO_2, partial pressure of oxygen in arterial blood; S_aO_2, saturation of haemoglobin with oxygen in arterial blood.

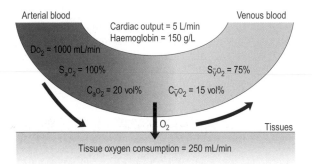

Fig. 3.1 Tissue oxygen delivery and consumption. S_aO_2, arterial oxygen saturation; C_aO_2, arterial oxygen content; DO_2, oxygen delivery; $C_{\bar{v}}O_2$, mixed venous oxygen content; $S_{\bar{v}}O_2$, mixed venous oxygen saturation. Adapted from Kumar P, Clark M 2005 Clinical Medicine 6E Elsevier with permission.

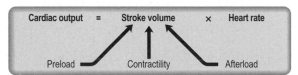

Fig. 3.2 The determinants of cardiac output. Adapted from Kumar P, Clark M 2005 Clinical Medicine 6E Elsevier with permission.

Extreme bradycardias and tachycardias can cause cardiac output to fall.

■ *As heart rate increases*, the duration of systole remains essentially unchanged, whereas diastole, and therefore the time available for ventricular filling, becomes progressively shorter, and stroke volume eventually falls. In the normal heart this occurs at rates greater than about 160 beats/min, but in those with cardiac pathology, especially when this restricts ventricular filling (e.g. mitral stenosis), stroke volume may fall at much lower heart rates. Furthermore, tachycardias cause marked increases in myocardial oxygen consumption (VmO_2) and this may precipitate ischaemia in areas of myocardium with restricted coronary perfusion. It is therefore most important to control tachyarrhythmias, but it must be recog-

nized that the majority have an underlying cause such as hypokalaemia, which should be diagnosed and treated before instituting specific therapy (see Chapter 9).

■ *When heart rate falls*, on the other hand, a point is reached at which the increase in stroke volume is insufficient to compensate for the bradycardia and again cardiac output falls. Under these circumstances overdistension of the ventricles may impair myocardial performance and jeopardize subendocardial perfusion.

Alterations in heart rate are often caused by disturbances of rhythm in which atrial transport is lost (e.g. atrial fibrillation, complete heart block or nodal rhythm), thereby further reducing ventricular filling and stroke volume. In this situation, catastrophic reductions in cardiac output may occur and urgent treatment is then required (see Chapter 9).

STROKE VOLUME

The volume of blood ejected by the ventricle in a single contraction is the difference between the ventricular end-diastolic volume (VEDV) and end-systolic volume (VESV) (i.e. stroke volume = VEDV − VESV).

The *ejection fraction* describes the stroke volume as a percentage of VEDV (i.e. ejection fraction = VEDV − VESV/VEDV × 100%) and is an indicator of myocardial performance.

Three interdependent factors determine the stroke volume: preload, myocardial contractility and afterload.

Preload

Preload is defined as the tension of the myocardial fibres at end-diastole, just before the onset of ventricular contraction, and is therefore related to their degree of stretch (**Fig. 3.3**). The main factor influencing preload is the venous return to the heart. According to *Starling's law*, 'the force of myocardial contraction is directly proportional to the initial fibre length'. Therefore, as the filling pressure, and consequently the VEDV, increases, tension in the myocardial fibres is increased and stroke volume rises (**Fig. 3.4**). If, however, the ventricle is overstretched, excessive dilatation and thinning of the myocardium, combined with the mechanical disadvantage caused by the reduced curvature of the almost spherical left ventricle (Laplace's law – see below), may cause stroke volume to fall (**Fig. 3.5**). There is also a risk of pulmonary oedema when left ventricular filling pressures increase.

Achieving the optimal preload improves cardiac output by increasing stroke volume without affecting the main determinants of myocardial oxygen requirements (i.e. heart rate and afterload; **Table 3.2**). Consequently, VmO_2 increases only slightly and manipulation of preload is therefore in this respect the most efficient way of improving cardiac output.

Myocardial contractility

Myocardial contractility refers to the ability of the heart to perform work, independent of changes in preload and afterload. The state of myocardial contractility, which is mainly

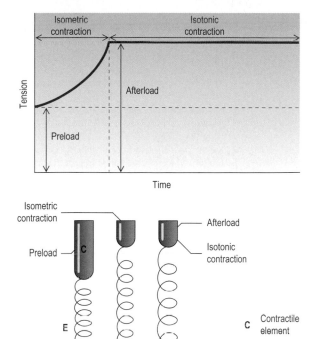

Fig. 3.3 The relationship between myocardial tension and contraction. 'Preload' is the tension of the myocardial fibres prior to the onset of systole and depends on the degree to which they are passively stretched. During isometric contraction, the tension in the contractile elements increases; the tension required to open the aortic or pulmonary valve and eject blood from the ventricle is the 'afterload'.

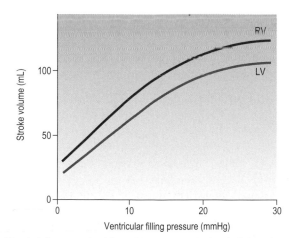

Fig. 3.4 In normal subjects the left ventricular (LV) function curve is displaced downwards because the left ventricle is less compliant and is working against a higher afterload than the right ventricle (RV).

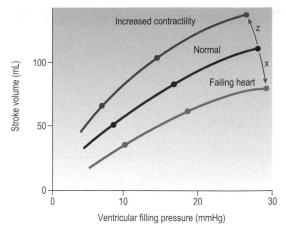

Fig. 3.5 The Frank–Starling relationship: as preload is increased, stroke volume rises. If the ventricle is overstretched, stroke volume will fall (x). In myocardial failure, the curve is depressed and flattened. Increasing contractility, e.g. due to sympathetic stimulation, shifts the curve upwards and to the left (z).

Table 3.2 The determinants of myocardial oxygen consumption	
Major effect	Heart rate Afterload
Intermediate effect	Ventricular wall tension Contractility
Least effect	Preload Stroke volume

influenced by extrinsic factors (neural, hormonal and chemical) therefore determines the response of the ventricles to changes in preload and afterload. Contractility is often reduced in intensive care patients as a result of either pre-existing myocardial damage (e.g. ischaemic heart disease) or the acute disease process itself (e.g. sepsis). Changes in myocardial contractility alter the slope and position of the ventricular function curve; worsening ventricular performance is manifested as a depressed, flat curve (see Fig. 3.5). Therefore, for a given preload, stroke volume is lower and increasing filling pressures leads to only limited improvement in cardiac output. Under these circumstances, cardiac output can be maintained only by increasing heart rate, with an associated rise in Vm_{O_2}.

Alterations in myocardial performance can also be appreciated by understanding the pressure changes which occur during the cardiac cycle (Fig. 3.6), by examining changes in the ventricular pressure–volume loops and by further analysis of pressure–volume curves (Fig. 3.7).

Afterload

Afterload is defined as the myocardial wall tension developed during systolic ejection (see Fig. 3.3) and is a

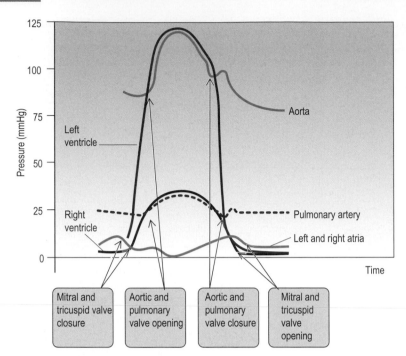

Fig. 3.6 The cardiac cycle. Left ventricular contraction begins slightly before right ventricular contraction. Once ventricular pressures exceed those in the atria, the mitral and tricuspid valves close. There then follows a period of isovolumetric contraction until the pressures in the right and left ventricle exceed the pulmonary arterial and aortic pressures respectively, at which point the pulmonary and aortic valves open and ventricular ejection occurs. As the ventricles relax intraventricular pressures fall to below those in the pulmonary artery and aorta. Aortic and pulmonary valve closure is followed by isovolumetric relaxation. Once ventricular pressures have fallen below the right and left atrial pressure, the tricuspid and mitral valves open. Adapted from Kumar P, Clark M 2005 Clinical Medicine 6E Elsevier with permission.

significant determinant of left ventricular performance. From *Laplace's law* the ventricular wall tension (T) is given by:

$$T = P_{tM} \times R/2H$$

where P_{tM} is the transmural pressure, R is the ventricular radius and H is the ventricular wall thickness.

Left ventricular afterload will therefore be increased by:

- ventricular dilatation;
- an increase in intraventricular pressure;
- a negative intrathoracic pressure.

Conversely, afterload will be reduced by:

- a positive intrathoracic pressure;
- decreased intraventricular pressure;
- increased ventricular wall thickness.

Other important determinants of left ventricular afterload are:

- the resistance imposed by the aortic valve and the peripheral vasculature;
- the elasticity of major blood vessels.

Decreasing afterload can increase the stroke volume achieved at a given preload (**Fig. 3.8**), while at the same time ventricular wall tension and VmO_2 are reduced. The reduction in wall tension may produce an increase in coronary blood flow, thereby improving the myocardial oxygen supply:demand ratio. An increase in afterload, on the other hand, can cause a fall in stroke volume, particularly in those with myocardial dysfunction, and is a potent cause of increased VmO_2.

Right ventricular afterload is normally negligible because the resistance of the pulmonary circulation is very low. In patients with stenosis of the pulmonary valve or pulmonary hypertension, however, right ventricular afterload may become the dominant influence on overall cardiac performance.

OXYGEN CONTENT

The oxygen content of arterial blood (C_aO_2) depends on the amount of Hb present per unit volume of blood, its oxygen capacity and its percentage saturation with oxygen (see **Table 3.1**). Maintenance of an 'adequate' Hb concentration is therefore essential in critically ill patients. Tissue oxygenation is, however, also dependent on blood flow. This in turn is determined not only by the cardiac output and its distribution, but also by the viscosity of the blood, which depends largely on the packed cell volume.

OXYHAEMOGLOBIN DISSOCIATION CURVE

The saturation of Hb with oxygen is determined by the PO_2 in the blood; the relationship between the two is described by the *oxyhaemoglobin dissociation curve* (**Fig. 3.9**). The sigmoid shape of this curve is clinically important for a number of reasons:

- Modest falls in P_aO_2 may be tolerated (since oxygen content is relatively unaffected) provided percentage saturation remains above about 90%.
- Increasing P_aO_2 to above normal has only a minimal effect on oxygen content unless hyperbaric oxygen is administered (when the amount of oxygen in solution in plasma becomes significant).
- Once on the steep portion of the curve (percentage saturation below about 90% – the 'slippery slope'), a small

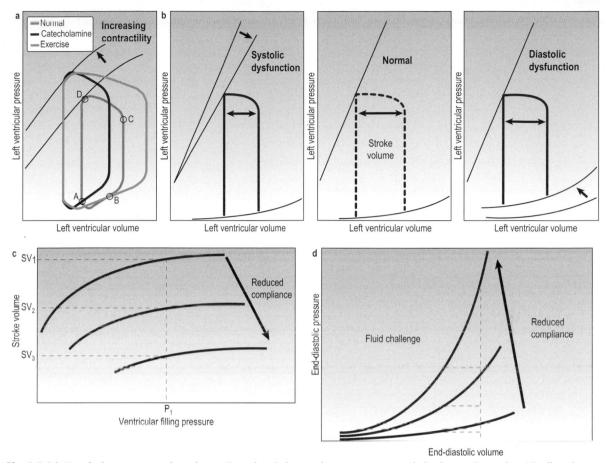

Fig. 3.7 (a) Ventricular pressure–volume loops. Normal and changes in response to catecholamines and exercise. AB, diastole: ventricle filling; BC, systole: isovolumetric ventricular contraction; CD, systole: ventricle emptying; DA, diastole: isovolumetric ventricular relaxation. (b) Effects of systolic and diastolic myocardial dysfunction on the ventricular pressure–volume curves. Systolic dysfunction: ventricular contractility is impaired, with a reduced ability of the myofibrils to shorten against a load. Ejection fraction is reduced. Diastolic dysfunction: ejection fraction and ventricular volume are relatively normal. The fundamental abnormality is a reduction in ventricular compliance leading to increased filling pressures with an essentially unchanged end-diastolic volume. (c) Effect of progressive reductions in ventricular compliance on ventricular function curves. If blood pressure remains constant, a similar end diastolic pressure will generate progressively lower stroke volumes (SV) as ventricular compliance decreases. (d) Ventricular end-diastolic pressure–volume relationships. As compliance decreases, an increase in end-diastolic volume produced by a fluid challenge will generate a greater increase in end-diasolic pressure, leading to venous congestion and oedema.

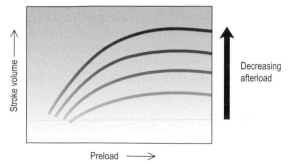

Fig. 3.8 The effect of changes in afterload on the ventricular function curve. Adapted from Kumar P, Clark M 2005 Clinical Medicine 6E Elsevier with permission.

decrease in P_aO_2 can cause large falls in oxygen content. Conversely, increasing P_aO_2 only slightly (e.g. by administering 28% oxygen to a patient with chronic obstructive pulmonary disease) can lead to a useful increase in oxygen saturation and content.

In contrast, *the carbon dioxide dissociation curve* is virtually linear over the range normally encountered in clinical practice so that alterations in P_{CO_2} cause proportional changes in carbon dioxide content (**Fig. 3.10**).

The arterial oxygen tension is influenced by the alveolar oxygen tension ($P_{A}O_2$), the efficiency of pulmonary gas exchange and the mixed venous PO_2 ($P_{\bar{v}}O_2$).

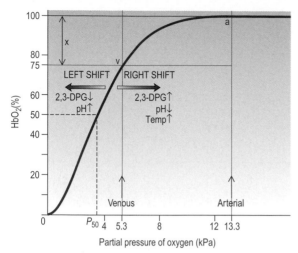

Fig. 3.9 The oxyhaemoglobin dissociation curve: a, arterial point; v, venous point; x, arteriovenous oxygen content difference. HbO_2 (%) is the percentage saturation of haemoglobin with oxygen. The curve will move to the right in the presence of acidosis (metabolic or respiratory), pyrexia or an increased red cell 2,3-DPG concentration. For a given arteriovenous oxygen content difference, the mixed venous PO_2 will then be higher. Furthermore, if the mixed venous PO_2 is unchanged, the arteriovenous oxygen content difference increases and more oxygen is offloaded to the tissues. The P_{50} (the PO_2 at which haemoglobin is 50% saturated with oxygen) is a useful index of these shifts – the higher the P_{50} (i.e. shift to the right), the lower the affinity of haemoglobin for oxygen. Adapted from Kumar P, Clark M 2005 Clinical Medicine 6E Elsevier with permission.

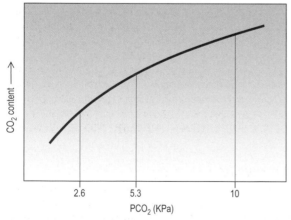

Fig. 3.10 The carbon dioxide dissociation curve: note that in the physiological range the curve is essentially linear. The curve is shifted to the right by increases in SO_2. Adapted from Kumar P, Clark M 2005 Clinical Medicine 6E Elsevier with permission.

PULMONARY VENTILATION AND GAS EXCHANGE

ALVEOLAR VENTILATION AND DEAD SPACE

The volume of effective alveolar ventilation per unit time ($\dot{V}_A$) is determined by the expired minute volume ($\dot{V}_E$),

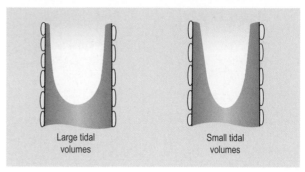

Fig. 3.11 The cone front effect: as tidal volume falls, the volume of stationary gas increases, thereby reducing the effective dead space.

reduced by the amount 'wasted' in terms of gas exchange (the *physiological, or total, dead space*, V_D).

The latter consists of '*anatomical*' *dead space* (the conducting airways) and *alveolar dead space* (ventilated alveoli, which are either not perfused or relatively underperfused; see below under ventilation/perfusion mismatch), i.e.:

$$\dot{V}_A = \dot{V}_E - V_D \qquad 3.1$$

For a single breath, this can be rewritten as:

$$\dot{V}_A = V_T - V_D \qquad 3.2$$

where V_T is the tidal volume.

In practice, however, V_D varies in proportion to the tidal volume. This is due to the *cone front effect* (**Fig. 3.11**). Because gas flow in the large airways is laminar, the leading front is conical, with the gas in the centre moving more rapidly than that towards the periphery; indeed, gas close to the walls of the conducting airways may be stationary. This reduces the effective volume of the dead space. As V_T falls, the amount of stationary gas increases and V_D is reduced (Briscoe *et al.*, 1954). In clinical practice it is therefore preferable to refer to the V_D/V_T ratio.

Calculation of V_D/V_T

Since no gas exchange takes place in the conducting airways and there is essentially no carbon dioxide in inspired air, all the carbon dioxide in the mixed expired gas must originate from gas-exchanging areas of the lung. Therefore:

$$\dot{V}_E \times F_ECO_2 = \dot{V}_A \times F_ACO_2 \qquad 3.3$$

where F_ECO_2 and F_ACO_2 are the fractional concentrations of carbon dioxide in mixed expired and alveolar gas respectively.

Then, substituting from equation **3.1** for V_A:

$$\dot{V}_E \times F_ECO_2 = (\dot{V}_E - V_D) \times F_ACO_2 \qquad 3.4$$

Substituting partial pressures for fractional concentrations and V_T for $\dot{V}_E$:

$$V_T \times P_ECO_2 = (V_T - V_D) \times P_ACO_2 \qquad 3.5$$

Finally, in an 'ideal' alveolus, P_ACO_2 can be assumed to be identical to P_aCO_2, and rearranging the equation:

$$V_D/V_T = P_aCO_2 - P_ECO_2/P_aCO_2 \qquad 3.6$$

This is the *Bohr equation*. In normal subjects the V_D/V_T ratio is less than 0.3.

Relationship between alveolar ventilation and arterial carbon dioxide tension

The amount of carbon dioxide excreted per unit time ($\dot{V}CO_2$) is clearly determined by the volume of the expired gas and the concentration of carbon dioxide in that gas:

$$\dot{V}CO_2 = \dot{V}_E \times F_ECO_2 \qquad 3.7$$

Substituting from equation 3.3:

$$\dot{V}CO_2 = \dot{V}_A \times F_ACO_2 \qquad 3.8$$

Substituting partial pressure for fractional concentration and rearranging:

$$\dot{V}_A = K \times \dot{V}CO_2/P_ACO_2 \qquad 3.9$$

where K is a constant.

As before, P_aCO_2 can be substituted for P_ACO_2 and therefore rearranging gives:

$$P_aCO_2 \propto \dot{V}CO_2/V_A \qquad 3.10$$

If $\dot{V}CO_2$ remains constant, P_aCO_2 is determined solely by alveolar ventilation (i.e. V_T and V_D), while for a given level of alveolar ventilation, P_aCO_2 is proportional to carbon dioxide production.

The alveolar air equation

DERIVATION

The amount of oxygen taken up through the lungs per unit time (the oxygen consumption, $\dot{V}O_2$) must be given by the difference between the volume of oxygen breathed in and the volume breathed out. Therefore:

$$\dot{V}O_2 = (\dot{V}_A \times F_IO_2) - (\dot{V}_A \times F_AO_2) \qquad 3.11$$

where F_IO_2 and F_AO_2 are the fractional concentrations of oxygen in inspired air and expired alveolar gas respectively.

Rearranging gives:

$$F_AO_2 - F_IO_2 - \dot{V}O_2/V_A \qquad 3.12$$

Substituting for V_A from equation 3.8:

$$F_AO_2 = F_IO_2 - (F_ACO_2 \times \dot{V}O_2/\dot{V}CO_2) \qquad 3.13$$

$\dot{V}O_2/\dot{V}CO_2$ is, of course, the inverse respiratory exchange ratio R, and therefore:

$$F_AO_2 = F_IO_2 - F_ACO_2/R \qquad 3.14$$

Fractional concentrations can be converted to partial pressures:

$$P_AO_2 = P_IO_2 - P_ACO_2/R \qquad 3.15$$

In clinical practice it is usual to measure F_IO_2 and multiply this by the barometric pressure to obtain P_IO_2. Furthermore, P_ACO_2 is considered to be identical to P_aCO_2 and R is usually assumed to be 0.8. Therefore:

$$P_AO_2 = (F_IO_2 \times PB) - P_aCO_2/0.8 \qquad 3.16$$

where PB = barometric pressure.

COMPOSITION OF ALVEOLAR GAS

Room air contains 20.93% oxygen, so that the F_IO_2 is 0.21 and, for a normal barometric pressure of 101 kPa (760 mmHg), the P_IO_2 is 21.2 kPa (159 mmHg) (Fig. 3.12). There is virtually

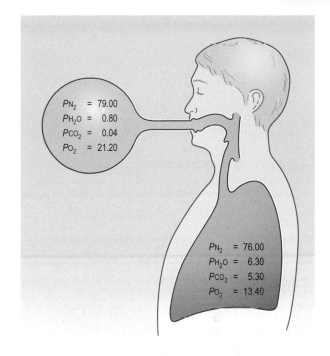

$$PN_2 = 79.00$$
$$PH_2O = 0.80$$
$$PCO_2 = 0.04$$
$$PO_2 = 21.20$$

$$PN_2 = 76.00$$
$$PH_2O = 6.30$$
$$PCO_2 = 5.30$$
$$PO_2 = 13.40$$

Fig. 3.12 The composition of inspired and alveolar gas (partial pressures in kPa).

no carbon dioxide in inspired air, and the amount of water vapour is relatively small, so the remainder is largely nitrogen. However, by the time the inspired gases reach the alveoli they are fully saturated with water vapour at body temperature (37°C), which has a partial pressure of 6.3 kPa (47 mmHg), and carbon dioxide has been added at a partial pressure of approximately 5.3 kPa (40 mmHg). The P_AO_2 is thereby reduced to approximately 13.4 kPa (100 mmHg).

The clinician can therefore influence P_AO_2 by altering the F_IO_2, or the barometric pressure (i.e. administering hyperbaric oxygen). Because of the reciprocal relationship between the partial pressures of oxygen and carbon dioxide in the alveoli, a small increase in P_aO_2 can be achieved by lowering the P_aCO_2.

THE ALVEOLI (Fig. 3.13)

There are approximately 150 million alveoli in each lung, with a total surface area of 40–80 m². The epithelial lining consists predominantly of *type I pneumocytes* which have an extremely attenuated, extended cytoplasm and are connected to each other by tight junctions that limit movement of fluid across the alveolar–capillary barrier. Type I cells are derived from *type II pneumocytes* which, although slightly more numerous, cover less of the epithelial lining. The type II cells are generally found in the borders of the alveolus and are the source of surfactant (see below). Holes in the alveolar wall (the pores of Kohn) allow communication between alveoli in adjoining lobules. Macrophages are also present in the alveoli and play an important role in pulmonary defence mechanisms.

THE ALVEOLAR–CAPILLARY BARRIER
Structure

Alveolar gas is separated from blood in the pulmonary capillaries by the alveolar–capillary barrier, the detailed structure of which has been demonstrated by Weibel (1984) and others using electron microscopy (**Fig. 3.13**). The pulmonary capillaries lie asymmetrically within the walls of the alveoli so that, on one side, where there is a single basement membrane, the alveolar–capillary membrane is extremely thin (i.e. < 0.5 μm in cross-section), allowing rapid gas transfer, while on the opposite 'thick' side, there is an interstitial space lying between the basement membranes of the capillary endothelium and the alveolar epithelium. This is the major site for fluid and solute exchange in the lungs and extends to surround the smaller blood vessels and airways from where fluid is drained by the terminal branches of the lymphatics.

Surfactant

Conventionally it is believed that the alveoli are lined by a continuous film of fluid, or aqueous hypophase, and that they therefore behave as one-sided bubbles, having an inherent tendency to collapse until the internal pressure exceeds the external by a difference, which can be quantified by the Laplace equation:

$$\Delta P = 2T/r$$

where r is the radius of curvature of the bubble, and T is the surface tension.

In order to minimize the tendency for alveoli to collapse, a monomolecular layer of a surface-active phospholipid (predominantly dipalmitoyl phosphatidylcholine), secreted as *lamellar bodies* by the type II alveolar cells, is located at the liquid–air interface. This surfactant, it is suggested, acts as a detergent to lower surface tension, thereby stabilizing the alveoli and reducing the pressure differential required to inflate the lung. Nevertheless, in this model the interconnecting fluid-lined alveoli remain inherently unstable since the smaller 'bubbles' will always have a tendency to empty into their larger neighbours. Indeed, this would be an accelerating process because the pressure differences would increase progressively as one alveolus collapses into another.

Considerable controversy has surrounded the role of surfactant in excluding fluid from the alveoli. In the conventional model outlined above, it is claimed that surfactant reduces the negative pressure in the aqueous lining, thereby minimizing the tendency for fluid to be sucked directly into the alveolus. This reduction in negative pressure would also reduce the chances of neighbouring alveoli collapsing and drawing fluid into the adjacent interstitial space.

An alternative proposal is that surfactant is directly adsorbed on to the epithelium, with no intervening aqueous layer, rendering the epithelial surface hydrophobic (Hills, 1990). It is suggested that the surfactant acts as a water-repellent layer capable of impeding the penetration of water from the pulmonary capillary into the alveolus with a force well in excess of normal capillary hydrostatic pressure.

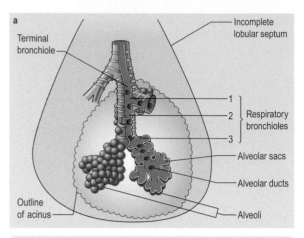

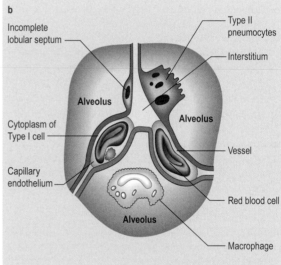

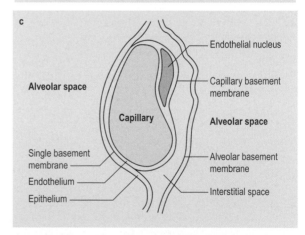

Fig. 3.13 (a) Branches of a terminal bronchiole terminating in the alveolar sacs. (b) The structure of alveoli, showing the pneumocytes and capillaries. (c) Structure of the alveolar–capillary barrier. Adapted from Kumar P, Clark M 2005 Clinical Medicine 6E Elsevier with permission.

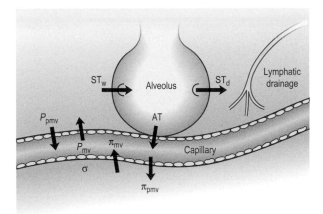

Fig. 3.14 Factors governing fluid flux in the lungs. P_{pmv}, perimicrovascular hydrostatic pressure; P_{mv}, microvascular hydrostatic pressure; π_{pmv}, perivascular colloid osmotic pressure; π_{mv}, microvascular colloid osmotic pressure; σ, reflection coefficient; ST_w, surface tension. (wet): ST_d, surface tension (dry); AT, active transport.

Surface tension forces water to collect as convex droplets at the angles of the alveoli, where they act as self-regulating 'corner pumps', which force fluid back into the pulmonary capillaries and interstitial spaces. This model of a 'dry' alveolus overcomes the problems associated with inherently unstable fluid-lined alveoli.

Surfactant may also be important in determining solute transport across the alveolar–capillary barrier. Depletion of surfactant is therefore associated not only with alveolar instability, but also with an increase in solute and water permeability of the alveolar–capillary barrier (Evander et al., 1987). Finally, surfactant contains a number of surfactant-specific proteins (Sp-A, -B, -C and – D) which contribute to the biophysical functions, anti-inflammatory and antimicrobial properties of this alveolar lining fluid.

Starling forces
The factors governing fluid flux (Q_f) across a semipermeable membrane such as the pulmonary capillary endothelium can be described by the modified Starling equation (Fig. 3.14):

$$Q_f = K_f \left([P_{mv} - P_{pmv}] - \sigma \left[\pi_{mv} - \pi_{pmv} \right] \right)$$

The membrane filtration coefficient (K_f) describes the permeability of the membrane to water. The direction and rate of fluid flux depend on the balance between the hydrostatic pressure gradient (i.e. the difference between microvascular and perimicrovascular pressures or $P_{mv} - P_{pmv}$) and the colloid osmotic pressure (COP) gradient (i.e. the difference between the COP in capillary blood and that in the interstitial space or $\pi_{mv} - \pi_{pmv}$), modified by the permeability of the membrane to protein – the reflection coefficient σ. When $\sigma = 1$, the membrane is perfectly semipermeable; when $\sigma = 0$ it is completely permeable. For albumin, the reflection coefficient of the pulmonary endothelium is normally about 0.6.

These Starling forces do not take into account the influence on overall lung fluid balance of lymphatic drainage or the surface area over which filtration takes place.

The Starling equation predicts a constant flow of protein and water across the capillary endothelium and into the interstitial space.

It has been estimated that in normal lungs the hydrostatic pressure falls from approximately 14 mmHg in the pulmonary artery to about 8 mmHg in the pulmonary capillary and 5 mmHg in the pulmonary vein. Since the hydrostatic pressure in the interstitial space is thought to be slightly subatmospheric (i.e. −2 mmHg), there is a net transendothelial hydrostatic pressure gradient of the order of 10 mmHg. This is counterbalanced by the difference between the COP in capillary blood (about 25 mmHg) and the interstitial COP, which has been estimated to be approximately 19 mmHg. There is therefore a transmural gradient of about 4 mmHg, which produces about 10–20 mL of fluid per hour. There is also a pressure gradient between the perimicrovascular interstitial space (−2 mmHg) and the peribronchovascular interstitium (−8 mmHg), which promotes movement of fluid towards the lymphatics.

OEDEMA FORMATION
If capillary hydrostatic pressure rises (e.g. in cardiac failure), there is a proportional increase in fluid flux across the endothelial membrane. Accumulation of extravascular lung water (EVLW) is, however, limited by:

- increased lymphatic drainage, which has a reserve capacity of approximately 10 times basal flow;
- a dilutional reduction in the perimicrovascular COP (the capillary endothelium retains its barrier function);
- a rise in hydrostatic pressure as fluid accumulates in the extravascular space.

Moreover, the interstitial compartment can accommodate a moderate increase in lung water (up to about 7 mL/kg) without directly interfering with gas exchange because the 'thin' side of the alveolar–capillary barrier remains dry.

In normal lungs these compensatory mechanisms are overwhelmed at hydrostatic pressures above about 18 mmHg and interstitial oedema begins to form at pressures of around 20 mmHg; marked increases in EVLW are seen when pressures exceed 25 mmHg. The intercellular junctions between the alveolar epithelial cells are, however, approximately 10 times 'tighter' (less permeable) than those of the endothelium, and the alveoli are therefore protected until the late stages of oedema formation. Eventually the mechanical stress of fluid distension causes a sudden disruption of the epithelial barrier and the alveoli are flooded. This is thought to occur in an 'all-or-none' fashion – either an alveolus is flooded or it is completely dry.

A fall in COP (e.g. due to a reduction in serum albumin levels) rarely in itself precipitates pulmonary oedema because of a concomitant fall in interstitial COP and increased lymphatic drainage. Nevertheless both reductions in plasma

COP and falls in the reflection coefficient, as occurs in acute respiratory distress syndrome (see Chapter 8), will reduce the threshold hydrostatic pressure for oedema formation.

Active transport of sodium across the alveolar barrier, accompanied by the passive movement of chloride and water, also plays an important role in the clearance of fluid from the lungs. The ability of the epithelium to transport sodium actively, combined with its low permeability, explains the large osmotic gradients that can be sustained across this membrane.

Electrostatic charge

The distribution of electrostatic charges within the alveolar–capillary membrane also has an important influence on the movement of fluid and solutes. The epithelial basement membrane has approximately five times more fixed negative electrostatic charge than the capillary basement membrane; in fact it has been suggested that the latter is predominantly positively charged. This distribution of charge ensures that diffusion of anionic molecules such as albumin into the alveolar space is inhibited, while movement into the interstitial spaces and thence into the lymphatics is relatively unimpeded. In addition the charges are predominantly negative within the interstitial space so that negatively charged proteins are likely to be repelled from interstitial structures, enhancing their movement into the lymphatics.

PULMONARY GAS EXCHANGE (Appendix 3)

If lung function was perfect, alveolar gas would completely equilibrate with arterial blood and P_aO_2 would equal P_AO_2. Even in normal individuals, however, there is a small pressure gradient between the oxygen in the alveoli and that in the arterial blood (the *alveolar–arterial oxygen difference*, $P_{A-a}O_2$) and this difference increases with age. Any disease of the lung parenchyma will interfere with oxygen transfer and cause an abnormal increase in $P_{A-a}O_2$. Three causes of the $P_{A-a}O_2$ can be identified: diffusion defects, right-to-left shunts and ventilation/perfusion mismatch.

Diffusion defects

Normally there is a very small pressure gradient (0.133 kPa or 1 mmHg) between oxygen in the alveoli and that in end-pulmonary capillary blood. Diffusion defects are probably not, however, an important cause of hypoxaemia, even in diseases such as fibrosing alveolitis, in which the alveolar–capillary membrane is considerably thickened, except possibly during exercise when pulmonary capillary transit time is markedly reduced or when P_AO_2 is very low (e.g. at altitude). Because carbon dioxide is so much more soluble than oxygen, its excretion is not influenced by diffusion defects.

Right-to-left shunts

Normally, a small amount of venous blood bypasses the lungs via the bronchial and Thebesian veins. Although this amounts to only 2% of total cardiac output, it is one cause of the $P_{A-a}O_2$ in normal subjects. In some diseases of the lung,

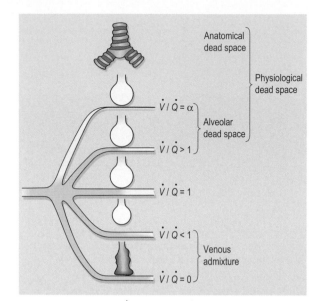

Fig. 3.15 Ventilation ($\dot{V}$)/perfusion ($\dot{Q}$) relationships.

such as lobar collapse, and with certain cardiac lesions, such as Fallot's tetralogy, a much larger proportion of the cardiac output passes to the left side of the heart without taking part in gas exchange, thereby causing significant arterial hypoxaemia. This hypoxaemia cannot be corrected by administering oxygen to increase P_AO_2, because blood leaving normal alveoli is already fully saturated with oxygen and further increases in P_AO_2 will not significantly affect the oxygen content. When this fully saturated blood is mixed with the shunted blood, arterial oxygen content, and therefore P_aO_2, falls proportionately. On the other hand, because of the shape of the carbon dioxide dissociation curve (see **Fig. 3.10**), the high PCO_2 of the shunted blood can be compensated by overventilating patent alveoli and thereby lowering the carbon dioxide content of the effluent blood. Indeed, many patients with acute right-to-left shunts hyperventilate, so that P_aCO_2 is normal or low.

Ventilation/perfusion mismatch (West, 1977)

In a perfect lung each alveolus would be perfused with a quantity of blood exactly equal to its volume of ventilation (i.e. the ventilation ($\dot{V}$)/perfusion ($\dot{Q}$) ratio would be unity ($\dot{V}/\dot{Q} = 1$; **Fig. 3.15**). If alveoli are ventilated, but not perfused ($\dot{V}/\dot{Q} = \alpha$), or if ventilation is excessive relative to their perfusion ($\dot{V}/\dot{Q} > 1$), then a proportion of this ventilation is wasted, and behaves as alveolar dead space. On the other hand, if an alveolus is well perfused, but poorly ventilated ($\dot{V}/\dot{Q} < 1$), complete oxygenation of the blood in contact with that alveolus is impossible. Finally, alveoli that are perfused, but not ventilated ($\dot{V}/\dot{Q} = 0$), behave as true shunts.

DISTRIBUTION OF VENTILATION

Even in normal subjects, inspired gas is not evenly distributed throughout the lungs. Studies using inhaled radioactive xenon have demonstrated that ventilation increases from

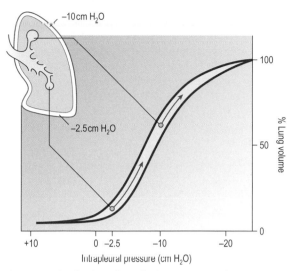

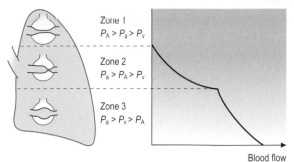

Fig. 3.18 Distribution of blood flow. Because of the hydrostatic effect, the pressure in the pulmonary vessels increases from the apex to the base of the lungs. Consequently, in zone I, alveolar pressure (P_A) exceeds both pulmonary arterial (P_a) and venous (P_v) pressures; the vessels are therefore collapsed and there is no blood flow (in fact, zone 1 does not exist in normal subjects). In zone 2, P_a exceeds P_A, which in turn is greater than P_v. Flow is therefore determined by the difference between P_A and P_a; since the former remains constant, flow increases progressively from the top to the bottom of this zone. In zone 3, both P_a and P_v exceed P_A. Flow therefore depends on the difference between P_a and P_v. Because of distension of the capillaries, blood flow increases slightly down this zone. A further zone, zone 4, may exist at the bases in which blood flow falls, due to compression of extra-alveolar vessels by poorly inflated lung tissue. Redrawn from West (2005), with permission. © 2005, Lippincott, Williams and Wilkins Co., Baltimore.

Fig. 3.16 Distribution of ventilation. Because of the weight of the lungs, intrapleural pressure is less negative at the base than at the apex. Consequently, there is less expansion of basal alveoli, which are on the steep portion of their compliance curve. For the same change in intrapleural pressure, therefore, these alveoli expand more than those at the apex. Alveolar ventilation therefore increases from the apex to the base of the lungs. Redrawn from West (2005), with permission. © 2005, Lippincott, Williams and Wilkins Co., Baltimore.

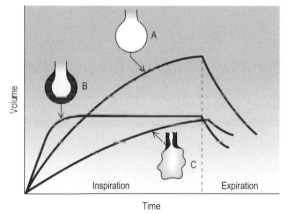

Fig. 3.17 Time constants. One time constant = compliance × resistance. For a normal alveolus (A): 0.6 s = 0.21/cm H_2O × 3 cm H_2O/l per second and by definition an alveolus is 95% filled in three time constants (i.e. 1.8 s). A non-compliant alveolus (B) will have a short time constant, whereas the time constant will be prolonged in those with airway narrowing (C). Redrawn from West (2005), with permission. © 2005, Lippincott, Williams and Wilkins Co., Baltimore.

this phenomenon is illustrated in **Figure 3.16**. Furthermore, especially in diseased lungs, ventilation may be unevenly distributed due to variations in the time constants of individual respiratory units (**Fig. 3.17**). Finally, although air is moved through the conducting airways by convection, gas transfer in distal lung segments occurs by molecular diffusion. This diffusion may be incomplete, particularly in abnormal lungs, and may further contribute to an uneven distribution of ventilation.

DISTRIBUTION OF PERFUSION (West et al., 1964)

In the normal lung, blood flow also increases downwards, but does so to a rather greater extent than does ventilation (**Fig. 3.18**). Normally, the overall $\dot{V}/\dot{Q}$ ratio is approximately 0.8. This has an effect equivalent to a right-to-left shunt of less than 3% of cardiac output and causes a $P_{A-a}O_2$ of no more than 0.7 kPa (5 mmHg) in normal subjects.

Conventionally gravity has been thought to be predominantly responsible for determining regional differences in blood flow and the distribution of ventilation. Recent evidence, however, suggests that the underlying structure of the bronchial and pulmonary vascular anatomy is an important factor, in both health and disease (Galvin *et al.*, 2007).

Diseases of the lung parenchyma interfere with the distribution of both ventilation and perfusion, causing an increased 'scatter' of $\dot{V}/\dot{Q}$ ratios. This produces an increase in alveolar V_D and hypoxaemia. As discussed above, the former can be compensated by increasing overall ventilation. *In contrast to the hypoxia resulting from a true right-to-left shunt, that due to areas of low $\dot{V}/\dot{Q}$ can be partially corrected*

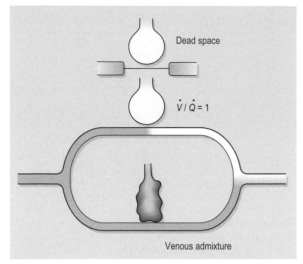

Fig. 3.19 The three-compartment model of pulmonary gas exchange.

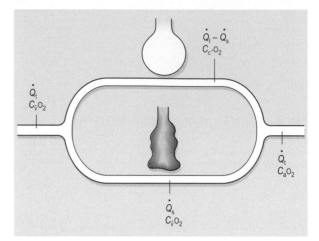

Fig. 3.20 Derivation of the shunt equation. The total amount of oxygen entering the systemic circulation per unit time must be equal to the sum of the amount leaving the ideal alveolus and the amount in the shunted blood. Therefore:

$$\dot{Q}_t \times C_aO_2 = [(\dot{Q}_t - \dot{Q}_s) \times C_cO_2] + [\dot{Q}_s \times C_{\bar{v}}O_2]$$

This can be rearranged to give:

$$\dot{Q}_s/\dot{Q}_t = C_cO_2 - C_aO_2/C_cO_2 - C_{\bar{v}}O_2$$

where $\dot{Q}_t$ = total flow (i.e. the cardiac output); $\dot{Q}_s$ = flow through the shunt; $(\dot{Q}_t - \dot{Q}_s)$ = flow through ideal alveolus; C_aO_2 = arterial oxygen content; $C_{\bar{v}}O_2$ = mixed venous oxygen content; C_cO_2 = end-capillary oxygen content in the ideal alveolus.

by administering oxygen and thereby increasing P_AO_2, even in poorly ventilated areas of lung.

Hypoxic pulmonary vasoconstriction

The degree of hypoxaemia produced by $\dot{V}/\dot{Q}$ mismatch or a right-to-left shunt is limited by the direct vasoconstrictor effect of alveolar hypoxia on the pulmonary vasculature. In acute lung injury in which capillary permeability is increased (see Chapter 8), this response may also limit oedema formation. The constriction occurs in the small arteries and arterioles (< 200 μm in diameter) when the alveolar PO_2 decreases to below about 8 kPa (60 mmHg). The exact mechanism is unclear, but may be a direct effect on the vascular smooth muscle or an indirect effect via the release of vasoactive mediators from lung parenchyma. This response occurs in only about two-thirds of healthy people and is much more pronounced in the young.

The three-compartment model of pulmonary gas exchange *(Riley and Cournand, 1949) (Fig. 3.19)*

In clinical practice it is often convenient to consider the lungs as if they consisted of three compartments:

- physiological dead space;
- perfectly matched $\dot{V}/\dot{Q}$;
- venous admixture.

The *dead-space compartment* (wasted ventilation) includes both the anatomical and the alveolar dead space, the latter consisting of 'true' dead space and lung units with $\dot{V}/\dot{Q}$ ratios > 1 (see **Fig. 3.15**).

Venous admixture combines all sources of 'wasted blood flow' (i.e. diffusion defects, right-to-left shunts and $\dot{V}/\dot{Q}$ ratios < 1; see **Fig. 3.15**) and treats them as if a given proportion of the cardiac output bypasses the lungs altogether. *Venous admixture* is then expressed as a percentage of the cardiac output – $\dot{Q}_s/\dot{Q}_t\%$, where $\dot{Q}_s$ is the flow per unit time

through the shunt and $\dot{Q}_t$ is the total flow (i.e. the cardiac output). Both total dead space and venous admixture can be calculated relatively easily in clinical practice and, by administering 100% oxygen to correct any hypoxaemia due to $\dot{V}/\dot{Q}$ inequalities, the relative contribution of true right-to-left shunt and $\dot{V}/\dot{Q}$ inequalities to the total venous admixture can be determined. This information is, however, of limited clinical relevance and administration of high concentrations of oxygen, even for short periods, may adversely affect lung function. This is because alveolar nitrogen, which is not absorbed, is replaced by oxygen, which is rapidly taken up by pulmonary capillary blood, thereby rendering alveoli unstable and liable to collapse.

$\dot{Q}_s/\dot{Q}_t\%$ can be calculated from the shunt equation (**Fig. 3.20**).

Oxygen content can be derived from oxygen saturation and the Hb concentration (see **Table 3.1** and Chapter 6, p. 151). If a pulmonary artery catheter is not in place, true mixed venous blood cannot be obtained, but some authorities suggest that, since in general only changes in venous admixture are of interest, central venous blood is adequate. Of course it is difficult to obtain true end pulmonary capillary blood; it is usual, therefore, to calculate P_AO_2 from the alveolar air equation (see equation **3.16**) and assume that equilibration in the ideal alveolus is complete, so that $P_cO_2 = P_AO_2$. Percentage saturation of Hb with oxygen is then calculated using a standard formula to represent the dissociation curve. Lastly, $C_{C'}O_2$ is derived from the Hb concentration. The V_D/V_T ratio can be calculated from the Bohr equation (**3.6**). This requires measurement of P_aCO_2 and determination of the concentration of carbon dioxide in expired gas (F_ECO_2).

MIXED VENOUS OXYGEN TENSION

If mixed venous oxygen tension ($P_{\bar{v}}O_2$) and therefore mixed venous oxygen content falls, the effect of a given degree of venous admixture on arterial oxygenation will be exacerbated (Kelman *et al.*, 1967). If cardiac output, and therefore oxygen delivery, falls and/or oxygen requirements increase, more oxygen has to be extracted from each unit volume of blood arriving at the tissues and $P_{\bar{v}}O_2$ falls. Worsening arterial hypoxaemia therefore does not necessarily indicate deterioration in pulmonary function, but may instead reflect a fall in cardiac output and/or a rise in oxygen consumption. Similarly, an increase in carbon dioxide production, if not compensated by increased alveolar ventilation, will cause P_aCO_2 to rise (see equation **3.10**).

The extent to which $P_{C'}O_2$ is altered by a reduction in $P_{\bar{v}}O_2$ depends on the $\dot{V}/\dot{Q}$ ratio of the lung unit in question. The effect will be most marked when there is a right-to-left shunt, while for ventilated units the impact of falls in $P_{\bar{v}}O_2$ will be greatest when the $\dot{V}/\dot{Q}$ ratio is low. Overall, the reduction in P_aO_2, which follows a fall in $P_{\bar{v}}O_2$ will depend on the $\dot{V}/\dot{Q}$ distribution of the whole lung (i.e. the greater the $\dot{V}/\dot{Q}$ mismatch, the larger the fall in P_aO_2).

The $P_{\bar{v}}O_2$ is also influenced by the position of the oxyhaemoglobin dissociation curve (see **Fig. 3.9**). Therefore, if the arteriovenous oxygen content difference remains constant, a shift of the curve to the right, which occurs with acidosis, hypercarbia, pyrexia and a rise in red cell 2,3-diphosphoglycerate (2,3-DPG) levels, may cause $P_{\bar{v}}O_2$ to rise. If, on the other hand, $P_{\bar{v}}O_2$ remains unchanged, more oxygen will be unloaded at tissue level. Conversely, a shift of the curve to the left will cause a fall in $P_{\bar{v}}O_2$, unless the arteriovenous oxygen difference falls. It might be argued then that under certain circumstances an acidosis may be beneficial in terms of tissue oxygenation, provided that the fall in pH is not sufficiently severe to interfere with cardiac function. It is probable though that shifts of the dissociation curve are of limited clinical significance.

The position of the oxyhaemoglobin dissociation curve is conventionally described by specifying the PO_2 at which Hb is 50% saturated with oxygen (the P_{50}) (see **Fig. 3.9**).

LUNG VOLUMES (see Appendix 3)

Normally individuals breathe in and out from the resting end-expiratory position with a *tidal volume* (V_T) of approximately 500 mL. A maximal inspiration, followed by a maximal expiration, is the *vital capacity* (VC) and comprises

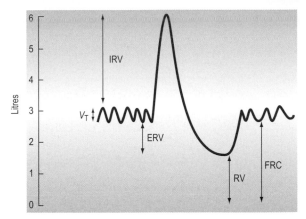

Fig. 3.21 Lung volumes. (V_T, tidal volume; IRV, inspiratory reserve volume; ERV, expiratory reserve volume; RV, residual volume; FRC, functional residual capacity.)

the V_T, the *inspiratory reserve volume* (IRV) and the *expiratory reserve volume* (ERV) (**Fig. 3.21**).

At the end of a forced expiration, intrapleural pressure becomes positive, overcoming the elastic forces that normally keep the distal airways patent so that the terminal airways collapse. The amount of gas thereby trapped in the lungs is called the *residual volume* (RV). The volume of gas remaining in the lungs at the end of a normal quiet expiration is the *functional residual capacity* (FRC) and consists of the ERV plus the RV. The *closing volume* (CV) is defined as the lung volume at which airway closure first begins.

LUNG MECHANICS AND WORK OF BREATHING (see Appendix 3)

To achieve normal ventilation, the respiratory muscles have to perform work against the *elastic* and *resistive forces* of the lungs and chest wall (**Fig. 3.22**); viscoelastic and *plastoelastic* forces must also be overcome. A negligible amount of work is expended in combating *inertial forces* (which depend on the mass of gases and tissues), *gravitational forces* and the *compressibility of intrathoracic gases*, as well as in *distorting the chest wall* from its relaxed configuration. *Hyperventilation* is associated with an additional workload due to asynchronous or paradoxical motion of the ribcage and abdomen, particularly in those with pulmonary disease.

In the presence of *airway obstruction and hyperinflation*, further work is expended in compressing gas within the lungs and airways.

Since work = force × distance moved, the amount of work performed by the respiratory system per breath is determined by the transpulmonary pressure gradient and V_T. At rest the metabolic cost of the work of breathing is small and constitutes only 1–3% of total oxygen consumption. In respiratory disease, however, there is an increase in

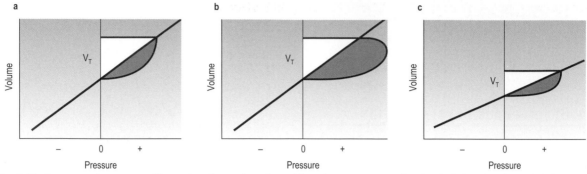

Fig. 3.22 Pressure–volume curves illustrating the work performed in order to overcome the elastic (□) and resistive (■) forces in the lungs. V_T, tidal volume. (a) Normal lung mechanics; (b) increased airway resistance; (c) decreased compliance.

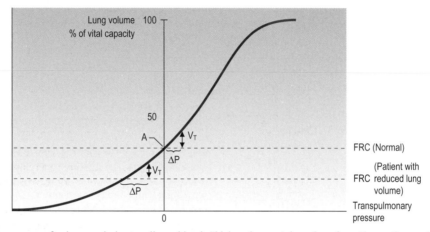

Fig. 3.23 Compliance curve for lung and chest wall combined. Tidal exchange takes place from the resting end-expiratory position (A), at which the tendency for the lungs to collapse is exactly counterbalanced by the tendency for the chest wall to expand (i.e. transpulmonary pressure is zero). It can be seen that this is also the steepest part of the curve, where small changes in pressure produce large changes in volume (i.e. compliance is greatest). However, as functional residual capacity (FRC) falls, the curve becomes flatter (i.e. the lungs become stiffer and compliance falls). V_T, tidal volume; ΔP, change in pressure.

the elastic and resistive forces, a larger transpulmonary gradient has to be generated to achieve the same V_T and the work of breathing increases. Under these circumstances respiratory effort may account for as much as 25–30% of total body oxygen consumption.

COMPLIANCE

Compliance (elastic opposing forces) is defined as the change in lung volume produced by a given change in airway pressure ($\Delta V/\Delta P$). It is possible to determine the compliance of the lungs and chest wall separately by measuring intrapleural pressure changes (approximated by oesophageal pressure), but in clinical practice it is more usual to consider both together. Normal lung compliance is approximately 200 mL/cm H_2O whereas total thoracic compliance is around 70–100 mL/cm H_2O. Reductions in total thoracic compliance may be caused by disorders affecting the thoracic cage or by reductions in the number of functioning lung units (e.g. due to lung resection, pneumothorax, pneumonia or pulmonary

oedema). Any reduction in overall lung volume, reflected by a fall in FRC, is associated with a fall in compliance (**Fig. 3.23**).

Effective dynamic compliance includes the influence of inspiratory airways resistance and is calculated as the ratio between the V_T delivered and the change in airway pressure (peak inspiratory pressure – end expiratory pressure; **Fig. 3.24**).

Static compliance is calculated from the change in volume produced by a given change in pressure *at a time of zero flow*. In practice if the inspiratory pause is sufficiently prolonged, the dynamic component is eliminated and 'quasistatic' or 'effective static' compliance is obtained (see **Fig. 3.24**). Alternatively the expiratory tubing can be briefly occluded.

In general, dynamic compliance is about 10–20% lower than compliance measured at plateau pressure. If dynamic compliance falls to a greater extent than total thoracic compliance, this suggests an increase in airway resistance. This approach, however, only measures compliance within the

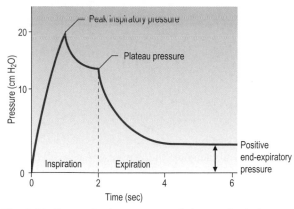

Fig. 3.24 Changes in airway pressure during mechanical ventilation. Effective dynamic compliance is calculated using peak inspiratory pressure – end expiratory pressure. Quasistatic or effective static compliance is calculated at time of zero flow (i.e. using plateau pressure – end expiratory pressure).

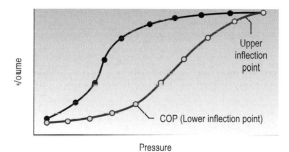

Fig. 3.25 Static pressure–volume curve illustrating a critical opening pressure (COP) during lung inflation (○) and a similar 'elbow' at a lower pressure in the deflationary curve (●).

range of tidal volumes normally employed and the value obtained may therefore alter depending on V_T and the level of positive end-expiratory pressure (see Chapter 7). An alternative is to perform a prolonged stepwise inspiratory–expiratory manoeuvre to obtain a true static pressure–volume loop. Sometimes this pressure–volume curve is found to be non-linear and points can be identified on both the inspiratory and expiratory curves at which the slope suddenly changes (**Fig. 3.25**). It is suggested that during inflation this 'elbow', where compliance suddenly increases, may be caused by re-expansion of a large number of previously collapsed alveoli as a *critical opening pressure* is reached. The upper inflection point may indicate the end of recruitment or the onset of overdistension. During deflation, at a pressure generally lower than the opening pressure, these same alveoli collapse with a sudden reduction in compliance. Some have suggested that this phenomenon of recruitment should be used as a basis for selecting the optimal level of positive end-expiratory pressure, although in practice this approach is associated with a number of difficulties (see Chapter 8, pp. 229–230).

RESISTANCE

Airway resistance is expressed as the airway pressure required to generate a given gas flow rate (cm H_2O/l per second). The relationship between the flow resistance of the total respiratory system (R_{rs}) and flow at a fixed lung volume is given by:

$$R_{rs} = R_t + K_1 + K_2 V$$

where R_t is the flow resistance of the thoracic tissues and K_1 and K_2 are empirical constants that describe the relationship between airway resistance (R_{aw}) and flow – $R_{aw} = K_1 + K_2 V$.

At a given lung volume therefore, R_{rs} will rise as flow increases. Moreover, at a given flow, R_{rs} will fall as lung volume rises because of a decrease in both R_{aw} and R_t. The former reflects airway dilatation, whereas the latter is a result of a decrease in the linear velocity of thoracic tissues and therefore a reduction in flow-dependent pressure losses.

An increase in airway resistance will require greater transpulmonary pressures to achieve the same V_T and will increase the work of breathing (see **Fig. 3.22**).

CONTROL OF BREATHING
(Richter *et al.*, 1992)

Breathing is normally precisely controlled by a tightly integrated feedback loop with three components: the respiratory control centres, the respiratory sensors and the respiratory effectors.

By balancing V_T and respiratory frequency to achieve the desired minute ventilation, this complex system maintains blood gas tensions within narrow limits despite marked fluctuations in V_{O_2} and V_{CO_2}, while at the same time minimizing the work of breathing. The body's capacity to store carbon dioxide far exceeds its ability to store oxygen and therefore changes in ventilation produce greater and more rapid changes in PO_2 than in PCO_2 or pH.

RESPIRATORY CONTROL CENTRES

The traditional concept of a single respiratory centre has been superseded. It is now appreciated that there are several localized regions of respiratory regulation, which, although situated at different levels within the brainstem, are highly interrelated by multilevel feedback connections. Functionally it is useful to consider two major centres of respiratory regulation, the *medullary centres* and the *groups of pontine neurones*, both of which can be overridden during wakefulness by projections from the *cerebral cortex*. The two phases of ventilation are controlled by three neural phases: inspiration (I phase), postinspiration (PI phase, passive expiration) and stage 2 expiration (E2 phase, active expiration).

Medullary centres

Respiratory rhythm originates in the medulla, possibly due to the interactive function of individual inspiratory and expiratory neurones, although separate respiratory pacemaker cells may also exist. In isolation the respiratory rhythm generated by this centre is not necessarily regular. There are two major groups of respiratory neurones in the medullary region: *the dorsal respiratory group* (DRG) and the *ventral respiratory group* (VRG).

DORSAL RESPIRATORY GROUP

The DRG is situated in the dorsomedial region of the medulla and is primarily composed of inspiratory neurones, which connect to the spinal inspiratory motor neurones of the phrenic and intercostal nerves. It seems likely that the DRG is the source of rhythmic respiratory drive, which is then transmitted to other regions, including the VRG, for modulation.

VENTRAL RESPIRATORY GROUP

The VRG is located ventrolaterally in the medulla and contains both inspiratory and expiratory neurones, which project to intercostal, abdominal and phrenic motor neurones, as well as to branches of the vagus, which supply the accessory muscles of respiration.

OTHER PARTICIPATING NEURONES

In addition there are other neurones in the vicinity of the DRG and VRG that may participate in some other aspects of inspiration, expiration and generation of respiratory rhythm.

Pontine neurones. Pontine neurones may be responsible for 'fine-tuning' respiratory adjustments. There are two major centres in this region: the *apneustic centre* in the lower pons and the *pneumotactic centre* in the upper pons.

Midpontine transection disinhibits the apneustic centre and produces a sustained inspiratory spasm, called *apneusis*. The pneumotactic centre regulates the relative duration of inspiration and expiration, although it is not essential for respiratory rhythmicity.

Cortical modulation. Cortical neurones project via corticobulbar and corticospinal pathways allowing conscious modulation of the respiratory neurones during activities such as speech and eating. In sleep the cortical drive to respiration is diminished and ventilation becomes more closely linked to the afferent input from chemoreceptors and vagal intrapulmonary receptors (see Chapter 8, sleep-related respiratory disturbances).

RESPIRATORY SENSORS

Respiratory sensors consist of the *chemoreceptors*, which are sensitive to changes in blood gas tensions and acid–base status, and sensory *mechanoreceptors*, within the lung and chest wall.

Central chemoreceptors

The central chemoreceptors are located on the ventral surface of the medulla oblongata. They respond rapidly to an increase in the H^+ ion concentration $[H^+]$ within the cerebrospinal fluid (CSF) by a linear increase in ventilation. Because carbon dioxide diffuses rapidly into the CSF, increasing its $[H^+]$, increases in P_aCO_2 produce an immediate ventilatory response. Changes in systemic pH, on the other hand, produce a delayed response because H^+ ions and HCO^-_3 diffuse more slowly into the CSF. The central chemoreceptors are depressed by hypoxia.

Peripheral chemoreceptors

The peripheral chemoreceptors are located at the bifurcation of the carotid arteries and along the aortic arch where they are exposed to a very high blood flow. They mainly respond to hypoxaemia and are activated to a much lesser extent by increases in PCO_2 and $[H^+]$, although the effects of combined hypoxaemia and hypercarbia are synergistic. The response to hypoxia is non-linear; as P_aO_2 falls below about 10 kPa (75 mmHg) there is an exponential increase in respiratory stimulation.

Under normal circumstances, therefore, carbon dioxide has a greater influence on the control of ventilation than oxygen. The peripheral chemoreceptors respond to changes in partial pressure, not oxygen content, and in carbon monoxide poisoning, for example, there is therefore no increase in ventilation, unless there is an accompanying acidosis. The peripheral chemoreceptors are also sensitive to reductions in blood pressure; this may partly account for the hyperventilation often seen in the early stages of shock.

Chest wall mechanoreceptors

Chest wall mechanoreceptors measure and modulate the forces generated by inspiratory effort. They respond to stretch of the respiratory muscles and reflexly modify the rate and depth of breathing. The *tendon receptors* within the intercostal muscles and diaphragm inhibit motor activity when the force of contraction is excessive. The *muscle spindles*, which are abundant in the intercostals, but more sparsely distributed in the diaphragm, may help to maintain V_T when chest wall movement is impeded (e.g. by changes in posture).

Pulmonary mechanoreceptors

The V_T and respiratory rate may also be influenced by stimuli arising in pulmonary receptors. *Irritant receptors*, which are located within the epithelium of the airways, respond to chemical or physical stimuli (e.g. mechanical deformation) to produce an increase in ventilation and bronchoconstriction. They are also involved in coughing.

The *pulmonary stretch receptors* are located in the smooth muscle of the airways and respond to changes in lung volume. The *Hering–Breuer reflex*, for example, is a vagally mediated reflex that normally terminates inspiration once a certain volume threshold has been reached. It is inoperative during quiet breathing, but is activated when V_T increases to about twice normal.

The *juxtacapillary (J) receptors* are found in the interstitium of the alveolar wall and are stimulated by distortion of the interstitial space as may occur with vascular engorgement, congestion or fibrosis. Stimulation of these receptors may explain the rapid shallow breathing seen in many patients with parenchymal lung disease.

RESPIRATORY EFFECTORS
Spinal pathways
The cortical pathways descend separately from the involuntary neuronal projections; there may also be spatial separation between the descending inspiratory and expiratory pathways.

Respiratory muscles
There are three major groups of respiratory muscles: the intercostal and accessory muscles, the diaphragm and the abdominal musculature.

The contractile properties of the respiratory muscles are governed by the same factors as those that control all striated muscles and their force of contraction is therefore influenced by force–length, force–velocity and force–frequency relationships. The greatest tension is generated when the muscle is at its resting optimal length when there is maximum overlap of the cross-bridges between the thick and thin filaments. An increase in lung volume will therefore lead to shortening of the respiratory muscles and a marked reduction in the tension generated (see Chapter 8). As the frequency of contraction increases there is a steep rise in the force of contraction, which plateaus at a rate of about 60 cycles/s, while increasing velocity of contraction is associated with a reduction in force.

There are three types of respiratory muscle fibre:

1. Slow-twitch type 1 fibres have the highest resistance to fatigue, with a low glycolytic and high oxidative capacity. These fibres are best suited to sustained tonic activity and constitute about 50% of the diaphragm.
2. Type II A fast-twitch red fibres are very resistant to fatigue and are suitable for sustained phasic activity.
3. Type II B fast-twitch white fibres have a poor oxidative capacity and the least resistance to fatigue. They are used for fast and powerful, but short-term activity.

DIAPHRAGM
The diaphragm is the major inspiratory muscle. It consists of a costal portion arising from the inner aspect of the lower six ribs and a crural portion originating from the upper lumbar vertebrae. In general, diaphragmatic contraction pushes down against the abdominal contents, leading to a rise in intra-abdominal pressure, and uses the resisting abdomen as a fulcrum to elevate the chest wall. The costal portion is capable of performing both these functions, while the major role of the crural portion is to increase intra-abdominal pressure. Diaphragmatic contraction therefore produces an outward movement of the anterior abdominal wall.

The efficiency with which the diaphragm translates its contraction into lung inflation depends on the ability of the abdominal wall to resist outward motion and create a positive pressure within the abdomen. Paradoxical inward movement of the abdomen during inspiration is a sign of diaphragmatic paralysis. Increases in lung volume will decrease the resting length of the diaphragm, thereby reducing its ability to develop tension. Moreover, the diaphragmatic fibres may come to lie at right angles to the chest wall and in this situation contraction may serve only to decrease the diameter of the inferior margin of the thoracic cage (see Chapter 8). Nevertheless contraction of the diaphragm continues to fulfil a useful function because it fixes the lower boundary of the thorax.

INTERCOSTALS
Intercostals fulfil both an inspiratory and an expiratory function, with the external intercostals being predominantly active during inspiration.

ABDOMINAL MUSCLES
The abdominal muscles are the major muscles of expiration and generate the increased intrathoracic pressures needed for coughing. They also act to facilitate inspiration, as described above.

MUSCLE WEAKNESS
Muscle weakness can be defined as an impaired ability of a rested muscle to generate force.

MUSCLE FATIGUE
Muscle fatigue can be defined as a situation in which muscle loses its ability to generate and sustain a required force or velocity of contraction. It is the result of muscle activity under load and is reversible by rest. It is likely to be due to depletion of energy stores, but recovery is slow and may take as long as 24 hours. The long-lasting component of fatigue is thought to be the result of impaired excitation–contraction coupling. Fatigue is generally a relatively acute phenomenon; little is known about chronic fatigue, in which muscle has not recovered from previous activity and there is a failure to generate a force, as opposed to sustaining a force. Central fatigue is considered to be present when a voluntary effort generates less force than electrical stimulation.

The respiratory muscles are relatively resistant to fatigue because they are continually active but, under extreme circumstances, they will eventually fail. Normal subjects are able to sustain minute ventilations less then 50–60% of maximum indefinitely. As the demand exceeds 60%, however, endurance times rapidly fall. Inspiratory resistive loads of less than 40% of maximum can be sustained indefinitely, but at higher loads the diaphragm fails as a pressure generator (Roussos and Macklem, 1977).

THE BRONCHIAL CIRCULATION
(Deffebach *et al.*, 1987)
The lung is perfused by two circulations.

The *pulmonary circulation* receives the entire venous return and is the major site for gas exchange. The much smaller *bronchial circulation* fulfils an important role in sustaining vital airway defences, fluid balance and metabolic activity in the lungs. It is the *systemic blood supply to the lungs,* supplying not only the bronchi, but also the trachea, the distal airways, the bronchoalveolar bundles, nerves, supporting structures, regional lymph nodes and visceral pleura. It also supplies, as the vasa vasorum, the walls of the pulmonary arteries and veins.

The bronchial veins draining the upper airways join the systemic veins to the right heart via the azygous and hemiazygous veins, while blood from the lower airways and lung parenchyma drains via the pulmonary veins into the left heart. This latter portion of the bronchial circulation is known as the *pulmonary collateral, bronchopulmonary anastomatic* or *bronchial systemic to pulmonary* flow. Branches from medium-sized bronchial arteries anastomose with the pulmonary alveolar microvasculature and with the pulmonary veins.

Bronchial blood flow is reduced by:

- systemic hypotension;
- raised intrathoracic pressure;
- increased lung volume;
- increases in pulmonary vascular pressures.

Systemic hypoxaemia increases both anastomotic and total bronchial blood flow. Although alveolar hypoxia may increase bronchial blood flow, in some situations simultaneous hypoxic pulmonary vasoconstriction may elevate downstream pressures and reduce flow. Systemic hypercarbia increases bronchial blood flow.

The bronchial circulation enlarges in response to lung injury and may provide the blood supply necessary for inflammation and subsequent healing in circumstances when pulmonary blood flow is often reduced. Moreover, significant gas exchange may be possible (e.g. during pulmonary artery occlusion) via the bronchial circulation, across either the bronchial or the alveolar epithelium, downstream of its anastomosis with the pulmonary circulation. The volume of gas exchange via the first route is likely to be small, but overall the bronchial circulation can contribute as much as 37% of total carbon dioxide output, and oxygen uptake may also occur in the presence of systemic hypoxia.

REFERENCES

Briscoe WA, Forster RE, Comroe JH Jr (1954) Alveolar ventilation at very low tidal volumes. *Journal of Applied Physiology* 7: 27–30.

Deffebach ME, Charan NB, Lakshminarayan S, *et al.* (1987) The bronchial circulation. Small, but a vital attribute of the lung. *American Review of Respiratory Disease* 135: 463–481.

Evander E, Wollmer P, Jonson B, *et al.* (1987) Pulmonary clearance of inhaled 99m Tc-DTPA: effects of surfactant depletion by lung lavage. *Journal of Applied Physiology* 62: 1611–1614.

Galvin I, Drummond GB, Mirmalan M (2007) Distribution of blood flow and ventilation in the lung: gravity is not the only factor. *British Journal of Anaesthesia* 98: 420–428.

Hills BA (1990) The role of lung surfactant. *British Journal of Anaesthesia* 65: 13–29.

Kelman GR, Nunn JF, Prys-Roberts C, *et al.* (1967) The influence of cardiac output on arterial oxygenation: a theoretical study. *British Journal of Anaesthesia* 39: 450–458.

Richter DW, Ballanyi K, Schwarzacher S (1992) Mechanisms of respiratory rhythm generation. *Current Opinion in Neurobiology* 2: 788–793.

Riley RL, Cournand A (1949) 'Ideal' alveolar air and the analysis of ventilation–perfusion relationships in the lungs. *Journal of Applied Physiology* 1: 825–847.

Roussos C, Macklem PT (1977) Diaphragmatic fatigue in man. *Journal of Applied Physiology* 43: 189–197.

Weibel ER (1984) *The Pathway for Oxygen: Structure and Function in the Mammalian Respiratory System.* Cambridge, Massachusetts: Harvard University Press.

West JB (1977) State of the art: ventilation–perfusion relationships. *American Review of Respiratory Disease* 116: 919–943.

West JB (2005) *Respiratory Physiology, The Essentials.* Lippincott, Williams and Wilkins: Baltimore.

West JB, Dollery CT, Naimark A (1964) Distribution of blood flow in isolated lung; relation to vascular and alveolar pressures. *Journal of Applied Physiology* 19: 713–724.

4 Assessment and monitoring of cardiovascular function

The ability to monitor patients continuously, to recognize the significance of changes in monitored variables and to respond rapidly and appropriately to such changes is fundamental to the successful management of the critically ill. To be effective and safe such monitoring requires the presence of an adequate number of appropriately trained nursing and medical staff at, or near, the bedside and is thus a defining characteristic of the intensive care or high-dependency environment.

As well as allowing early recognition of changes in the patient's condition, monitoring can also be used to establish or confirm a diagnosis, to gauge the severity of the condition, to follow the evolution of the illness, to guide interventions and to assess the response to treatment. When misapplied, however, invasive monitoring may delay or impede treatment, confuse rather than clarify diagnosis and management or even encourage the use of potentially dangerous interventions (for example, see Chapter 5, pp. 118–119). It is also important to appreciate that many monitored variables are only surrogates for the variable of primary interest.

Invasive monitoring is generally indicated in the more seriously ill patients and in those who fail to respond to initial treatment. These techniques are, however, associated with a significant risk of complications, as well as additional costs and patient discomfort. Invasive devices should therefore only be used when the potential benefits outweigh the dangers and should be removed as soon as possible.

Correct interpretation of monitored variables depends on an ability to recognize noise and artefacts, as well as to understand the limitations of the method (accuracy, precision, reproducibility, bias, response time). Thus, when the objective is to recognize trends, precision and reproducibility are more important than absolute accuracy, whereas for guiding treatment aimed at specific targets (e.g. goal-directed therapy, see Chapter 5) the requirement is for minimal bias and narrow limits of agreement. For titration of fluids or vasoactive drugs bias is less important than correlation.

The importance of combining the intelligent use of monitoring devices with frequent, astute clinical assessment cannot be overemphasized.

HEART RATE

As discussed in Chapter 3, heart rate is an important determinant of cardiac output and *continuous electrocardiographic (ECG) monitoring* is invariably indicated. Not only can changes in heart rate be observed immediately, but arrhythmias may be detected, diagnosed and treated. Moreover, changes in the ECG pattern may suggest the presence of electrolyte disturbances such as hypo- or hyperkalaemia and hypo- or hypercalcaemia (see Chapter 11) and allow the detection of episodes of myocardial ischaemia (ST-segment/T-wave changes) (see Chapter 9).

BLOOD PRESSURE

Alterations in blood pressure are often interpreted as reflecting changes in cardiac output but if the patient is vasoconstricted, with a high peripheral resistance, blood pressure may be normal, or occasionally high, even when cardiac output is low. Conversely the vasodilated patient may be hypotensive despite a very high cardiac output.

The absolute level of blood pressure is also important since hypotension may jeopardize perfusion of vital organs, while excessively high pressure increases myocardial work and can cause bleeding from arterial suture lines or precipitate a cerebrovascular accident. *The adequacy of blood pressure in individual patients must always be assessed in relation to their premorbid value.*

MEASURING BLOOD PRESSURE

Blood pressure can be measured intermittently using a sphygmomanometer cuff and auscultation. Automated instruments are now available, which automatically record and digitally display blood pressure and heart rate at intervals of 1–15 minutes. They are reliable and accurate and have the advantage of being non-invasive.

Arterial cannulation

If rapid alterations in blood pressure are a possibility, continuous monitoring using an *intra-arterial cannula* is advisable. An additional advantage of an indwelling arterial cannula is that repeated sampling for blood gas analysis can be performed without multiple arterial punctures, which can be more traumatic than prolonged cannulation.

APPROACHES

Percutaneous puncture of the radial artery (**Fig. 4.1**) is usually preferred because this superficial vessel is readily accessible, sterility of the insertion site is easily maintained, pressure can be applied to control bleeding and there is minimal restriction of patient mobility. Moreover, there is usually an adequate collateral circulation.

Some feel that cannulation of a larger vessel such as the femoral artery carries less risk of occlusive complications since good blood flow continues around the cannula. Femoral artery cannulation has been recommended as a safer alternative to difficult percutaneous radial artery cannulation or a surgical cut-down, both of which carry an increased risk of complications (Russell *et al.*, 1983). Certainly, cannulation of the femoral artery is relatively easy and is a useful approach in an emergency, particularly if the patient is hypotensive and other pulses are difficult to palpate. In difficult cases the brachial or dorsalis pedis arteries may be cannulated. In children the axillary artery can be used.

CANNULAE

Relatively small (20-gauge for adults, 22-gauge for children) short parallel-sided cannulae allow blood flow to continue past the cannula, and those made of Teflon are less irritant than, for example, those made of polypropylene or polyvinyl chloride; the use of such cannulae is therefore considered to minimize the risk of thrombosis.

SOURCES OF ERROR

It is important that the clinician is aware of some common sources of error in intra-arterial pressure measurement. If the arterial trace is overdamped, the recorded systolic pressure will be less than the actual systolic pressure (**Fig. 4.2**). This can occur if the cannula is kinked or partially obstructed by blood clot, if its tip is against the vessel wall or if there are air bubbles in the manometer line or transducer system. Compliant manometer lines can also produce a damped signal. Conversely, an underdamped trace will over-read, particularly at high pressures (see **Fig. 4.2**). Long manometer lines (more than 1–1.5 m) can also introduce inaccuracies since the natural resonant frequency of the system is decreased until it approaches the harmonics of the input signal, accentuating the recorded pressure. The mean arterial pressure is not influenced by either damping or resonance.

It is also important to appreciate that in peripheral vessels the systolic pressure is 1.1–1.3 times higher than in the ascending aorta (probably because of resonance in the arterial system) and that the diastolic pressure is lower by up to 5 mmHg. Conversely, early after cardiopulmonary bypass and in hypotensive septic patients receiving high-dose vasopressors, radial artery pressure significantly underestimates central pressure (Dorman *et al.*, 1998).

Catheter tip transducers have a number of advantages, including:
- artefacts due to catheter movement are avoided;
- there is no fluid-filled tubing;
- the frequency response is improved;
- correct positioning of the transducer is simplified.

Nevertheless these devices are not widely used in clinical practice.

TECHNIQUE

- The procedure is explained to the patient and if possible consent is obtained.
- The arm should be supported, with the wrist extended, by an assistant (see **Fig. 4.1a**).
- Assessment of the ulnar collateral circulation using Allen's test is no longer recommended since a normal result does not preclude ischaemia, neither does an abnormal result reliably predict this complication. Regular inspection of the cannulated hand is more likely to prevent ischaemic damage.
- Gloves should be worn.
- Clean the skin with chorhexidine.
- Palpate the radial artery where it arches over the head of the radius and make a small skin incision over the proposed puncture site. In conscious patients, raise a wheal of local anaesthetic, taking care not to puncture the vessel or obscure its pulsation.
- Insert the cannula over the point of maximal pulsation and advance in line with the direction of the vessel, at an angle of approximately 30°. 'Flashback' of blood indicates that the radial artery has been punctured.
- To ensure that the shoulder of the cannula enters the vessel, lower the needle and cannula, advance a few millimetres into the vessel and then thread the cannula off the needle into the vessel.
- Following withdrawal of the needle, connect the cannula to a non-compliant manometer line filled with heparinized saline. This is then connected via a disposable transducer and continuous-flush device to a flat-screen display (see **Fig. 4.1b**). The transducer should be zeroed.
- Cover the cannulation site with an occlusive dressing.
- The manometer line should be changed every 72–96 hours and the cannulation site may need to be changed approximately every 4–5 days, although routine replacement of the cannula is not recommended.

Some prefer to transfix the artery. When there is difficulty advancing the cannula into the vessel, a guidewire may prove useful. If cannulation fails, digital compression should be applied to the vessel for about 3 minutes. In some cases this may result in vasospasm, in which case the return of a good-volume pulse should be awaited (usually around 15 minutes) or cannulation should be attempted at another site.

COMPLICATIONS (Table 4.1)

Loss of arterial pulsation occurs in a significant proportion of patients and *digital ischaemia* is the most serious common complication of arterial cannulation. Fortunately, however,

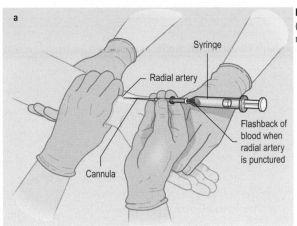

Fig. 4.1 (a) Percutaneous cannulation of the radial artery. (b) Cannula connected to monitor via fluid-filled, non-complaint manometer line, transducer and continuous flush device.

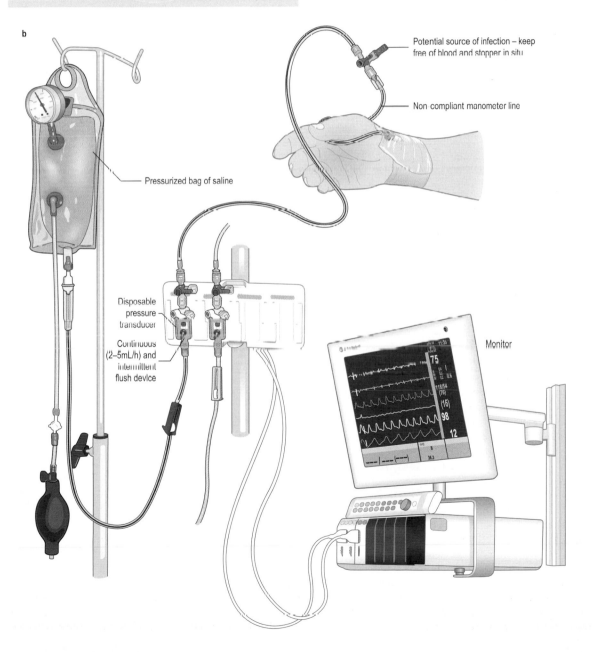

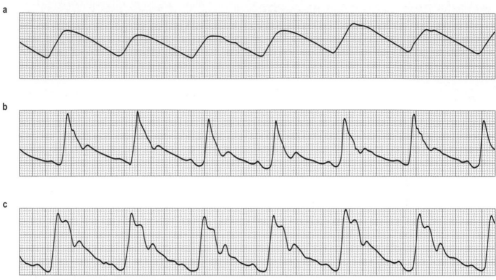

Fig. 4.2 Intra-arterial pressure recordings: (a) excessively damped; (b) critically damped to provide accurate readings; (c) underdamped.

Table 4.1 Complications of arterial cannulation
Bruising and haematoma
Occlusive complications (loss of arterial pulsation, digital ischaemia, digital necrosis)
Infection
Accidental injection of drugs
Disconnection
Arteriovenous fistula
Aneurysm/pseudoaneurysm

the much-feared complication of necrosis of one or more digits is rare, provided ischaemia is recognized early and the cannula is then removed promptly (Russell *et al.*, 1983). Transfixion of the artery does not increase the incidence of ischaemia. Persistent ischaemia may require aggressive management (e.g. brachial plexus or stellate ganglion block or even surgical exploration). Risk factors for ischaemia include:

- prolonged cannulation;
- low cardiac output;
- administration of vasoconstrictors;
- pre-existing peripheral vascular disease.

Also ischaemia is commoner:

- in females;
- following multiple attempts at cannulation;
- if a haematoma develops.

Some consider that there is an increased risk of *infection* with the femoral approach (Band and Maki, 1979), while others contend that the difference is insignificant (Thomas *et al.*,

1983); the overall complication rate is similar for both radial and femoral artery cannulation (7.5% and 6.9%, respectively) (Russell *et al.*, 1983). The incidence of catheter-related bacteraemia associated with arterial catheters seems to be similar to that attributable to central venous cannulation (Traoré *et al.*, 2005).

Other important complications associated with intra-arterial cannulation include:

- *accidental injection of drugs*, which can cause widespread vascular occlusion with the development of gangrene distally;
- *disconnection* or *accidental decannulation*, which, if unnoticed, can rapidly lead to exsanguination, particularly in children.

The risk of these complications can be minimized by clearly labelling the arterial line, ensuring fixation is secure and leaving the cannulation site exposed at all times so that disconnection is immediately recognized.

The development of an *arteriovenous fistula* and formation of an *aneurysm* or *pseudoaneurysm* are unusual, while *bruising* and *haematomas* are common.

PRELOAD

As discussed in the preceding chapter, the force with which myocardial fibres contract is dependent on the degree to which they are stretched prior to the onset of systole. This is in turn dependent on the ventricular end-diastolic volume (VEDV), which is related to the ventricular end-diastolic pressure (VEDP). The latter can, of course, be measured by direct catheterization of the ventricle, but in clinical practice it is more usual to measure the pressure in the

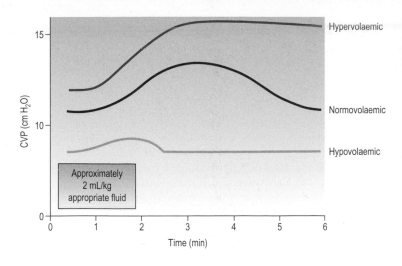

relevant atrium as this is nearly always closely related to VEDP. Importantly, the relationship between VEDV and VEDP depends on ventricular compliance; thus a stiff ventricle will need a higher EDP to achieve an adequate VEDV – a situation frequently encountered in the critically ill. Moreover, atrial pressure will not equal VEDP when there is an obstruction, such as a stenosed valve, between the two chambers. It is also important to appreciate that measuring dynamic changes in stroke volume, descending aortic flow and caval diameters (so-called *fluid responsiveness*) is a better guide to fluid requirements than the traditional approach of measuring filling pressures (see below).

CENTRAL VENOUS PRESSURE

In the case of the right ventricle the pressure within one of the large veins in the thorax is usually measured – the filling pressure of the right ventricle. This is a fairly simple, but approximate method of gauging the adequacy of a patient's circulating volume and the contractile state of the myocardium. It is important to realize that the absolute value of the central venous pressure (CVP) is not as important as its response to a fluid challenge (Fig. 4.3) (Sykes, 1963). Moreover, changes in CVP should always be interpreted in conjunction with other monitored variables (e.g. heart rate, blood pressure, urine flow, stroke volume and cardiac output) and with clinical assessment (e.g. skin colour, peripheral temperature and perfusion). The hypovolaemic patient will initially respond to transfusion with little or no change in CVP, together with some cardiovascular improvement (falling heart rate, rising blood pressure, resolving acidosis, improving urine output and increased peripheral temperature). As the normovolaemic state is approached, the CVP usually rises slightly and stabilizes, while other cardiovascular values begin to normalize. At this stage transfusion should be slowed, or even stopped, to avoid volume overload, which results in an abrupt and sustained rise in CVP, often accompanied by some deterioration in the patient's condition.

The CVP may be read:

- intermittently with a manometer system, which is only used when facilities for transducing the pressure are not available (e.g. on a general ward);
- continuously using a transducer connected to a flat-screen display as for intra-arterial pressure monitoring (see Fig 4.1b).

Whichever method is used, there are several common pitfalls when interpreting CVP measurements, many of which also apply to interpretation of other intravascular pressure measurements. These are:

- catheter obstructed;
- failure to refer the recorded pressure to the level of the right atrium;
- failure to zero the transducer;
- measuring the CVP while an infusion is in progress through the same lumen;
- taking a measurement when the catheter tip is in the right ventricle;
- misinterpreting the effect of respiratory oscillations.

Catheter obstruction. Catheter obstruction will result in a sustained high reading with a damped trace, which often does not correlate with the patient's overall clinical state. Check that a venous waveform and respiratory oscillations are present and that venous blood can be easily aspirated. A chest radiograph should be taken to confirm satisfactory positioning of the catheter (see below).

Pressure recording not referred to level of the right atrium. The recorded pressure is a combination of the pressure within the right atrium and a hydrostatic pressure caused by any difference in vertical height between the right atrium and the point of measurement. To allow meaningful comparisons between patients and between repeated readings obtained in the same patient, it is essential that the pressure recorded is always related to the level of the right atrium. Failure to adjust the level of the manometer or transducer after changing the patient's position is therefore a common cause of erroneous readings. Various landmarks are advocated to indicate the level of the right atrium, but it is largely immaterial which is chosen as long as it is used consistently and the readings are obtained with the patient in the appropriate position, i.e. sternal notch when the patient is supine or sternal angle when the patient is at 45°C. The axillary fold or the midpoint between the anteroposterior diameter of the thorax above the level of the fourth intercostal space can be used in either position.

Incorrect calibration. If an electronic transducer is used, it is important that the system is carefully zeroed before use and that the zero is checked if clinically doubtful values are obtained.

Infusion(s) in progress. If central venous access is at a premium, the CVP lumen may be used for other infusions and the pressure measured intermittently. If these infusions continue to be administered via a three-way tap while the pressure is read, a falsely high reading will result. Moreover, if the infusions contain inotropic or vasodilator agents, these may be interrupted and/or flushed into the patient when the CVP is measured. This can cause sudden episodes of cardiovascular instability.

Catheter tip in right ventricle. If the catheter is advanced too far it may enter the right ventricle. This should be suspected when an unexpectedly high pressure is recorded, particularly if oscillations are pronounced, and is easily recognized when the waveform is displayed.

Influence of respiratory oscillations. Respiratory oscillations may be particularly pronounced when patients are in respiratory distress and during mechanical ventilation. Pressures should be taken at end-expiration (i.e. when intrathoracic pressure is close to ambient pressure) in both spontaneously breathing and mechanically ventilated patients.

Central venous cannulation
INDICATIONS
The indications for central venous cannulation are:

■ to monitor right ventricular filling pressure;
■ to administer drugs (e.g. inotropes, antibiotics, cytotoxics, concentrated potassium);
■ to administer parenteral nutrition;
■ for cardiac pacing or pulmonary artery catheterization;
■ to allow rapid fluid administration;
■ when peripheral venous access is difficult;
■ for haemofiltration, dialysis and plasmapharesis.

APPROACHES AND POSITIONING THE CATHETER
The aim is to position a catheter with its tip in the superior vena cava (SVC), the upper right atrium or the innominate vein. This is usually achieved by percutaneous puncture of a central vein such as the *internal jugular* or *subclavian*. An advantage of the internal jugular approach is that pressure can be applied in the event of haemorrhage or inadvertent carotid artery puncture, although accidental arterial puncture may be more likely with this approach. The infraclavicular approach to the subclavian vein is also popular. It is ideal for long-term cannulation and is often preferred for the administration of parenteral nutrition, but probably carries a higher risk of pneumothorax and haemothorax (McGee and Gould, 2003), although this has not been the case in all studies (Ruesch *et al.,* 2002). It is therefore sensible to avoid this approach if possible in those with significant hypoxaemia. Less commonly, the *external jugular* veins may be used.

The *femoral* approach can be useful in those with a coagulopathy and when a head-down tilt is contraindicated. Haematoma and arterial puncture are common during femoral venous catheterization. There is also some evidence to suggest that cannulation of the femoral vein is associated with a higher incidence of infectious and thrombotic complications than the subclavian approach (Merrer *et al.,* 2001), although this has not been a consistent finding (Deshpande *et al.,* 2005). A technique in which a long femoral catheter is placed in the inferior vena cava, close to the right atrium, under ECG guidance has been described (Joynt *et al.,* 1996). The intra-abdominal CVP measurements obtained showed sufficient agreement with intrathoracic values to be clinically useful. Even when shorter catheters are used to measure femoroiliac pressures, agreement with SVC pressures seems to be sufficiently close for clinical purposes (Dillon *et al.,* 2001). Alternatively a long line may be inserted via an *antecubital vein*, although frequently it proves impossible to advance the catheter into a satisfactory position. Finally, if the chest is open, a cannula can be inserted *directly into the innominate vein*.

The risk of perforation of the great veins or the heart is reduced by correct positioning of the catheter. There is evidence that the more perpendicular the catheter is to the wall of the vessel or heart, especially if the catheter tip abuts the wall, the greater is the risk of perforation. Left-sided catheters pose a particular problem because the innominate vein forms a near right angle with the SVC. Catheters entering the SVC from the left therefore have a tendency to impinge on the lateral wall of this vein, with a well-documented risk of perforation. Atrial or ventricular perforation and subsequent cardiac tamponade can be avoided by ensuring that the catheter tip lies outside the pericardial sac and certainly placement deep in the right atrium or into the right ventricle must be avoided. On the other hand, placement in the upper SVC or above is associated with an increased risk of thrombosis.

It has been suggested, therefore, that, on balance, the low SVC/upper right atrium is the most suitable site for the tip of flexible catheters introduced from any access point in the upper body, provided the catheter tip does not abut the atrial wall end-on, is not in contact with the tricuspid valve and does not pass into the coronary sinus. The upper SVC is considered to be an acceptable tip position only for catheters placed via the internal jugular vein, while the midpoint of the innominate vein is an appropriate site for the tip of catheters introduced from the left internal jugular or subclavian vein (Fletcher and Bodenham, 2000).

CANNULAE

The relatively short and rigid *catheter-over-needle* devices, which are merely long intravenous cannulae, are easy to use and are particularly useful in an emergency. They have the disadvantage that the needle protrudes beyond the end of the catheter, making it possible to aspirate blood even when the catheter itself is outside the vein. Furthermore, the catheters need to be fairly sharp and rigid, since they have to be pushed through the skin and subcutaneous tissues. Consequently, they are associated with a significant risk of perforation. These devices are therefore only safe when inserted via the right internal jugular vein so that the catheter lies in a straight line with its tip in the SVC or high right atrium. They are now rarely used except in an emergency.

Long *catheter-through-cannula* devices are particularly useful when using a vein in the anticubital fossa. With these, venepuncture is first performed using a standard intravenous cannula. The needle is then withdrawn and a soft, flexible catheter is advanced through the cannula into the vein. The cannula is then removed. An important disadvantage of this technique is that the hole in the vein is larger than the catheter so there is a risk of bleeding around the puncture site.

Techniques using a *guidewire* (**Fig. 4.4**) are safer and less traumatic. They can be used in conjunction with a vein dilator for inserting *introducers for pulmonary artery catheters* (see below), *double-lumen cannulae for blood purification and multilumen catheters.* The latter are now used extensively in intensive care units, almost to the exclusion of other devices, because they allow CVP monitoring and the safe administration of multiple infusions through the various separate lumens of a single catheter. The rate of catheter-related complications is not increased by the use of multilumen catheters (McGee and Gould, 2003).

THE PROCEDURE

The general principles of a safe technique are common to all the approaches to central venous cannulation and should be learnt from instruction and demonstration in patients by an expert. The low anterior approach to the internal jugular vein will be described (**Fig. 4.5**), since this is probably the safest and most consistently successful route to use in an emergency. A technique in which the head is maintained in the neutral position has been proposed for internal jugular venous cannulation in trauma patients with suspected cervical instability (Willeford and Reitan, 1994).

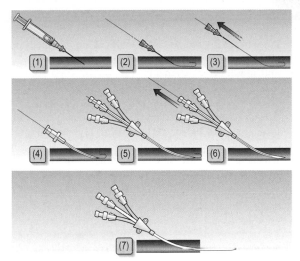

Fig. 4.4 Insertion of a catheter over a guidewire (Seldinger technique). (1) Puncture vessel; (2) advance guidewire; (3) remove needle; (4) dilate vessel then remove dilator; (5) advance catheter over guidewire; (6) remove guidewire; (7) catheter in situ. Adapted from Kumar P, Clark M 2005 Clinical Medicine 6E Elsevier with permission.

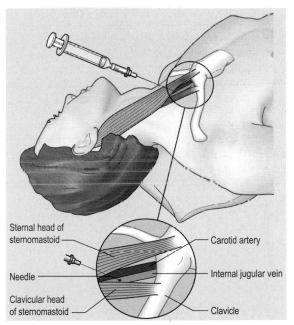

Fig. 4.5 Cannulation of the right internal jugular vein (see text). Adapted from Kumar P, Clark M 2005 Clinical Medicine 6E Elsevier with permission.

■ If the patient is conscious the procedure must be fully explained and should be carried out with the best sterile precautions compatible with the urgency of the situation. Normally the operator should scrub up and wear a sterile gown and gloves, but in extremely urgent cases (e.g. cardiac arrest), a no-touch technique can be acceptable, although gloves (preferably sterile) should always be worn for protection.

■ Place the patient in the head-down position so that the central veins are distended; this makes cannulation easier and minimizes the risk of air embolism. This position will, however, exacerbate any respiratory difficulty, particularly if due to cardiac failure. The head-down position is also potentially dangerous in patients with raised intracranial pressure.

■ Clean the skin over the proposed puncture site with an antiseptic solution, such as chlorhexidine, and place sterile towels in position.

■ Turn the patient's head away from the proposed site of entry. Usually, the right side is chosen because this approach is technically easier for a right-handed operator, correct placement of the catheter (see above) is more likely and on the left there is a danger of damaging the thoracic duct.

■ Palpate the apex of the triangle formed by the two heads of sternomastoid, with the clavicle as its base and raise a wheal of 2% plain lidocaine over this point.

■ Determine the position of the carotid artery to minimize the risk of accidental arterial puncture.

■ Make a small incision in the anaesthetized skin, through which the cannula or introducing needle is inserted, directed laterally downwards and backwards, aiming for the nipple, at an angle of about 20° so that the vein is punctured just beneath the skin, deep to the lateral head of sternomastoid. If the vein is not encountered, the needle must not be advanced more than a few centimetres because of the risk of a pneumothorax. Failure suggests that either the vein is not sufficiently distended or the cannula is being misdirected. The anatomical landmarks should be checked and the patient can be placed more steeply head-down before the attempt is repeated.

■ Once the catheter has been inserted and is thought to be correctly positioned, venous blood should be easily aspirated; then, the CVP manometer line can be connected. There is always a risk of air embolism whenever the catheter is open to air, so necessary periods of disconnection should be as short as possible and Luer locks must be used on all connections.

■ It is important to check that the fluid level in the manometer falls rapidly and fluctuates with respiration because this indicates that the tip of the catheter is in an intrathoracic vein. Similarly, when transduced, there should be a clear venous waveform with respiratory oscillations.

■ The application of antibiotic ointments to catheter insertion sites increases the rate of catheter colonization by fungi, promotes the emergence of antibiotic resistant bacteria and has not been shown to reduce the rate of catheter-related bloodstream injections (McGee and Gould, 2003). Because data on the optimum type of dressing (gauze or transparent) and the frequency of dressing changes are conflicting, evidence-based rec-

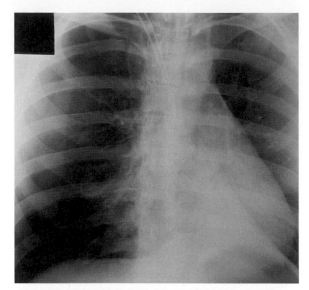

Fig. 4.6 Pneumothorax following insertion of two central venous cannulae via the internal jugular vein. Note also the collapsed left lower lobe (sail-shaped shadow behind the heart obscuring the outline of the elevated left hemidiaphragm; the mediastinum is deviated to the left).

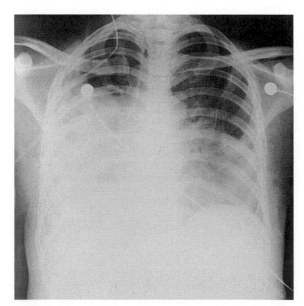

Fig. 4.7 Fluid has been infused into the right pleural space via an incorrectly positioned catheter. There is also bilateral consolidation in the left mid and lower zones.

ommendations cannot be made (McGee and Gould, 2003).

■ Obtain a chest radiograph as soon as possible to verify that the tip of the catheter is correctly positioned, and to exclude the presence of a pneumothorax (Gladwin *et al.*, 1999) (**Fig. 4.6**). This is particularly important before infusing large volumes of fluid (**Fig. 4.7**).

COMPLICATIONS

Complications may occur in more than 15% of patients who undergo central venous catheterization. Mechanical complications have been reported in 5–19% of patients, infectious complications in 5–26% and thrombotic complications in 2–26% (McGee and Gould, 2003).

The complications of central venous cannulation include:

- arterial puncture (haematoma, arteriovenous fistula, stroke) (Mainland *et al.*, 1997); } most common complications
- pneumothorax (see **Fig. 4.6**);
- vascular perforation (stiff catheters, positioning, mobility of tip, guidewire, fluids infused under pressure or at high flows);
- thrombosis (particularly with the femoral approach and high placement of the catheter tip; subclavian vein catheterization may be associated with the lowest risk) and pulmonary embolism;
- catheter-related bloodstream infections (a clear relationship with thrombosis: remove catheters as soon as they are no longer required) (see Chapter 12);
- septic thrombophlebitis;
- air embolism.

Less common complications include:

- catheter embolism;
- pericardial tamponade;
- haemothorax or hydrothorax (see **Fig 4.7**);
- haemomediastinum or hydromediastinum;
- injury to the brachial plexus, phrenic nerve or recurrent laryngeal nerve;
- puncture endotracheal tube cuff;
- damage to the thoracic duct;
- Horner's syndrome.

Cardiac arrhythmias and endocardial damage may occur, but are more commonly associated with pulmonary artery catheterization (see below). It has been shown that the overall incidence of failed cannulation and complications is related not to the approach used (internal jugular or subclavian), but to operator experience (Sznajder *et al.*, 1986). The failure rate was 10.1% for experienced and 19.4% for inexperienced operators, while the incidence of complications was 5.4% and 11% respectively. The incidence of failed attempts is higher in the obese and those who have undergone major surgery in the region of attempted cannulation or in whom the vein has previously been cannulated. Complications are strongly associated with failed attempts (Mansfield *et al.*, 1994).

Ultrasound-guided puncture has been recommended for difficult cases and to reduce the incidence of failed/multiple attempts and complications. Certainly ultrasound guidance can be useful when difficulties or complications have been encountered or are anticipated (Hatfield and Bodenham, 1999) and may be helpful for inexperienced operators.

Moreover the authors of a recent meta-analysis concluded that two-dimensional ultrasound guidance reduces the failure rate and complications associated with central venous cannulation (Hind *et al.*, 2003). Some therefore recommend that ultrasound imaging should be used routinely. Others emphasize that all anaesthetists and intensivists should become skilled in blind central venous cannulation and suggest that ultrasound guidance should be reserved for those in whom cannulation is anticipated to be difficult and complications could be serious, as well as a back-up after failed attempts (Muhm, 2002).

ARTERIAL PRESSURE VARIATION AS A GUIDE TO HYPOVOLAEMIA (Stoneham, 1999)

Systolic arterial pressure decreases during the inspiratory phase of intermittent positive-pressure ventilation. The magnitude of this cyclical variability has been shown to correlate more closely with hypovolaemia than other monitored variables, including CVP. *Systolic pressure variation* during mechanical ventilation can therefore be used as a simple and reliable guide to the adequacy of the circulating volume. In mechanically ventilated patients with acute circulatory failure related to sepsis, analysis of the respiratory change in *pulse pressure* has been shown to be a simple method for predicting and assessing the haemodynamic effects of volume expansion, and to be a more reliable predictor of fluid responsiveness than changes in systolic pressure (Michard *et al.*, 2000).

OTHER TECHNIQUES FOR ASSESSING INTRAVASCULAR VOLUME

Respiratory changes in inferior vena cava diameter and SVC collapsibility measured by echocardiography may accurately predict fluid responsiveness in mechanically ventilated septic patients (Barbier *et al.*, 2004; Vieillard-Baron *et al.*, 2004). The response to fluid loading can also easily be predicted by observing the changes in pulse pressure during passive leg raising (Boulain *et al.*, 2002). It has also been shown that standardized scoring of the portable chest radiograph and in particular measurement of the vascular pedicle width can assist clinicians in the assessment of fluid balance and intravascular volume (Martin *et al.*, 2002).

LEFT ATRIAL PRESSURE

In uncomplicated cases careful interpretation of the CVP provides a reasonable guide to the filling pressures of both sides of the heart. In many critically ill patients, however, this is not the case and there is a *disparity in ventricular function*. Usually left ventricular performance is most impaired so that the left ventricular function curve is displaced downward and to the right (**Fig. 4.8**). This situation is encountered in many patients with clinically significant ischaemic heart disease and has also been reported in multisystem trauma, sepsis, peritonitis, hepatic failure, valvular heart disease and after cardiac surgery. High right ventricular filling pressure with normal or low left atrial pressure (LAP) is less common,

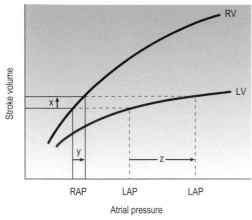

Fig. 4.8 Left (LV) and right (RV) ventricular function curves in a patient with left ventricular dysfunction. Since the stroke volume of the two ventricles must be the same (except perhaps for a few beats during a period of circulatory adjustment), left atrial pressure (LAP) must be higher than right atrial pressure (RAP). Moreover, an increase in stroke volume (x) produced by intravascular volume expansion will be associated with a small rise in RAP (y), but a marked increase in LAP (z).

but may occur in situations in which pulmonary vascular resistance (i.e. right ventricular afterload) is raised, such as acute respiratory failure and pulmonary hypertension, as well as in those with right ventricular ischaemia. These discrepancies between right and left ventricular performance can be exacerbated by the use of inotropic and vasoactive drugs. If there is a disparity in ventricular function after cardiac surgery the left atrium can be cannulated directly, but if the thorax is not open, some other means of determining left ventricular filling pressure is required.

PULMONARY ARTERY PRESSURE

In 1953 pulmonary artery catheterization with a balloon-tipped, flow-directed catheter was pioneered in the animal laboratory (Lategola and Rahn, 1953). Seventeen years later Swan and colleagues described the use of a similar catheter in humans (Swan *et al.*, 1970). This *balloon flotation catheter* allowed prompt and reliable catheterization of the pulmonary artery without the need for screening, and minimized the incidence of arrhythmias. Later, a catheter with a slightly increased diameter, a larger balloon, a proximal lumen for CVP measurement and a thermistor located near the tip was introduced, the thermistor allowing determination of cardiac output by the thermodilution technique (see below) (Forrester *et al.*, 1972). Balloon flotation catheters have since been modified for other purposes, including cardiac pacing, pulmonary angiography, continuous monitoring of mixed venous oxygen saturation and determination of right ventricular ejection fraction (Zink *et al.*, 2004). More recently methods have been developed for the continuous measurement of cardiac output (see later).

Approaches

Pulmonary artery catheters can be inserted centrally, through the femoral vein or via a vein in the antecubital fossa. The latter route is perhaps the most comfortable, but it may be difficult to advance the catheter beyond the shoulder region. Furthermore secure fixation is not easily achieved and involves some degree of immobilization of the arm. On the other hand, the complication rate, particularly the risk of pneumothorax, is reduced. The left infraclavicular approach to the subclavian vein conforms most closely to the natural curvature of the catheter, and secure fixation is more easily achieved at this site. Catheterization of the right internal jugular vein is, however, safer and is the shortest and most direct route to the right side of the heart.

The procedure

Because pulmonary artery catheters have to be introduced through a wide-bore cannula, a guidewire technique is used (see **Fig. 4.4**).

- First an incision is made in the anaesthetized skin and the vein is punctured with a needle or a standard intravenous cannula.
- A guidewire with a flexible, J-shaped tip is then introduced and the cannula or needle is removed.
- A tapered vein dilator is passed over the guidewire to ease subsequent passage of the cannula.
- The dilator carrying the wide-bore cannula is inserted over the guidewire, which is then withdrawn. (If the original skin incision is not sufficiently large and deep, pushing the dilator and cannula through the skin and subcutaneous tissues may prove difficult.)
- The dilator is then removed and the pulmonary artery catheter passed through the introducer into the vein. The introducer incorporates a valve mechanism, which prevents air embolism and spillage of blood after the dilator is removed and during insertion of the catheter. This introducer cannula should be left *in situ* and provides an additional central venous access point. A plastic sleeve is provided with most introducer kits, which protects a length of catheter, thereby maintaining its sterility. This can subsequently be manipulated if the catheter becomes misplaced, without risking contamination.

PRECAUTIONS

Before the pulmonary artery catheter is inserted:

- The balloon should be inflated with the recommended volume of air to check for leaks and to ensure that inflation is symmetrical.
- Confirm that the thermistor is functioning.
- The oximeter, if present, should be calibrated.
- The various lumens should be flushed with heparinized saline.

The technique must be learnt under supervision because complications are inversely related to operator experience.

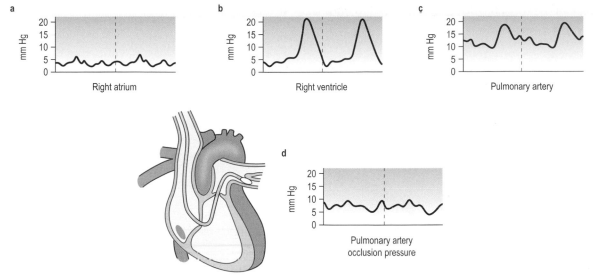

Fig. 4.9 Pressure waveforms as a pulmonary artery catheter is passed through the chambers of the heart into the wedge position. (a) Once in the thorax, respiratory oscillations are seen. The catheter should be advanced further towards the lower superior vena cava/right atrium when oscillations become more pronounced (15–20 cm of catheter inserted). The balloon should then be inflated and the catheter advanced. (b) In the right ventricle (25–35 cm) there is no dicrotic notch and the diastolic pressure is close to zero. *The patient should be returned to the horizontal, or slight head-up, position before advancing the catheter further.* (c) In the pulmonary artery (35–50 cm) a dicrotic notch appears and there is elevation of the diastolic pressure. The catheter should be advanced further with the balloon inflated. (d) Reappearance of a venous waveform indicates that the catheter is wedged. Stop advancing. The balloon should be deflated to obtain pulmonary artery pressure, and then inflated intermittently to obtain pulmonary artery wedge or occlusion pressure.

INTRODUCING THE CATHETER

■ Passage of the catheter from the major veins, through the chambers of the heart into the pulmonary artery and the wedge position, is monitored and guided by the pressure waveforms recorded from the distal lumen (**Fig. 4.9**).

■ The catheter should not be advanced too rapidly since redundant loops may form in the right atrium or ventricle, with a risk of knotting.

■ Radiographic control must be used if any difficulty is encountered and is most often required in those with a low cardiac output and/or a large heart.

■ A chest radiograph should always be obtained to check the position of the catheter; the tip should be within 2 cm of the cardiac silhouette (**Fig. 4.10**). Some recommend a lateral chest radiograph taken when the patient is supine to ensure that the tip of the catheter is in a posterior vessel.

PRESSURE MEASUREMENTS

Once in position, the balloon is deflated and pulmonary artery systolic pressure, end-diastolic pressure (PAEDP) and mean pulmonary artery pressure (PAP) can be obtained. The balloon is then inflated intermittently with the recommended volume of air (0.8–1.5 mL), thereby propelling the catheter distally where it will impact in a medium-sized pulmonary artery and record pulmonary artery occlusion pressure (PAOP) (see **Fig. 4.11**). If a PAOP is obtained when the balloon is inflated with less than 0.8 mL of air, the catheter

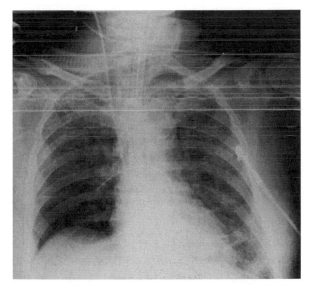

Fig. 4.10 Pulmonary artery flotation catheter correctly positioned in a patient with acute respiratory distress syndrome.

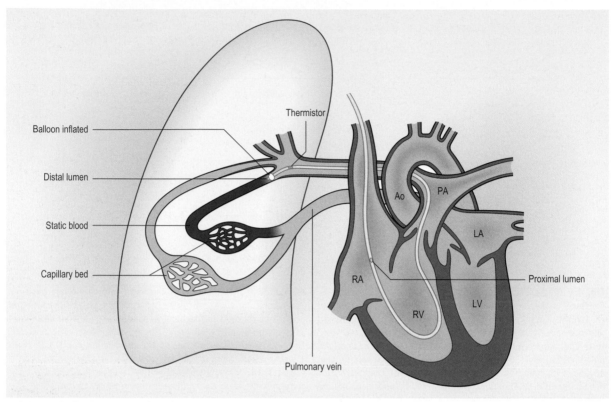

Fig. 4.11 Balloon flotation pulmonary artery catheter in the wedged position. There is now a continuous column of static blood between the tip of the catheter and the left atrium; pulmonary artery occlusion pressure (PAOP) is therefore usually closely related to left atrial pressure. LA, left atrium; LV, left ventricle; PA, pulmonary artery; RA, right atrium; RV, right ventricle.

should be withdrawn a few centimetres to reduce the risk of pulmonary artery rupture or infarction (see later).

All intravascular pressures should be measured relative to atmospheric pressure and should therefore be obtained at end-expiration. The digital pressure display does not provide an accurate end-expiratory value; occlusion pressure should therefore be determined from a continuous recording of the waveform using a cursor and inbuilt algorithms. In patients receiving a positive end-expiratory pressure (PEEP) (see Chapter 7), the recorded pressure will be incremented by an amount proportional to the level of PEEP. This effect is, however, difficult to quantify in the individual patient and depends on a number of factors, including lung compliance. PEEP should not be discontinued while obtaining pressure measurements because this alters the haemodynamic conditions unpredictably, there may be a sudden increase in venous return and there is usually a significant fall in P_aO_2. It is important to remember that in obstructive airways disease there may be an intrinsic PEEP (see Chapter 8).

INTERPRETATION

When the pulmonary artery catheter is in the wedge position, flow ceases in the isolated segment of pulmonary vasculature and the pressure in the occluded vessels equilibrates with pulmonary venous pressure (**Fig. 4.11**). PAOP is therefore usually closely related to LAP. The measurement of

PAOP is, however, prone to errors and misinterpretation. It is clearly essential to *establish that a genuine PAOP reading has been obtained*. When the catheter 'wedges':

- a relatively damped venous waveform should appear;
- respiratory oscillations should be apparent;
- the PAOP should be a few mmHg less than PAEDP;
- some check that it is possible to withdraw arterialized blood, although as much as 20–40 mL of blood may have to be aspirated to obtain a fully oxygenated sample.

Occasionally, when the balloon is inflated, a PAOP trace is obtained only intermittently. This *transitional waveform* can occur when the fluctuations in PAP cause the catheter to 'wedge and unwedge' in a branch of the pulmonary artery. The recorded PAOP may be higher than PAEDP if:

- the balloon is overinflated;
- the balloon inflates eccentrically and/or the catheter tip abuts the vessel wall;
- the waveform is abnormal (e.g. large V waves in mitral regurgitation or cannon waves in complete heart block).

Once a genuine PAOP has been obtained, a number of *potential causes of misinterpretation* remain. The assumptions are that:

PAOP = LAP = LVEDP = LVEDV

As discussed above, the relationship between LVEDP and LVEDV depends on the compliance of the ventricles, which is altered in many critically ill patients. Furthermore, LAP may not accurately reflect LVEDP in the presence of mitral valve disease, left atrial myxoma or severe left ventricular dysfunction. Finally, PAOP will only be equivalent to LAP when there is a continuous column of blood between the catheter tip and the left atrium (i.e. West's zone 3 conditions prevail; see Chapter 3). This will not be the case when the intervening pulmonary vessels are collapsed by intra-alveolar pressures that are higher than pulmonary venous pressure. This can occur in ventilated patients requiring high inflation pressures or extrinsic PEEP, and in those with airway obstruction, particularly if they are hypovolaemic and/or the catheter is in the upper zones of the lungs (West's zones 1 and 2; see Chapter 3). Under these circumstances the pressure recorded is a reflection of intra-alveolar, rather than left atrial, pressure. Non-zone 3 conditions are suggested:

- by the absence of normal cardiac oscillations in the PAOP trace;
- when PAOP exceeds PAEDP;
- if, during the application of increasing levels of PEEP, PAOP increases by more than half the PEEP increment.

It has also been suggested that in sepsis Starling resistor effects in the pulmonary venous system may lead to a dissociation between PAOP and LAP, with PAOP tending to overestimate left ventricular filling pressures (Fang et al., 1996).

In the supine patient a lateral chest radiograph taken with the catheter wedged can determine whether the tip is correctly positioned at or below left atrial level. Fortunately, because the catheter enters the right ventricle anteriorly through the tricuspid valve and leaves it to enter the pulmonary artery in a posterior direction, the curve on the catheter usually causes it to enter a posterior branch of the pulmonary artery supplying the right lower lobe. Also blood flow is greatest in zone 3, increasing the likelihood of the catheter 'floating' into this region of the lung.

The PAOP may also overestimate LVEDP if there is a tachycardia because premature closure of the mitral valve will increase the atrioventricular pressure gradient and there is limited time for equilibration between PAOP and LAP.

If it proves impossible to obtain a satisfactory PAOP (e.g. if the balloon ruptures), it has been suggested that PAEDP can provide a reasonable guide to LAP. There is, however, normally a gradient of 1–3 mmHg between PAEDP and PAOP, and this is increased in the presence of pulmonary hypertension, in those with tachycardias and during rapid transfusion (Lappas et al., 1973). In general, PAEDP is an unreliable guide to left ventricular filling pressures in the critically ill.

It must be emphasized that, as with CVP measurement, the response of PAEDP and PAOP to a fluid challenge is often of more significance than the absolute value. Also, as

Table 4.2 Complications of pulmonary artery catheterization
Haemorrhage/haematoma
Pneumothorax
Arrhythmias (during passage of catheter through the right ventricle, usually benign, can often be prevented with lidocaine)
Sepsis (at insertion site, bacteraemia)
Endocarditis (seldom recognized clinically)
Knotting (catheter coils in right ventricle)
Valve trauma (catheter withdrawn with balloon inflated, valves repeatedly closing on catheter)
Thrombosis/embolism
Pulmonary infarction (embolism or catheter remains in 'wedge' position)
Pulmonary artery rupture (frequently fatal)
Balloon rupture/leak/embolism

mentioned earlier in this chapter, it is important to appreciate that in general PAOP and CVP are rather poor guides to ventricular filling, intravascular volume, cardiac performance and the response to volume infusion, even in normal subjects (Kumar et al., 2004).

COMPLICATIONS

There are a large number of complications associated with the use of pulmonary artery catheters, some of which may be extremely serious and even fatal (Table 4.2).

Arrhythmias. These are more common when the larger thermodilution catheters are used and there is a higher incidence in patients with electrolyte disorders, acidosis or myocardial ischaemia. It is important to inflate the balloon to the recommended volume to conceal the tip of the catheter and prevent it irritating the endocardium during its passage through the right ventricle. Although fatal ventricular tachycardia has been reported (Sise et al., 1981), these arrhythmias are usually transient and consist of a few benign ventricular premature contractions, which stop as soon as the catheter enters the pulmonary artery. If troublesome, they can usually be suppressed with intravenous lidocaine, although in some very unstable patients it may be safer to abandon the procedure. Transient right bundle branch block occurs in up to 5% of patients, but usually resolves within 24 hours. In the presence of pre-existing left bundle branch block, this may precipitate complete atrioventricular block or asystole.

Knotting. To avoid knotting, which is more common in those with enlarged cardiac chambers and in low-flow states, the catheter should not be advanced by more than 30 cm without observing a change in waveform (see **Fig. 4.9**).

Heart valve damage. Heart valves can be severely damaged if the operator withdraws the catheter without deflating the balloon. In the longer term, valve cusps can be progressively traumatized by repeated closure against the catheter.

Pulmonary infarction. This may be related to thrombus formation in and around the catheter, but will also occur if the catheter remains in the wedge position for any length of time. The latter can be avoided by continuously displaying the PAP so that the spontaneous appearance of a wedge pressure (caused by softening and migration of the catheter) can be detected and remedied immediately. It is also important to minimize the length of time for which the catheter is intentionally wedged.

Pulmonary artery rupture. Although rare, pulmonary artery rupture may be fatal due to intractable haemorrhage. This complication appears to be commoner in the elderly, particularly in those with pulmonary hypertension, and in those receiving anticoagulants. Pulmonary artery rupture is usually due to either continuous impaction of the catheter tip with erosion of the vessel wall, or rapid inflation of a distally placed balloon. It may also occur if the catheter is advanced with the balloon deflated or if a wedged catheter is flushed by hand. Management may include reversal of anticoagulation, application of high levels of PEEP, selective endobronchial intubation, transcatheter embolization and early surgical intervention, perhaps involving pulmonary resection. Mortality has been reported to be between 25 and 83%.

Infection. Infections are more common with internal jugular placement, if the catheter remains in place for more than 4 days and when a catheter is reinserted at an old site. Infection of catheter-associated thrombosis can produce systemic sepsis in the absence of local inflammation. Infective endocarditis attributable to pulmonary artery catheterization is a rare event.

Overview of the complications. Despite this rather formidable list of potential hazards, in practice haemodynamic monitoring using pulmonary artery catheters has an acceptably low morbidity and mortality (Sise et al., 1981). The majority of complications are closely related to user inexperience and their incidence has fallen as worldwide expertise has increased. There is now some concern, however, that the recent reduction in the use of pulmonary artery catheters may be associated with an increase in the incidence of complications due to lack of user experience.

BLOOD VOLUME AND LUNG WATER MEASUREMENTS (Hudson and Beale, 2000)
COLD (circulation, oxygenation, lung water and liver function diagnosis) technique
Cannulae are placed in the femoral, brachial or axillary artery, the pulmonary artery and/or a central vein. Thermodilution cardiac output measurements can be made by injecting a bolus of cold fluid into a central vein and recording from a thermistor incorporated into the tip of the arterial catheter. Such transpulmonary thermodilution measurements tend to overestimate cardiac output because of loss of indicator into

the lungs. They are, however, more repeatable than the conventional method because the normal respiratory variation in stroke volume is integrated. The arterial catheter also has an optional oximetry probe for measurement of S_aO_2 and a similar catheter can be placed in the pulmonary artery for monitoring S_vO_2 and measuring cardiac output by thermodilution. A fibreoptic reflectance densitometer built into the arterial catheter measures changes in indocyanine green concentration following bolus injection, allowing an assessment of liver function based on the rate of disappearance of the dye. Since indocyanine green is bound to albumin and is therefore retained in the intravascular compartment, whereas cold distributes to the extravascular space, extravascular lung water (EVLW) and intrathoracic blood volume (ITBV) can be determined by the double-indicator technique. Global end-diastolic volume (i.e. the sum of the diastolic volumes of both left and right atria and ventricles) can also be estimated. Changes in global end-diastolic volume and ITBV correlate well with changes in cardiac output. This device is no longer available commercially.

Pulse-induced continuous cardiac output (PiCCO) technique
This more recent development allows measurement of EVLW and ITBV, as well as calculation of global end-diastolic volume, by analysing only the transpulmonary thermodilution curve recorded from a thermistor-tipped cannula sited in the femoral or brachial artery. The device also provides continuous estimates of cardiac output by pulse contour analysis (see below), with automatic recalibration being performed by intermittent thermodilution. The device is relatively non-invasive and can be used in conscious patients.

Given the well-recognized limitations of pulmonary artery catheterization discussed elsewhere in this chapter, the concept of using direct estimates of cardiac filling and lung water to guide volume replacement and the administration of inotropes and vasoactive agents is undoubtedly attractive. In the light of experience with pulmonary artery catheters, however (see below), some are sceptical about the potential of these monitoring devices to improve outcome. Further studies are clearly required to establish the precise indications for these techniques and their influence on clinically relevant outcome measures.

CARDIAC OUTPUT AND MYOCARDIAL FUNCTION

As discussed in Chapter 3, cardiac output is a major determinant of oxygen delivery and is therefore one of the most clinically relevant haemodynamic variables.

NON-INVASIVE TECHNIQUES FOR ASSESSING CARDIAC FUNCTION
Over the years, there have been many attempts to develop clinically viable, non-invasive techniques for determining

cardiac output and myocardial function when pulmonary artery catheterization is either unavailable or considered unwarranted. These have included impedance cardiography, Doppler ultrasound, echocardiography and various radio-isotope techniques. The value of these non-invasive methods in the more seriously ill patients may, however, be limited because they do not allow sampling of mixed venous blood, continuous monitoring of mixed venous oxygen saturation, the measurement of PAPs or estimation of EVLW.

Impedance cardiography

Electrical conductors are placed around the patient's neck and thorax. Some of the electrodes are supplied with a current, while others detect voltage changes produced by the alterations in thoracic bioimpedance caused by ventricular ejection. Stroke volume can then be calculated from the magnitude of the voltage fluctuations. This method tends to overestimate low cardiac outputs and underestimate high values. Furthermore, other factors such as sweating, lung volume and oedema fluid influence thoracic bioimpedance, and limit the accuracy of the technique, particularly in the critically ill. In patients with sepsis, for example, the bioimpedence method overestimated low cardiac outputs, markedly underestimated high cardiac outputs and was too insensitive for clinical monitoring of changes in cardiac output in individual patients (Young and McQuillan, 1993).

Aortic Doppler ultrasound (Singer and Bennett, 1991; Singer et al., 1991)

When transmitted sound waves are reflected from a moving object their frequency is shifted by an amount proportional to the relative velocity between object and observer. This effect, originally described by Doppler, can be represented by the equation:

$$V = C\,fd/2\,f_1\,\cos\theta$$

where V is the blood flow velocity, C is speed of sound in tissue, fd is the Doppler frequency shift, f_T is the frequency of transmitted sound and $\cos\theta$ is the cosine of the angle between the ultrasound beam and the direction of flow.

Therefore, provided the frequency of the transmitted sound and the angle of interrogation remain constant, the flow velocity will be proportional to the shift in frequency. The Doppler effect is greater the smaller the angle between the beam and the velocity vector; when the beam is perpendicular to the direction of flow, no shift can be detected, whereas maximal shift is seen with a parallel beam. Best results are obtained when the angle of interrogation is less than 20°.

The *Doppler ultrasound technique* uses an acoustic wave with a frequency exceeding the upper range of human audibility, which may be transmitted continuously or in pulses (*pulse-wave Doppler*). Back-scattered Doppler signals can be processed to produce velocity–time waveforms, which are visually displayed (**Fig. 4.12**).

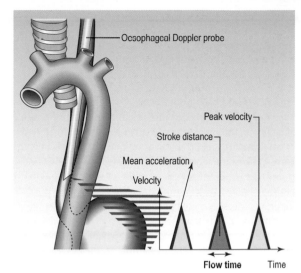

Fig. 4.12 Stylized velocity waveform traces obtained using oesophageal Doppler ultrasonography. (Reproduced from Singer et al. (1991), with permission © 1991 The Williams and Wilkins Co. Baltimore.)

DERIVED AND MEASURED VARIABLES

A number of derived or measured variables can be obtained from the velocity waveform (see **Fig. 4.12**).

In order that changes in the velocity waveform can be used as an estimate of proportional changes in stroke volume, the velocity profile must be flat, flow should be laminar and it has to be assumed that the aortic cross-sectional area remains constant throughout systole. Although the aortic diameter increases slightly in early systole, these conditions are largely fulfilled over a wide range of flow, pressure and temperature. The angle of interrogation must also be known and remain constant.

Stroke distance. The distance that a column of blood travels along the aorta with each ventricular contraction can be calculated by integrating the velocity–time waveform. The product of stroke distance and cross-sectional area (calculated using a nomogram based on the patient's age, height and weight) gives an estimate of the volume of blood passing along the aorta with each ventricular ejection. In the case of the ascending aorta this is the left ventricular stroke volume.

Minute distance. Multiplying stroke distance by heart rate provides an estimate of cardiac output.

Flow time is related to circulating volume and peripheral resistance.

The rate of change of velocity during systole (*acceleration*) and *peak velocity* provide some indication of left ventricular function.

SUPRASTERNAL SITE

This site has the advantage of being entirely non-invasive, but it is often difficult to achieve an interrogation angle of less than 20° and good signals cannot be obtained in about 5% of patients (e.g. after cardiac surgery and in those with emphysema). It is also difficult to achieve secure fixation of the probe for continuous beat-to-beat monitoring and there may be interference from breathing or patient movement.

OESOPHAGEAL SITE

A flexible Doppler probe with a diameter of about 6 mm is passed into the oesophagus until it lies approximately 30–40 cm from the teeth. In this position velocity waveforms from descending aortic blood flow can be continuously monitored. The sensor is securely positioned and high-quality signals with minimal artefact are usually easily obtained. Measurements are unaffected by mediastinal air and the technique can be used during and after cardiac surgery. Oesophageal Dopplers are unreliable, however, when aortic flow is turbulent, for example in the presence of an intra-aortic balloon pump and in those with coarctation of the aorta. Oesophageal Dopplers can be left in place for up to 2 weeks (Gan and Arrowsmith, 1997) but, because of discomfort, are generally only suitable for patients who are sedated and mechanically ventilated. Oesophageal Dopplers are not associated with major complications but, because of the risk of oesophageal perforation or haemorrhage, they should not be used in patients with known pharyngo-oesophagogastric pathology or a bleeding diathesis. Clearly these devices are not suitable for those undergoing oesophageal surgery.

When using the oesophageal approach it has to be assumed that blood flow in the descending aorta remains a fixed proportion of total left ventricular output over a wide range of flows and pressures. Approximately 75% of the total cardiac output passes through the descending aorta and this proportion is little changed in high-output states; in those with low cardiac outputs, however, the proportion falls by about 10%.

The interobserver variability with oesophageal Doppler is less than 2% and there is a reasonable correlation, at least in adults, between Doppler and thermodilution determinations of cardiac output, although absolute values are generally underestimated.

Aortic Doppler ultrasound is a safe, non-invasive and reliable means of continuous haemodynamic monitoring. Although reasonable estimates of stroke volume and cardiac output can be obtained, the technique is best used for trend analysis rather than for making absolute volumetric measurements. A recent systematic review concluded that, when estimating absolute values of cardiac output, oesophageal Doppler monitoring has minimal bias but limited agreement with thermodilution measurements. On the other hand the technique had high validity for monitoring changes in cardiac output (Dark and Singer, 2004). Oesophageal Doppler monitoring is particularly valuable for perioperative optimization of the circulating volume and cardiac performance (see Chapter 5), when it can be used as an alternative to right heart catheterization (Gan and Arrowsmith, 1997).

Echocardiography (Poelaert et al., 1998)

Transthoracic echocardiography (TTE) is a non-invasive technique in which the ultrasound beam is transmitted via a transducer positioned on the chest wall. More recently, the semi-invasive technique of transoesophageal echocardiography (TOE) has been introduced into intensive care practice. Both methods allow high-quality intermittent real-time imaging of the heart, great vessels and mediastinal structures, as well as qualitative and quantitative blood flow assessments, at the patient's bedside. They provide immediate diagnostic information about cardiac structure and function (**Figs 4.13–4.22**). Portable devices are now available, although currently the images obtained can be suboptimal (Ashrafian et al., 2004).

In *two-dimensional (2D) echocardiography* the beam is moving continuously to produce a cross-sectional slice through the heart and great vessels; this image is displayed in real time. Initially TOE probes scanned only in the transverse plane or in two planes but now multiplane devices, which allow scanning through 180°, are normally used. An *M-mode examination* can also be performed in which the heart is examined by a single beam of ultrasound to obtain measurements of ventricular wall thickness, size of the ventricular cavities and valve leaflet excursions. M-mode echocardiography is better than 2D for detecting rapid intravascular movements and for quantitation of temporal relationships. Additional information can be derived using *Doppler echocardiography* (pulsed or continuous-wave), which allows determination of the direction and velocity of blood flow. This can be combined with *colour flow mapping* in which normal and abnormal flows are colour-coded and shown as real-time 2D images. Future developments are likely to include three-dimensional reconstructions which will allow additional important diagnostic information to be derived.

The quality of information obtained with echocardiography depends on the skill and experience of the operator. To locate a suitable *acoustic window* through which to image the heart, transthoracic examinations are best performed in the left recumbent position; this may be difficult in some critically ill patients. In others access to the precordium may be obscured (e.g. by dressings or chest wounds). The beam may also be interrupted by overexpanded lungs, and this can lead to difficulties, particularly in those receiving mechanical ventilation and especially when levels of PEEP in excess of 10 cm H_2O are used.

Unlike the transthoracic approach, TOE provides an imaging window which is not obscured by intervening structures. Moreover, because the oesophagus is in close proximity to the heart and great vessels, high-frequency probes, which provide higher-resolution images than conventional transthoracic probes, can be used. Although the clarity of the images obtained with TOE means that they are easier to interpret, considerable training and experience are still required. The probe is mounted on a flexible, steerable endoscope which is passed into the oesophagus through the

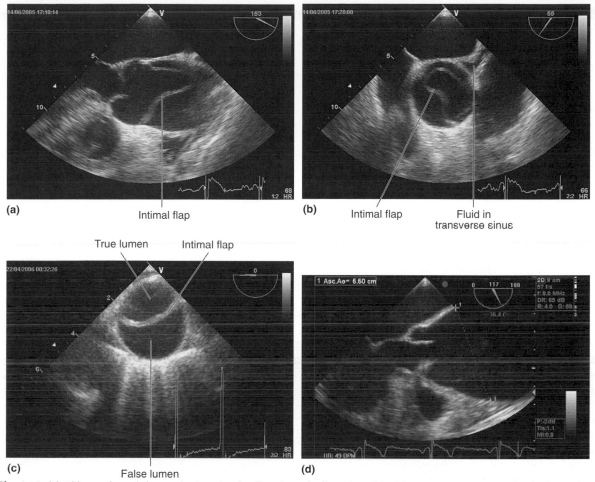

(a) Intimal flap

(b) Intimal flap   Fluid in transverse sinus

True lumen   Intimal flap

(c) False lumen

(d)

Fig. 4.13 (a) Mid oesophageal, long axis view showing Type A aortic dissection. (b) Mid oesophageal, short axis view showing Type A aortic dissection with fluid in transverse sinus. (c) Short axis view of descending aorta showing intimal flap with false and true lumen.(d) Mid oesophageal, long axis view of ascending aorta showing aneurysmal dilatation. (Courtesy of Dr C. Rathwell.)

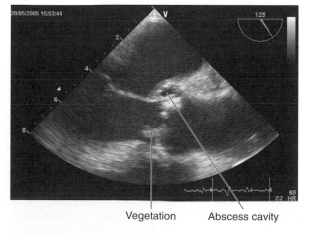

Vegetation   Abscess cavity

Fig. 4.14 Mid oesophageal, long axis view showing vegetation on right coronary cusp and associated root abscess in a patient with endocarditis. (Courtesy of Dr C. Rathwell.)

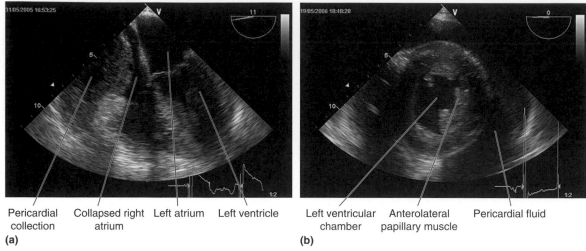

Pericardial   Collapsed right   Left atrium   Left ventricle
collection   atrium

(a)

Left ventricular   Anterolateral   Pericardial fluid
chamber   papillary muscle

(b)

Fig. 4.15 (a) Mid oesophageal four-chamber view demonstrating cardiac tamponade with right atrial collapse. (b) Transgastric mid-papillary view of left ventricle showing large pericardial collection. (Courtesy of Dr C. Rathwell.)

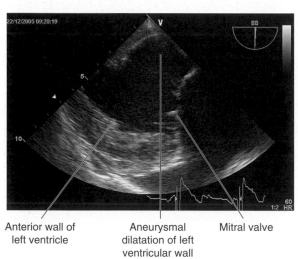

Anterior wall of   Aneurysmal   Mitral valve
left ventricle   dilatation of left
                ventricular wall

Fig. 4.16 Transgastric two-chamber view demonstrating inferobasal left ventricular aneurysm. (Courtesy of Dr C. Rathwell.)

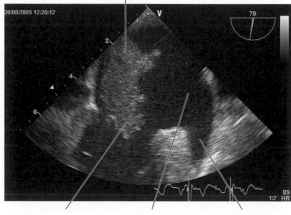

Attachment of myxoma
to interatrial septum

Myxoma prolapsing   Left atrium   Left atrial appendage
through mitral valve

Fig. 4.17 Mid oesophageal two-chamber view of left atrium showing left atrial myxoma. (Courtesy of Dr C. Rathwell.)

mouth, protected by a bite guard. Occasionally the transnasal approach is used. With either approach the probe can be maintained in a stable position, allowing real-time monitoring of cardiac function over prolonged periods. The awake, non-intubated patient should be fasted, lightly sedated and placed in the left lateral position. Topical lidocaine (10%) is used to provide local anaesthesia of the tongue, pharynx and larynx. In mechanically ventilated patients small doses of midazolam or propofol can be administered intravenously; occasionally a laryngoscope is required to displace the tongue and allow insertion of the probe.

TOE appears to be remarkably safe with an overall complication rate (bleeding, oesophageal damage or laceration) in the order of a fraction of 1% in most series. Transient bacteraemia has been reported but antibiotic prophylaxis against endocarditis is currently considered unnecessary. Contraindications to TOE include oesophageal tumours, stenoses and diverticula, while oesophageal varices are a relative contraindication.

INDICATIONS FOR ECHOCARDIOGRAPHY IN THE CRITICALLY ILL

Indications for echocardiography in the critically ill include:

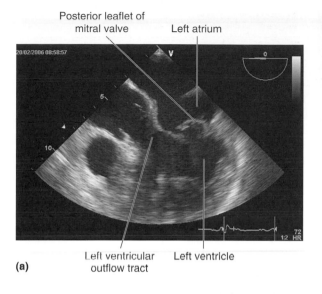

(a)

Posterior leaflet of mitral valve

Left atrium

Left ventricular outflow tract

Left ventricle

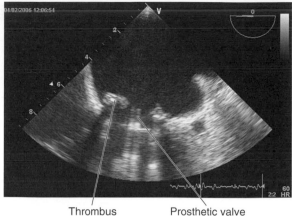

Thrombus   Prosthetic valve

Fig. 4.19 Mid oesophageal four-chamber view showing mechanical bileaflet prosthetic mitral valve with attached thrombus. (Courtesy of Dr C. Rathwell.)

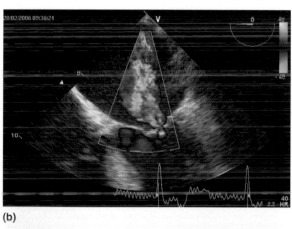

(b)

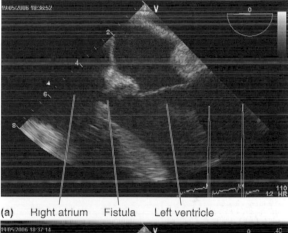

(a)   Right atrium   Fistula   Left ventricle

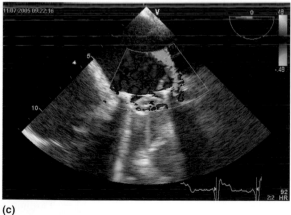

(c)

Fig. 4.18 (a) Mid oesophageal five-chamber view showing prolapse of posterior leaflet of mitral valve. (b) Mid oesophageal four-chamber view demonstrating mitral regurgitation using colour flow Doppler. (c) Mid oesophageal four-chamber view of mechanical bileaflet mitral valve with paraprosthetic leak. (Courtesy of Dr C. Rathwell.)

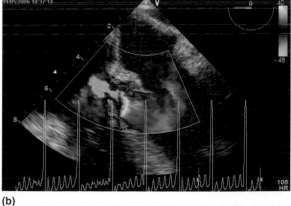

(b)

Fig. 4.20 (a) Mid oesophageal four-chamber view showing traumatic postoperative fistula between left ventricle and right atrium. (b) Fistula demonstrated by colour flow Doppler. (Courtesy of Dr C. Rathwell.)

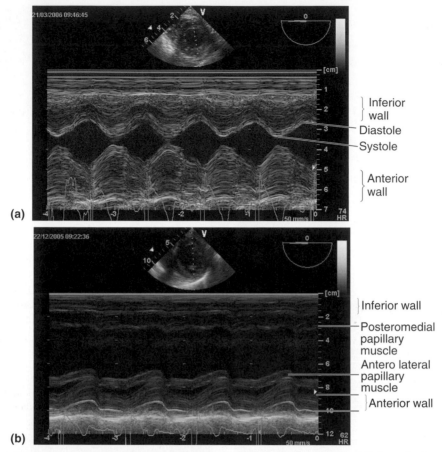

Fig. 4.21 (a) Normal M-mode examination of left ventricle. (b) M-mode examination showing inferior wall akinesia. (Courtesy of Dr C. Rathwell.)

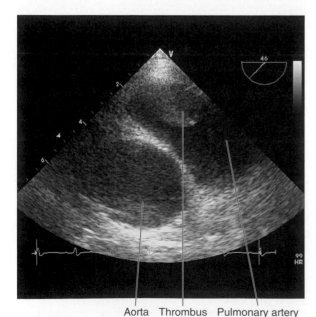

Aorta   Thrombus   Pulmonary artery

Fig. 4.22 Upper oesophageal short-axis view of the asending aorta showing large thrombus in right pulmonary artery. (Courtesy of Dr C. Rathwell.)

- Assessment of systolic and diastolic ventricular function and preload (e.g. to determine the cause of refractory hypotension). Echocardiography can be used to determine left ventricular end-diastolic and end-systolic diameters, from which a reasonable estimate of ejection fraction can be derived. Visualization of the ventricles may reveal segmental hypokinesia, dyskinesia or akinesia (Fig 4.21b), cavity enlargement or paradoxical septal motion. Contractility and ventricular filling can be assessed.
- Assessment of myocardial ischaemia and infarction. Echocardiography can be used to diagnose and assess the extent of myocardial ischaemia or infarction and to detect complications of ischaemia such as left ventricular aneurysm, mitral regurgitation or ventricular septal defect (Figs 4.16, 4.18, 4.20). Right ventricular infarction may also be diagnosed.
- Diagnosis of valvular heart disease and malfunction of prosthetic valves. (Figs 4.18, 4.19)
- Confirmation of infective endocarditis. Vegetations may be visualized, thereby confirming the diagnosis, although a negative echocardiogram does not exclude endocarditis. Complications of endocarditis such as valvular incompetence may be detected. (Fig 4.14)

- Diagnosis of congenital heart disease.
- Distinction between hypertrophic, congestive and restrictive cardiomyopathies.
- Detection and location of pericardial effusions. Compression of the right atrium or ventricle is indicative of cardiac tamponade. Echocardiography can be used to guide pericardiocentesis. (**Fig. 4.15**).
- Diagnosis of diseases of the aorta (e.g. aortic dissection) (**Fig. 4.13**).
- Diagnosis of pulmonary embolism. Signs of right ventricular failure, tricuspid regurgitation and visualization of thrombus in the main pulmonary trunk or arteries (**Fig. 4.22**) (see Chapter 5).
- Detection of intracardiac thrombus or myxoma (**Figs 4.17, 4.19**).
- Positioning of intra-aortic balloon pumps and other support devices.

Although TTE is non-invasive, can be performed immediately and can be frequently repeated, in many situations TOE is the preferred technique, mainly because of the superior image clarity (**Table 4.3**). Also Doppler TOE is a reasonable alternative method for assessing stroke volume and cardiac output. When used by intensive care clinicians, TOE is a safe procedure which provides useful information for the evaluation and management of critically ill patients (Colreavy *et al.*, 2002). TOE appears to be of particular value in the assessment of patients after blunt chest trauma, allowing early diagnosis of, for example, myocardial contusions, traumatic valvular injuries and aortic disruption. In general, however, TTE remains the first-choice investigation in critically ill patients, with TOE being reserved for those in whom insufficient information has been obtained. In some centres TTE or TOE is used routinely for rapid diagnosis and assessment of haemodynamics, as well as for monitoring the initial response to treatment. Only when prolonged continuous monitoring is required because of persistent haemodynamic instability or failure to respond to treatment is more invasive monitoring such as pulmonary artery catheterization considered.

Nuclear cardiac imaging

Radionuclide techniques can be performed at the bedside using a portable gamma camera to detect intravenously administered radioisotopes.

FIRST-PASS TECHNIQUE

A high-speed scintillation camera follows the transit of a bolus of radionuclide (e.g. technetium-99m) as it passes through the chambers of the heart.

EQUILIBRATION TECHNIQUE

Human serum albumin or red blood cells are labelled with technetium-99m and allowed to equilibrate in the blood pool for 8–10 min. The detection of the emitted radiation is timed, or 'gated', to end-systole and end-diastole using the ECG and performed repeatedly (*multigated technique or Muga scan*). Counts can then be averaged over several cardiac cycles. Ejection fraction is calculated as:

$$\text{end-diastolic counts} - \text{end-systolic counts/end-diastolic counts}$$

and corrected for background activity.

For accurate results, heart rhythm and function must be relatively stable. By using multiple projections, regional wall motion abnormalities can be detected.

PERFUSION IMAGING

By using an isotope such as thallium-20, which is concentrated in viable myocardium by active transport via $Na^+/K^+/$ ATPase, the ventricular muscle can be directly visualized. Ischaemia or infarction will appear as areas of low uptake.

Although non-invasive, these techniques do expose the patient to radioactivity, therefore limiting the number of occasions on which the investigation can be performed, and they cannot be used for continuous monitoring. Moreover, portable gamma cameras are extremely expensive.

Non-imaging radionuclide detectors

An alternative radionuclide technique involves the use of a non-imaging detector (or *nuclear stethoscope*) to provide continuous online monitoring of ejection fraction derived from end-diastolic and end-systolic counts. This technique seems to be a practical, relatively low-cost bedside method for estimating ejection fraction in critically ill patients (Timmins *et al.*, 1994), but has been largely superseded by the techniques just described.

INVASIVE TECHNIQUES
Direct fick method

Fick's principle states that, if an indicator is added to a column of flowing liquid at a constant rate, then the flow of that liquid is equal to the amount of substance entering the

Table 4.3 Situations in which transoesophageal echocardiography may be superior to transthoracic echocardiography

Diagnosis of vegetations/endocarditis
Visualization of thrombus, especially in the left atrial appendage
Assessment of prosthetic valve function
Assessment of structural or functional abnormalities of native valves, including following surgical repair
Diagnosis of thoracic aortic dissection
Cardiac tamponade
Acute perioperative haemodynamic derangements
Detection of perioperative myocardial ischaemia
Ventilated patients, especially prone ventilation
Obesity, emphysema or skeletal deformity
Intraoperatively

stream divided by the difference between the concentration of the indicator either side of the entry point. The principle is also valid for the removal of a substance and can therefore be applied to the consumption of oxygen by the body (V_{O_2}). Thus:

$$\dot{Q}_t = \dot{V}_{O_2}/C_aO_2 - C_{\bar{v}}O_2 \qquad \qquad 4.1$$

where Q_t is cardiac output, C_aO_2 is arterial oxygen content, and $C_{\bar{v}}O_2$ is mixed venous oxygen content.

Conceptually, it may be easier to appreciate that the amount of oxygen consumed by the body can be calculated from the product of the flow of blood to the tissues and the amount of oxygen extracted from each unit of blood. Thus:

$$\dot{V}_{O_2} = \dot{Q}_T \times (C_aO_2 - C_{\bar{v}}O_2) \qquad \qquad 4.2$$

and this can be rearranged in order to derive Q_T as above. This formula can be used clinically to calculate V_{O_2}.

To obtain cardiac output by the direct Fick method, arterial and mixed venous oxygen contents and V_{O_2} have to be measured directly, as described in Chapter 6. In practice, however, a number of difficulties limit the clinical application of this method (see Chapter 6) and it is in fact rarely used in intensive care units.

Indicator dilution techniques

Indicator dilution techniques are based on a modification of the Fick principle in which a substance is added to the central circulation as a bolus, rather than continuously. The appearance and disappearance of this substance are then recorded at a distal site. The cardiac output is calculated from the total amount of indicator injected divided by its average concentration and the time taken to pass the recording site.

DYE DILUTION

In this technique a bolus of dye (usually indocyanine green) is injected into the pulmonary artery. Its subsequent passage through the systemic circulation is recorded at a downstream site (usually the radial artery) by continuously aspirating blood through a densitometer. This records the changing concentration of dye, thereby describing an *indicator dilution curve,* as shown in **Figure 4.23**. (It is essential that the dye mixes completely with the blood, which might not occur if dye is injected into, for example, the right atrium with sampling from the pulmonary artery.)

The amount of dye injected is known, while the transit time and average concentration can be determined by analysing the dilution curve. As illustrated in **Figure 4.23**, recirculation of dye causes a second peak, which interferes with accurate determination of transit time. This is overcome by plotting the curve logarithmically, so that the exponential disappearance of dye becomes a straight line, which can be extrapolated to the baseline. The average concentration of dye is determined by integrating the area under the curve.

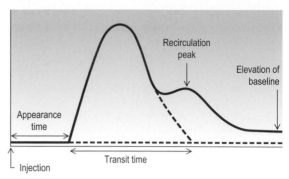

Fig. 4.23 Indicator dilution curve obtained using indocyanine green.

Unfortunately, dye accumulates in the circulation, causing a progressive elevation of the baseline, and this limits the number of times the measurement can be performed. Also the technique is less accurate when cardiac output is low since the curve is flat, the recirculation peak is more evident and the shape of the curve is difficult to define.

Finally, the densitometer has first to be calibrated by mixing a sample of the patient's blood with a known amount of dye.

THERMODILUTION

Many of the problems associated with dye dilution can be overcome by using cold liquid as the indicator (Branthwaite and Bradley, 1968; Forrester *et al.*, 1972), a technique which has been used extensively in critically ill patients.

In practice, a modified pulmonary artery catheter, with a lumen opening in the right atrium and a thermistor located a few centimetres from its tip, is inserted as described above. A known volume of liquid at a known temperature is injected as a bolus into the atrium. Subsequently, the injectate, which is completely mixed with blood during its passage through the right atrium and ventricle, passes into the pulmonary artery, where the fall in temperature is detected by the thermistor (**Fig. 4.24**). The dilution curve is usually analysed by a computer, which provides a direct readout of cardiac output.

Withdrawal of blood is not required and, because the cold is rapidly dissipated in the tissues, there is no recirculation peak and no elevation of the baseline. Measurements can therefore be repeated as often as required. Furthermore, thermodilution is more accurate than dye dilution in low-flow states, and the catheters are precalibrated.

Accuracy. The larger the volume of the injectate, and the lower its temperature, the greater is the signal-to-noise ratio. This increases accuracy (Schmid *et al.*, 1999) and may be particularly important in ventilated patients in whom pulmonary artery temperature fluctuates during the respiratory cycle. Therefore, although it is possible to use as little as 5 mL of room temperature injectate, it is more usual to inject 10 mL of ice-cold 5% dextrose. The injectate is normally cooled in a container of iced water. Its temperature is mea-

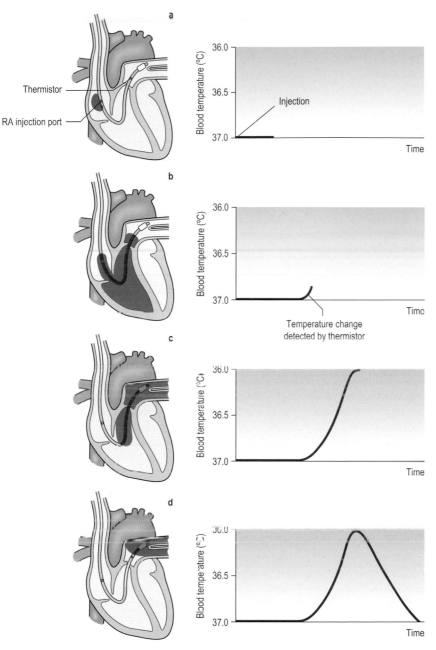

Fig. 4.24 Thermodilution method for cardiac output determination. Cold fluid injected into the right atrium (RA):(a) passes through the right ventricle and into the pulmonary artery, where the temperature change is detected by the thermistor (b, c and d). Notice the absence of a recirculation peak and that there is no elevation of the baseline.

sured by a thermistor placed just beyond the syringe. It is important to avoid warming the injectate by handling the barrel of the syringe. Inevitably, the injectate absorbs heat during its passage through the catheter and the necessary corrections are therefore incorporated into the formulae used to calculate cardiac output. For similar reasons, the first of each series of measurements should be rejected since the injectate will include warm fluid from within the catheter lumen.

Accuracy also depends on a *smooth injection*; it is therefore usual to record the shape of the dilution curve and to reject uneven curves. The mean of three consecutive cardiac output determinations that do not differ by more than 10% should be calculated. The repeatability of the method should be within ± 10% but, with care, greater accuracy can usually be achieved. Although repeatability can be improved by timing injections to coincide with the same point in the respiratory cycle, values obtained in this way are probably not a true reflection of overall cardiac output. To obtain a truly accurate value for mean cardiac output it may be necessary to perform a series of four measurements spread equally throughout the ventilatory cycle.

The technique is inaccurate in the presence of *intracardiac shunts* and *incompetence of the pulmonary or tricuspid valves* and tends to overestimate low cardiac outputs (Tournadre *et al.*, 1997). Also, it seems that inaccuracies may occur if injectate refluxes up the sidearm of the introducer sheath. Errors are greater when the injectate port is close to the tip of the introducer or is within the sheath, and are further increased when the sidearm of the sheath is open. It is therefore recommended that the injectate port should be located well downstream of the introducer sheath (i.e. the catheter should be inserted to a depth of > 45 cm) and that the introducer sidearm should be closed (Boyd *et al.*, 1994).

Complications. Bradycardia and supraventricular tachycardias have been reported in association with the injection of cold fluid. It is important to note the volumes of 5% dextrose injected, especially when cardiac output is measured repeatedly, in order to avoid inadvertent water overload.

CONTINUOUS CARDIAC OUTPUT DETERMINATION

A 10-cm thermal filament is mounted on the pulmonary artery catheter close to the CVP lumen. Low heat energy is transmitted into the surrounding blood according to a pseudo-random binary sequence. The heat signal in the blood is processed over time and a thermodilution curve is reconstructed from the temperature changes. A computer system produces a continuously updated (every 30–60 s) value for cardiac output which is averaged over several minutes. Agreement with thermodilution cardiac output measurements appears to be sufficiently close for most clinical applications (Boldt *et al.*, 1994) and continuous measurement of cardiac output has largely superseded intermittent cold injectate thermodilution. Nevertheless, in view of the reduced precision of the continuous method, intermittent cold injectate thermodilution is still preferred by some for research (Schmid et al., 1999).

LITHIUM DILUTION (LiDCO)

Transpulmonary lithium indicator dilution does not require pulmonary artery catheterization and is suitable for use in conscious patients. A bolus of lithium chloride (0.15–0.3 mmol) is normally administered via a central venous catheter (although injection via an antecubital vein gives acceptable accuracy) and the change in arterial plasma lithium concentration is detected by a lithium-sensitive electrode. This sensor can be connected to any existing arterial cannula via a three-way tap. A small battery-powered peristaltic pump is used to create a constant blood flow through the sensor and over the electrode tip. The electrode contains a reference material which provides a constant ionic environment and supports a membrane which is selectively permeable to lithium ions. The potential difference across the membrane is related to the plasma lithium concentration, as described by the Nernst equation. A correction for sodium is therefore required because this is the main determinant of potential difference at baseline. A correction for packed cell volume is also applied because lithium is distributed throughout the plasma.

Administration of positively charged non-depolarizing muscle relaxants (e.g. atracurium and vecuronium) may interfere with the lithium ion-sensitive electrode and thereby prevent cardiac output determination for up to 45 minutes. Lithium chloride is safe in the doses used and the maximum dose is rarely a limiting factor. Administration of lithium intravenously is not recommended in patients who weigh less than 40 kg, are pregnant or are receiving oral lithium therapy. In the latter instance the increased background concentration will result in an overestimation of cardiac output. The presence of intracardiac shunts can also lead to significant measurement errors. When compared to both continuous and bolus thermodilution, this technique appears to be safe, simple and at least as accurate as bolus thermodilution (Linton *et al.*, 1997).

PULSE CONTOUR ANALYSIS (Linton and Linton, 2001)

The characteristics of the arterial pressure waveform are determined by both cardiac function and the peripheral circulation; the forward pressure wave produced by ventricular contraction is reflected back from the peripheries and the magnitude of the reflected wave varies according to changes in systemic vascular resistance and the compliance of the arterial vascular tree. Complex mathematical analysis is therefore required to determine accurately volume changes from the arterial pressure waveform. This approach is only reliable when used to calculate changes in stroke volume rather than absolute values, and calibration against a standard method is required (lithium dilution with LiDCO, thermodilution with PiCCO). As would be anticipated, cardiac output estimated by pulse contour analysis can be profoundly altered by changes in the damping coefficient of the arterial pressure-transducing system (see earlier in this chapter); in some cases the arterial cannula has to be replaced. The morphology of the arterial waveform will also be altered by changes in vascular compliance caused, for example, by the administration of vasoactive drugs. Under these circumstances calibration may be required more frequently than the 8-hour intervals recommended by the manufacturer. Performance may also be compromised in patients with severe peripheral arterial vasoconstriction, in those undergoing intra-aortic balloon counterpulsation and in the presence of aortic regurgitation.

The PulseCO Haemodynamic Monitor System calculates changes in stroke volume by power analysis of the first harmonic of the arterial pressure waveform, whereas the PiCCO system (see earlier in this chapter) utilizes only the area under the systolic portion of the curve. The systemic vascular resistance can be estimated from the diastolic pressure decay.

The LiDCO plus system combines LiDCO and Pulse CO to provide continuous haemodynamic assessment (Pearse *et al.*, 2004). Derived parameters include systolic pressure variation, pulse pressure variation, cardiac index, stroke volume and systemic vascular resistance. This device is therefore useful for assessing preload responsiveness (see above) and seems to be sufficiently accurate to guide goal-directed therapy.

FLOTRAC SENSOR AND VIGILEO MONITORING SYSTEM

With this system calculations are based entirely on arterial waveform characteristics in conjunction with patient demographic data. Unlike other arterial waveform cardiac output monitoring systems, it has been claimed that this technique does not require calibration by another method.

DERIVED HAEMODYNAMIC AND OXYGEN TRANSPORT VARIABLES

Measurement of cardiac output, intravascular pressures and heart rate permits calculation of a number of clinically important haemodynamic and oxygen transport variables (see Appendices 1 and 2).

Determination of *pulmonary and systemic vascular resistances* may contribute to establishing a diagnosis (e.g. a low peripheral resistance is characteristic of septic shock), and provides a useful estimate of changes in right and left ventricular afterload. Calculation of the work performed by each ventricle (*right and left ventricular stroke work*) gives some indication of myocardial performance, especially if a *ventricular function curve* is constructed by relating changes in PAOP to alterations in stroke work. Construction of a ventricular function curve has also been used as a guide to the adequacy of a patient's circulating volume; fluid replacement can be considered to be optimal when further increases in PAOP do not improve left ventricular stroke work. It is worth noting, however, that assessments of ventricular performance derived from haemodynamic data correlate poorly with estimates based on images obtained by TOE (Bouchard *et al.*, 2004).

Haemodynamic assessment of a critically ill patient can be supplemented by analysis of arterial and mixed venous blood for blood gas tensions, acid–base status, the percentage saturation of haemoglobin with oxygen and oxygen contents (see Chapter 6). It is then possible to calculate oxygen delivery (DO_2) and oxygen consumption ($\dot{V}O_2$), which are important determinants of outcome from critical illness, as well as the arteriovenous oxygen content difference ($C_{a-v}O_2$), which, together with the mixed venous oxygen saturation ($S_{\bar{v}}O_2$), provides a guide to the relationship between tissue oxygen supply and demand.

INDICATIONS FOR HAEMODYNAMIC MONITORING WITH A PULMONARY ARTERY CATHETER

Although it is usually reasonable to assess a patient's response to treatment before making the decision to employ more invasive monitoring, it is clearly important not to delay until the situation has become irretrievable. In general, pulmonary artery catheters can help to establish the nature of the haemodynamic problem, they enable the clinician to optimize cardiac output and DO_2 while minimizing the risk of pulmonary oedema, and they allow the rational use of ino-

tropes and vasoactive drugs. Although the current trend is to use less invasive techniques, *specific indications for pulmonary artery catheterization* have included the following.

- Myocardial infarction – haemodynamically unstable, unresponsive to initial therapy. To differentiate between hypovolaemia and cardiogenic shock.
- Shock – unresponsive to simple measures or when there is diagnostic uncertainty. To guide administration of fluid, inotropes and vasoactive agents and to optimize DO_2 and VO_2*.
- Pulmonary embolism – to establish the diagnosis, assess severity and to guide haemodynamic support.
- Pulmonary oedema – to differentiate cardiogenic from non-cardiogenic pulmonary oedema, to enable optimization of DO_2 and VO_2* in acute respiratory distress syndrome (particularly when haemodynamically unstable and in those with ventricular dysfunction), and to guide haemodynamic support in cardiac failure.
- Haemodynamic instability when the diagnosis is unclear.
- High-risk surgical patients, particularly those with left ventricular dysfunction and/or ischaemic heart disease and those in whom massive volume losses are anticipated (e.g. routine use is often recommended in liver transplantation). To optimize DO_2 and VO_2*.
- Major trauma – to guide volume replacement. To optimize DO_2 and VO_2*.
- Pre-eclampsia with hypertension, pulmonary oedema or oliguria.
- Chronic obstructive airways disease – patients with cardiac failure, to exclude reversible causes of failure to wean from mechanical ventilation.
- Cardiac surgery in selected cases only; routine use is unnecessary.

BENEFITS AND RISKS OF HAEMODYNAMIC MONITORING WITH A PULMONARY ARTERY CATHETER

There can be no doubt that pulmonary artery catheters have made an enormous contribution to our understanding of the pathophysiology of critical illness and its treatment, but their clinical value, and in particular their influence on outcome, remains in doubt (Hall, 2005). Although it is clear that clinical haemodynamic assessment is frequently inaccurate, that pulmonary artery catheterization improves diagnostic accuracy, and that clinically relevant information is obtained, which often prompts changes in treatment (Bailey *et al.*, 1990; Eisenberg *et al.*, 1984; Marinelli *et al.*, 1999; Mimoz *et al.*, 1994), it has been less easy to demonstrate that this results in improved outcome – indeed, there is some evidence to suggest that pulmonary artery catheters may increase morbidity and mortality. In particular a prospective, observational cohort study in 15 intensive care units in the USA (Connors *et al.*, 1996) indicated that right heart catheterization might be associated with

*But see Chapter 5.

increased mortality and a greater utilization of resources. However, this study was not randomized, the investigators used a controversial propensity score for matching individual cases and it has been suggested that the findings may have reflected misuse of pulmonary artery catheters in some of the participating units (Vincent *et al.*, 1998). Certainly there is evidence that in both North America and Europe (Gnaegi *et al.*, 1997), misinterpretation of data derived from right heart catheterization, and hence potential misdirection of therapy, is disturbingly common. It is also clear that improved diagnostic accuracy can only influence survival when unequivocally effective treatment is available for the underlying disorder and that more sophisticated haemodynamic manipulation, even when appropriately guided by right heart catheterization, may not necessarily influence the final outcome. Indeed, more aggressive therapy with administration of large volumes of fluid and high-dose inotropes/vasoactive agents could be harmful (see Chapter 5), an observation that might explain the finding that the use of right heart catheters was associated with a higher net positive fluid balance and increased morbidity, including congestive heart failure, in patients undergoing non-cardiac surgery (Polanczyk *et al.*, 2001). On the other hand some investigations have indicated that catheter-prompted changes in therapy may improve outcome in refractory shock (Mimoz *et al.*, 1994) and a later single-centre prospective study using a comprehensive and relevant propensity score did not demonstrate an increased mortality attributable to the use of pulmonary artery catheters (Murdoch *et al.*, 2000). There is also some evidence to suggest that pulmonary artery catheters can decrease mortality in severely injured patients (see Chapter 10) and in the most severely ill, whereas their use in less seriously ill patients may worsen outcome (Chittock *et al.*, 2004).

More recently, a number of large randomized controlled trials have indicated that the use of pulmonary artery catheters does not significantly affect the outcome of patients with congestive cardiac failure (Binanay *et al.*, 2005) or acute lung injury or shock and/or the acute respiratory distress syndrome (see Chapter 8), whilst the risk of complications may be increased (Binanay *et al.*, 2005). Moreover a large, randomized, controlled, 'pragmatic' trial in the UK (which compared the pulmonary artery catheter with alternative monitoring devices and did not specify treatment protocols) could find no clear evidence of benefit (or harm) as a result of pulmonary artery catheterization in a large mixed population of intensive care patients (Harvey *et al.*, 2005). Similarly, the authors of a recent meta-analysis concluded that the use of the pulmonary artery catheter neither increased overall mortality or days in hospital, nor conferred benefit, perhaps because of the lack of evidence-based interventions which could be implemented in response to the haemodynamic information obtained (Shah *et al.*, 2005).

Despite these negative findings, there is insufficient evidence to conclude that pulmonary artery catheters are intrinsically harmful and further studies will be required to determine whether specific management protocols involving the use of pulmonary artery catheters can be effective in certain subgroups of critically ill patients. In the meantime, since the procedure seems to be safe in experienced hands (Harvey *et al.*, 2005; Shah *et al.*, 2005) and is comparatively cheap, many still believe that, when used selectively, and provided data are accurately collected, correctly interpreted and prompt appropriate interventions, pulmonary artery catheterization can be a valuable aid to the management of a few of the most seriously ill patients (perhaps especially those with pulmonary hypertension). There is no doubt, however, that the use of pulmonary artery catheters has decreased dramatically over the last few years (Weiner and Welch, 2007), an observation that has important implications for training and safe clinical care.

ASSESSMENT OF TISSUE PERFUSION AND OXYGENATION

CLINICAL EVALUATION

It is usually possible to gain a fairly accurate idea of tissue perfusion, and by implication cardiac output and circulating volume, from a thorough clinical examination. When perfusion is poor the skin is cold, pale and dusky blue with delayed capillary refill and an absence of visible veins in the hands and feet. In the more seriously ill patients this may be associated with profuse sweating and the skin then feels cold and clammy. A low pulse volume and oliguria are confirmatory signs, while blood pressure may be normal or low. Conversely, when the peripheries are pink and warm, with a strong pulse and rapid capillary refill, circulating volume and cardiac output are probably normal or high. If these signs are combined with a normal blood pressure, the absence of tachycardia and an adequate urine output, it is usually safe to assume that the patient has an *effective cardiac output* (Palazzo, 2001). Clinical examination can, however, be misleading (Bailey *et al.*, 1990), especially in patients with sepsis or septic shock, in whom significant haemodynamic abnormalities and tissue dysoxia (see Chapter 5) may be present despite apparently well-perfused extremities.

CORE–PERIPHERAL TEMPERATURE GRADIENT

A more objective assessment of peripheral perfusion can be obtained by recording peripheral temperature, usually from the extensor surface of the great toe (Joly and Weil, 1969). This non-invasive technique is cheap, safe and reliable and is conventionally thought to be a good guide to tissue perfusion, provided it is related to a reference value. Often the core temperature is measured simultaneously (e.g. from a nasopharyngeal probe or the thermistor of a pulmonary artery catheter), in which case an increased core–peripheral temperature gradient is considered to be indicative of poor perfusion. Others recommend that toe temperature should be related to room temperature. A fall in peripheral temperature is often the first sign of a deterioration in cardiovascular function and, because vasoconstriction is an early compensatory response, may occur before changes in other variables, such as heart rate, blood pressure or CVP. There is, however, evidence to suggest that in shock the core–peripheral temperature gradient is not a good guide to either the cardiac output or the systemic vascular resistance and that changes in this gradient do not correlate with alterations in either of these variables (Woods *et al.*, 1987).

CENTRAL AND MIXED VENOUS OXYGEN SATURATION ($S_{cv}O_2$, $S_{\bar{v}}O_2$), ARTERIOVENOUS OXYGEN CONTENT DIFFERENCE ($C_{a-v}O_2$) AND OXYGEN EXTRACTION RATIO (OER)

Venous oxygen saturation ($S_{\bar{v}}O_2$) can be determined intermittently using a bench oximeter or continuously using a modified fibreoptic pulmonary artery catheter (see Chapter 6). Because there is streaming of blood from the upper and lower halves of the body within the right atrium, true mixed venous blood can only be obtained from the pulmonary artery; central venous oxygen saturation is consistently higher than $S_{\bar{v}}O_2$ and the two measurements cannot be considered to be equivalent in critically ill patients (Chawla *et al.*, 2004). At the level of PO_2 encountered in venous blood, the oxyhaemoglobin dissociation curve is essentially linear and the normal range for $S_{\bar{v}}O_2$ is 70–85%.

In general $S_{\bar{v}}O_2$ is a reflection of tissue oxygenation. A fall implies that the supply of oxygen to the tissues is inadequate; values less than 50% are commonly associated with the onset of anaerobic metabolism. Reductions in $S_{\bar{v}}O_2$ frequently precede changes in other monitored variables and it has been suggested that continuous $S_{\bar{v}}O_2$ monitoring can provide a useful early indication of decompensation. Nevertheless, the clinical indications for continuous $S_{\bar{v}}O_2$ monitoring have not been clearly defined. The main sources of error with this approach are malposition of the catheter and the oximeter abutting the vessel wall.

Changes in $S_{\bar{v}}O_2$ require careful interpretation, they must not be considered in isolation and should prompt measurement of other variables to ascertain the cause. The various possibilities can easily be appreciated by rearranging the Fick equation to give:

$$C_{\bar{v}}O_2 = C_aO_2 - \dot{V}O_2/\dot{Q}_t$$

A fall in $S_{\bar{v}}O_2$ may therefore be secondary to arterial hypoxaemia, a reduction in haemoglobin concentration, a fall in cardiac output, an increase in oxygen consumption or any combination of these.

Monitoring $S_{\bar{v}}O_2$ can be misleading. In sepsis, for example, cellular hypoxia is largely due to impaired extraction or utilization of oxygen and $S_{\bar{v}}O_2$ is therefore frequently normal or high. In addition, at a critical level of DO_2 below which the tissues are unable to extract more oxygen, further reductions in DO_2 are associated not with the expected fall in $S_{\bar{v}}O_2$, but with a reduction in VO_2. It seems that in some critically ill patients this relationship may apply at levels of DO_2 normally considered adequate – *pathological supply dependency* (see Chapter 5). Under these circumstances maintenance of a

normal $S_{\bar{v}}O_2$ does not necessarily indicate that tissue oxygenation is satisfactory. It must also be appreciated that $S_{\bar{v}}O_2$ is the weighted average of blood draining all the various vascular beds, and hypoxia in one region may be masked by luxury perfusion in another. Finally, a high $S_{\bar{v}}O_2$ may be the result of a left-to-right intracardiac shunt.

The normal $C_{a-v}O_2$ is approximately 4–5 vol%. A widening $C_{a-v}O_2$ indicates that the tissues are receiving insufficient oxygen to satisfy their requirements, whereas a narrow $C_{a-v}O_2$ is seen in high-output states and those with impaired tissue oxygen utilization, for example in sepsis.

The OER is the proportion of delivered oxygen extracted by the tissues:

$$(C_aO_2 - C_{\bar{v}}O_2)/C_aO_2$$

the normal value being 0.22–0.30. This index has the advantage of taking into consideration both the haemoglobin concentration and arterial oxygenation; it is therefore influenced only by changes in cardiac output and oxygen consumption. An increased OER indicates inadequate oxygen supply, while a narrow OER suggests a reduced metabolic rate or impaired oxygen utilization/extraction.

GASTROINTESTINAL TONOMETRY

The earliest compensatory response to hypovolaemia or a low cardiac output and the last to resolve following resuscitation is splanchnic vasoconstriction, whilst in sepsis gut mucosal ischaemia may be precipitated by disturbed microcirculatory flow combined with increased oxygen requirements (see Chapter 5). Theoretically, therefore, the development of a mucosal acidosis should be a valuable early sign of compensated shock, which might precede other signs of impaired tissue perfusion; therefore changes in mucosal pH might provide a good guide to the adequacy of resuscitation. Moreover, a persistently low intramucosal pH is likely to be a marker of the ischaemic gut mucosal injury which seems to predispose patients to the development of sepsis and multiple organ failure (see Chapter 5), a suggestion supported by studies showing that a low mucosal pH in the intraoperative period is associated with an increased risk of postoperative complications (Mythen and Webb, 1994), and that persistent mucosal acidosis is related to major morbidity after abdominal aortic surgery (Björck and Hedberg, 1994).

Intramucosal pH (pHi) can be estimated by placing a catheter with a saline-filled, Silastic balloon at its tip in either the sigmoid colon, as originally described or, more usually in clinical practice, in the stomach (*gastric* tonometry: Fig. 4.25). In the latter instance some recommend administration of an H_2-receptor antagonist to minimize gastric acid secretion. The PCO_2 of the saline within the balloon equilibrates with intraluminal fluid, and hence with mucosal PCO_2 over a period of about 30 minutes. The carbon dioxide tension in samples of saline withdrawn from the balloon can be determined intermittently. Low-flow states and tissue ischaemia are associated with a rise in mucosal PCO_2 due to

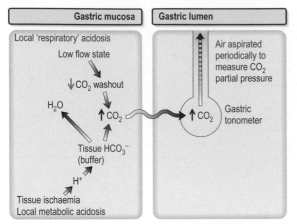

Fig. 4.25 Gastric tonometry. A Silastic balloon is passed into the stomach. Equilibration of carbon dioxide partial pressure between mucosa and balloon takes up to 30 minutes. Low flow states and tissue ischaemia are associated with a rise in carbon dioxide partial pressure. From Singer M, Grant I (eds) (1999) *ABC of Intensive Care*. BMJ Books: London, with permission. Adapted from Kumar P, Clark M 2005 Clinical Medicine 6E Elsevier with permission.

a combination of reduced washout and increased production, the latter being a consequence of the buffering action of bicarbonate on the excess hydrogen ion. It is assumed that the bicarbonate concentration in arterial blood approximates that in the tissues and that pHi can be derived using the Henderson–Hasselbalch equation.

Estimating pH in this way underestimates the severity of the acidosis in low-flow states because of the discrepancy between tissue and arterial bicarbonate which may develop under these circumstances. Moreover, considerable experience and familiarity with the technique are required to obtain accurate and repeatable results. Largely because of these difficulties gas tonometry, in which CO_2 equilibrates with an air-filled tonometer and gastric mucosal P_{CO_2} is referenced to systemic P_{CO_2} ('the CO_2 gap'), has superseded saline tonometry. With both techniques it is important to appreciate that tonometry more accurately reflects changes in the superficial than in the deeper layers and that gut ischaemia may be more reliably detected by placing the balloon in the small bowel. Automated methods have been developed using an infrared analyser which allow frequent calculation of the gastric mucosal to end-tidal P_{CO_2} difference and it has been proposed that this technique could be used in clinical practice as a semi-continuous indicator of the adequacy of splanchnic perfusion (Uusaro *et al.*, 2000).

Gastric tonometry has proved to be a sensitive but not very specific predictor of outcome from critical illness, in that those patients who are able to achieve or maintain a normal pHi are more likely to survive than those who cannot. In patients with acute circulatory failure, for example,

gastric pHi was found to be a more reliable guide to the adequacy of tissue oxygenation than arterial pH, base deficit or lactate levels, and only gastric pHi at 24 hours independently predicted outcome (Maynard *et al.*, 1993). Similarly, in patients with sepsis, only gastric pHi contributed to the prediction of both multiple-organ failure and death (Marik, 1993). Although there is some evidence to support the suggestion that the use of gastric tonometry to guide therapy can improve outcome in critically ill patients (Gutierrez *et al.*, 1992), including trauma victims (Ivatury *et al.*, 1996), a more recent controlled trial (Gomersall *et al.*, 2000) failed to confirm these earlier findings. The clinical utility of gastric tonometry remains uncertain and in practice this technique is now rarely used.

LACTIC ACIDOSIS

Ultimately the consequence of impaired tissue perfusion is cellular hypoxia, anaerobic glycolysis and the production of lactic acid (see Chapters 5 and 6). The development of a metabolic acidosis and elevated blood lactate levels may therefore indicate an imbalance between oxygen supply and demand. This is, however, a relatively late and insensitive marker of reduced perfusion, and the absence of a metabolic acidosis does not exclude regional blood flow abnormalities. It is also important to appreciate that in many critically ill patients, especially those with sepsis, lactic acidosis is caused by metabolic disorders unrelated to tissue hypoxia and may be exacerbated by reduced clearance due to hepatic or renal dysfunction.

DIRECT VISUALIZATION OF THE MICROCIRCULATION

Orthogonal polarization spectral (OPS) imaging utilizes a small hand-held device that illuminates an area of interest with polarized light, while imaging the remitted light through a second polarizer (analyser) oriented in a plane precisely orthogonal to the plane of illumination. The chosen wavelength within the haemoglobin absorption spectrum (548 nm) is selected so that red blood cells appear dark and white blood cells may be visible as refringent bodies. Because vessel walls are not visualized directly, the vasculature can only be seen by virtue of the presence of circulating erythrocytes (Mathura *et al.*, 2001). This technique allows semiquantitative analysis of microcirculatory flow and provides a reproducible means of directly monitoring and evaluating the microcirculation in critically ill patients, especially those with sepsis (Boerma *et al.*, 2005) (see Chapter 5).

Sidestream dark-field illumination is a novel technique which uses a method of reflectance avoidance in which the illuminating and reflected light travel by different pathways. The light from green (530 nm) light-emitting diodes is absorbed by haemoglobin, whilst penetrating green light illuminates the microcirculation. With this technique, resolution seems to be considerably better than that achieved with OPS.

REFERENCES

Ashrafian H, Bogle RG, Rosen SD, *et al.* (2004) Portable echocardiography. *British Medical Journal* 328: 300–301.

Bailey JM, Levy JH, Kopel MA, *et al.* (1990) Relationship between clinical evaluation of peripheral perfusion and global hemodynamics in adults after cardiac surgery. *Critical Care Medicine* 18: 1353–1356.

Band JD, Maki DG (1979) Infections caused by arterial catheters used for hemodynamic monitoring. *American Journal of Medicine* 67: 735–741.

Barbier C, Loubières Y, Schmit C, *et al.* (2004) Respiratory changes in inferior vena cava diameter are helpful in predicting fluid responsiveness in ventilated septic patients. *Intensive Care Medicine* 30: 1740–1746.

Binanay C, Calliff RM, Hasselblad V, *et al.* (2005) Evaluation study of congestive heart failure and pulmonary artery catheterization effectiveness. The ESCAPE trial. *Journal of the American Medical Association* 294: 1625–1633.

Björck M, Hedberg B (1994) Early detection of major complications after abdominal aortic surgery: predictive value of sigmoid colon and gastric intramucosal pH monitoring. *British Journal of Surgery* 81: 25–30.

Boerma EC, Mathura KR, van der Voort PH, *et al.* (2005) Quantifying bedside-derived imaging of microcirculatory abnormalities in septic patients: a prospective validation study. *Critical Care* 9: R601–R606.

Boldt J, Menges T, Wollbruck M, *et al.* (1994) Is continuous cardiac output measurement using thermodilution reliable in the critically ill patient? *Critical Care Medicine* 22: 1913–1918.

Bouchard M-J, Denault A, Couture P, *et al.* (2004) Poor correlation between hemodynamic and echocardiographic indexes of left ventricular performance in the operating room and intensive care unit. *Critical Care Medicine* 32: 644–648.

Boulain T, Achard J-M, Teboul J-L, *et al.* (2002) Changes in BP induced by passive leg raising predict response to fluid loading in critically ill patients. *Chest* 121: 1245–1252.

Boyd O, Mackay CJ, Newman P, *et al.* (1994) Effects of insertion depth and use of the sidearm of the introducer sheath of pulmonary artery catheters in cardiac output measurement. *Critical Care Medicine* 22: 1132–1135.

Branthwaite MA, Bradley RD (1968) Measurement of cardiac output by thermal dilution in man. *Journal of Applied Physiology* 24: 434–438.

Chawla LS, Zia H, Gutierrez G, *et al.* (2004) Lack of equivalence between central and mixed venous oxygen saturation. *Chest* 126: 1891–1896.

Chittock DR, Dhingra VK, Ronco JJ, *et al.* (2004) Severity of illness and risk of death associated with pulmonary artery catheter use. *Critical Care Medicine* 32: 911–915.

Colreavy FB, Donovan K, Lee KY, *et al.* (2002) Transesophageal echocardiography in critically ill patients. *Critical Care Medicine* 30: 989–996.

Connors AF, Speroff T, Dawson NV, *et al.* (1996) The effectiveness of right heart catheterization in the initial care of critically ill patients. *Journal of the American Medical Association* 276: 889–897.

Dark PM, Singer M (2004) The validity of trans-esophageal Doppler ultrasonography as a measure of cardiac output in critically ill adults. *Intensive Care Medicine* 30: 2060–2066.

Deshpande KS, Hatem C, Ulrich HL, *et al.* (2005) The incidence of infectious complications of central venous catheters at the subclavian, internal jugular, and femoral sites in an intensive care unit population. *Critical Care Medicine* 33: 13–20.

Dillon PJ, Columb MO, Hume DD (2001) Comparison of superior vena caval and femoroiliac venous pressure measurements during normal and inverse ratio ventilation. *Critical Care Medicine* 29: 37–39.

Dorman T, Breslow MJ, Lipsett PA, *et al.* (1998) Radial artery pressure monitoring underestimates central arterial pressure during vasopressor therapy in critically ill surgical patients. *Critical Care Medicine* 26: 1646–1649.

Eisenberg PR, Jaffe AS, Schuster DP (1984) Clinical evaluation compared to pulmonary artery catheterization in the hemodynamic assessment of critically ill patients. *Critical Care Medicine* 12: 549–553.

Fang K, Krahmer RL, Rypins EB, *et al.* (1996) Starling resistor effects on pulmonary artery occlusion pressure in endotoxin shock provide inaccuracies in left ventricular compliance assessments. *Critical Care Medicine* 24: 1618–1625.

Fletcher SJ, Bodenham AR (2000) Safe placement of central venous catheters: where should the tip of the catheter lie? *British Journal of Anaesthesia* 85: 188–191.

Forrester JS, Ganz W, Diamond G, *et al.* (1972) Thermodilution cardiac output determination with a single flow-directed catheter. *American Heart Journal* 83: 306–311.

Gan TJ, Arrowsmith JE (1997) The oesophageal Doppler monitor. *British Medical Journal* 315: 893–894.

Gladwin MT, Slonim A, Landucci DL, *et al.* (1999) Cannulation of the internal jugular vein: is postprocedural chest radiography always necessary? *Critical Care Medicine* 27: 1819–1823.

Gnaegi A, Feihl F, Perret C (1997) Intensive care physicians' insufficient knowledge of right-heart catheterization at the bedside: time to act? *Critical Care Medicine* 25: 213–220.

Gomersall CD, Joynt GM, Freebairn RC, *et al.* (2000) Resuscitation of critically ill patients based on the results of gastric tonometry: a prospective, randomized, controlled trial. *Critical Care Medicine* 28: 607–614.

Gutierrez G, Palizas F, Doglio G, *et al.* (1992) Gastric intramucosal pH as a therapeutic index of tissue oxygenation in critically ill patients. *Lancet* 339: 195–199.

Hall JB (2005) Searching for evidence to support pulmonary artery catheter use in critically ill patients. *Journal of the American Medical Association* 294: 1693–1694.

Harvey S, Harrison DA, Singer M, *et al.* (2005) Assessment of the clinical effectiveness of pulmonary artery catheters in management of patients in intensive care (PAC-MAN): a randomised controlled trial. *Lancet* 366: 472–477.

Hatfield A, Bodenham A (1999) Portable ultrasound for difficult central venous access. *British Journal of Anaesthesia* 82: 822–826.

Hind D, Calvert N, McWilliams R, *et al.* (2003) Ultrasonic locating devices for central venous cannulation: meta-analysis. *British Medical Journal* 327: 361.

Hudson E, Beale R (2000) Lung water and blood volume measurements in the critically ill. *Current Opinion in Critical Care* 6: 222–226.

Ivatury RR, Simon RJ, Islam S, *et al.* (1996) A prospective randomized study of end points of resuscitation after major trauma: global oxygen transport indices versus organ-specific gastric mucosal pH. *Journal of the American College of Surgeons* 183: 145–154.

Joly HR, Weil MH (1969) Temperature of the great toe as an indication of the severity of shock. *Circulation* 39: 131–138.

Joynt GM, Gomersall CD, Buckley TA, *et al.* (1996) Comparison of intrathoracic and intra-abdominal measurements of central venous pressure. *Lancet* 347: 1155–1157.

Kumar A, Ariel R, Bunnell E, *et al.* (2004) Pulmonary artery occlusion pressure and central venous pressure fail to predict ventricular filling volume, cardiac performance, or the response to volume infusion in normal subjects. *Critical Care Medicine* 32: 691–699.

Lappas D, Lell WA, Gabel JC, *et al.* (1973) Indirect measurement of left-atrial pressure in surgical patients – pulmonary capillary wedge and pulmonary artery diastolic pressures compared with left-atrial pressure. *Anesthesiology* 38: 394–397.

Lategola M, Rahn H (1953) A self guiding catheter for cardiac and pulmonary arterial catheterization and occlusion. *Proceedings of the Society for Experimental Biology and Medicine* 84: 667–668.

Linton NW, Linton RA (2001) Estimation of changes in cardiac output from the arterial blood pressure waveform in the upper limb. *British Journal of Anaesthesia* 86: 486–496.

Linton R, Band D, O'Brien T, *et al.* (1997) Lithium dilution cardiac output measurement: a comparison with thermodilution. *Critical Care Medicine* 25: 1796–1800.

McGee DC, Gould MK (2003) Preventing complications of central venous catheterization. *New England Journal of Medicine* 348: 1123–1133.

Mainland P-A, Tam W-H, Law B, *et al.* (1997) Stroke following central venous cannulation. *Lancet* 349: 921.

Mansfield PF, Hohn DC, Fornage BD, *et al.* (1994) Complications and failures of subclavian-vein catheterization. *New England Journal of Medicine* 331: 1735–1738.

Marik PE (1993) Gastric intramucosal pH. A better predictor of multiorgan dysfunction syndrome and death than oxygen-derived variables in patients with sepsis. *Chest* 104: 225–229.

Marinelli WA, Weinert CR, Gross CR, *et al.* (1999) Right heart catheterization in acute lung injury: an observational study. *American Journal of Respiratory and Critical Care Medicine* 160: 69–76.

Martin GS, Ely EW, Carroll FE, *et al.* (2002) Findings on the portable chest radiograph correlate with fluid balance in critically ill patients. *Chest* 122: 2087–2095.

Mathura KR, Vollebregt KC, Boer K, *et al.* (2001) Comparison of OPS imaging and conventional capillary microscopy to study the human microcirculation. *Journal of Applied Physiology* 91: 74–78.

Maynard N, Bihari D, Beale R, et al. (1993) Assessment of splanchnic oxygenation by gastric tonometry in patients with acute circulatory failure. *Journal of the American Medical Association* **270**: 1203–1210.

Merrer J, De Jonghe B, Golliot F, et al. (2001) Complications of femoral and subclavian venous catheterization in critically ill patients. *Journal of the American Medical Association* **286**: 700–707.

Michard F, Boussat S, Chemla D, et al. (2000) Relation between respiratory changes in arterial pulse pressure and fluid responsiveness in septic patients with acute circulatory failure. *American Journal of Respiratory and Critical Care Medicine* **162**: 134–138.

Mimoz O, Rauss A, Rekik N, et al. (1994) Pulmonary artery catheterization in critically ill patients: a prospective analysis of outcome changes associated with catheter prompted changes in therapy. *Critical Care Medicine* **22**: 573–579.

Muhm M (2002) Ultrasound guided central venous access. *British Medical Journal* **325**: 1373–1374.

Murdoch SD, Cohen AT, Bellamy MC (2000) Pulmonary artery catheterization and mortality in critically ill patients. *British Journal of Anaesthesia* **85**: 611–615.

Mythen MG, Webb AR (1994) Intra-operative gut mucosal hypoperfusion is associated with increased post-operative complications and cost. *Intensive Care Medicine* **20**: 99–104.

Palazzo M (2001) Circulating volume and clinical assessment of the circulation. *British Journal of Anaesthesia* **86**: 743–746.

Pearse R, Ikram K, Barry J (2004) Equipment review: an appraisal of the LiDCO plus method of measuring cardiac output. *Critical Care* **8**: 190–195.

Poelaert J, Schmidt C, Colardyn F (1998) Transoesophageal echocardiography in the critically ill. *Anaesthesia* **53**: 55–68.

Polanczyk CA, Rohde LE, Goldman L, et al. (2001) Right heart catheterization and cardiac complications in patients undergoing noncardiac surgery: an observational study. *Journal of the American Medical Association* **286**: 309–314.

Ruesch S, Walder B, Tramer MR (2002) Complications of central venous catheters:
internal jugular versus subclavian access – a systematic review. *Critical Care Medicine* **30**: 454–460.

Russell JA, Joel M, Hudson RJ, et al. (1983) Prospective evaluation of radial and femoral artery catheterization sites in critically ill adults. *Critical Care Medicine* **11**: 936–939.

Schmid ER, Schmidlin D, Tornic M, et al. (1999) Continuous thermodilution cardiac output: clinical validation against a reference technique of known accuracy. *Intensive Care Medicine* **25**: 166–172.

Shah MR, Hasselblad V, Stevenson LW, et al. (2005) Impact of the pulmonary artery catheter in critically ill patients; meta-analysis of randomized clinical trials. *Journal of the American Medical Association* **294**: 1664–1670.

Singer M, Bennett ED (1991) Noninvasive optimization of left ventricular filling using esophageal Doppler. *Critical Care Medicine* **19**: 1132–1137.

Singer M, Allen MJ, Webb AR, et al. (1991) Effects of alterations in left ventricular filling, contractility, and systemic vascular resistance on the ascending aortic blood velocity waveform of normal subjects. *Critical Care Medicine* **19**: 1138–1145.

Sise MJ, Hollingsworth P, Brimm JE, et al. (1981) Complications of the flow-directed pulmonary artery catheter: a prospective analysis in 219 patients. *Critical Care Medicine* **9**: 315–318.

Stoneham MD (1999) Less is more . . . using systolic pressure variation to assess hypovolamia. *British Journal of Anaesthesia* **83**: 550–551.

Swan HJC, Ganz W, Forrester J, et al. (1970) Catheterization of the heart in man with use of a flow-directed balloon-tipped catheter. *New England Journal of Medicine* **283**: 447–451.

Sykes MK (1963) Venous pressure as a clinical indication of adequacy of transfusion. *Annals of the Royal College of Surgeons of England* **33**: 185–197.

Sznajder JI, Zveibil FR, Bitterman H, et al. (1986) Central vein catheterization. Failure and complication rates by three percutaneous approaches. *Archives of Internal Medicine* **146**: 259–261.

Thomas F, Burke JP, Parker J, et al. (1983) The risk of infection related to radial *vs* femoral sites for arterial catheterization. *Critical Care Medicine* **11**: 807–812.

Timmins AC, Giles M, Nathan AW, et al. (1994) Clinical validation of a radionuclide detector to measure ejection fraction in critically ill patients. *British Journal of Anaesthesia* **72**: 523–528.

Tournadre JP, Chassard D, Muchada R (1997) Overestimation of low cardiac output measured by thermodilution. *British Journal of Anaesthesia* **79**: 514–516.

Traoré O, Liotier J, Souweine B (2005) Prospective study of arterial and central venous catheter colonization and of arterial and central venous catheter-related bacteremia in intensive care units. *Critical Care Medicine* **33**: 1276–1280.

Uusaro A, Lahtinen P, Parviainen I, et al. (2000) Gastric mucosal end-tidal PCO_2 difference as a continuous indicator of splanchnic perfusion. *British Journal of Anaesthesia* **85**: 563–569.

Vieillard-Baron A, Chergui K, Rabiller A, et al. (2004) Superior vena caval collapsibility as a gauge of volume status in ventilated septic patients. *Intensive Care Medicine* **30**: 1734–1739.

Vincent J-L, Dhainaut J-F, Perret C, et al. (1998) Is the pulmonary artery catheter misused? A European view. *Critical Care Medicine* **26**: 1283–1287.

Weiner RS, Welch HG (2007) Trends in the use of the pulmonary artery catheter in the United States, 1993–2004. *Journal of the American Medical Association* **298**:423–429.

Willeford KL, Reitan JA (1994) Neutral head position for placement of internal jugular vein catheters. *Anaesthesia* **49**: 202–204.

Woods I, Wilkins RG, Edwards JD, et al. (1987) Danger of using core/peripheral temperature gradient as a guide to therapy in shock. *Critical Care Medicine* **15**: 850–852.

Young JD, McQuillan P (1993) Comparison of thoracic electrical bioimpedance and thermodilution for the measurement of cardiac index in patients with severe sepsis. *British Journal of Anaesthesia* **70**: 58–62.

Zink W, Nöll J, Rauch H, et al. (2004) Continuous assessment of right ventricular ejection fraction: new pulmonary artery catheter versus transoesophageal echocardiography. *Anaesthesia* **59**: 1126–1132.

5 Shock, sepsis and multiple-organ failure

DEFINITION

The word 'shock' probably entered the English language in the sixteenth century, derived from the French word *choc*, meaning a sudden or violent blow between two armed forces or warriors. It was not used medically until 1743 in the French text of le Dran's 'A treatise of reflections drawn from experiences with gunshot wounds', and later, in 1831, Latto used the term to describe the effects of cholera on circulatory function.

In current medical practice, shock can be defined as 'acute circulatory failure with inadequate or inappropriately distributed tissue perfusion resulting in generalized cellular hypoxia and/or inability of the cells to utilize oxygen'. The various causes of shock can be classified as shown in **Table 5.1**. (See pp. 100–102 and 123 for definitions of sepsis and multiple-organ failure (MOF).)

CAUSES

Abnormalities of tissue perfusion may result from:

- failure of the heart to act as an effective pump;
- mechanical impediments to forward flow;
- loss of circulating volume;
- abnormalities of the peripheral circulation;
- a combination of these factors.

CARDIOGENIC SHOCK

In cardiogenic shock, cardiac output is reduced (in the presence of a normal intravascular volume) because of an abnormality of the heart itself, most commonly as a result of an *acute myocardial infarction*. Cardiogenic shock may develop if more than 40% of the left ventricular myocardium is damaged, while infarction of more than 70% is usually rapidly fatal. Pre-existing conditions such as valvular stenosis, prior myocardial infarction or cardiomyopathy may render the heart more susceptible to the insult of acute ischaemia. Cardiogenic shock may also occur as a result of:

- acute aortic incompetence;
- acute ischaemic mitral regurgitation, ventricular septal defect or myocardial rupture;

- left ventricular aneurysm;
- myocarditis;
- severe disturbance of cardiac rhythm.

Cardiogenic shock remains a major cause of death amongst patients with acute coronary syndromes. It may also be seen after cardiac surgery and as a result of traumatic myocardial contusion. Myocardial depression may also complicate other forms of shock.

OBSTRUCTIVE SHOCK

In obstructive shock, the fall in cardiac output is caused by a mechanical obstruction to the circulation (e.g. a *pulmonary embolus*), or by restriction of cardiac filling, as occurs in *tamponade* or *tension pneumothorax*.

HYPOVOLAEMIC SHOCK

In hypovolaemic shock, the circulating volume is reduced, venous return to the heart falls and there is a reduction in stroke volume, cardiac output and blood pressure. Hypovolaemia may be due to *exogenous losses*, as occurs with haemorrhage and burns, or *endogenous losses*. In the latter, fluid is lost into the interstitial spaces through leaky capillaries or into body cavities such as the bowel (e.g. intestinal obstruction).

DISTRIBUTIVE SHOCK

Vascular dilatation, sequestration of blood in venous capacitance vessels, maldistribution of flow and abnormalities of the microcirculation may lead to shock due to relative hypovolaemia, a reduction in peripheral resistance and impaired oxygen extraction, as occurs for example in those with *sepsis* and *anaphylaxis*. True hypovolaemia usually supervenes because of the fluid losses caused by the increase in microvascular permeability. In sepsis and other shock conditions, a later phase of disturbed cellular metabolism and bioenergetics follows, affecting the ability of the tissues to utilize oxygen.

PATHOPHYSIOLOGY

SYMPATHOADRENAL RESPONSE TO SHOCK

Hypotension stimulates the baroreceptors and, to a lesser extent, the chemoreceptors, causing increased sympathetic nervous activity with 'spillover' of noradrenaline (norepinephrine) into the circulation. Later, this is augmented by the release of catecholamines (predominantly adrenaline (epinephrine)) from the adrenal medulla. The resulting vasoconstriction, together with positive inotropic and chronotropic effects, helps to restore blood pressure and cardiac output (**Fig. 5.1**).

The reduction in perfusion of the renal cortex stimulates the juxtaglomerular apparatus to release renin. This converts angiotensinogen to angiotensin I, which is in turn converted to the potent vasoconstrictor, angiotensin II, in the lungs. In addition, angiotensin II stimulates secretion of aldosterone by the adrenal cortex, causing sodium and water retention. This helps to restore the circulating volume (**Fig. 5.2**).

Opioid peptides containing the enkephalin sequence, which are widely distributed throughout the body, particularly within the sympathetic nervous system, have been identified within the same chromaffin cells as catecholamines and are also released into the circulation in shock (Evans *et al.*, 1984).

ACTIVATION OF THE HYPOTHALAMIC–PITUITARY–ADRENAL (HPA) AXIS IN SHOCK

The HPA axis is activated in response to stress by, for example, cytokines (see below) which stimulate release of corticotrophin-releasing hormone (CRH) from the hypothalamus, as well as directly activating the pituitary and adrenals. Circulating levels of adrenocorticotrophic hormone (ACTH), growth hormone (GH), prolactin and vasopressin (antidiuretic hormone, ADH) are therefore increased in early shock and sepsis, but may fall later if shock is prolonged. β-endorphin is derived from the same precursor molecule as ACTH (pro-opiomelanocortin) and plasma levels of this peptide also increase in response to stressful stimuli. CRH and β-endorphin may also be released from cells of the immune system; both endogenous opioid peptides and exogenous opioids modulate immune function (Webster, 1998). As well as their role as natural analgesics, β-endorphins and other endogenous opioid peptides (e.g. the enkephalins), may be partly responsible for some of the cardiovascular changes seen in shock.

Table 5.1 Causes of shock

Cardiogenic ('pump failure')
Obstructive (e.g. pulmonary embolus, cardiac tamponade)
Hypovolaemic (exogenous losses, endogenous losses)
Distributive (vascular dilatation, sequestration, maldistribution of flow, e.g. sepsis, anaphylaxis)

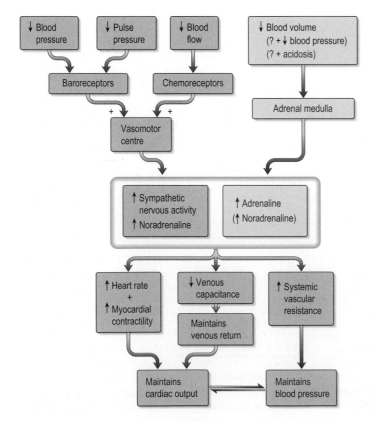

Fig. 5.1 The sympathoadrenal response to shock.

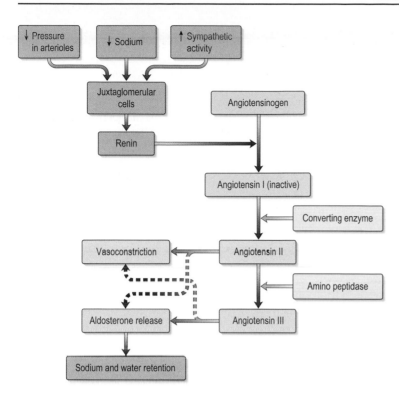

Fig. 5.2 The renin–angiotensin system in shock.

Adrenocortical function in sepsis/septic shock

Endogenous corticosteroids have a number of important regulatory functions which may be overwhelmed in severe shock. These include:

- modulation of the inflammatory response;
- maintenance of endothelial integrity and vascular permeability;
- inhibition of inducible nitric oxide (NO) synthases;
- maintenance of vascular tone and responsiveness to adrenergic stimulation;
- maintenance of myocardial function and responsiveness to adrenergic stimulation;
- influencing the distribution of fluid and electrolytes;
- increasing gluconeogenesis.

Characteristically, plasma cortisol increases markedly in early shock, and the normal circadian rhythm is lost. A reduction in corticosteroid-binding globulin may contribute to increases in plasma levels of free cortisol. Clearance of cortisol from the circulation may also be decreased, for example because of hepatic dysfunction. On the other hand, cytokines can reduce the affinity of cortisol for its receptor.

The extent and duration of the rise in cortisol levels are generally related to the severity of illness, although there is often considerable variation and the precise relationship between circulating levels and outcome remains unclear. Whereas several studies have shown that higher plasma cortisol levels are associated with a worse prognosis (Annane et al., 2000), others have found that circulating cortisol levels are lower in non-survivors than in survivors. In some studies there was no correlation between plasma cortisol and outcome.

Although absolute adrenocortical insufficiency (due, for example, to bilateral adrenal haemorrhage or necrosis) seems to be rare, there is evidence that patients with sepsis often have a blunted response to exogenous ACTH (Annane et al., 2000; Briegel et al., 1996; Rothwell et al., 1991) (so-called relative or occult adrenal insufficiency) and that this may be associated with an impaired pressor response to noradrenaline (Annane et al., 1998) and a worse prognosis (Annane et al., 2000; Rothwell et al., 1991). It has been suggested that the incidence of occult adrenal insufficiency in septic shock may be as high as 54%, although many of the patients in this study had previously received etomidate, which suppresses cortisol production (Annane et al., 2000). These authors also defined three patterns of activation of the HPA axis in a large group of patients with septic shock, each being associated with a different prognosis. In one-third of their patients, activation of the HPA axis was considered to be appropriate (basal cortisol < 34 µg/dL (938 nmol/L) and a cortisol response to corticotrophin > 9 µg/dL (248 nmol/L)); in this group 28-day mortality was only 26%. The highest mortality rate (82%) was seen in the 20% of patients in whom high basal cortisol levels were combined with occult adrenal insufficiency. Patients in the third group, comprising more than half the total, had either a low basal cortisol with a blunted response to corticotrophin or a high basal cortisol with an adequate response to stimulation. In this intermediate group 28-day mortality was

67%. In a more recent study of a larger cohort of patients baseline control levels were higher, and the cortisol response lower in non-survivors. Etomidate influenced the ACTH response and was associated with a worse outcome (Lipiner-Friedman et al 2007). Nevertheless, further studies are required to refine the diagnosis of adrenal insufficiency in the critically ill (Lipiner-Friedman et al 2007) and there is uncertainty whether relative adrenal insufficiency contributes to the poor outcome in these cases or is simply a marker of the severity of illness. Lastly, it is important to appreciate that in critically ill patients with hypoproteinaemia, free cortisol levels are consistently elevated, despite reduced baseline and ACTH-stimulated levels of serum total cortisol (Hamrahian *et al.*, 2004).

The causes of occult adrenocortical insufficiency in shock are also not clear, but may be related to altered adrenal perfusion, ischaemic injury, mediator-induced adrenal damage, receptor downregulation, drugs (e.g. etomidate) or a combination of these. In some cases the adrenals may simply be maximally stimulated whereas in others there may be hypothalamic or pituitary abnormalities, including reduced responsiveness to CRH (Schroeder *et al.*, 2001).

THE INNATE IMMUNE/INFLAMMATORY RESPONSE

Severe infection, the presence of large areas of damaged tissue (e.g. following major trauma, burns or extensive surgery), major blood loss, hypoxia or prolonged episodes of hypoperfusion can trigger an inflammatory response with systemic activation of leukocytes and release of a variety of potentially damaging mediators. Although clearly beneficial when targeted against local areas of infection or necrotic tissue, dissemination of this highly conserved *innate immune response* is responsible for the haemodynamic changes, microvascular abnormalities, mitochondrial dysfunction and tissue injury which can culminate in organ dysfunction (**Fig. 5.3**). Characteristically, the initial episode of overwhelming inflammation is followed by a period of immune suppression, which in some cases may be profound and during which the patient is at increased risk of developing secondary infections (see later).

Microorganisms and their toxic products

In sepsis/septic shock the innate immune system and inflammatory cascade are triggered by the recognition of *pathogen-associated molecular patterns* (PAMPs), including cell wall components, flagellin, fimbriae and intracellular motifs released during bacterial lysis, such as heat-shock proteins (HSPs) and DNA fragments. In other forms of shock, ischaemia/reperfusion injury to the bowel mucosa may be associated with translocation of bacteria and their cellular components into the circulation (see later).

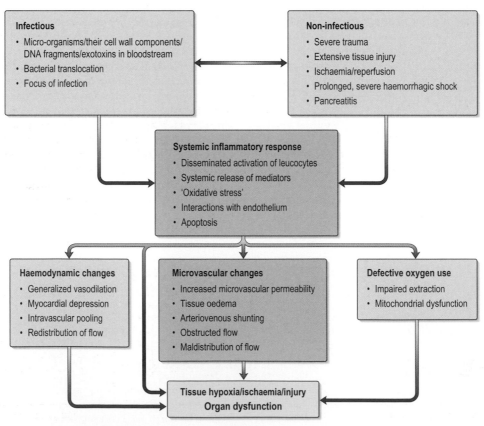

Fig. 5.3 Aetiology of multiple-organ dysfunction syndrome (MODS).

Lipopolysaccharide (LPS), or bacterial *endotoxin*, is derived from the cell wall of Gram-negative bacteria and is considered to be one of the most important triggers of sepsis/septic shock. Certainly, administration of endotoxin to both animals and humans (Suffredini *et al.*, 1989) can reproduce many of the manifestations of septic shock. Also intermittent endotoxaemia is common in those with septic shock and is associated with the more severe manifestations of the syndrome, including myocardial depression and MOF (Danner *et al.*, 1991). These authors also detected endotoxin in the blood of some patients with septic shock due to Gram-positive bacteria or *Candida* and speculated that this may have been related to undetected Gram-negative bacteraemia or release of endotoxin from elsewhere (e.g. the bowel lumen; see later). Interestingly, depletion of endogenous antiendotoxin core antibody has been associated with non-survival in severe sepsis (Goldie *et al.*, 1995).

Endotoxin consists of (**Fig. 5.4**):

- a lipid moiety (lipid A), which is structurally highly conserved and is thought to be responsible for most, if not all, of its biological activity;
- a core polysaccharide;
- oligosaccharide side chains, which differ considerably between strains and confer '0'-antigen specificity to the molecule.

The lipid A portion of LPS can be bound by a protein normally present in human serum called *lipopolysaccharide-binding protein* (LBP), the concentration of which increases by around 100 times during the acute-phase response to infection. In the case of intact Gram-negative bacteria, binding of LBP to membrane LPS enhances opsonization by neutrophils and cells of the reticuloendothelial system (RES), whereas when LBP binds with free endotoxin it forms a complex which facilitates interaction with the cell surface marker CD14. The LPS/LBP/CD14 complex, combined with a secreted protein (MD2), attaches to a member of the Toll-like family of *pattern recognition receptors* (TLR4), which transduces the activation signal into the cell. Stimulated intracellular pathways lead to activation of nuclear transcription factors which pass into the nucleus where they bind to DNA and promote the synthesis of a wide variety of inflammatory mediators. The best-known nuclear transcription factor is NF-κB, which is released after specific kinases phosphorylate its inhibitory subunit, IκB (**Fig. 5.5**). LPS activation of cells which do not express membrane-bound CD14, such as those of the vascular endothelium, can take place following binding to soluble CD14 in the bloodstream. Other cell surface receptors, such as the integrin CD11/18 and the macrophage scavenger receptor (MSR), may also be involved in the response to endotoxin.

Cell wall components from Gram-positive bacteria, such as *lipoteichoic acid* (which is similar in structure to LPS) and *peptidoglycan*, can also trigger a systemic inflammatory response through similar, but not identical, pathways. For example, whereas TLR4 is required for the response to LPS, it seems that TLR2 is more important for binding to Gram-positive products. There is evidence that peptidoglycan can dramatically enhance the inflammatory response not only to lipoteichoic acid but also to LPS, providing a possible explanation for the poor prognosis associated with mixed Gram-positive and Gram-negative infections (Wray *et al.*, 2001).

Intracellular pattern recognition receptors may also be involved in the response to invading microorganisms. For example, the nucleotide-binding oligomerization domain (NOD)1 protein recognizes a peptidoglycan fragment that is almost exclusive to Gram-negative bacteria, whereas NOD2 detects a similar fragment, but also recognizes muramyl dipeptide, the smallest bioactive fragment common to all peptidoglycans.

The inflammatory cascade may also be triggered by the toxic products of microorganisms. Whereas some bacteria produce a single toxin that is principally responsible for the disease (e.g. tetanus, cholera and botulism), others (e.g. staphylococci and streptococci) produce an array of secreted proteins or *exotoxins*. These include the so-called superantigens produced by *Staphylococcus aureus* and *Streptococcus pyogenes* which can directly activate monocytes, macrophages and T cells, without intracellular processing, by cross-linking major histocompatibility complex class II molecules with subsets of T-cell receptors. Bacteria can also provoke a host response by causing cellular injury through the production of pore-forming toxins and a variety of proteolytic enzymes. Some of these proteases stimulate the immune system directly by cleavage of native substrates to active proinflammatory mediators (e.g. release of bradykinin from kininogen or

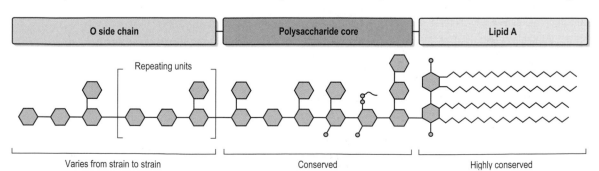

Fig. 5.4 Structure of endotoxin.

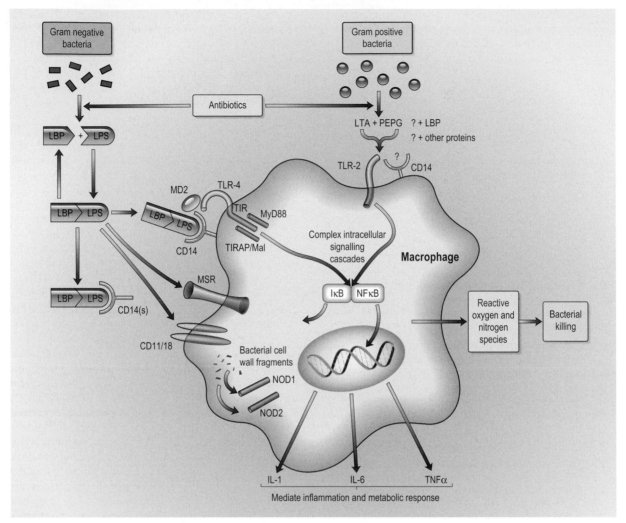

Fig. 5.5 Induction of the innate immune response by gram negative and gram positive bacteria. Please see text for explanation of abbreviations.

conversion of pro-IL-1 to active interleukin-1 (IL-1)) (**Table 5.2**). Some organisms also have the ability to defend themselves against the host response; for example, some group A streptococci can produce a protease that degrades IL-8 (Hidalgo-Grass *et al.*, 2004). Group A streptococci can also cause a *toxic shock syndrome*, in which deep tissue infection is associated with bacteraemia, vascular collapse and organ failure. It seems that in such cases M protein, a constituent of the streptococcal cell wall, forms a complex with fibrinogen which binds to integrins on the surface of polymorphonuclear leukocytes causing adherence, degranulation and a 'respiratory burst' (Brown, 2004).

Cytokines

Cytokines are polypeptide messengers released by activated lymphocytes, macrophages and endothelium which are important mediators of the inflammatory response in shock and sepsis. They influence thermoregulation, endocrine function and metabolic responses, and also play an important role in immune function.

Tumour necrosis factor (TNF) can be detected in the circulation shortly after the administration of endotoxin to human volunteers (Michie *et al.*, 1988a) and induces similar metabolic responses to endotoxin when given to humans (Michie *et al.*, 1988b). It is thought to play a pivotal role as an initiator of the host response to infection. TNF enhances phagocytosis and neutrophil adherence, and also activates neutrophil degranulation.

The *IL-1 response* occurs shortly after TNF release. IL-1 shares many of the biological properties of TNF and the two cytokines act synergistically, in part through induction of cyclooxygenase, platelet-activating factor (PAF) and NO synthase (NOS: see later). IL-1 stimulates helper T cells to produce IL-2, which promotes the growth and proliferation of cytotoxic T cells.

Subsequently, *other cytokines, including IL-6 and IL-8*, appear in the circulation. IL-6 is the major stimulant for hepatic synthesis of acute-phase proteins (see below), is a cause of myocardial dysfunction in sepsis (Pathan *et al.*, 2004) and is involved with other cytokines in the induction

Table 5.2 Some examples of microbial products implicated in the pathogenesis of sepsis/septic shock

	Microbial product	Bacterial source
Cell wall components	Lipopolysaccharide	Gram-negative bacteria
	Peptidoglycan	Gram-positive bacteria
	Lipoteichoic acid	
Secreted toxins		
Superantigens	Staphylococcal toxic shock syndrome toxin 1	*Staphylococcus aureus*
	Staphylococcal enterotoxin B	
	Streptococcal pyrogenic exotoxin A	*Streptococcus pyogenes*
Proteases	Phospholipase C	*Clostridium*
	Lipase	*Staphylococcus aureus*
	Nuclease	
	Neuraminidase	*Streptococcus pneumoniae*
	Streptococcal pyrogenic exotoxin B	*Streptococcus pyogenes*
Porins	α-Haemolysin	*Escherichia coli*
	Leukocidin	*Staphylococcus aureus*
	Catalase	
	Pneumolysin	*Streptococcus pneumoniae*
	Streptolysin S and O	*Streptococcus pyogenes*

of fever, anaemia and cachexia, whereas IL-8 is an important neutrophil chemoattractant. These cytokines are, however, less proinflammatory and may fulfil an important role as downregulators of TNF and IL-1 production. TNF, IL-1 and IL-6 also synergistically stimulate the HPA axis, although at higher concentrations they may downregulate pituitary–adrenocortical function. The behavioural changes that often accompany inflammation, including anorexia, somnolence and lethargy, are similarly induced by cytokines. More recently it has also been appreciated that the cytokine response activates the coagulation system and inhibits fibrinolysis (see pp. 94 and 95).

Macrophage migration inhibitory factor (MIF) was originally described as a soluble factor released by activated lymphocytes that inhibited the migration of macrophages in peritoneal fluid. MIF is now recognized as a potent proinflammatory cytokine which acts by modulating the expression of TLR-4, and thereby its downstream effects.

It is important to appreciate that the cytokine network is extremely complex, with widespread interactions with other systems and many self-regulating mechanisms. In particular, the proinflammatory response is counterbalanced not only by endogenous corticosteroids and catecholamines but also by the release of anti-inflammatory cytokines such as IL-10 and IL-4, and is associated with downregulation of human leukocyte antigen (HLA)-DR expression on monocytes. Moreover, cytokines can often downregulate their own synthesis. In the case of TNF, shedding of TNF receptors from the cell surface reduces cellular responsiveness and releases *soluble TNF receptors* (sTNFR 1 and 2) into the circulation where they may bind to, and diminish the biological activity of circulating TNF-α (although it is also possible that binding of TNF to sTNFR prolongs its half-life and perpetuates the

inflammatory response). An endogenous inhibitory protein that binds competitively to the IL-1 receptor (IL-1 receptor antagonist – IL-1-ra) has also been identified. Finally, *MIF* is released from the anterior pituitary gland and macrophages in shock and sepsis and counteracts the anti-inflammatory effects of glucocorticoids, as well as inhibiting the random migration of macrophages. High circulating levels of MIF and TNF have been associated with a poor outcome in patients with systemic inflammation (Gando *et al.*, 2001).

Although severe sepsis/septic shock is conventionally thought to be the result of an exaggerated proinflammatory response which overwhelms counterregulatory mechanisms, such a response is probably less frequent than was originally thought. Moreover, an anti-inflammatory cytokine profile with a high ratio of IL-10 to TNF-α (van Dissel *et al.*, 1998) and high circulating levels of s-TNFR1 and 2 (Goldie *et al.*, 1995) has been associated with a poor outcome from severe infections. Certainly, persistent immune hyporesponsiveness predisposes to nosocomial infection and death. On the other hand, high circulating levels of IL-6 are consistently associated with a higher mortality rate (Goldie *et al.*, 1995) and an increasing ratio of IL-6 to IL-10 was indicative of a poor outcome in patients with systemic inflammation (Taniguchi *et al.*, 1999).

Finally, it is important to appreciate that circulating levels of cytokines may not accurately reflect their local activity as intercellular and cell surface signalling molecules.

Acute-phase proteins and complement *(Gabay and Kushner, 1999) (Fig. 5.6)*

The term 'acute-phase response' encompasses a large number of behavioural, physiological, biochemical and nutritional

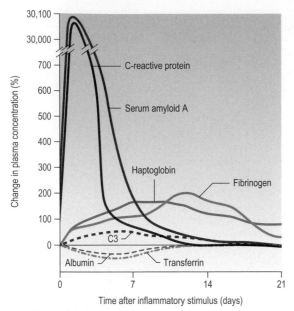

Fig. 5.6 Characteristic patterns of change in plasma concentrations of some acute-phase proteins after a moderate inflammatory stimulus. From Gabay C, Kushner I (1999) Acute-phase proteins and other systemic responses to inflammation. *New England Journal of Medicine* **340**: 448–454. © New England Journal of Medicine.

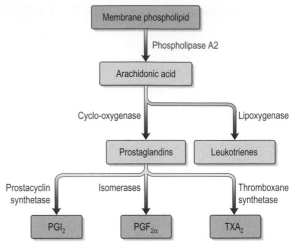

Fig. 5.7 Arachidonic acid metabolites. PG, prostaglandin; TXA$_2$, thromboxane A$_2$.

changes, distant from the site of inflammation, which can accompany tissue injury or infection. An acute-phase protein has been defined as one whose plasma concentration increases (positive acute-phase protein) or decreases (negative acute-phase protein) by at least 25% during inflammatory disorders. The fall in circulating levels of the negative acute-phase proteins, such as albumin and transferrin, is probably largely a reflection of diversion of available amino acids for the synthesis of other acute-phase proteins, although some of the changes may serve to modulate the inflammatory response. Important positive acute-phase proteins in humans include:

- C-reactive protein (CRP) – a component of the innate immune system which, when bound to foreign ligands, can activate complement. CRP acts as an opsonin and modulates the inflammatory response.
- Serum amyloid A (SAA) – a family of proteins which bind rapidly to high-density lipoproteins. The actions of SAA are largely unknown but they have the potential to influence cholesterol metabolism during inflammatory states and modulate inflammation.
- LBP – see above.
- Haptoglobin – an antioxidant.
- α_1 protease inhibitor – antagonizes the activity of proteolytic enzymes.
- Fibrinogen – can influence wound healing and modulate inflammation (see below).

Many of the classic components of the *complement system* can be considered to be acute-phase proteins. Recognition of PAMPs activates the complement cascade via three distinct pathways, leading to the generation of the membrane attack complex (C5b–C9). The *classic pathway* is triggered either by immunoglobulin M (IgM) antibodies that recognize particular PAMPs or IgG antibodies produced during a previous encounter with the pathogen. The *alternative pathway* directly recognizes PAMPs on the surface of bacteria or fungi. The *lectin-binding pathway* (mannose-binding lectin) recognizes and binds to foreign carbohydrate structures and recruits specific circulating serine proteases (e.g. mannose-binding lectin-associated serine proteases: MASP1 and 2) to activate the fourth component of complement. Mannose-binding lectin also acts as an opsonin. During the proteolytic activation of serum complement a number of ancillary mediators are produced. For example, fragments of C3 act as opsonins and as co-stimulatory molecules that assist lymphocytes with the adaptive immune response, while small cationic peptides derived from C3, C4 and C5 cause leukocyte chemotaxis, release of cytokines and increased vascular permeability.

Arachidonic acid metabolites

Arachidonic acid is an essential fatty acid, derived from the increased breakdown of membrane phospholipid catalysed by phospholipase A$_2$. It is metabolized via the cyclooxygenase pathways to form prostaglandins and thromboxanes and via the lipoxygenase pathway to produce leukotrienes (**Fig. 5.7**).

There are a large number of cyclooxygenase products, each of which has distinct physiological effects: some cause vasoconstriction, others are vasodilators, some activate platelets, others inhibit platelet aggregation. Some prostaglandins also increase vascular permeability. Those members of the family considered to be of particular importance in shock are:

- prostacyclin, which is a vasodilator and inhibits platelet aggregation;
- thromboxane (TX) A_2, which causes pulmonary vasoconstriction and activates platelets;
- prostaglandin (PG) $F_{2\alpha}$, which may be responsible for the early phase of pulmonary hypertension commonly seen in experimental septic shock.

Clearly, the net effect of the release of these substances in an individual patient depends on the relative concentrations of each particular cyclooxygenase product.

The role of leukotrienes in shock is less certain, but they may be responsible for increased vascular permeability, coronary vasoconstriction and a reduction in cardiac output.

Platelet-activating factor

PAF is a vasoactive lipid released by the hydrolysis of membrane phospholipids, catalysed by phospholipase A_2. Its effects, which are caused both directly and indirectly through the secondary release of other mediators, include:

- hypotension;
- increased vascular permeability;
- platelet aggregation.

Lysosomal enzymes

Lysosomal enzymes are released not only when cells die, but also in response to hypoxia, ischaemia, sepsis and acidosis. As well as being directly cytotoxic, they can cause myocardial depression and coronary vasoconstriction. Furthermore, lysosomal enzymes can convert *inactive kininogens*, which are usually combined with α_2-globulin, to *vasoactive kinins* such as bradykinin. These substances can cause:

- vasodilatation;
- increased capillary permeability;
- myocardial depression;
- activation of clotting mechanisms.

Heat-shock proteins

HSPs are highly conserved intracellular proteins ranging from 8 to 110 kDa that are classified into families based roughly on the molecular mass of a typical member. The best characterized are the HSP-70 family, which are found in inducible and constitutive forms in many cells. Inducible HSP-72, for example, is synthesized after exposure to various harmful stimuli such as heat, cytokines, hypoxia, endotoxin, various chemicals and oxygen free radicals. HSPs appear to be protective in sepsis, probably because they recognize and form complexes with denatured proteins, thus inducing correct protein folding and, where necessary, proteolytic degradation. They also appear to protect normal functional proteins against degradation and inhibit apoptosis. In recognition of these effects, HSPs are often referred to as

'molecular chaperones'. HSPs also play a role in antigen presentation to T lymphocytes.

High-mobility group box 1 (HMGB-1) protein

HMGB-1 is a nuclear factor and a secreted protein. It acts in the cell nucleus as an architectural chromatin-binding factor that bends DNA and promotes protein assembly on specific DNA loci. Outside the cell it activates inflammatory responses in immune cells and the endothelium and transduces cellular signals through RAGE (the receptor for advanced glycation end products) and other receptors such as TLR2 and TLR4. HMGB-1 is secreted by activated mononuclear cells and is passively released by necrotic or damaged cells. HMGB-1 appears to be a late mediator of sepsis and may therefore be particularly amenable to therapeutic intervention.

Adhesion molecules

Adhesion of neutrophils to the vessel wall with subsequent extravascular migration of activated leukocytes are likely to be key components of the sequence of events leading to endothelial injury, tissue damage and organ dysfunction. This process is mediated by inducible intercellular adhesion molecules (ICAMs) found on the surface of leukocytes and endothelial cells. Expression of these molecules can be induced by LPS and by inflammatory cytokines such as IL-1 and TNF. Three separate families of molecules are involved in promoting leukocyte–endothelial interaction:

- Selectins (P, E and L selectin): these are initial 'capture' molecules and initiate the process of leukocyte rolling on vascular endothelium.
- Immunoglobulin superfamily: ICAM-1, vascular cell adhesion molecule-1 (VCAM-1): these are involved in the formation of a more secure bond, which leads to leukocyte migration into the tissues.
- Integrins.

Soluble forms of adhesion molecules have been identified in peripheral blood and may serve as an indirect measure of the state of endothelial activation. Circulating levels of E-selectin, ICAM-1 and VCAM-1 have been found to be higher in patients with sepsis and organ dysfunction than in control patients. High levels of E-selectin, in particular, were associated with a very poor prognosis (Cowley *et al.*, 1994).

Endothelium-derived vasoactive mediators

It is now recognized that the vascular endothelium is not only a physical barrier between blood and the vessel wall, but is also a highly complex organ involved in the regulation of blood vessel tone, vascular permeability, coagulation, angiogenesis, leukocyte and platelet reactivity, phagocytosis of bacteria and the metabolism of many vascular mediators.

Endothelial cells synthesize a number of vasoactive mediators, which contribute to the regulation of blood vessel tone and the fluidity of the blood. These include:

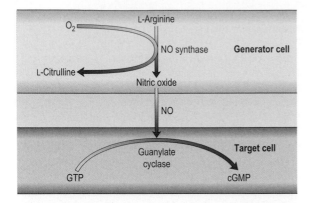

Fig. 5.8 Synthesis of nitric oxide (NO). cGMP, cyclic guanosine monophosphate; GTP, guanosine triphosphate. Adapted from Kumar P, Clark M 2005 Clinical Medicine 6E Elsevier with permission.

- prostacyclin;
- endothelin-1;
- NO – originally called endothelium-derived relaxing factor.

NO is synthesized from the terminal guanidino-nitrogen atoms of the amino acid L-arginine under the influence of NOS. NO has cytotoxic effects, inhibits mitochondrial respiration, inhibits platelet aggregation and adhesion and produces vasodilatation by activating guanylate cyclase in the underlying vascular smooth muscle to form cyclic guanosine monophosphate (cGMP) from guanosine triphosphate (GTP) (**Fig. 5.8**). There is now evidence for the existence of several distinct NOS isoforms:

- *Constitutive* or *endothelial* NOS (cNOS or eNOS), present in endothelial cells, is responsible for the basal release of NO and is involved in the physiological regulation of vascular tone, blood pressure and tissue perfusion.
- *Inducible* NOS (iNOS) is induced in vascular endothelial and smooth-muscle cells and monocytes within 2–18 hours of stimulation with certain cytokines, such as TNF-α and IL-1, and endotoxin. The resulting prolonged increase in NO formation is now believed to be one of the main factors responsible for the sustained vasodilatation, hypotension and hyporeactivity to adrenergic agonists ('vasoplegia') that characterizes septic shock and may contribute to myocardial dysfunction in these patients. This mechanism may also be involved in severe or prolonged haemorrhagic/traumatic shock. The NO generated by stimulated macrophages contributes to their role as highly effective killers of intracellular and extracellular pathogens, in part as a consequence of its ability to bind to cytochrome oxidase and other mitochondrial respiratory enzymes, thus inhibiting electron transport. NO can also combine with super-oxide anions to form the unstable radical peroxynitrite ($ONOO^-$), which is more toxic and has a more prolonged, and perhaps irreversible, effect compared to NO.
- *Neuronal* NOS (nNOS) The role of nerves containing nNOS is uncertain but they probably provide neurogenic vasodilator tone. In the central nervous system nNOS may be an important regulator of local cerebral blood flow as well as fulfilling a number of other physiological functions, such as signalling and the acute modulation of neuronal firing behaviour.

Circulating levels of *endothelin-1*, a potent endogenous vasoconstrictor, are increased in sepsis, cardiogenic shock and following severe trauma. The exact physiological and pathological roles of the endothelins are not yet well understood.

High-density lipoproteins (Wu et al., 2004)

High-density lipoproteins (HDLs) possess significant anti-inflammatory properties by virtue of their ability to bind and neutralize LPS (facilitated by LBP), inhibit adhesion molecule expression, stimulate the production of NOS and protect low-density lipoproteins against peroxidative damage (through associated enzymes such as paraoxonase). Typically, the inflammatory response is associated with increased hepatic synthesis of triglyceride-rich lipoproteins – 'the lipaemia of sepsis' – and a reduction in plasma cholesterol (especially HDL cholesterol), the magnitude of which is related to the severity of illness, lethality and susceptibility to infection. Moreover the acute-phase protein SAA (see above) is incorporated into HDLs where it displaces protective enzymes, such as paraoxonase, thereby modifying their anti-inflammatory properties and enhancing their catabolism. These changes in the levels, structure and function of HDLs are permissive for a proinflammatory response and reduce LPS-neutralizing capacity.

Redox imbalance

In health the balance between reducing and oxidizing conditions (redox) is controlled by antioxidants that may either prevent radical formation (e.g. transferrin and lactoferrin, which bind iron, a catalyst for radical formation) or remove/inactivate reactive oxygen and nitrogen species (e.g. enzymes such as superoxide dismutase, sulphydryl group donors such as glutathione, antioxidants such as vitamins C and E). There are also mechanisms to remove and repair oxidatively damaged molecules and preserve DNA integrity. In severe systemic inflammation the uncontrolled production of oxygen-derived free radicals and reactive nitrogen species (**Fig. 5.9**), particularly by activated polymorphonuclear leukocytes, can overwhelm these defensive mechanisms and cause:

- lipid and protein peroxidation;
- damage to cell membranes;
- increased capillary permeability;
- impaired mitochondrial respiration;

- DNA strand breakage;
- activation of the DNA repair enzyme poly-ADP ribose synthase (PARS);
- apoptosis (low levels of reactive oxygen species: ROS), oncosis and necrosis (high levels of ROS).

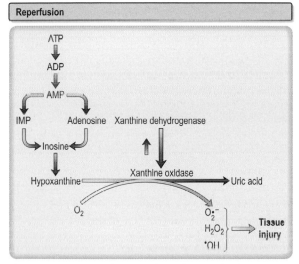

Fig. 5.9 Production of oxygen-derived free radicals and reactive nitrogen species during ischaemia/reperfusion. ADP, adenosine diphosphate; AMP, adenosine monophosphate; ATP, adenosine triphosphate; IMP, inosine monophosphate.

Apoptosis, oncosis, necrosis and programmed cell death *(Kam and Ferch, 2000)*

The term *apoptosis* is derived from the Greek word for 'falling off', a reference to the autumnal fall of leaves in anticipation of the damaging cold and darkness of winter. Specifically, apoptosis refers to an energy-dependent, asynchronous, genetically controlled process by which damaged, senescent or unnecessary individual cells self-destruct. During this process, which may take as little as 15 minutes, the cell shrinks and detaches from its substratum and neighbouring cells; the nucleus is broken down, the nuclear fragments and organelles condense and are packaged in membrane-bound vesides which are then exocytosed and ingested by surrounding cells. Membrane integrity is initially preserved and the remaining cell becomes a round smooth remnant or *apoptotic body*. Later, the cell membrane becomes permeable and the apoptotic body and membrane-bound buds may then be phagocytosed by macrophages. Death receptors known to initiate apoptosis include the fas receptor and the TNF receptors. Activation of the transmembrane fas receptor by binding of fas ligand (expressed on the surface of cytotoxic T lymphocytes) leads to the intracellular production of fas-associated death domain (FADD) molecules, whilst a TNF receptor-associated death domain (TRADD) has also been identified. The decision phase of apoptosis is genetically controlled (two genes, *BcL-2* and *p53*, are important) whilst the execution phase involves proteolysis and mitochondrial disruption, in part a consequence of activation of a family of cysteine-aspartate proteases termed *caspases*.

The absence of associated inflammation differentiates apoptotic cell death from *necrosis* (**Table 5.3**), which stimulates the immune system and causes widespread cell damage and *oncosis*, in which cell swelling caused by a lack of adenosine triphosphate (ATP) and failure of the membrane pumps is followed by nuclear fragmentation, breakdown by lysosomal enzymes, cell rupture, phagocytosis and inflammation. Apoptosis can be triggered by four main categories of stimuli (**Table 5.4**), many of which can also, when severe, precipitate oncosis/necrosis. *Programmed cell death* is a distinct process which does not require *de novo* gene expression

Table 5.3 Differences between apoptosis and necrosis	
Apoptosis	**Necrosis**
Physiological or pathological	Always pathological
Asynchronous process in single cells	Occurs synchronously in multiple cells
Genetically controlled	Caused by overwhelming noxious stimuli
Late loss of membrane integrity	Early loss of membrane integrity
Cell shrinkage	Generalized cell and nucleus swelling
Condensation of nuclear contents ('ladder' formation of chromatin)	Nuclear chromatin disintegration
No inflammatory reaction	Inflammatory reaction

Table 5.4 Stimuli for apoptosis

DNA (genome) damage	Ionizing radiation Anticancer drugs (e.g. alkylating agents)
Activation of death receptors	Binding of 'death receptors' (e.g. Fas receptor, tumour necrosis factor receptor) Withdrawal of growth factors (e.g. nerve growth factor, interleukin-3)
Stimulation of apoptotic pathway	Phosphatases, kinase inhibitors
Direct physical damage	Heat, ultraviolet light, reactive oxygen and nitrogen species

and is involved in normal embryological development and maturation of organs or tissues.

In sepsis, apoptosis is thought to be initiated by enhanced production of ROS and increased intracellular calcium levels and may contribute to the organ damage and immune hypo-responsiveness associated with this disorder (Hotchkiss *et al.*, 1999). In particular, the normal rapid turnover through apoptosis of lymphocytes and gastrointestinal epithelial cells is accelerated. On the other hand, granulocytes show delayed apoptosis during sepsis. It remains unclear why these white cell populations behave differently. Apoptotic cell death can limit the inflammatory response and may act as an important regulator of the balance between pro- and anti-inflammatory stimuli. For example, apoptosis is an important mechanism of lymphocyte death during viral and bacterial infections and granulocyte apoptosis contributes to resolution of the inflammatory response.

The influence of genetic variation

It has long been recognized that individuals vary considerably in their susceptibility to infection, as well as in their ability to recover from apparently similar infectious illnesses or traumatic insults. More than 20 years ago, it was convincingly demonstrated that premature death in adults, especially when due to infectious causes, is a strongly heritable trait (Sorensen *et al.*, 1988). Since then a number of relatively small studies have suggested that interindividual variations in susceptibility to, and outcome from, severe sepsis/septic shock can be partly explained by polymorphisms of the genes encoding proteins involved in mediating and controlling innate immunity and the inflammatory response. For example, individuals homozygous for an allele (TNFB2) located in an intron of the TNF locus were found to have higher circulating levels of TNF-α and an increased mortality if they develop severe sepsis, when compared to heterozygotes and individuals hormozygous for the TNFB1 allele (Stüber *et al.*, 1996). Similarly, the frequency of TNF2, a polymorphism within the promotor region of the TNF-α gene, was found to be higher among septic shock patients who died than in those who survived and the risk of death was significantly increased in patients with this allele (Mira *et al.*, 1999). Susceptibility to sepsis may also be influenced by such polymorphisms; for example, the TNF2 allele has been strongly associated with susceptibility to septic shock (Mira *et al.*, 1999) and variants of the gene for mannose-binding lectin (which are associated with reduced circulating levels of the encoded protein) have been linked to susceptibility to meningococcal disease (Hibberd *et al.*, 1999), as well as being more common in patients with severe sepsis/septic shock (Gordon *et al.*, 2006).

At present, however, such candidate gene association studies should be interpreted cautiously, not least because the functional importance of these polymorphisms is frequently uncertain and they may simply represent a genomic marker for other more functionally relevant genetic variations. Disappointingly, failure to replicate positive findings is a common experience and findings are often conflicting. Thus, for example, in a more recent study in a larger cohort of septic patients, there were no significant associations between a number of candidate TNF or TNF receptor polymorphisms and susceptibility to sepsis, illness severity or outcome (Gordon *et al.*, 2004). Much larger studies (thousands, rather than hundreds, of patients), with more comprehensive genotyping, replication and allied functional studies will be required to resolve these uncertainties.

HAEMODYNAMIC CHANGES
Cardiogenic shock *(Hasdai et al., 2000)*

The clinical features of cardiogenic shock are generally seen when the cardiac index falls to around 1.8 l/min per m^2 or less. Heart rate and systemic vascular resistance increase in an attempt to maintain blood pressure. This may lead to a vicious circle in which increasing myocardial oxygen consumption causes an extension of ischaemic areas and a decrease in myocardial compliance with a further reduction in cardiac output. Ventricular filling pressures are usually high, although relative hypovolaemia is sometimes precipitated by therapy with vasodilators or diuretics, combined with volume losses into the lungs, and may coexist with persisting chest radiographic evidence of pulmonary oedema. The patient may then benefit from cautious volume expansion. Cardiogenic shock may also be associated with a low pulmonary artery occlusion pressure (PAOP) in those with right ventricular infarction. In some cases of right ventricular infarction, however, PAOP may be unexpectedly high because of leftward shift of the intraventricular septum (reversed Bernheim effect) or concomitant left ventricular dysfunction. When cardiogenic shock is caused by a ventricular septal defect, valvular incompetence or a ventricular aneurysm, a proportion of ventricular ejection fails to reach the systemic circulation.

Obstructive shock
CARDIAC TAMPONADE
Increasing intrapericardial pressure progressively reduces ventricular volumes and increases diastolic pressures. This is associated with corresponding increases in right and left atrial pressures, although sometimes, for example following cardiac surgery, one or other filling pressure may rise earlier, and to a greater extent, than the other. Cardiac transmural pressures fall and in extreme tamponade may become negative, in which case the ventricles probably fill by diastolic suction. Ultimately, the ventricles may fill only during atrial systole, particularly at rapid heart rates. Reduced ventricular filling leads to a reduction in ventricular systolic pressure, stroke volume and cardiac output. There is a compensatory tachycardia and vasoconstriction, while ejection fraction is initially maintained or even increased. Eventually, compensation fails and blood pressure falls. In extreme tamponade the rise in diastolic pressures may precipitate myocardial ischaemia, although in less severe cases the reduction in coronary flow may be offset by decreased myocardial work.

PULMONARY EMBOLISM
See page 130.

Hypovolaemic shock
Cardiac output falls as a result of the reduction in ventricular preload and there is a compensatory rise in systemic vascular resistance, venoconstriction and tachycardia. Blood flow is diverted away from less important areas in order to maintain perfusion of vital organs. The pulse pressure is narrowed and tachycardia almost invariably precedes the development of hypotension. Blood pressure is usually maintained until the circulating blood volume is reduced by more than 20–25%. Ventricular filling pressures are usually low, although their response to a fluid challenge provides a more accurate assessment of the extent of volume losses. Later in the evolution of severe hypovolaemic shock there may be a paradoxical bradycardia. In some cases myocardial contractility is impaired by ischaemia, infarction, pre-existing cardiac disease or, later, by the effects of complicating sepsis (see later).

Distributive shock
ANAPHYLAXIS
See page 128.

SEPTIC SHOCK (Parrillo et al., 1990)
The dominant haemodynamic feature of septic shock is *peripheral vascular failure*; persistent vasodilation, refractory to vasoconstrictors, is characteristic of non-survivors (Groeneveld et al., 1986). Provided hypovolaemia has been corrected, cardiac output is usually high: a low cardiac index is relatively uncommon, even in the very late stages of septic

shock (Parrillo et al., 1990). Nevertheless it is now recognized that *myocardial depression* is a common feature and is usually manifested as a decreased ejection fraction, with a reduced left ventricular stroke work, which responds poorly to volume loading (Ellrodt et al., 1985; Ognibene et al., 1988; Parker et al., 1984; Suffredini et al., 1989). Despite the reduced ejection fraction, stroke volume is generally maintained by ventricular dilatation, probably related to increased myocardial compliance (Ognibene et al., 1988; Parker et al., 1984; Suffredini et al., 1989), and tachycardia is responsible for the high cardiac output.

As well as this global myocardial dysfunction, *reversible segmental left ventricular abnormalities* have also been noted in patients with septic shock, most often in those with underlying heart disease (Ellrodt et al., 1985). Although in this study there were no differences in left ventricular ejection fraction, left ventricular stroke work or the frequency of segmental dysfunction between survivors and non survivors (Ellrodt et al., 1985), others have noted that reversible ventricular dilatation with a reduced ejection fraction is seen more commonly in those who survive (Parrillo et al., 1990). The latter observation may be explained by a greater degree of myocardial oedema, or right ventricular distension, which could impede left ventricular dilatation in non-survivors. Moreover, extreme vasodilatation in non-survivors would tend to minimize the reduction in ejection fraction and the degree of ventricular dilatation. Similar abnormalities also affect the right ventricle in septic shock (Parker et al., 1990). The precise relationship between cardiac output and outcome from septic shock remains unclear. Whereas some authors have noted that cardiac output and oxygen delivery are higher in survivors (Tuchschmidt et al., 1989), and that myocardial depression characterizes non-survivors (Vincent et al., 1992), others have been unable to demonstrate such a relationship (Dhainaut et al., 1987).

It seems unlikely that these alterations in ventricular performance are attributable to global myocardial ischaemia since coronary blood flow is normal or increased and the myocardial oxygen content difference is narrowed in patients with septic shock (Cunnion et al., 1986). These findings do not, however, exclude focal myocardial ischaemia due to regional reductions in flow (Dhainaut et al., 1987) or microcirculatory abnormalities. Ischaemia may also occur in those with pre-existing coronary artery disease.

Ventricular performance may be impaired in septic shock by a circulating *myocardial-depressant substance*, the presence of which correlates quantitatively with the decrease in left ventricular ejection fraction (Parrillo et al., 1985). In the normal heart NO plays an important physiological role by regulating oxygen supply via changes in vascular tone and by altering determinants of oxygen demand such as heart rate, contractility, relaxation and ventricular filling. In sepsis, however, excess production of NO contributes to myocardial depression through increased production of cGMP and formation of peroxynitrite (Walley, 2000). On the other hand, increased NO production may contribute to the increase in ventricular diastolic compliance which is important for the maintenance of stroke volume in sepsis (see above). Other factors that may contribute to myocardial depression in shock include intracellular acidosis, hypoxaemia, myocardial oedema and downregulation of adrenergic receptors.

MICROCIRCULATORY CHANGES

In *septic shock* there is:

- vasodilatation;
- maldistribution of regional flow;
- abnormalities in the microcirculation:
  - 'stop-flow' capillaries (flow is intermittent);
  - 'no-flow' capillaries (capillaries are obstructed);
  - failure of capillary recruitment;
  - increased capillary permeability with interstitial oedema.

In patients with severe sepsis microvascular density was found to be reduced, especially amongst the small vessels, and there were a large number of non-perfused and intermittently perfused small vessels with marked heterogeneity. These abnormalities were more severe in non-survivors (De Backer *et al.*, 2002).

Endothelial injury is mediated by a number of factors, including intravascular thrombosis, microemboli, release of vasoactive compounds and complement activation, as well as by the adhesion and extravascular migration of leukocytes (see above and Chapter 8, acute respiratory distress syndrome). Capillary permeability is thereby increased so that fluid is lost into the interstitial space, causing further hypovolaemia, oedema and organ dysfunction. The detection of circulating endothelial cells in patients with septic shock supports the concept that widespread endothelial damage occurs in human sepsis (Mutunga *et al.*, 2001).

Although these *vascular and microcirculatory* abnormalities may partly account for the reduced oxygen extraction often seen in patients with sepsis, there is probably also a *primary defect in cellular oxygen utilization* due to mitochondrial dysfunction (Adrie *et al.*, 2001; Brealey *et al.*, 2002). These changes are associated with impaired utilization of available oxygen, a reduced arteriovenous oxygen content difference, an increased S_vO_2 and lactic acidosis (so-called *tissue dysoxia*) (see also Supply dependency, p. 95, and Goal-directed therapy, pp. 118–119). Vasodilatation and increased vascular permeability also occur in anaphylactic shock (see below).

In the initial stages of other forms of shock, and sometimes when hypovolaemia supervenes in sepsis and anaphylaxis, cardiac output is low and increased sympathetic activity causes constriction of precapillary arterioles and, to a lesser extent, the postcapillary venules. This helps to maintain systemic blood pressure. Furthermore, the hydrostatic pressure within the capillaries falls and fluid is mobilized from the extravascular space into the intravascular compartment. This *transcapillary refill*, combined with the salt and water retention described above, to some extent restores the circulating volume and promotes flow by reducing viscosity.

If shock persists, the accumulation of metabolites, such as lactic acid and carbon dioxide, combined with the release of vasoactive substances, causes relaxation of the precapillary sphincters, while the postcapillary venules, which are more sensitive to hypoxic damage, become relatively unresponsive to these substances and remain constricted. Blood is therefore sequestered within the dilated capillary bed and fluid is forced into the interstitial spaces. Combined with the increase in capillary permeability, this causes *interstitial oedema, haemoconcentration* and an *increase in viscosity*. Blood also becomes more viscous at low flow rates, since the streaming effect, which normally channels red blood cells (RBCs) down the centre of vessels, is reduced. In addition, erythrocyte and neutrophil deformability is decreased, impairing passage of these cells through the microcirculation. These changes are compounded by endothelial swelling, increased neutrophil adherence to the endothelium and aggregation of platelets, red cells and leukocytes with fibrin deposition. Shocked patients are therefore highly susceptible to procoagulant stimuli.

Activation of the coagulation system *(Fig. 5.10)*

The release of inflammatory mediators in response to shock, tissue injury and infection is associated with systemic activation of the clotting cascade (for example, through the expression of tissue factor) leading to *platelet aggregation* and *thrombosis* that is usually microvascular though, occasionally, macrovascular. The production of PGI_2 by the vascular endothelium may be impaired. Cell damage (for example, to the vascular endothelium) leads to exposure to tissue factor and the release of tissue thromboplastin, whilst activated factor XII cleaves factor XI to XIa. In severe cases these changes are compounded by elevated levels of plasminogen activator inhibitor type I, which impairs fibrinolysis, as well as by deficiencies in physiological inhibitors of coagulation (including antithrombin III, proteins C and S and tissue factor pathway inhibitor). Importantly, antithrombin III and protein C have a number of anti-inflammatory properties whereas thrombin is proinflammatory. This combination of procoagulant and inflammatory stimuli therefore provides a potent mechanism for initiating and perpetuating microvascular injury, intravascular coagulation, inadequate tissue perfusion and organ failure. Not surprisingly, high levels of plasminogen activator inhibitor type I and low levels of antithrombin III and protein C have been associated with a poor outcome from septic shock (Lorente *et al.*, 1993).

Ultimately, unregulated activation of the coagulation cascade can progress to *disseminated intravascular coagulation* (DIC), which is characterized by widespread microvascular thrombosis, and is associated with an increased risk of mortality. This hypercoagulable state leads to the depletion of clotting factors and platelets and a paradoxical coagulation defect (hence the alternative term for DIC of *consumption coagulopathy*). This is associated with abnormal bleeding (e.g. from surgical wounds or venepuncture sites), haematuria, bleeding from the nose or gums and ecchymoses. Plas-

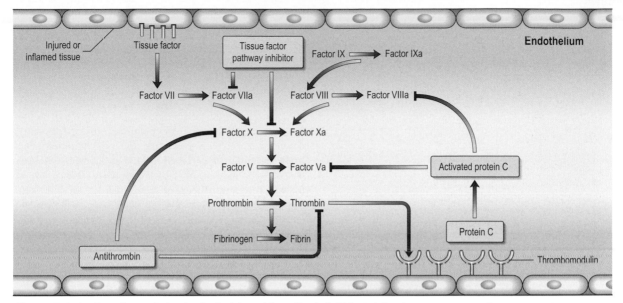

Fig. 5.10 Activation of coagulation in shock. Adapted from Marshall JC (2004) Sepsis: current status, future prospects. Current Opinion in Critical Care 10: 257.

minogen is converted to plasmin, which breaks down thrombus, liberating fibrin/fibrinogen degradation products (FDPs). Circulating levels of FDPs (e.g. D-dimers) are therefore increased, the platelet count and fibrinogen levels fall, and the prothrombin time, thrombin time and partial thromboplastin time are prolonged. Activation of the coagulation cascade can be confirmed by demonstrating increased levels of D-dimers. In some cases a *microangiopathic haemolytic anaemia* develops. DIC is particularly associated with severe sepsis/septic shock, especially when due to meningococcal infection.

Reperfusion injury (see Fig 5.9)

If resuscitation is successful and flow through the microcirculation is restored, tissue damage may be exacerbated by the generation of large quantities of ROS and activation of phospholipase A_2. The gut mucosa may be particularly vulnerable to this reperfusion injury (Schoenberg and Beger, 1993).

SUPPLY DEPENDENCY

A number of studies have suggested that, in apparently stable critically ill patients, especially those with the acute respiratory distress syndrome (ARDS), MOF and sepsis, oxygen consumption ($\dot{V}O_2$) often rises if oxygen delivery (DO_2) is actively increased (e.g. with fluid loading, prostacyclin, catecholamines or blood transfusion) and falls in response to reductions in oxygen transport (e.g. induced by the application of positive end-expiratory pressure: PEEP) (Danek *et al.*, 1980; Gilbert *et al.*, 1986; Kruse *et al.*, 1990). This linear relationship between $\dot{V}O_2$ and DO_2, termed *pathological supply dependency*, contrasts with normal physiology, where in resting subjects $\dot{V}O_2$ remains constant once a critical DO_2

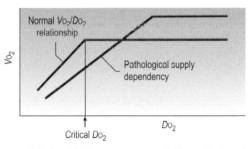

Fig. 5.11 Relationship between oxygen delivery (DO_2) and oxygen consumption ($\dot{V}O_2$).

is exceeded and exercise-induced increases in $\dot{V}O_2$ are met by an appropriate increase in DO_2 (**Fig. 5.11**).

Pathological supply dependency is probably largely a consequence of maldistribution of flow in the microcirculation, predominantly related to inappropriate vasodilation, but is likely to be exacerbated by microemboli, intravascular thrombosis, interstitial oedema and localized vasoconstriction (see above). These microcirculatory disturbances are often combined with defective cellular oxygen utilization. As a result, oxygen extraction is impaired, mixed venous oxygen saturation (SO_2) rises, arteriovenous oxygen content difference ($C_{a-v}O_2$) is narrowed, and the slope of the $\dot{V}O_2/DO_2$ relationship is flattened to the right, with an increase in the critical DO_2. In addition, $\dot{V}O_2$ may be increased as a result of the hypermetabolic response to illness or injury, although notably, $\dot{V}O_2$ may fall with increasing severity of illness.

It might be anticipated that these abnormalities would be associated with an oxygen debt. In some studies supply dependency has, as predicted, been accompanied by lactic acidosis (Gilbert *et al.*, 1986; Kruse *et al.*, 1990). Others, however, have not been able to confirm a relationship between supply dependency and lactic acidosis (Phang *et al.*, 1994). It has also proved difficult to demonstrate that the critical DO_2 can be exceeded (and the plateau attained) in apparently supply-dependent patients. Not surprisingly, therefore, this phenomenon has given rise to considerable controversy and for a number of reasons studies investigating $DO_2/\dot{V}O_2$ relationships should be interpreted cautiously:

■ DO_2 is calculated as the product of Q_t and C_aO_2. In many studies $\dot{V}O_2$ has been derived using the reverse Fick equation, that is, $\dot{V}O_2 = Q_t \times (C_aO_2 - C_vO_2)$. The presence of the shared variables Q_t and C_aO_2 may give rise to 'mathematical coupling' in which, for example, an erroneously high determination of Q_t will translate into increases in both DO_2 and $\dot{V}O_2$. Although the magnitude and relevance of this effect have been disputed, in one study of clinically resuscitated patients with ARDS there was evidence to suggest that mathematical coupling of random error in the measurement of shared variables could explain an apparent dependence of Fick derived $\dot{V}O_2$ on DO_2 (Phang *et al.*, 1994).

■ When adrenergic agents are used to boost DO_2, their calorigenic effect may directly increase $\dot{V}O_2$, leading to apparent supply dependency.

■ Importantly, $\dot{V}O_2$ may vary spontaneously (Villar *et al.*, 1990), as well as in response to minor disturbances and therapeutic interventions such as chest physiotherapy (Weissman and Kemper, 1991) and the associated appropriate increase in DO_2 may then be wrongly interpreted as indicating supply dependency.

■ In septic shock the $\dot{V}O_2$ response to an increase in oxygen transport may vary from time to time in the same patient (Palazzo and Suter, 1991).

■ It is unclear for how long patients could continue to accumulate an oxygen debt without succumbing.

■ The significance of lactic acidosis in patients with sepsis is not clear (see p. 105).

■ The critical DO_2 in critically ill patients may be considerably lower than previously reported and may not be altered by sepsis (Ronco *et al.*, 1993).

■ The relationship between pathological supply dependency and prognosis remains unclear (Palazzo and Suter, 1991).

Some have therefore questioned the relevance of supply dependency in stable, adequately resuscitated critically ill patients. Many now prefer to use the term *tissue dysoxia*, in which the ability of systemic tissues to extract or utilize the available oxygen is compromised and impaired oxidative metabolism is resistant to increases in DO_2 (Hayes *et al.*, 1997).

ORGAN DYSFUNCTION

The precise mechanisms responsible for the organ dysfunction often associated with sepsis remain unclear, as do the reasons for its persistence after the acute inflammatory response has resolved. Inflammation, apoptosis, toxin-induced cellular injury and tissue ischaemia/hypoxia caused by haemodynamic and microcirculatory abnormalities have all been implicated; indeed, persistent microcirculatory alterations have been associated with organ failure and death in patients with septic shock (Sakr *et al.*, 2004). There is, however, increasing evidence to suggest that the predominant defect may be tissue dysoxia and *bioenergetic failure* caused by mitochondrial dysfunction (Adrie *et al.*, 2001; Brealey *et al.*, 2002). For example, the mitochondrial membrane potential of peripheral blood monocytes has been shown to be reduced in sepsis (Adrie *et al.*, 2001), and in patients with septic shock mitochondrial dysfunction (inhibition of complex I activity) has been associated with NO overproduction, reduced levels of the antioxidant glutathione and ATP depletion (Brealey *et al.*, 2002). Further, these abnormalities were related to organ failure and outcome. The observation that histological abnormalities are often relatively minor given the degree of organ dysfunction, and that, in those who survive, organ function usually recovers rapidly, has led some to suggest that organ dysfunction in sepsis can be explained by 'cell hibernation' or 'cell stunning', during which cellular processes are reduced to basic 'housekeeping' roles (Hotchkiss and Karl, 2003).

Autoregulation of organ flow

The most vital organs of the body, such as the brain and heart, are relatively protected from the ill effects of alterations in blood pressure by their ability, within certain limits, to maintain blood flow at a constant level despite changes in perfusion pressure (**Fig. 5.12**). This *autoregulation* is an intrinsic property of some vascular smooth muscle and is independent of its innervation. It is lost when the vessels become rigid (e.g. due to atheroma), and the limits for autoregulation are reset at higher levels in those with pre-existing hypertension (see **Fig. 5.12**).

Because sympathetic tone is often high in shocked patients, the autoregulation curve is shifted to the right (i.e. tissue flow will fall at higher pressures than in normal subjects). Later in the evolution of shock and in sepsis, vasoparesis may occur (see above), and under these circumstances autoregulation may fail (i.e. flow becomes passive and pressure-dependent) (see Fig. 5.12). Furthermore, dilatation of healthy vessels in the presence of atheroma elsewhere may 'steal' blood from areas supplied by diseased vessels. This can cause, for example, symptoms of cerebral ischaemia, particularly in the elderly.

Heart

Despite the ability of the coronary circulation to autoregulate, and the reduction in myocardial oxygen consumption which usually occurs when perfusion falls, reversible myocardial dysfunction may develop during shock of any aetiology and may complicate a wide range of other severe illnesses associated with inflammation and metabolic stress such as trauma, pancreatitis, anaphylaxis, traumatic brain injury and ARDS (see above). *Myocardial ischaemia*, affecting par-

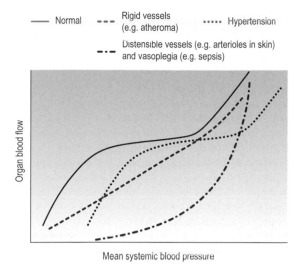

Fig. 5.12 Autoregulation of organ blood flow. Flow to vital organs is normally maintained constant over a wide range of perfusion pressures. When vessels are rigid (e.g. due to atheroma), flow is linearly related to pressure. Passive flow occurs in distensible vessels (e.g. normal arterioles in skin, sepsis) and those in ischaemic areas with toxic arteriolar paralysis. In hypertensive subjects the limits for autoregulation are reset at a higher level.

ticularly the vulnerable endocardial layer, may be an important cause of this reduction in cardiac performance, although its contribution to myocardial depression in septic shock is uncertain (see above). When systemic blood pressure falls below a certain critical level, myocardial blood flow is inevitably reduced, especially when the ability of the coronary circulation to autoregulate is impaired by atheroma. Myocardial ischaemia could be exacerbated by coronary steal, a reduction in the distensibility of collateral vessels and obstruction of capillary flow by myocardial oedema. Furthermore, the local effects of cellular hypoxia can cause abnormalities of excitation and contraction with the development of arrhythmias and impaired myocardial function. Circulating myocardial-depressant substances, free radicals, cytokines and ischaemia–reperfusion injury may also contribute to cardiac dysfunction in shock.

Lungs

In the early stages of shock, the reduction in pulmonary blood flow and perfusion pressure leads to $\dot{V}/\dot{Q}$ *inequalities* with an increased dead space, while in hyperdynamic patients the $\dot{V}/\dot{Q}$ ratio will be low. The patient usually develops a tachypnoea in response to metabolic acidosis and chemoreceptor stimulation, so that P_aCO_2 is often reduced whereas P_aO_2 may be either normal or low. Later, *respiratory muscle fatigue* may supervene, in part because of reduced perfusion; rarely a reduction in cerebral blood flow may *depress the respiratory centre.*

Patients in whom shock is severe and prolonged may develop respiratory failure 12–48 hours after the initial episode. Previously, this was referred to as the *shock lung syndrome*, and it is one cause of acute lung injury (ALI)/ ARDS (see Chapter 8). The development of ALI/ARDS in shock is almost invariably associated with sepsis and is a rare sequel of pure hypovolaemia. Similarly, sepsis is frequently associated with respiratory dysfunction.

Finally, respiratory failure associated with shock may be caused or exacerbated by other factors such as:

- aspiration of gastric contents;
- fluid overload;
- lung contusion;
- thermal inhalation injury;
- pulmonary infection;
- oxygen toxicity.

(These subjects are discussed elsewhere.)

Kidneys

Oliguria is almost invariable in the shocked patient and may be prerenal, renal or postrenal. Prerenal oliguria will respond to volume expansion; resuscitation should be achieved as rapidly as possible to prevent progression to established acute renal failure. In the early stages autoregulation maintains the glomerular filtration rate (GFR) and oliguria is related to increased circulating levels of ADH and aldosterone. Subsequently, oliguria may be exacerbated by a fall in GFR. Postrenal causes, such as *urethral damage in trauma patients*, must also be excluded (see Chapter 13). A few patients with severe sepsis/septic shock may develop an inappropriate polyuria despite hypovolaemia.

Central nervous system *(Papadopoulos et al., 2000)*

Although the central nervous system is well protected from the ill effects of hypotension by autoregulation and the cerebral vasodilation induced when patients are hypoxic or hypercarbic (see Chapter 15), reversible cerebral dysfunction is a common feature of shock.

Patients with severe sepsis are particularly liable to develop acute disturbances of cerebral function. This may present as restlessness, irritability, agitation, disorientation, confusion, lethargy, somnolence, stupor or even coma and may be due to:

- inadequate cerebral perfusion;
- renal or liver failure;
- metabolic disturbances – electrolyte imbalance, acid–base disorders, hypo- or hyperglycaemia, hypo- or hyperthermia, hypoxaemia, endocrine disturbances;
- the effects of drug administration;
- meningoencephalitis (occasionally);
- a specific encephalopathy.

Early or *septic encephalopathy* presents before the onset of MOF whereas late encephalopathy occurs in association with failure of other vital organs. Encephalopathy may occur in up to 70% of septic patients and is probably largely explained by the effects of inflammatory mediators on the cerebral microvasculature (see above). Damage to astrocytes and changes in the number and activity of receptors may also be important. There are, however, a number of striking similarities between the hypercatabolic response to sepsis and the metabolic changes associated with the encephalopathy of liver failure (see Chapter 14). There is some evidence that septic encephalopathy can be attributed to similar alterations in plasma and brain amino acid profiles. In sepsis, increased muscle protein breakdown combined with impaired hepatic metabolism leads to elevated plasma levels of sulphur-containing and aromatic amino acids (AAA), the increase in sulphur-containing amino acids being somewhat greater than in hepatic encephalopathy. Plasma levels of branched-chain amino acids (BCAA) are normal or, in some cases, slightly reduced, perhaps because of increased oxidation in muscle and fat. Combined with altered amino acid transport across the blood–brain barrier, these changes lead to increased concentrations of AAA within the brain. Consequently, the activity of serotinergic pathways is increased, cerebral concentrations of adrenergic neurotransmitters fall and levels of 'false neurotransmitters' such as octopamine and phenylethanolamine increase.

There is some evidence that administration of BCAA to patients with sepsis may normalize the plasma amino acid profile, as well as competing with AAAs for transport across the blood–brain barrier. Brain amino acid and neurotransmitter profiles may be returned to normal and this could potentially improve or reverse the encephalopathy.

There seems to be an association between the severity of the encephalopathy and prognosis in sepsis. In those who survive, however, full recovery of cerebral function can be anticipated unless hypotension is particularly severe and prolonged, there is pre-existing cerebrovascular disease or the patient has a cerebrovascular accident.

Liver

The liver is, to some extent, protected from ischaemic damage, not only by its ability to autoregulate, but also by its dual blood supply. Nevertheless, the reduction in hepatic arterial and portal flow frequently leads to a *benign and reversible conjugated hyperbilirubinaemia* and also *impairs the reticuloendothelial function* of the liver. The latter exacerbates bacteraemia/endotoxaemia. Hepatic dysfunction may also lead to increased lactate production, a raised blood ammonia and elevated aminotransferases. The liver is particularly vulnerable when hepatic venous congestion is combined with a reduction in arterial flow, as occurs for example in cardiac tamponade. In the most severe cases overt hepatic failure (see Chapter 14) may develop and, although rare, this is often irreversible.

Hepatosplanchnic circulation

The gut is the largest immune organ in the body and behaves as a unit with the liver anatomically, functionally and metabolically.

In *hypovolaemic* and *cardiogenic shock*, marked compensatory vasoconstriction in the splanchnic bed redistributes flow to more immediately vital organs and may increase the circulating blood volume by as much as 30%. These changes in splanchnic vascular resistance cause substantial alterations in total peripheral resistance and may account for almost all of the increase seen in hypovolaemic and cardiogenic shock. In *septic shock*, particularly when volume replacement has been adequate, splanchnic flow is markedly increased and parallels changes in cardiac output.

When the reduction in intestinal perfusion pressure and/or blood flow is only modest, autoregulation and a compensatory increase in oxygen extraction normally prevent mucosal injury; following brief episodes of more serious reductions in flow, damage may be limited to an increase in capillary permeability, caused largely by ROS generated during reperfusion (see above). More prolonged episodes of hypoperfusion are, however, associated with significant ischaemic injury, which is initially confined to the superficial layer of the mucosa. Characteristically, mucosal damage starts as a small lesion at the tip of the villus; the villi may then become denuded. Finally, the entire villous layer becomes necrotic. Gastrointestinal injury in low-output shock and following partial ischaemia occasionally involves the deeper layers and is substantially exacerbated by reperfusion (see above). *Complete vascular occlusion,* on the other hand, produces a rapid progression of injury from increased mucosal permeability seen after only about 30 minutes to complete loss of villi at 1 hour, transmucosal necrosis after 4 hours and transmural infarction within 8–16 hours. Reperfusion injury does not appear to play an important role.

Mucosal injury in *sepsis,* when splanchnic flow and $\dot{V}O_2$ are increased (Meier-Hellmann *et al.*, 1996), may be explained by maldistribution of microcirculatory flow, a cellular defect in oxidative metabolism and by a marked increase in splanchnic oxygen demand (Ruokonen *et al.*, 1993). As a result of the latter, oxygen extraction may rise and portal venous PO_2 falls, and this may contribute to hepatic hypoxia.

It has been suggested that, in severe shock of any aetiology, loss of mucosal integrity within the gastrointestinal tract may allow increased bacterial translocation and the passage of endotoxin and other bacterial cell wall components into the portal venous system. Activation of liver macrophages and systemic bacteraemia/endotoxaemia combine to amplify the systemic inflammatory response, thereby contributing to the development and persistence of sepsis and MOF (see later). This concept is supported by experimental investigations and by studies in humans suggesting that intestinal permeability may increase in sepsis and following burns or major trauma. Moreover, in these conditions endotoxin has been found in the systemic circulation. Nevertheless, the relevance of these findings to the pathogenesis of sepsis and organ failure has been questioned (Lemaire *et al.*, 1997).

Mucosal vasoconstriction (e.g. in response to hypovolaemia) increases the susceptibility of the gastric mucosa to acid-mediated damage and this may result in subclinical or, less often, frank bleeding. In sepsis, a reduction in gastric mucosal flow is not consistently found, but ischaemia may result from an increased oxygen demand and impaired oxygen extraction. Splanchnic ischaemia may also damage the pancreas (*shock pancreas*) (Lamy *et al.*, 1987) with the systemic release of pancreatic enzymes and myocardial-depressant factors.

METABOLIC RESPONSE (see also Chapters 11 and 17)

This is initiated and controlled by the neuroendocrine system and various cytokines (e.g. IL-6) acting in concert, and is characterized initially by an increase in energy expenditure (*hypermetabolism*). Gluconeogenesis is stimulated by increased glucagon and catecholamine levels, whilst hepatic mobilization of glucose from glycogen is increased. Catecholamines inhibit insulin release and reduce peripheral glucose uptake. Combined with elevated circulating levels of other insulin antagonists such as cortisol and downregulation of insulin receptors, these changes ensure that the majority of patients are hyperglycaemic (*insulin resistance*). Later hypoglycaemia may be precipitated by depletion of liver glycogen stores and inhibition of gluconeogenesis. Free fatty acid synthesis is also increased, leading to *hypertriglyceridaemia*.

Protein breakdown is initiated to provide energy from amino acids and hepatic protein synthesis is preferentially augmented to produce acute-phase reactants (see above). The conditionally essential amino acid glutamine is mobilized from muscle for use as a metabolic fuel by rapidly dividing cells such as leukocytes and enterocytes. Glutamine is also required for hepatic production of the antioxidant glutathione. When severe and prolonged, this *catabolic response* can lead to considerable weight loss. Protein breakdown is associated with wasting and weakness of skeletal and respiratory muscle, prolonging the need for mechanical ventilation and delaying mobilization. Tissue repair, wound healing and immune function may also be compromised.

CLINICAL FEATURES OF SHOCK

HYPOVOLAEMIC SHOCK

The aetiology of hypovolaemic shock is usually clinically obvious (e.g. trauma, surgery, burns or intestinal obstruction), although gastrointestinal haemorrhage may be concealed, at least initially.

Signs of inadequate tissue perfusion in shock include:

- cold, pale, slate-grey skin – 'clammy';
- slow capillary refill;
- oliguria or anuria;
- drowsiness, confusion and irritability (in severe cases).

Increased sympathetic activity produces vasoconstriction, which, although helping to maintain blood pressure, further reduces tissue blood flow and causes:

- tachycardia;
- a narrowed pulse pressure, 'weak' or 'thready' pulse;
- sweating.

Sometimes, pre-existing heart disease or the administration of β-blockers limits the tachycardia. As shock becomes more severe, the skin changes spread further proximally and *extreme hypovolaemia may be associated with bradycardia*. Hypotension is an unreliable sign, particularly in hypovolaemic shock, since blood pressure may be maintained despite the loss of up to 35% of the circulating volume in young people. On the other hand, such a patient will exhibit all the signs of compensatory sympathetic activity just described. It is therefore not adequate simply to restore blood pressure in shock and treatment must be continued until the tachycardia has settled, peripheral perfusion is improved and urine flow is adequate.

In the initial stages of shock, the patient is often *tachypnoeic*, either due to associated chest or lung injury or in an attempt to compensate for a metabolic acidosis. The development of a tachypnoea some time after the onset of shock is often the first sign of the development of ALI/ARDS or, occasionally, the fat embolism syndrome.

CARDIOGENIC SHOCK (Hasdai *et al.*, 2000)

Cardiogenic shock has been defined as a systolic blood pressure less than 80 or 90 mmHg (or a fall of more than 30 mmHg from the premorbid value) with evidence of reduced perfusion such as oliguria (urine output < 0.5 ml/kg per hour), impaired mental function and peripheral vasoconstriction caused by cardiac dysfunction. Hypotension due to vasovagal reactions, serious arrhythmias, drug reactions or hypovolaemia must first be excluded.

The clinical features of cardiogenic shock are the same as those described for hypovolaemic shock with the addition of the signs of cardiac failure. These may include:

- an elevated jugular venous pressure (JVP);
- basal end-inspiratory crepitations;
- pulsus alternans;
- a triple rhythm.

In some cases there may be frank pulmonary oedema with severe dyspnoea and central cyanosis. Clinical examination may also reveal the aetiology of cardiogenic shock (e.g. a pansystolic murmur appearing after a myocardial infarction suggests mitral regurgitation or a new ventricular septal defect).

There is some evidence that the death rate among patients with cardiogenic shock has fallen over the last decade from more than 70% to less than 60%.

OBSTRUCTIVE SHOCK
Cardiac tamponade

The clinical features of cardiac tamponade resemble those of congestive cardiac failure, except that the lungs are nearly always clear (probably because the reduction in right ventricular output prevents pulmonary engorgement). Most patients are relatively or absolutely hypotensive and the neck veins are distended. When tamponade is due to massive haemorrhage (e.g. due to penetrating cardiac injury or aortic rupture), shock is the dominant feature.

Heart sounds are usually muffled, but are often better heard over the base of the heart. Sometimes there is relative accentuation of the pulmonary component of the second heart sound and in those with inflammatory or neoplastic lesions there may be a pericardial rub. The apex beat may be impalpable. *Kussmaul's sign* (inspiratory expansion of the neck veins) should be absent unless there is epicardial constriction as well as fluid in the pericardium. The possibility of constrictive pericarditis should also be suspected if a third heart sound is heard before or after drainage. In those with clinically significant tamponade without extreme hypotension, *pulsus paradoxus* (a decline in systolic blood pressure which exceeds 10 mmHg on a spontaneous inspiratory effort) is normally detectable on arterial palpation. Pulsus paradoxus may be absent or minimal when there is significant constriction and in those with left ventricular hypertrophy, severe left heart failure, atrial septal defect or severe aortic regurgitation. Right heart tamponade, which may be caused by loculated blood after cardiac surgery, is generally not associated with pulsus paradoxus.

Pulmonary embolism *(see p. 130)*

DISTRIBUTIVE SHOCK
Anaphylaxis *(see p. 128)*
Sepsis and septic shock
Sepsis can be defined as the systemic inflammatory response to a documented infection; it is now one of the commonest causes of death in non-coronary adult intensive care units (ICUs) and is being diagnosed with increasing frequency (Martin *et al.*, 2003; Dombrovskiy *et al.*, 2007). Although the increasing incidence of sepsis may be partly explained by a greater awareness of the condition, there has undoubtedly been a dramatic increase in the true incidence of sepsis caused by a progressive and continuing rise in the number of susceptible patients due to:

- an enlarging older population (the average age of patients with sepsis has increased consistently over time);
- increased use of cytotoxics, corticosteroids and radiotherapy;
- prolonged survival of patients with diseases that compromise immunity, such as malignancy, infection with human immunodeficiency virus (HIV), diabetes mellitus and critical illness, as well as transplant recipients;
- the more widespread use of invasive techniques such as intravascular cannulation, parenteral nutrition, urinary tract instrumentation and radical surgery;
- increasing microbial resistance.

For reasons that are at present unclear, but which may include genetic differences and social factors, the risk of developing sepsis is greater in non-whites and in males. In particular the risk is considerably increased among black men, the group in which sepsis occurs at the youngest age and is associated with the highest mortality (Martin *et al.*, 2003).

Recent estimates suggest that in the USA there may be as many as 750 000 cases of severe sepsis a year (Angus *et al.*, 2001). The estimated incidence of severe sepsis has varied from 77 to 300 cases per 100 000 of the population (Angus *et al.*, 2001; Brun-Buisson *et al.*, 2004; Finfer *et al.*, 2004a; Martin *et al.*, 2003). The in-hospital incidence of severe sepsis in academic medical centres has been conservatively estimated at 2 per 100 admissions (Sands *et al.*, 1997) and the incidence amongst patients in French ICUs at around 6 per 100 admissions (Brun-Buisson *et al.*, 1995). More recently, the frequency of septic shock in French ICUs was reported to have increased from 7.0 to 9.1 per 100 admissions between 1993 and 2000 (Annane *et al.*, 2003). In the UK, around 27% of adult ICU admissions meet the criteria for severe sepsis in the first 24 hours after admission, approximating to 51 per 100 000 of the population (Padkin *et al.*, 2003) and in the USA the age-adjusted rate of hospitalisation for severe sepsis increased from around 67 to about 132 per 100 000 of the population from 1993–2003 (Dombrovskiy *et al.*, 2007).

Mortality rates, which are closely related to the severity of illness and the number of organs which fail (Brun-Buisson *et al.*, 1995; Martin *et al.*, 2003; Pittet *et al.*, 1996) are high (20–60%). There may be more than 200 000 deaths from severe sepsis every year in the USA (Angus *et al.*, 2001). The impact on health care expenditure and resource utilization has been considerable (annual total hospital costs for these patients in the USA has been estimated at approximately $17 billion and in Europe at €7.6 billion). Furthermore, for those who survive, the risk of death is increased for up to 5 years after the septic episode (Quartin *et al.*, 1997) and quality of life is significantly reduced (see Chapter 2). There is, however, some evidence to suggest that, despite an increase in the average age of patients with sepsis and in the proportion of those with organ failure, mortality rates have declined during the 1990s from 28% to 18% in those with sepsis (Martin *et al.*, 2003) from 46% to 38% in those with severe sepsis (Dombrovskiy *et al.*, 2007) and from 62% to 56% in those with septic shock (Annane *et al.*, 2003). These reductions in mortality are probably largely explained by non-specific improvements in standards of care, as well as the introduction and dissemination of management guidelines.

The success of attempts to reduce the high mortality associated with sepsis hinges on early recognition of life-threatening infection. Prompt institution of specific treatment and supportive measures (see later) may then prevent the development of dangerous sequelae such as shock and vital organ failure, and improve outcome.

Signs of sepsis include:

- pyrexia or hypothermia;
- rigors;
- sweating;

- nausea;
- vomiting;
- tachypnoea;
- tachycardia;
- hyperdynamic circulation (warm, pink peripheries, rapid capillary refill and a bounding pulse);
- occasionally, signs of cutaneous vasoconstriction.

Other manifestations of sepsis include:

- leukocytosis, leukopenia, a leukaemoid reaction, eosinopenia;
- hyperglycaemia, and, in more severe cases, hypoglycaemia.

It has been recommended that the term *severe sepsis* (previously called 'sepsis syndrome'; Bone, 1991) be used when these signs are combined with hypotension or evidence of hypoperfusion and organ dysfunction such as hypoxaemia, oliguria, lactic acidosis or altered mental function (confusion, irritability, lethargy and coma) (Bone *et al.*, 1992; Members of the American College of Chest Physicians/ Society of Critical Care Medicine Consensus Conference Committee, 1992).

Mild *liver dysfunction* with jaundice and a coagulopathy with thrombocytopenia/DIC often complicate more serious cases. The clinical signs of DIC include excessive bleeding from wounds and vascular cannulation sites, sometimes combined with a purpuric rash. Particularly severe DIC classically occurs in meningococcal sepsis and may very occasionally be associated with bilateral adrenal haemorrhage, hypoadrenalism and profound hypotension (see Chapter 17).

The diagnosis of sepsis is often difficult and a high index of suspicion is required if cases are not to be missed or diagnosed too late. The classical signs may not be present, particularly in the elderly, and mild confusion, tachycardia, tachypnoea, glucose intolerance and a rising plasma creatinine, for example, may be the only clues; sometimes these signs are associated with unexplained hypotension.

SEPTIC SHOCK
Septic shock can be defined as hypotension complicating severe sepsis despite adequate fluid resuscitation.

Patients with septic shock are usually clinically hyperdynamic ('warm shock'), but occasionally there is cutaneous vasoconstriction with cold, pale, blue extremities. Conventionally this clinical picture of 'cold shock' is interpreted as indicating a low-output state related to hypovolaemia or myocardial depression with compensatory vasoconstriction, but invasive monitoring may sometimes reveal a low total systemic vascular resistance and a high cardiac output. Nevertheless, in some patients volume replacement, combined with inotropic support when indicated, is associated with an increased cardiac output and improved peripheral perfusion. It has been suggested that the terms 'warm' and 'cold' shock are unhelpful and should be discarded (Bone, 1991).

Much of the confusion in the literature, particularly in relation to the outcome of septic shock, has been attributed

to a failure to distinguish between readily reversible episodes of hypotension and the much more serious *refractory shock*. The latter has been defined as shock unresponsive to conventional therapy (intravenous fluids with inotropic and/or vasoactive agents) within 1 hour (Bone, 1991).

SYSTEMIC INFLAMMATORY RESPONSE SYNDROME
The clinical signs of sepsis may or may not be associated with bacteraemia (defined as the presence of viable bacteria in the circulating blood). Some cases may be related to infection with fungi, pathogenic viruses or *Rickettsia*, but similar or even identical physiological responses can be produced by non-infectious processes such as pancreatitis, severe trauma, extensive tissue injury, and following prolonged, severe haemorrhagic shock. It has been recommended, therefore, that the term *systemic inflammatory response syndrome* (*SIRS*) be used to describe the disseminated inflammation that can complicate this diverse range of disorders and that the term 'sepsis' should be reserved for those patients with SIRS who have a documented infection (**Fig. 5.13**).

COMPENSATORY ANTI-INFLAMMATORY RESPONSE SYNDROME
The body attempts to control the inflammatory cascade by mounting a counterregulatory anti-inflammatory response (see earlier in this chapter) (sometimes called the *compensatory anti-inflammatory response syndrome* – CARS) (Bone, 1996) which, when inadequate, is associated with uncontrolled systemic inflammation and, when excessive, can produce immune hyporesponsiveness. The patient's progress and outcome following an inciting event are to some extent determined by the balance between pro- and anti-inflammatory influences, as well as their ability to activate and deactivate the inflammatory response appropriately (**Figs 5.14 and 5.15**). In some cases the patient may alternate between pro- and anti-inflammatory phases, perhaps

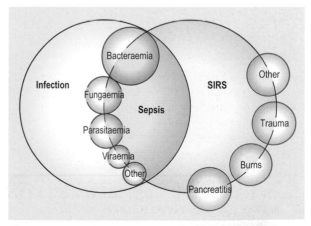

Fig. 5.13 Systemic inflammatory response syndrome (SIRS), sepsis and infection. From the Members of the American College of Chest Physicians/Society of Critical Care Medicine Consensus Conference, 1992.

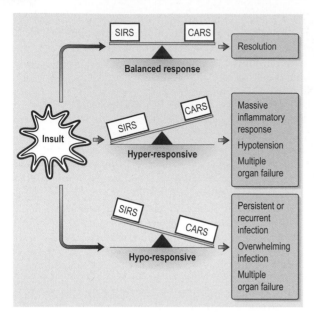

Fig. 5.14 Patterns of systemic inflammatory response. CARS, compensatory anti-inflammatory response syndrome; SIRS, systemic inflammatory response syndrome.

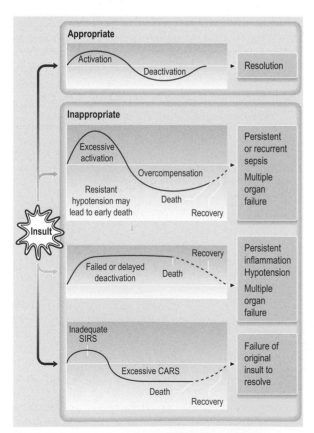

Fig. 5.15 Patterns of systemic inflammatory response. CARS, compensatory anti-inflammatory response syndrome.

gradually diminishing in intensity in those who survive (the *mixed antagonistic response syndrome* – MARS). It is also possible that the more severe the initial inflammatory response, the more likely it is to be followed by an excessive CARS. More recently it has been suggested that, outside the affected tissues, the usual response is immediate activation of anti-inflammatory mechanisms, resulting in systemic immune suppression even in the early stages of sepsis (Munford and Pugin, 2001). In an individual patient the nature of the response is influenced by a number of factors, including the virulence of the organism, the size of the inoculum, comorbidities, nutritional status, age and, probably, genetic factors.

To avoid confusion, ensure reliable communication and allow meaningful evaluation of the efficacy of new treatments, standard terminology for SIRS, sepsis, severe sepsis, septic shock and refractory shock has been proposed (**Table 5.5**). It has also been suggested that septi-

Table 5.5 Recommended standard terminology
Infection
Invasion of microorganisms into a normally sterile site, often associated with an inflammatory host response
Bacteraemia
Viable bacteria in the bloodstream
Systemic inflammatory response syndrome (SIRS)
The systemic inflammatory response to a variety of severe clinical insults. The response is manifested by two or more of the following:
■ Temperature > 38°C or < 36°C
■ Heart rate > 90 beats/min
■ Respiratory rate > 20 breaths/min or $P_a\text{CO}_2 < 4.3$ kPa
■ White cell count > 12 000 cells/mm³, <4000 cells/mm³ or > 10% immature forms
Sepsis
SIRS resulting from documented infection
Severe sepsis
Sepsis associated with organ dysfunction, hypoperfusion or hypotension. Hypoperfusion and perfusion abnormalities may include, but are not limited to, lactic acidosis, oliguria or an acute alteration in mental state
Septic shock
Severe sepsis with hypotension (systolic blood pressure < 90 mmHg or a reduction of > 40 mmHg from baseline) in the absence of other causes for hypotension, despite adequate fluid resuscitation. (Patients receiving inotropic or vasopressor agents may not be hypotensive when perfusion abnormalities are documented)
Compensatory anti-inflammatory response syndrome (CARS)
The counterregulatory response to proinflammatory stimuli
Mixed antagonistic response syndrome (MARS)
Alternating pro- and anti-inflammatory responses

Table 5.6 The PIRO (predisposition, infection, response, organ dysfunction) system for staging sepsis

Domain	Present	Future	Rationale
Predisposition	Premorbid illness with reduced probability of short-term survival. Cultural or religious beliefs, age, gender	Genetic polymorphisms in components of inflammatory response; enhanced understanding of specific interactions between pathogens and host diseases	At present premorbid factors impact on the potential attributable morbidity and mortality of an acute insult; deleterious consequences of insult may depend on genetic predisposition
Insult (infection)	Culture and sensitivity of infecting pathogens: detection of disease amenable to source control	Assay of microbial products (lipopolysaccharide, mannan, bacterial DNA); gene transcript profiles	Specific therapies directed against inciting insult require demonstration and characterization of that insult
Response	Systemic inflammatory response syndrome, other signs of sepsis, shock, C-reactive protein	Non-specific markers or activated inflammation (e.g. procalcitonin or interleukin-6) or impaired host responsiveness (e.g. HLA-DR); specific detection of target of therapy (e.g. protein C, tumour necrosis factor, platelet-activating factor)	Both mortality risk and potential to respond to therapy vary with non-specific measures of disease severity (e.g. shock); specific mediator-targeted therapy is predicated on presence and activity of mediator
Organ dysfunction	Organ dysfunction as number of failing organs or composite score (e.g. multiple-organ dysfunction syndrome, Sequential Organ Failure Assessment)	Dynamic measures of cellular response to insult: apoptosis, cytopathic dysoxia, cell stress	Response to pre-emptive therapy (e.g. targeting microorganism or early mediator) not possible if damage already present; therapies targeting the injurious cellular process require that it be present

caemia is an imprecise term and to avoid confusion should no longer be used (Bone, 1991; Bone *et al.*, 1992; Members of the American College of Chest Physicians/Society of Critical Care Medicine Consensus Conference Committee, 1992).

Although undoubtedly useful in epidemiological studies, the value of this terminology in clinical practice and when used as criteria for enrolment in clinical trials has been questioned (Abraham *et al.*, 2000; Vincent, 1997). The definition of SIRS, for example, is now widely considered to be too sensitive and non-specific (Vincent, 1997) and it is generally accepted that the frequent failure of sepsis trials to demonstrate benefit may be in part related to the use of these descriptive definitions to recruit large, heterogeneous groups of patients. It has been suggested, therefore, that in the future more precise mechanistic definitions, which would include specific immunological or biochemical criteria as well as the nature and site of infection, should be used to define more homogeneous populations in whom the intervention in question is most likely to be effective (Abraham *et al.*, 2000). To this end a system for characterizing sepsis on the basis of predisposing factors and premorbid conditions (P), the nature of the underlying infection (I), the characteristics of the host response (R) and and the extent of the resulting organ dysfunction (O) has been described – PIRO (Levy *et al.*, 2003) (**Table 5.6**).

MONITORING AND LABORATORY INVESTIGATIONS IN SHOCK (Table 5.7)

Monitoring is discussed in Chapters 4 and 6, but some particular aspects of monitoring the shocked patient will be mentioned here.

CARDIOVASCULAR MONITORING AND INVESTIGATIONS

If mistakes are to be avoided, frequent clinical examination is essential, even in the most fully monitored patients. It is usually possible to make some assessment of volume losses in hypovolaemic shock, although such approximations can be grossly inaccurate; in major trauma, for example, losses are often considerably underestimated.

Examination of skin colour, temperature, capillary refill time and the presence or absence of sweating, together with the rate and character of the pulse provides a rapid guide to the severity of shock and the response to treatment. In straightforward cases, such as a fit young man with mild to moderate haemorrhage following a road traffic crash, invasive monitoring may be unnecessary. Clinical assessment combined with frequent blood pressure measurement using a sphygmomanometer may be sufficient. An electrocardiogram (ECG) is non-invasive and allows detection of arrhythmias and myocardial ischaemia.

Table 5.7 Monitoring and laboratory investigations in shock

Cardiovascular

Clinical assessment	Peripheral perfusion
	Rate and character of pulse
	Mental status
Non-invasive monitoring	Electrocardiogram
	Blood pressure
	Core–peripheral temperature gradient
	Oesophageal Doppler
	Echocardiography
Invasive monitoring	Intra-arterial blood pressure
	Central venous pressure
	Urine output
	Pulmonary artery flotation catheter (in selected patients including some of those with major haemorrhage, severe trauma, septic shock, massive pulmonary embolus, myocardial dysfunction, acute lung injury/acute respiratory distress syndrome) or other dye/thermal dilution catheter (e.g. PiCCO, lithium dilution)

Respiratory

Clinical assessment	Respiratory rate
Investigations	Chest radiograph
	Blood gas analysis

Investigations

Biochemistry	Acid–base
	Blood lactate
	Urea and electrolytes
	Blood sugar
	Liver function tests
Haematology	Haemoglobin concentration/packed cell volume
	Coagulation studies
	White blood cell count
Microbiology (in sepsis/septic shock)	Blood cultures
	Urine, sputum, cerebrospinal fluid (in selected cases) and pus for microscopy, culture and sensitivities. In some cases polymerase chain reaction may be useful
Markers of the inflammatory response to infection	Procalcitonin, C-reactive protein

PiCCO, pulse-induced continuous cardiac output.

The more seriously ill and those who fail to respond to initial treatment will require invasive monitoring, including *central venous pressure (CVP) measurement* and *intra-arterial pressure* recording. As discussed in Chapter 4, measurement of the *core–peripheral temperature gradient* (or the big-toe temperature related to ambient temperature), together with the *hourly urine output*, provides a useful guide to the adequacy of cardiac output and tissue perfusion in hypovolaemic shock. Use of the *oesophageal Doppler, pulmonary artery catheterization*, or one of the newer techniques for monitoring cardiac output may be indicated in selected cases, including patients with:

- major haemorrhage (e.g. > 8 units transfusion);
- severe multiple trauma;
- septic shock;

- myocardial dysfunction;
- ALI/ARDS;
- massive pulmonary embolism.

In patients wth severe sepsis, however, pulmonary artery catheter use does not seem to influence overall mortality or resource utilization (Yu *et al.*, 2003) (see also Chapter 4).

Echocardiography (preferably transoesophageal) may be used to assess ventricular filling and myocardial performance, as well as to exclude complications such as mitral valve prolapse (see Chapter 4).

RESPIRATORY MONITORING AND INVESTIGATIONS

The *respiratory rate* must be recorded at frequent intervals and should gradually decrease as any metabolic acidosis resolves. The subsequent development of tachypnoea is an indication that all is not well, and may herald the onset of fat embolism or ALI/ARDS.

A *chest radiograph* must always be taken and may initially reveal:

- unsuspected rib fractures;
- pneumothorax;
- haemothorax;
- widening of the mediastinum (suggestive of aortic dissection).

The onset of ALI/ARDS will be associated at first with ill-defined diffuse shadowing or a ground-glass appearance on the chest radiograph, which may later progress to a mottled appearance with areas of consolidation in an alveolar pattern. Air bronchograms may also be seen (see Chapter 8).

Blood gas analysis may reveal hypoxaemia with a normal or low P_aCO_2. A rising P_aCO_2, severe hypoxaemia, increasing tachypnoea and exhaustion suggest that respiratory support will be required.

BIOCHEMICAL INVESTIGATIONS

Conventionally, the development of a lactic acidosis is attributed to anaerobic glycolysis caused by cellular hypoxia. Particularly in sepsis, however, a variety of other factors may contribute to raised blood lactate levels, including inhibition of pyruvate dehydrogenase, adrenaline-induced increases in aerobic glycolysis (see below), mitochondrial dysfunction and decreased clearance by the liver and kidney. Recent evidence suggests that skeletal muscle is an important source of lactate in sepsis as a result of accelerated glycolysis caused by stimulation of $Na^+/K^+ATPase$ (Levy et al., 2005). Moreover the relationship between increased blood lactate levels and acidosis is complex. Some have argued, therefore, that lactate is an unreliable indicator of hypoxia in injury or sepsis (James et al., 1999). Nevertheless serial determination of *blood lactate levels* provides a guide to the severity of shock, the response to therapy and the prognosis (Bakker et al., 1991) and prolonged hyperlactatcaemia is a good predictor of the development of MOF (Bakker et al., 1996). In view of these observations, many recommend that blood lactate measurement should be a routine investigation in the assessment of acutely ill or injured patients (Bakker, 2001), although it should not be regarded as proof of an oxygen debt requiring increases in systemic or regional oxygen transport.

A proportion of patients will have a *metabolic alkalosis*. In some, this may be related to identifiable causes such as massive blood transfusion or hypokalaemia, but in others the aetiology is unclear.

Urea and electrolytes should always be measured since they provide a baseline, which may be useful in the event of subsequent deterioration. They may also reveal unsuspected problems such as pre-existing renal dysfunction, as well as abnormalities such as hyper- or hypokalaemia, hypo- or hypercalcaemia and hypo- or hypermagnesaemia. Shocked patients may also develop either hypo- or hyperglycaemia (see above) and *blood sugar* levels should always be measured.

Liver function tests are of importance since pre-existing liver disease, in particular cirrhosis, predisposes to sepsis, acute respiratory failure and subsequent acute liver failure and is associated with increased mortality (Foreman et al., 2003) (see Chapter 14). Hepatic dysfunction may follow a period of impaired perfusion. The breakdown of transfused blood and haematomas may also increase bilirubin levels. Total protein and albumin levels should be measured regularly because the albumin concentration is an important determinant of plasma colloid osmotic pressure (COP) which may influence the development of pulmonary oedema (see Chapter 3). COP can be measured directly using an oncometer, although in routine practice this measurement is now rarely performed. Use of artificial colloids will dilute the albumin concentration yet can still maintain an adequate COP.

HAEMATOLOGICAL INVESTIGATIONS

The *haemoglobin (Hb) concentration* and *packed cell volume (PCV)* (microhaematocrit) should always be measured, although they do not provide a reliable guide to the extent of blood and fluid losses because of the variable degree of haemoconcentration that may occur. They are, however, useful when deciding which solution to use for volume replacement (see later).

Thrombocytopenia and *coagulopathies* may occur, either as a result of transfusing large amounts of stored blood or excessive consumption. A falling platelet count is often the first indication of the latter and the diagnosis can be confirmed by measuring the thrombin time and circulating levels of fibrinogen and FDPs.

In septic shock, the *white blood cell count* is often raised, with a left shift and toxic granulation, although sometimes the patient is leukopenic – a poor prognostic sign. A rising white cell count some time after an episode of shock may indicate the development of septic complications (e.g. an intra-abdominal abscess in a patient with multiple injuries), though neither sensitivity nor specificity is high.

MICROBIOLOGICAL INVESTIGATIONS

In patients with sepsis or septic shock, every effort must be made to identify the source of infection and the causative organism. Samples of urine, sputum, cerebrospinal fluid (when indicated) and pus from drainage sites should be sent to the laboratory for microscopy and culture. In meningococcal sepsis serogroup-specific *Neisseria meningitidis* DNA can be detected using polymerase chain reaction (PCR). This technique has the advantage of not requiring live organisms for a positive result. *Lumbar puncture need not be performed in patients with an obvious clinical diagnosis of meningococcal disease* (the yield is higher from skin lesion aspirates).

Blood cultures should always be performed, although they may be negative even when the clinical diagnosis is beyond doubt in patients with severe sepsis or septic shock (Sands *et al.*, 1997). The lung is the most common site of infection (up to 30% of patients), followed by the abdomen and the urinary tract, but in about 5% of cases a definite site of infection cannot be identified (Brun-Buisson *et al.*, 1995). In patients who develop infection whilst in ICU, catheter-related infections are the commonest source. It should be remembered that shock may be the result of infection with rickettsiae, viruses or fungi, as well as bacteria. Gram-positive infections are now a more common cause of sepsis than Gram-negative bacteria in developed countries, and the incidence of polymicrobial infections, as well as sepsis due to fungi and multi-drug-resistant organisms, continues to increase (Annane *et al.*, 2003; Martin *et al.*, 2003).

In some cases, the presence of endotoxin in the circulation can be detected using the *Limulus lysate test*, even when blood cultures are negative. This test uses an extract of amoebocytes present in the haemolymph of the horseshoe crab (*Limulus polyphemus*), which forms a solid gel within 24 hours of being exposed to endotoxin. This technique has been modified by the introduction of synthetic substrates, which bypass the gelation steps and release a chromophore. Although the use of these chromogenic substrates increases the sensitivity and specificity of the method, it is rarely used in clinical practice. New endotoxin assays are being developed.

MARKERS OF THE PRESENCE AND SEVERITY OF THE INFLAMMATORY RESPONSE TO INFECTION
(Reinhart *et al.*, 2000) (see also Chapter 12)
C-reactive protein
This acute-phase protein has been used to assess the presence and severity of an inflammatory response, although the value of CRP measurement in clinical practice is limited because plasma levels:

- are also elevated during non-infectious inflammatory states;
- remain elevated for up to several days after the infection has been eliminated;
- do not reflect the severity of infection and do not distinguish survivors from non-survivors;
- do not increase for up to 24 hours after the onset of inflammation.

Trends are considered to be more useful than absolute values.

Procalcitonin (PCT)
PCT, a propeptide of calcitonin, is normally produced in the C cells of the thyroid gland. In health, circulating levels of PCT are extremely low, but in sepsis PCT is produced by extrathyroid tissues, such as monocytes and the liver, and plasma concentrations increase dramatically. The pathophysiological role of PCT is unclear. Plasma levels of PCT:

- are claimed to increase approximately 20 hours earlier than CRP;

- may be a useful marker of severe infection and sepsis;
- are related to the severity of systemic inflammation;
- are related to prognosis, particularly changes over time.
- can be used to assess the effectiveness of treatment to eradicate infection;
- are not usually raised when infection is localized and not accompanied by systemic inflammation;
- may also increase, but not usually to the same extent, in response to non-infectious inflammation (e.g. major trauma, extensive surgery);
- may also increase in cardiogenic shock, perhaps in response to endotoxaemia/bacteraemia, although levels are lower than in septic shock;
- may help to differentiate between infectious and non-infectious causes of ARDS, between rejection and infection in transplant recipients, and to identify infection in pancreatitis.

The authors of a recent systematic review and meta-analysis, however, concluded that PCT cannot reliably differentiate sepsis from other non-infectious causes of a systemic inflammatory response (Tang *et al.*, 2007).

Triggering receptor expressed on myeloid cells-1 (TREM-1)
TREM-1 is a member of the immunoglobulin superfamily. Following bacterial invasion, tissues are infiltrated with polymorphonuculear leukocytes and monocytes that express TREM-1, whereas this receptor is only weakly expressed in patients with non-infectious inflammatory disorders. A soluble form of TREM-1 (sTREM-1) can be measured in various body fluids, probably reflecting receptor shed from the membranes of activated phagocytes. Measurement of plasma levels of sTREM-1 seems to be a useful means of identifying patients with an infectious cause of SIRS, and may be a better marker of sepsis than both CRP and PCT (Gibot *et al.*, 2004) (see also Chapter 7, diagnosis of ventilator-associated pneumonia, p. 168).

MANAGEMENT (Dellinger *et al.*, 2008)

GENERAL CONSIDERATIONS
In all forms of shock, the aim of treatment is to restore perfusion pressure and oxygen delivery to the tissues (**Fig. 5.16**; see Chapter 3), while at the same time correcting the underlying cause (e.g. by surgical intervention to arrest haemorrhage or eradicate infection). Delay in making the diagnosis and initiating treatment, as well as suboptimal resuscitation, contributes to the development of the peripheral vascular failure and irreversible tissue dysoxia which can culminate in vital organ dysfunction. Epidemiological evidence confirming that some patients progress from sepsis, through severe sepsis to septic shock and MOF over a period of hours to days highlights the potential benefits of early therapeutic intervention (Rangel-Frausto *et al.*, 1995) as does a recent study in which early institution of a 'goal-directed' treatment pro-

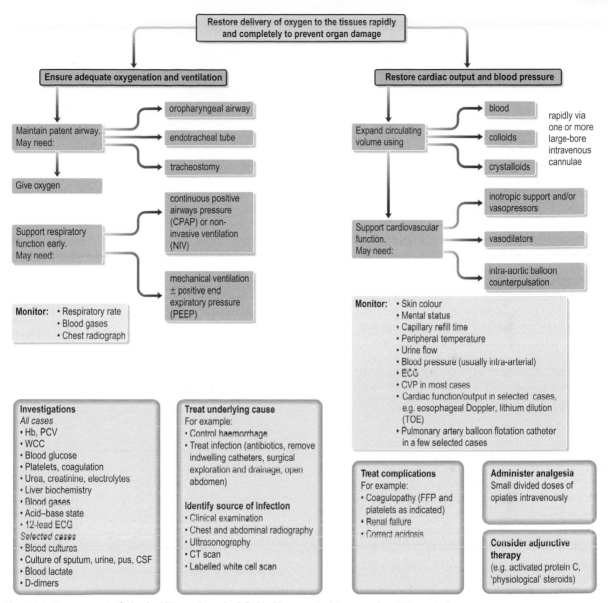

Fig. 5.16 Management of shock. CSF, cerebrospinal fluid; CT, computed tomography; CVP, central venous pressure; ECG, electrocardiogram; FFP, fresh frozen plasma; Hb, haemoglobin; PCV, packed cell volume; TOE, transoesophageal echocardiography; WCC, white cell count. Adapted from Kumar P, Clark M 2005 Clinical Medicine 6E Elsevier with permission.

tocol in the emergency department significantly improved outcome in severe sepsis/septic shock (Rivers *et al.*, 2001).

It is important to remember that shocked patients may require *analgesia* since this is easily overlooked in the heat of the moment. Because of the sluggish muscle blood flow, opiates should be administered in small divided doses intravenously (e.g. morphine 2–4 mg i.v.).

Sepsis/septic shock

A thorough *clinical examination* should be performed to identify the source of infection, followed by conventional chest and abdominal *radiography*. In difficult cases, more sophisticated imaging techniques may prove useful. For example, portable real-time *ultrasonography* is non-invasive and can be used at the bedside to localize fluid collections in the chest and abdomen. It can also demonstrate gallstones, obstruction to the biliary tree and pyonephrosis. Once a collection has been identified, the ultrasound image can be used to guide diagnostic and therapeutic needle aspiration. This can be particularly useful in the case of a loculated empyema. Unfortunately, the ultrasound image is often distorted by neighbouring gas-filled structures such as the stomach and large bowel. Consequently, although ultrasound can visualize a right subphrenic abscess satisfactorily, it is less valuable when fluid is suspected in the left sub-phrenic or paracolic regions. Under these circumstances, a *computed tomography (CT) scan* may be more useful, although this will involve moving the patient from the ICU and can therefore be hazardous for unstable patients. CT scanning can also be used to guide percutaneous needle aspiration of fluid collections. *Gallium-67 citrate and indium-labelled white cells* have been used to detect inflammatory foci. They do not, however, differentiate between a sterile inflammatory response and bacterial infection, nor is localization sufficiently accurate to allow needle aspiration. It has been suggested that the use of the synthetic broad-spectrum antibiotic ciprofloxacin linked to the radiochemical technetium^{99m} confers greater specificity combined with ease of administration (Vinjamuri *et al.*, 1996).

In patients with intra-abdominal sepsis or abscess formation in any site, an aggressive approach to *surgical exploration/radiological intervention* and *drainage of pus* must be adopted. If there is any doubt about the origin of sepsis, all intravascular catheters should be removed and their tips sent for culture. In *toxic shock syndrome*, the tampon, if present, must be removed. This alone may lead to resolution of infection. In *necrotizing fasciitis* and *gas gangrene* (see Chapter 12), radical surgical excision of infected tissue is essential. There is evidence that an *open-abdomen* approach to the management of severe intra-abdominal sepsis, perhaps with daily laparotomies using a 'zipper' in the abdominal wall, can improve outcome.

Appropriate antibiotic therapy is vital in sepsis and should be guided by the source of infection, whether it was acquired in the hospital, in a health care institution (e.g. nursing home) or in the community, and known local patterns of sensitivity (see Chapter 12). In patients with septic shock, administration of effective antimicrobial therapy within the first hour of documented hypertension has been associated with increased survival to hospital discharge; mortality rates increased progressively with increasing delays in instituting treatment (Kumar *et al.*, 2006). **The Surviving Sepsis guidelines (Dellinger *et al.*, 2008) recommend that intravenous antibiotic therapy should be started as early as possible and within 1 hour of the recognition of severe sepsis and septic shock, after appropriate cultures have been obtained.**

RESPIRATORY SUPPORT

The first priority in all acutely ill patients is to *secure the airway*. This often simply requires insertion of an oropharyngeal airway, but in some cases tracheal intubation may be necessary. The latter also protects the lungs from aspiration of blood, vomit and other debris and is often essential in those with severe facial injuries. Very rarely, emergency cricothyrotomy (see Chapter 7) may be required.

All shocked patients should receive supplementary oxygen, and those with severe chest and/or head injuries may require immediate intubation and *mechanical ventilation*. Because of the adverse haemodynamic effects of positive-pressure ventilation (Chapter 7), it is important (when time

allows) to optimize the patient's cardiovascular performance (e.g. by restoring circulating volume) before instituting mechanical ventilation. Patients who later develop ALI/ARDS will also require respiratory support (see Chapter 8).

Because mechanical ventilation abolishes or minimizes the work of breathing, reduces oxygen consumption and improves oxygenation, early respiratory support has been considered to be beneficial in patients with severe shock, including those with cardiogenic shock complicated by pulmonary oedema. Indeed, in the 1970s it was suggested that the introduction of a standardized treatment regimen that included the early institution of mechanical ventilation and aggressive surgery could improve outcome from septic shock (Ledingham and McArdle, 1978). More recent evidence indicates, however, that a more conservative approach to mechanical ventilation (use of non-invasive respiratory support when possible, low tidal volume ventilation, spontaneous breathing modes) should be adopted in order to avoid ventilator-induced lung injury and exacerbation of the inflammatory response (see Chapters 7 and 8).

CARDIOVASCULAR SUPPORT

Whatever the aetiology of the haemodynamic disturbance, tissue blood flow must be restored by achieving and maintaining an adequate cardiac output as well as by ensuring that systemic blood pressure is sufficient to maintain perfusion of vital organs. Traditionally, a mean arterial pressure (MAP) ≥ 60 mmHg or a systolic blood pressure ≥ 80 mmHg has been considered to be adequate, although some have suggested that a MAP ≥ 80 mmHg may be a more appropriate target, while others advocate targeting the patient's pre-morbid blood pressure. In a small study of patients with septic shock, there was no evidence that increasing MAP from 65 to 85 mmHg with noradrenaline improved tissue perfusion, but neither was there any indication that such a strategy was deleterious (LeDoux *et al.*, 2000). **The Surviving Sepsis guidelines (Dellinger *et al.*, 2008) advocate targeting a MAP > 65 mmHg, CVP 8–12 mmHg, urine output > 0.5 mL/kg per hour and a central venous oxygen saturation ≥ 70% (or mixed venous oxygen saturation ≥ 65%) as the initial goals of resuscitation.**

As well as controlling heart rate, the three determinants of stroke volume (preload, contractility and afterload) must be manipulated appropriately.

Preload and volume replacement

Optimization of preload is the most efficient way of increasing cardiac output and is a prerequisite for restoring tissue perfusion. Volume replacement is obviously of primary importance in hypovolaemic shock, but is also required in anaphylaxis (see below) and sepsis because of vasodilatation, sequestration of blood and loss of circulating volume due to the increase in microvascular permeability. In many cases volume depletion is exacerbated by reduced oral intake and increased losses due to, for example, vomiting and sweating. In obstructive shock, high filling pressures may be required to maintain an adequate stroke volume, while even in cardiogenic shock, careful volume expansion may lead to a useful increase in cardiac output. On the other hand, patients with severe cardiac failure in whom ventricular filling pressures may be markedly elevated can benefit from measures to reduce preload (and afterload), such as the administration of vasodilators and diuretics (see later). Adequate perioperative volume replacement also reduces morbidity and mortality in high-risk surgical patients (see later).

A crude clinical assessment of the extent of the volume deficit in hypovolaemic shock is usually possible, although, as mentioned previously, these estimates can be very inaccurate. Blood losses are often underestimated, particularly when there are scalp and facial wounds, because bandaging merely disguises the extent of the haemorrhage in these extremely vascular areas. Measurement of Hb, PCV and urea and electrolytes is usually unhelpful in the early stages of resuscitation.

The clinical response to transfusion (slowing heart rate, improved tissue perfusion, increased urine output and rising blood pressure) may be a sufficient guide to the volume required, but monitoring of CVP is usually required. In some cases oesophageal Doppler monitoring or pulmonary artery catheterization and monitoring of cardiac output and SvO_2, as well as left ventricular filling pressures, is indicated (see Chapter 4). Volume replacement can be titrated to achieve optimal stroke volume or the PAOP that produces optimum ventricular stroke work. When interpreting these variables, it is important to recognise that ventricular compliance is often reduced in shock. It is also important to appreciate that isolated readings of CVP or PAOP do not provide a meaningful measure of the circulating volume and that other methods of predicting fluid responsiveness, such as systolic pressure variation, are often more helpful (see also Chapters 3 and 4). In view of the increased microvascular permeability, particularly in those with sepsis, it is sometimes sensible to limit volume requirements by the addition of inotropic support and vasopressors to achieve the desired cardiac output and MAP.

The circulating volume must be replaced as quickly as possible (i.e. within minutes, not hours) since rapid restoration of cardiac output and perfusion pressure reduces the chances of serious organ damage, particularly the development of acute renal failure. Therefore, in patients with severe haemorrhagic shock, for example, two or more large-bore intravenous cannulae may be required so that fluid can be transfused rapidly under pressure. Careful monitoring will ensure that, despite this aggressive approach, volume overload does not occur.

Failure to respond to fluid replacement should prompt a careful search for complications such as tension pneumothorax, cardiac tamponade or significant continued bleeding.

The clinical use of a 'G-suit' (*military antishock trousers – MAST*) to limit blood loss and reduce venous pooling in victims of massive trauma was first described in Vietnam. Although the application of MAST helps to maintain blood pressure, it can interfere with ventilation, and deflation may be associated with profound hypotension. The use of MAST remains controversial, but they may help to tamponade intra-abdominal haemorrhage, especially in those with pelvic fractures or severe retroperitoneal haemorrhage.

CHOICE OF FLUID FOR VOLUME REPLACEMENT

The choice of intravenous fluid for resuscitation of critically ill patients, and the relative merits of blood, crystalloids or colloids, remains controversial, despite the large number of comparative studies performed since the 1960s and, more recently, several meta-analyses (see below).

Blood. Donor blood is normally separated into its various components (red cells, platelet concentrates, fresh frozen plasma and cryoprecipitate) and in many countries, including the UK, is invariably leukodepleted. It is therefore necessary to transfuse concentrated red cells to maintain adequate levels of Hb (conventionally 9–10 g/dl in septic shock – but see below), and use plasma or a plasma substitute or crystalloids for volume replacement.

Standard red cell concentrates are being replaced by *supplemented red cell concentrates* in which most of the plasma is removed and the red cells are suspended in 100 mL of nutrient additive solution. In this way plasma extraction from donor blood is maximized, the shelf-life of the red cell suspensions is prolonged and transfusion is facilitated by the reduction in viscosity. The most commonly used additive is SAG (saline, adenine, glucose), to which mannitol (M) is added to reduce spontaneous lysis (SAGM blood). The haematocrit of supplemented red cell concentrates is about 57%. In extreme emergencies, uncross-matched O-negative blood can be used, but an emergency cross-match can be performed in less than 30 minutes and is almost as safe as the standard procedure.

Blood transfusion may be complicated by:

- incompatibility reactions (transfusion of the wrong blood remains by far the commonest cause of blood transfusion-related morbidity and mortality; although rare, fatal acute haemolytic reactions continue to occur);
- immune suppression (probably caused by mediators released from stored leukocytes);
- pyrexia due to contained pyrogens;
- bacterial contamination with fever, sepsis, shock and sometimes death;
- transmission of diseases such as viral hepatitis, HIV and new variant Creutzfeldt–Jakob disease (vCJD);
- transfusion-related acute lung injury (TRALI).

In the mid-1990s it was estimated that in the USA the risk of HIV transmission was 1 for every 450 000–660 000 donations of screened blood (Lackritz *et al.*, 1995). Most recipients of HIV-infected blood become seropositive but in the UK the risk of transmission has now been reduced to less than 1 in 8 million. The risk of transmission of hepatitis B is 1 in 900 000 and of hepatitis C is less than 1 in 30 million. Recent concern about the theoretical risk of transmission of vCJD disease has led to the universal leukodepletion of donated blood and donor screening.

TRALI is characterized by dyspnoea and hypoxaemia due to non-cardiogenic pulmonary oedema, occurring within about 4 hours of transfusion. The estimated frequency is approximately 1 in 5000 transfusions and TRALI is the third most common cause of transfusion-related death. In some cases TRALI is thought to be caused by a reaction between antibodies in the donor blood and the recipient's leukocytes, whilst in others reactive lipid products that arise from donor red cell membranes during storage have been implicated. Such donors should be removed from the donor panel. In some cases transfusion of fresh frozen plasma or platelets has been implicated. Diagnosis can be difficult and depends on excluding other causes of ALI. The diagnosis can be supported by identifying neutrophil or human leukocyte antigen antibodies in the donor or recipient plasma. Management is supportive as for other causes of ALI (see Chapter 8). TRALI is self limiting and clinical improvement usually occurs within 48–96 hours. At least 90% of patients with TRALI recover (Looney *et al.*, 2004).

Other special problems may arise when large volumes of stored blood are transfused rapidly. These include:

- *Hypothermia.* Bank blood is stored at $4° \pm 2°C$ and, if large volumes are transfused, the patient will become hypothermic. Furthermore, peripheral venoconstriction may slow the rate of the infusion, and cold blood transfused rapidly through a centrally placed cannula can induce arrhythmias. If possible, blood should be warmed during massive transfusion and in those at risk of hypothermia (e.g. during prolonged major surgery with open body cavity).
- *Coagulopathy.* Stored blood has essentially no effective platelets and is deficient in clotting factors. Consequently, with large transfusions, a coagulation defect may develop. This should be treated by replacing clotting factors with fresh frozen plasma and the administration of platelet concentrates. Occasionally, cryoprecipitate may be required.
- *Metabolic acidosis/alkalosis.* Stored blood is now collected in citrate/phosphate/dextrose (CPD) anticoagulant, which is less acidic than the acid/citrate/dextrose (ACD) solution used previously, and metabolic acidosis attributable solely to blood transfusion is unusual. Patients will often develop a metabolic alkalosis 24–48 hours after a large blood transfusion, probably partly due to citrate metabolism, and this will be exacerbated if a preceding acidosis has been corrected with intravenous sodium bicarbonate.
- *Hypocalcaemia.* Stored blood is anticoagulated using citrate, which binds calcium ions. During rapid transfusions excess citrate may reduce total body ionized calcium levels, causing myocardial depression. This is uncommon in practice, but if necessary can be corrected by administering 10 mL of 10% calcium chloride intravenously. Routine administration of calcium is not recommended.
- *Increased oxygen affinity.* As mentioned in Chapter 3, the position of the oxyhaemoglobin dissociation curve is influenced by the concentration of 2,3-diphosphoglycerate (DPG) in the red cell. In stored blood, the red cell 2,3-DPG content is reduced so that the curve is shifted to the left. The oxygen affinity of Hb is therefore increased and oxygen unloading to the tissues is impaired. This effect is less marked with CPD blood. Red cell levels of 2,3-DPG are substantially restored within 12 hours of transfusion.
- *Hyperkalaemia.* Potassium levels in stored blood rise progressively. When the blood is warmed prior to transfusion, however, the cells begin to metabolize, the sodium pump becomes active and potassium levels fall. Hyperkalaemia is rarely a problem with massive transfusion.
- *Microembolism.* The microaggregates in stored blood may be filtered out in the pulmonary vasculature. This process was thought by some to contribute to the development of TRALI. The use of 40-μm filters is, however, no longer considered to be necessary.

Concern about the supply, cost and safety of blood, including the risk of disease transmission and immune suppression, has encouraged a conservative approach to blood transfusion. It has long been recognized that previously fit patients who have an episode of haemorrhagic shock can survive with extremely low Hb concentrations provided their circulating volume, and thus their ability to maintain an adequate cardiac output, is maintained. It has also been generally accepted that limited normovolaemic haemodilution (PCV 25–30%) can improve tissue oxygen delivery since the reduction in oxygen-carrying capacity may be offset by an increase in cardiac output and improved distribution of flow through the microcirculation. Moreover, there is evidence that transfusing old RBCs to patients with sepsis fails to improve oxygen uptake and may precipitate splanchnic ischaemia, perhaps because poorly deformable transfused cells cause microvascular occlusion (Marik and Sibbald, 1993). More recent evidence suggests that in normovolaemic critically ill patients a restrictive strategy of red cell transfusion (Hb maintained at 7.0–9.0 g/dL) is at least as effective as, and may be safer than, a liberal approach (Hb maintained at 10–12 g/dL), especially in younger, less severely ill patients (Hebert *et al.*, 1999). Additional support for a restrictive transfusion policy is provided by a large, prospective, observational study which demonstrated an association between blood transfusion and increased mortality (Vincent *et al.*, 2002) and by the observation that red cell transfusions are associated with ICU-acquired bloodstream infections (Shorr *et al.*, 2005). It has been suggested that the adverse affect of blood transfusion on outcome may be largely related to immune suppression and that leukodepleted blood might be safer in this respect. Some groups of patients (e.g. the elderly, those with significant cardiac or respiratory disease and patients with acute myocardial infarction and unstable angina) may benefit from a higher threshold for transfusion, although one study suggested that a restrictive red cell transfusion strategy is safe in most critically ill patients, with the possible exception of those with acute myocardial infarction and angina (Hebert et al., 2001).

As well as adopting a generally conservative approach to blood transfusion in the critically ill, specific measues to reduce the use of donated blood have included *preoperative autologous donation* and *intraoperative cell salvage*, although these techniques are still not widely employed. The value of *acute normovolaemic haemodilution* during surgery remains uncertain whilst attempts to develop oxygen-carrying *blood substitutes* have met with little success. Diaspirin cross-linked Hb (DCLHb), for example, consisted of stroma-free Hb cross-linked at a specific site between the alpha subunits with *bis* (3, 5-dibromosalicyl) fumarate to prevent dissociation of the Hb molecule into dimers. The intravascular half-life of the tetramer was thereby increased and oxygen-binding affinity decreased, theoretically improving oxygen delivery to the tissues. Unfortunately, the use of DCLHb in severe traumatic haemorrhagic shock was associated with a significant increase in mortality, perhaps related to scavenging of NO and consequent vasoconstriction (Sloan et al., 1999). This compound is no longer manufactured. Administration of recombinant human *erythropoietin* (40 000 units weekly) to critically ill patients did not reduce the incidence of red-cell transfusion, and may have been associated with an increase in the incidence of thrombotic events, although mortality may have been reduced in trauma victims (Corwin et al., 2007).

Crystalloid solutions. Although crystalloid solutions are cheap, convenient to use and free of immediate side-effects, the use of large volumes of these fluids should, in general, be avoided. They are rapidly distributed across the intravascular and interstitial spaces, and volumes of crystalloid 2–4 times that of colloid are required to achieve an equivalent haemodynamic response (Rackow et al., 1983). Moreover, volume expansion is transitory, COP is reduced, fluid accumulates in the interstitial spaces, and pulmonary oedema may be precipitated (Rackow et al., 1983). It has also been suggested that the development of peripheral oedema may impair tissue oxygenation, delay wound healing and decrease gastrointestinal motility and absorptive capacity. There is also evidence to suggest that even large volumes of crystalloid may fail to restore microcirculatory flow. Usually, however, any excess fluid is rapidly mobilized once the stress response abates. Moreover, in hypovolaemic shock, both the interstitial and intracellular compartments are eventually depleted as fluid moves into the intravascular space and crystalloid solutions can be used to correct these deficits. Nevertheless, a recent large prospective, randomized, controlled trial (PRCT) has demonstrated that in a heterogeneous group of critically ill patients the use of either 0.9% saline or 4% albumin for fluid resuscitation resulted in similar outcomes (Finfer et al., 2004b).

It is worth noting that 5% dextrose distributes throughout the total pool of body water and is useless for expanding the intravascular compartment. Conversely, *hyperosmotic sodium chloride* draws large volumes of intracellular water into the extracellular space and some have suggested that this fluid may be valuable in the early stages of resuscitation (see also Chapter 15). There is, however, little evidence that it is more effective than conventional fluid replacement in shock and major limiting factors include hypernatraemia, reduced intracellular volume, hyperosmolality and the possibility of an increased risk of bleeding.

Colloidal solutions. These produce a greater and more sustained increase in plasma volume with associated improvements in cardiovascular function, oxygen transport and oxygen consumption. They also increase COP (Rackow et al., 1983) and, if the circulating volume is promptly restored with colloids, depletion of the interstitial and intravascular spaces can be avoided. When capillary permeability is increased, however, colloids may escape from the intravascular compartment and increase interstitial oncotic pressure, thereby enhancing oedema formation and slowing its resolution.

Despite the theoretical advantages of colloidal solutions, one systematic review suggested that resuscitation with colloids rather than crystalloids may be associated with an increased risk of death (Schierhout and Roberts, 1998). Many were unconvinced by this controversial review, not least because the trials included used a variety of fluid preparations in relatively small, disparate patient groups in predominantly historical studies. In fact, this review is perhaps more correctly interpreted as confirming the uncertainty of other meta-analyses (Choi et al., 1999; Velanovich, 1989), thereby emphasizing the urgent need for PRCTs in clearly defined patient populations. In the meantime, although volume replacement with predominantly crystalloid solutions is advocated by some for the uncomplicated previously healthy patient with traumatic or perioperative hypovolaemia, a more reasonable approach is to use crystalloids initially, but to use colloids if there is a continued need for volume replacement in excess of about 1 litre. Until more definitive evidence becomes available we believe that in most categories of critically ill patients requiring volume expansion, colloids should be used in preference to administering large volumes of crystalloid. Unfortunately, not only does the crystalloid/colloid controversy continue but there is still considerable debate about the relative merits of the various colloidal solutions (Boldt, 2000).

Natural colloids—Human albumin solution (HAS) is prepared by fractionating pooled donor plasma and is heat-treated to inactivate contaminating viruses. HAS has until now been widely available, although expensive, but the impact of the decision to discontinue the pooling of donated blood for the production of blood products, including albumin, in the UK remains to be seen.

The 4.5% solution is iso-oncotic and, in normal subjects, will expand the circulating volume by an amount roughly equivalent to the volume infused. It has a half-life in the circulation of 10–15 days, although in those with increased microvascular permeability this is considerably reduced.

HAS has the same sodium content as plasma, which may be a disadvantage in those at risk of developing hypernatraemia. Allergic reactions are rare.

In one randomized comparison the use of albumin rather than 3.5% polygeline (see below) for volume replacement had no influence on mortality, length of stay in intensive care or the incidence of pulmonary oedema and renal failure (Stockwell *et al.*, 1992a, b), whereas a later systematic review controversially suggested that the administration of HAS to patients with hypovolaemia, burns or hypoalbuminaemia might increase mortality (Cochrane Injuries Group Albumin Reviewers, 1998). Suggested explanations for this unexpected observation have included exacerbation of interstitial oedema (see above), adverse immunological effects and extravascular binding of heavy metals and drugs in the presence of capillary leak. Many were sceptical of these findings, however, especially since they were not replicated in other meta-analyses (Wilkes and Navickis, 2001) and a recent large PRCT has demonstrated the overall safety of 4% albumin in a heterogeneous group of critically ill patients (Finfer *et al.*, 2004b). In the latter study, there was a non-significant trend towards reduced mortality with albumin in the septic subgroup and a suggestion that mortality may be increased in the albumin group in those with traumatic brain injury. These findings from subgroup analysis need to be confirmed or refuted in PRCTs (see Chapter 15).

Although apparently safe, HAS should probably not be used for routine volume replacement, particularly if losses are continuing, since other cheaper solutions are equally effective in the short term. Clinically significant hypoalbuminaemia may be associated with hypovolaemia, oedema, pleural effusions and ascites. Under these circumstances some have recommended administration of albumin in combination with diuretics. There is also some evidence to suggest that HAS may be beneficial in cirrhotic patients with ascites requiring paracentesis and may reduce the incidence of renal impairment and death when such patients develop spontaneous bacterial peritonitis (Sort *et al.*, 1999). A recent PRCT suggested that albumin administration may improve organ function in hypoalbuminaemic critically ill patients (Dubois *et al.*, 2006) although a subgroup analysis of the Saline versus Albumin Fluid Evaluation (SAFE) study indicated that outcomes of resuscitation with albumin or saline are similar irrespective of the patient's baseline serum albumin concentration (Saline versus Albumin Fluid Evaluation Study Investigators, 2006). In those who are hypernatraemic and/or at risk of fluid overload, concentrated 20% or 25% albumin may be used. HAS is also an appropriate replacement fluid for patients undergoing plasma exchange, and is used extensively in patients with burns and by many in children with septic shock.

Dextrans—These are polymolecular polysaccharides contained in either 5% dextrose or normal saline. Low-molecular-weight dextran (40 kDa) has a powerful osmotic effect so that fluid moves from the extravascular to the intravascular compartment, thereby expanding the circulating volume by approximately twice the volume infused. Micro-circulatory flow may be improved by the reduction in viscosity, decreased erythrocyte and platelet sludging and reduced leukocyte adherence, although this may be offset by a decrease in the flexibility of the red cells. Dextran 40 is rapidly excreted by the kidneys and its effect is therefore relatively short-lived. Dextran 40 also coats the red cell membrane so that blood must be taken for cross-matching before it is given. Dextran 70 (70 kDa) is also hyperoncotic, although less so than dextran 40, and also interferes with cross-matching. It has a longer half-life, however, and is probably the most suitable dextran for routine use. Dextrans can induce a coagulopathy, probably by reducing von Willebrand factor and inhibiting platelet function. There is a small risk of delayed allergic reactions to all the dextrans. Anaphylactic reactions, which can be extremely violent and life-threatening, are increasing in frequency. Because of the availability of other, safer plasma expanders, dextrans are now rarely used in the UK and they are not currently available in the USA.

Gelatin solutions (Haemaccel, Gelofusine)—These have an average molecular weight of 35 kDa and are iso-oncotic with plasma. Haemaccel consists of urea-linked gelatin, whereas Gelofusine is a succinylated gelatin, but the only important difference between the two solutions is that Haemaccel has about 10 times more calcium (6.3 mmol/L) and potassium (5.1 mmol/L) than Gelofusine. The electrostatic charge of succinylated preparations differs from that of other gelatin solutions, but the clinical implications of this difference are unclear. Gelatins do not interfere with cross-matching. It appears that large volumes of gelatins can be given with relative impunity as clinically significant coagulation defects are unusual and they do not impair renal function, although they can interfere with platelet aggregation and compromise clot quality. They are also reasonably cheap. Because they readily cross the glomerular basement membrane their half-life in the circulation is only 4–5 hours and they can promote an osmotic diuresis. There is also some evidence that high-molecular-weight gelatin complexes may leak out of the capillaries, exacerbating pulmonary oedema. Moreover, administration of large volumes of gelatin represents a considerable saline load and, if Haemaccel is used, can precipitate hyperkalaemia and exacerbate hypernatraemia. These solutions are particularly useful during the acute phase of resuscitation, especially when volume losses are continuing but, in many patients, colloids with a longer half-life may be required later to achieve haemodynamic stability. The incidence of anaphylactic reactions is high compared to alternative colloid solutions and appears to be more common with urea-linked preparations.

Hydroxyethyl starches (HES)—These are high-polymeric glucose compounds manufactured by hydrolysis and subsequent hydroxyethylation of amylopectin, a highly branched starch. They are rather more expensive than the gelatins but cheaper than HAS. Numerous preparations are now available, characterized by their concentrations (3%, 6%, 10%), mean molecular weight (low 70 kDa, medium 200–270 kDa, high 450 kDa) and the level of substitution with hydroxyethyl groups (0.5, 0.62, 0.7). Thus the first-generation high-molecular-weight HES Hetastarch has a concentration of 6%, a mean molecular weight of 450 kDa and a molar substitution of 0.7, whereas Elohaes, for example, has a mean molecular weight of 200 kDa and a molar substitution of 0.62. The half-life of these HES solutions is between 12 and 24 hours, whilst that of the low-molecular-weight solutions (e.g. Pentaspan) is 4–6 hours. Elimination of HES occurs primarily via the kidneys following hydrolysis by amylase.

HES are stored in the reticuloendothelial system, apparently without causing functional impairment, but skin deposits have been associated with persistent pruritus (Morgan and Berridge, 2000). This pruritis can be generalized or localized, can have a delayed onset of up to several weeks and may be precipitated by warmth or mechanical irritation. It is frequently persistent, lasting months or even years, and is usually refractory to treatment. HES, especially the higher molecular weight fractions, reduce factor VIII activity and inhibit platelet aggregation; although these anticoagulant properties are rarely implicated in clinical bleeding, many therefore recommend limiting the volume of HES administered. Preparations with a low molecular weight and low degree of substitution may be safer in this regard. Finally, there is some evidence from animal models to suggest that HES are more effective in avoiding or reducing increased capillary permeability ('plugging the capillaries') than other preparations. On the other hand in a recent study of patients with severe sepsis or septic shock the use of Elohaes as opposed to gelatin was an independent risk factor for the development of acute renal failure, although the mechanism is unknown (Schortgen et al., 2001). Moreover in a recent randomised controlled trial the use of a low molecular weight starch to resuscitate patients with severe sepsis was associated with a higher rate of acute renal failure and renal replacement therapy than was Ringer's lactate (Brunkhorst et al., 2008). In patients undergoing abdominal aortic aneurysm surgery, perioperative lung function was better in those receiving HES compared to those given Gelofusine (Rittoo et al., 2004). Anaphylactic reactions are less common than with the gelatins.

Inotropic and vasoactive agents

If the signs of shock persist despite adequate volume replacement, and perfusion of vital organs is jeopardized, inotropic or vasoactive agents may be administered to improve cardiac output and blood pressure. Vasopressor therapy may also be required to maintain perfusion in those with life-threatening hypotension, even when volume replacement is incomplete. It is also important at this stage to identify and if possible correct any of the various associated abnormalities that can impair cardiac performance and vascular responsiveness. These include:

- hypoxaemia;
- hypocalcaemia;
- the effects of some drugs (e.g. β-blockers, angiotensin-converting enzyme (ACE) inhibitors, antiarrhythmics and sedatives).

CORRECTION OF METABOLIC ACIDOSIS

Conventionally, extreme acidosis is said to depress myocardial contractility and limit the response to vasopressor agents, although there is little evidence to support this contention. Moreover, attempted correction of acidosis with intravenous sodium bicarbonate may be detrimental. Additional carbon dioxide is generated and, as carbon dioxide but not bicarbonate readily diffuses across the cell membrane, intracellular and, in some cases, extracellular, pH may be paradoxically further reduced. Other potential disadvantages of bicarbonate therapy include sodium overload, hyperosmolality, a left shift of the oxyhaemoglobin dissociation curve and hypokalaemia. Also ionized calcium levels may be reduced and, in combination with the fall in intracellular pH, may contribute to impaired myocardial performance.

In a prospective, randomized, controlled, cross-over clinical study both sodium bicarbonate and sodium chloride produced slight increases in PAOP and cardiac output, while MAP was unchanged. Sodium bicarbonate significantly increased pH and plasma bicarbonate but, unlike sodium chloride, decreased ionized calcium and increased both P_aCO_2 and end-tidal carbon dioxide. The response to infused catecholamines was unaffected (Cooper et al., 1990). In general, therefore, treatment of lactic acidosis should concentrate on correcting the cause. In the absence of hard data, some believe that acidosis may be most safely controlled by hyperventilation; others suggest that administration of bicarbonate may be indicated as a temporizing measure, and to provide a margin of safety, in those with severe persistent metabolic acidosis (pH < 7.15). Bicarbonate therapy is still considered to be useful in renal tubular acidosis and in acidosis due to gastrointestinal losses of bicarbonate.

CHOICE OF INOTROPIC/VASOACTIVE AGENT

The rational selection of an appropriate pressor agent depends on a thorough understanding of the cardiovascular effects of the available drugs (**Table 5.8**), combined with an accurate assessment of the haemodynamic disturbance. The effects of a particular agent in an individual patient are unpredictable and the response must therefore be closely monitored so that the regimen can be altered appropriately if necessary. In many cases this requires measurement of cardiac output, monitoring of venous oxygen saturation and calculation of derived variables (see Chapter 4). In some patients, inodilators are administered to redistribute blood flow (e.g. dopexamine to improve splanchnic perfusion) and, in others, inotropic support can be usefully combined with the administration of a vasodilator (see below). All inotropic agents should be given via a large central vein. Although it is recognized that β-agonists have anti-inflammatory properties, mediated by reduced degradation of IκB and increased intracellular concentrations of cyclic adenosine monophosphate, the clinical importance of the immune-modulating activities of adrenergic agents remains uncertain.

Table 5.8 Adrenergic agents

	β_1	β_2	α_1	α_2	DA1	DA2	Dose dependence
Adrenaline (epinephrine)							++++
Low-dose	++	+	+	±	–	–	
Moderate-dose	++	+	++	+	–	–	
High-dose	++(+)	+(+)	++++	+++	–	–	
Noradrenaline (norepinephrine)	++	0	+++	+++	–	–	+++
Isoprenaline	+++	+++	0	0	–	–	
Dopamine							+++++
Low-dose	±	0	±	+	++	+	
Moderate-dose	++	+	++	+	++(+)	+	
High-dose	+++	++	+++	+	++(+)	+	
Dopexamine	+	+++	0	0	++	+	++
Dobutamine	++	+	±	?	0	0	++

Receptor	Action
β_1 – postsynaptic	Positive inotropism and chronotropism Renin release
β_2 – presynaptic	Stimulates noradrenaline release
β_2 – postsynaptic	Positive inotropism and chronotropism Vascular dilatation Relaxes bronchial smooth muscle
α_1 – postsynaptic	Constriction of peripheral, renal and coronary vascular smooth muscle Positive inotropism Antidiuresis
α_2 – presynaptic	Inhibition of noradrenaline release, vasodilatation
α_2 – postsynaptic	Constriction of coronary arteries Promotes salt and water excretion
DA1 – postsynaptic	Dilates renal, mesenteric and coronary vessels Renal tubular effect (natriuresis, diuresis)
DA2 – presynaptic	Inhibits adrenaline release

ADRENALINE (EPINEPHRINE)

Adrenaline stimulates both α- and β-receptors but, at low doses, β effects seem to predominate. This produces a tachycardia with an increase in stroke volume and cardiac index; peripheral resistance may fall. As the dose is increased, α-mediated vasoconstriction develops. If this is associated with an increase in perfusion pressure, urine output may improve. Particularly at higher doses and in severe septic shock, however, adrenaline can cause excessive vasoconstriction, with potentially worrying reductions in splanchnic flow and associated falls in gastric mucosal pH, indicative of gut mucosal ischaemia (De Backer *et al.*, 2003; Levy *et al.*, 1997a; Meier-Hellmann *et al.*, 1997). Renal blood flow may fall with adrenaline and prolonged high-dose administration can cause peripheral gangrene. Adrenaline may also precipitate tachyarrhythmias. Lactic acidosis is a common complication of adrenaline administration (Day *et al.*, 1996) and is probably explained by β_2-mediated accelerated glycolysis, often combined with other causes of increased lactate production and, in many cases, exacerbated by impaired lactate clearance (see above). The prognostic significance of adrenaline-induced lactic acidosis is unclear, but this phenomenon emphasizes the limitations of using blood lactate levels as a guide to tissue hypoxia in shock, especially in those receiving adrenaline. In an experimental septic shock model adrenaline administration was associated with dose-related reductions in cardiac index, ejection fraction and pH, as well as increases in systemic vascular resistance and creatinine. Adrenaline also adversely affected systemic perfusion, organ function and survival when compared to noradrenaline and vasopressin (Minneci *et al.*, 2004b).

Despite these disadvantages, adrenaline can be a useful agent in patients with refractory hypotension. It is very potent and may prove successful when other agents have failed, particularly following cardiac surgery, perhaps because it stimulates myocardial α-receptors. Adrenaline is still preferred by some as a cheap, effective means of reversing hypotension and increasing oxygen delivery in septic shock (Bollaert et al., 1990), especially when haemodynamic monitoring is not available or is considered unwarranted. In order to avoid adverse effects the minimum effective dose should be used, and its administration should be discontinued as soon as possible

NORADRENALINE (NOREPINEPHRINE)

Noradrenaline has both α- and β-adrenergic actions, but the α-mediated vasoconstrictor effect predominates. Noradrenaline is particularly useful in those with unresponsive hypotension associated with a low systemic vascular resistance and an adequate cardiac output, for example in septic shock resistant to dopamine. It is also increasingly used to maintain blood pressure in vasodilated patients post cardiac surgery. Administration of noradrenaline to patients with vasodilatory shock is associated with an increase in systemic vascular resistance and MAP, while cardiac output usually falls in line with the increased afterload. In some cases, however, cardiac output is unchanged and in patients with dobutamine-resistant septic shock noradrenaline has been shown to improve cardiac output and left ventricular stroke work, as well as increasing systemic vascular resistance and MAP (Martin et al., 1999). These findings indicate that noradrenaline can sometimes exert a positive inotropic effect in septic shock, probably via stimulation of cardiac α and β receptors or possibly as a consequence of improved coronary perfusion (Martin et al., 1999). Moreover, provided cardiac output does not fall, restoration of blood pressure with noradrenaline may be associated with maintained or improved splanchnic perfusion and oxygenation (Marik and Mohedin, 1994; Meier-Hellmann et al., 1996) and reductions in blood lactate levels, as well as increases in urine flow and creatinine clearance (Martin et al., 1990). PAOP and mean pulmonary artery pressure are usually either unchanged or slightly increased. In some cases, large doses may be required to overcome α-receptor downregulation but there is a risk of producing excessive vasoconstriction and masking hypovolaemia, with impaired organ perfusion, peripheral ischaemia and increased afterload. Administration of high doses of noradrenaline has been implicated as a contributory factor in the development of symmetrical peripheral gangrene (Hayes et al., 1992). Noradrenaline administration must, therefore, be accompanied by close haemodynamic monitoring and, certainly when higher doses are used, determination of cardiac output.

ISOPRENALINE

This β-stimulant has both inotropic and chronotropic effects, and also reduces peripheral resistance by dilating skin and muscle blood vessels. This latter effect means that much of the increased flow is diverted away from vital organs such as the kidneys and may account for the oliguria that can be associated with its use. Most of the increase in cardiac output produced by isoprenaline is due to the tachycardia and this, together with the development of arrhythmias,

seriously limits its value. There are now few indications for isoprenaline in the critically ill adult, except, perhaps, as a treatment for bradycardia after cardiac surgery.

DOPAMINE

Dopamine is a natural precursor of noradrenaline that acts on β_1 and, to a lesser extent, β_2 receptors, α receptors (via noradrenaline release) and dopaminergic DA1 and DA2 receptors. When used in low doses (1–3 μg/kg per min) dopaminergic vasodilatory receptors in the cerebral, coronary and splanchnic circulations are activated (DA1 receptors are located on postsynaptic membranes and mediate vasodilatation, whereas DA2 receptors are presynaptic and potentiate these vasodilatory effects by preventing the release of noradrenaline). Peripheral resistance falls, renal and hepatic blood flow increase, and urine output, GFR, fractional excretion of sodium and creatinine clearance can be improved. The importance of the renal vasodilator effect of dopamine has, however, been questioned and it has been suggested that the increased urine output is largely attributable to a rise in cardiac output and blood pressure, combined with a decrease in aldosterone concentrations and inhibition of tubular sodium reabsorption mediated via DA1 stimulation. Despite the increase in urine output, low-dose dopamine has no effect on the need for renal replacement therapy or mortality in patients with, or at risk of, acute renal dysfunction (Friedrich et al., 2005) (see also Chapter 13).

As the dose of dopamine is increased (3–10 μg/kg per min), β_1-adrenergic effects predominate, producing an increase in heart rate and cardiac contractility. Dopamine also increases noradrenaline release contributing to its cardiac effects, and at higher doses (> 10 μg/kg per min), vasoconstriction occurs, increasing blood pressure and afterload and raising ventricular filling pressures. This can be dangerous in patients with cardiac failure in whom filling pressures are already high. There is also some evidence to suggest that in septic shock the use of high dose dopamine to achieve a target MAP > 75 mmHg may precipitate gut mucosal ischaemia, perhaps by redistributing flow, whereas noradrenaline can improve splanchnic oxygenation (Marik and Mohedin, 1994). In another study dopamine (5 μg/kg per min) was associated with a reduction in gastric mucosal blood flow and pH (Neviere et al., 1996). Dopamine consistently increases pulmonary shunt fraction and in some patients the dose of dopamine is limited by β effects such as tachycardia and arrhythmias. In septic shock dopamine restores MAP primarily by increasing stroke volume and cardiac index, with minimal effect on heart rate and systemic vascular resistance. Central venous, pulmonary artery and PAOPs are usually unchanged. At doses higher than 20 μg/kg per min, however, right heart pressures may increase and this dose should not normally be exceeded. The median dose of dopamine required to restore blood pressure in septic shock is 15 μg/kg per min (Task Force of the American College of Critical Care Medicine, Society of Critical Care Medicine, 1999).

Dopamine also suppresses the circulating concentrations of all the anterior pituitary-dependent hormones except cortisol (Van den Berghe and de Zegher, 1996). Although the clinical implications of this effect are unclear, such changes are unlikely to be beneficial and suggest that long-term administration of dopamine to critically ill patients should be avoided. Indeed an observational study has suggested that dopamine administration may be associated with increased mortality rates in shock (Sakr *et al.*, 2006).

DOPEXAMINE

Dopexamine is an analogue of dopamine which activates β_2 receptors as well as DA1 and DA2 receptors. It is more potent at DA1 than DA2 receptors, is a weak β_1 agonist and inhibits neuronal reuptake of noradrenaline. Dopexamine is a very weak positive inotrope, but is a powerful splanchnic vasodilator, reducing afterload and improving cardiac output and blood flow to vital organs, including the kidneys. It is an effective natriuretic and diuretic agent. At higher doses a fall in diastolic pressure and MAP may reduce regional blood flow. In septic shock, dopexamine can increase cardiac index and heart rate, but causes further reductions in systemic vascular resistance (Colardyn *et al.*, 1989) and the dose may be limited by tachycardia. Although some early studies suggested that dopexamine can improve gut mucosal perfusion, in a later study in patients with severe sepsis (who were already receiving dobutamine) dopexamine only increased splanchnic oxygen delivery in proportion to the increase in cardiac output and caused a dose-dependent reduction in intramucosal pH (Meier-Hellmann *et al.*, 1999). Moreover, in patients with septic shock receiving noradrenaline, the addition of dopexamine failed to improve hepatosplanchnic haemodynamics, oxygen exchange and energy balance, despite increases in oxygen delivery (Kiefer *et al.*, 2000). It has been suggested that dopexamine is likely to be most useful in the management of low-output left ventricular failure, but this agent is not generally recommended for the management of sepsis/septic shock.

DOBUTAMINE

Dobutamine is a racemic mixture of two isomers, a D-isomer with β_1 and β_2 activity and an L-isomer with β_1- and α_1-adrenergic actions. Dobutamine causes less tachycardia and arrhythmias than isoprenaline but when compared with dopamine the relative effects of the two agents on heart rate and rhythm are a matter of dispute. An advantage of dobutamine is its ability to reduce systemic resistance, as well as improve cardiac performance, thereby decreasing both afterload and ventricular filling pressures. Dobutamine is therefore useful in patients with cardiogenic shock and cardiac failure, although the associated vasodilatation may be complicated by hypotension. In septic shock dobutamine increases heart rate, stroke volume, ventricular stroke work, cardiac output, DO_2 and VO_2 while, in some cases, systemic vascular resistance falls (Vincent *et al.*, 1990). Dobutamine may be particularly useful in septic patients with fluid overload or myocardial failure (Jardin *et al.*, 1981). In adrenaline-treated patients with septic shock, the addition of dobutamine (5 µg/kg per min) selectively improved gastric mucosal perfusion without altering systemic haemodynamics (Levy *et al.*, 1997b) and in another study the same dose of dobutamine improved gastric mucosal perfusion in septic patients, whereas dopamine was deleterious in this respect (Neviere *et al.*, 1996). Dobutamine has no specific effect on the renal vasculature or dopamine receptors, although urine output and, in some cases, creatinine clearance often increase as cardiac output and blood pressure improve.

PHOSPHODIESTERASE INHIBITORS (E.G. AMRINONE, MILRINONE, ENOXIMONE)

These agents have both inotropic and vasodilator properties. They inhibit phosphodiesterase type III (PDE III), thereby increasing concentrations of cyclic adenosine monophosphate (AMP) and improving cardiac contractility, whilst inhibition of other PDE isoforms increases cGMP and produces vasodilatation. Cardiac index and stroke work indices usually increase, whilst systemic and pulmonary vascular resistances fall. Vasopressors such as noradrenaline may be required to counteract excessive vasodilatation. These agents have a relatively long half-life (e.g. 4–7 hours for enoximone) and are usually administered as a loading dose followed by a continuous infusion, although single doses may be sufficient for weaning from cardiopulmonary bypass. Because PDE III inhibitors bypass the β-adrenergic receptor they do not cause significant tachycardia, are considerably less arrhythmogenic than sympathomimetic agents and can potentiate the effects of β-agonists. PDE III inhibitors may be particularly useful in patients with adrenergic receptor downregulation, those receiving β-blockers, for weaning patients from cardiopulmonary bypass, and for patients with cardiac failure. In vasodilated septic patients, however, they may precipitate or worsen hypotension, an effect which can be prolonged. Although PDE III inhibitors are not generally recommended for patients with sepsis/septic shock, they can occasionally be useful in combination with adrenergic agents. Indeed, one study suggested that enoximone could improve hepatosplanchnic function in fluid-resuscitated septic shock patients in whom MAP was maintained with noradrenaline, perhaps in part by inhibiting the inflammatory response, as well as by improving regional perfusion (Kern *et al.*, 2001).

VASOPRESSIN

Vasopressin is an ADH with thermoregulatory, haemostatic and gastrointestinal effects which also acts as a potent vasopressor via activation of V1 receptors on vascular smooth muscle. Its antidiuretic action is mediated via V2 receptor activation in the renal collecting duct system. In addition, vasopressin, at low concentrations, mediates vasodilatation in coronary, cerebral and pulmonary arterial circulations. Although circulating levels of vasopressin are usually increased in response to stress, inappropriately low levels have been described in patients with septic shock, possibly because of impaired secretion or depletion of vasopressin stores in the neurohypophysis (Landry *et al.*, 1997; Sharshar *et al.*, 2002). Moreover, in contrast to the blunted response to adrenergic agents, patients with vasodilatory shock appear to be hypersensitive to the pressor effects of exogenous vasopressin and administration of vasopressin to these patients potentiates the vasoconstrictor effects of noradrenaline. In a randomized double-blind study, a short-term vasopressin infusion reduced the requirement for conventional vasopressors and improved renal function (Patel *et al.*, 2002). Cardiac index was maintained whilst ventricular filling pressures, pulmonary artery pressures, pulmonary vascular resistance and heart rate were unchanged, as was gastric mucosal perfusion. The increase in urine output and creatinine clearance following vasopressin administration may be a consequence of increased systemic blood pressure combined with preferential constriction of renal efferent arterioles leading to increased glomerular perfusion pressure. Also vasopressin may directly activate oxytocin receptors, causing natriuresis and diuresis, as well as releasing atrial natriuretic peptide. At high doses, however, there is a danger that vasopressin will precipitate excessive renal, coronary, mesenteric and systemic vasoconstriction, as well as causing a significant reduction in cardiac output. A recent randomised controlled trial, however, found that low dose vasopressin did not reduce mortality rates when compared to noradrenaline, although there was a suggestion of benefit in those with less severe septic shock (Russell *et al.*, 2008).

Vasopressin is relatively contraindicated in hypovolaemia, heart failure and in those with a history of coronary artery disease, although there are studies showing utility in cardiogenic shock. An alternative is to use terlipressin, a cheaper, longer-acting, synthetic analogue of vasopressin. Small doses (0.25–0.5 mg), repeated at 20-minute intervals to a maximum of 2 mg, should be used with close observation for signs of peripheral ischaemia and with cardiac output monitoring. In sepsis patients a single dose is often sufficient to improve blood pressure, reduce vasopressor requirements and improve renal function (Leone *et al.*, 2004).

Angiotensin has been used in resistant septic shock (Wray and Coakley, 1995) but there is a danger of excessive vasoconstriction with associated falls in cardiac output and tissue perfuison. This agent is no longer available in the UK.

INHIBITION OF NITRIC OXIDE SYNTHESIS

Experimental studies have demonstrated that the vascular hyporeactivity to adrenergic agonists and the peripheral vascular failure associated with endotoxaemia can be reversed by inhibiting NO synthesis with L-arginine analogues, and prevented by inhibiting the induction of inducible NOS with dexamethasone. There is evidence that NO production is increased in human sepsis (Evans *et al.*, 1993) and preliminary studies in patients with septic shock suggested that administration of the non-selective NOS inhibitor *N*-monomethyl-L-arginine hydrochloride (L NMMA) was safe and could restore vasomotor tone and maintain blood pres-

sure (Grover *et al.*, 1999). At higher doses, however, cardiac output and oxygen delivery fell, although oxygen consumption was maintained by an increase in oxygen extraction. There were also concerns about the effects of inhibiting NO production on regional perfusion, the microcirculation, the pulmonary vasculature, coagulation, free radical injury and immune function. These concerns were highlighted when a phase III study of L-NMMA was terminated prematurely because of excess mortality in the treatment group, perhaps partly explained by the inclusion of patients with hypodynamic septic shock in this trial and the deleterious effect of higher doses of NOS inhibitor (Lopez *et al.*, 2004).

Methylene blue inhibits guanylate cyclase and possibly also NOS. Administration of methylene blue to patients with septic shock can increase arterial blood pressure, although stroke volume, left ventricular stroke work and oxygen delivery are unchanged (Kirov *et al.*, 2001). Further studies are required to determine whether this agent has a role in routine clinical practice.

LEVOSIMENDAN

This novel agent sensitizes troponin C to calcium, thereby improving myocardial contractility, and causes vasodilation by opening ATP-sensitive potassium channels. Myocardial oxygen demand is not increased. In patients with severe low-output heart failure, levosimendan improved haemodynamic performance more effectively than dobutamine and was associated with a lower mortality (Follath *et al.*, 2002).

RECEPTOR DOWNREGULATION

Many of the most seriously ill patients become increasingly resistant to the effects of pressor agents, an observation attributed to downregulation of adenergic receptors. This may be due to a reduction in receptor numbers, a decreased affinity of the receptor for its ligand induced by overstimulation, or a direct effect of inflammatory mediators on signal transduction either at or distal to the receptor. This affects intracellular calcium levels and the resultant vascular hypo reactivity to both endogenous and exogenous catecholamines is a particular feature of septic shock.

Guidelines for the use of inotropic and vasopressor agents *(Task Force of the American College of Critical Care Medicine, Society of Critical Care Medicine, 1999)*

Many still consider dopamine in low to moderate doses to be the first-line agent for restoring blood pressure, although others favour dopexamine as a means of increasing cardiac output and organ blood flow. High-dose dopamine is usually best avoided. Dobutamine is particularly indicated in patients in whom the vasoconstriction caused by dopamine could be dangerous (i.e. patients with cardiac disease, those with a low cardiac output after fluid resuscitation and septic patients with fluid overload or myocardial failure). The combination of dobutamine and noradrenaline is currently popular for the management of patients who are hypotensive with a low systemic vascular resistance (e.g. septic shock). Dobutamine is given to maintain an appropriate cardiac output and improve organ perfusion, whilst noradrenaline is used to restore an adequate blood pressure by reducing vasodilatation. In some vasodilated patients with a high cardiac output, noradrenaline is used alone. **The Surviving Sepsis campaign guidelines (Dellinger *et al.*, 2008) recommend either dopamine or noradrenaline as first-choice vasopressor agents to correct hypotension in septic shock and dobutamine as the first-choice inotrope.** Adrenaline, because of its potency, remains a useful agent in patients with refractory hypotension, although adverse effects are relatively common. Recent evidence, however, suggests that there is no difference in the efficacy and safety of adrenaline when compared to a noradrenaline/dobutamine combination for the management of septic shock (Annane *et al.*, 2007). PDE inhibitors are most often used for patients with heart failure, especially when complicating cardiac surgery; they have little place in the management of septic shock, except perhaps in combination with vasoconstrictors. The value of alternative vasopressors such as vasopressin in septic shock remains uncertain.

TARGETING SUPRANORMAL VALUES FOR CARDIAC INDEX, DO_2 AND $\dot{V}O_2$ (Hinds and Watson, 1995)

Although resuscitation has conventionally been aimed at achieving normal haemodynamics, it is clear that survival of patients with septic or traumatic shock (as well as following major surgery and those with ARDS) is associated with elevated values for cardiac output, DO_2 and $\dot{V}O_2$ (Russell *et al.*, 1990; Shoemaker *et al.*, 1973; Tuchschmidt *et al.*, 1989).

HIGH-RISK SURGICAL PATIENTS (Table 5.9)

It has been suggested that treatment in high-risk surgical patients should be directed at increasing cardiac output, DO_2 and $\dot{V}O_2$ until they equal or exceed the median maximum values found in survivors (i.e. cardiac index > 4.5 L/min per m², DO_2 > 600 mL/min per m² and $\dot{V}O_2$ > 170 mL/min per m²) in order to replenish tissue oxygen and prevent organ dysfunction (Shoemaker *et al.*, 1973). In one study, early institution of treatment aimed at achieving these survivor values was found to improve survival after major surgery (Shoemaker *et al.*, 1988), and in another the use of dopexamine to increase perioperative oxygen delivery reduced

mortality in high-risk surgical patients (Boyd *et al.*, 1993). Other studies have also indicated that preoperative optimization of oxygen delivery might reduce the risk associated with major elective surgery (Wilson *et al.*, 1999), whilst aggressive intraoperative volume expansion alone, guided by the oesophageal Doppler, has been shown to improve outcome after repair of proximal femoral fracture (Sinclair *et al.*, 1997) and following cardiac surgery (Mythen and Webb, 1995). Similarly, a nurse-delivered protocol guided by the oesophageal Doppler and aimed at achieving a stroke volume of more than 35 mL/m² reduced hospital stay in patients after cardiac surgery (McKendry *et al.*, 2004). Moreover, during repair of proximal femoral fracture, repeated colloid fluid challenges guided by either CVP or oesophageal Doppler shortened time to being medically fit for discharge (Venn *et al.*, 2002) and intraoperative oesophageal Doppler-guided fluid management reduced hospital length of stay after major bowel surgery (Wakeling *et al.*, 2005). More recently *postoperative* institution of treatment aimed at achieving a DO_2 of at least 600 mL/min per m² using fluids and dopexamine (guided by lithium indicator dilution cardiac output monitoring) was associated with reductions in postoperative complications and duration of hospital stay (Pearse *et al.*, 2005).

Although these high-risk surgical patients undoubtedly benefit from intensive perioperative haemodynamic monitoring and support, especially optimal expansion of the circulating volume, as well as postoperative management in a high-dependency or ICU, the value of *preoperative* admission to intensive care for optimization of DO_2, the targeting of survivor values for DO_2 and $\dot{V}O_2$ and the routine use of inodilators such as dopexamine remains unclear. Moreover, there is considerable doubt as to the benefit of pulmonary artery catheterization in such cases (Sandham *et al.*, 2003) (see Chapter 4). There is also uncertainty as to which is the most effective inotrope/vasopressor in these circumstances. Interestingly, the routine use of dopexamine, in doses which increased cardiac output and oxygen delivery, failed to influence the overall outcome after major abdominal surgery compared to fluid optimization alone (Takala *et al.*, 2000). This study did, however, indicate that the most high-risk cases might benefit from such treatment and there is some evidence to suggest that dopexamine reduces the incidence of acute inflammation in the gut mucosa of these patients (Byers *et al.*, 1999). Indeed, it has been suggested that the anti-inflammatory actions of catecholamines might explain the beneficial effects of targeting high levels of DO_2 in critically ill surgical patients (Uusaro and Russell, 2000).

CRITICALLY ILL PATIENTS

It seemed possible that elevation of DO_2 and $\dot{V}O_2$ to levels that some have called 'supranormal' might also improve outcome in patients with septic shock (Tuchschmidt *et al.*, 1992), as well as in heterogeneous groups of critically ill patients (Yu *et al.*, 1993) and trauma victims (Fleming *et al.*, 1992). Disappointingly, subsequent PRCTs have demonstrated that, at least when instituted following admission to intensive care or after a significant delay, treatment aimed at

---

Table 5.9 High-risk surgery: patients at risk of developing perioperative multiorgan failure

Patients with compromised cardiorespiratory function

Patients with trauma to two body cavities requiring multiple blood transfusions

Patients undergoing surgery involving extensive tissue dissection, e.g. oesophagectomy, pancreatectomy, aortic aneurysm surgery

Patients undergoing emergency surgery for intra-abdominal or intrathoracic catastrophic states, e.g. faecal peritonitis, oesophageal perforation

Modified from Shoemaker *et al.* (1988).

achieving survivor values (or at maintaining S_vO_2) is of no benefit (Alia *et al.*, 1999; Gattinoni *et al.*, 1995; Hayes *et al.*, 1994) and might even be harmful (Alia *et al.*, 1999; Hayes *et al.*, 1994) in such patients. Although there is no doubt that the prognosis for those who do achieve survivor values in response to fluids alone or only moderate inotropic support is excellent, in a significant number (often the older or more severely ill patients) it proves impossible to achieve target values, even with high-dose inotropic support (Alia *et al.*, 1999; Gattinoni *et al.*, 1995; Hayes *et al.*, 1994) and in such patients mortality rates are extremely high (Hayes *et al.*, 1993, 1997). The failure of these non-survivors to respond to aggressive haemodynamic support is in part related to reduced responsiveness of the myocardium to inotropes but is particularly associated with peripheral vascular failure, resistance to vasopressors and an impaired ability of the tissues to extract or utilize the increased amounts of delivered oxygen and/or to metabolize aerobically (Hayes *et al.*, 1997) – so-called 'tissue dysoxia' (see above).

Nevertheless, it remains possible that earlier institution of some form of 'goal-directed' treatment might prevent progression to refractory shock, tissue hypoxia and organ failure and thereby improve outcome. In patients admitted with severe sepsis or septic shock, for example, early goal-directed therapy in the emergency room aimed at maintaining central venous oxygen saturation at more than 70% significantly reduced in-hospital mortality (Rivers *et al.*, 2001). On the other hand, institution of treatment aimed at achieving 'supranormal' values for CI, DO_2 and $\dot{V}O_2$ immediately after admission failed to improve outcome in critically injured patients (Velmahos *et al.*, 2000). These authors concluded, as have others (Hayes *et al.*, 1997), that the ability to achieve the recommended target values simply indicates an adequate physiological reserve, with preserved cellular function and therefore a good prognosis. This suggestion is supported by studies demonstrating the prognostic value of the responses of DO_2 and $\dot{V}O_2$ to a short-term infusion of dobutamine in patients with sepsis syndrome and normal lactate levels (Vallet *et al.*, 1993), and in patients with sepsis, severe sepsis or septic shock (Rhodes *et al.*, 1999).

In conclusion, although **The Surviving Sepsis Guidelines do not recommend aggressive targeting of 'survivor values' for CI, DO_2 and $\dot{V}O_2$ for critically ill patients after admission to intensive care (Dellinger *et al.*, 2008), early resuscitation, aimed especially at achieving an adequate circulating volume (see above), combined with the rational use of inotropic and/or vasoactive agents to maintain blood pressure and an appropriate cardiac output, is essential.** Resuscitation may be more effective when guided by monitoring of venous oxygen saturation, or cardiac output, e.g. by oesophageal Doppler, but the value of routine pulmonary artery catheterization is increasingly in doubt (see Chapter 4).

Vasodilator therapy, afterload and preload reduction

In selected patients, afterload reduction may be used to increase stroke volume and decrease myocardial oxygen requirements by reducing systolic wall tension. Vasodilatation also decreases heart size and diastolic ventricular wall tension so that coronary blood flow is improved. The relative magnitude of the falls in preload and afterload depends on the pre-existing haemodynamic disturbance, concurrent volume replacement, the agent selected and the dose used (see later). There is also reason to believe that, in some circumstances, specific vasodilators may improve microcirculatory flow (see later).

Vasodilator therapy can be particularly helpful in patients with cardiac failure in whom the ventricular function curve is flat, so that falls in preload have only a limited effect on stroke volume. This form of treatment, combined in selected cases with inotropic support, can therefore sometimes be useful in cardiogenic shock and in patients with cardiogenic pulmonary oedema, mitral regurgitation or an acute ventricular septal defect. In such cases, nitrate vasodilators are usually used. Furthermore, because of their ability to improve the myocardial oxygen supply:demand ratio, nitrates can be used to control angina and limit ischaemic damage following myocardial infarction. Vasodilators may also be valuable for controlling hypertension in post cardiac surgery patients, as well as for the treatment of hypertensive emergencies, dissecting aneurysm, accelerated hypertension of pregnancy and in pulmonary hypertension.

Vasodilator therapy is potentially dangerous and vasodilatation should be achieved cautiously, usually guided by invasive haemodynamic monitoring. The circulating volume must be adequate before treatment is started and, except in those with cardiac failure, falls in preload should be prevented to avoid serious reductions in cardiac output and blood pressure. If diastolic pressure is allowed to fall, coronary blood flow may be jeopardized and myocardial ischaemia may be precipitated, particularly if a reflex tachycardia develops in response to the hypotension. Provided myocardial performance is not impaired, it is therefore sometimes appropriate to control the tachycardia with a β-blocker. Other side-effects of vasodilators include:

- hypoxaemia;
- vertigo;
- flushing;
- nausea and vomiting;
- headache;
- rebound hypertension.

The selection of an appropriate agent in an individual patient depends on a careful assessment of the haemodynamic disturbance and on whether the effect required is predominantly a reduction in preload, afterload or both.

NITRIC OXIDE DONORS
Sodium nitroprusside (SNP). This agent dilates both arterioles and venous capacitance vessels, as well as the pulmonary vasculature. SNP therefore reduces the afterload and preload of both ventricles and can improve cardiac output and the myocardial oxygen supply:demand ratio. Some authorities

have suggested, however, that SNP can exacerbate myocardial ischaemia by producing a 'steal' phenomenon in the coronary circulation. The increased cardiac output is preferentially distributed to musculoskeletal regions. If arterial pressure falls, hepatic and renal blood flow are unchanged, whereas if pressure is maintained, splanchnic flow increases slightly.

The effects of SNP are rapid in onset and spontaneously reversible within a few minutes of discontinuing the infusion. Moreover, tachyphylaxis is not a problem. SNP is most commonly used to control resistant hypertension after cardiac surgery and in malignant hypertension. SNP has been shown to improve cardiac function rapidly in patients with decompensated heart failure due to severe left ventricular systolic dysfunction and severe aortic stenosis (Khot et al., 2003).

An *overdose* of SNP can cause cyanide poisoning with histotoxic hypoxia caused by inhibition of cytochrome oxidase, the terminal enzyme of the respiratory chain. This is manifested as a metabolic acidosis and a fall in the arteriovenous $(C_{a-v}O_2)$ oxygen content difference. These effects should not inhibit the clinical use of SNP since they are only seen when a gross overdose has been administered and are easily avoided with care. In the short term (a few hours) infusions should be limited to a total dose of 1.5 mg/kg. There is only limited information concerning the safe dosage for long-term administration (several hours to days, or even weeks), although it has been suggested that maximum infusion rates of approximately 4 µg/kg per min (certainly less than 8 µg/kg per min) and a total dose of 70 mg SNP/kg over periods of up to 2 weeks are the maximum allowable without risking toxic effects (Vesey and Cole, 1985). Although thiocyanate accumulation is not a concern during hypotensive anaesthesia, high plasma levels may be achieved during long-term administration, with possible toxic consequences. Monitoring of thiocyanate levels has therefore been recommended during infusions lasting more than 3 days, particularly in the presence of renal insufficiency (Vesey and Cole, 1985). Treatment of cyanide toxicity is discussed in Chapter 19. SNP is broken down during prolonged exposure to light; this problem can be avoided by making up the solution in relatively small quantities or by protecting it with silver foil.

Nitroglycerine (glyceryl trinitrate, GTN) and isosorbide dinitrate (ISDN). At low doses these agents are predominantly venodilators but as the dose is increased they produce arterial dilatation, thereby decreasing both preload and afterload; cardiac output may increase, although most of the additional flow is distributed to musculoskeletal regions. Nitrates are particularly useful in the treatment of acute cardiac failure with pulmonary oedema and are conventionally used in combination with intravenous furosemide. In these circumstances the reduction in right ventricular volume and preload may lead to an increase in left ventricular volume and an improvement in stroke volume, with relief of pulmonary oedema. The reduction in preload may also reduce ventricular wall tension and improve coronary perfusion. With higher doses of nitrate the reduction in afterload might increase cardiac output and further reduce pulmonary congestion, whereas furosemide can activate both the sympathetic and renin–angiotensin systems, potentially increasing afterload and reducing stroke volume. Moreover, the majority of patients presenting in acute heart failure are hypovolaemic as a result of vomiting, sweating, reduced fluid intake and extracellular fluid shifts. This hypovolaemia will be exacerbated by the diuresis induced by furosemide, leading to vasoconstriction and further reductions in cardiac output. Indeed, many patients will benefit from judicious expansion of the circulating volume in conjunction with vasodilator therapy. There is evidence that the use of high-dose ISDN (given as a 3-mg intravenous bolus every 5 minutes after low-dose frusemide) is more effective than high-dose furosemide with low-dose ISDN (Cotter et al., 1998). In particular, the need for mechanical ventilation and the frequency of subsequent myocardial infarction were significantly reduced by high-dose ISDN.

Because nitrates can reverse myocardial ischaemia by increasing and redistributing coronary blood flow, as well as reducing ventricular wall tension, they can be used to control angina, prevent myocardial infarction and limit infarct size. GTN and ISDN are usually used in preference to SNP in patients with cardiac failure and/or myocardial ischaemia. Both GTN and ISDN reduce pulmonary vascular resistance, an effect that can occasionally be exploited in patients with a low cardiac output secondary to pulmonary hypertension. Finally, recent evidence suggests that in patients with septic shock who have been volume-resuscitated, cautious administration of GTN can improve microvascular flow (Spronk et al., 2002).

ADRENERGIC BLOCKERS
Adrenergic blockers predominantly dilate arterioles and therefore mainly influence afterload. Phenoxybenzamine is unsuitable for use in the critically ill because of its slow onset (1–2 hours to maximum effect) and prolonged duration of action (2–3 days). Phentolamine is very potent with a rapid onset and short duration of action (15–20 minutes). It can be used to control blood pressure acutely in hypertensive crises, but may produce a marked tachycardia and is expensive to administer as a continuous infusion. Labetalol is an $α_1$- and β-blocking agent which can be given as a continuous infusion. It is particularly indicated for control of blood pressure in patients with dissecting thoracic aortic aneurysms in whom the reduction in shear stress consequent on β-blockade may be an advantage. Side-effects include bradycardia, heart block and bronchostriction. It is contraindicated in asthma and chronic obstructive pulmonary disease.

HYDRALAZINE
This agent predominantly affects arterial resistance vessels. It therefore reduces afterload and blood pressure while cardiac output and heart rate increase. Renal and limb blood

flow are also increased. Hydralazine can be administered orally to patients with chronic cardiac failure, but in intensive care practice it is usually given as an intravenous bolus (5–10 mg) to control acute increases in blood pressure, particularly after cardiac surgery.

CALCIUM ANTAGONISTS

The calcium channel blocker nifedipine can be administered orally or sublingually to control hypertension. It is a particularly potent peripheral smooth-muscle relaxant that causes a reduction in systemic vascular resistance and an increase in cardiac output. Most of the increased flow is distributed to musculoskeletal beds, with lesser increases in hepatic, splanchnic and renal flow.

ANGIOTENSIN-CONVERTING ENZYME INHIBITORS

ACE inhibitors such as captopril and enalapril reduce systemic vascular resistance and generally increase renal blood flow by reducing angiotensin-induced arteriolar tone. This effect is, however, more pronounced in the efferent vessels, and GFR may therefore remain unchanged or fall despite the increased flow. Nevertheless, sodium excretion usually increases, largely due to a reduction in aldosterone release. ACE inhibitors can be useful when weaning patients with cardiac failure from intravenous vasodilators.

Note: when used in patients with respiratory failure most inotropes and vasoactive agents increase venous admixture; this may be due simply to passive opening of pulmonary vessels by the increased flow and pressure or to a specific reversal of the hypoxic vasoconstrictor response.

Mechanical circulatory assistance
INTRA-AORTIC BALLOON COUNTERPULSATION

Various techniques for mechanically supporting the failing myocardium have been described; of these, intra-aortic balloon counterpulsation (IABCP) has proved most practical and is now widely used.

A catheter with an inflatable sausage-shaped balloon is inserted via a femoral artery using a percutaneous Seldinger technique and passed into the aorta until its tip lies just distal to the left subclavian artery (**Fig. 5.17**). If the Seldinger

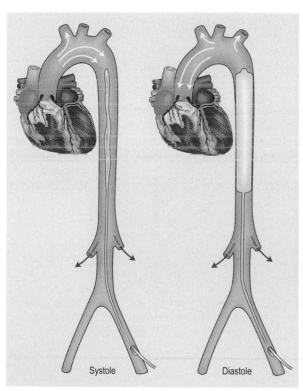

Systole   Diastole

(a)

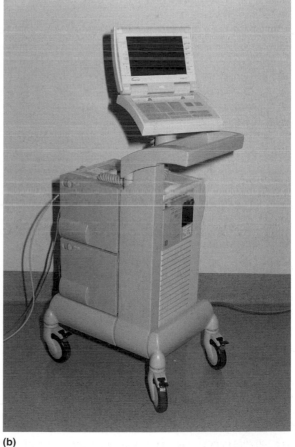

(b)

Fig. 5.17 Intra-aortic balloon counterpulsation (IABCP). (a) Rapid deflation of the balloon occurs at the onset of systole and causes a reduction in afterload. Early in diastole the balloon is rapidly inflated to increase the pressure in the aortic root and enhance coronary blood flow. (b) An intra-aortic balloon pump and console.

technique fails, an open surgical approach can be used. Fluoroscopy makes insertion safer and allows accurate positioning of the catheter tip. In the absence of fluoroscopy the position of the catheter must be verified by chest X-ray. Occasionally, the balloon is inserted via the ascending aorta in those undergoing cardiac surgery, whilst in other cases the axillary or sublcavian arteries are used.

Early in diastole, the balloon is rapidly inflated so that the pressure in the aortic root rises and coronary blood flow is increased. Rapid deflation of the balloon is timed to occur at the onset of systole (usually triggered by the R wave on the ECG) and this leads to a reduction in afterload and left ventricular wall tension. Preload, pulmonary artery pressure and pulmonary vascular resistance may also be reduced. Heart rate is usually unchanged. The reduction in left ventricular work reduces myocardial oxygen requirements and this, combined with the increased coronary blood flow, may result in a reversal of ischaemic changes and limitation of infarct size. IABCP may not, however, increase coronary blood flow distal to significant stenoses. Improved myocardial performance, together with the reduction in afterload, can lead to an increased cardiac output. Inflation and deflation of the balloon must be precisely timed to achieve effective counterpulsation (**Fig. 5.18**).

The only absolute *contraindications* to IABCP are *aortic aneurysms* (or other severe disease of the descending aorta) and *significant aortic regurgitation*. Relative contraindications include arrhythmias and extreme tachycardias, both of which limit the ability of the device to trigger balloon deflation accurately, and severe peripheral vascular disease.

IABCP is associated with significant morbidity. *Complications* include:

- failure to pass the balloon (usually in those with severe atheromatous disease);
- arterial dissection;
- limb ischaemia;
- thrombosis;
- embolism;

- infection;
- a distally positioned balloon may intermittently occlude the renal vasculature;
- balloon rupture is rare.

In order to minimize the risk of thrombosis on the surface of the balloon the patient should be heparinized to achieve a partial thromboplastin time of about $1\frac{1}{2}$ times normal and the balloon should be kept in motion. Because there is a tendency to develop thrombocytopenia, the platelet count should be carefully monitored.

IABCP has proved most useful for weaning patients from cardiopulmonary bypass and for those who develop myocardial ischaemia in the perioperative period. It may also be used to support patients in cardiogenic shock who have surgically correctable lesions, such as ischaemic ventricular septal defects or mitral regurgitation, while they are being prepared for surgery. In patients with severe ischaemia (e.g. those with unstable angina) IABCP may relieve pain and possibly prevent infarction while preparations are made for coronary artery bypass grafting or percutaneous transluminal coronary angioplasty (PTCA) (see Chapter 9). The use of IABCP for the treatment of cardiogenic shock complicating myocardial infarction without a surgically correctable lesion has been less successful, although some feel that this may be due partly to delay in instituting IABCP and extension of the infarct caused by the prior use of inotropes. Although there are no PRCT data to indicate that IABCP can improve outcome in cardiogenic shock, it has been suggested that the technique might be beneficial when used in conjunction with revascularization, either surgically or by coronary angioplasty (Hasdai *et al.*, 2000).

IABCP may also be indicated in patients with a failing transplanted heart and in those with viral myocarditis. IABCP is occasionally used prophylactically in patients undergoing high-risk cardiac surgery or PTCA. There is only limited experience with the use of IABCP in myocardial failure complicating septic shock, but it seems that the technique may be life-saving in those with reversible global myo-

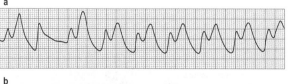

a

Balloon initially inflating on alternate beats (1:2) then 1:1

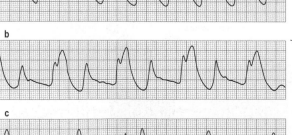

b

c

Balloon inflating on alternate beats (1:2)

Fig. 5.18 (a) The effect of intra-aortic balloon counterpulsation (IABCP) on the arterial pressure trace. Note the increased diastolic pressure, the slight fall in systolic pressure (due to afterload reduction) and reduced end-diastolic pressure (due to rapid balloon deflation). (b) It is important that the balloon inflates immediately the aortic valve closes (i.e. on the dicrotic notch). In this case the balloon is inflating too early. This impedes left ventricular ejection. (c) In this case balloon inflation is delayed.

cardial dysfunction complicating anaphylaxis (Raper and Fisher, 1988).

OTHER VENTRICULAR ASSIST DEVICES

Centrifugal pumps can be used to bypass and 'off-load' the right or, more often, the left ventricle while maintaining adequate systemic blood flow. Such devices are usually used as a means of discontinuing cardiopulmonary bypass in the hope that ventricular function will improve significantly over the ensuing 48–72 hours. They may also be used as a 'bridge' to cardiac transplantation. Alternative devices include *mechanical hearts*, used to support potential cardiac transplant recipients and *arteriovenous pumps*.

HAEMATOLOGICAL PROBLEMS

The most commonly encountered haematological problem in shock is a coagulation defect, usually due to massive blood transfusion and/or consumption coagulopathy (DIC), the latter being particularly common in sepsis (see above). This can usually be corrected with transfusions of fresh frozen plasma, occasionally combined with platelets, or cryoprecipitate. DIC should be prevented or reversed by aggressive treatment of the underlying condition. Heparinization has been recommended, but this is potentially extremely dangerous, particularly in trauma victims and postoperative patients, and is rarely indicated. Later, coagulation may be impaired secondary to the development of renal and/or hepatic failure.

RENAL FUNCTION

Prevention of acute intrinsic renal failure is best achieved by restoring cardiac output, blood pressure and renal blood flow as rapidly as possible, combined with early and aggressive management of oliguria (see Chapter 13).

MULTIPLE-ORGAN FAILURE

Although it is now usually possible to support patients through the early stages of shock, trauma or other life-threatening illnesses, a disappointingly high proportion subsequently develop progressive failure of several vital organs (Barton and Cerra, 1989; DeCamp and Demling, 1988). Mortality is high and correlates with the number of organs which fail; those with prolonged three-system failure have a mortality rate exceeding 50%, whilst more than 90% of those with prolonged six-system failure die. Sequential MOF is now the commonest mode of death in intensive care patients, accounting for as many as 75% of all deaths in surgical ICUs (Barton and Cerra, 1989). Moreover, these patients spend long periods in intensive care and consume a large proportion of available resources.

DEFINITION

Currently there is no consensus on the definition of the MOF syndrome and criteria for failure of individual organs differ. Because the extent of organ dysfunction can vary both between patients and within the same patient over time, the term *multiple-organ dysfunction syndrome* (MODS) has been suggested to indicate the wide range of severity and dynamic nature of this disorder (Bone *et al.*, 1992; Members of the American College of Chest Physicians/Society of Critical Care Medicine Consensus Conference, 1992). Organ dysfunction is defined as '*the presence of altered organ function in an acutely ill patient such that homeostasis cannot be maintained without intervention*'. Transient impairment of organ function rapidly responsive to short-term measures should probably be excluded from this definition.

AETIOLOGY AND CAUSES (see also pp. 96–99)

There are two distinct, but not mutually exclusive, pathways by which MODS may develop (**Fig. 5.19**).

- In *primary MODS* there is a direct insult to an individual organ (e.g. pulmonary aspiration, lung contusion or renal damage due to rhabdomyolysis), which fails early as the result of an inflammatory response that is confined, at least in the early stages, to the affected organ.
- The aetiology of *secondary MODS* is complex but, in general terms, organ damage is thought to be precipitated by systemic dissemination of a poorly controlled inflammatory/anti-inflammatory response associated with haemodynamic disturbance, microcirculatory abnormalities and defective oxygen utilization, as described earlier in this chapter. However, the precise mechanisms responsible for organ damage have yet to be determined. Secondary MODS can therefore be viewed as a complication of SIRS (see above) and can be considered as representing the more severe end of the spectrum of illness of patients with SIRS/sepsis/septic shock. Secondary MODS usually evolves after a latent period from the initiating event, which is most commonly infectious (usually bacterial, but sometimes viral, fungal or parasitic), but may be non-infectious (e.g. the presence of extensive wounds or necrotic tissue). Secondary MODS may therefore follow sepsis, trauma, shock, major surgery and many other serious illnesses (e.g. pancreatitis, perforation of the gastrointestinal tract, pneumonia), or may arise in response to SIRS precipitated by primary MODS.

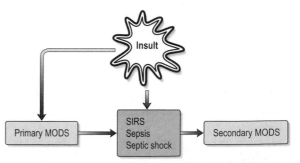

Fig. 5.19 Pathways for the development of multiple-organ dysfunction syndrome (MODS). SIRS, systemic inflammatory response syndrome.

CLINICAL FEATURES

Characteristic features of patients with MODS include:

- an increased metabolic rate (at least, in the early stages of the syndrome);
- a hyperdynamic circulation;
- hyperventilation;
- an impaired immune response;
- evidence of persistent or recurrent sepsis with fever (almost invariable);
- hypotension (common).

Sequential failure of vital organs occurs progressively over days to weeks, although the pattern and speed of development of organ dysfunction are highly variable. In most cases the lung is the first organ to be affected, usually with the development of ALI/ARDS (see Chapter 8), in association with cardiovascular instability and deteriorating renal function. Secondary pulmonary infection (ventilator-associated pneumonia – see Chapter 7) frequently acts as a further stimulus to the inflammatory response. Gastrointestinal failure is common, with an inability to tolerate enteral feeding, large gastric aspirates, abdominal distension due to paralytic ileus and diarrhoea. Gastrointestinal haemorrhage, ischaemic colitis, acalculous cholecystitis and pancreatitis may also occur, as may coagulopathies (see above) and bone marrow depression. Hepatic metabolism is markedly increased in the early stages, but later liver dysfunction, partly attributable to Kupffer cell activation, is associated with jaundice, elevated liver enzymes and a decreased albumin level. Frank hepatic failure is unusual, however. On the other hand, renal dysfunction or failure is common. Features of central nervous system dysfunction (see above) include an impaired conscious level, agitation and confusion progressing to coma. Critical illness polyneuropathy is almost invariable (see Chaper 15). In one study the organs that failed most frequently in patients with sepsis were the lungs (in 18% of patients) and the kidneys (in 15% of patients); less frequent were cardiovascular failure (7%), haematological failure (6%), metabolic failure (4%) and neurological failure (2%) (Martin et al., 2003).

Disruption of the muscosal barrier (see above) allows bacteria within the gut lumen, or their cell wall components to gain access to the portal, lymphatic, and hence systemic circulations. The liver defences, which are often compromised by poor perfusion, are overwhelmed and the lungs and other organs are exposed to bacterial toxins and inflammatory mediators released by liver macrophages. Some have therefore called the gut the 'motor of multiple-organ failure', although the role of translocation in the pathogenesis of MOF remains controversial (Lemaire et al., 1997).

The metabolic derangement is associated with elevated blood sugar levels, catabolism and wasting. Although characteristically these patients initially have a hyperdynamic circulation, eventually cardiovascular collapse supervenes, culminating in hypometabolism and failure of tissue oxygenation.

TREATMENT

Treatment of established MODS is essentially supportive. The principles of cardiovascular support are discussed earlier in this chapter, and respiratory, renal, hepatic and nutritional support in the relevant chapters elsewhere. Prevention of organ failure in those at risk is crucial. Aggressive early resuscitation is essential, and activation of the inflammatory response must be prevented or minimized by early excision of devitalized tissue and drainage of infection. Preservation of the integrity of the gut mucosal barrier by maximizing splanchnic perfusion and early enteral feeding is also important, as is strict normalization of blood sugar levels (see Chapter 17). Early recognition of organ dysfunction and prompt intervention may be associated with reversal of organ impairment and an improved outcome. Improvements in the prevention, control and eradication of infection, in techniques of cardiovascular, respiratory and renal support and in the provision of adequate nutrition, may have contributed to better outcomes. It is now often possible to support these patients for weeks or months; many now die following a decision to withdraw or not to escalate treatment (see Chapter 2).

ADJUNCTIVE THERAPY IN SHOCK, SEPSIS AND ORGAN FAILURE

The persistently high mortality associated with sepsis and organ failure has stimulated a search for additional forms of treatment that, when used in conjunction with conventional therapy, would assist shock reversal, prevent or minimize organ damage and improve outcome. Because many of the manifestations of severe sepsis, including the haemodynamic changes and vital organ damage, are mediated by an uncontrolled dissemination of the inflammatory and coagulation cascades, it has been postulated that mortality might be reduced by inhibiting the mediators of this response (see above) or by neutralizing bacterial cell wall components.

Despite encouraging results in animal models, however, this approach has proved generally disappointing. To some extent this failure to achieve a demonstrable improvement in outcome with adjunctive therapies, despite many years of intensive research, can be explained by the limitations of some of the large PRCTs that have been performed so far. Methodological difficulties have included:

- the definitions used for sepsis;
- the heterogeneity and wide range of illness severity of the patients studied;
- the influence of comorbidities;
- the criteria used to diagnose infection;
- the use of concomitant therapy (especially antibiotics);
- the timing of treatment;
- the question of attributable mortality;
- the choice of outcome measures.

Nevertheless, there is no doubt that the development of successful strategies to modulate inflammation/coagulation has been hampered by our limited understanding of the extremely complex mechanisms which trigger and regulate these responses and of the factors that can interfere with normal homeostasis, as well as the uncritical extrapolation of results obtained in animal models to clinical practice. There has also been a naïve assumption that mortality could be reduced by temporarily neutralizing just one component of the proinflammatory pathway. Finally, it is now well understood that suppression of inflammatory pathways can prevent the beneficial as well as the adverse effects of mediators and could, for example, impair the patient's ability to eradicate infection, thereby increasing susceptibility to recurrent sepsis. Further, anti-inflammatory strategies are likely to be harmful when, as often seems to be the case, immune suppression is the predominant abnormality. Indeed, such patients might be expected to benefit from treatment designed to enhance the function of the innate or adaptive immune systems.

CORTICOSTEROIDS

Corticosteroids are powerful anti-inflammatory agents that have a number of potentially beneficial actions in shock, including:

- inhibition of complement-induced granulocyte activation;
- reduction in the liberation of free arachidonic acid, and hence prostaglandins, from membrane phospholipid;
- inhibition of the release of PAF;
- inhibition of cytokine synthesis via suppression of NF-κB;
- inhibition of adhesion molecule expression;
- inhibition of inducible NOS;
- restoration of vascular reactivity;
- improved myocardial function;
- attenuation of adrenergic receptor downregulation;
- compensation for downregulation of glucocorticoid receptors and relative adrenal insufficiency.

The use of high-dose corticosteroids (usually methylprednisolone 30 mg/kg intravenously) in shock has been extensively investigated. Experimental investigations suggested that pharmacological doses of corticosteroids could reduce mortality, particularly in septic shock, provided they were administered sufficiently early (Hinshaw et al., 1980). Initial clinical studies, albeit much criticized, were also encouraging (Schumer, 1976). For many years, therefore, high-dose corticosteroids were widely used in the management of shock. Later, large well-designed clinical trials demonstrated that high doses of methylprednisolone did not improve outcome in severe sepsis or septic shock, even when administered within a few hours of the diagnosis (Bone et al., 1987; Veterans Administration Systemic Sepsis Cooperative Study Group, 1987). Indeed, in one of these studies there was evidence that, in some cases, mortality may be increased (Bone et al., 1987), probably because of a higher incidence of deaths attributable to infective complications in those given corticosteroids. A more recent meta-analysis has confirmed that pharmacological doses of corticosteroids do not improve survival rates in patients with sepsis or septic shock and indicated that their use may be associated with increased mortality. Although there was no difference in infection rates, there was a trend towards increased mortality from secondary infections in patients receiving corticosteroids (Cronin et al., 1995). It is, however, important to note that high-dose steroids may improve outcome in some specific infectious illnesses such as typhoid fever (Hoffman et al., 1984) and bacterial meningitis (see Chapter 15).

It is therefore generally accepted that pharmacological doses of corticosteroids should not be administered to patients in the early phases of shock or sepsis but there is now considerable interest in the possibility that so-called 'stress doses' of hydrocortisone administered later in the course of shock and over a longer timescale may be beneficial (see also Chapter 17). The administration of relatively low doses of hydrocortisone (100 mg i.v. 8 hourly) for 5 days to patients with septic shock requiring catecholamines increased the speed and likelihood of shock reversal, in association with an increase in the systemic vascular resistance. There was also a trend toward a reduction in 28-day mortality (Bollaert et al., 1998). Interestingly, in this study reversal of shock in the treatment group appeared to be unrelated to the presence of occult adrenocortical insufficiency (see pp. 83–84), suggesting that other mechanisms (see above) may explain the benefits of hydrocortisone in these patients.

A subsequent study confirmed that modest doses of hydrocortisone (in this case 100 mg i.v. followed by a continuous infusion of 0.18 mg/kg per hour, reduced when shock had been reversed to 0.08 mg/kg per hour and continued for 6 days) can increase systemic vascular resistance and reduce the time to cessation of vasopressor therapy in septic shock. This restoration of vascular reactivity was associated with a trend to earlier resolution of sepsis-induced organ dysfunction (Briegel et al., 1999). A later study confirmed that in septic shock 'low-dose' hydrocortisone increases systemic vascular resistance and blood pressure and reduces noradrenaline requirements (Keh et al., 2003). These haemodynamic changes were associated with reduced NO production and anti-inflammatory effects (Keh et al., 2003). Subsequently, a large PRCT demonstrated that administration of low-dose hydrocortisone and fludrocortisone significantly reduced the risk of death in those patients with relative adrenocortical insufficiency (Annane et al., 2002).

Recent meta-analyses have concluded that, although short courses of high-dose corticosteroids decrease survival in sepsis, a 5–7-day course of low-dose hydrocortisone increases shock reversal and improves outcome in patients with vasopressor-dependent septic shock (Annane et al., 2004; Minneci et al., 2004a). Recently, however, a randomised controlled trial found that low dose hydrocortisone therapy did not decrease mortality in a general population of patients with septic shock, even though shock reversal was more rapid. The failure to improve outcome in this study may have been related to an increased incidence of secondary infections. Further, no benefit was seen in a subgroup of patients who had no response to corticotrophin (Sprung *et al.*, 2008). It is acknowledged that some authorities use a 250-μg ACTH stimulation test to identify responders, in whom they then discontinue hydrocortisone. This is not a requirement of the guidelines, in which it is emphasized that clinicians should not delay steroid administration while waiting for the results of the stimulation test. More recently uncertainty surrounding the diagnosis of relative adrenocortical insufficiency and the efficacy and safety of low dose hydrocortisone have led to the suggestion that in clinical practice low dose steroids should perhaps be reserved for the management of severe, refractory septic shock. **The Surviving Sepsis guidelines (Dellinger *et al.*, 2008) suggest that intravenous hydrocortisone be given only to adult septic patients when hypotension remains poorly responsive to adequate fluid resuscitation and vasopressors. An ACTH stimulation text is not recommended to identify the subset of adults with septic shock who should receive hydrocortisone. It is also suggested that steroid therapy may be weaned once vasopressors are no longer required.**

NON-STEROIDAL ANTI-INFLAMMATORY AGENTS

Inhibition of cyclooxygenase with non-steroidal anti-inflammatory agents (NSAIDs), such as aspirin, indomethacin or ibuprofen, limits formation of eicosanoids from arachidonic acid and has been associated with beneficial effects in animal shock models. These agents are, however, relatively unselective and will inhibit formation of eicosanoids with potentially advantageous actions (e.g. prostacyclin) as well as those with deleterious effects such as the thromboxanes and leukotrienes. In a large multicentre PRCT of patients with severe sepsis, intravenous ibuprofen reduced circulating levels of prostacyclin and thromboxane and decreased fever, tachycardia, oxygen consumption and lactic acidosis. Disappointingly, however, the development of shock or ARDS was not prevented and survival was not improved (Bernard *et al.*, 1997).

PROSTAGLANDINS

Some of the vasodilator eicosanoids (such as PGE_1 and prostacyclin) could theoretically be beneficial in patients with sepsis/MODS by virtue of their ability to inhibit platelet aggregation and their anti-inflammatory properties. Nevertheless, there are no data to support the use of these agents in shock or sepsis (see also Chapter 8 for studies in ARDS).

PENTOXIFYLLINE

Pentoxifylline is a xanthine derivative that increases intracellular cyclic AMP levels and inhibits TNF production by mononuclear cells. Pentoxifylline might, therefore, be expected to have beneficial effects in sepsis. In a PRCT in patients with severe sepsis, however, this agent failed to influence cytokine levels or mortality (Staubach *et al.*, 1998).

PLATELET-ACTIVATING FACTOR ANTAGONISTS

Administration of PAF antagonists can produce beneficial effects in animal models of shock, including reversal of hypotension. In a PRCT, administration of a PAF-receptor antagonist failed to reduce mortality in patients with severe sepsis, although outcome was significantly improved in the subgroup with Gram-negative sepsis. A later confirmatory trial failed to demonstrate benefit in a prospectively defined group of patients with severe Gram-negative bacterial sepsis (Dhainaut *et al.*, 1998).

FREE RADICAL SCAVENGERS

N-acetylcysteine (NAC) has antioxidant properties and being a sulphydryl donor may contribute to the regeneration of NO and glutathione. In liver failure NAC can increase cardiac output, DO_2, $\dot{V}O_2$ and oxygen extraction (see Chapter 14), and in patients with septic shock seemed to improve tissue oxygenation in about half of those treated (Spies *et al.*, 1994). In a more recent PRCT, prolonged infusion of NAC failed to prevent the development of organ failure in consecutively admitted critically ill patients. Moreover, treatment with NAC initiated more than 24 hours after the initial insult was associated with a worse prognosis (Molnar *et al.*, 1999). Further studies, perhaps focussing on early or preventive treatment, are required. The role of other free radical scavengers, such as vitamins E and C and selenium, in the treatment of shock and sepsis, also require further investigation.

ANTICYTOKINE THERAPIES

It was hoped that the development of monoclonal antibodies, which can be precisely targeted against individual mediators or their receptors and thus have reduced potential for side-effects, might allow more effective manipulation of the systemic inflammatory response. In early studies pretreatment with monoclonal antibodies to TNF produced encouraging results in some animal models of septic shock (Tracey *et al.*, 1987) although, in others, administration of TNF antagonists had no effect or proved deleterious. Initial human studies also suggested that a murine monoclonal antibody to human TNF-α (TNF-α MAb) might improve outcome in the subgroup of patients with septic shock, although it was ineffective in those with severe sepsis. Disappointingly, a large PRCT found no improvement in survival of patients with septic shock treated with TNF-α MAb (Abraham *et al.*, 1998). Likewise, administration of a murine monoclonal anti-TNF-α antibody fragment failed to improve outcome significantly in patients with severe sepsis and high circulating levels of IL-6 (Reinhart *et al.*, 2001), although the results of a later trial were more encouraging (Panacek *et al.*, 2004).

The recognition that the proinflammatory effects of cytokines such as TNF-α might be naturally regulated by 'shedding' of TNF receptors from the cell surface into the circulation (see above) led to the suggestion that administration of soluble receptor fusion constructs might be an effective anti-inflammatory treatment for sepsis. Unfortunately, treatment with the extracellular portion of the type II (p75) receptor joined to the F_c portion of a human IgG antibody molecule not only failed to reduce mortality in patients with septic shock but, at higher doses, worsened outcome. Possible reasons include the soluble receptor being toxic or that it acted as an intravascular carrier for TNF-α, thereby pro-longing the inflammatory response, or because complete neutralization of TNF-α was deleterious (Fisher *et al.*, 1996). Similarly, administration of a p55 TNF receptor fusion protein failed to improve outcome in patients with severe sepsis or early septic shock (Abraham *et al.*, 2001). Another approach is to administer recombinant cytokine receptor antagonists. For example, a recombinant human IL-1 receptor antagonist (rh IL-1ra) reduced mortality in experimental shock, although in a multicentre PRCT in patients with severe sepsis or septic shock, it failed to improve outcome significantly (Opal *et al.*, 1997).

In general, because cytokines play an important role in host resistance, inhibition could, as with steroids, impair the patient's immune capabilities. Conversely, inhibiting only one of the many cytokines involved in the response to infection may not be sufficient in itself to influence outcome.

ANTIENDOTOXIN STRATEGIES

An alternative approach, which might overcome some of these problems, could be to target the toxic products of the infecting organism, rather than the mediators of the inflammatory response.

Studies in the early 1980s indicated that immunotherapy with human *polyclonal antiserum or plasma* directed against endotoxin core determinants could reduce mortality in Gram-negative bacteraemia (Ziegler *et al.*, 1982) and protect high-risk patients from septic shock (Baumgartner *et al.*, 1985). The use of polyclonal antiserum was, however, limited by the variability of the antibody content, the potential for transmitting infection and the fact that an individual can donate serum only once. These difficulties were circumvented by the production of *monoclonal antibodies* such as HA-1A, a human monoclonal IgM antibody that binds to lipid A. In a PRCT (Ziegler *et al.*, 1991), HA-1A significantly reduced 28-day mortality, but only in the subgroup of patients with Gram-negative bacteraemia. Similarly, initial results suggested that the murine antilipid A antibody E5 could reduce mortality and enhance the resolution of organ failure in patients with Gram-negative sepsis, but only in the subgroup who were not shocked (Greenman *et al.*, 1991). Disappointingly, subsequent trials failed to confirm benefit (McCloskey *et al.*, 1994). It then emerged that HA-1A was probably binding non-specifically to Gram-negative bacteria and that these antibodies are probably incapable of effectively preventing the proinflammatory effects of endotoxin. More recently, however, a meta-analysis has suggested that polyclonal intravenous immunoglobulin may improve outcome from sepsis (Turgeon *et al.*, 2007).

Bactericidal/permeability-increasing (BPI) *protein* is a member of a group of naturally occurring proteins released from granules within polymorphonuclear leukocytes, which bind and neutralize endotoxin, as well as being cytotoxic for Gram-negative bacteria. In a randomized trial administration of rhBPI to children with meningococcal sepsis was associated with a trend towards improvement in all primary outcome variables, but as mortality was low in both groups, this difference was not statistically significant (Levin *et al.*, 2000).

In general, antiendotoxin strategies are limited by difficulties in identifying patients with Gram-negative bacteraemia/endotoxaemia before initiating treatment (except those with meningococcal sepsis), and by the reduced efficacy associated with delays in therapy.

HIGH-DENSITY LIPOPROTEINS (Wu *et al.*, 2004)

As described above, HDLs bind endotoxin and exert potent anti-inflammatory effects. Reconstituted HDL has been shown to reduce the degree of inflammation, organ dysfunction and mortality in experimental models of endotoxaemia, haemorrhagic shock and ischaemia–reperfusion injury. The results of trials in patients with severe sepsis/septic shock are awaited.

STATINS

Although the main action of the statins is to lower cholesterol levels, these agents have a large number of other potentially beneficial effects, including anti-inflammatory, immune-modulating, antioxidant, antithrombotic and endothelium-stabilizing properties. There is some evidence to suggest that statins may reduce the risk of sepsis (Hackam *et al.*, 2006), but large PRCTs are required to confirm this preventive effect and to evaluate the therapeutic value of these agents in patients with established sepsis.

INHIBITORS OF COAGULATION

The recognition that DIC is likely to play a role in the pathogenesis of organ damage in sepsis, together with a greater understanding of the complex interactions between the coagulation and inflammatory pathways (see above), has prompted studies investigating the potential of naturally occurring anticoagulant molecules such as antithrombin III (AT III), tissue factor pathway inhibitor (TFPI) and activated protein C (APC) in the treatment of severe sepsis. In a PRCT, administration of recombinant TFPI was associated with an increased risk of bleeding and failed to influence all-cause mortality (Abraham *et al.*, 2003). Similarly, in another large PRCT, AT III failed to improve overall outcome, with high-dose AT III being associated with an increased risk of haemorrhage when administered with heparin. There was, however, some evidence to suggest a treatment benefit in the subgroup of patients who were not receiving heparin (Warren *et al.*, 2001). More encouragingly, a PRCT investigating administration of a continuous infusion of rhAPC (which promotes fibrinolysis whilst inhibiting thrombosis and inflammation) to patients with severe sepsis was associated with a fall in circulating levels of D-dimer and IL-6 (confirming its antithrombotic and anti-inflammatory actions) and a significant reduction in the relative risk of death at 28 days by almost 20% (Bernard *et al.*, 2001). There are, however, a number of concerns and uncertainties about the application of these findings to routine clinical practice, in particular with regard to patient selection and minimizing the risk of bleeding (Hinds, 2001). Importantly, in patients with severe sepsis and a low risk of death (single-organ failure or Acute Physiology and Chronic Health Evaluation (APACHE) score < 25), rhAPC failed to influence mortality positively and was associated with an increased incidence of serious bleeding (Abraham *et al.*, 2005). Consequently, administration of APC is not recommended for such cases. **The Surviving Sepsis guidelines (Dellinger *et al.*, 2008) suggest that rhAPC be considered in adult patients with sepsis-induced organ dysfunction with clinical assessment of high risk of death (typically APACHE II ≥ 25 or multiple organ failure) if there are no contraindications. It is recommended that adult patients with severe sepsis and low risk of death (e.g. APACHE II ≤ 20 or one organ failure) should not receive rhAPC.** It is possible that the concurrent administration of heparin may mask some of the treatment benefits of APC and promote bleeding. Heparin should therefore be avoided during infusion of APC. Whether heparin is itself beneficial in sepsis remains unclear.

PLASMA EXCHANGE/HAEMOFILTRATION
(Grooteman and Groeneveld, 2000)
It has been suggested that haemofiltration or plasma exchange might benefit patients with sepsis and organ failure by removing various toxins, pro-/anti-inflammatory mediators and vasoactive substances. Other effects, unrelated to solute and water removal, include reductions in fever, consumption of platelets and activation of white cells, as well as removal of lactate, correction of acidosis and attenuation of oedema. The anticoagulants given to prolong filter life may also have useful therapeutic effects. Many observational, uncontrolled studies have documented potentially beneficial effects of haemofiltration, such as a decrease in vasopressor requirements, a variable increase in systemic vascular resistance, blood pressure and cardiac output and improvements in oxygenation. There is, however, no evidence that such treatment improves outcome.

Modifications designed to increase clearance of toxins and mediators have included high-volume haemofiltration, haemodiafiltration, high-flux dialysis and adsorption techniques, for example, using the endotoxin binder polymyxin B. Although, theoretically, plasmapheresis or plasma exchange might be more efficacious, a PRCT of plasma exhange using a large-pore haemofilter failed to demonstrate a mortality difference, despite attenuation of the acute-phase response (Reeves *et al.*, 1999). On the other hand a small PRCT of plasmapheresis suggested that mortality might be reduced by this intervention (Busund *et al.*, 2002).

EXTRACORPOREAL SUPPORT
Extracorporeal membrane oxygenation has been used to support patients with intractable cardiorespiratory failure due to meningococcal disease (Goldman *et al.*, 1997).

'TIGHT GLYCAEMIC CONTROL'
The Surviving Sepsis guidelines (Dellinger *et al.*, 2008) suggest using a validated protocol for insulin dose adjustment aiming to keep blood glucose < 8.3 mmol/L. A recent randomised controlled trial, however, found that intensive insulin therapy (target blood glucose 6.2 mmol/L) was associated with a higher rate of severe hypoglycaemia and adverse events than conventional therapy (target blood glucose 8.4 mmol/L) and that mortality did not differ significantly between the groups (Brunkhorst *et al.*, 2008).

THE POTENTIAL OF GENOMICS
In the future it may be possible to genotype individual patients, as well as to examine patterns of gene expression, enabling us to identify those at high risk of developing sepsis and organ dysfunction, as well as those with a particularly poor prognosis. It may also be possible to tailor treatment to the individual and time interventions more appropriately.

Gene therapy is in its infancy but offers some promise for the future, in particular because it may allow treatment to be targeted to individual organs and the effects of a single administration can be prolonged for a number of days.

■ ANAPHYLACTIC SHOCK

PATHOGENESIS
Anaphylactic shock is an acute reaction to a foreign substance to which the patient has already been sensitized (immediate, or type I, hypersensitivity) and commonly follows the administration of a drug, blood product, plasma substitute or contrast media. It may also occur in response to an insect sting or the ingestion of a particular food (peanut and tree nut allergy are particularly dangerous) or food additive. Clinically indistinguishable anaphylactoid reactions in which the mechanism of mast cell or basophil degranulation is non-immunological or undetermined may also occur. Similar symptoms may also be produced by direct drug effects, physical factors or exercise. In some cases, a causative agent cannot be identified.

Sensitization follows exposure to an allergenic substance, which, either alone or in combination with a hapten, stimulates synthesis of IgE; this binds to the surface of mast cells or basophils. On re-exposure the antigen interacts with the IgE on the cell surface, leading to mast cell degranulation and release of histamine. Other mediators involved in anaphylaxis include PAF, bradykinin and various cytokines. Intravenous hypnotic agents and contrast media may activate the alternative complement pathway. As well as haemodynamic changes, these mediators may precipitate smooth-muscle contraction and increased glandular secretion.

CLINICAL FEATURES
The clinical manifestations of anaphylaxis are variable. There is often a latent period between exposure and the

development of symptoms, which is usually less than 30 minutes if the agent has been given parenterally, but may be delayed for a few hours. Reactions may be transient, protracted, or rarely biphasic and vary in severity from mild to fatal.

The commonest feature is *profound vasodilatation* with *hypotension* and *tachycardia*. The combination of vasodilatation and hypovolaemia due to *increased capillary permeability* leads to a reduction in ventricular filling pressures and a fall in cardiac output. Myocardial function may also be impaired. These haemodynamic changes may occur in isolation, but are often accompanied by *dyspnoea* and *cutaneous manifestations* such as:

- an erythematous blush;
- generalized urticaria;
- angioedema;
- conjunctival injection;
- pallor and cyanosis.

Loss of protein-rich fluid into the tissues through the 'leaky' microvasculature appears as *oedema*, often most obvious in the face but, more dangerously, may cause laryngeal obstruction with *stridor*. There may also be:

- bronchospasm;
- rhinitis;
- nausea;
- vomiting;
- abdominal cramps;
- diarrhoea.

Other features may include:

- pulmonary oedema;
- coughing;
- arthralgia;
- paraesthesiae, convulsions, coma;
- clotting abnormalities;
- arrhythmias.

The patient may complain of a metallic taste, a choking sensation and apprehension or a sense of impending doom. If symptoms are restricted to a single system the diagnosis may be difficult.

MANAGEMENT (Hughes and Fitzharris, 1999) (Table 5.10)

The drug of first choice for severe anaphylactic reactions is *adrenaline* (500 μg of a 1:1000 solution intramuscularly is safe and can be repeated within 5 minutes if there is no improvement or the patient's condition deteriorates) (McClean-Tooke *et al.*, 2003). If muscle blood flow is thought to be compromised by shock, a slow intravenous injection of 300–500 μg adrenaline of a 1:10 000 (*never* 1:1000) solution can be given over 5 minutes. This may be followed by a continuous intravenous infusion. It should be recognized that the intravenous route is more hazardous and ECG monitoring is mandatory. Devices for self-administration

Table 5.10 Management of anaphylaxis

Adrenaline

500 μg of a 1:1000 solution intramuscularly, repeated within 5 minutes if there is no improvement or the patient deteriorates (or as a slow intravenous injection of 500 μg of a 1:10 000 solution given over 5 minutes. This may be followed by a continuous intravenous infusion)

Oxygen and airway (may require tracheal intubation/cricothyrotomy)

Establish venous access

Expand circulating volume

May require mechanical ventilation (with positive end-expiratory pressure in those with pulmonary oedema)

Antihistamine used routinely to help counter histamine-mediated vasodilatation

Intravenous aminophylline for bronchospasm unresponsive to adrenaline

Noradrenaline for profound refractory vasodilatation

Steroids after severe attacks

Consider intra-aortic balloon counterpulsation for severe myocardial failure

of adrenaline are now available (e.g. EpiPen). Adrenaline increases intracellular levels of cyclic AMP in leukocytes and mast cells and inhibits further release of histamine and slow-reacting substance of anaphylaxis (SRS-A). Adrenaline will also increase myocardial contractility and peripheral vascular tone, and relax bronchial smooth muscle. Occasionally, cardiopulmonary resuscitation (see Chapter 9) will be required.

If bronchospasm is unresponsive to parenteral adrenaline alone, *nebulized salbutamol* or adrenaline is indicated; *aminophylline* can be administered as a slow intravenous bolus (see treatment of asthma: Chapter 8). *Noradrenaline* can be given for profound refractory vasodilatation. Consensus guidelines in the UK (Chamberlain, 1999) recommend routine administration of an antihistamine (chlorpheniramine) 10–20 mg by intramuscular or slow intravenous injection to help counter histamine-mediated vasodilatation and administration of hydrocortisone (100–500 mg by slow intravenous or intramuscular injection) after severe or recurrent attacks and in those with asthma to help avert late sequelae. Steroids are also indicated in those with asthma. Others emphasize that neither antihistamines nor steroids are first-line drugs for the treatment of anaphylaxis, whilst some consider aminophylline given with adrenaline to be dangerous. Patients receiving β-blockers may suffer particularly severe reactions and are often resistant to treatment with adrenaline, as are those with an epidural in place. Adequate expansion of the circulating volume with colloid is essential.

Ideally, 10 mL of clotted blood should be taken within 45–60 minutes after the reaction for retrospective confirmation of the diagnosis, for example by measurements of specific IgE antibody or mast cell tryptase. The serum should be separated and stored at −20°C. Follow-up of these patients is essential. The responsible agent must be determined or confirmed by *in vitro* or *in vivo* testing. Desensitization should be considered for food, pollen and bee sting allergies. The patient should wear a Medic-Alert bracelet and be given a note stating the nature of the reaction and the causative agent. Patients and their next of kin can be given appropriate drugs and be instructed in their use.

PULMONARY EMBOLISM
(Goldhaber, 2004)

Pulmonary emboli usually originate from thromboses in the deep veins of the lower limbs, pelvis or inferior vena cava. Much less often, thrombi in the upper limbs, right atrium or ventricle may be the source. Frequently, these venous thrombi are asymptomatic. Risk factors, which are present in 80–90% of those with proven pulmonary embolism, include:

- heart failure;
- chronic obstructive pulmonary disease;
- diabetes mellitus;
- high blood pressure;
- cancer;
- surgery, trauma;
- hip fractures;
- varicose veins;
- prolonged bedrest/immobilization/long-haul air travel;
- increasing age;
- obesity;
- pregnancy;
- oestrogen therapy/oral contraceptives;
- genetic predisposition (e.g. factor V Leiden mutation);
- cigarette smoking.

Usually emboli lodge in second-, third- or fourth-order pulmonary vessels, although occasionally a very large embolus may lodge at the bifurcation of the pulmonary artery (*saddle embolus*).

SYMPTOMS
Symptoms include a sudden onset of dyspnoea, chest pain (substernal or pleuritic), apprehension and a non-productive cough. Massive pulmonary embolism may precipitate syncope. Later pulmonary infarction may be associated with pleuritic pain, cough and haemoptysis.

HAEMODYNAMIC AND RESPIRATORY CHANGES
Massive pulmonary embolism precipitates systemic hypotension and shock. Cardiac output falls, systemic vascular resistance is increased, and there is usually a tachycardia; bradycardia is an ominous sign. Pulmonary arterial obstruction and the release by platelets of vasoactive agents such as serotonin lead to a rise in pulmonary vascular resistance.

The consequent increase in alveolar dead space and redistribution of pulmonary blood flow result in ventilation/perfusion mismatch and impaired gas exchange. Profound hypoxaemia may also occur if there is right-to-left shunting through a patent foramen ovale. Combined with stimulation of irritant receptors, this causes tachypnoea. There may also be reflex bronchoconstriction and a reduction in lung compliance caused by pulmonary oedema, haemorrhage and loss of surfactant. Right ventricular afterload increases, tension in the right ventricular wall rises and there may be dilatation, dysfunction and ischaemia of the right ventricle. The CVP is elevated whereas the PAOP is often low. The interventricular septum may be displaced to the left, decreasing left ventricular diastolic filling and end-diastolic volume. A finding of right ventricular hypokinesis in the presence of a normal systemic blood pressure is associated with a poor outcome. Death is usually a consequence of right ventricular infarction and circulatory arrest.

PHYSICAL SIGNS AND INVESTIGATIONS
The diagnosis of pulmonary embolus can be difficult and the differential diagnosis is extensive (**Table 5.11**). The classical symptoms and signs are often absent. The diagnosis is easily missed in those with concurrent cardiorespiratory disease (e.g. pneumonia, heart failure), the elderly and those presenting with isolated dyspnoea. Physical signs include tachypnoea, cyanosis and tachycardia. The rise in pulmonary artery pressure may be associated with splitting of the second heart sound and a loud pulmonary component, right ventricular heave and a gallop rhythm. The JVP may be elevated. There may be clinical evidence of deep-vein thrombosis and a slight fever.

A normal *ECG* is usual in acute pulmonary embolus. The commonest ECG finding is non-specific ST depression

Table 5.11 Differential diagnosis of pulmonary embolism
Pneumonia
Asthma
Exacerbation of chronic obstructive pulmonary disease
Myocardial infarction
Pulmonary oedema
Anxiety
Aortic dissection
Pericardial tamponade
Lung cancer
Primary pulmonary hypertension
Rib fracture
Pneumothorax
Costochondritis
Musculoskeletal pain

and T-wave inversion in the anterior leads, especially V_1–V_4, P pulmonale, right bundle branch block and atrial arrhythmias may also be seen. The widely quoted pattern of S_1, Q_3, T_3 is unusual. *Blood gas analysis* should be performed and will usually reveal hypoxaemia with respiratory alkalosis and a metabolic acidosis if organ perfusion is compromised.

The chest radiograph may be normal or may show oligaemic lung field(s). There may be an enlarged heart, localized infiltrates, consolidation, a wedge-shaped density due to pulmonary infarction, a raised diaphragm, pleural effusion or large pulmonary arteries. The chest radiograph cannot be used to diagnose or exclude pulmonary embolus but is useful to exclude some of the differential diagnoses, such as pneumonia, pneumothorax, rib fractures and heart failure.

Although raised D-*dimer concentrations* are not specific for patients with pulmonary embolus, normal levels have a very high negative predictive value. Chest CT and lung scans are therefore not indicated for most patients with normal D-dimer concentrations and low clinical pretest probability of pulmonary embolus. Raised *troponin* levels are associated with a worse prognosis, presumably because they reflect myocardial, and particularly right ventricular, damage. High concentrations of *brain natriuretic peptide* also predict a poor outcome.

In the stable patient venous Doppler ultrasonography and a $\dot{V}/\dot{Q}$ scan should be performed. A normal result on venous ultrasonography does not, of course, rule out pulmonary embolism. Although entirely normal $\dot{V}/\dot{Q}$ scans or findings indicating a high probability of embolism are extremely helpful, intermediate results are difficult to interpret. The ability of a negative CT scan to rule out pulmonary embolus is similar to that reported for conventional pulmonary angiography (Quiroz et al., 2005); contrast-enhanced spiral CT has largely replaced lung scanning for the investigation of acute pulmonary embolus and is highly sensitive for emboli in the proximal pulmonary vasculature down to the third-order arteries.

Visualization of segmental and subsegmental pulmonary arteries is substantially better with the use of multidetector scanners for CT angiography, and diagnostic sensitivity is further improved when this technique is combined with venous-phase imaging to detect acute deep-vein thrombosis (Stein et al., 2006). Magnetic resonance pulmonary angiography is a promising new technique, which uses safer contrast agents and does not involve ionizing radiation (Oudkerk et al., 2002). For a patient presenting with collapse or in shock, echocardiography is the investigation of choice and will identify proximal emboli, as well as right ventricular dysfunction. Transoesophageal echocardiography is particularly useful in critically ill patients suspected of having pulmonary embolism. In some cases echocardiography may reveal another cause for the clinical presentation. Contrast pulmonary angiography (the traditional 'gold standard' for the diagnosis of pulmonary embolus) can be reserved for those cases where diagnostic uncertainty persists. In most cases the diagnosis can be made, or excluded, by combining the history, physical examination and clinical setting with ECG, chest radiography, D-dimer testing and chest CT–angiography.

TREATMENT (Table 5.12)
Resuscitation
Oxygen should be administered in high concentrations; patients with severe respiratory distress may require mechanical ventilation. Haemodynamic support centres on maintaining right ventricular output. Expansion of the circulating volume should therefore be combined with inotropic support using an agent that will maintain systemic blood pressure and thereby preserve right ventricular perfusion in the face of elevated right ventricular pressures.

Definitive treatment
Definitive treatment is directed towards preventing further thrombus formation and proximal embolization. Low-risk patients have an excellent prognosis with anticoagulation alone. Thrombolysis and, rarely, physical removal of emboli may be indicated in high-risk cases.

HEPARIN
Administration of unfractionated heparin (an intravenous bolus of 5000–10 000 units followed by a continuous intravenous infusion at 1000–1600 units/hour) accelerates the action of AT III, thereby inhibiting new thrombus formation and allowing endogenous fibrinolysis to dissolve the clot. The dose should be adjusted to maintain the activated partial thromboplastin time at 1.5–2.5 times the control value. Adequate anticoagulation can be achieved more rapidly by the use of nomograms, most of which are weight-based. Heparin administration has the additional advantage of limiting the rise in pulmonary artery pressure by inhibiting the release of serotinin and histamine from platelets.

Newer low molecular-weight heparins have several theoretical advantages, including:

- easier to administer (weight-adjusted twice-daily subcutaneous injection);
- higher bioavailability after subcutaneous injection;
- longer half-life;
- lower propensity to induce thrombocytopenia;
- lower risk of haemorrhagic complications;
- laboratory monitoring not required except in the obese, those with renal insufficiency and during pregnancy.

Such treatment seems to be as safe and effective as unfractionated heparin in the treatment of the early phase of acute pulmonary embolism in hospital (Simonneau et al., 1997). In certain circumstances, however, it is sensible to use intravenous heparin because it can be discontinued abruptly, for example in those at high risk of bleeding.

Treatment with heparin may be complicated by thrombocytopenia (*heparin-induced thrombocytopenia* – HIT). This condition usually develops 5–14 days after initial heparin exposure, although patients who have received heparin within the previous 100 days can develop HIT

Table 5.12　Management of pulmonary embolism	
Resuscitation	Oxygen and airway May require mechanical ventilation Expand circulating volume Inotrope/vasopressor to maintain right ventricular coronary perfusion
Definitive treatment	Heparin (intravenous bolus 5000–10 000 units, followed by 1000–1600 units/hour for 7–10 days), 　or low-molecular-weight heparin by subcutaneous injection and warfarin (overlapping by at least 　5 days) (loading dose of around 10 mg/day for 2 days, followed by maintenance dose of 3–9 mg/ 　day) Thrombolytic therapy (e.g. streptokinase 250 000 units intravenously over 30 minutes, followed by 　infusion of 100 000 units/h for 12–24 hours) should be considered in massive pulmonary embolism 　with haemodynamic instability and possibly in those with right ventricular dysfunction. An 　alternative is tissue plasminogen activator. Commence heparin infusion when streptokinase is 　discontinued (usually after 24 hours, but 3–7 days of streptokinase may be more effective) Percutaneous catheter fragmentation/removal may be indicated in patients with acute massive 　pulmonary embolism in whom thrombolysis is contraindicated or unsuccessful Vena caval filter if there are recurrent pulmonary emboli despite anticoagulation or if pulmonary 　embolism occurs in the presence of active bleeding. Filters may also be used if the patient cannot 　tolerate anticoagulation, or following pulmonary embolectomy Pulmonary embolectomy may be indicated if the patient is profoundly shocked due to massive embolus 　when thrombolysis is contraindicated or fails

within 24 hours of re-exposure to heparin. Delayed-onset HIT, occurring more than 2 weeks after heparin exposure is increasingly being recognized. HIT is caused by an immune response directed against heparin/platelet factor 4 complexes. It is difficult to diagnose because patients receiving heparin are often seriously ill and may develop thrombocytopenia for many other reasons. Laboratory tests based on bioassay or immunoassay are neither sensitive nor specific and management decisions often have to be made before the results are available. Because HIT is paradoxically associated with severe thrombosis, heparin must be immediately withdrawn when the diagnosis is suspected. Alternative anticoagulants include the heparinoid danaparoid and the new antithrombin hirudin. Two recombinant forms of the latter are now available, lipirudin and desirudin, the former being used in those with HIT. Hirudins are excreted by the kidney and must be used with caution in renal failure, particularly as they are long-acting and have no direct antidote.

WARFARIN

Usually heparin is continued for 7–10 days, overlapping by at least 5 days with warfarinization to counteract the hypercoagulability that may occur during the early stages of warfarin treatment. The loading dose of warfarin is normally around 10 mg/day for 2 days followed by a maintenance dose of about 3–9 mg/day. The dose must, however, be closely monitored and adjusted to maintain the prothrombin time at about 2–3 times the control value. Oral warfarin therapy should be continued for 1.5–2 months in those with deep-vein thrombosis, for 3–6 months following pulmonary embolism, and for longer in particularly high-risk cases. If acute reversal of warfarin therapy is essential it is best achieved by administering fresh frozen plasma. Longer-lasting reversal of anticoagulation can be produced by giving vitamin K.

THROMBOLYTIC THERAPY

Thrombolysis can be life-saving in massive pulmonary embolism with hypotension and/or cardiogenic shock. The role of thrombolysis in submassive pulmonary embolism is less clear and controversy persists regarding the use of thrombolytic therapy in patients with stable systemic blood pressure but right ventricular dysfunction identified by echocardiography. In a recent PRCT, alteplase (see below) given in conjunction with heparin improved the clinical course of such patients and prevented clinical deterioration requiring escalation of treatment in hospital (Konstantinides et al., 2002). Nevertheless, because mortality was unaffected, some believe that, for the time being at least, thrombolysis should be restricted to those with massive pulmonary embolism. In all cases the potential benefit must be weighed against the risk of major haemorrhage.

A loading dose of 250 000 units of streptokinase should be administered intravenously over 30 minutes, followed by an infusion of 100 000 units/hour for 12–24 hours. There is, however, some evidence that a longer period of treatment (3–7 days) may be more effective. Treatment should be monitored using the thrombin time, which should be maintained at 2–4 times the control value. A heparin infusion should be started when the streptokinase is discontinued.

Streptokinase is pyrogenic and antigenic. Immunological reactions can be controlled with antihistamines and hydrocortisone; adrenaline and resuscitation equipment should be immediately available. There is also a significant risk of haemorrhage with streptokinase. If serious bleeding occurs streptokinase should be discontinued, fresh frozen plasma should be administered and the fibrinolytic activity of streptokinase antagonized by ε-aminocaproic acid or aprotinin.

So called 'clot-specific' thrombolytic agents such as recombinant tissue-type plasminogen activator (e.g. alteplase) may cause less systemic fibrinogenolysis and may have some advantage. Tissue-type plasminogen activator can be given at a dose of 100 mg over 2 hours as a peripheral intravenous infusion. Regional (directed) infusion of these agents may achieve more rapid clearance of thrombi.

PERCUTANEOUS CATHETER FRAGMENTATION/REMOVAL

In patients with acute massive pulmonary embolism in whom thrombolysis is contraindicated or unsuccessful, it may be possible to restore cardiac output rapidly by breaking up the embolus and dispersing the fragments distally using a cardiac catheter. More recently, suction catheter embolectomy has been employed.

VENA CAVAL FILTERS

In patients who have either recurrent pulmonary emboli despite intensive and prolonged anticoagulation or pulmonary embolism in the presence of active haemorrhage, a filter can be positioned in the inferior vena cava to prevent further pulmonary embolism. Filters may also be used in patients who cannot tolerate anticoagulation and immediately following pulmonary embolectomy. Filters appear to offer no advantage in those with free-floating thrombi in the ileofemoral veins. The introduction of retrievable vena caval filters has provided the option of inserting these devices temporarily. Such filters must be removed within a few weeks, otherwise they endothelialize and can become permanent.

PULMONARY EMBOLECTOMY

The value of pulmonary embolectomy is uncertain. It may be indicated in a patient who is profoundly shocked due to massive pulmonary embolism when thrombolysis is contraindicated or fails. Patients with chronic thrombotic involvement of large pulmonary arteries and cor pulmonale may be candidates for pulmonary thromboendarterectomy.

REFERENCES

Abraham E, Anzueto A, Gutierrez C, et al. (1998) Double-blind randomised controlled trial of monoclonal antibody to human tumour necrosis factor in treatment of septic shock. Lancet 351: 929–933.

Abraham E, Matthay MA, Dinarello CA, et al. (2000) Consensus conference definitions for sepsis, septic shock, acute lung injury and acute respiratory distress syndrome: time for a reevaluation. Critical Care Medicine 28: 232–235.

Abraham E, Laterre P-F, Garbino J, et al. (2001) Lenercept (p55 tumor necrosis factor receptor fusion protein) in severe sepsis and early septic shock: a randomized, double-blind placebo-controlled multicenter phase III trial with 1,342 patients. Critical Care Medicine 29: 503–510.

Abraham E, Reinhart K, Opal S, et al. (2003) Efficacy and safety of tifacogin (recombinant tissue factor pathway inhibitor) in severe sepsis. A randomized controlled trial. Journal of the American Medical Association 290: 238–247.

Abraham E, Laterre P-F, Garg R, et al. (2005) Drotrecogin alfa (activated) for adults with severe sepsis and a low risk of death. New England Journal of Medicine 353: 1332–1341.

Adrie C, Bachelet M, Vayssier-Taussat M, et al. (2001) Mitochondrial membrane potential and apoptosis in peripheral blood monocytes in severe human sepsis. American Journal of Respiratory and Critical Care Medicine 164: 389–395.

Alia I, Esteban A, Gordo F, et al. (1999) A randomized and controlled trial of the effect of treatment aimed at maximizing oxygen delivery in patients with severe sepsis or septic shock. Chest 115: 453–461.

Angus DC, Linde-Zwirble WT, Lidicker J, et al. (2001) Epidemiology of severe sepsis in the United States: analysis of incidence, outcome and associated costs of care. Critical Care Medicine 29: 1303–1310.

Annane D, Bellissant E, Sébille V, et al. (1998) Impaired pressor sensitivity to noradrenaline in septic shock patients with and without impaired adrenal function reserve. British Journal of Clinical Pharmacology 46: 589–597.

Annane D, Sèbille V, Troché G, et al. (2000) A 3-level prognostic classification in septic shock based on cortisol levels and cortisol response to corticotrophin. Journal of the American Medical Association 283: 1038–1045.

Annane D, Sébille V, Charpentier C, et al. (2002) Effect of treatment with low doses of hydrocortisone and fludrocortisone on mortality in patients with septic shock. Journal of the American Medical Association 288: 862–871.

Annane D, Aegerter P, Jars-Guincestre MC, et al. (2003) Current epidemiology of septic shock. The CUB-Réa Network. American Journal of Respiratory and Critical Care Medicine 168: 165–172.

Annane D, Bellissant PE, Bollaert PE, et al. (2004) Corticosteroids for severe sepsis and septic shock: a systematic review and meta-analysis. British Medical Journal 329: 480.

Annane D, Vignon P, Renault A, et al. for the CATS Study Group (2007) Norepinephrine plus dobutamine versus epinephrine alone for the management of septic shock: a randomised trial. Lancet 370:676–684.

Bakker J (2001) Lactate: may I have your votes please? Intensive Care Medicine 27: 6–11.

Bakker J, Coffernils M, Leon M, et al. (1991) Blood lactate levels are superior to oxygen-derived variables in predicting outcome in human septic shock. Chest 99: 956–962.

Bakker J, Gris P, Coffernils M, et al. (1996) Serial blood lactate levels can predict the development of multiple organ failure following septic shock. American Journal of Surgery 171: 221–226.

Barton R, Cerra FB (1989) The hypermetabolism, multiple organ failure syndrome. Chest 96: 1153–1160.

Baumgartner J-D, Glauser MP, McCutchan JA, et al. (1985) Prevention of Gram negative shock and death in surgical patients by antibody to endotoxin core glycolipid. Lancet 2: 59–63.

Bernard GR, Wheeler AP, Russell JA, et al. (1997) The effects of ibuprofen on the physiology and survival of patients with sepsis. New England Journal of Medicine 336: 912–918.

Bernard GR, Vincent J-L, Laterre P-F, et al. (2001) Efficacy and safety of recombinant human activated protein C for severe sepsis. New England Journal of Medicine 344: 699–709.

Boldt J (2000) Volume therapy in the intensive care patient – we are still confused, but . . . Intensive Care Medicine 26: 1181–1192.

Bollaert PE, Bauer P, Audibert G, et al. (1990) Effects of epinephrine on hemodynamics and oxygen metabolism in dopamine-resistant septic shock. Chest 98: 949–953.

Bollaert PE, Charpentier C, Levy B, et al. (1998) Reversal of late septic shock with supraphysiologic doses of hydrocortisone. Critical Care Medicine 26: 645–650.

Bone RC (1991) Sepsis, sepsis syndrome, multi-organ failure: a plea for comparable definitions. Annals of Internal Medicine 114: 332–333.

Bone RC (1996) Sir Isaac Newton, sepsis, SIRS and CARS. Critical Care Medicine 24: 1125–1128.

Bone RC, Fisher CJ Jr, Clemmer TP, et al. (1987) A controlled clinical trial of high-dose methylprednisolone in the treatment of severe sepsis and septic shock. New England Journal of Medicine 317: 653–658.

Bone RC, Sprung CL, Sibbald WJ (1992) Definitions for sepsis and organ failure. Critical Care Medicine 20: 724–726.

Boyd O, Grounds RM, Bennett ED (1993) A randomized clinical trial of the effect of deliberate perioperative increase of oxygen delivery on mortality in high-risk surgical patients. Journal of the American Medical Association 270: 2699–2707.

Brealey D, Brand M, Hargreaves I, et al. (2002) Association between mitochondrial dysfunction and severity and outcome of septic shock. Lancet 360: 219–223.

Briegel J, Schelling G, Haller M, et al. (1996) A comparison of the adrenocortical response during septic shock and after complete recovery. Intensive Care Medicine 22: 894–899.

Briegel J, Forst H, Haller M, et al. (1999) Stress doses of hydrocortisone reverse hyperdynamic septic shock: a prospective randomized, double-blind, single-center study. Critical Care Medicine 27: 723–732.

Brown EJ (2004) The molecular basis of streptococcal toxic shock syndrome. New England Journal of Medicine 350: 2093–2094.

Brun-Buisson C, Doyon F, Carlet J, et al. (1995) Incidence, risk factors and outcome of severe sepsis and septic shock in adults. Journal of the American Medical Association 274: 968–974.

Brun-Buisson C, Meshaka P, Pinton P, et al. (2004) EPISEPSIS: a reappraisal of the epidemiology and outcome of severe sepsis in French intensive care units. Intensive Care Medicine 30: 580–588.

Brunkhorst FM, Engel C, Bloos F, et al. for the German Competence Network Sepsis (SepNet) (2008) Intensive insulin therapy and pentastarch resuscitation in severe sepsis. New England Journal of Medicine 358: 125–139.

Busund R, Koukline V, Utrobin U, et al. (2002) Plasmapheresis in severe sepsis and septic shock: a prospective, randomised, controlled trial. Intensive Care Medicine 28: 1434–1439.

Byers RJ, Eddleston JM, Pearson RC, et al. (1999) Dopexamine reduces the incidence of acute inflammation in the gut mucosa after abdominal surgery in high risk patients. Critical Care Medicine 27: 1787–1793.

Chamberlain D (1999) Emergency medical treatment of anaphylactic reactions. Project Team of the Resuscitation Council (UK). Journal of Accident and Emergency Medicine 16: 243–247.

Choi P, Yip G, Quinonez LG, et al. (1999) Crystalloids vs. colloids in fluid resuscitation: a systematic review. Critical Care Medicine 27: 200–210.

Cochrane Injuries Group Albumin Reviewers (1998) Human albumin administration in critically ill patients: systematic review of randomised controlled trials. British Medical Journal 317: 235–240.

Colardyn FC, Vandenbogaerde JF, Vogelaers DP, et al. (1989) Use of dopexamine hydrochloride in patients with septic shock. Critical Care Medicine 17: 999–1003.

Cooper DJ, Walley KR, Wiggs BR, et al. (1990) Bicarbonate does not improve hemodynamics in critically ill patients who have lactic acidosis. A prospective, controlled clinical study. Annals of Internal Medicine 112: 492–498.

Corwin HL, Gettinger A, Fabian TC, et al. for the EPO Critical Care Trials Group (2007) Efficacy and safety of epoietin alfa in critically ill patients. New England Journal of Medicine 357:956–976.

Cotter G, Metzkor E, Kaluski E, et al. (1998) Randomised trial of high-dose isosorbide dinitrate plus low-dose furosemide versus high dose furosemide plus low dose isosorbide dinitrate in severe pulmonary oedema. Lancet 351: 389–393.

Cowley HC, Heney D, Gearing AJ, et al. (1994) Increased circulating adhesion molecule concentrations in patients with the systemic inflammatory response syndrome: a prospective cohort study. Critical Care Medicine 22: 651–657.

Cronin L, Cook DJ, Carlet J, et al. (1995) Corticosteroid treatment for sepsis: a critical appraisal and meta-analysis of the literature. Critical Care Medicine 23: 1430–1439.

Cunnion RE, Schaer GL, Parker MM, et al. (1986) The coronary circulation in human septic shock. Circulation 73: 637–644.

Danek SJ, Lynch JP, Weg JG, et al. (1980) The dependence of oxygen uptake on oxygen delivery in the adult respiratory distress syndrome. American Review of Respiratory Disease 122: 387–395.

Danner RL, Elin RJ, Hosseini JM, et al. (1991) Endotoxemia in human septic shock. Chest 99: 169–175.

Day NP, Phu NH, Bethell DP, et al. (1996) The effects of dopamine and adrenaline infusions on acid–base balance and systemic haemodynamics in severe infection. Lancet 348: 219–223.

De Backer D, Creteur J, Preiser J-C, et al. (2002) Microvascular blood flow is altered in patients with sepsis. American Journal of Respiratory and Critical Care Medicine 166: 98–104.

De Backer D, Creteur J, Silva E, et al. (2003) Effects of dopamine, norepinephrine, and epinephrine on the splanchnic circulation in septic shock: which is best? Critical Care Medicine 31; 1659–1667.

DeCamp MM, Demling RH (1988) Posttraumatic multisystem organ failure. Journal of the American Medical Association 260: 530–534.

Dellinger RP, Levy MM, Carlet JM, et al. (2008) Surviving Sepsis Campaign International guidelines for management of severe sepsis and septic shock: 2008 Critical Care Medicine 36: 296–327.

Dhainaut JF, Huyghebaert MF, Monsallier JF, et al. (1987) Coronary hemodynamics and myocardial metabolism of lactate, free fatty acids, glucose, and ketones in patients with septic shock. Circulation 75: 533–541.

Dhainaut JF, Tennaillon A, Hemmer M, et al. (1998) Confirmatory platelet-activating factor receptor antagonist trial in patients with severe gram-negative bacterial sepsis: a phase III, randomized, double-blind, placebo-controlled, multicenter clinical trial. Critical Care Medicine 26: 1963–1971.

Dombrovskiy VY, Martin AA, Sunderram J, Paz HL (2007) Rapid increase in hospitalization and mortality rates for severe sepsis in the United States: a trend analysis from 1993–2003. Critical Care Medicine 35:1244–1250.

Dubois MJ, Orellana-Jimenez C, Melot C, et al. (2006) Albumin administration improves organ function in critically ill hypoalbuminemic patients: a prospective, randomized, controlled, pilot study. Critical Care Medicine 34: 2536–2540.

Ellrodt AG, Riedinger MS, Kimchi A, et al. (1985) Left ventricular performance in septic shock: reversible segmental and global abnormalities. American Heart Journal 110: 402–409.

Evans T, Carpenter A, Kinderman H, et al. (1993) Evidence of increased nitric oxide production in patients with the sepsis syndrome. Circulatory Shock 41: 77–81.

Finfer S, Bellomo R, Lipman J, et al. (2004a) Adult population incidence of severe sepsis in Australian and New Zealand intensive care units. Intensive Care Medicine 30; 589–596.

Finfer S, Bellomo R, Boyce N, et al. (2004b) A comparison of albumin and saline for fluid resuscitation in the intensive care unit. New England Journal of Medicine 350: 2247–2256.

Fisher CJ, Agosti JM, Opal SM, et al. (1996) Treatment of septic shock with the tumor necrosis factor receptor: Fc fusion protein. New England Journal of Medicine 334: 1697–1702.

Fleming A, Bishop M, Shoemaker W, et al. (1992) Prospective trial of supranormal values as goals of resuscitation in severe trauma. Archives of Surgery 127: 1175–1181.

Follath F, Cleland JG, Just H, et al. (2002) Efficacy and safety of intravenous levosimendan compared with dobutamine in severe low output heart failure (the LIDO study): a randomised double-blind trial. Lancet 360: 196–202.

Foreman MG, Mannino DM, Moss M (2003) Cirrhosis as a risk factor for sepsis and death: analysis of the National Hospital Discharge Survey. Chest 124: 1016–1020.

Friedrich JO, Adhikari N, Herridge MS, et al. (2005) Meta-analysis: low-dose dopamine increases urine output but does not prevent renal dysfunction or death. Annals of Internal Medicine 142: 510–524.

Gabay C, Kushner I (1999) Acute-phase proteins and other systemic responses to inflammation. New England Journal of Medicine 340: 448–454.

Gando S, Nishihira J, Kobayashi S, et al. (2001) Macrophage migration inhibitory factor is a critical mediator of systemic inflammatory response syndrome. Intensive Care Medicine 27: 1187–1193.

Gattinoni L, Brazzi L, Pelosi P, et al. (1995) A trial of goal-oriented hemodynamic therapy in critically ill patients. New England Journal of Medicine 333: 1025–1032.

Gibot S, Kolopp-Sarda M-N, Béné MC, et al. (2004) Plasma level of a triggering receptor expressed on myeloid cells-1: its diagnostic accuracy in patients with suspected sepsis. Annals of Internal Medicine 141: 9–15.

Gilbert EM, Haupt MT, Mandanas RY, et al. (1986) The effect of fluid loading, blood transfusion, and catecholamine infusion on oxygen delivery and consumption in patients with sepsis. American Review of Respiratory Disease 134: 873–878.

Goldhaber SZ (2004) Pulmonary embolism. Lancet 363: 1295–1305.

Goldie AS, Fearon KC, Ross JA, et al. (1995) Natural cytokine antagonists and endogenous antiendotoxin core antibodies in sepsis syndrome. Journal of the American Medical Association 274: 172–177.

Goldman AP, Kerr SJ, Butt W, et al. (1997) Extracorporeal support for intractable cardiorespiratory failure due to meningococcal disease. Lancet 349: 466–469.

Gordon AC, Lagan AL, Aganna E, et al. (2004) TNF and TNFR polymorphisms in severe sepsis and septic shock: a prospective multicentre study. Genes and Immunity 5: 631–640.

Gordon AC, Waheed U, Hansen TK, et al. (2006) Mannose-binding lectin polymorphisms in severe sepsis: relationship to levels, incidence and outcome. Shock 25: 88–93.

Greenman RL, Schein RM, Martin MA, et al. (1991) A controlled clinical trial of E5 murine monoclonal IgM antibody to endotoxin in the treatment of gram-negative sepsis. Journal of the American Medical Association 266: 1097–1102.

Groeneveld AB, Bronsveld W, Thijs LG (1986) Hemodynamic determinants of mortality in human septic shock. *Surgery* **99**: 140–153.

Grooteman MP, Groeneveld AB (2000) A role for plasma removal during sepsis? *Intensive Care Medicine* **26**: 493–495.

Grover R, Zaccardelli D, Colice G, et al. (1999) An open-label dose escalation study of the nitric oxide synthase inhibitor, N(G)-methyl-L-arginine hydrochloride (546C88), in patients with septic shock. *Critical Care Medicine* **27**: 913–922.

Hackam DG, Mamdani M, Li P, et al. (2006) Statins and sepsis in patients with cardiovascular disease: a population-based cohort analysis. *Lancet* **367**: 413–418.

Hamrahian AH, Oseni TS, Arafah BM (2004) Measurements of serum free cortisol in critically ill patients. *New England Journal of Medicine* **350**: 1629–1638.

Hasdai D, Topol EJ, Califf RM, et al. (2000) Cardiogenic shock complicating acute coronary syndromes. *Lancet* **356**: 749–756.

Hayes MA, Yau EH, Hinds CJ, et al. (1992) Symmetrical peripheral gangrene: association with noradrenaline administration. *Intensive Care Medicine* **18**: 433–436.

Hayes MA, Yau EH, Timmins AC, et al. (1993) Response of critically ill patients to treatment aimed at achieving supranormal oxygen delivery and consumption. Relationship to outcome. *Chest* **103**: 886–895.

Hayes MA, Timmins AC, Yau EH, et al. (1994) Elevation of systemic oxygen delivery in the treatment of critically ill patients. *New England Journal of Medicine* **330**: 1717–1722.

Hayes MA, Timmins AC, Yau EH, et al. (1997) Oxygen transport patterns in patients with sepsis syndrome or septic shock: influence of treatment and relationship to outcome. *Critical Care Medicine* **25**: 926–936.

Hebert PC, Wells G, Blajchman MA, et al. (1999) A multicenter, randomized, controlled clinical trial of transfusion requirements in critical care. *New England Journal of Medicine* **340**: 409–417.

Hebert PC, Yetisir E, Martin C, et al. (2001) Is a low transfusion threshold safe in critically ill patients with cardiovascular diseases? *Critical Care Medicine* **29**: 227–234.

Hibberd ML, Sumiya M, Summerfield IA, et al. (1999) Association of variants of the gene for mannose-binding lectin with susceptibility to meningococcal disease. *Lancet* **353**: 1049–1053.

Hidalgo-Grass C, Dan-Goor M, Maly A, et al. (2004) Effect of a bacterial pheromone peptide on host chemokine degradation in group A streptococcal necrotising soft-tissue infections. *Lancet* **363**: 696–703.

Hinds CJ (2001) Treatment of sepsis with activated protein C. *British Medical Journal* **323**: 881–882.

Hinds C, Watson D (1995) Manipulating hemodynamics and oxygen transport in critically ill patients. *New England Journal of Medicine* **333**: 1074–1075.

Hinshaw LB, Archer LT, Beller-Todd BK, et al. (1980) Survival of primates in LD100 septic shock following steroid/antibiotic therapy. *Journal of Surgical Research* **28**: 151–170.

Hoffman SL, Punjabi NH, Kumala S, et al. (1984) Reduction of mortality in chloramphenicol-treated severe typhoid fever by high-dose dexamethasone. *New England Journal of Medicine* **310**: 82–88.

Hotchkiss RS, Karl IE (2003) The pathophysiology and treatment of sepsis. *New England Journal of Medicine* **348**; 138–150.

Hotchkiss RS, Swanson PE, Freeman BD, et al. (1999) Apoptotic cell death in patients with sepsis, shock and multiple organ dysfunction. *Critical Care Medicine* **27**: 1230–1251.

Hughes G, Fitzharris P (1999) Managing acute anaphylaxis. *British Medical Journal* **319**: 1–2.

James JH, Luchette FA, McCarter FD, et al. (1999) Lactate is an unreliable indicator of tissue hypoxia in injury or sepsis. *Lancet* **354**: 505–508.

Jardin F, Sportiche M, Bazin M, et al. (1981) Dobutamine: a hemodynamic evaluation in human septic shock. *Critical Care Medicine* **9**: 329–332.

Kam PC, Ferch NI (2000) Apoptosis: mechanisms and clinical implications. *Anaesthesia* **55**: 1081–1093.

Keh D, Boehnke T, Weber-Cartens S, et al. (2003) Immunologic and hemodynamic effects of 'low-dose' hydrocortisone in septic shock. A double-blind, randomized, placebo-controlled, crossover study. *American Journal of Respiratory and Critical Care Medicine* **167**: 512–520.

Kern H, Schröder T, Kaulfuss M, et al. (2001) Enoximone in contrast to dobutamine improves hepatosplanchnic function in fluid-optimized septic shock patients. *Critical Care Medicine* **29**: 1519–1525.

Khot UN, Novaro GM, Popovic ZB, et al. (2003) Nitroprusside in critically ill patients with left ventricular dysfunction and aortic stenosis. *New England Journal of Medicine* **348**: 1756–1763.

Kiefer P, Tugtekin I, Wiedeck H, et al. (2000) Effect of a dopexamine-induced increase in cardiac index on splanchnic hemodynamics in septic shock. *American Journal of Respiratory and Critical Care Medicine* **161**: 775–779.

Kirov MY, Evgenov OV, Evgenov NV, et al. (2001) Infusion of methylene blue in human septic shock: a pilot, randomized, controlled study. *Critical Care Medicine* **29**: 1860–1867.

Konstantinides S, Geibel A, Heusel G, et al. (2002) Heparin plus alteplase compared with heparin alone in patients with submassive pulmonary embolism. *New England Journal of Medicine* **347**: 1143–1150.

Kruse JA, Haupt MT, Puri VK, et al. (1990) Lactate levels as predictors of the relationship between oxygen delivery and consumption in ARDS. *Chest* **98**: 959–962.

Kumar A, Roberts D, Wood KE, et al. (2006) Duration of hypotension before initiation of effective antimicrobial therapy is the critical determinant of survival in human septic shock. *Critical Care Medicine* **34**: 1589–1596.

Lackritz EM, Satten GA, Aberle-Grasse J, et al. (1995) Estimated risk of the transmission of the human immunodeficiency virus by screened blood in the United States. *New England Journal of Medicine* **333**: 1721–1725.

Lamy M, Faymonville ME, Deby-Dupont G (1987) Shock pancreas: a new entity? In: Vincent JL (ed) *Update in Intensive Care and Emergency Medicine*, pp. 148–154. Springer-Verlag: Berlin.

Landry DW, Levin HR, Gallant EM, et al. (1997) Vasopressin pressor hypersensitivity in vasodilatory septic shock. *Critical Care Medicine* **25**: 1279–1282.

Ledingham IM, McArdle CS (1978) Prospective study of the treatment of septic shock. *Lancet* **1**: 1194–1197.

LeDoux D, Astiz ME, Carpati CM, et al. (2000) Effects of perfusion pressure on tissue perfusion in septic shock. *Critical Care Medicine* **28**: 2729–2732.

Lemaire LC, van Lanschot JJ, Stoutenbeek CP, et al. (1997) Bacterial translocation in multiple organ failure: cause or epiphenomenon still unproven. *British Journal of Surgery* **84**: 1340–1350.

Leone M, Albanèse J, Delmas A, et al. (2004) Terlipressin in catecholamine-resistant septic shock patients. *Shock* **22**: 314–319.

Levin M, Quint PA, Goldstein B, et al. (2000) Recombinant bactericidal/permeability-increasing protein (rBPI₂₁) as adjunctive treatment for children with severe meningococcal sepsis: a randomised trial. *Lancet* **356**: 961–967.

Levy B, Bollaert PE, Charpentier C, et al. (1997a) Comparison of norepinephrine and dobutamine to epinephrine for hemodynamics, lactate metabolism and gastric tonometric variables in septic shock: a prospective, randomized study. *Intensive Care Medicine* **23**: 282–287.

Levy B, Bollaert PE, Lucchelli J-P, et al. (1997b) Dobutamine improves the adequacy of gastric mucosal perfusion in epinephrine-treated septic shock. *Critical Care Medicine* **25**: 1649–1654.

Levy MM, Fink MP, Marshall JC (2003) 2001 SCCM/ESICM/ACCP/ATS/SIS International Sepsis Definitions Conference. *Intensive Care Medicine* **29**: 530–538.

Levy B, Gibot S, Franck P, et al. (2005) Relation between muscle Na⁺/K⁺ ATPase activity and raised lactate concentrations in septic shock: a prospective study. *Lancet* **365**: 871–875.

Lipiner-Friedman D, Sprung CL, Laterre PF, et al. (2007) Adrenal function in sepsis: the retrospective corticus cohort study. *Critical Care Medicine* **35**: 1012–1018.

Looney MR, Gropper MA, Matthay MA (2004) Transfusion-related acute lung injury: a review. *Chest* **126**: 249–258.

Lopez A, Lorente JA, Steingrub J, et al. (2004) Multiple-center, randomized, placebo-controlled, double-blind study of the nitric oxide synthase inhibitor 546C88: effect on survival in patients with septic shock. *Critical Care Medicine* **32**: 21–30.

Lorente JA, Garcia-Frade LJ, Landin L, et al. (1993) Time course of hemostatic abnormalities in sepsis and its relation to outcome. *Chest* **103**: 1536–1542.

McClean-Tooke AP, Bethune CA, Fay AC, et al. (2003) Adrenaline in the treatment of anaphylaxis: what is the evidence? *British Medical Journal* **327**: 1332–1335.

McCloskey RV, Straube RC, Sanders C, et al. (1994) Treatment of septic shock with human monoclonal antibody HA-1A. A randomized double-blind, placebo-controlled trial. *Annals of Internal Medicine* **121**: 1–5.

McKendry M, McGloin H, Saberi D, et al. (2004) Randomised controlled trial assessing the impact of a nurse delivered, flow monitored protocol for optimisation of circulatory status after cardiac surgery. *British Medical Journal* **329**: 258.

Marik PE, Mohedin M (1994) The contrasting effects of dopamine and norepinephrine on systemic and splanchnic oxygen utilization in hyperdynamic sepsis. *Journal of the American Medical Association* **272**: 1354–1357.

Marik PE, Sibbald WJ (1993) Effect of stored blood transfusion on oxygen delivery in patients with sepsis. *Journal of the American Medical Association* **269**: 3024–3029.

Martin C, Eon B, Saux P, et al. (1990) Renal effects of norepinephrine used to treat septic shock patients. *Critical Care Medicine* **18**: 282–285.

Martin C, Viviand X, Arnaud S, et al. (1999) Effects of norepinephrine plus dobutamine or norepinephrine alone on left ventricular performance of septic shock patients. *Critical Care Medicine* **27**: 1708–1713.

Martin GS, Mannino DM, Eaton S, et al. (2003) The epidemiology of sepsis in the United States from 1979 through 2000. *New England Journal of Medicine* **348**: 1546–1554.

Meier-Hellmann A, Specht M, Hannemann L, et al. (1996) Splanchnic blood flow is greater in septic shock treated with norepinephrine than in severe sepsis. *Intensive Care Medicine* **22**: 1354–1359.

Meier-Hellmann A, Reinhart K, Bredle DL, et al. (1997) Epinephrine impairs splanchnic perfusion in septic shock. *Critical Care Medicine* **25**: 399–404.

Meier-Hellmann A, Bredle DL, Specht M, et al. (1999) Dopexamine increases splanchnic blood flow but decreases gastric mucosal pH in severe septic patients treated with dobutamine. *Critical Care Medicine* **27**: 2166–2171.

Members of the American College of Chest Physicians/Society of Critical Care Medicine Consensus Conference Committee (1992) Definitions for sepsis and organ failure and guidelines for the use of innovative therapies in sepsis. *Critical Care Medicine* **20**: 864–874.

Michie HR, Manogue KR, Spriggs DR, et al. (1988a) Detection of circulating tumor necrosis factor after endotoxin administration. *New England Journal of Medicine* **318**: 1481–1486.

Michie HR, Spriggs DR, Manogue KR, et al. (1988b) Tumor necrosis factor and endotoxin induce similar metabolic responses in human beings. *Surgery* **104**: 280–286.

Minneci PC, Deans KJ, Banks SM, et al. (2004a) Meta-analysis: the effect of steroids on survival and shock during sepsis depends on the dose. *Annals of Internal Medicine* **141**: 47–56.

Minneci PC, Deans KJ, Banks SM, et al. (2004b) Differing effects of epinephrine, norepinephrine, and vasopressin on survival in a canine model of septic shock. *American Journal of Physiology* **287**: H2545–H2554.

Mira J-P, Cariou A, Grall F, et al. (1999) Association of TNF2, a TNF-α promoter polymorphism, with septic shock susceptibility and mortality. *Journal of the American Medical Association* **282**: 561–568.

Molnar Z, Shearer J, Lowe D (1999) N-Acetylcysteine treatment to prevent the progression of multisystem organ failure: a prospective, randomised, placebo-controlled study. *Critical Care Medicine* **27**: 1100–1104.

Morgan PW, Berridge JC (2000) Giving long-persistent starch as volume replacement can cause pruritus after cardiac surgery. *British Journal of Anaesthesia* **85**: 696–699.

Munford RS, Pugin J (2001) Normal responses to injury prevent systemic inflammation and can be immunosuppressive. *American Journal of Respiratory and Critical Care Medicine* **163**: 316–321.

Mutunga M, Fulton B, Bullock R, et al. (2001) Circulating endothelial cells in patients with septic shock. *American Journal of Respiratory and Critical Care Medicine* **163**: 195–200.

Mythen MG, Webb AR (1995) Perioperative plasma volume expansion reduces the incidence of gut mucosal hypoperfusion during cardiac surgery. *Archives of Surgery* **130**: 423–429.

Neviere R, Mathieu D, Chagnon J-L, et al. (1996) The contrasting effects of dobutamine and dopamine on gastric mucosal perfusion in septic patients. *American Journal of Respiratory and Critical Care Medicine* **154**: 1684–1688.

Ognibene FP, Parker MM, Natanson C, et al. (1988) Depressed left ventricular performance. Response to volume infusion in patients with sepsis and septic shock. *Chest* **93**: 903–910.

Opal SM, Fisher CJ, Dhainaut J-F, et al. (1997) Confirmatory interleukin-1 receptor antagonist trial in severe sepsis: a phase III, randomized, double-blind, placebo-controlled, multicenter trial. *Critical Care Medicine* **25**: 1115–1124.

Oudkerk M, van Beek EJ, Wielopolski P, et al. (2002) Comparison of contrast-enhanced magnetic resonance angiography and conventional pulmonary angiography for the diagnosis of pulmonary embolism: a prospective study. *Lancet* **359**: 1643–1647.

Padkin A, Goldfrad C, Brady AR, et al. (2003) Epidemiology of severe sepsis occurring in the first 24 hrs in intensive care units in England, Wales and Northern Ireland. *Critical Care Medicine* **31**: 2332–2338.

Palazzo MG, Suter PM (1991) Delivery dependent oxygen consumption in patients with septic shock: daily variations, relationship with outcome and the sick-euthyroid syndrome. *Intensive Care Medicine* **17**: 325–332.

Panacek EA, Marshall JC, Albertson TE, et al. (2004) Efficacy and safety of the monoclonal anti-tumor necrosis factor antibody F(ab')₂ fragment afelimomab in patients with severe sepsis and elevated interleukin-6 levels. *Critical Care Medicine* **32**: 2173–2182.

Papadopoulos MC, Davies DC, Moss RF, et al. (2000) Pathophysiology of septic encephalopathy: a review. *Critical Care Medicine* **28**: 3019–3024.

Parker MM, Shelhamer JH, Bacharach SL, et al. (1984) Profound but reversible myocardial depression in patients with septic shock. *Annals of Internal Medicine* **100**: 483–490.

Parker MM, McCarthy KE, Ognibene FP, et al. (1990) Right ventricular dysfunction and dilatation, similar to left ventricular changes, characterize the cardiac depression of septic shock in humans. *Chest* **97**: 126–131.

Parrillo JE, Burch C, Shelhamer JH, et al. (1985) A circulating myocardial depressant substance in humans with septic shock. *Journal of Clinical Investigation* **76**: 1539–1553.

Parrillo JE, Parker MM, Natanson C, et al. (1990) Septic shock in humans. Advances in the understanding of pathogenesis, cardiovascular dysfunction and therapy. *Annals of Internal Medicine* **113**: 227–242.

Patel BM, Chittock DR, Russell JA, et al. (2002) Beneficial effects of short-term vasopressin infusion during severe septic shock. *Anesthesiology* **96**: 576–582.

Pathan N, Hemingway CA Alizadeh AA, et al. (2004) Role of interleukin 6 in myocardial dysfunction of meningococcal septic shock. *Lancet* **363**: 203–209.

Pearse R, Dawson D, Fawcett J, et al. (2005) Early goal-directed therapy after major surgery reduces complications and duration of hospital stay. A randomised, controlled trial. *Critical Care* **9**: R687–R693.

Phang PT, Cunningham KF, Ronco JJ, et al. (1994) Mathematical coupling explains dependence of oxygen consumption on oxygen delivery in ARDS. *American Journal of Respiratory and Critical Care Medicine* **150**: 318–323.

Pittet D, Thievent B, Wenzel RP, et al. (1996) Bedside prediction of mortality from bacteremic sepsis. A dynamic analysis of ICU patients. *American Journal of Respiratory and Critical Care Medicine* **153**: 684–693.

Quartin AA, Schein RM, Kett DH, et al. (1997) Magnitude and duration of the effect of sepsis on survival. *Journal of the American Medical Association* **277**: 1058–1063.

Quiroz R, Kucher N, Zou KH, et al. (2005) Clinical validity of a negative computed tomography scan in patients with suspected pulmonary embolism: a systematic review. *Journal of the American Medical Association* **293**: 2012–2017.

Rackow EC, Falk JL, Fein IA, et al. (1983) Fluid resuscitation in circulatory shock: a comparison of the cardiorespiratory effects of albumin, hetastarch, and saline solutions in patients with hypovolemic and septic shock. *Critical Care Medicine* **11**: 839–850.

Rangel-Frausto MS, Pittet D, Costigan M, et al. (1995) The natural history of the systemic inflammatory response syndrome (SIRS). *Journal of the American Medical Association* **273**: 117–123.

Raper RF, Fisher MM (1988) Profound reversible myocardial depression after anaphylaxis. *Lancet* **1**: 386–388.

Reeves JH, Butt WW, Shann F, et al. (1999) Continuous plasmafiltration in sepsis syndrome. *Critical Care Medicine* **27**: 2096–2104.

Reinhart K, Karzai W, Meisner M (2000) Procalcitonin as a marker of the systemic inflammatory response to infection. *Intensive Care Medicine* **26**: 1193–1200.

Reinhart K, Menges T, Gardlund B, et al. (2001) Randomized, placebo-controlled trial of the anti-tumor necrosis factor antibody fragment afelimomab in hyperinflammatory response during severe sepsis: the RAMSES study. *Critical Care Medicine* **29**: 765–769.

Rhodes A, Lamb FJ, Malagon I, et al. (1999) A prospective study of the use of a dobutamine stress test to identify outcome in patients with sepsis, severe sepsis or septic shock. *Critical Care Medicine* **27**: 2361–2366.

Rittoo D, Gosling P, Burnley S, et al. (2004) Randomized study comparing the effects of hydroxyethyl starch solution with Gelofusine on pulmonary function in patients undergoing abdominal aortic aneurysm surgery. *British Journal of Anaesthesia* **92**: 61–66.

Rivers E, Nguyen B, Havstad S, et al. (2001) Early goal-directed therapy in the treatment of severe sepsis and septic shock. *New England Journal of Medicine* **345**: 1368–1377.

Ronco JJ, Fenwick JC, Tweeddale MG, et al. (1993) Identification of the critical oxygen delivery for anaerobic metabolism in critically ill septic and nonseptic humans. *Journal of* the American Medical Association **270**: 1724–1730.

Rothwell PM, Udwadia ZF, Lawler PG (1991) Cortisol response to corticotrophin and survival in septic shock. *Lancet* **337**: 582–583.

Ruokonen E, Takala J, Kari A, et al. (1993) Regional blood flow and oxygen transport in septic shock. *Critical Care Medicine* **21**: 1296–1303.

Russell JA, Ronco JJ, Lockhat D, et al. (1990) Oxygen delivery and consumption and ventricular preload are greater in survivors than in nonsurvivors of the adult respiratory distress syndrome. *American Review of Respiratory Disease* **141**: 659–665.

Russell JA, Walley KR, Singer J, et al. for the VASST Investigators (2008) Vasopressin versus norepinephrine infusion in patients with septic shock. *New England Journal of Medicine* **358**: 877–887.

Sakr Y, Dubois M-J, De Backer D, et al. (2004) Persistent microcirculatory alterations are associated with organ failure and death in patients with septic shock. *Critical Care Medicine* **32**: 1825–1831.

Sakr Y, Reinhart K, Vincent J-L, et al. (2006) Does dopamine administration in shock influence outcome? Results of the Sepsis Occurrence in Critically Ill Patients (SOAP) study. *Critical Care Medicine* **34**:589–597.

Saline versus Albumin Fluid Evaluation Study Investigators (2006) Effect of baseline serum albumin concentration on outcome of resuscitation with albumin or saline in patients in intensive care units; analysis of data from the saline versus albumin fluid evaluation (SAFE) study. *British Medical Journal* **333**: 1044.

Sandham JD, Hull RD, Brant RF, et al. (2003) A randomized, controlled trial of the use of pulmonary-artery catheters in high-risk surgical patients. *New England Journal of Medicine* **348**: 5–14.

Sands KE, Bates DW, Lanken PN, et al. (1997) Epidemiology of sepsis syndrome in 8 academic medical centers. *Journal of the American Medical Association* **278**: 234–240.

Schierhout G, Roberts I (1998) Fluid resuscitation with colloid or crystalloid solutions in critically ill patients: a systematic review of randomised trials. *British Medical Journal* **316**: 961–964.

Schoenberg MH, Beger HG (1993) Reperfusion injury after intestinal ischemia. *Critical Care Medicine* **21**: 1376–1386.

Schortgen F, Lacherade J-C, Bruneel F, et al. (2001) Effects of hydroxyethylstarch and gelatin on renal function in severe sepsis: a multicentre randomised study. *Lancet* **357**: 911–916.

Schroeder S, Wichers M, Klingmüller D, et al. (2001) The hypothalamic–pituitary–adrenal axis of patients with severe sepsis: altered response to corticotrophin-releasing hormone. *Critical Care Medicine* **29**: 310–316.

Schumer W (1976) Steroids in the treatment of clinical septic shock. *Annals of Surgery* **184**: 333–341.

Sharshar T, Carlier R, Blanchard A, et al. (2002) Depletion of neurohypophyseal content of vasopressin in septic shock. *Critical Care Medicine* **30**: 497–500.

Shoemaker WC, Montgomery ES, Kaplan E, et al. (1973) Physiologic patterns in surviving and nonsurviving shock patients. *Archives of Surgery* **106**: 630–636.

Shoemaker WC, Appel PL, Kram HB, et al. (1988) Prospective trial of supranormal values of survivors as therapeutic goals in high risk surgical patients. *Chest* **94**: 1176–1186.

Shorr AF, Jackson WL, Kelly KM, et al. (2005) Transfusion practice and blood stream infections in critically ill patients. *Chest* **127**: 1722–1728.

Simonneau G, Sors H, Charbonnier B, et al. (1997) A comparison of low-molecular-weight heparin with infractionated heparin for acute pulmonary embolism. *New England Journal of Medicine* **337**: 663–669.

Sinclair S, James S, Singer M (1997) Intraoperative intravascular volume optimisation and length of hospital stay after repair of proximal femoral fracture: randomised controlled trial. *British Medical Journal* **315**: 909–912.

Sloan EP, Koenigsberg M, Gens D, et al. (1999) Diaspirin cross-linked hemoglobin (DCLHb) in the treatment of severe traumatic hemorrhagic shock. A randomized controlled efficacy trial. *Journal of the American Medical Association* **282**: 1857–1864.

Sorensen TI, Nielsen GG, Andersen PK, et al. (1988) Genetic and environmental influences on premature death in adult adoptees. *New England Journal of Medicine* **318**: 727–732.

Sort P, Navasa M, Arroyo V, et al. (1999) Effect of intravenous albumin on renal impairment and mortality in patients with cirrhosis and spontaneous bacterial peritonitis. *New England Journal of Medicine* **341**: 403–409.

Spies CD, Reinhart K, Witt I, et al. (1994) Influence of N-acetylcysteine on indirect indicators of tissue oxygenation in septic shock patients: results from a prospective, randomized, double-blind study. *Critical Care Medicine* **22**: 1738–1746.

Spronk PF, Ince C, Gardien MJ, et al. (2002) Nitroglycerin in septic shock after intravascular volume resuscitation. *Lancet* **360**: 1395–1396.

Sprung CL, Annane D, Keh D, et al. for the CORTICUS Study Group (2008) Hydrocortisone therapy for patients with septic shock. *New England Journal of Medicine* **358**: 111–124.

Staubach KH, Schröder J, Stüber F, et al. (1998) Effect of pentoxifylline in severe sepsis: results of a randomized, double-blind, placebo-controlled study. *Archives of Surgery* **133**: 94–100.

Stein PD, Fowler SE, Goodman LR, et al. (2006) Multidetector computed tomography for acute pulmonary embolism. *New England Journal of Medicine* **354**: 2317–2327.

Stockwell MA, Soni N, Riley B (1992a) Colloid solutions in the critically ill. A randomised comparison of albumin and polygeline. 1. Outcome and duration of stay in the intensive care unit. *Anaesthesia* **47**: 3–6.

Stockwell MA, Scott A, Day A, et al. (1992b) Colloid solutions in the critically ill. A randomised comparison of albumin and polygeline 2. Serum albumin concentration and incidences of pulmonary oedema and acute renal failure. *Anaesthesia* **47**: 7–9.

Stüber F, Petersen M, Bokelmann F, et al. (1996) A genomic polymorphism within the tumor necrosis factor locus influences plasma tumor necrosis factor-α concentrations and outcome of patients with severe sepsis. *Critical Care Medicine* **24**: 381–384.

Suffredini AF, Fromm RE, Parker MM, et al. (1989) The cardiovascular response of normal humans to the administration of endotoxin. *New England Journal of Medicine* **321**: 280–287.

Takala J, Meier-Hellmann A, Eddleston J, et al. (2000) Effect of dopexamine on outcome after major abdominal surgery: a prospective, randomized, controlled multicenter study. *Critical Care Medicine* **28**: 3417–3423.

Tang BMP, Eslick GD, Craig JC, McLean AS (2007) Accuracy of procalcitonin for sepsis diagnosis in critically ill patients: systematic review and meta-analysis. *Lancet* **7**:210–217.

Taniguchi T, Koido Y, Aiboshi J, et al. (1999) Change in the ratio of interleukin-6 to interleukin-10 predicts a poor outcome in patients with systemic inflammatory response syndrome. *Critical Care Medicine* **27**: 1262–1264.

Task Force of the American College of Critical Care Medicine, Society of Critical Care Medicine (1999) Practice parameters for hemodynamic support of sepsis in adult patients with sepsis. *Critical Care Medicine* **27**: 639–660.

Tracey KJ, Fong Y, Hesse DG, et al. (1987) Anti-cachectin/TNF monoclonal antibodies prevent septic shock during lethal bacteraemia. *Nature* **330**: 662–664.

Tuchschmidt J, Fried J, Swinney R, et al. (1989) Early hemodynamic correlates of survival in patients with septic shock. *Critical Care Medicine* **17**: 719–723.

Tuchschmidt J, Fried J, Astiz M, et al. (1992) Elevation of cardiac output and oxygen delivery improves outcome in septic shock. *Chest* **102**: 216–220.

Turgeon AF, Hutton B, Fergusson DA, et al. (2007) Meta-analysis: intravenous immunoglobulin in critically ill adult patients with sepsis. *Annals of Internal Medicine* **146**: 193–203.

Uusaro A, Russell JA (2000) Could anti-inflammatory actions of catecholamines explain the possible beneficial effects of supranormal oxygen delivery in critically ill surgical patients? *Intensive Care Medicine* **26**: 299–304.

Vallet B, Chopin C, Curtis SE, et al. (1993) Prognostic value of the dobutamine test in patients with sepsis syndrome and normal lactate values: a prospective, multicenter study. *Critical Care Medicine* **21**: 1868–1875.

Van den Berghe G, de Zegher F (1996) Anterior pituitary function during critical illness and dopamine treatment. *Critical Care Medicine* **24**: 1580–1590.

van Dissel JT, van Langevelde P, Westendorp RG, et al. (1998) Anti-inflammatory cytokine profile and mortality in febrile patients. *Lancet* **351**: 950–953.

Velanovich V (1989) Crystalloid versus colloid fluid resuscitation. A meta-analysis of mortality. *Surgery* **105**: 65–71.

Velmahos GC, Demetriades D, Shoemaker WC, et al. (2000) Endpoints of resuscitation of critically injured patients: normal or supranormal? A prospective randomized trial. *Annals of Surgery* **232**: 409–418.

Venn R, Steele A, Richardson P, et al. (2002) Randomised controlled trial to investigate influence of the fluid challenge on duration of hospital stay and perioperative morbidity in patients with hip fractures. *British Journal of Anaesthesia* **88**: 65–71.

Vesey CJ, Cole PV (1985) Blood cyanide and thiocyanate concentrations produced by long-term therapy with sodium nitroprusside. *British Journal of Anaesthesia* 57: 148–155.

Veterans Administration Systemic Sepsis Cooperative Study Group (1987) Effect of high-dose glucocorticoid therapy on mortality in patients with clinical signs of systemic sepsis. *New England Journal of Medicine* 317: 659–665.

Villar J, Slutsky AS, Hew E, *et al.* (1990) Oxygen transport and oxygen consumption in critically ill patients. *Chest* 98: 687–692.

Vincent J-L (1997) Dear SIRS, I'm sorry to say that I don't like you . . . *Critical Care Medicine* 25: 372–374.

Vincent J-L, Roman A, Kahn RJ (1990) Dobutamine administration in septic shock: addition to a standard protocol. *Critical Care Medicine* 18: 689–693.

Vincent J-L Gris P, Coffernils M, *et al.* (1992) Myocardial depression characterizes the fatal course of septic shock. *Surgery* 111: 660–667.

Vincent J-L, Baron J-F, Reinhart K, *et al.* (2002) Anemia and blood transfusion in critically ill patients. *Journal of the American Medical Association* 288: 1499–1507.

Vinjamuri S, Hall AV, Solanki KK, *et al.* (1996) Comparison of ^{99m}Tc infection imaging with radiolabelled white-cell imaging in the evaluation of bacterial infection. *Lancet* 347: 233–235.

Wakeling HG, McFall MR, Jenkins CS, *et al.* (2005) Intraoperative oesophageal Doppler guided fluid management shortens postoperative hospital stay after major bowel surgery. *British Journal of Anaesthesia* 95: 634–642.

Walley KR (2000) Many roles of nitric oxide in regulating cardiac function in sepsis. *Critical Care Medicine* 28: 2135–2137.

Warren BL, Eid A, Singer P, *et al.* (2001) High-dose antithrombin III in severe sepsis: a randomized controlled trial. *Journal of the American Medical Association* 286: 1869–1878.

Webster NR (1998) Opioids and the immune system. *British Journal of Anaesthesia* 81: 835–836.

Weissman C, Kemper M (1991) The oxygen uptake–oxygen delivery relationship during ICU interventions. *Chest* 99: 430–435.

Wilkes MM, Navickis RJ (2001) Patient survival after human albumin administration. A meta-analysis of randomized, controlled trials. *Annals of Internal Medicine* 135: 149–164.

Wilson J, Woods I, Fawcett J, *et al.* (1999) Reducing the risk of major elective surgery: randomised controlled trial of preoperative optimisation of oxygen delivery. *British Medical Journal* 318: 1099–1103.

Wray GM, Coakley JH (1995) Severe septic shock unresponsive to noradrenaline. *Lancet* 346: 1604.

Wray G, Foster SJ, Hinds CJ, *et al.* (2001) A cell wall component of gram positive bacteria (peptidoglycan) synergises with endotoxin to cause the release of tumour necrosis factor-α, nitric oxide production, shock and multiple organ injury/dysfunction in the rat. *Shock* 15: 135–142.

Wu A, Hinds CJ, Thiemermann C (2004) High-density lipoproteins in sepsis and septic shock: metabolism, actions and therapeutic applications. *Shock* 21: 210–221.

Yu M, Levy MM, Smith P, *et al.* (1993) Effect of maximizing oxygen delivery on morbidity and mortality rates in critically ill patients: a prospective, randomized controlled study. *Critical Care Medicine* 21: 830–838.

Yu DT, Platt R, Lanken PN, *et al.* (2003) Relationship of pulmonary artery catheter use to mortality and resource utilization in patients with severe sepsis. *Critical Care Medicine* 31: 2734–2741.

Ziegler EJ, McCutchan JA, Fierer J, *et al.* (1982) Treatment of Gram-negative bacteremia and shock with human antiserum to a mutant *Escherichia coli*. *New England Journal of Medicine* 307: 1225–1230.

Ziegler EJ, Fisher CJ Jr, Sprung CL, *et al.* (1991) Treatment of Gram-negative bacteremia and septic shock with HA-1A human monoclonal antibody against endotoxin. *New England Journal of Medicine* 324: 429–436.

6 Assessment and monitoring of respiratory function

Important management decisions, both on admission (such as the institution of mechanical ventilation) and later (such as when to start weaning the patient from respiratory support), depend on a reliable and accurate assessment of respiratory function. Respiratory monitoring is also required to evaluate the patient's response to treatment and optimize respiratory support.

Clinical assessment is of the utmost importance. Signs of severe respiratory distress include (see Chapter 8):

■ the use of accessory muscles of respiration;
■ suprasternal and intercostal recession;
■ paradoxical or asynchronous movement of the ribcage and abdomen;
■ respiratory alternans (an increase in the breath-to-breath variation in the relative contribution of the ribcage and abdomen to tidal volume);
■ tachypnoea;
■ tachycardia;
■ sweating;
■ pulsus paradoxus (an exaggeration of the normal fall in systolic blood pressure and pulse pressure during inspiration);
■ inability to speak in sentences.

Together with a subjective assessment of the degree of exhaustion, these clinical signs are often the best guides to the need for respiratory support.

The most sensitive indicator of increasing respiratory difficulty is a rising respiratory rate, although when respiratory frequency is determined by observing chest wall movement over 15 seconds and multiplying the number of excursions by four, errors of up to 4 breaths/min may easily occur (Tobin, 1992). Signs of carbon dioxide retention include a bounding pulse, warm, vasodilated peripheries, a tremor of the outstretched hand and an impaired conscious level, but the presence or absence of cyanosis is an unreliable guide to the adequacy of oxygenation.

The history and clinical examination can be supplemented by regular measurements of the pulse rate, blood pressure and respiratory rate, as well as, in selected cases, tidal volume (V_T) and vital capacity (VC). Repeated blood gas analysis is essential and a chest radiograph should always be obtained. In some cases maximum mouth pressures may

be helpful, and in those with airways obstruction, maximum expiratory flow rates should be recorded. An assessment of lung mechanics can also be valuable in selected cases. More sophisticated investigations, such as the determination of ventilation/perfusion relationships and alveolar–capillary permeability are usually confined to research applications.

These techniques for assessing respiratory function are performed intermittently. Continuous monitoring (e.g. with pulse oximetry and capnography) is required to detect the rapid changes that may sometimes occur, for example in response to alterations in treatment or when there is rapid decompensation.

MEASUREMENT OF LUNG VOLUMES
(see also Chapter 3)

VITAL CAPACITY AND TIDAL VOLUME
VC provides an indication of the patient's ability to inspire deeply, maintain lung expansion and cough. It is particularly useful when assessing patients with respiratory inadequacy due to neuromuscular weakness. The VC depends on:

■ the power of the respiratory muscles;
■ the elastic properties of the chest wall and lung parenchyma;
■ the size and patency of the airways at low lung volumes;
■ the volume of the lungs, which varies with sex and body size.

There are many causes of a reduced VC (Table 6.1), all of which can, if severe, eventually lead to a fall in V_T, the latter being a less sensitive indicator of deterioration than the former. In respiratory failure minute ventilation (the product of V_T and respiratory rate) rises initially and falls precipitously only at a late stage when the patient is exhausted.

The normal VC is 65–75 mL/kg and the normal V_T is 7 mL/kg (about 500 mL). In general a $V_T < 5$ mL/kg or a VC < 15 mL/kg is indicative of serious respiratory difficulty.

FUNCTIONAL RESIDUAL CAPACITY
Functional residual capacity (FRC) can be measured using helium dilution, nitrogen washout or a body

Table 6.1 Causes of a reduced vital capacity

Diseases of chest wall, pleura, lung parenchyma, nerves, muscles

Pleural effusion, haemothorax, pneumothorax

Loss of lung tissue (e.g. lung resection)

Replacement of lung tissue (e.g. tumour)

Premature airway closure (e.g. chronic airflow limitation)

Abdominal distension

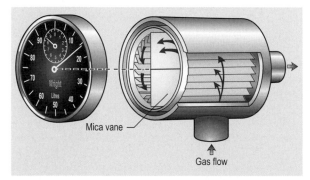

Fig. 6.1 Wright's respirometer. Gas flowing into the device is channelled through a series of tangential slits and rotates the light-weight mica vane. The latter is connected to the pointer on the dial by gears.

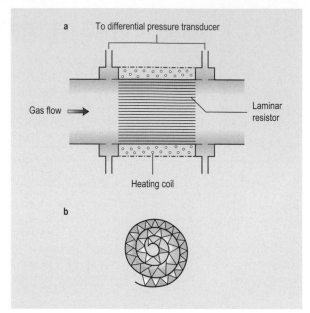

Fig. 6.2 Fleisch pneumotachograph head (see text). (a) Longitudinal section. (b) Cross-section to show corrugated foil wound into spiral. From Sykes MK, Vickers MD (1973) *Principles of Measurement for Anaesthetists*. Blackwell Scientific Publications: Oxford, pp. 126, 131, with permission.

plethysmograph. These techniques are difficult or impossible in ventilated intensive care patients and are generally used only for research. FRC falls when:

- the abdomen is distended;
- there are painful thoracic or abdominal wounds;
- in the supine position;
- lung volume is reduced by pulmonary pathology.

WRIGHT'S RESPIROMETER

The V_T, minute volume and VC can be measured at the bedside using a Wright's respirometer (**Fig. 6.1**). Access to the airway is required, but this is easily achieved in intubated patients by attaching the device to the catheter mount. In the spontaneously breathing, unintubated patient a mouthpiece can be used or a mask can be closely applied to the patient's face. There is therefore inevitably some interference with the patient's airway, which has the disadvantage of interrupting the oxygen supply, as well as potentially altering the respiratory pattern.

The Wright's respirometer is a delicate instrument and is easily damaged if dropped. Because of the inertia of the vane and the resistance of the device, it under-reads at low flows. Conversely, at high flows, the momentum of the vane causes the instrument to overread. Accuracy is also affected by condensation of water vapour and, to a lesser extent, by alterations in the composition of respired gas. Nevertheless, in clinical practice errors are rarely greater than ±10%. The

dead space and resistance of the device are low and it is therefore well tolerated by spontaneously breathing patients. Electronic versions are also available.

PNEUMOTACHOGRAPH

Whereas the Wright's respirometer is a unidirectional device that only measures expired volumes, pneumotachographs record flows in both inspiration and expiration (**Fig. 6.2**). Flow rates are calculated from the measured pressure difference across the fixed resistance; inspired and expired volumes are obtained by integrating these flows.

One of the best known of the original designs is the *Fleisch head*, in which the resistance is formed by a piece of corrugated foil wound into a spiral. This creates a large number of parallel-sided tubes, which ensure laminar flow. Condensation of water vapour on the foil, which could alter its resistance and create turbulent flow, is prevented by surrounding the device with a heating coil. Mucus traps are also required to prevent obstruction. Although alterations in the composition and temperature of the gas mixture interfere with the measurement, when used carefully an accuracy of ±5% is possible.

Considerable care and attention to detail are required when using such devices and they have not proved suitable for routine clinical use. Alternatives have therefore been described. These have included the use of a *heated wire mesh* to provide the resistance (in which case, flow is turbulent and sophisticated electronics are required to produce a linear output), and light-weight devices with a *variable orifice*, which are unaffected by water vapour, allow tracheal secretions to pass easily and are relatively insensitive to temperature changes.

HOT WIRE ANEMOMETER

Another approach to the measurement of inspired and expired volume is to place a heated wire through which a known current is passed in the gas stream. The magnitude of temperature changes, and hence alterations in resistance, reflect the gas flow rates.

ULTRASONIC FLOWMETERS

With these devices an ultrasonic signal is sent upstream and downstream. The time difference provides a measure of gas flow.

VORTEX SPIROMETER

The vortex spirometer generates vortices in the gas stream. These are detected and counted by an ultrasonic beam, the number of vortices being dependent on gas flow rate. These vortex spirometers are said to be accurate over a wide range of flows and are largely unaffected by gas composition, humidity or temperature.

ASSESSING AIRWAYS OBSTRUCTION

Clinical evaluation of the severity of airflow obstruction is notoriously inaccurate. The patient's progress, and in particular response to treatment, can be assessed objectively by serial measurement of *expiratory flow rates*. These depend not only on the resistance of the intrathoracic airways, but also on lung elastic recoil; they are therefore greatest at high lung volumes (when airways resistance is least and elastic recoil maximal) and decrease progressively throughout expiration. Because increasing expiratory force leads to collapse of the distal airways, flow rates are largely independent of muscular effort. Expiratory flow rates are, however, reduced by extreme weakness. Improvement in expiratory flow rates following administration of bronchodilators distinguishes reversible from irreversible airways obstruction.

TIMED MEASUREMENTS OF A FORCED VITAL CAPACITY

Timed measurements of forced vital capacity (FVC) can be performed at the bedside using a *vitalograph* and provide an accurate, reproducible measure of airway calibre. The portion of the FVC exhaled in the first second is termed the *forced expiratory volume in one second (FEV$_1$)*, which is best expressed as a percentage of the FVC.

Normally the FEV$_1$ is 50–60 mL/kg and represents 70–80% of the FVC. In those with airways obstruction the FEV$_1$ is reduced to a greater extent than the FVC and the FEV$_1$/FVC ratio falls below 70%. In restrictive disorders, on the other hand, both FEV$_1$ and FVC are reduced and the ratio is unchanged or increased.

THE WRIGHT'S PEAK FLOW METER

The Wright's peak flow meter (**Fig. 6.3a**) is a cheap and convenient means of assessing airways obstruction at the bedside. Newer, relatively cheap, light-weight, hand-held

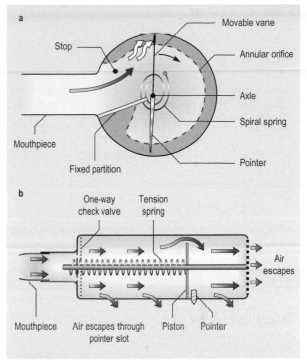

f06-03-S2596.eps

Fig. 6.3 (a) Wright's peak flow meter. The patient makes a forced expiration. The expired gas is deflected on to the rotating vane, which is moved against the resistance offered by the spiral spring. As the vane rotates the annular orifice opens progressively, allowing gas to escape to the outside. The maximum deflection of the vane depends on the peak flow rate. The vane is maintained in this position by a ratchet. From Sykes MK, Vickers MD (1973) *Principles of Measurement for Anaesthetists*. Blackwell Scientific Publications: Oxford, pp 126, 131, with permission. (b) Lightweight, hand-held device for measuring peak flow.

devices which operate on a similar principle are now more commonly used (**Fig. 6.3b**). *Peak expiratory flow rate (PEFR)* is, however, relatively effort-dependent and is less reproducible than the FEV$_1$. Although it is useful for assessing the severity of airways obstruction and the response to treatment, it is not sufficiently specific to be diagnostic of airflow limitation. The normal PEFR is 450–700 L/min in adult males and 300–500 L/min in adult females. In severe airways obstruction, values as low as 60 L/min may be recorded.

MAXIMUM MOUTH PRESSURES

Maximum inspiratory and expiratory pressures can be measured at the mouth or via an endotracheal/tracheostomy tube using an aneroid manometer or a pressure transducer. They are useful indices of the power of the inspiratory and expiratory muscles respectively, although they do depend on patient cooperation.

■ Maximum expiratory pressure is not often measured in intensive care patients.

■ *Maximum inspiratory pressure* (MIP) is usually measured during a maximum inspiratory effort against an occluded airway at residual volume or FRC.

The normal value for MIP varies with age and sex, exceeding −90 cm H_2O in young females and −130 cm H_2O in young males. Values less than −20 to −25 cm H_2O suggest that the patient is unlikely to be able to sustain adequate spontaneous ventilation (see Chapter 7).

FLOW–VOLUME AND PRESSURE–VOLUME LOOPS

Many modern mechanical ventilators continuously measure pressure, volume and flow and display the resultant waveforms. In general, pressure–volume (PV) relationships of the lung and chest wall can be used to assess changes in compliance, whereas flow–volume curves provide an indication of alterations in airways resistance.

Pressure–volume curves

During mechanical ventilation it is possible to determine the shape of the PV curve and, provided the patient is relaxed and flow during inspiration is constant, effective static compliance (C_{es}) (see Chapter 3) can then be calculated from:

$$C_{es} = V_{et}/P_{plat} - PEEP_A - PEEP_i$$

where V_{et} is exhaled tidal volume, P_{plat} is plateau airway pressure, $PEEP_A$ is applied positive end-expiratory pressure (PEEP) and $PEEP_i$ is intrinsic PEEP.

Dynamic compliance (C_{dyn}) (see Chapter 3) is given by:

$$C_{dyn} = V_{et}/PIP - PEEP_A - PEEP_i$$

where PIP is peak inspiratory pressure.

The stiffness of the lung and chest wall can also be assessed by performing a series of small inflations (e.g. 200 mL) from a large (1.5 litre) calibrated syringe, each inflation being followed by a measurement of pressure when flow has ceased. The lung is deflated in similar steps and the pressure is again recorded at intervals (**Fig. 6.4**). The PV curve obtained in this way can be used to identify the pressure required to open collapsed lung units (the lower inflection point) and an upper inflection point, which in normal lungs corresponds to maximum lung volume (see Chapter 3). Compliance can be calculated from the linear portion of the PV slope. In acute respiratory distress syndrome (ARDS), for example, the first change is the appearance of a lower inflection point, indicative of alveolar collapse, whilst later the slope of the PV curve becomes less steep as compliance decreases and hysteresis (**Fig. 6.4**) increases. This technique does, however, require specialized equipment and the patient has to be disconnected from respiratory support, although it is possible to obtain a quasistatic PV curve using automated single-volume steps without the need for ventilator disconnection (Sydow *et al.*, 1991).

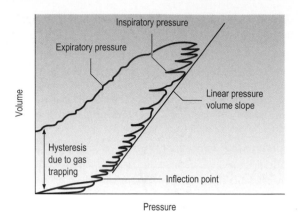

Fig. 6.4 Pressure–volume (*PV*) loop in a patient with ARDS (see text for explanation). Adapted from Webb *et al.*, 1999 Oxford Textbook of Critical Care, Oxford Medical Publications with permission.

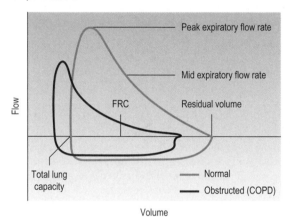

Fig. 6.5 Flow–volume loops from residual volume to total lung capacity for a normal subject and a patient with chronic obstructive pulmonary disease (COPD). In COPD the lung volume is inflated (offset to the left), total lung capacity is increased and expiratory flow is reduced. FRC, functional residual capacity. Adapted from Webb *et al.*, 1999 Oxford Textbook of Critical Care, Oxford Medical Publications with permission.

Flow–volume curves

Flow–volume loops can be used to assess the effects of changes in airways resistance in cooperative subjects in a respiratory function laboratory (**Fig. 6.5**). In intubated patients flow–volume loops are not normally performed over the total lung volume range, forced manoeuvres are rarely performed and exhalation is usually passive. Nevertheless, if the patient is relaxed the expiratory flow can be used to assess airways resistance and visual inspection of the flow–volume loop can demonstrate bronchodilatation and reductions in auto-PEEP (see Chapter 8). The level of external PEEP required to overcome intrinsic PEEP, without worsening hyperinflation, can be assessed by ensuring that the flow–volume loop is not shifted along the volume axis.

Airway resistance (R_{aw}) can be calculated from:

$$R_{aw} = PIP - P_{plat}/peak flow$$

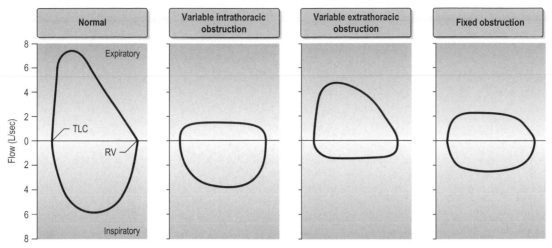

Fig. 6.6 Characteristic flow–volume loops in a normal subject and patients with various forms of upper-airway obstruction. RV, residual volume; TLC, total lung capacity.

Flow–volume loops can also be useful in the assessment of the site of the lesion in patients with upper-airways obstruction (**Fig. 6.6**).

MEASURING THE WORK OF BREATHING

Measurement of the work of breathing requires simultaneous determination of the transpulmonary pressure change (i.e. airway pressure – intrapleural pressure) and V_T. Because an oesophageal balloon has to be inserted, the work of breathing is rarely measured in routine practice; a clinical estimate is usually considered to be adequate.

NON-INVASIVE MONITORING OF VENTILATION

There have been a number of attempts to develop a satisfactory method for continuously monitoring respiratory function that does not intrude on the airway. One example, which can be used in the spontaneously breathing patient, is the *inductance plethysmograph* (Tobin, 1992). The inductive elements are formed by two coils of insulated wire sewn on to bands placed around the ribcage and abdomen. Changes in thoracic and abdominal volumes alter the inductance of the coil. Provided the device is correctly calibrated, it can provide accurate measurements of respiratory timing and thoracic abdominal coordination, as well as a reasonably accurate assessment of changes in V_T (Tobin, 1992). Changes in impedance detected by *ECG electrodes* can be used to continuously monitor respiratory rate.

When using such non-invasive devices, the most valuable information is obtained by analysing changes in the pattern of respiration (e.g. the increasing respiratory rate, the later reduction in V_T and the loss of the normal breath-to-breath

variation in V_T which is seen during the onset of acute respiratory failure). The reverse trend may be seen during weaning from mechanical ventilation.

MONITORING INSPIRED AND EXPIRED GAS COMPOSITION

OXYGEN

Usually the inspired oxygen concentration (F_iO_2), which is expressed as a decimal fraction of 1, is measured using either a polarographic or a fuel cell method. Determination of the expired oxygen fraction is less frequently required.

Fuel cells produce a voltage that is proportional to the partial pressure of oxygen (PO_2) to which they are exposed. They are unaffected by water vapour, but have a slow response time and are relatively inaccurate. Furthermore, they are depleted by continued exposure to oxygen and this limits their lifespan.

Polarographic electrodes also have a slow response time, although this can be increased electronically to allow breath-by-breath analysis.

Paramagnetic analysers are extremely accurate, but require careful calibration. They are affected by water vapour and, again, the response time is slow. They are only suitable for the intermittent analysis of discrete samples of dried gas and consequently their use is generally confined to research.

Mass spectrometers are also very accurate and have the added advantages of a rapid response time and the ability to analyse multiple gas concentrations in the presence of water vapour. They are therefore well suited to the continuous analysis of both inspired and expired gas concentrations in ventilated patients, but are expensive, bulky and require considerable expertise during operation and maintenance. These difficulties have limited their introduction into clinical intensive care practice.

a

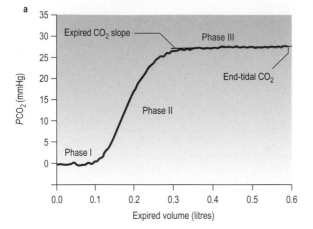

b

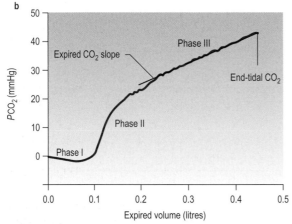

Fig. 6.7 Expired capnograms from mechanically ventilated patients: (a) normal; (b) during an episode of airway obstruction in a patient with chronic obstructive pulmonary disease. Note progressive increase in the concentration of CO_2 in expired gas and increased slope during phase III due to delayed emptying of poorly ventilated lung units. Adapted from Webb *et al.* 1999 Oxford Textbook of Critical Care, Oxford Medical Publications with permission.

CARBON DIOXIDE

Traditionally, the fractional concentration of carbon dioxide in mixed expired gas ($F_E\text{CO}_2$) was determined by analysing a Douglas bag collection with an infrared carbon dioxide analyser. $F_E\text{CO}_2$ has to be measured in order to determine V_D/V_T and the amount of carbon dioxide excreted per unit time ($\dot{V}\text{CO}_2$), as described in Chapter 3.

Capnography (Fig. 6.7)

Continuous breath-by-breath analysis of expired carbon dioxide, using either an infrared analyser or a mass spectrometer, also provides clinically useful information. The infrared absorption technique is inexpensive and simple to use. Expired gas is either sampled from a sidestream port and analysed by a remote sensor or the sensor is positioned in the mainstream of expired gas. The disadvantage of side-stream sampling is that the tubing may become occluded by

mucus and water vapour. Mainstream sensors also have a faster response time.

Absence of a carbon dioxide waveform indicates misplacement of the tracheal tube, usually due to oesophageal intubation, or poor/absent pulmonary perfusion (e.g. cardiac arrest or massive pulmonary embolism). Variations in the carbon dioxide waveform can indicate:

- changes in the production or transport of carbon dioxide;
- alterations in lung function;
- apparatus malfunction;
- altered cardiac output when ventilation is constant.

Changes in the waveform are not, however, diagnostic and other clinical observations are usually required to determine the underlying cause.

The end-tidal carbon dioxide tension ($P_E\text{CO}_2$) can be considered to reflect the partial pressure of alveolar carbon dioxide ($P_A\text{CO}_2$) and therefore the partial pressure of arterial carbon dioxide ($P_a\text{CO}_2$). $P_E\text{CO}_2$ can therefore be used as an immediate guide to the patient's ventilation requirements, bearing in mind the normal gradient between alveolar and arterial carbon dioxide tensions. The discrepancy between $P_E\text{CO}_2$ and $P_a\text{CO}_2$ does, however, increase as lung function deteriorates and changes in $P_E\text{CO}_2$ may also be caused by alterations in the distribution of ventilation or in the ventilatory pattern. It has been suggested that capnography may be a useful non-invasive means of assessing alveolar ventilation during weaning from mechanical ventilation (Saura *et al.*, 1996).

MEASUREMENT OF RESPIRATORY GAS EXCHANGE

Direct measurements of oxygen consumption ($\dot{V}\text{O}_2$) and $\dot{V}\text{CO}_2$ by analysing respiratory gases can be used to estimate energy expenditure and to calculate alveolar/dead-space ventilation and cardiac output by the Fick principle (see Chapters 3 and 4). Determination of respiratory $\dot{V}\text{O}_2$ may also be indicated when evaluating the relationship between oxygen supply and demand (see Chapter 5).

Traditionally $\dot{V}\text{O}_2$ has been determined by collecting expired gas in a Douglas bag over a timed period. The volume of gas in the bag can be measured most accurately using a wet gas meter. $F_I\text{O}_2$ and $F_E\text{O}_2$ are determined using one of the methods already described (e.g. a paramagnetic analyser). If the subject is breathing air, $F_I\text{O}_2$ is, of course, known to be 20.98% and need not be measured. Often, the inspired volume is not measured directly, but is derived using a standard formula. $\dot{V}\text{O}_2$ is then calculated from:

$$\dot{V}\text{O}_2 = (V_I \times F_I\text{O}_2) - (V_E \times F_E\text{O}_2)$$

This technique is, however, relatively complicated and time-consuming and the principle on which the method is based only applies under steady-state conditions, when respiratory

$\dot{V}_{O_2}$ is identical to tissue $\dot{V}_{O_2}$. This is extremely difficult to achieve clinically, particularly in mechanically ventilated subjects. Also determination of $\dot{V}_{O_2}$ becomes progressively less accurate as F_IO_2 increases.

Various alternative means of measuring $\dot{V}_{O_2}$ which overcome some of these difficulties are available and may be more appropriate for clinical use. For example, a pneumotachnograph can be used to measure inspired and expired volumes continuously, as described previously. This can be combined with continuous determination of F_IO_2 and F_EO_2 to obtain $\dot{V}_{O_2}$. $\dot{V}_{CO_2}$ can also be determined if F_ECO_2 is measured (F_ICO_2 can be assumed to be zero). This allows calculation of the respiratory quotient (RQ).

A suitable device for use in critically ill patients is the *Deltatrac* (Datex/Instrumentarium, Helsinki, Finland). This system measures the difference between F_IO_2 and F_EO_2 using a fast-response, paramagnetic differential oxygen sensor; F_ECO_2 is measured with an infrared carbon dioxide analyser. Expired air is collected through an inbuilt mixing chamber and flow is measured by gas dilution. Spontaneously breathing patients can be studied using a canopy system (Takala *et al.*, 1989).

BLOOD GAS ANALYSIS AND ACID–BASE DISTURBANCES

In the early days of intensive care, blood gas analysis was performed using the equilibration technique. This method, developed over 40 years ago by Professor Astrup, was a relatively time-consuming procedure and required a degree of technical expertise. Combined with the reluctance of clinicians to puncture arteries, this meant that blood gas analysis was performed only rarely.

The original Astrup trolleys consisted of a pH electrode and a microtonometer, but some of the later versions also included a direct-reading Clark electrode for the determination of blood oxygen tension. Subsequently, the equilibration technique was superseded by the commercial development of the direct-reading P_{CO_2} electrode and all three were then sufficiently miniaturized to be incorporated in a single cuvette, allowing measurements to be performed on one blood sample. Following the introduction of the microprocessor, automation of most of the processes involved became feasible and modern automated blood gas analysers were soon available commercially. At the same time, there was an increasing acceptance of the ease and relative safety of arterial puncture and cannulation. Consequently, arterial blood gas analysis is now one of the most commonly performed objective tests of respiratory function.

As well as direct measurements of H^+ activity (expressed as pH or $[H^+]$), P_{O_2} and P_{CO_2}, other values relevant to the assessment of the patient's oxygenation and acid–base status are measured or calculated. Most analysers include the option to incorporate ion-sensitive electrodes for measurement of Na^+, K^+, Cl^-, and Ca^{2+}, as well as lactate. Some also include an oximeter for measurement of haemoglobin concentration and oxygen saturation.

More recently the traditional electrodes have been miniaturized and reformed into electrochemical sensors that can be imprinted on a card and combined with a disposable cartridge containing a supply of calibrating reagents, allowing analysis to be performed at the bedside (point-of-care analysers). There is, however, some concern about the reliability and accuracy of these devices, especially in relation to the measurement of haemoglobin and oxygen saturation.

ACCURACY OF BLOOD GAS ANALYSIS

Automation of measurement, calculation and display can give a false impression of reliability and accuracy. This may lead to an uncritical acceptance of the results obtained. The clinician must therefore be aware of the potential sources of error when performing blood gas analysis and of the ways in which these can be minimized.

Sampling

In the past, it was recommended that glass syringes should be used to obtain the arterial sample. These were said to have two advantages:

- the plunger moves freely, allowing arterial blood to flow into the syringe under its own pressure;
- glass is an efficient barrier to diffusion of gases out of the sample.

In fact, most clinicians find an ordinary plastic syringe, with a continuous negative pressure applied to the plunger, quite satisfactory, and in practice diffusion of gases into the wall of the syringe is not a problem. Purpose-designed, pre-heparinized plastic syringes are also available, but are expensive.

Continuing metabolism of white blood cells, and to a lesser extent reticulocytes, can cause significant reductions in P_{O_2} and pH, combined with increases in P_{CO_2}, particularly when the initial gas tension is high. If the sample cannot be analysed immediately (within a few minutes), metabolism can be slowed by immersing the syringe in iced water, having first sealed the end with a plastic cap (Biswas *et al.*, 1982).

To prevent clot formation within the analyser, the sample must be adequately anticoagulated. On the other hand, *excessive dilution of the blood with heparin*, which is acidic, will significantly reduce its P_{CO_2}, although dilution probably has little effect on pH or P_{O_2} (Bradley, 1972). Therefore, heparin should be used in a concentration of 1000 u/mL, and the volume limited to that contained within the dead space of the syringe (i.e. approximately 0.1 mL). Although this will adequately anticoagulate a 2-mL sample, it is not sufficient for the unnecessarily large volumes of blood sometimes presented for analysis.

Even with the most careful technique, air almost inevitably enters the sample. The gas tensions within these *air bubbles* will equilibrate with those in the blood, thereby lowering the P_{CO_2} and usually raising the P_{O_2} of the sample.

Provided they are ejected immediately, however, their effect is insignificant. Nevertheless, errors will arise if bubbles taking up more than 0.5–1% of the sample volume are not removed, particularly if the sample is stored at room temperature (Biswas *et al.*, 1982).

Measurement errors

pH ELECTRODES

Although the traditional pH notation is still used extensively, many now refer to the hydrogen ion concentration ($[H^+]$) in nmol/L. The measurement of H^+/pH is prone to error, the commonest cause of erroneous readings being contamination of the electrode with blood proteins.

PCO_2 ELECTRODES

PCO_2 measurements are generally very accurate. When errors do arise they are usually associated with the development of holes in the electrode membrane or, less often, loss of the silver chloride coating on the reference electrode. The membrane can be replaced relatively easily, but in the latter instance a new electrode is required. Since holes in the membrane occur fairly frequently, there is usually no time for protein contamination to become a problem.

PO_2 ELECTRODES

The current output of the oxygen electrode is less for blood than for a gas with an identical PO_2. This discrepancy is called the blood gas factor and is peculiar to oxygen electrodes. It is thought to be due to consumption of oxygen by the electrode from blood immediately adjacent to the tip of the cathode. This generates a gradient of oxygen tension across the sample and causes the electrode to under-read. The blood gas factor has a proportionately greater effect on the absolute value of PO_2 at higher oxygen tensions. Furthermore, loss of oxygen into the plastic walls of the cuvette and tubing increases as PO_2 rises; therefore, considerable care is necessary to obtain accurate measurements of oxygen tension when PO_2 is high. As with the other electrodes, protein contamination may also cause problems.

Quality control and maintenance

It is essential that on-site equipment that is used extensively out of hours by both medical and nursing staff is subject to strict quality control procedures and regular maintenance. Although automated blood gas analysers are self-calibrating, they should be checked regularly with quality control material, preferably daily. Ampoules containing buffered liquid of known pH and blood gas tensions are available for this purpose. The discrepancy between the measured and the known standard values can then be recorded. Any deviation of these figures outside the predetermined limits indicates a significant fault in the relevant electrode. This can then be remedied (e.g. by replacing the membrane). In practice, however, it is more usual to avoid problems by changing the membranes according to the manufacturer's instructions or when prompted by the analyser. Although buffered liquids can detect the majority of errors associated with the O_2 and

Table 6.2 Normal values for measurements obtained when blood gas analysis is performed

Variable	Normal value
H^+	35–45 nmol/L (7.35–7.45 pH units)
PO_2 (breathing room air)	10.6–13.3 kPa (80–100 mmHg)
PCO_2	4.8–6.1 kPa (36–46 mmHg)
Actual HCO_3^-	22–26 mmol/L
Standard HCO_3^-	22–26 mmol/L
Base deficit	± 2.5
Percentage saturation of haemoglobin with oxygen	95–100%

CO_2 electrodes, they may fail to demonstrate protein contamination of the pH electrode. The latter can be avoided by cleaning the electrode at regular intervals.

INTERPRETATION OF BLOOD GASES AND ACID–BASE STATUS

The range of normal values obtained when blood gas analysis is performed are shown in **Table 6.2**.

Total or actual bicarbonate concentration

Total or actual bicarbonate concentration is influenced by alterations in the amount of carbon dioxide, and by metabolic changes in the amounts of acid and alkali in the blood. It is calculated from the Henderson–Hasselbalch equation (see later).

Standard bicarbonate

The standard bicarbonate concentration can be derived to assess the contribution of metabolic factors, disregarding changes due to alterations in PCO_2. The standard bicarbonate is the amount of bicarbonate that would be present in the sample if the PCO_2 was 5.3 kPa (40 mmHg), the temperature was 37°C and the blood was fully oxygenated at sea level.

Base deficit

Base deficit is simply a convenient number for calculating the amount of sodium bicarbonate required to correct a metabolic acidosis. It is calculated as the amount of base that needs to be added to or subtracted from each litre of extracellular fluid to return the pH to a value of 7.4 at a PCO_2 of 5.3 kPa (40 mmHg) at 37°C. Most often, the clinician is given the base excess, which is negative if there is a base deficit (i.e. a metabolic acidosis) and positive if there is a metabolic alkalosis.

Saturation of haemoglobin with oxygen

Automated blood gas analysers can also calculate the saturation of haemoglobin with oxygen using one of the mathematical formulae describing the oxyhaemoglobin dissociation curve. This calculation is usually performed assuming that the curve is normally positioned, although in some shifts caused by pH changes are taken into account. Percentage saturation is closely related to the oxygen content of the blood, which, as discussed in Chapter 3, can be of more clinical relevance than the PO_2. Some analysers will also calculate oxygen content, either assuming a value for the haemoglobin concentration or by using a value entered by the operator. Others measure haemoglobin concentration optically. The calculation also assumes that all the haemoglobin is available to bind oxygen, (i.e. there is no met- or carboxyhaemoglobin present). Increasingly, modern automated blood gas analysis measures the haemoglobin concentration and the saturation of haemoglobin with oxygen, as well as carboxy – and met – haemoglobin directly using an oximeter.

The interpretation of these results can be considered in two separate parts: disturbances of carbon dioxide homeostasis and acid–base balance, and alterations in oxygenation. In all cases, the following information is essential for correct interpretation:

- the history;
- the age of the patient;
- the F_IO_2;
- any other relevant treatment (e.g. the administration of sodium bicarbonate and the ventilator settings for those on mechanical ventilation).

DISTURBANCES OF ACID–BASE BALANCE

All enzymatically driven biological reactions have optimum values for pH at which the reaction proceeds most rapidly. Alterations in pH can, therefore, lead to a state of 'metabolic chaos' in which some reactions proceed faster than they should, while others slow down. The pH also affects the degree of ionization of various molecules (e.g. an alkalosis causes ionized calcium to bind to protein and may precipitate tetany), as well as altering hydrogen bonding and protein structure. The distribution of ions across cell membranes is also influenced by the quantity of H^+ ions in the body. Severe metabolic acidosis can cause cerebral and myocardial depression, while the respiratory centre is stimulated initially, but is subsequently depressed as the acidosis becomes more severe. A marked metabolic alkalosis may combine with an associated hypokalaemia to depress cardiac function. As discussed in Chapter 3, changes in both pH and PCO_2 cause shifts of the oxyhaemoglobin dissociation curve.

The body therefore resists changes in pH using a variety of buffer systems, as well as by regulating the renal excretion of non-volatile acids and bases and adjusting minute ventilation to control the arterial carbon dioxide tension.

Buffer systems

A buffer is a mixture of a weak acid (which, in contrast to a strong acid, is only partially dissociated in water) and its conjugate base. In the body, the main buffer systems are carbonic acid/bicarbonate, phosphates and proteins.

- For the phosphate system: $H_2PO_4 \rightleftharpoons H^+ + HPO_4^{2-}$;
- For the carbonic acid/bicarbonate system: $H_2CO_3 \rightleftharpoons H^+ + HCO_3^-$

At equilibrium the law of mass action applies and states that the product of the concentrations of H^+ and HCO_3^- divided by the concentration of H_2CO_3 will remain constant. That is:

$$K = [H^+] [HCO_3^-]/[H_2CO_3]$$

Henderson rearranged this equation to allow calculation of the $[H^+]$:

$$[H^+] = K[H_2CO_3]/[HCO_3^-]$$

Later Hasselbalch modified this equation using the pH nomenclature:

$$pH = pK + \log [HCO_3^-]/[H_2CO_3]$$

Buffer systems are most effective when they are maximally dissociated, that is, when the pH is close to their dissociation constant (pK). Protein is an effective intracellular buffer because its pK is similar to the intracellular pH (7.0), while the pK of haemoglobin is 7.4. The pK of the phosphate system is 6.8, but that of the bicarbonate system is only 6.1. Nevertheless, the latter is of particular interest to clinicians because it is present in large amounts, its components can be measured and it is influenced by renal and respiratory compensatory mechanisms.

$$H^+ + HCO_3^- \xrightleftharpoons[\text{Ionic dissociation}]{} H_2CO_3 \xrightleftharpoons[\text{Carbonic anhydrase}]{} CO_2 + H_2O \quad (\text{in solution}) \quad \textit{Kidneys}$$
$$\downarrow$$
$$CO_2 (\text{gas phase}) \quad \textit{Lungs}$$

Alterations in minute ventilation can rapidly compensate for metabolic abnormalities by adjusting P_aCO_2, while renal mechanisms operate over a longer time course and can also compensate for respiratory disturbances. Renal regulation of H^+ balance is achieved by reabsorption or excretion of filtered HCO_3^-, excretion of ammonia or excretion of titratable acidity. Electrical neutrality is usually maintained by reabsorption of Na^+.

The haemoglobin within circulating red blood cells also acts as a buffering system. Carbon dioxide in plasma diffuses into red cells down a concentration gradient. Within erythrocytes CO_2 is converted to HCO_3^-, which diffuses back into the plasma, in a reaction catalysed by carbonic anhydrase. The H^+ generated in this reaction is buffered by combination with haemoglobin. Electrical neutrality is maintained by the movement of Cl^- ions from plasma into the cells (*chloride shift*).

Since $[H_2CO_3]$ is proportional to the P_aCO_2, the Henderson–Hasselbalch equation can be rewritten as:

$$[H^+] \propto PCO_2/[HCO_3^-]$$

PCO_2 can therefore be plotted against $[H^+]$ (or pH) and the various acid–base disturbances described in relation to this diagram (**Fig. 6.8**). Both acidosis and alkalosis can occur, and

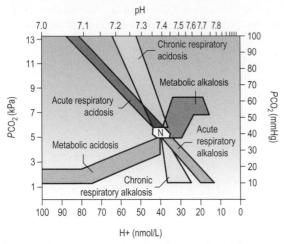

Fig. 6.8 Diagram representing disturbances of acid–base balance (95% confidence limits). The area of normal values is labelled N. From Goldberg *et al.* (1973), with permission. © 1973, American Medical Association.

either may be metabolic (i.e. primarily affecting the bicarbonate component of the system) or respiratory (i.e. primarily affecting P_{CO_2}). Compensatory changes may also be apparent. In clinical practice, arterial $[H^+]$ values outside the range 18–126 nmol/L (pH 6.9–7.7) are very rarely encountered. There is no scientific justification for routinely temperature-correcting blood gas measurements when body temperature is altered, although some recommend correction during hypothermic cardiopulmonary bypass.

Respiratory acidosis

Respiratory acidosis is caused by retention of carbon dioxide; the P_{CO_2} and $[H^+]$ rise (see **Fig. 6.8**). Sometimes there is a small increase in HCO_3^-. A chronically raised P_{CO_2} is compensated by renal retention of bicarbonate and $[H^+]$ returns towards normal. A constant arterial bicarbonate concentration is then usually established within 2–5 days. This represents a primary respiratory acidosis with a compensatory metabolic alkalosis. It is worth recognizing that because treatment such as the administration of diuretics can exacerbate hypochloraemia and produce further retention of bicarbonate, $[H^+]$ may be on the low side of normal, even when carbon dioxide retention is the primary abnormality.

Common causes of respiratory acidosis include ventilatory failure and chronic obstructive pulmonary disease (COPD, type II respiratory failure: see Chapter 8).

Respiratory alkalosis

In respiratory alkalosis the reverse occurs, with a fall in P_{CO_2} and $[H^+]$ (see **Fig. 6.8**), often with a small reduction in bicarbonate concentration. If hypocarbia persists some degree of renal compensation may occur, producing a metabolic acidosis, although in practice this is unusual. A respiratory alkalosis is often produced intentionally or unin-

tentionally when patients are mechanically ventilated; this abnormality may also be seen in hypoxaemic (type I) respiratory failure (see Chapter 8) and in those living at altitude.

Metabolic acidosis

Metabolic acidosis may be due to excessive acid production, most commonly lactic acid, during an episode of shock or following cardiac arrest. Another common cause is diabetic ketoacidosis. A metabolic acidosis may also develop in chronic renal failure, or following either the administration of acid substances, or the loss of large amounts of alkali (e.g. from the lower gastrointestinal tract or in renal tubular acidosis). Respiratory compensation for a metabolic acidosis is usually slightly delayed because the blood–brain barrier initially prevents the respiratory centre from sensing the increased blood $[H^+]$. Following this short delay, however, the patient hyperventilates and 'blows off' carbon dioxide to produce a compensatory respiratory alkalosis. As can be seen from **Figure 6.8**, there is a limit to this respiratory compensation since values for P_aCO_2 less than about 1.5 kPa (11 mmHg) are in practice rarely achieved. It should also be noted that the patient cannot produce respiratory compensation if ventilation is controlled, although the clinician can induce hypocarbia by appropriate adjustment of the ventilator settings.

ANION GAP

When the aetiology of a metabolic acidosis is not clinically obvious, calculation of the anion gap may help to differentiate between the various causes. This is calculated as the difference between the sum of the bicarbonate and chloride concentrations and the sum of the sodium and potassium concentrations. Normally the anion gap, which reflects the sum of the unmeasured anions (sulphates, phosphates, plasma proteins and anions of organic acids), is positive and ranges from 5 to 12 mmol/L. When the acidosis is due to a loss of base, the anion gap will be normal. Conversely, a metabolic acidosis with an increased anion gap is the result of a gain of acid (e.g. in ketoacidosis, renal failure, poisoning with methanol, salicylates or ethylene glycol, and in lactic acidosis).

A number of confounding factors may, however, limit the usefulness of the anion gap, in particular alterations in plasma protein concentrations. In critical illness, for example, reduced plasma albumin concentrations will lead to a reduction in the calculated anion gap. Correction of the anion gap for serum albumin can improve the accuracy of the calculation.

LACTIC ACIDOSIS

Lactic acidosis may be due to increased production and/or decreased removal of lactic acid. The principal sources of lactic acid are skeletal muscle, brain and erythrocytes; lactate ions are converted to glucose or oxidized by the liver and kidney. Two types of lactic acidosis have been described, designated type A and type B.

Type A lactic acidosis. This is more common and is due to inadequate tissue perfusion, cellular hypoxia and anaerobic glycolysis. The ability of the liver to remove the excess lactic acid is often impaired by underperfusion, as well as by severe acidosis, and in extreme cases the liver may actually produce, rather than consume, lactate. The clinical picture is usually dominated by the underlying cause and treatment is directed at reversing tissue hypoxia (see Chapter 5).

Type B lactic acidosis. This occurs in the absence of tissue hypoxia. In the past, the most common cause was the administration of phenformin to patients with impaired renal or hepatic function. Other causes include diabetic ketoacidosis (see Chapter 17), severe liver disease (see Chapter 14), intravenous infusion of sorbitol or fructose, ethanol ingestion, methanol poisoning (see Chapter 19), acute infections and rare hereditary disorders (e.g. glucose-6-phosphate dehydrogenase deficiency). Renal failure is commonly present, but is probably not a cause in itself. The patient usually presents with marked hyperventilation, which may progress to drowsiness, vomiting and eventually coma. Blood pressure is normal, there is no cyanosis and the patient is well perfused.

Treatment of severe type B lactic acidosis involves removal of the precipitating cause and the intravenous administration of sodium bicarbonate; it may prove to be extremely difficult to reverse the acidosis and very large amounts of bicarbonate may be required (e.g. 1000 mmol). Therefore, some recommend that the first 2–3 litres are given as an isotonic (1.4%) solution, followed by 8.4% sodium bicarbonate. The large volumes of fluid required may precipitate volume overload and pulmonary oedema. Haemodiafiltration has been advocated for resistant cases.

Metabolic alkalosis

Metabolic alkalosis can be caused by loss of acid (e.g. from the stomach with nasogastric suction or in high intestinal obstruction) or by excessive administration of absorbable alkali. Overzealous treatment with intravenous sodium bicarbonate is sometimes implicated. In such causes of metabolic alkalosis the urinary chloride concentration is usually low. Some less common causes of metabolic alkalosis in which urinary chloride is high include hyperaldosteronism, Cushing's syndrome, ingestion of liquorice and severe potassium deficiency. Depletion of the extracellular fluid volume and a reduction in total body potassium are both important precipitating factors in the development of metabolic alkalosis. Contraction of the extracellular compartment causes increased sodium reabsorption in exchange for hydrogen ions. The latter are lost in the urine and bicarbonate reabsorption is increased. Similarly, potassium depletion stimulates the kidneys to retain potassium in exchange for hydrogen ions. Diuretics are frequently implicated in both extracellular fluid volume depletion and hypokalaemia.

Respiratory compensation for a metabolic alkalosis is often slight and it is rare to encounter a $P_aCO_2 > 6.5$ kPa (50 mmHg), even with severe alkalosis.

Treatment consists of correcting the underlying cause; specific treatment is rarely required. If severe alkalosis persists, despite restoring the extracellular fluid volume and correction of potassium depletion, the carbonic anhydrase inhibitor acetazolamide or, very occasionally, intravenous hydrochloric acid may be indicated. There is evidence that a single intravenous dose of acetazolamide 500 mg is as effective as 250 mg every 6 hours for a total of four doses, and reverses metabolic alkalosis for a prolonged period (Mazur *et al.*, 1999).

Interpreting the acid–base status
Proceed as follows (**Table 6.2**):

- Look at the pH to see whether the patient is acidotic or alkalotic.
- Look at the PCO_2 to determine whether there is a respiratory component. If the PCO_2 is high, there is a respiratory acidosis; if it is low, there is a respiratory alkalosis.
- Look at the standard bicarbonate and the base excess. If the standard bicarbonate is low and the base excess is negative (i.e. there is a base deficit), there is a metabolic acidosis. If the standard bicarbonate is high and the base excess is positive, there is a metabolic alkalosis.
- Although the primary abnormality is often indicated by the direction of the pH change, this is not always the case. The nature of the primary abnormality can then only be determined by considering the clinical context in which it has arisen.

It should be noted that, during cardiac arrest and in severe circulatory failure, carbon dioxide tension may be considerably higher and pH markedly lower in venous blood than in arterial blood. This discrepancy is particularly marked when P_aCO_2 is controlled by mechanical ventilation and may be exacerbated by the administration of sodium bicarbonate (Adrogué *et al.*, 1989). Therefore, it has been suggested that a widened arteriovenous PCO_2 difference may be a useful indicator of circulatory failure and that analysis of venous blood may provide a better guide to tissue acid–base status.

AN ALTERNATIVE APPROACH TO UNDERSTANDING ACID–BASE PHYSIOLOGY (Sirker *et al.*, 2002)
Because the Henderson–Hasselbalch approach to analysing acid–base disorders is relatively easy to understand and apply, this method is still by far the most widely used in clinical practice. There are, however, some problems with interpretation. These include the supposition that HCO_3^- and P_aCO_2 are independently adjusted variables that ultimately determine pH and the assumption that the dissociation equilibrium for carbonic acid is used as the control system for setting pH (Sirker *et al.*, 2002). Another limitation of the traditional approach is that the various possible causes of a metabolic acidosis can only be distinguished by calculating the anion gap (see above).

Stewart (1983) therefore proposed an alternative approach which used fundamental principles of physical chemistry to identify factors that must determine the pH of biological solutions. The principles employed were those of electrical neutrality and the conservation of mass, combined with the requirement that the dissociation equilibria of all incompletely dissociated substances must be satisfied at all times. These principles were then applied to the various components which constitute fluids in the human body (i.e. water, strong ion solutions in water, weak acid or buffer solutions in water and solutions containing carbon dioxide). Stewart was able to show that three *independent variables* determine pH in plasma by altering the degree of dissociation of water into H^+ ions. These three directly measurable, independent variables were:

1. The strong ion difference (SID). (A strong ion is defined as an ion which is effectively fully dissociated in biological solutions.) The SID is the net charge difference between the sum of the measured strong plasma cations (Na^+, K^+, Ca^{2+} and Mg^{2+}) and strong plasma anions (Cl^-, lactate$^-$). In a patient with a normal acid–base status the SID is usually 38–42 mEq/L. This charge difference is called the effective SID;
2. Total weak acid (A_{TOT}) (mainly albumin and inorganic phosphate);
3. Carbon dioxide in solution (P_{CO_2}).

This approach postulates that both HCO_3^- and H^+ are dependent variables and that HCO_3^- cannot be independently adjusted to regulate pH.

Using the Stewart approach the direct contribution of unmeasured anions to a metabolic acidosis can be accurately quantified, thus defining the cause, and acid–base disorders can be classified on the basis of alterations in the independent variables. Thus, as with the traditional approach, respiratory disorders are those primarily attributable to changes in carbon dioxide, whilst changes in SID represent the compensatory response. A metabolic alkalosis will occur if there is an increase in plasma SID or a fall in [A_{TOT}], whereas an increase in [A_{TOT}] or a decrease in plasma SID will cause a metabolic acidosis.

The kidneys are the most important regulators of SID for acid–base purposes; because [Na^+] and [K^+] must be tightly controlled for other functions (e.g. maintenance of intravascular volume and neuromuscular function respectively), the kidneys use Cl^- to regulate acid–base status without interfering with other important homeostatic mechanisms. Thus, for example, compensation for a respiratory acidosis involves urinary excretion of Cl^- (together with ammonium cations) which increases the SID, whereas correction of an alkalosis is achieved by renal tubular resorption of Cl^-, with a consequent reduction in SID. Similarly, the chloride shift in red cells described above can raise plasma SID and help to compensate for increased plasma carbon dioxide concentration. This approach emphasizes the importance of chloride in acid–base disturbances and can explain the metabolic acidosis commonly observed in patients who have received large volumes of normal saline, which, unlike plasma, contains equal amounts of sodium and chloride. The resulting hyperchloraemia reduces plasma SID and causes an increase in [H^+]. Similarly, the loss of large amounts of Cl^- in gastric fluid will increase plasma SID and cause a metabolic alkalosis. Because there are no known mechanisms that control (A_{TOT}) for the purpose of acid–base regulation, some authorities do not classify alterations in pH caused by changes in [A_{TOT}] as acid–base disorders.

The strong ion difference gap (SIG) is calculated as the difference between the SID and the effective SID. The normal range for the SIG is zero, implying that there are very few strong ions other than Na^+, K^+, Ca^{2+}, Mg^{2+} and Cl^- in the plasma of healthy individuals. The ions which may increase the SIG are the same as those which can cause an elevated anion gap or normochloraemic metabolic acidosis (see above), as well as a number of other unidentified strong anions which can be detected in critically ill patients. In critical illness the relationship between the SIG and the anion gap can be improved by correcting the latter for the charge contribution from protein and phosphate.

Although Stewart's approach provides useful insights into the mechanisms by which the body regulates pH and the causes of acid–base disturbances (particularly the relevance of Cl^- ion homeostasis), the cumbersome mathematical equations required have so far limited the introduction of this method into routine clinical practice, although a simplified approach suitable for use in clinical practice has recently been described (Story *et al.*, 2004).

ALTERATIONS IN OXYGENATION

Having interpreted the acid–base state, the adequacy of oxygenation can be evaluated. When interpreting the P_{O_2} it is important to remember that it is often the oxygen content of the arterial blood (C_aO_2) that is most relevant clinically; this is determined by the percentage saturation of haemoglobin with oxygen. The latter is related to the P_{O_2} by the oxyhaemoglobin dissociation curve. The clinical significance of the dissociation curve is discussed in Chapter 3, but it is most important to consider the P_{O_2} in conjunction with the percentage saturation of haemoglobin with oxygen; in general, if the latter is greater than 95%, oxygenation can be considered to be adequate. Remember that P_aO_2 is influenced by factors other than pulmonary function, including alterations in the mixed venous oxygen tension (P_vO_2) caused by changing metabolic rate and/or cardiac output, and shifts in the position of the dissociation curve (see Chapter 3). Also the normal range for P_aO_2 decreases with age, although in subjects more than 74 years old there is a tendency for this trend to reverse. In the age group 40–74 years, P_aO_2 is influenced by age, body mass index (BMI) and P_aCO_2 such that: P_aO_2 (mmHg) $= 143.6 - (0.39 \times age) - (0.56 \times BMI) - (0.57 \times P_aCO_2)$ (Cerveri *et al.*, 1995).

DETERMINATION OF OXYGEN CONTENT

As discussed above, the calculated values for oxygen content produced by automated blood gas analysers are subject to considerable error. Direct measurement of oxygen content, or its calculation from accurately determined values for haemoglobin and oxygen saturation, is therefore sometimes required, for example, in order to derive other important variables such as DO_2, $\dot{V}O_2$ and percentage venous admixture.

In clinical practice, oxygen content is usually calculated from accurately determined values for haemoglobin and oxygen saturation. These can be measured using a *photometric technique*. The automated bench oximeters designed for this purpose are relatively robust and easy to operate and can therefore be used on-site by staff who have been instructed in their use. They measure the optical absorbance of haemolysed blood at least at four separate wavelengths, thereby providing values for carboxy- and methaemoglobin as well as oxyhaemoglobin. These values, together with derived oxygen content, are then displayed digitally. It is now more usual to integrate the oximeter into a blood gas analyser.

IN VIVO BLOOD GAS MEASUREMENT

There are obvious potential clinical advantages in monitoring blood gas tensions continuously rather than intermittently. The instantaneous detection of changes in blood gas tensions allows rapid evaluation and adjustment of therapy, as well as immediate recognition of deteriorating cardiorespiratory function. The effects of potentially dangerous manoeuvres (e.g. hypoxaemia occurring during tracheal suction) or accidents such as circuit disconnection are also immediately apparent.

Intravascular blood gas tensions can be monitored continuously using miniaturized electrodes, while oxygen saturation can be determined using fibreoptic oximeters. Blood gas tensions and oxygen saturation can also be estimated continuously using transcutaneous electrodes or oximetry.

ELECTRODE SYSTEMS

Techniques for continuous *in vivo* determination of oxygen tension are usually based on miniaturized Clark electrodes. These devices often incorporate a lumen to allow discrete samples of arterial blood to be obtained intermittently.

Although the linear response of these electrodes is good when compared with bench analysis, they have a tendency to drift and are influenced by changes in body temperature. They therefore have to be calibrated at regular intervals against conventionally analysed arterial samples. Because fresh blood is continuously flowing past the electrode membrane, the blood gas factor is normally small and can be ignored, although in low-flow states this may become a significant source of error.

Such electrodes have been widely used to monitor P_aO_2 continuously in neonates, in whom it is essential to control P_aO_2 within narrow limits at all times to avoid cerebral hypoxia on the one hand and retrolental fibroplasia on the other. They have also been used for continuous monitoring of venous oxygen tension. In critically ill adults a sustained fall in P_vO_2 to below 5.3 kPa (40 mmHg) was found to be a reliable indicator of respiratory or cardiovascular deterioration, which was not always clinically obvious (Armstrong *et al.*, 1978). Despite the potential advantages of intravascular PO_2 electrodes, their use has not become established in adult intensive care practice.

The development of intravascular electrodes for determining PCO_2 has been beset by technical problems that have prevented their introduction into the intensive care unit for long-term monitoring, although they have been used for limited periods in anaesthetized subjects.

FIBREOPTIC SPECTROPHOTOMETRY

The technique of *in vivo* oximetry uses an intravascular fibreoptic catheter and is based on the same principles as those used in the bench oximeters described above. A beam of light consisting of two or three precisely known wavelengths is generated, usually by a light-emitting diode, and transmitted down one of two bundles of optical fibres. Light reflected from the red cells is returned to a photodiode detector along the other bundle of fibres. In this way, the percentage saturation of haemoglobin with oxygen can be measured continuously and accurately *in vivo*. Fibreoptic spectrophotometers are, however, prone to drift and the signal may be distorted by deposition of fibrin, or if the tip of the catheter impinges on the vessel wall. As with all optical methods for measuring haemoglobin oxygen saturation, there is the possibility of interference from other optically active compounds (see below).

These devices can be positioned relatively easily in the pulmonary artery and have been used successfully for continuous determination of mixed venous and central venous oxygen saturation (S_vO_2, $S_{cv}O_2$). Fibreoptic oximeters have been incorporated into pulmonary artery and central venous catheters and this has facilitated their introduction into routine clinical practice.

TRANSCUTANEOUS BLOOD GAS MEASUREMENT
(Eberhard *et al.*, 1981; Shoemaker and Vidyasagar, 1981)
Transcutaneous Po₂ ($P_{tc}O_2$)
As with continuous intravascular PO_2 determination, most of the initial experience with measurement of $P_{tc}O_2$ was gained in neonates. The method is based on the principle of increasing the diffusion of oxygen from the blood in the subdermal capillary loops to the skin surface, where its partial pressure can be measured with a conventional Clark electrode housed behind a membrane. The oxygen tension

gradient from capillary to skin surface is clearly dependent on P_aO_2 but is also influenced by many other factors, including:

- skin thickness;
- tissue blood flow;
- tissue oxygen consumption;
- the position of the oxyhaemoglobin dissociation curve.

Transcutaneous electrodes therefore incorporate a heating element, which is maintained at 44°C and warms the underlying skin to approximately 43°C. This increases skin permeability and blood flow, and also facilitates unloading of oxygen from haemoglobin by shifting the dissociation curve to the right. These effects are, however, to some extent offset by a local increase in $\dot{V}O_2$. Nevertheless, provided tissue blood flow is adequate, it is usually possible to obtain a reasonable linear correlation between $P_{tc}O_2$ and P_aO_2.

Accurate results are very dependent on adequate skin blood flow so that in patients with low cardiac output $P_{tc}O_2$ is a poor indicator of P_aO_2. Although in neonates $P_{tc}O_2$ usually closely reflects P_aO_2, many feel that in adults, even when peripheral perfusion is good, $P_{tc}O_2$ should only be used as an indicator of trends in P_aO_2 and perhaps changes in tissue oxygenation.

Although the response time is rapid in infants (10–15 seconds), this increases to 45–60 seconds in adults and the reading will take 5–15 minutes to reach a plateau following application of the electrode. Finally the area of skin underlying the electrode can be damaged by excessive heating.

Polarographic oxygen sensors

A polarographic oxygen sensor that can be applied to the conjunctiva has been described (Fatt and Deutsch, 1983). These devices eliminate the need to heat the skin and have a faster response time than transcutaneous electrodes. Although it was initially thought that conjunctival sensors would be less dependent on perfusion, they have since been found to be sensitive to local and systemic alterations in flow. Some consider them to be of use during resuscitation and transport but in general they have been superseded by pulse oximetry.

Transcutaneous P_{CO_2} ($P_{tc}CO_2$)

Most transcutaneous carbon dioxide electrodes consist of a conventional glass pH electrode combined with a heating element. Carbon dioxide is, of course, more soluble than oxygen and is produced, rather than consumed, by the tissues. Furthermore, heating the skin increases local carbon dioxide production and capillary P_{CO_2}. Therefore $P_{tc}CO_2$ is consistently higher than P_aCO_2 and the difference between the two varies considerably from patient to patient depending on skin characteristics. However, changes in $P_{tc}CO_2$ do follow the trend of alterations in P_aCO_2, although in shock

$P_{tc}CO_2$ can be very high and the discrepancy between P_aCO_2 and $P_{tc}CO_2$ is increased.

PULSE OXIMETRY (Taylor and Whitwam, 1986)

Light-weight oximeters that measure the differential change in light absorption at a red wavelength (e.g. 660 nm) and an infrared wavelength (e.g. 940 nm) in pulsating arterial blood can be applied to an earlobe or finger to provide a continuous, non-invasive assessment of arterial oxygen saturation (S_pCO_2) (Yoshiya *et al.*, 1980). These devices are reliable, do not require calibration, are easy to use and have superseded transcutaneous blood gas electrodes for continuous monitoring of oxygenation in adult intensive care practice. They automatically compensate for variations in skin thickness, slight differences in skin pigmentation and small changes in peripheral perfusion. The signal is, however, very susceptible to noise; electrical interference, excessive, fluctuating ambient light and movement artefact may all cause difficulties.

The accuracy of oximeters varies, but in general the 95% confidence limits are roughly ±4% when S_aO_2 is greater than 80%; below this value they tend to overread. A reduction in arterial pulsation, due to poor peripheral perfusion, hypotension, cold extremities, oedema, venous congestion or a combination of these, can lead to inaccuracies. Importantly, it has been shown that in critically ill patients the discrepancy between S_pO_2 and S_aO_2 may be large and that the reproducibility of S_pO_2 is poor. The accuracy of S_pO_2 measurements appeared to be influenced by the type of oximeter, the presence of hypoxaemia and the requirement for vasoactive drugs (Van de Louw *et al.*, 2001). Also, because pulse oximeters use light of only two wavelengths and assume that haemoglobin is present only in either the reduced or oxygenated form, values for S_pO_2 will be erroneous in the presence of abnormal haemoglobins (e.g. met- or carboxyhaemoglobin). Importantly, elevated carboxyhaemoglobin levels, as may be found in those with carbon monoxide poisoning and recently admitted heavy smokers, result in falsely high readings for S_pO_2. Jaundice, on the other hand, may cause S_pO_2 to be falsely low. Multi-wavelength pulse oximeters (or pulse co-oximeters), that can measure the concentration of abnormal haemoglobins and correct the S_pO_2 reading accordingly, are now available.

Transoesophageal pulse oximetry has been shown to produce more consistent readings than surface pulse oximetry, and is less influenced by changes in blood pressure or body temperature (Vicenzi *et al.*, 2000).

It is important to appreciate that pulse oximetry is not a sensitive guide to changes in oxygenation because, assuming an error of ± 4%, a reading of 95% could represent either a true value of 91% (i.e. P_aO_2 approximately 8 kPa) or 99% (i.e. P_aO_2 approximately 20 kPa); S_pO_2 becomes a useful indicator of P_aO_2 only when it has fallen below 90% (a P_aO_2 of about 8 kPa), and pulse oximetry cannot be used to monitor P_aO_2 when the upper level of P_aO_2 is critical (e.g. in neonates). Clearly an S_pO_2 within normal limits in a patient receiving supplemental oxygen in no way excludes the possibility of hypoventilation (Hutton and Clutton-Brock, 1993).

Nevertheless pulse oximetry has been shown to improve the anaesthetist's ability to detect hypoxaemia and related events in the operating theatre/recovery area and the use of this device has been associated with a reduced rate of myocardial ischaemia (Moller et al., 1993), as well as a reduction in the number of unanticipated intensive care unit admissions (Cullen et al., 1992).

Dual oximetry (Räsänen et al., 1987)

Continuous monitoring of S_aO_2 and S_vO_2 has been advocated as a means of obtaining real-time assessment of changes in peripheral oxygen extraction and pulmonary gas exchange. Thus, for example, the development of hypoxaemia with convergence of S_aO_2 and S_vO_2 indicates worsening gas exchange with a fall in extraction, whereas divergence of S_aO_2 and S_vO_2 implies increased peripheral oxygen use.

OTHER INDICES OF PULMONARY OXYGEN TRANSFER AND LUNG FUNCTION

In the more complex or seriously ill patients (e.g. those with acute lung injury/ARDS) and for research, more objective indices of pulmonary gas exchange and lung function may prove useful (e.g. in following a patient's progress and response to therapy or deciding whether to initiate specific forms of therapy or when to wean a patient from mechanical ventilation).

ALVEOLAR–ARTERIAL OXYGEN TENSION DIFFERENCE ($P_{A-a}O_2$)

$P_{A-a}O_2$ can be determined by measuring P_aO_2 and calculating P_AO_2 from the alveolar air equation (see Chapter 3). This requires accurate determination of the F_IO_2, barometric pressure and P_aCO_2. The RQ can be assumed to be 0.8. The $P_{A-a}O_2$ has limitations as an index of pulmonary function because:

- It is influenced by the P_AO_2 so that even in normal subjects $P_{A-a}O_2$ increases as F_IO_2 rises.
- It is influenced by the arteriovenous oxygen content difference (i.e. it will alter if cardiac output, metabolic rate, oxygen extraction or the position of the dissociation curve changes).

Some feel that it is useful to determine the $P_{A-a}O_2$ with the patient breathing 100% oxygen. This can then be compared with predicted values under these circumstances and with values obtained in the same patient breathing air. Breathing pure oxygen, even for short periods, can, however, impair lung function and this practice should in general be avoided.

THE P_aO_2/F_IO_2 RATIO

The P_aO_2/F_IO_2 ratio has gained widespread acceptance as a simple index of the severity of lung dysfunction for clinical and research purposes. The accuracy with which this ratio reflects $\dot{Q}_s/\dot{Q}_T$ is, however debatable. Certainly P_aO_2/F_IO_2 is influenced by F_IO_2, especially when F_IO_2 is low and the relationship becomes more complex when $C_{(a-v)}O_2$ is reduced, as may be the case in sepsis, for example (Nirmalan et al., 2001). Some argue that the P_aO_2/F_IO_2 ratio is not a reliable measure of pulmonary oxygen transfer in patients with haemodynamic and metabolic instability and must therefore be interpreted with caution in ARDS (Nirmalan et al., 2001).

Other indices, such as the calculated oxygen content difference between end-capillary and arterial blood (C_cO_2–C_aO_2), the arterial/alveolar ratio of PO_2 (P_aO_2/P_AO_2), and the respiratory index ($P_{(A-a)}O_2/P_aO_2$) are also limited by the influence of changes in F_IO_2 and $C_{(a-v)}O_2$.

PERCENTAGE VENOUS ADMIXTURE, DEAD SPACE AND V/Q DISTRIBUTIONS

Because of the limitations of the relatively simple oxygen tension-based indices, calculation of percentage venous admixture is considered by many to be a much better measure of pulmonary oxygen transfer (Nirmalan et al., 2001). Physiological dead space can be calculated at the same time to provide the three-compartment analysis of respiratory function described in Chapter 3.

This analysis does not, however, provide any information about the relative contribution of true shunt and V/Q disturbance to the total venous admixture, nor does it describe the nature of the V/Q inequality. Moreover, calculated $\dot{Q}_s/\dot{Q}_T$ can vary with changes in F_IO_2 (although these changes are usually clinically insignificant and depend on the proportion of the cardiac output perfusing alveolar units with a low V/Q ratio) and the shunt equation does assume that alveolar gas exchange is in a steady state and that blood flow is continuous. Methods have been developed using the intravenous injection of inert tracer gases of different solubilities, which can, when analysed by computer, produce a description of alveolar V/Q distributions. These multiple inert-gas elimination techniques are generally not used in clinical practice.

ALVEOLAR–CAPILLARY PERMEABILITY

Techniques for determining alveolar–capillary permeability have been developed largely as research tools and are rarely used clinically.

Epithelial permeability can be assessed by recording the clearance of an inhaled aerosol of technetium[99m]-diethylene triamine pentaacetic acid (Tc[99m]-DTPA) from the lungs using a gamma camera or an externally placed scintillation counter. Tc[99m]-DTPA is an inert γ-emitter with a short half-life of about 6 hours; it is assumed that the endothelium is freely permeable to this small molecule and that changes in clearance therefore reflect alterations in epithelial integrity. Tc^{99m}-DTPA clearance is increased in smokers, as well as in ARDS, and the technique has been used to distinguish cardiogenic from non-cardiogenic pulmonary oedema (see Chapter 8).

Endothelial permeability can be assessed by measuring the accumulation in the lung of an intravascular radiotracer such as Tc^{99m} or iodine[131]-labelled albumin or transferrin. In ARDS this method appears to be less sensitive, but more specific than the measurement of DTPA clearance. Specificity and sensitivity can be increased by using a double-isotope technique (e.g. by simultaneously labelling red blood cells to provide an intravascular marker).

A less sensitive and more invasive technique is to measure the accumulation of I^{131}-labelled albumin in bronchoalveolar secretions.

EXTRAVASCULAR LUNG WATER (see Chapter 4, p. 64) (Staub, 1986)

The ideal method for measuring lung water should be accurate, sensitive, reproducible, non-invasive, convenient and inexpensive (Staub, 1986). None of the currently available methods fulfil all these requirements. Gravimetric measurement of lung water is a postmortem technique, clinical examination can be misleading and the interpretation of chest radiographic appearances is inconsistent. The indicator dilution technique for measurement of lung water relies on the central injection of two indicators and their detection in the femoral artery. One (the diffusible indicator) distributes between the intravascular and extravascular spaces, while the other (the non-diffusible indicator) remains confined to the intravascular compartment. Dilution curves can be generated at the femoral artery for both indicators from which their volume of distribution can be calculated, allowing determination of lung water by simple subtraction. Cold can be used as the diffusible indicator and indocyanine green as the non-diffusible indicator. Lung water can also be measured by transpulmonary thermodilution alone and by a number of densitometric techniques such as computed tomographic (CT) scanning and positron tomography. The value of extravascular lung water measurement in clinical practice remains unclear.

VENTILATION–PERFUSION SCANS

Lung perfusion can be assessed by determining the distribution of intravenous Tc^{99m}-labelled microspheres. Although segmental perfusion defects in the appropriate clinical setting are suggestive of pulmonary embolism, hypoxic pulmonary vasoconstriction in lung regions where ventilation is reduced or absent (e.g. in areas of collapse and/or consolidation) may complicate interpretation. The diagnosis of pulmonary embolism is supported by excluding obvious lung pathology in the region of interest on plain chest radiography or by demonstrating normal ventilation in areas of reduced perfusion using, for example, aerosolized xenon[133] (*V/Q* scan). Ventilation scanning can, however, be difficult, if not impossible, in critically ill patients, especially when an endotracheal tube is in place.

IMAGING

The value of ultrasound and CT imaging of the lungs, pleura, mediastinal structures and thoracic wall has been increasingly recognized. Ultrasound can be used to identify and direct drainage of pleural effusions, whilst CT scans are valuable in the management of patients with ARDS and in the diagnosis of pulmonary embolism (see Chapters 5, 7 and 8).

REFERENCES

Adroguè HJ, Rashad MN, Gorin AB, *et al.* (1989) Assessing acid–base status in circulatory failure. Differences between arterial and central venous blood. *New England Journal of Medicine* **320**: 1312–1316.

Armstrong RF, Walker JS, Andrew DS, *et al.* (1978) Continuous monitoring of mixed venous oxygen tension P_vO_2 in cardiorespiratory disorders. *Lancet* **1**: 632–634.

Biswas CK, Ramos JM, Agroyannis B, *et al.* (1982) Blood gas analysis: effect of air bubbles in syringe and delay in estimation. *British Medical Journal* **284**: 923–927.

Bradley JG (1972) Errors in the measurement of blood PCO_2 due to dilution of the sample with heparin solution. *British Journal of Anaesthesia* **44**: 231–232.

Cerveri I, Zoia MC, Fanfulla F, *et al.* (1995) Reference values of arterial oxygen tension in the middle-aged and elderly. *American Journal of Respiratory and Critical Care Medicine* **152**: 934–941.

Cullen DJ, Nemeskal AR, Cooper JB, *et al.* (1992) Effect of pulse oximetry, age and ASA physical status on the frequency of patients admitted unexpectedly to a postoperative intensive care unit and the severity of their anesthesia-related complications. *Anesthesia and Analgesia* **74**: 181–188.

Eberhard P, Mindt W, Schafer R (1981) Cutaneous blood gas monitoring in the adult. *Critical Care Medicine* **9**: 702–705.

Fatt I, Deutsch TA (1983) The relation of conjunctival PO_2 to capillary bed PO_2. *Critical Care Medicine* **11**: 445–448.

Goldberg M, Green SB, Moss ML, *et al.* (1973) Computer-based instruction and diagnosis of acid–base disorders. A systematic approach. *Journal of the American Medical Association* **223**: 269–275.

Hutton P, Clutton-Brock T (1993) The benefits and pitfalls of pulse oximetry. *British Medical Journal* **307**: 457–458.

Mazur JE, Devlin JW, Peters MJ, *et al.* (1999) Single versus multiple doses of acetazolamide for metabolic alkalosis in critically ill medical patients: a randomized, double-blind trial. *Critical Care Medicine* **27**: 1257–1261.

Moller JT, Johannessen NW, Espersen K, *et al.* (1993) Randomized evaluation of pulse oximetry in 20 802 patients: II perioperative events and postoperative complications. *Anesthesiology* **78**: 445–453.

Nirmalan M, Willard T, Columb MO, *et al.* (2001) Effect of changes in arterial-mixed venous oxygen content difference ($C_{(a-v)}O_2$) on indices of pulmonary oxygen transfer in a model ARDS lung. *British Journal of Anaesthesia* **86**: 477–485.

Räsänen J, Downs JB, Malec DJ, *et al.* (1987) Estimation of oxygen utilization by dual oximetry. *Annals of Surgery* **206**: 621–623.

Saura P, Blanch L, Lucangelo U, *et al.* (1996) Use of capnography to detect hypercapnic episodes during weaning from mechanical ventilation. *Intensive Care Medicine* **22**: 374–381.

Shoemaker WC, Vidyasagar D (1981) Physiological and clinical significance of $P_{tc}O_2$ and $P_{tc}CO_2$ measurements. *Critical Care Medicine* **9**: 689–690.

Sirker AA, Rhodes A, Grounds RM, *et al.* (2002) Acid–base physiology: the 'traditional' and the 'modern' approaches. *Anaesthesia* **57**: 348–356.

Staub NC (1986) Clinical use of lung water measurements. Report of a workshop. *Chest* **90**: 588–594.

Stewart PA (1983) Modern quantitative acid–base chemistry. *Canadian Journal of Physiology and Pharmacology* **61**: 1444–1461.

Story DA, Morimatsu H, Bellomo R (2004) Strong ions, weak acids and base excess; a simplified Fencl–Stewart approach to clinical acid–base disorders. *British Journal of Anaesthesia* **92**: 54–60.

Sydow M, Burchardi H, Zinserling J, *et al.* (1991) Improved determination of static compliance by automated single volume steps in ventilated patients. *Intensive Care Medicine* **17**: 108–114.

Takala J, Keinänen O, Väisänen P, *et al.* (1989) Measurement of gas exchange in intensive care: laboratory and clinical validation of a new device. *Critical Care Medicine* **17**: 1041–1047.

Taylor MB, Whitwam JG (1986) The current status of pulse oximetry. *Anaesthesia* **41**: 943–949.

Tobin MJ (1992) Breathing pattern analysis. *Intensive Care Medicine* **18**: 193–201.

Van de Louw A, Cracco C, Cerf C, *et al.* (2001) Accuracy of pulse oximetry in the intensive care unit. *Intensive Care Medicine* **27**: 1606–1613.

Vicenzi MN, Gombotz H, Krenn H, *et al.* (2000) Transesophageal versus surface pulse oximetry in intensive care unit patients. *Critical Care Medicine* **28**: 2268–2270.

Yoshiya I, Shimada Y, Tanaka K (1980) Spectrophotometric monitoring of arterial oxygen saturation in the fingertip. *Medical and Biological Engineering and Computing* **18**: 27–32.

7 Respiratory support

Although orotracheal intubation was first used to facilitate anaesthesia by MacEwen, a Glasgow surgeon, as long ago as 1878, it only became a routine procedure following the work of Magill and others in the 1920s. Using tracheal intubation, anaesthetists were able to control their patient's ventilation and, in the 1940s, neuromuscular blockade with intermittent positive-pressure ventilation (IPPV), usually performed manually, became a standard anaesthetic technique. Nevertheless, mechanical ventilation for therapeutic purposes was initially performed using negative-pressure devices. Not only were morbidity and mortality high with this technique, but it was much less successful in those with abnormal lungs. It was therefore used infrequently except in the treatment of ventilatory failure due to poliomyelitis; when polio became a rare disease, its use declined further. During the polio epidemic in Copenhagen in 1952 the advantages of positive-pressure ventilation had been clearly demonstrated (Lassen, 1953) and in 1955 the use of IPPV for the treatment of acute exacerbations of chronic obstructive pulmonary disease (COPD) was described (Bjorneboe et al., 1955). Subsequently, clinicians increasingly accepted that IPPV could be used to treat patients with a variety of diseases affecting the lung parenchyma, as well as those with neuromuscular weakness.

The various techniques of respiratory support currently available are shown in **Table 7.1**.

NEGATIVE-PRESSURE VENTILATION

TANK VENTILATORS ('iron lungs')

At one time, tank ventilators (**Fig. 7.1**) were widely used for the treatment of ventilatory failure complicating polio. They are still used very occasionally for nocturnal ventilation of patients with chronic respiratory failure due to neuromuscular disease, skeletal deformity or sleep-related respiratory disturbances.

The patient's body is enclosed in an airtight tank within which a negative pressure is created intermittently by a separate pump. During the negative-pressure phase, the patient's thorax expands, drawing air into the lungs. Expiration then occurs passively. Although patients who are conscious can

speak and swallow in time with the ventilator, this technique has a number of disadvantages. Firstly, the ventilator itself is very bulky and access to the patient is restricted, making it difficult to perform nursing and medical procedures. Secondly, the patient's airway is unprotected and there is no route for endotracheal suction. This technique is therefore only suitable for those with competent swallowing, laryngeal and cough reflexes, and even then pulmonary aspiration can be a problem. Lastly, because the negative pressure is applied to the whole body, the normal inspiratory pressure gradient is lost, venous return is reduced and cardiac output may fall.

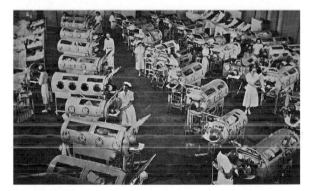

Fig. 7.1 Tank ventilators in use during an epidemic of poliomyelitis.

CUIRASS VENTILATORS

Cuirass ventilators, which encase only the thorax, were originally used most frequently during the recovery phase of poliomyelitis. They are inefficient and difficult to use, a particular problem being the creation of an airtight seal around the lower thorax and abdomen, especially in those with musculoskeletal deformity. Skin chafing may therefore be a problem. Nevertheless, such devices can be useful in those with borderline respiratory function when used to assist ventilation, particularly during sleep. The *Tunnicliffe jacket* and the *pulmowrap* are more efficient alternatives. They incorporate an inner framework of metal or plastic which is covered with an airtight jacket with seals around the neck, arms and thighs.

Table 7.1 Techniques for respiratory support

Negative-pressure ventilation	Tank ventilators Cuirass ventilators
Intermittent positive-pressure ventilation (IPPV)	
Controlled mechanical ventilation (CMV)	ZEEP (NEEP) PEEP (CPPV) IRV Pressure-limited or volume-controlled pressure-limited Low tidal volume (± 'permissive hypercarbia')
Synchronized intermittent mandatory ventilation (SIMV) Mandatory minute volume (MMV) Assist control ventilation (ACV) Pressure support ventilation (PSV) Automatic tube compensation (ATC) Proportional assist ventilation (PAV) Airway pressure release ventilation (APRV) Biphasic positive airway pressure (BiPAP)	
Independent lung ventilation	
High-frequency jet or oscillatory ventilation (HFJV or HFOV)	
Non-invasive respiratory support	Nasal mask Face mask
Continuous positive airway pressure (CPAP)	Endotracheal tube, mask or hood
Extracorporeal techniques	ECMO $ECCO_2$-R

CPPV, continuous positive-pressure ventilation; ECMO, extracorporeal membrane oxygenation; ECCO2-R, extracorporeal CO2 removal; IRV, inverse-ratio ventilation; NEEP, negative end-expiratory pressure; PEEP, positive end-expiratory pressure; ZEEP, zero end-expiratory pressure.

ROCKING BEDS

Rocking beds can be used for those patients with neuromuscular disease whose respiratory reserve is limited, but who only develop significant hypercapnia when they fall asleep. The rocking motion of the bed causes the abdominal contents to push the diaphragm in and out of the thorax, thereby assisting tidal exchange.

Non-invasive ventilation (NIV) via a nasal mask (see below) has now largely replaced the use of these devices in the management of chronic hypercapnic respiratory failure caused by chest wall deformity, neuromuscular disease or impaired central respiratory drive.

EXTERNAL HIGH-FREQUENCY OSCILLATION (EHFO) (Fig. 7.2)

In 1990 Hayek and Schonfeld developed a cuirass device connected to a high-frequency oscillator which oscillates the chest around a variable, subatmospheric pressure. In contrast to negative-pressure devices both inspiratory and expiratory phases are active and as a result respiratory rate is not limited. End-expiratory chamber pressure can be positive, atmospheric or negative so that ventilation can be achieved below, at or above functional residual capacity (FRC). Carbon dioxide elimination increases with increasing minute ventilation up to a frequency of 180 cycles/minute. Oxygenation often improves, sputum clearance is encouraged and

weaning times may be reduced. EHFO has been used in patients with exacerbations of COPD and acute respiratory failure, as well as in combination with conventional mechanical ventilation in patients with acute lung injury/acute respiratory distress syndrome (ALI/ARDS). The role of this technique in the management of respiratory failure remains to be established (Al-Saady et al., 1995).

POSITIVE-PRESSURE VENTILATION

During positive-pressure ventilation pulmonary gas exchange is achieved by intermittently inflating the lungs with a positive pressure applied via an endotracheal tube, a tracheostomy or a tight-fitting mask. As mentioned above, IPPV has a number of important advantages over negative-pressure ventilation. In particular:

- the airway is secured and protected;
- secretions can be aspirated more easily;
- the technique can be used more successfully in those with diseases involving the lung parenchyma;
- access to and movement of the patient is relatively unrestricted.

IPPV has therefore largely superseded the use of negative-pressure devices. More recently there have been a number of

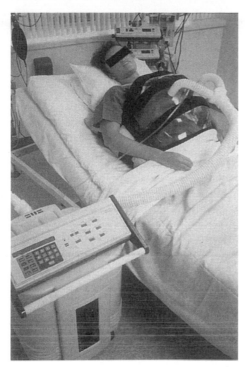

Fig. 7.2 External high-frequency oscillation: chest cuirass, wide-bore hose and power unit. Reproduced from Webb et al 1999 Oxford Textbook of Critical Care, Oxford Medical Publications with permission.

refinements and modifications to the manner in which positive pressure is applied to the airway and in the interplay between the patient's respiratory effort and mechanical assistance. These will be discussed in more detail later in this chapter. They include:

- Modifications to conventional controlled mechanical ventilation (CMV):
  - application of an appropriate level of positive end-expiratory pressure (PEEP);
  - inverse-ratio ventilation (IRV);
  - pressure-limited or volume-controlled, pressure-limited ventilation;
  - low tidal volume (± permissive hypercarbia).
- Techniques in which intermittent mechanical breaths supplement unassisted spontaneous breathing:
  - synchronized intermittent mandatory ventilation (SIMV);
  - mandatory minute volume (MMV).
- Techniques in which every respiratory effort is mechanically supported by the ventilator:
  - assist control ventilation (ACV);
  - pressure support ventilation (PSV);
  - proportional assist ventilation (PAV);
  - automatic tube compensation (ATC).
- Techniques in which alveolar ventilation is achieved by cycling between two levels of positive airway pressure:

- airway pressure release ventilation (APRV);
- biphasic positive airway pressure (BiPAP).
- Hybrid modes, for example:
  - SIMV + PSV or ATC with PEEP.

CLASSIFICATION OF POSITIVE-PRESSURE VENTILATORS

A mechanical ventilator has to perform four operations during each respiratory cycle:

1. Inflate the lungs.
2. Cycle from inspiration to expiration.
3. Allow expiration to take place.
4. Cycle expiration to inspiration.

Mechanical ventilation can therefore be described according to the method used to inflate the lungs (the driving mechanism) and the means by which they change from one phase of the respiratory cycle to the other (cycling).

Pressure-controlled (preset) ventilation

A preset pressure is generated. The magnitude and shape of the set inspiratory pressure waveform produced by the ventilator are therefore uninfluenced by changes in lung mechanics, whereas the pattern of flow during inflation depends on the interaction between the generated pressure pattern and the mechanical properties of the lung and chest wall. Therefore, if pulmonary compliance falls or resistance increases, there will be a reduction in the delivered tidal volume (V_T) unless the operator increases the inflation pressure. Pressure preset ventilation compensates for small leaks in the circuit.

Volume-controlled (preset) ventilation

A fixed V_T is delivered regardless of alterations in lung mechanics; if, for example, the lungs become stiffer, there will be a compensatory increase in inflation pressure and there will be only a small reduction in V_T due to the increased volume of gas compressed within the ventilator circuit. This type of ventilation does not compensate for leaks in the circuit.

Minute volume dividers

Some ventilators can be considered as minute volume dividers. With these devices the minute volume depends on the total flow delivered by the gas source, while the ventilation rate is determined by the preset V_T and inflation pressure. Such ventilators are now obsolete and rarely encountered.

Cycling

The change from inspiration to expiration is usually time-cycled, while inspiration is nearly always time-cycled and/or patient-triggered (by flow or pressure). Ventilation can also be volume-, pressure- or flow-cycled from inspiration to expiration. With volume-cycled ventilation the inspiration:expiration (I:E) ratio is indirectly determined by regulating V_T, frequency and inspiratory flow rate.

SELECTING A SUITABLE MECHANICAL VENTILATOR FOR USE IN THE INTENSIVE CARE UNIT (ICU)

A large number of mechanical ventilators are now available, most of which are complex and extremely expensive. *Cost* and *user-friendliness* are therefore important considerations. There is some advantage in restricting the number of different types of ventilator available on a particular unit since familiarity with the equipment generates confidence and reduces the incidence of mishaps.

The provision of *comprehensive monitoring, a high-pressure relief valve* and *suitable alarms* are fundamental safety requirements. The alarms should be activated in the event of disconnection or obstruction and if the gas or power supply fails, although the ventilator should in any case continue to function in either of these latter eventualities. It should be possible to provide safe, effective *humidification* and to *nebulize* drugs. Some ventilators incorporate *nitric oxide delivery systems* (but see Chapter 8).

It should also be possible to select *optimal patterns of ventilation* for all clinical circumstances and age groups. The ability to adjust the duration of both the inspiratory and expiratory phases, as well as the ratio of one to the other, and the inspiratory flow rate are fundamental requirements.

The ventilator should deliver an accurate stable *inspired oxygen concentration* from 30 to 100%. In addition, it should be possible to *apply PEEP* (see later). Other features that are often incorporated, but are not of proven benefit, include *sigh functions* and a *selection of inspiratory wave-forms*. Ventilators should be *robust, reliable* and *easy to maintain*.

These criteria are adequately fulfilled by most current, microprocessor-controlled, electronic ventilators (**Fig. 7.3**). These devices use analogue-to-digital converters to digitize pressure and flow signals, as well as analogue inputs from the control panel, before they are transmitted to the microprocessor which interprets the information and executes instructions. The digital output from the microprocessor is in turn converted to analogue signals which control the various functions of the mechanical ventilator, including the accurate, high-speed operation of the inspiratory and expiratory valves. Some ventilators use a *servocontrol* system in which the output of the microprocessor is influenced by the input from the monitoring devices. Such systems are designed to minimise differences (errors) between the control panel settings and the quantified output produced by the interaction of the ventilator with the patient.

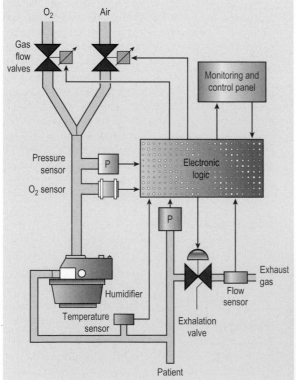

(a)

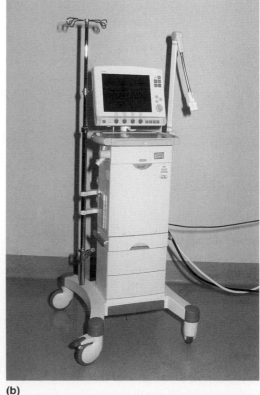

(b)

Fig. 7.3 (a) Schematic illustration of the basic elements of an electronic ventilator. P, pressure. Reproduced from Webb et al 1999 Oxford Textbook of Critical Care, Oxford Medical Publications with permission. (b) An electronic "servocontrol" ventilator.

HUMIDIFICATION

Inspired gas is normally warmed, filtered and moistened during its passage through the upper airways, a process which is prevented by tracheal intubation and tracheostomy. Exposing the lungs and airways to dry cold gas has a number of adverse effects, including:

- loss of heat and moisture;
- an increase in mucus viscosity;
- depressed ciliary activity, destruction of ciliated epithelium;
- obstruction of the airways by tenacious secretions;
- increased risk of infection;
- decreased surfactant production.

Artificial humidification of inspired gases is therefore essential when the upper respiratory tract is bypassed.

Humidifiers should be simple to use and maintain. Their performance should be unaffected by variations in gas flow and they must ensure that gas delivered to the trachea is at a temperature of 32–36°C with a water content of 33–43 g/m^3. The temperature of the humidifier should be constantly controlled at the set value and the humidifier should incorporate alarms and safety mechanisms to prevent overheating, overhydration and electrocution. Ideally humidifiers should be suitable for use during spontaneous as well as controlled ventilation and therefore their dead space, resistance and compliance should all be as low as possible.

Cold-water humidifiers

Cold-water, air and bubble humidifiers are inefficient and there is a risk of bacterial contamination. They are sometimes used to humidify supplemental oxygen administered via a facemask, although many consider that usually humidification is unnecessary under these circumstances.

Heated humidifiers

The fresh gas is passed over or through a water reservoir heated to 45–60°C so that it leaves the humidifier with a water content of more than 43 g/m^3. Although at this stage it is not fully saturated, cooling in the ventilator tubing causes the relative humidity to approach 100%. The heater is thermostatically controlled to ensure that the temperature of the fully saturated inspired gas is close to 37°C. These devices are efficient, but their performance depends on the fresh gas flow, the water temperature and the surface area available for vaporization. They also have the following disadvantages:

- They cause condensation in the ventilator tubing. Water traps are therefore required. Overhydration may occur.
- There is a risk of infection from bacteria, especially *Pseudomonas*, contaminating the water reservoir. They multiply rapidly at 45°C, but infection can be controlled by operating the device at 60°C or by adding 0.02% chlorhexidine gluconate.
- If the thermostat fails and the temperature of the inspired gas exceeds 41°C, damage to the tracheal mucosa is likely. Close observation is therefore essential.

More sophisticated devices are available that include a heating element in the inspiratory limb of the circuit to minimize condensation. A thermometer at the Y-piece controls the temperature of the inspired gas.

Nebulizers

Nebulizers produce an aerosol of variously sized microdroplets suspended in the inspired gas. Droplets smaller than 1 μm are thought to reach the alveoli, those of about 5 μm are deposited in the bronchi and larger particles of 7–10 μm are deposited in the nose or oropharynx.

Ultrasonic nebulizers are the most efficient and can produce supersaturation of inspired gas with the risk of overhydration, especially in children. There is a danger of bacterial contamination and infection with these devices. Sterile water should be used to fill the reservoir and the nebulizer should be replaced and sterilized daily. Nebulizers are now rarely used in clinical practice.

Heat and moisture exchangers (HMEs)

These small, light-weight devices consist of a hydrophobic membrane or contain various hygroscopic materials and chemicals arranged as pleated or corrugated sheets or sponges. When placed in the breathing circuit close to the airway they retain by condensation the heat and moisture in expired gas. Inspired gas is then warmed and humidified as it passes through the filter. These devices provide up to 30 mg H_2O/L of ventilation at 27–30°C and are suitable for most patients undergoing long-term ventilation, although a heated humidifier may be preferred for hypothermic patients, when minute ventilation is ≥10 l/min and for those with viscid secretions. It seems that airway obstruction with inspissated secretions is more likely to occur when hydrophobic HMEs are used at high minute volumes. HMEs also act as efficient bacterial filters, avoiding the need to sterilize breathing systems or decontaminate ventilators, and they offer substantial advantages as regards cost, ease of use and patient safety. In one study the use of an HME was associated with a reduction in bacterial contamination of the breathing circuit when compared to a heated-water device. Humidification was clinically adequate, the resistance to breathing was low and costs were reduced (Boots *et al.*, 1997).

BENEFICIAL EFFECTS OF MECHANICAL VENTILATION

The objectives of mechanical ventilation are primarily to reduce the work of breathing and to reverse life-threatening hypoxaemia or acute progressive respiratory acidosis (Tobin, 2001).

IMPROVED OXYGENATION

The percentage of venous admixture generally falls slightly when mechanical ventilation is instituted, but this effect is variable and therefore usually of only marginal benefit. Indeed, in the absence of PEEP, prolonged mechanical ventilation with small tidal volumes has been associated with an increase in venous admixture and a deterioration in lung function, which in the early days of mechanical ventilation prompted the use of intermittent large tidal volumes or 'sighs' (see later). Because ventilated patients are connected to a leak-free circuit it is possible to administer high concentrations of oxygen (up to 100%) accurately, and to apply PEEP. In selected patients, the latter may reduce shunt and increase arterial oxygen tension (P_aO_2) (see later).

REDUCED WORK OF BREATHING

Importantly, mechanical ventilation can, if applied appropriately, decrease or abolish the work of breathing, relieve exhaustion and rest the respiratory muscles. In those with severe pulmonary parenchymal disease, the lungs may be very stiff and the work of breathing is therefore greatly increased (the inspiratory effort expended by patients with acute respiratory failure is about four times normal and may increase to around six times normal in some cases); institution of mechanical ventilation may then significantly reduce oxygen consumption ($\dot{V}O_2$). This reduction in oxygen requirements may allow mixed venous oxygen tension ($P_{\bar{v}}O_2$), and consequently arterial oxygen tension (P_aO_2), to rise.

IMPROVED CARBON DIOXIDE ELIMINATION

Using mechanical ventilation, the carbon dioxide that accumulates in some patients with respiratory failure can be removed and the arterial carbon dioxide tension (P_aCO_2) returned to within normal limits. Because of the operation of the alveolar air equation (see Chapter 3), the reduction in alveolar carbon dioxide tension (P_ACO_2) inevitably leads to a rise in alveolar oxygen tension (P_AO_2) and improved arterial oxygenation. By adjusting the delivered minute volume, it is possible to compensate for changes in the patient's dead space (V_D) and/or carbon dioxide production. Under certain circumstances, improved distribution of inspired gases may lead to a fall in V_D and further benefit may accrue from abolishing the work of breathing, thereby reducing carbon dioxide production.

INDICATIONS FOR MECHANICAL VENTILATION

RESPIRATORY FAILURE

The commonest indication for mechanical ventilation, accounting for 66% of cases in one series (Esteban *et al.*, 2000), is *acute respiratory failure* due to a variety of causes, including ARDS, pneumonia, cardiac failure, sepsis, the complications of surgery and trauma. Mechanical ventilation may also be indicated in those with *acute exacerbations of COPD* and in respiratory failure due to *neuromuscular disorders*.

PROPHYLACTIC MECHANICAL VENTILATION

Mechanical ventilation can also be used to prevent the development of respiratory failure in susceptible patients. For example, prophylactic *postoperative ventilation* is now a well-established practice in high-risk patients in whom some degree of respiratory failure might otherwise be anticipated. Ventilatory support may also be used prophylactically in patients with *neuromuscular or skeletal abnormalities*. In these patients, a fall in vital capacity (VC) impairs the ability to cough, sigh and take deep breaths; consequently, retention of secretions and progressive alveolar collapse eventually lead to respiratory failure, often in association with secondary infection. This sequence of events can be prevented by instituting respiratory support when the VC has fallen to approximately one-quarter of the predicted value (see Chapter 8).

Mechanical ventilation may also be instituted to prevent deterioration in those with *severe thoracic or upper abdominal injuries*, especially when associated with a *head injury* (see Chapters 10 and 15).

By no means all patients with respiratory failure and/or a reduced VC require ventilation, however, and clinical assessment of each individual case is essential. Factors such as the patient's general condition, degree of exhaustion and level of consciousness are at least as important as blood gas values (see Chapter 8).

RAISED INTRACRANIAL PRESSURE, CEREBRAL ISCHAEMIA, CEREBROVASCULAR ACCIDENT

In patients with intracranial hypertension (e.g. following severe head injury), it is most important to avoid hypercarbia and/or hypoxia, since both will increase intracranial blood volume and exacerbate cerebral oedema. Furthermore, elective hyperventilation, even in those not in respiratory failure, can temporarily decrease cerebral blood flow and, secondarily, intracranial pressure, although the value of such treatment remains uncertain (see Chapter 15). Mechanical ventilation may also be indicated in some patients following an episode of cerebral ischaemia (see Chapter 9 and 15) or a cerebrovascular accident.

DANGERS OF MECHANICAL VENTILATION
(Table 7.2)

GENERAL

Mechanically ventilated patients are exposed to the dangers and complications inherent in *tracheal intubation or tracheostomy* (see later). In addition, *disconnection* from the ventilator and accidental or self-*extubaton* are ever-present dangers. *Failure of gas or power supplies* and *mechanical faults* are unusual, but equally dangerous, and a suitable means of manually ventilating the patient with oxygen must always be available by the bedside.

Table 7.2 Dangers of mechanical ventilation	
General	Tracheal intubation/ tracheostomy
	Disconnection/accidental or self-extubation
	Failure of gas or power supply
	Mechanical faults
Cardiovascular depression	
Respiratory changes and ventilator-associated lung injury	Maldistribution of inspired gases
	Collapse of distal lung units
	Decreased surfactant activity
	Damage to alveolar/capillary membrane
	Barotrauma
	Bronchiolectasis
	Nosocomial pneumonia
Psychological	
Venous thrombosis/embolism	
Ileus	
Hepatic dysfunction	
Water retention	

CARDIOVASCULAR

The application of positive pressure to the lungs and thoracic wall *reduces venous return* and distends alveoli, thereby 'stretching' the pulmonary capillaries and causing a *rise in pulmonary vascular resistance and right ventricular afterload*. Both these mechanisms can produce a *fall in cardiac output* in response to positive-pressure ventilation.

In *normal subjects*, the fall in cardiac output is limited by constriction of capacitance vessels, which restores venous return. *Hypovolaemia, pre-existing pulmonary hypertension, right ventricular failure* and *autonomic dysfunction* (e.g. in Guillain–Barré syndrome, acute spinal cord injury and diabetes) can exacerbate the haemodynamic disturbance. Expansion of the circulating volume, on the other hand, can often restore cardiac output. In some cases, inotropic support is required in addition to volume expansion.

In patients with *cardiac failure*, a paradoxical rise in blood pressure and cardiac output may occur in response to institution of positive-pressure ventilation with or without PEEP. This may be due to reversal of hypoxia and a reduction in $\dot{V}O_2$, both of which will reduce the burden on a failing heart. Moreover, afterload falls as a result of the increased pressure gradient between the intra- and extrathoracic vascular beds and this is associated with an increase in stroke volume. The reduction in afterload and preload reduces ventricular wall tension, allowing increased coronary blood flow and improved myocardial function. Finally, when the ventricular function curve is flat, the reduction in preload has little effect on stroke volume, while stiff lungs limit the transmission of

high inflation pressures to the great veins and pulmonary capillaries. There should therefore be no hesitation in instituting positive-pressure ventilation in patients with cardiogenic pulmonary oedema who have severe respiratory distress and exhaustion (see also Chapter 8).

RESPIRATORY CHANGES AND VENTILATOR-ASSOCIATED LUNG INJURY (Pinhu *et al.*, 2003)

During spontaneous breathing, ventilation is preferentially distributed to the lower lung zones and is matched by a similar pattern of blood flow (see Chapter 3). During positive-pressure ventilation, however, there is *maldistribution of inspired gas*, with ventilation being more evenly distributed throughout the lungs, leading to an increase in the overall V/Q ratio. This effect is enhanced when high intra-alveolar pressure (high inflation pressures, PEEP) and/or a reduced pulmonary artery pressure (PAP) divert blood flow away from apical lung regions. Positive-pressure ventilation therefore normally increases V_D/V_T, but this effect is variable and usually of little clinical significance.

In the early days of IPPV it was soon recognized that patients ventilated with small tidal volumes became progressively more hypoxic, with a reduction in FRC and compliance. This was probably mainly due to *collapse of distal lung units* and could be prevented by using larger tidal volumes (10–15 mL/kg) and reducing the respiratory rate to avoid hypocarbia, or by the application of PEEP. Some ventilators incorporate a 'sigh' mechanism, which regularly hyperinflates the lungs in an attempt to re-expand distal lung segments and prevent hypoxia. The benefits of 'sigh functions' have not, however, been established and they may damage the lung parenchyma (see Chapter 8).

There is evidence that *high airway pressures* (e.g. peak inspiratory pressure, or, more importantly, plateau pressure, which reflects transpulmonary pressure, > 30–35 cm H_2O) may overdistend compliant alveoli in aerated areas of lung, leading to progressive impairment of pulmonary mechanics and lung function associated with reduced surfactant activity and pulmonary oedema. The latter is attributable to an increase in both microvascular permeability and the filtration pressure across the pulmonary vasculature (due to the rise in PAP), especially when the inspiratory phase is prolonged or PEEP is applied. High airway pressures and overdistension may also disrupt the alveolar epithelium, lowering the threshold for alveolar flooding. This damage to the alveolar–capillary membrane seems to be related to both circumferential stress (vascular pressures) and longitudinal stress (lung volume). Large tidal volumes and overdistension (*volutrauma*) are probably more important than high inflation pressures (*barotrauma*). Lung injury may be exacerbated by *shear stress* caused by repeated opening and closure of distal airways if lung volume, which is largely dependent on mean airway pressure and PEEP, is allowed to fall below a critical point. Increased release of inflammatory mediators may contribute to the development of this ventilator-

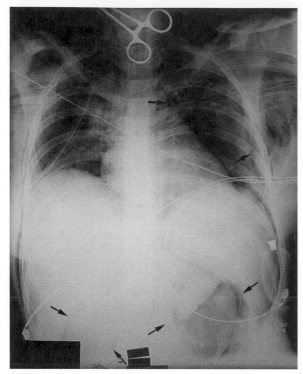

Fig. 7.4 Pulmonary barotrauma. Note subcutaneous air, left pneumothorax, right pleural drain, pneumomediastinum (air outlining aortic arch) and retroperitoneal air outlining left and right kidneys. (Courtesy of Prof. KM Hillman.)

associated lung injury (see Chapter 8). It is important to appreciate that when chest wall compliance is reduced, as can occur in patients with non-pulmonary ARDS, which is often associated with raised intra-abdominal pressure, intrapleural pressures may be higher and plateau inflation pressures of > 35 cm H_2O may not then cause alveolar overdistension.

Barotrauma

Overdistension of the lungs with high airway pressures has also been associated with alveolar rupture, causing air to dissect centrally along the perivascular sheaths. This *pulmonary interstitial air* is difficult to detect, but can sometimes be seen on a good-quality chest radiograph as linear or circular perivascular collections or, most specifically, subpleural blebs (Rohlfing *et al.*, 1976). In some cases, this progresses to produce pneumomediastinum, pneumoperitoneum, air in the retroperitoneal space, subcutaneous emphysema and pneumothorax (when gas under pressure in the pulmonary ligament penetrates the thin visceral pleura or a subpleural bleb ruptures) (**Fig. 7.4**). Each of these may occur in isolation or in combination with any of the others. Pneumomediastinum, pneumoperitoneum and subcutaneous emphysema can all precede the appearance of a pneumothorax and their presence should alert the clinician to an increased risk of this complication. Intra-abdominal air

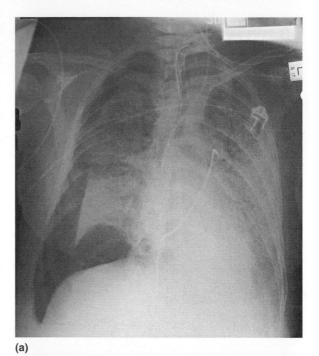

(a)

(b)

Fig. 7.5 (a) and (b) Recurrent pneumothoraces in a patient with acute respiratory distress syndrome receiving high levels of PEEP.

originating in the lungs is probably always associated with pneumomediastinum; this can help distinguish pneumoperitoneum due to barotrauma from a ruptured viscus.

Conventionally the incidence of barotrauma has been related to the use of excessively high inflation pressures and levels of PEEP (**Fig. 7.5**). In one study of patients with sepsis-induced ARDS, however, there were no correlations between high ventilatory pressures or volumes and the development of pneumothorax or other air leaks. Nor was the development of pneumothorax or other air leaks associated with

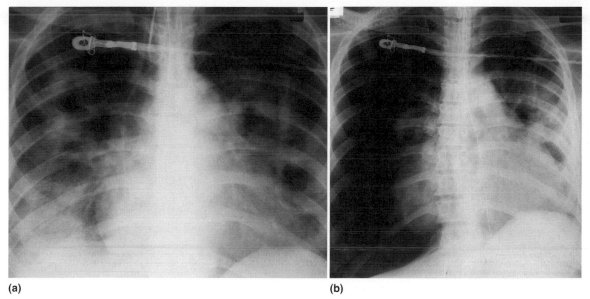

Fig. 7.6 (a) Bilateral consolidation with multiple cavities. (b) The same patient has developed a right tension pneumothorax, displacing the right hemidiaphragm inferiorly and the mediastinum to the left.

increased mortality (Weg *et al.*, 1998). The risk of pneumothorax is increased in those with destructive lung disease (e.g. necrotizing pneumonia, acid aspiration, emphysema), asthma or fractured ribs (**Fig. 7.6**). Barotrauma may also be the result of endotracheal tube obstruction, intubation of a main bronchus or overvigorous manual ventilation.

Pneumothorax

Because a life-threatening *tension pneumothorax* (see **Fig. 7.6**) can develop extremely quickly in mechanically ventilated patients and may be rapidly fatal, facilities for chest drain insertion should be immediately available. Intensive care personnel must always be alert to the possibility of this complication. Suggestive signs include:

- the sudden development or worsening of hypoxia;
- cyanosis;
- fighting the ventilator;
- an unexplained increase in inflation pressure;
- hypotension and tachycardia;
- a rising central venous pressure.

Examination may reveal reduced expansion on one side of the chest, mediastinal shift (deviated trachea, displaced apex beat) and hyperresonance of one hemithorax. Although breath sounds are traditionally diminished over the pneumothorax, this sign can be misleading in ventilated patients. If there is time, the diagnosis can be confirmed by chest radiography.

TREATMENT

In an extreme emergency, the tension can be relieved by inserting a large-bore intravenous cannula anteriorly through the second intercostal space in the mid-clavicular line. Otherwise a chest drain should be inserted.

Some recommend the second or third intercostal space in the mid-clavicular line as the safest site for emergency insertion of chest drains by the inexperienced. Generally, however, it is preferable to place the drain through the sixth or seventh intercostal space in the mid-axillary line. In this position both fluid and air can be removed, and it is cosmetically more acceptable. The drain should not be inserted posteriorly since in this position it is very uncomfortable and easily kinked. If the patient is conscious, the procedure should be explained and, when possible, consent should be obtained. Additional sedation and analgesia may be required.

TECHNIQUE (Fig. 7.7)

- The patient is positioned supine or semirecumbent, with the affected side slightly elevated and the arm flexed over the head.
- The chest wall is prepared and draped as a sterile field; a gown, mask and gloves should be worn if time allows.
- Chest drain insertion can be a very painful procedure and generous amounts of local anaesthetic should be used (20 mL 1% lidocaine).
- A skin incision should be made over the proposed site of insertion.
- A purse string suture should be placed around, and a retaining suture adjacent to this incision.
- The pleural space should be entered using blunt dissection with, for example, a large artery clip close to the top of the rib to avoid the neurovascular bundle on the underside of the rib above.

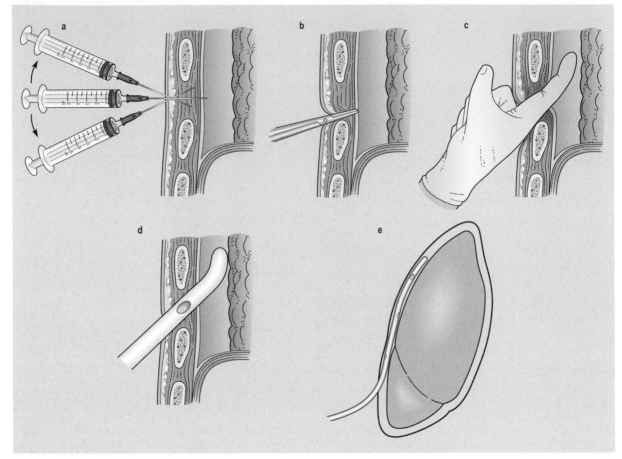

Fig. 7.7 Chest drain insertion. (a) Infiltration of skin, muscle and periosteum of upper border of rib below with local anaesthetic. Pleura may be punctured with needle. (b) Blunt dissection. (c) Digital exploration of pleural cavity. (d) Chest drain, with introducer withdrawn, guided into position. (e) Chest drain correctly positioned.

- The chest drain (with introducer tip withdrawn) is then guided into position with an index finger, which has gently explored the pleural space.
- The chest tube is passed up to the apex of the chest wall to drain a pneumothorax, while the lowest side hole is positioned only 1–2 cm into the chest to drain fluid.
- The drain is then secured with the retaining suture and connected to the underwater seal.
- A sterile dressing is applied and the tubing taped to the skin.
- A chest radiograph is obtained to check the position of the drain and the adequacy of drainage.
- When the drain is removed, the purse string suture is pulled tight to close the wound.

An air leak that persists for more than 24 hours following insertion of a chest drain suggests the development of a *bronchopleural fistula*. This will be associated with loss of minute ventilation and PEEP, as well as failure of lung re-expansion and a risk of pleural infection. Management involves minimizing airway pressures or discontinuing mechanical ventilation as soon as possible. Independent lung ventilation or high-frequency ventilation may be useful (see later). The presence of a persistent bronchopleural fistula is an ominous sign with a high mortality rate.

Bronchiolectasis

Bronchiolectasis is a term that has been applied to the pronounced dilatation of terminal and respiratory bronchioles that has been described in adults who die following a period of positive-pressure ventilation with sustained high levels of PEEP (Slavin *et al.*, 1982). These changes were associated with an increased V_D/V_T ratio. The authors felt that oxygen toxicity was unlikely to be important in the pathogenesis of the lung lesions, and a subsequent study suggests that the changes are reversible in those who survive (Navaratnarajah *et al.*, 1984).

Ventilator-associated pneumonia
(Young and Ridley, 1999)

Ventilator-associated pneumonia (VAP) is a nosocomial infection occurring in patients who have been mechanically ventilated for more than 48 hours. *Early-onset VAP* occurs between 48 and 72 hours after instituting mechanical ventilation and is thought to result mainly from aspiration during the process of tracheal intubation. Risk factors for developing pneumonia within 48 hours of intubation include (Rello *et al.*, 1999a):

- large-volume aspiration;
- sedation;
- intubation following respiratory or cardiac arrest/cardiopulmonary resuscitation;
- Glasgow Coma Scale < 9;

VAP developing beyond 72 hours is considered to be *late-onset*. The reported incidence of VAP varies from around 10% to more than 30%, depending on case-mix and the diagnostic criteria. In one study the incidence of VAP was higher in those with ARDS (36.5%) than in those without ARDS (23%) (Markowicz *et al.*, 2000). VAP is the most prevalent infection in European ICUs and accounts for almost half of all infections acquired in the ICU. The development of VAP prolongs intensive care and hospital stay, increases costs and may independently increase mortality (the mortality directly attributable to VAP has been estimated at 27%). Other investigators, however, have been unable to demonstrate an increase in attributable mortality after controlling for confounding factors (Papazian *et al.*, 1996) and it is likely that many patients die with, rather than because of, VAP. In patients with ARDS, for example, the occurrence of VAP was responsible for a nearly threefold increase in the duration of mechanical ventilation but did not seem to be associated with an increased mortality (Markowicz *et al.*, 2000).

PATHOGENESIS

The development of late-onset VAP is usually a consequence of aspiration of infected secretions from the aerodigestive tract into the distal airway. Whereas in health the oropharynx is colonized by non-pathogenic bacteria and the stomach is sterile, during critical illness the stomach, oropharynx, periodontal areas and sinuses become colonized with pathogenic organisms including aerobic Gram-negative bacteria, *Staphylococcus* spp. and *Pseudomonas* spp. Subsequently infected secretions pooling in the oropharynx and the laryngeal opening leak past the cuff of the tracheal tube and are dispersed distally. The almost invariable presence of a nasogastric tube is thought to predispose patients to gastric reflux and increase the potential for aspiration. Moreover the inner lumen of the tracheal tube rapidly develops a viscous, adhesive layer of accretions containing pathogenic organisms (biofilm), particles of which may be dislodged and propelled deeper into the lungs. Direct inoculation from contaminated respiratory apparatus or the ventilator circuit is an unusual cause of VAP.

The vulnerability of mechanically ventilated patients to the development of nosocomial pneumonia is further increased by compromised defence mechanisms, including impaired cough and decreased mucociliary clearance. Mucosal injury at the level of the tracheal tube cuff and tip (perhaps exacerbated by aspiration of bile and gastric fluid) and damage to the mucosa by suction catheters expose the basement membrane, thereby facilitating bacterial adhesion and colonization. Finally alveolar damage and loss of surfactant further impair lung defences. Recognized risk factors for the development of VAP include:

- mechanically ventilated for > 7 days;
- supine body position (Drakulovic *et al.*, 1999);
- nasogastric tube *in situ*;
- need for reintubation;
- enteral nutrition;
- previous exposure to antibiotics;
- decreased conscious level/excessive sedation;
- smoking;
- acute or chronic respiratory conditions;
- severe burns;
- more seriously ill.

Some studies and meta-analyses have suggested that the use of pH-lowering drugs such as H_2 receptor antagonists as prophylaxis against gastrointestinal haemorrhage predisposes to gastric colonization and hence VAP (Cook *et al.*, 1996). On the other hand a more recent large, multicentre study comparing ranitidine with the surface-active agent sucralfate found no significant differences in VAP rates, length of ICU stay or mortality. There was, however, a trend towards lower VAP rates with sucralfate, although, importantly, clinically significant gastrointestinal bleeding was significantly less common in those treated with ranitidine (1.7% versus 3.8%) (Cook *et al.*, 1998). Surprisingly, in a study of patients with ARDS, those given sucralfate seemed to be at greater risk of developing pulmonary infection (Markowicz *et al.*, 2000), a tendency also seen in one other study (Drakulovic *et al.*, 1999) (see Chapter 11).

DIAGNOSIS

The diagnosis of VAP depends on:

- fever > 38°C, leukocytosis or leucopenia;
- deterioration in gas exchange;
- radiographic appearance of new and persistent infiltrates;
- grossly purulent tracheobronchial secretions.

Unfortunately, these signs lack specificity in critically ill, mechanically ventilated patients. For example, while pulmonary infiltrates are considered essential for the diagnosis of VAP, the cause of such infiltrates is frequently non-infective and histological/microbiological evidence of pneumonia may be found without new and persistent infiltrates on the chest X-ray. Also fever is commonplace and purulent secretions can be caused by tracheobronchitis. Confirmation of the diagnosis therefore depends on positive culture of an appropriate specimen, preferably obtained before the initiation of antibiotic therapy. Straightforward endotracheal aspirates are often contaminated with organisms colonizing the upper airways or inner surface of the tracheal tube and results obtained by non-quantitative culture of such specimens often reflect colonization, rather than invasive infection. Invasive diagnostic techniques such as bronchoscopic bronchoalveolar lavage (BAL), mini-BAL or protected specimen brushing (PSB) and non-bronchoscopic PSB or BAL may, when combined with quantitative culture, increase diagnostic accuracy, reduce antibiotic use and improve outcome (Pittet and Bonten, 2000). There is, however, some evidence that in clinical practice quantitative culture of endotracheal aspirates can be as useful as BAL and PSB for the diagnosis of VAP and as a guide to appropriate antibiotic therapy. In particular, although invasive sampling may prompt alterations in the antibiotic regime, length of ICU stay and mechanical ventilation and mortality may not be reduced by the use of bronchoscopic diagnostic tests (Ruiz et al., 2000; Shorr et al., 2005), not least because of the delay in obtaining the results of BAL (Luna et al., 1997). In one recent study quantitative culture of BAL fluid and non-quantitative culture of endotracheal aspirate were associated with similar clinical outcomes and overall use of antibiotics (Canadian Critical Care Trials Group, 2006). Advantages of endotracheal aspirates when compared with more invasive techniques include simplicity, fewer delays in sampling and therefore more expedient antibiotic therapy, fewer complications (hypoxaemia, bleeding and pneumothorax) and reduced costs (Ruiz et al., 2000). The presence of soluble triggering receptor expressed on myeloid cells in BAL fluid may be useful for establishing the diagnosis of bacterial or fungal pneumonia (Gibot et al., 2004).

TREATMENT (see Chapter 12)

Inappropriate or delayed antibiotic therapy adversely influences prognosis, whereas early administration of appropriate antibiotics seems to reduce the mortality attributable to VAP (Iregui et al., 2002; Luna et al., 1997). The immediate choice of antibiotic depends on whether the VAP is early- or late-onset and is influenced by the results of previous cultures of respiratory specimens and recent antibiotic treatment, as well as the presence of underlying chronic lung disease, neutropenia or immunosuppressive treatment. Early-onset VAP is most likely to be caused by *Staphylococcus aureus*, *Haemophilus influenzae*, *Streptococcus* spp. or *Enterobacteriaceae* spp. and methicillin-resistant *Staphylococcus aureus* (MRSA). Conventionally anaerobic organisms are thought to be an unusual cause of VAP, although colonization of the lower airways by potentially pathogenic anaerobic bacteria is common in intubated patients (Agvald-Öhman et al., 2003). It must be recognized, however, that causative organisms and resistance patterns differ between institutions and antimicrobial prescribing practices should be based on local knowledge (Rello et al., 1999b). Nevertheless, in general, severe early-onset VAP can usually be treated adequately by monotherapy with high doses of a β-lactam/β-lactamase inhibitor combination or a second- or third-generation cephalosporin. Severe late-onset VAP normally requires high-dose combination therapy with an aminoglycoside and antipseudomonal cover with, for example, a quinolone, ceftazidime or piperacillin/tazobactam. If patients have received a cephalosporin in the previous 7–10 days a carbapenem or a quinolone can be prescribed. In those with VAP due to MRSA, initial therapy with linezolid may be more effective than initial vancomycin treatment (Kollef et al., 2004). Following laboratory identification of the pathogen and determination of sensitivities it may be possible to change to narrower-spectrum antibiotic treatment. An 8-day course of antibiotics is likely to be as effective as a 15-day regime (Chastre et al., 2003). Routine prophylactic antibiotics are not recommended.

PREVENTION (Kollef, 1999)

The introduction of a programme to prevent VAP, coordinated by a dedicated individual or group, can improve outcome and reduce costs. In addition to normal infection control measures, such as handwashing and microbiological surveillance, recommended preventive measures include:

- minimize the unnecessary use of antibiotics;
- semirecumbent positioning of the patient to minimize regurgitation of gastric contents and aspiration (Drakulovic et al., 1999);
- avoidance of tracheal intubation by using non-invasive respiratory support (see later in this chapter);
- early removal of tracheal and nasogastric tubes;
- avoidance of accidental extubation/reintubation;
- oropharyngeal decontamination with chlorhexidine (Brun-Buisson, 2007; DeRiso et al., 1996);
- oral rather than nasal intubation (to reduce the risk of sinusitis);
- scheduled drainage of condensate from ventilator circuits;
- maintenance of adequate pressure in the endotracheal tube cuff;
- limit stress ulcer prophylaxis to high-risk patients.

Although early institution of enteral nutrition has been identified as a risk factor for the development of VAP (Ibrahim et al., 2002a), the provision of *adequate nutritional support*, especially via the enteral route, is thought to reduce the incidence of nosocomial infection and improve outcome (see Chapter 11). Enteral nutrition should therefore be administered in a manner that minimizes the risk of colonization of the aerodigestive tract and subsequent aspiration. In particular, gastric overdistension must be avoided, if necessary by using the jejunal route. The use of fine-bore nasogastric tubes does not appear to reduce gastro-oesophageal reflux or microaspiration (Ferrer et al., 1999).

In one study the use of a modified endotracheal tube, with a separate lumen opening above the cuff through which pooled secretions can be aspirated from the subglottic space, reduced the incidence of VAP, although outcome was not improved (Smulders et al., 2002). A recent meta-analysis concluded that subglottic secretion drainage effectively prevents early-onset VAP (Dezfulian et al., 2005). Leakage of fluid past high-volume low-pressure tracheal tube cuffs can be reduced, at least temporarily, by lubrication and the application of PEEP. Interestingly, a new pressure-limited, high-volume low-pressure cuff appears to provide complete protection against aspiration whilst tracheal wall pressure is controlled at 30 cm H_2O; this device requires further evaluation (Young *et al.*, 1999). The use of HMEs with bacteriological filters and regular postural changes may also help to prevent VAP, whereas the value of kinetic beds is uncertain and chest physiotherapy is probably ineffective as a preventive measure. Frequent (e.g. every 2 days) changing of the ventilator circuit may actually increase the risk of VAP and closed suctioning systems appear to be ineffective in this regard (Lorente *et al.*, 2005). Oral decontamination with topical antibiotics alone can reduce the incidence of VAP (Bergmans *et al.*, 2001) but the role of selective decontamination of the digestive tract remains controversial and is considered in more detail in Chapter 12.

GASTROINTESTINAL

Initially, many mechanically ventilated patients will develop an *ileus* and abdominal distension. The cause is unknown, although electrolyte disturbances and the administration of opiates may be partly responsible.

HEPATIC DYSFUNCTION

Hepatic dysfunction is usually related to the underlying disease, but the reduction in splanchnic flow associated with positive pressure ventilation, combined with the effects of raised intra-abdominal pressure on portal vein pressure, hepatic venous flow and biliary drainage, may contribute to liver impairment.

WATER RETENTION

Positive-pressure ventilation, particularly with PEEP, is associated with a reduction in renal blood flow, glomerular filtration rate, urinary output and sodium excretion. These changes are probably largely related to the reduction in cardiac output and systemic blood pressure combined with increased sympathetic activity and renin release (Payen *et al.*, 1987). Restoration of renal blood flow by enhancing venous return does not, however, abolish the reduction in urine volume and natriuresis (Farge *et al.*, 1995), suggesting that other mechanisms may be involved. The role of increased antidiuretic hormone levels and decreased release of atrial natriuretic peptide in ventilation-induced salt and water retention is unclear (Leithner *et al.*, 1987; Payen *et al.*, 1987; Teba *et al.*, 1990). For reasons outlined above, this fluid retention is often particularly noticeable in the lungs, and may cause a deterioration in pulmonary function (see Chapter 11 for discussion of fluid and electrolyte management).

PSYCHOLOGICAL SEQUELAE (see Chapter 11)

Mechanically ventilated patients are subjected to a wide variety of stressful experiences, including pain, fear, anxiety, lack of sleep, inability to speak/communicate, loss of control, nightmares and loneliness. Stressful experiences associated with the presence of the endotracheal tube seem to be strongly associated with spells of terror, feeling nervous when left alone and poor sleep patterns (Rotondi *et al.*, 2002). Measures to reduce stressful experiences, such as

adequate analgesia/sedation, communication and reassurance, are an important aspect of managing mechanically ventilated patients.

DEEP-VEIN THROMBOSIS (DVT) (see Chapter 11)

DVT is common in patients undergoing mechanical ventilation (24% in one series) despite the use of conventional prophylactic measures (Ibrahim *et al.*, 2002b).

INSTITUTION OF INVASIVE RESPIRATORY SUPPORT

Intubating patients in severe respiratory failure is hazardous and should only be performed by experienced staff. The patient is usually hypoxic and may be hypercarbic, with increased sympathetic activity; the oxygen mask has to be removed to allow intubation, although nasal cannulae can be left *in situ*. Under these circumstances, the stimulus of laryngoscopy followed by intubation can precipitate dangerous arrhythmias and even cardiac arrest. When only inexperienced staff are present and respiratory arrest is thought to be imminent, bag-mask ventilation is usually the safest option. An alternative is insertion of a laryngeal mask airway.

Except in an extreme emergency, therefore, the *electrocardiogram (ECG) and oxygen saturation should be monitored throughout*. When available, *capnography* can confirm tracheal intubation. *Resuscitation drugs* should be immediately available. Many patients are hypotensive and most are hypovolaemic. If time allows, the *circulating volume should be optimized* and, if necessary, *inotropes* commenced before attempting intubation. In some cases it may be appropriate to establish *intra-arterial and central venous pressure monitoring* before instituting mechanical ventilation, although many patients will not tolerate the supine or head-down position for central venous cannulation.

The patient should be *preoxygenated* or *ventilated* with added *oxygen* using a facemask and a self-inflating bag before laryngoscopy. In some deeply comatose patients, no sedation will be required, although when there is a possibility of intracranial hypertension, an *intravenous anaesthetic agent* should be administered to prevent surges in intracranial pressure. In the majority of patients, a short-acting intravenous anaesthetic agent followed by *muscle relaxation* will be necessary. In those at risk of regurgitation and aspiration of stomach contents, preoxygenation should be followed by administration of an intravenous anaesthetic agent and a rapidly acting muscle relaxant (e.g. suxamethonium or a rapidly acting non-depolarizing agent such as rocuronium) (see also Chapter 11). *Cricoid pressure* should be applied as soon as the patient loses consciousness and should not be released until the endotracheal tube is in place with the cuff inflated. It must be remembered that there is a considerable risk of precipitating dangerous hyperkalaemia when suxamethonium is used in those with burns, renal failure, spinal cord injury, prolonged immobility or neuromuscular disease, including critical illness polyneuropathy. Indeed some believe that in view of the risk of extreme bradycardia and cardiac arrest, suxamethonium has no place in the management of critically ill patients. Some institutions favour *awake intubation*, although this practice is very unusual in the UK.

Following tracheal intubation, it is important to avoid the temptation to hyperventilate the patient, since this can lead to dynamic hyperinflation of the lungs and a fall in cardiac output, particularly in those with airway obstruction.

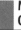 ## MANAGEMENT OF PATIENTS ON VENTILATORS

GENERAL
Because the upper respiratory tract has been bypassed, the inspired gases must be artificially warmed, humidified and filtered (see above). Patients on ventilators are unable to cough effectively, sigh or take deep breaths and therefore regular physiotherapy, manual hyperinflation of the lungs and endotracheal suction are normally employed. (For further discussion of the general aspects of managing these patients, see Chapters 8 and 11.)

SETTLING THE PATIENT ON THE VENTILATOR
It is important that patients who require CMV do not 'fight the ventilator'. Not only does this increase VO_2 and carbon dioxide production, but the rise in mean intrathoracic pressure can reduce cardiac output. It is also distressing for the patient, relatives and staff.

Frequent explanation, reassurance and encouragement are essential for all alert patients. Manual hyperventilation with 100% oxygen will often assist initial synchronization with the ventilator by ensuring adequate oxygenation and a degree of hypocarbia. Most ventilated patients will require sedation. In the majority, the drug of first choice is a *parenteral narcotic*, which also provides analgesia and some respiratory depression. Many patients will also need an anxiolytic agent and usually a *benzodiazepine* is administered in combination with the opiate. For short-term sedation *propofol* may be preferred (see Chapter 11). In most cases – provided the P_aO_2 is within normal limits, there is moderate hypocarbia and sedation/analgesia is adequate – the patient will not fight the ventilator.

Causes of persistent failure to synchronize with the ventilator include:

- hypoxia/hypercarbia;
- obstructed ventilation;
- severe pulmonary parenchymal disease (e.g. ARDS);
- bladder or abdominal distension;
- metabolic acidosis;
- raised intracranial pressure.

If specific treatment is not possible, heavy sedation with opiates and benzodiazepines, and occasionally *muscle relaxation*, may be required. Muscle relaxants should, however,

only be used as a last resort, or in certain special situations (e.g. in those with severe hypoxia or life-threatening airway obstruction). In patients with ARDS the administration of neuromuscular-blocking agents has been associated with sustained improvements in oxygenation (Gainnier *et al.*, 2004). The administration of muscle relaxants must always be accompanied by adequate sedation and analgesia to avoid the situation of a patient who is aware and possibly in pain, but unable to move.

Clearly, bolus administration of sedatives and analgesics will produce wide fluctuations in conscious level and often precipitates hypotension. *Continuous infusions of intravenous anaesthetic agents* such as propofol, or a benzodiazepine such as midazolam, usually combined with opiates, are therefore preferred to provide a consistent level of sedation and analgesia (see Chapter 11). It is, however, questionable whether it is desirable to anaesthetize ventilated patients for long periods, except in certain specific situations such as traumatic coma. In addition, by using the newer, spontaneous or assisted modes of respiratory support, perhaps combined with early tracheostomy (see later), the requirements for sedatives can be dramatically reduced and the need for muscle relaxants can be obviated.

SELECTING THE PATTERN OF VENTILATION
The aim is to achieve optimal gas exchange while minimizing the adverse effects of positive-pressure ventilation on haemodynamics, the respiratory system and vital organ function.

IPPV with negative end-expiratory pressure (NEEP)
To minimize the fall in cardiac output that occurs with IPPV, it was at one time suggested that the application of NEEP might increase venous return and restore cardiac output. Although this is in fact the case, NEEP is no longer used because it also causes progressive alveolar collapse.

IPPV with zero end-expiratory pressure (ZEEP)
As discussed above, IPPV alone may improve oxygenation by re-expanding collapsed alveoli and reducing oxygen requirements. To prevent progressive alveolar collapse, tidal volumes of 10–12 mL/kg have conventionally been used in those without serious lung pathology and who are not at risk for acute lung injury/ARDS (see above). It may, however, be prudent to limit tidal volumes and avoid overdistension and high airway pressures in all mechanically ventilated patients since potentially injurious ventilator settings have been implicated in the subsequent development of ARDS (Gajic *et al.*, 2005). The length of the *inspiratory phase* should be sufficient to allow filling of all distal lung segments. Since an alveolus will be 95% filled in three time constants (i.e. on average within 1.8 seconds in a normal lung), inspiration is normally timed to last for 1.5–2.0 seconds (see Chapter 3). In order to minimize the fall in cardiac output, the *expiratory phase* should be at least twice as long as inspiration (I : E ratio of 1 : 2). In those with severe lung disease, however, there is

an increased 'scatter' of time constants and it may therefore be beneficial to prolong the inspiratory phase further (see below). In some cases, *extending inspiration* so that the I:E ratio is reversed, sometimes to as much as 4:1, can improve gas distribution, recruit or stabilize alveoli and increase P_aO_2. The obvious danger of reversing the I:E ratio is that it could lead to gas trapping with 'auto-PEEP' and severe cardiovascular depression; in this respect the same considerations apply as during continuous positive-pressure ventilation (CPPV: see below). In addition, this 'inverse ratio ventilation' is uncomfortable and the use of heavy sedation and even paralysis is often necessary.

The influence of the *shape of the inspiratory waveform* on the efficiency of gas exchange is less certain and probably of little clinical relevance (**Fig. 7.8**). A decelerating inspiratory flow waveform is produced when a constant pressure is applied to the airway. This pattern of ventilation may lower airway resistance and peak pressure, as well as producing optimal distribution of inspired gas and improving oxygenation (Al-Saady and Bennett, 1985). It is also thought to be the most effective pattern for re-expanding collapsed lung. Mean intrathoracic pressure is, however, highest with this 'square-wave' pattern of positive-pressure ventilation and it therefore causes the greatest reduction in cardiac output. In contrast, the pressure wave required to produce a constant flow pattern is associated with a relatively low mean intrathoracic pressure and minimal cardiovascular depression. An accelerating flow pattern appears to offer little clinical advantage and may increase V_D.

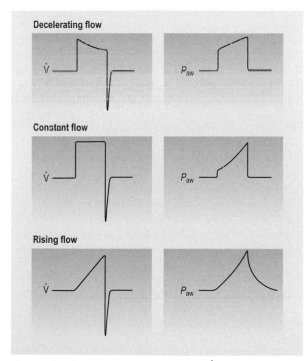

Decelerating flow

Constant flow

Rising flow

Fig. 7.8 Inspiratory waveforms (see text). $\dot{V}$, flow; P_{aw}, airway pressure.

IPPV with PEEP (also referred to as continuous positive-pressure ventilation)

Traditionally the application of PEEP was only considered if it proved impossible to achieve adequate oxygenation of arterial blood (e.g. > 90% saturation of haemoglobin with oxygen) without raising the F_IO_2 to potentially dangerous levels (conventionally, $F_IO_2 > 0.5$) and CPPV was therefore confined to those with severe acute respiratory failure. Now, however, many consider a low level of PEEP to be physiological in intubated patients and low to moderate levels of PEEP are frequently used in those with basal atelectasis, for example postoperatively, and in selected cases with airflow obstruction (see later and Chapter 8), even in the absence of severe hypoxaemia. Although at one time it was suggested that the early or prophylactic use of PEEP in those at risk of developing ARDS could decrease the incidence and severity of subsequent pulmonary complications, a later controlled study demonstrated that the early application of PEEP had no effect on the incidence of ARDS or other associated complications (Pepe *et al.*, 1984).

The rational use of PEEP is based on a knowledge of its physiological effects and of the pathophysiology of the patient's pulmonary disease.

RESPIRATORY EFFECTS OF PEEP

The application of PEEP expands underventilated lung units and *increases FRC*. Provided that shunting is due to alveolar collapse, this will *reduce venous admixture* and improve arterial oxygenation (Ashbaugh and Petty, 1973). It has been suggested that the improvement in oxygenation with PEEP may also be partly related to an increase in the alveolar surface available for gas exchange caused by distension of lung units which were already open. Provided the rise in arterial oxygen content (C_aO_2) is not offset by a fall in cardiac output (see below), oxygen delivery (DO_2) also improves. In general, the worse the shunt, the greater the response to PEEP, while patients with pulmonary causes of ARDS, such as pneumonia, are less responsive to PEEP than those with non-pulmonary ARDS. The effect of PEEP on *lung water* remains uncertain. Theoretically, the rise in PAP which can be caused by the application of PEEP might be expected to enhance oedema formation by increasing filtration pressure across the pulmonary vasculature, and alveolar overdistension is associated with an increase in alveolar–capillary permeability. On the other hand, moderate levels of PEEP may protect the lung from ventilator-induced lung damage (Dreyfuss *et al.*, 1988), perhaps by preventing collapse of distal airways during expiration and thereby avoiding high shear stresses when they reopen during inspiration (see earlier in this chapter and Chapter 8). Moreover, there is some evidence that in hydrostatic pulmonary oedema PEEP may limit the increase in extravascular lung water and increase lymphatic drainage (Fernandez Mondéjar *et al.*, 1996), thereby maintaining the blood–gas interface. In some cases, the application of excessive PEEP may be associated with overdistension of non-dependent regions, with an *increase in alveolar dead space.* This effect may be exacerbated by PEEP-induced decreases in cardiac output.

HAEMODYNAMIC EFFECTS OF PEEP

The inevitable rise in mean intrathoracic pressure that follows the application of PEEP may further *reduce venous return and increase pulmonary vascular resistance* and therefore *reduce cardiac output* (Ashbaugh and Petty, 1973; Qvist *et al.*, 1975). This effect may be proportional to lung compliance (i.e. the stiffer the lungs, the less the fall in cardiac output). At levels of PEEP higher than about 10 cm H_2O the rise in pulmonary vascular resistance and therefore right ventricular afterload may be associated with *dilatation of the right ventricle.* Because lateral expansion is restricted by the pericardium, the interventricular septum is displaced and encroaches on the left ventricular cavity. This is thought to restrict left ventricular filling and reduce stroke volume, despite a slight increase in myocardial contractility (Jardin *et al.*, 1981). Left ventricular volume may be further limited as a result of compression by the distended lungs.

The fall in cardiac output can usually be ameliorated by *volume loading* (Qvist *et al.*, 1975), although in some cases *inotropic support* may be required. As mentioned above, CPPV is often beneficial in patients with cardiac failure and low cardiac output since the reduction in preload and afterload can decrease ventricular wall tension, improve the balance between myocardial oxygen supply and demand, and increase stroke volume.

Although arterial oxygenation is often improved by the application of PEEP, a simultaneous fall in cardiac output can lead to a reduction in DO_2. This reduction in cardiac output is associated with a redistribution of blood flow to vital organs such as the brain, heart and kidneys, which may precipitate ischaemia of other organs such as stomach, pancreas and liver. In one study, CPPV produced a *fall in hepatic flow*, which was related to the level of PEEP and proportional to the reduction in cardiac output; hepatic DO_2 fell to an even greater extent, mainly due to a decrease in portal venous oxygen content (Sha *et al.*, 1987). Although total renal blood flow is preserved, oliguria with salt and water retention is often observed and may be due to *intrarenal redistribution of blood flow* exacerbated by increased sympathetic activity and renin release. The application of PEEP may also be associated with reductions in bronchial blood flow (Baile *et al.*, 1984), and this may limit the delivery of oxygen and nutrients to the lung parenchyma.

CLINICAL IMPLICATIONS

The net effect of PEEP in an individual patient is therefore unpredictable and dependent on a balance of many factors, including the extent of any reduction in FRC, the severity of the shunt and the nature of the pulmonary lesion, as well as cardiovascular performance, in particular left ventricular preload and right ventricular function (Schulman *et al.*, 1988). Although it is clear that patients with ARDS are likely to benefit from the judicious application of PEEP (see Chapter 8), it is usually of limited value in those with fibrotic lung disease and is potentially dangerous in those with emphysema, asthma or COPD. There is now evidence, however, that low levels of PEEP may reduce expiratory resistance and the work of breathing in patients with severe airflow obstruction, without substantially increasing the hazards of hyperinflation (Smith and Marini, 1988; Sydow *et al.*, 1995) (see Chapter 8). In patients with clearly localized areas of diseased lung (e.g. lobar pneumonia, unilateral aspiration pneumonia), high levels of PEEP may adversely affect oxygenation by overexpanding normal lung tissue and diverting blood to underventilated lung units. On the other hand, the use of low-level PEEP (e.g. 5–10 cm H_2O) is an extremely effective and safe means of improving oxygenation in hypoxic postoperative patients with basal atelectasis and many believe that the vast majority of mechanically ventilated patients benefit from the application of a 'physiological' level of about 5 cm H_2O PEEP. In most cases the adverse effects of PEEP can be minimized by using an appropriate V_T and limiting inspiratory airway pressures (see Chapter 8). Temporary removal of PEEP should be avoided if possible since P_aO_2 falls almost immediately, while following its reapplication arterial oxygenation may take up to 60 minutes to return to previous levels.

Thus it is important to select a level of PEEP which produces the greatest improvement in oxygenation and prevents cyclical opening and closing of alveoli, whilst avoiding overdistension of open lung units and haemodynamic compromise (see Chapter 8). In difficult cases pulmonary artery catheterization may be considered, although it seems that the use of this form of invasive monitoring may not influence outcome (see Chapters 4 and 8). Oesophageal Doppler ultrasonography may be a satisfactory non-invasive technique for optimizing PEEP (Singer and Bennett, 1989) and one study has suggested that in ventilated patients with acute lung injury respiratory changes in arterial pulse pressure may be useful in predicting and assessing the haemodynamic effects of PEEP and fluid loading (Michard *et al.*, 1999).

Mechanical ventilation with low tidal volumes
(see also Chapter 8)

With *low-volume pressure-limited* ventilation a constant preset inspiratory pressure is delivered for a prescribed time, generating low tidal and minute volumes and reducing peak inspiratory pressures. When combined with *IRV* and *low levels of PEEP*, this may provide optimal improvement in oxygenation while minimizing peak airway pressures, although mean airway pressure may be unchanged or even increase (Tharratt *et al.*, 1988). An alternative is to use volume-controlled ventilation with low V_T (e.g. 6–8 mL/kg). Both techniques can be used with SIMV. Although respiratory rate can be increased (e.g. up to 30 breaths/min) to limit the rise in P_aCO_2, some degree of hypercarbia is often unavoidable; this is generally well tolerated and can be accepted (*permissive hypercarbia*) (see Chapter 8). Severe hypercapnia can have adverse effects, however, including increased intracranial pressure, decreased myocardial contractility, pulmonary hypertension and decreased renal blood flow. On the other hand there is evidence that 'therapeutic' hypercapnia alone can decrease the severity of ventilator-associated lung injury and protect against ischaemia/reperfusion-induced lung injury (Laffey *et al.*, 2000; Sinclair *et al.*, 2002). The reduction in tidal volume may also lead to a decrease in the volume of aerated lung and a consequent worsening of oxygenation. This loss of lung volume can be minimized by using *sighs* or *recruitment manoeuvres*, although in some circumstances these techniques may exacerbate lung injury as a result of alveolar overdistension (see Chapter 8). The more usual approach is to counteract the decrease in oxygenation by applying a higher level of PEEP, but again there is a danger of overdistending normally aerated lung.

High-frequency ventilation

Surprisingly, it is possible to achieve adequate oxygenation and carbon dioxide elimination by injecting gas into the trachea at rates of between 60 and several thousand breaths per minute with tidal volumes of only 1–5 mL/kg.

HIGH-FREQUENCY JET VENTILATION (HFJV)

Although it is known that adequate oxygenation can be produced by apnoeic diffusion, it is unclear how carbon dioxide elimination is achieved with this technique. Some consider the explanation to be the reduction in V_D that is known to occur as V_T falls (see Chapter 3). Others feel that conventional physiology cannot account for the removal of carbon dioxide, particularly at higher frequencies, and attribute the gas exchange produced with this technique to *augmented or facilitated diffusion and gas dispersion* in more proximal small airways. Cross-ventilation between lung units with different time constants (pendelluft) also contributes to effective gas exchange. Convection is thought to be less important. When compared to conventional ventilation, HFJV results in more uniform distribution of gas throughout the lungs.

During HFJV short pulses of gas are accelerated into the airway through a jet nozzle placed in a T-piece (**Fig. 7.9**). The T-piece provides both a route for expiration and a source of fresh gas entrainment. New devices employ very-rapid-response solenoid valves so that the gas pulse is delivered with a square pressure wave, allowing optimal entrainment and maintenance of mean airway pressure if required. These ventilators operate at frequencies of 60–600 breaths/min. Modern machines also provide continuous analysis of ventilator function and airway pressure profiles as well as safety-monitoring alarms. With HFJV, airway pressure and oxygenation are influenced by inspiratory time and driving pressure. Inspiratory time has little effect on CO_2 clearance, which is most influenced by driving pressure and frequency. Typical settings when ventilating normal lungs would be a frequency of 60–120 breaths/min, a driving pressure of 1–1.5 atm and an inspiratory time of 15–20%. By contrast, in ARDS the frequency might be set at 250–350 breaths/min, the driving pressure to 2–3 atm and the inspiratory time to 36–40%. With these new devices external

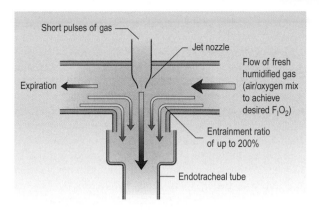

Fig. 7.9 High-frequency jet ventilation.

application of PEEP is usually unnecessary because intrinsic PEEP is an inherent feature of HFJV.

Potential advantages of HFJV are largely related to the low peak airway pressures and possibly a reduction in mean airway pressure, as a consequence of which venous return may be preserved, changes in pulmonary vascular resistance can be minimized and cardiac output may be well maintained. Furthermore, the risk of barotrauma in patients with stiff lungs may be reduced and it is possible that ventilator-associated lung injury is minimized. Also physiotherapy and tracheal suctioning can be performed without disconnection from the ventilator, thereby maintaining lung recruitment at all times. Importantly, permissive hypercapnia may not be necessary during HFJV, a feature which may be particularly advantageous in patients with renal failure, metabolic acidosis, cardiac insufficiency or central neurological disorders. Another possible advantage is that HFJV appears to suppress respiratory drive and unobstructed spontaneous respiration can take place via the T-piece circuit. Many alert patients therefore find this form of mechanical ventilation particularly easy to tolerate, and weaning from ventilatory support can normally be achieved relatively smoothly by gradually reducing driving pressure, frequency and inspiratory time.

Although it is clear that this technique is valuable in the management of patients with large air leaks (e.g. those with bronchopleural fistulae or lung lacerations) who require ventilatory support (Derderian *et al.*, 1982), and may be useful in the management of tracheal laceration (Brimioulle *et al.*, 1990), the place of HFJV in the management of patients with acute respiratory failure is less certain. Early prospective randomized evaluations suggested that neither HFJV nor high-frequency percussive ventilation (Hurst *et al.*, 1990) offers tangible advantages compared to CMV (see also Chapter 8), although newer devices with greater ventilatory capacity may prove to be more effective. In one study such a device produced significant improvements in oxygenation and reductions in peak and mean airway pressures, with excellent CO_2 clearance in patients with severe ARDS (Gluck *et al.*, 1993). Finally it is important to be aware that in patients with airflow limitation HFJV may rapidly precipitate extreme hyperinflation with barotrauma and cardiovascular collapse.

HIGH-FREQUENCY OSCILLATION (HFO)

With HFO there is no bulk flow of gas; rather gas oscillates to and fro at rates of 60–3000 cycles/min with a V_T of 1–3 mL/kg. Both inspiration and expiration are actively controlled with a sine-wave pump. The mechanism of gas exchange with HFO is still not clearly defined, but is probably largely related to *augmented dispersion*. Lung volume is well maintained. Experience with this technique in adults is limited, although in one study in severe ARDS oxygenation was improved by HFO, without compromising DO_2 (Fort *et al.*, 1997), and a recent prospective trial suggested that HFO might be a safe and effective intervention for severely hypoxaemic patients with ARDS (see Chapter 8).

HIGH-FREQUENCY POSITIVE-PRESSURE VENTILATION (HFPPV)

Gas from a high-pressure source is delivered via an endotracheal tube at a frequency of around 60–120 breaths/min with a V_T of approximately 3–5 mL/kg and an I : E ratio less than 0.3. This technique is mainly used during laryngoscopy and bronchoscopy with a narrow-bore endotracheal tube, but may have advantages in patients with non-compliant lungs.

High-frequency ventilation has yet to find an established role in adult intensive care practice but enthusiasts believe that wider availability of the new technology, combined with a better understanding of the principles underlying the effective use of the technique, will lead to an increase in the use of HFJV over the next few years.

Independent lung ventilation

Occasionally, a patient with predominantly unilateral lung disease (e.g. following aspiration of gastric contents) will require positive-pressure ventilation. Under these circumstances, conventionally delivered respiratory support may fail to achieve satisfactory gas exchange. The normal compliant lung tends to become overinflated, while the stiff, diseased lung collapses progressively, causing further mechanical deterioration. Furthermore, pulmonary blood flow is diverted away from normal alveoli to underventilated areas of lung and shunt is increased. The application of PEEP in an attempt to re-expand the diseased lung may simply exacerbate the situation. Finally, the 'good' lung is exposed to the high concentrations of oxygen required to combat hypoxia, as well as high airway pressures and overdistension, and as a result may itself be damaged.

In such cases, it is possible to ventilate each lung independently, using separate ventilators, through a double-lumen endotracheal tube (**Fig. 7.10**). The diseased lung can then be ventilated using higher inflation pressures, an increased F_1O_2 and, if indicated, PEEP or a reversed I : E ratio. The good lung is ventilated conventionally and is therefore protected from the adverse effects of exposure to high airway pressures and potentially toxic concentrations of oxygen.

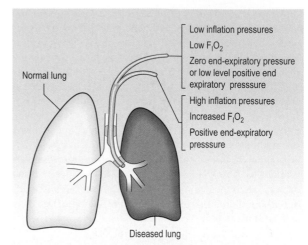

Fig. 7.10 Independent lung ventilation.

Initially, it was thought that to avoid marked reductions in cardiac output, both lungs should inflate and deflate synchronously. It is possible to achieve this by linking two ventilators electronically, but it is not, in fact, necessary to do so (Hillman and Barber, 1980). Numerous variations of the technique have been described, including the application of continuous positive airway pressure (CPAP: see below) or HFJV (see above) to the diseased lung.

Spontaneous modes of respiratory support

The potential advantages of maintaining spontaneous breathing during mechanical respiratory support include:

- improved distribution of inspired gases with reductions in V/Q mismatch and improved oxygenation (Putensen *et al.*, 1999);
- avoidance of the progressive deterioration in gas exchange seen with CMV;
- work of breathing can be reduced by CPAP, PSV and ATC (see below);
- reduction in cardiovascular side-effects with increases in cardiac index and DO_2 (Putensen *et al.*, 2001);
- avoidance of the need to suppress or abolish spontaneous breathing by heavy sedation, muscle relaxation and hyperventilation (Putensen *et al.*, 2001);
- preservation of respiratory muscle function.

Moreover, when compared to an initial period of CMV for 72 hours followed by weaning, maintenance of spontaneous breathing with APRV throughout is associated with significantly fewer days of mechanical ventilation, and a shorter length of ICU stay (Putensen *et al.*, 2001).

The optimal balance between preservation of some inspiratory effort to prevent muscle wasting and reducing the work of breathing to prevent respiratory muscle fatigue has not yet been determined. Significant reductions in inspiratory effort are only achieved when the ventilator cycles are in unison with the patient's central respiratory rhythm. Difficulties with synchronization can arise at the onset of inspiratory effort, at the onset of flow delivery by the ventilator, during the period of ventilator-induced inflation and at the switch between inspiration and expiration (Tobin, 2001). With these assisted modes of mechanical ventilation the patient's own respiratory effort triggers the ventilator, usually at a threshold for airway pressure selected by the clinician (set sensitivity) of -1 to -2 cm H_2O. Because inspiratory neurones do not switch off once the threshold is reached, the patient may expend considerable respiratory effort throughout the machine-assisted inflation. Moreover at high levels of mechanical assistance, up to one-third of a patient's inspiratory efforts may fail to trigger an assisted inflation, adding an additional burden to the already stressed respiratory muscles (Tobin, 2001).

Assisted mechanical ventilation (AMV)

Also known as *ACV*, this technique, in which the patient's own respiratory efforts trigger the delivery of a set tidal volume, is widely used in some centres, particularly in North America, as an alternative to CMV. Using ACV, it is not necessary to abolish the patient's respiratory efforts, and the use of heavy sedation and paralysis can often be avoided. If a spontaneous respiratory effort does not occur within a preset period, the ventilator will deliver an untriggered V_T. Hyperventilation is common with this technique, and the work of breathing can be considerable.

Intermittent mandatory ventilation (IMV)

Originally introduced as a technique for weaning patients from mechanical ventilation (Downs *et al.*, 1973), IMV is now frequently used in preference to conventional IPPV (either CMV or ACV). IMV allows the patient to breathe spontaneously between the mandatory tidal volumes delivered by the ventilator. It is important that the mandatory breaths are timed to coincide with the patient's own inspiratory effort (SIMV), and IMV can be used with or without PEEP/CPAP and PSV (see below).

When used to wean patients from mechanical ventilation, the frequency of the mandatory breaths is progressively reduced so that spontaneous respiration accounts for an increasing proportion of the total minute volume (see later).

A disadvantage of IMV is that increased ventilatory demand does not automatically lead to an increase in the level of mechanical support. Also patients often find it difficult to adjust to the intermittent nature of the mandatory breaths and the extent of the reduction in the work of breathing may be less than optimal. Clearly as the respiratory rate is increased, the opportunity for spontaneous breaths diminishes. Lastly the potential advantages of IMV are less clear when compared with AMV/ACV rather than CMV.

Mandatory minute volume (Hewlett et al., 1977)

This modification of IMV ensures that the patient always receives the preset minute volume despite moment-to-moment variations in the level of spontaneous ventilation.

Although MMV is inherently safer than SIMV, it is rarely used in clinical practice.

Pressure support ventilation (Brochard et al., 1987)

With this technique spontaneous breaths are augmented by a constant preset positive pressure (usually between 5 and 20 cm H_2O) triggered by the patient's spontaneous inspiratory effort and applied for a given fraction of inspiratory time or until inspiratory flow decreases below a specified level (e.g. to 25% of the peak flow). Respiratory frequency, inspiratory time and inspiratory flow rate are controlled by the patient, while V_T is determined by the level of PSV, patient effort and lung mechanics. Patients may find this form of respiratory support particularly easy to tolerate, although patients with COPD, in whom gas flow is restricted, may begin to exhale before ventilator-assisted inflation has ceased and volunteers appear to find ATC more comfortable than PSV (see below). PSV can reduce the work of breathing, in part by counteracting the load imposed by the endotracheal tube and ventilator circuit. The level of pressure support is usually adjusted according to the patient's respiratory rate, although the respiratory frequency which indicates a satisfactory degree of muscle rest has not been clearly defined and recommendations range from 16 to 30 breaths/ min. An excessive level of PSV, on the other hand, risks pulmonary hyperinflation and barotrauma. Another important consequence of excessive pressure assistance is the appearance of ineffective muscle contraction, probably largely as a consequence of hyperinflation and high levels of intrinsic PEEP.

PSV can be used with SIMV and, by gradually reducing the level of pressure support, for weaning (see later in this chapter).

Proportional assist ventilation

During PAV the inspiratory support pressure is dynamically adjusted in linear proportion to the patient's inspiratory efforts. Increased ventilatory demand can be met by an increase in tidal volume, whereas during PSV patients may have to increase their respiratory rate (Ranieri *et al.*, 1996). This method of ventilatory support is rarely used in the UK.

Automatic tube compensation

To compensate for the resistance imposed by the endotracheal tube the ventilator automatically increases the airway pressure during inspiration and reduces airway pressure during expiration, the intention being to maintain a constant pressure at the distal end of the tube throughout the respiratory cycle. ATC may compensate for the resistance of the endotracheal tube more effectively than PSV (Fabry *et al.*, 1997). ATC may also be more comfortable than PSV, perhaps because lung overinflation is avoided (Guttmann *et al.*, 1997). The role of ATC in clinical practice is not yet established.

Airway pressure release ventilation, biphasic positive airway pressure

Alveolar ventilation is achieved by the time-cycled switching between two levels of CPAP. Inspiratory and expiratory pressure levels and times are set independently and unhindered spontaneous breathing is possible in any phase of the mechanical ventilatory cycle. APRV as originally described employs very high I:E ratios with a short expiratory time. With BiPAP the I:E ratio and flow rates can be varied over a wide range. BiPAP can also be patient-triggered. Changes in ventilatory demand do not result in alterations in the level of mechanical support. Peak airway pressures are minimized and theoretically the risk of barotrauma is reduced. BiPAP is now widely used, especially during NIV (see below).

Continuous positive airway pressure
CARDIORESPIRATORY EFFECTS OF CPAP

CPAP achieves for the spontaneously breathing patient what PEEP does for the ventilated patient. Not only can it *improve oxygenation* by the same mechanism, but *lung mechanics improve, breathing becomes easier, respiratory rate falls, V_T increases* and both *VC* and *inspiratory force* have been shown to improve (Feeley *et al.*, 1975; Katz and Marks, 1985; Venus *et al.*, 1979).

The cause of the increased compliance can be appreciated by referring to **Figure 3.23** (Chapter 3), which shows the compliance curve for the lung and chest wall combined. Normally, tidal exchange takes place from the resting expiratory position at which the propensity for the lungs to collapse is exactly counterbalanced by the tendency of the chest wall to expand. It can be seen that this is also the steepest point on the curve, where relatively small changes in pressure produce a large change in volume (i.e. compliance is greatest and the work of breathing least). As lung volume falls, however, the curve becomes flatter (i.e. the lungs become stiffer and the work of breathing increases). The application of positive airway pressure re-expands the lungs and compliance increases. If the lungs are overexpanded, however, compliance will again fall.

Because mean intrathoracic pressure is lower with CPAP than with IPPV plus PEEP, cardiovascular depression is minimized (Simonneau *et al.*, 1982; Venus *et al.*, 1979), renal perfusion is maintained and the incidence of barotrauma may be reduced. Furthermore, heavy sedation is unnecessary. A circuit suitable for applying CPAP is shown in **Figure 7.11a**.

CLINICAL USE OF CPAP

CPAP can be used as the primary treatment in patients with acute hypoxaemic respiratory failure who are not exhausted and in whom alveolar ventilation is adequate (Venus *et al.*, 1979). The use of a *tight-fitting facemask* (**Fig 7.11b**) allows the application of CPAP without the need for tracheal intubation or tracheostomy (Greenbaum *et al.*, 1976). This technique has been used extensively in the belief that clinical deterioration might be prevented, tracheal intubation could be avoided and outcome might be improved. This approach is supported by a study in which mask CPAP was shown to produce early physiological improvement as well as to reduce the need for intubation and mechanical ventilation in patients with severe hypercapnic cardiogenic pulmonary oedema (Bersten *et al.*, 1991). CPAP is particularly useful in the management of postoperative respiratory failure associated with basal lung collapse/consolidation (see Chapter 8) and is indicated in the management of selected patients with chest trauma who remain hypoxic despite adequate analgesia and high-flow oxygen. In a randomized, controlled trial, however, application of CPAP by full facemask failed to reduce the need for tracheal intubation or improve outcome in patients with acute hypoxaemic, nonhypercapnic respiratory insufficiency due to acute lung injury (Delclaux *et al.*, 2000). Worryingly, in this study there were four cardiac arrests in the CPAP group, compared to none in the standard therapy group: three occurred at the time of intubation and one when the mask was removed, precipitating extreme hypoxia. It may be that mask CPAP is most useful when the underlying cause of the respiratory failure is readily reversible, as is the case in cardiogenic pulmonary oedema or collapsed basal lung segments, but is less likely to be beneficial when the lung pathology is progressive and/or slow to resolve. Although there is some evidence that CPAP may benefit patients with acute exacerbations of COPD, NIV is now the treatment of choice in such patients (see below and Chapter 8).

CPAP masks are uncomfortable to wear for prolonged periods and the technique is only suitable for those who are alert, able to clear secretions and protect their airway. Gastric distension, vomiting and aspiration are a potential risk and a nasogastric tube should be inserted in most patients receiving mask CPAP.

Nasal masks may be better tolerated and safer, but mouth breathing renders them less effective. They are most useful when applied at night in patients with obstructive sleep apnoea and nocturnal hypoventilation (Jenkinson *et al.*, 1999). Recently *helmets* that surround the patient's head and neck have been introduced; these may be better tolerated than masks.

CPAP is also useful for weaning patients from mechanical ventilation since it prevents the alveolar collapse and hypoxia that may otherwise occur (Feeley *et al.*, 1975). In general, therefore, patients who have required CPAP should not be allowed to breathe spontaneously through an endotracheal tube with ZEEP, but rather should be extubated directly from 5 cm H_2O PEEP. Once extubated, patients provide their own 'physiological PEEP'.

Non-invasive ventilation

NIV involves the provision of mechanical respiratory support without invading the patient's upper airway and can be delivered using either a nasal or full facial mask. Although nasal masks are generally better tolerated they require a cooperative

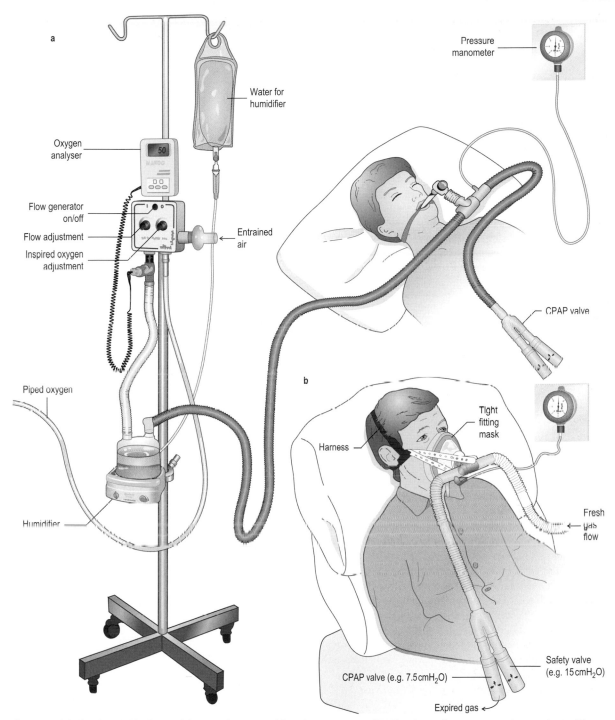

Fig. 7.11 (a) Circuit suitable for applying continuous positive airway pressure (CPAP) using a flow generator in a patient with an endotracheal tube in place. (b) CPAP can be applied using a tight-fitting facemask.

patient who is able to maintain mouth closure to be effective. In general alveolar ventilation, and consequently the reduction in P_aCO_2, is greater with full facemasks which are therefore the most appropriate choice for patients with acute respiratory failure. Nasal plugs or 'pillows' can also be effective but

are often poorly tolerated. The application of non-invasive positive-pressure ventilation via a 'helmet' is also feasible but is not as effective in terms of carbon dioxide elimination (Antonelli *et al.*, 2004). Most modern ventilators can provide NIV, but they are often unnecessarily complicated and portable non-invasive devices are now widely used, both on intensive care/high-dependency units and on respiratory wards. The most popular ventilators for this purpose are those providing BiPAP, which are simple to use, cheap and flexible. Alternatively ACV, volume control or PSV, with or without PEEP, can be delivered using a conventional mechanical ventilator.

Successful application of NIV requires considerable attention to detail, particularly in the first few hours, in order to ensure that the mask is comfortable, with minimal leaks, and that the ventilatory pattern is optimal (Brochard, 2000). Achieving a good mask fit is crucial both for patient comfort and to ensure effective ventilatory support; simply overtightening the headgear in an attempt to eliminate leaks is uncomfortable for the patient and increases the risk of skin damage. A better fit is obtained if dentures are left in place.

The patient's response to NIV should be assessed by clinical evaluation, including patient comfort, conscious level, chest wall motion, accessory muscle use, coordination of respiratory effort with the ventilator, respiratory rate and heart rate and by continuous pulse oximetry supplemented by repeated blood gas analysis. The patient should be reviewed regularly to optimize ventilator settings.

Institution of NIV can rest the respiratory muscles, reduce respiratory acidosis and restlessness, improve clearance of secretions and re-expand collapsed lung segments. NIV may be undertaken as a therapeutic trial, recognizing that in the event of failure tracheal intubation will be required, or as the ceiling of treatment in patients who are not candidates for invasive respiratory support or admission to intensive care.

Advantages of NIV include:

- avoidance of tracheal intubation and associated complications, especially VAP;
- improved patient comfort and avoidance of sedation;
- preservation of airway defence mechanisms;
- spontaneous coughing and expectoration are not hampered;
- ventilatory assistance can be provided intermittently, allowing normal eating, drinking and communication (periods of NIV as short as 6–8 hours a day can be effective), as well as facilitating gradual weaning;
- ventilation can be interrupted to allow administration of nebulized medications, physiotherapy, coughing and expectoration;
- early mobilization is facilitated;
- patient morale is maintained;
- ventilatory support can be initiated at an earlier stage and in some cases admission to intensive care can be avoided.

Disadvantages include the absence of a route for endotracheal suction and the lack of airway protection. *Complications* include nasal bridge and facial ulceration, nasal congestion and eye irritation. Air swallowing is common and most patients receiving NIV should have a nasogastric tube in place. More serious complications, such as aspiration of gastric contents, cardiovascular instability and pneumothorax, are fortunately rare.

Contraindications to NIV include:

- recent facial or upper-airway surgery, burns or trauma;
- fixed obstruction of the upper airway;
- vomiting;
- recent upper gastrointestinal surgery or bowel obstruction;
- uncooperative patient, coma, confusion or agitation;
- inability to protect the airway or to cough and expectorate effectively;
- copious respiratory secretions;
- focal consolidation on chest X-ray;
- life-threatening hypoxaemia;
- haemodynamic instability;
- severe comorbidity.

NIV is most clearly indicated in the management of selected patients with an acute exacerbation of COPD who are not severely hypoxaemic and in whom a respiratory acidosis persists despite maximum medical treatment and controlled oxygen therapy. In this situation NIV has been used successfully both in intensive care/high-dependency units (Brochard *et al.*, 1990, 1995, Girou *et al.*, 2000; Martin *et al.*, 2000; Meduri *et al.*, 1991) and on general respiratory wards (Bott *et al.*, 1993; Plant *et al.*, 2000, 2001, 2003). Taken together these studies have demonstrated that in such patients appropriately applied NIV can reduce the need for tracheal intubation, the length of hospital stay, costs and the in-hospital mortality rate, a conclusion supported by a meta-analysis (Peter *et al.*, 2002). The improved outcome with NIV seems to be at least partly explained by a reduction in the incidence of complications, especially VAP and other nosocomial infections (Brochard *et al.*, 1995; Girou *et al.*, 2000). Long-term survival is sufficiently good to lend further support to the use of NIV in this category of patient (Plant *et al.*, 2001).

The role of NIV in the management of acute respiratory failure unrelated to COPD is less clear, however (Peter *et al.*, 2002). In one study of patients with unresponsive acute respiratory failure and severe hypoxaemia non-invasive positive-pressure ventilation reduced the rate of serious complications and, in survivors, the length of ICU stay (Antonelli *et al.*, 1998), whilst in another study the rate of tracheal intubation was reduced (Martin *et al.*, 2000), although improved survival was only seen in those with COPD. Similarly, Confalonieri *et al.* (1999) found that in selected patients with acute respiratory failure caused by community-acquired pneumonia NIV was associated with a significant reduction in the rate of tracheal intubation and duration of ICU stay. Again 2-month survival was only improved in those with COPD. In a more recent study, the use of NIV prevented intubation, reduced the incidence of septic shock and improved survival in patients with severe hypoxaemic respiratory failure, except in those with ARDS (Ferrer *et al.*, 2003b).

Non-invasive PSV has also been shown to lead to more rapid improvement in oxygenation and reduction in respiratory rate when compared to conventional oxygen therapy in acute cardiogenic pulmonary oedema (Masip *et al.*, 2000; Nava *et al.*, 2003; Park *et al.*, 2004), although in some studies outcome was not improved (Masip *et al.*, 2000; Nava *et al.*, 2003) and it is unclear whether NIV/BiPAP is more efficacious than CPAP in this condition (Park *et al.*, 2004). Indeed, a recent meta-analysis indicated that, compared with standard therapy, CPAP reduces mortality in acute cardiogenic pulmonary oedema but there was only a suggestion of a trend towards a reduction in mortality with bilevel NIPPV (Peter *et al.*, 2006). There is even some suggestion that CPAP or NIV may reduce the need for tracheal intubation in selected patients with severe asthma (Fernández *et al.*, 2001), although currently this approach cannot be recommended. Finally NIV may be particularly indicated in the management of immunocompromised patients with acute respiratory failure, in whom the rates of tracheal intubation and serious complications may be reduced and survival improved (Hilbert *et al.*, 2001).

In conclusion, current evidence supports the use of NIV in acute hypercapnic respiratory failure associated with COPD, provided that the patient is not profoundly hypoxaemic, and suggests that the technique may also be useful in selected patients with acute hypoxaemic respiratory failure of various aetiologies. NIV may also be useful as an aid to early extubation of patients who cannot sustain unsupported spontaneous ventilation (Girault *et al.*, 1999), although the influence of this approach on length of stay and survival is unclear (Girault *et al.*, 1999; Nava *et al.*, 1998). NIV is also the treatment of choice in decompensated ventilatory failure due to chest wall deformity or neuromuscular disease and has been used successfully in decompensated sleep apnoea (see Chapter 8).

Extracorporeal gas exchange

EXTRACORPOREAL MEMBRANE OXYGENATION (ECMO)

The technique of ECMO using venoarterial bypass was introduced in an attempt to save the lives of some patients who would otherwise inevitably have died from severe progressive acute respiratory failure. It was based on the premise that the lungs of such patients would eventually recover provided death from hypoxia could be avoided. This proved not to be the case since in the majority of cases the lung lesion continued to progress, culminating in irreversible pulmonary fibrosis. When a prospective randomized study demonstrated that the mortality of patients with severe ARF was similar whether or not ECMO was used (Zapol *et al.*, 1979), its use in adults was largely abandoned.

LOW-FREQUENCY POSITIVE-PRESSURE VENTILATION WITH EXTRACORPOREAL CARBON DIOXIDE REMOVAL (Gattinoni et al., 1980, 1986)

This technique uses a venovenous bypass, with low flows of only 20–30% of the cardiac output, to remove carbon dioxide. The lungs are ventilated at a very low frequency and oxygenation is maintained by applying a positive pressure to the airways and adjusting the F_1O_2. Although alveolar oxygen concentrations may be high, the combination of normal pulmonary perfusion and minimum ventilation may avoid ventilator-associated lung injury, rest the lungs and provide optimal conditions for lung healing.

The major complication of this technique is bleeding, which is potentially fatal. The incidence of bleeding can be reduced by using surface heparinized extracorporeal circuits or by the simultaneous administration of aprotinin with heparin. In general, however, extracorporeal techniques are contraindicated in patients at risk of haemorrhage. In contrast to the use of ECMO, thromboembolic complications have not been reported and the technique is simplified by the use of percutaneous venous cannulation.

A later randomized controlled trial indicated that this technique may not improve outcome, especially when compared to protocol-driven ventilatory strategies designed to minimize levels of PEEP and F_1O_2 (Morris *et al.*, 1994).

Nevertheless, some authorities remain convinced that, when used by experienced teams in specialist centres, extracorporeal gas exchange can significantly reduce the mortality associated with severe ARDS, and that further technical improvements will facilitate the more widespread application of this technique.

DISCONTINUING AND WEANING VENTILATORY SUPPORT (MacIntyre et al., 2001)

In view of the numerous complications associated with invasive respiratory support it is important to discontinue mechanical ventilation, and, if possible, to extubate the patient as soon as possible. On the other hand, premature attempts at weaning may be deleterious and can adversely affect the morale of conscious patients; during weaning a fine balance must be drawn between proceeding too quickly and unnecessarily prolonging the process.

Following a prolonged period of mechanical respiratory support ventilatory function may be compromised by:

- decreased central drive;
- weakness and wasting of skeletal muscle and the diaphragm;
- critical-illness polyneuromyopathy (see Chapter 15);
- pathological changes in muscle, including corticosteroid-induced myopathy (Douglass *et al.*, 1992);
- chest wall instability;
- operative or traumatic damage to the phrenic nerves;
- abdominal distension with upward displacement of the diaphragm.

The role of respiratory muscle fatigue is poorly understood but there is usually some persisting abnormality of gas exchange and lung mechanics, including, for example, dynamic hyperinflation. In patients who have been ventilated for any length of time, therefore, spontaneous respiration normally has to be resumed gradually.

Criteria for discontinuing mechanical ventilation
CLINICAL CRITERIA

Clinical assessment is of paramount importance when deciding whether a patient is ready to be weaned from the ventilator. The patient's conscious level, psychological state, metabolic function, the effects of drugs, cardiovascular performance, lung mechanics, pulmonary gas exchange and ventilatory function must all be taken into account.

An altered *level of consciousness* does not necessarily prevent weaning, but patients should not be extubated until they can cough, cooperate with physiotherapy and protect their own airway. Attempts should be made to re-establish a normal sleep–wake cycle and to treat depression/demotivation (see below). Weaning will, however, often prove difficult in those who are *restless, confused* and *uncooperative*. Some patients who have undergone a prolonged period of respiratory support become *psychologically dependent* on the ventilator (see Chapter 11) and will require particular care and continual reassurance throughout the weaning period.

Malnourished patients may have difficulty in sustaining adequate alveolar ventilation. For this, and many other reasons (see Chapter 11), malnutrition should if possible be prevented or corrected by providing an adequate protein and energy intake during the patient's hospitalization and by correcting any specific deficiencies, in particular *hypophosphataemia, hypocalcaemia, hypomagnesaemia* and *hypokalaemia*. On the other hand, some patients with borderline respiratory function may be unable to excrete the large quantities of carbon dioxide produced by the metabolism of high-energy carbohydrate feeds, although it remains unclear whether the use of high-fat feeds can facilitate weaning in difficult cases. Similarly, *increased oxygen demands* (e.g. in response to fever or shivering) and *impaired oxygen uptake*, as may occur in sepsis, can prevent successful weaning. *Hypothyroidism* is associated with impaired diaphragmatic function and blunted ventilatory responses to hypercapnia and hypoxia.

It is also important to correct any significant abnormalities of *acid–base balance*; although a metabolic alkalosis increases muscle strength, it can blunt the respiratory drive and cause carbon dioxide retention, while metabolic acidosis decreases muscle strength and stimulates respiration. In patients with COPD and chronic hypercarbia inappropriate overventilation, with consequent correction of a long-standing compensatory metabolic alkalosis, may inhibit weaning because the patient is unable to maintain arterial carbon dioxide tension at the level required to achieve a normal pH.

In patients who prove difficult to wean, especially those with COPD, correction of *anaemia* may facilitate discontinuation of respiratory support (Schönhofer *et al.*, 1998).

Pain must be controlled but the possibility that the residual *effects of drugs* are impairing respiration must also be considered. Of most importance in this respect are the opiates and the non-depolarizing muscle relaxants; both are a particular problem in the presence of renal failure. In particular, morphine metabolites such as morphine-6-glucuronide can accumulate in patients with renal impairment, and the long-term administration of vecuronium may be especially likely to cause persistent paralysis, perhaps due to the accumulation of a metabolite (Segredo *et al.*, 1992).

Cardiovascular stability is another important prerequisite for successful weaning. In particular, weaning is likely to be difficult in those with left ventricular failure and a low cardiac output. This is partly because the low cardiac output is associated with a reduction in PAP, which increases the number of relatively underperfused alveoli; V_D/V_T ratio therefore rises. Also DO_2 is limited and may be insufficient for the increase in VO_2 associated with resumption of respiratory efforts. Venous return and afterload both increase and catecholamine release may exacerbate the situation by causing vasoconstriction and tachycardia. In some cases myocardial ischaemia may be precipitated. In difficult cases a pulmonary artery catheter or other means of monitoring cardiac output may be used to guide haemodynamic support during and after the weaning period. Life-threatening arrhythmias and bleeding likely to require surgical intervention (e.g. after cardiac surgery) are also contraindications to discontinuing ventilation. On the other hand, provided the patient is stable, dependence on inotropes, vasopressors or intra-aortic balloon counterpulsation is not a contraindication to commencing cautious weaning. Indeed, some patients with borderline cardiopulmonary function may benefit from elective maintenance of inotropic support during the weaning process.

Finally, *mechanical factors* likely to impair ventilation, such as residual pulmonary oedema, pneumothorax, abdominal distension and pleural effusions, should, if possible, be corrected. *Ultrasound-guided drainage of pleural effusions* has been shown to be effective, safe and relatively easy in mechanically ventilated patients (Lichtenstein *et al.*, 1999).

A subjective evaluation of the patient's response to a short period of spontaneous respiration by an experienced clinician (*spontaneous breathing trial*: SBT) remains the most reliable predictor of weaning success or failure. Asynchronous or paradoxical respiration, respiratory alternans, use of accessory muscles, tachypnoea and low tidal volumes all suggest incipient decompensation. Recent evidence suggests that weaning from mechanical ventilation and discharge from hospital can be accelerated, and mortality reduced, by combining daily awakening with daily spontaneous breathing trials (Girard *et al.*, 2008).

OBJECTIVE CRITERIA (Table 7.3)

Although many objective criteria for predicting the ability to wean have been suggested (Sahn and Lakshminarayan, 1973; Skillman *et al.*, 1971), these often prove misleading (Krieger *et al.*, 1989) and may even prolong the weaning time when incorporated into a weaning protocol (Tanios *et al.*, 2006). In most cases, a clinical assessment, as outlined above, together with blood gas analysis (considered in conjunction with the F_IO_2 and the minute volume) and an assessment of the mechanical properties of the patient's lungs will be sufficient to make the correct decision. The various quantitative criteria that have been recommended for predicting the

Table 7.3 Objective criteria for weaning

Gas exchange

$P_aO_2 > 10$ kPa (80 mmHg) with an $F_IO_2 < 0.5$ or
$P_aO_2 > 8$ kPa (60 mmHg) with an $F_IO_2 = 0.4$
$P_aO_2/F_IO_2 \times 150–200$ with PEEP $\leq 5–10$ cm H_2O
$P_{A–a}O_2 < 40–47$ kPa (300–350 mmHg) with an $F_IO_2 = 1.0$
Percentage venous admixture < 15%
V_D/V_T ratio < 0.58–0.60
pH $\geq 7.3–7.5$

Mechanical

Vital capacity > 10–15 mL/kg
Negative inspiratory force −20 to −30 cm H_2O
Maximum inspiratory pressure > −15 to −30 cm H_2O
Respiratory rate < 30–38 breaths/min
V_T 4–6 mL/kg

f/V_T ratio ≤ 105 breaths/min per litre
CROP index ≥ 13 mL/breath per min

CROP, compliance, respiratory rate, arterial oxygenation and Pimax.

outcome of weaning are best used as adjuncts to clinical assessment in difficult cases.

The gas exchanging properties of the lungs may be considered adequate for weaning if the P_aO_2 is > 10 kPa (80 mmHg) with an $F_IO_2 < 0.5$ (some suggest a $P_aO_2 > 8$ kPa (60 mmHg) with an F_IO_2 of 0.4, or a P_aO_2/F_IO_2 ratio > 150–200 with PEEP $\leq 5–10$ cm H_2O), if the $P_{A–a}O_2$ is < 40–47 kPa (300–350 mmHg) with an $F_IO_2 = 1.0$, if the percentage venous admixture is <15% and if the V_D/V_T ratio is < 0.58–0.6 (Feeley and Hedley-Whyte, 1975; Skillman et al., 1971) (Table 7.3).

The strength of the respiratory muscles in relation to the mechanical properties of the lungs can be assessed by measuring VC, which should be higher than 10–15 mL/kg to commence weaning, and the maximum inspiratory pressure (P_{imax}), which should be more than −20 cm H_2O, although these tests are dependent on the ability of the patient to cooperate. In one study, all those patients who were able to produce a peak negative pressure of more than −30 cm H_2O weaned successfully, while a resting minute volume of less than 10 l/min and the ability to double this voluntarily correlated well with the ability to wean (Sahn and Lakshminarayan, 1973). Measuring the airway occlusion pressure 0.1 seconds after the onset of inspiration ($P_{0.1}$), and its response to a hypercapnic challenge may also prove to be a useful means of predicting the likely outcome of weaning attempts (Montgomery et al., 1987). If the cardiac index can be measured, it should be higher than 2 l/min per m^2 at least and preferably within the normal range. Finally, the pH should be 7.3–7.5.

The use of these traditional objective criteria is, however, associated with a high incidence of false-positive or false-negative results. A study conducted in medical patients (Yang and Tobin, 1991) demonstrated that the most accurate predictor of failure to wean was rapid, shallow, spontaneous unsupported breathing, as reflected by the f/V_T ratio, although a more recent study concluded that f/V_T should not be used routinely to predict ability to wean (Tanios et al., 2006). P_{imax} and expired minute volume were poor predictors, whereas an index that integrated thoracic compliance, respiratory rate, arterial oxygenation and P_{imax} (called CROP) was considerably more accurate. Of the primary indices, V_T was the most accurate predictor of weaning outcome.

Techniques for discontinuing respiratory support

Uncomplicated patients who have undergone mechanical ventilation for less than 24–48 hours (e.g. electively after major surgery) can usually resume spontaneous respiration abruptly and no weaning process is required. They should be connected to a T-piece or CPAP circuit and provided with humidified fresh gas of an appropriate F_IO_2 (**Fig. 7.12**). This procedure can also be adopted for patients with readily reversible causes of respiratory failure. Those who sustain adequate ventilation, without signs of distress (see above) during this SBT can be extubated, provided there are no other contraindications (see below).

The *traditional method of weaning* in difficult cases is to allow patients to breathe entirely spontaneously for a short time (e.g. 10 minutes in the first instance), following which they are reconnected to the ventilator. The periods of spontaneous breathing are gradually increased in duration and frequency. Initially, it is usually advisable to provide ventilatory support at night. This method can be stressful and tiring for patients and is time-consuming for the staff, but may prove successful when other methods have failed. It is now usual to rest the patient between periods of unassisted breathing using a spontaneous mode of respiratory support, rather than CMV. It has been suggested that *SIMV* can provide a smoother, more controlled method of weaning, and may enable weaning to commence at an earlier stage than is possible using the traditional method. There is, however, evidence that the use of SIMV may contribute to respiratory muscle fatigue and can unnecessarily prolong weaning times. The application of *inspiratory pressure support* has been shown to prevent diaphragmatic fatigue and limit hyperinflation during weaning from mechanical ventilation (Brochard et al., 1989) and is now a popular technique, often used in combination with SIMV/CPAP. Weaning by gradually reducing the level of PSV (by 2–4 cm H_2O twice a day) with no mandatory breaths has been shown to be superior to withdrawing ventilatory support using gradually increasing fixed periods of spontaneous breathing or SIMV (Brochard et al., 1994).

An alternative approach is to allow the patient to breathe spontaneously through a T-piece circuit for up to 2 hours once each day and to extubate those who tolerate the SBT without signs of distress. Full ventilatory support, for example with ACV, is provided between SBTs. In a group of patients who were difficult to wean this technique led to more rapid extubation than either SIMV or pressure support reduction and was as effective as multiple daily SBTs (Esteban et al., 1995). More recently, half-hour SBTs have been shown

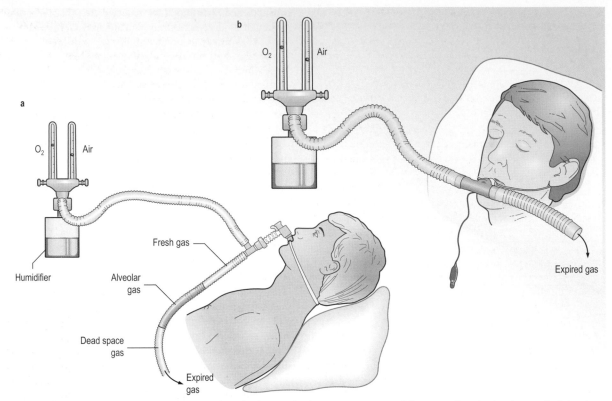

Fig. 7.12 (a) A T-piece circuit: situation at end expiration. Expired gases are prevented from entering the inspiratory limb by the flow of fresh gas. During the end-expiratory pause fresh gas enters the expiratory limb, pushing the expired gases distally. At peak inspiration, when the fresh gas flow may be insufficient, fresh gas can be entrained from the expiratory limb of the T-piece. In order to prevent rebreathing of alveolar gas, the fresh gas flow must exceed 2½ times the patient's minute volume. In order to prevent entrainment of air, the volume of the expiratory limb must be greater than the patient's tidal volume. (b) When it is not essential to provide a constant inspired oxygen concentration a short expiratory unit can be used.

to be as effective as 2-hour trials (Esteban *et al.*, 1999). Similarly, a two-stage approach to weaning, in which systematic measurement of predictors, including f/V_T, is followed by a single daily trial of spontaneous breathing, has been shown to be superior to conventional management (Ely *et al.*, 1996). Although injudicious prolongation of a failing trial of spontaneous breathing could theoretically be hazardous, in practice this approach appears to be extremely safe. Because the detrimental effects of ventilatory muscle overload usually become obvious in the early stages of the trial, close monitoring is essential during the first few minutes. It also seems that the outcome of these trials is not significantly affected by whether they are performed on CPAP, with low levels of pressure support or using a simple T-piece. Some believe that this approach is not only simpler but may also be the most effective method for reconditioning respiratory muscles. On the other hand, the reintubation rate can be disturbingly high (around 23%). In general it seems likely that the pace of weaning is influenced more by the manner in which the technique is applied than by the method chosen. What remains unclear is whether daily SBTs coupled with gradual reduction of respiratory support have any advan-

tages compared to maintenance of a stable level of support between SBTs.

The *application of CPAP* can prevent the alveolar collapse, hypoxaemia and fall in compliance that may otherwise occur when patients start to breathe spontaneously (Feeley *et al.*, 1975). It is therefore often used during weaning with SIMV/ PSV and in spontaneously breathing patients before extubation, particularly when the patient was previously receiving CPPV. CPAP may also assist weaning in patients with severe airflow obstruction by decreasing the work of breathing and their sensation of breathlessness (Petrof *et al.*, 1990), and there are good arguments for using at least 3–5 cm H_2O CPAP during weaning in all bedridden patients receiving mechanical respiratory support. It is also important to provide sufficient inspiratory pressure support during spontaneous breaths to overcome the resistance of the ventilator circuit and endotracheal tube (about 6–8 cm H_2O).

To discourage atelectasis and encourage adequate lung inflation during weaning, patients should remain as upright and mobile as possible, and should be encouraged to take deep breaths periodically. It is important to avoid overtaxing the respiratory muscles because recovery from fatigue may take 24 hours or more and sufficient ventilatory support should be provided at night to allow the patient to sleep. The value of *training the respiratory muscles* remains in doubt, but reconditioning of respiratory muscles, the return of coordinated muscular activity and the matching of ventilation to requirements are important adjustments during successful weaning. Indeed, weaning time can be reduced by using tidal volume and relaxation biofeedback techniques (Holliday and Hyers, 1990). In difficult cases the use of mask CPAP, non-invasive ventilatory support and augmentation of gas exchange by tracheal catheterization may assist the transition to independence.

Although protocols directed by nursing and respiratory care staff can expedite weaning from mechanical ventilation, it seems that such an approach may be unnecessary in closed ICUs, in which patients are managed by an adequate complement of specialist clinicians who perform structured, system-based ward rounds (Krishnan *et al.*, 2004). On the other hand computer-driven protocolized weaning may reduce the duration of mechanical ventilation and length of ICU stay when compared with a physician-controlled weaning process (Lellouche *et al.*, 2006).

Failure to wean

In patients who fail to wean from mechanical ventilation the act of spontaneous breathing seems to be associated with worsening respiratory mechanics. In one study respiratory resistance increased progressively, reaching about seven times the normal value by the end of the trial of spontaneous breathing, whilst lung compliance fell approximately five-fold. There was an associated increase in gas trapping (Jubran and Tobin, 1997a). Respiratory rate usually increases considerably and tidal volume falls. Interestingly, respiratory mechanics before weaning are similar in patients who fail to wean and those who are weaned successfully (Jubran and Tobin, 1997b) and in general the mechanisms underlying the acute changes in respiratory mechanics during weaning are poorly understood (Tobin, 2001). The rise in P_aCO_2 which accompanies weaning failure in some patients is not usually a consequence of a decrease in minute ventilation but rather is a result of rapid, shallow breathing which causes an increase in dead-space ventilation. In a few patients hypercapnia may be due to central respiratory depression.

Failure to wean from mechanical ventilation is also frequently associated with cardiovascular dysfunction. Pulmonary arterial and systemic blood pressure can increase considerably and cardiac output fails to increase to meet the additional oxygen demands of spontaneous breathing. Oxygen extraction is therefore increased and the consequent fall in mixed venous oxygen saturation contributes to the arterial hypoxaemia that is seen in some patients.

Prolonged weaning from mechanical ventilation accounts for a considerable proportion of the workload of ICU staff, has implications for the use of resources and costs and is associated with increased morbidity and mortality. Inadequate nurse-to-patient ratios have been associated with pro-

longed weaning times (Thorens *et al.*, 1995). Patients who remain ventilator-dependent despite resolution of their acute illness and aggressive attempts to discontinue respiratory support may benefit from transfer to a long-term weaning facility. These are potentially more cost-effective and better suited to the needs of such patients. Usually those who have undergone prolonged mechanical ventilation (sometimes defined as requiring ventilator support for more than 21 days) will require a slow wean with gradual reduction of partial support (e.g. SIMV/PSV), followed later by self-breathing trials of increasing duration.

Finally prolonged ventilatory support does not preclude a satisfactory recovery and an acceptable perceived quality of life. Long-term outcome is influenced more by the aetiology of the respiratory failure, the reversibility of the acute illness and associated comorbidities than the need for prolonged respiratory support *per se* (Chatila *et al.*, 2001).

Extubation

Extubation should not be considered until patients can cough effectively, swallow, protect their own airway and are sufficiently alert to be cooperative. Patients who fulfil these criteria can be extubated provided their respiratory function has improved sufficiently to sustain spontaneous ventilation indefinitely. A simple, reproducible method for predicting successful extubation in patients who have passed a SBT has been described (Salam *et al.*, 2004). This involves an assessment of cough, peak flow, the volume of tracheal secretions and ability to perform four simple tasks (open eyes, follow with eyes, grasp hand, protrude tongue).

A pressure support of 6–8 cm H_2O is widely used to compensate for the resistance imposed by the endotracheal tube and circuit. Many clinicians will then extubate patients who can breathe comfortably with this level of support. In some cases, however, swelling of the upper airways may impose a similar degree of respiratory work as breathing through an endotracheal tube (Straus *et al.*, 1998) and under these circumstances the use of pressure support may be misleading.

It has been suggested that the use of mask CPAP or non-invasive mechanical ventilation might prevent deterioration following extubation and non-invasive mechanical ventilation has been used to enable early extubation of patients with COPD who could not sustain spontaneous breathing (Nava *et al.*, 1998). There is also evidence that the use of NIV to achieve earlier extubation is associated with shorter periods of mechanical ventilation and hospital and ICU stays, less need for tracheostomy and improved survival (Ferrer *et al.*, 2003a). On the other hand non-invasive positive-pressure ventilation failed to prevent reintubation or reduce mortality in unselected patients who developed respiratory failure following extubation; indeed, delays in reintubation actually correlated with worse survival rates (Esteban *et al.*, 2004).

As many as 10–25% of patients may require reintubation (Brochard *et al.*, 1994; Esteban *et al.*, 1995). This adverse event is associated with a considerable increase in mortality (Esteban *et al.,* 1999), although the need for reintubation may simply be a marker of the severity of the underlying illness. Although the acceptable reintubation rate has not been defined, a figure of between 5 and 15% has been suggested. Unplanned extubation (self-extubation and accidental extubation) and reintubation after weaning have been associated with longer periods of mechanical ventilation and prolonged ICU and hospital stays, although mortality rates were unaffected (de Lassence *et al.,* 2002). Accidental extubation increased the risk of VAP (de Lassence *et al.,* 2002).

Extubation failure may be a result not only of respiratory failure but also of upper-airway obstruction or an inability to protect the airway and clear secretions. The risk of postextubation upper-airway obstruction increases with the duration of mechanical ventilation, female gender, trauma and repeated or traumatic intubation. Treatment is with steroids and/or nebulized adrenaline. Although in one study routine administration of hydrocortisone 1 hour before extubation did not influence the development of postextubation stridor (Ho *et al.,* 1996), in a more recent study methylprednisolone given 12 hours before extubation and every 4 hours until tube removal reduced the incidence of postextubation laryngeal oedema and reintubation (Francois *et al.,* 2007). In patients with upper-airway obstruction it is generally accepted that the safety of extubation is best determined by demonstrating a leak around the endotracheal tube when the cuff is deflated. Although the presence of such a leak suggests that extubation is likely to be successful, a failed cuff leak test does not preclude uneventful extubation and if used in isolation may prolong the period of intubation or lead to unnecessary tracheostomy (Fisher and Raper, 1992).

It is important to recognize that prolonged tracheal intubation impairs the swallowing reflex, perhaps contributing to the development of aspiration pneumonia following extubation. Significant improvement is seen within about 7 days (de Larminat *et al.,* 1995). There is also a significant incidence of sleep-related breathing disorders in such patients following discharge from intensive care and overnight oxygen desaturation is common (Chishti *et al.,* 2000).

TRACHEAL INTUBATION

INDICATIONS
Apart from providing a route for mechanical respiratory support, tracheal intubation may be required to secure and maintain a clear airway, to protect the lungs from aspiration and to allow control of bronchial secretions with tracheal suction.

COMPLICATIONS
Early
Rarely tracheal intubation may prove difficult or impossible, but more often may be complicated by trauma, for example to the lips, teeth, gums or trachea. Many of the common

immediate hazards of tracheal intubation cause difficulty with inflation of one or both lungs. It is therefore essential to ensure that both sides of the chest are expanding equally and adequately at all times and that the inflation pressure is not excessive.

A common mistake is *intubation of one or other bronchus*, usually the right, since this is most directly in line with the trachea; in one series this occurred in 9% of all tracheal intubations (Stauffer *et al.,* 1981). As a result, the left lung, and often the right upper lobe, collapse and the patient becomes hypoxic. Therefore, the position of the endotracheal tube must always be checked on the chest radiograph; if the tip is close to or beyond the carina, the tube should be withdrawn.

In the absence of capnography accidental *intubation of the oesophagus* can occasionally be surprisingly difficult to recognize. Hypoxia with gaseous distension of the stomach may then develop rapidly. Endotracheal tubes can *migrate out of the trachea* so that they come to lie in the oropharynx; this process is often accelerated by overinflation of the cuff in an attempt to abolish the leak that inevitably develops when the cuff herniates between the vocal cords. A leak around the tube is usually clearly audible and will also develop if the *cuff ruptures*.

Obstruction may be due to inspissated secretions, kinking, biting on the tube, cuff herniation, compression of the tube by an overinflated cuff or the bevel of the tube impinging on the tracheal wall or carina.

All these acute complications are potentially extremely dangerous; they must be recognized promptly and dealt with appropriately. If at any time the tube becomes obstructed – indicated by the patient becoming distressed and/or cyanosed with inadequate or absent expansion of one or both sides of the chest, accompanied by a rise in inflation pressures and activation of the ventilator alarm – the following procedure should be adopted:

- Attempt manual inflation with 100% oxygen.
- Check and adjust position of tube.
- If the position of the tube appears to be correct, carry out endotracheal suction, which may confirm or relieve obstruction.
- Check that the tube is not kinked in the oropharynx.
- Deflate cuff (relieves obstruction if due to cuff herniation or tube compression).
- Change endotracheal tube (the tube can be changed over a bougie). Sedation, with or without muscle relaxation may be required.

If a significant leak develops that cannot be abolished by reinflating the cuff, either the endotracheal tube has been dislodged or the cuff has ruptured. If the tube has become misplaced and cannot easily be repositioned, it should be removed and the patient ventilated using a facemask or laryngeal mask airway and rebreathing bag before reintubation. If the cuff is leaking, the endotracheal tube should be replaced electively.

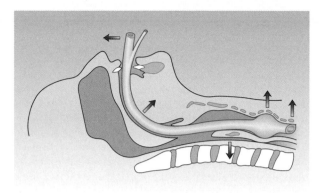

Fig. 7.13 Points at which excessive pressure is exerted by an endotracheal tube. From Lindholm and Grenvik (1977), with permission.

Late

Prolonged pressure on the structures of the upper respiratory tract, caused by either the tube itself or the cuff, causes *mucosal oedema*, which may then progress to *ulceration*. This later heals by *granulation* with the development of *fibrotic scar* tissue and tracheal narrowing. The points at which excessive pressure may occur are shown in **Figure 7.13**. At the level of the glottis, the posterior aspect of the vocal cords, the arytenoid cartilages and the cricoarytenoid joints may be damaged, while in some patients the lesions extend down into the subglottic space (Stauffer *et al.*, 1981). Damage may also occur at the level of the cuff, often anteriorly; this may be extensive with complete loss of mucosa and exposure of underlying tracheal cartilage. Granuloma formation is unusual (Stauffer *et al.*, 1981). The ways in which this damage may be minimized are as follows:

■ *Tube size*. To avoid the risk of circular subglottic stenosis, a tube with an external diameter well below the internal diameter of the cricoid ring should be used.
■ *Tube material*. Endotracheal tubes are made of thermo labile material so that once in place they conform to the shape of the airway. Otherwise undue force is exerted, particularly on the medial aspects of the arytenoid cartilages and on both sides of the midline at the cricoid plate (see **Fig. 7.13**). Tubes are made of non-irritant (implant-tested) material.
■ *Movements of the larynx*. Coughing and straining on the tube are thought to increase the risk of mucosal damage; the arytenoid cartilages are again particularly vulnerable.
■ *Tube cuff*. In the early days of intensive care high pressures were required to inflate the cuffs of red rubber endotracheal tubes and because their shape did not conform to that of the trachea, this high pressure was concentrated on a small area of the tracheal wall, impairing capillary blood flow in the underlying tracheal mucosa. In addition, prolonged high cuff pressures can lead to distension of the trachea, with eventual erosion of the cartilaginous rings. It has been shown that by using *high-volume, pre-*

shaped, low-pressure cuffs made of *non-irritant material*, the severity of tracheal injury can be minimized. It is important that these cuffs are not overinflated since, once a seal has been created, further inflation causes a steep rise in intracuff pressure. Inflation of the cuff beyond this point can be avoided by monitoring the intracuff pressure or by using a pressure-limiting valve. In this way the incidence of cuff-related complications may be reduced. Theoretically the pressure exerted by the cuff on the tracheal mucosa should not exceed the capillary perfusion pressure (i.e. about 30 mmHg).

Other factors thought to increase the risk of mucosal damage include:

■ prolonged intubation;
■ episodes of hypotension during which mucosal blood flow is further compromised;
■ the administration of corticosteroids;
■ tracheitis due to pooling of infected material above the cuff.

Despite the relatively high incidence of laryngeal injury detected at autopsy, including posterior glottic ulceration and laryngeal haematoma, late laryngeal sequelae of prolonged tracheal intubation are rare in survivors. Subglottic stenosis is more common, and in one series was detected in 19% of cases following tracheal intubation. The incidence was even higher after tracheostomy (65%), but in most of these patients tracheal narrowing occurred at stomal, rather than cuff, level. However, only one patient with tracheal stenosis had symptoms of upper-airway obstruction (Stauffer *et al.*, 1981).

ORAL OR NASAL TRACHEAL INTUBATION?

Many patients find it difficult to tolerate oral endotracheal tubes. This applies particularly to those who are fully conscious and require prolonged intubation. In these cases, the nasal route may sometimes be preferred since it is more comfortable, secure fixation of the tube is more easily achieved and the tube is less likely to kink. Furthermore, damage to, or occlusion of, the tube by the teeth is avoided. Nasal tracheal intubation does, however, have a number of important disadvantages, including:

■ epistaxis;
■ damage to the nasopharyngeal mucosa (including submucosal insertion of the tube);
■ erosion of the alar cartilages;
■ necrosis of the nasal septum;
■ difficulty with bronchial suction (due to the greater length and increased angle of curvature);
■ increased resistance to gas flow, which may delay or prevent weaning.

Importantly, nasal intubation is associated with an increased risk of *sinusitis* (Bach *et al.*, 1992), as well as *otis media*, and is contraindicated in patients with adjacent facial or skull fractures. On the other hand, ulceration of the corners of the mouth and superadded fungal infection may complicate the

Table 7.4 Indications for tracheostomy
Upper-airway obstruction
Prolonged mechanical ventilation
To facilitate bronchopulmonary toilet
To maintain and protect the airway

use of oral tubes. Also laryngeal injury may be more common with oral, as opposed to nasal, intubation (Stauffer *et al.*, 1981). The choice of route in an individual patient often depends largely on the experience and preference of a particular unit, but currently the oral route is usually preferred in adults.

TRACHEOSTOMY

INDICATIONS (Table 7.4)

The only indication for immediate tracheostomy is a life-threatening obstruction of the upper respiratory tract that cannot be bypassed with an endotracheal tube. Tracheostomy performed under these circumstances can be extremely hazardous, mainly because of engorgement of the blood vessels in the neck. An emergency tracheostomy may also be necessary to secure the airway in patients with head and neck injuries, including burns to the face and upper airway.

As well as providing a secure artificial airway for prolonged respiratory support, tracheostomy may be required for the long-term control of excessive bronchial secretions, particularly in those with a reduced conscious level, and/or to maintain an airway and protect the lungs in those with impaired pharyngeal and laryngeal reflexes. It is important to appreciate that, when patients are extubated following an extended period of translaryngeal intubation, their ability to cough may be impaired by oedema and rigidity of the vocal cords. This may influence the decision to perform a tracheostomy, particularly in those who continue to produce excessive secretions and/or are unable to cooperate fully with physiotherapy.

Potential benefits of tracheostomy include:

- reduced oropharyngeal and laryngeal injury;
- reduced dead space and airway resistance with reduction in the work of breathing;
- facilitates control of secretions;
- improved patient comfort and communication;
- reduced requirement for sedation;
- facilitates mobilization to chair and ambulation;
- oral nutrition may be possible.

Conventionally translaryngeal tracheal intubation is recommended for up to 10 days, whilst tracheostomy is preferred when the need for an artificial airway exceeds 21 days. There is now some evidence, however, that earlier tracheostomy

(within 7 days) may be beneficial by reducing sedation requirements and days on the ventilator and in intensive care (Griffiths *et al.*, 2005). The increasing use of percutaneous tracheostomy (see below) may encourage this approach. Certainly when prolonged dependence on an artificial airway can be confidently predicted (e.g. traumatic cervical cord injury, severe ARDS) early tracheostomy (within 3–5 days) should be seriously considered. The appropriate timing of tracheostomy has, nevertheless, yet to be precisely defined. In an individual patient the decision is governed by a number of considerations, including the presence of relative contraindications to tracheostomy, the degree of discomfort caused by the presence of the endotracheal tube, the extent of difficulties related to tracheal toilet and the anticipated duration of the need for an artificial airway.

CONTRAINDICATIONS

Relative contraindications to tracheostomy include:

- local inflammation, infection or burns injury;
- severe coagulopathy;
- cardiovascular or respiratory instability.

COMPLICATIONS

The incidence of the large number of adverse events which can complicate tracheostomy varies widely between different reports. Many authors have reported a small but significant perioperative mortality associated with tracheostomy (up to 3%), although more recently deaths directly attributable to tracheostomy have become extremely rare (Dulguerov *et al.*, 1999). Potentially lethal perioperative events include *hypoxaemia, hypotension, cardiac arrhythmias, immediate or delayed haemorrhage*.

Early complications

The tracheostomy tube is easily *misplaced* in the pretracheal subcutaneous tissue, particularly during emergency reinsertion in the early postoperative period, leading to mediastinal or subcutaneous emphysema. This danger may be minimized by using a Bjork flap (see below). The tube may *obstruct* if tilted, and *leaks* around the cuff can give rise to *surgical emphysema. Pneumothorax, pneumomediastinum* and *perioperative haemorrhage* are other well-recognized complications (Stauffer *et al.*, 1981).

Intermediate complications

As with translaryngeal tracheal intubation, ulceration of the tracheal mucosa may occur at the level of the cuff and, because a tracheostomy tube is prone to tilting, the mucosa may also be damaged by the tip of the tube. Erosion of the tracheal cartilages and neighbouring structures may lead to fatal *haemorrhage* from the innominate artery or to a *tracheo-oesophageal fistula*.

Tracheostomy wounds are usually colonized with resident bacteria which are often resistant to the commonly used antibiotics. These may cause local *infection*, sometimes with extensive necrosis of the anterior neck, with or without systemic sepsis.

Late complications

Tracheal *narrowing* or *stenosis* may occur at the level of the stoma, the cuff or the tip of the tube; sometimes, the *tracheal rings collapse* at stomal level, a *tracheal granuloma* may develop or there may be *delayed healing* with a *persistent sinus* at the tracheostomy stoma. Cosmetic deformity is common. The incidence of these complications may be decreased by preserving as much tracheal cartilage as possible at operation, correct positioning of the tube and minimizing movement of the tube relative to the trachea.

TECHNIQUES
Surgical

It is important to avoid damaging the cricoid cartilage or first tracheal ring since this renders the larynx unstable. On the other hand, a low tracheostomy increases the risk of erosion of the innominate artery. The trachea should therefore be opened through the second, third and fourth tracheal rings. Ligation and division of the thyroid isthmus are not usually necessary. Duke's modification of the *Bjork flap*, in which an inverted U incision is made in the trachea and the flap is sutured to the lower skin edge, remains a popular technique. It has the advantages of supporting the tracheostomy tube, thereby minimizing erosion of the lower border of the trachea and facilitating reinsertion. Alternatively, a simple *window* of tracheal wall can be removed. Both these methods weaken the tracheal wall and a *vertical slit* is now preferred, the edges of which are held apart with hooks while the tracheostomy tube is inserted. Some use a *T-shaped incision*. In general, however, there are a large number of surgical approaches and there is little information concerning the influence of these various techniques on the incidence of long-term complications. Although most surgeons prefer to perform the procedure in an operating theatre, surgical tracheostomy can be performed safely at the bedside in the ICU.

Percutaneous tracheostomy

Elective percutaneous tracheostomy should be performed with the patient heavily sedated and following administration of a muscle relaxant. Analgesia and sedation may be supplemented by local infiltration with lidocaine. The patient is positioned with a roll between the shoulders to extend the neck; the anterior neck is then cleansed and painted with antiseptic. A transverse incision (approximately 2.5 cm) is made through the skin and subcutaneous tissues midway between the cricoid cartilage and the sternal notch. Curved forceps can be used for blunt dissection of the cervical fascia anterior to the trachea. When using the *sequential dilatation technique* the trachea is punctured with an introducer needle (e.g. 16–17G) between the first and second or second and third tracheal rings. After introducing the catheter into the tracheal lumen the needle is withdrawn and a

J-tipped guidewire is threaded through the catheter. It is recommended that the position and depth of the tracheal puncture, as well as the position of the guidewire, are checked by an assistant with a bronchoscope. A guiding catheter can then be advanced over the guidewire, followed by *serial dilatation* of the stoma with dilators of increasing size. Finally the tracheostomy tube, preloaded on to a dilator of the appropriate size, is advanced over the guidewire and guiding catheter into the tracheal lumen. More recently, a single tapered (conic dilator – the *Blue Rhino*) has been introduced and has been shown to be safe, with an acceptably low incidence of major complications (Fikkers *et al.*, 2002).

The *forceps dilatational technique* involves introducing the forceps over the guidewire and opening the handles of the forceps with the blades in the soft tissue anterior to the trachea. The forceps are then inserted into the trachea and the stoma fully dilated. The tracheostomy tube, mounted on a plastic trochar, is then passed over the guidewire into the trachea. With the *translaryngeal technique* the guidewire is passed retrogradely into the oropharynx, parallel to or within the endotracheal tube. The patient is then reintubated using the small internal diameter tube provided and the wire is connected to the pointed head of the tracheal cannula. The cannula is advanced through the pharynx into the trachea; the pointed head is pulled through the tracheal wall and skin. The pointed head is then cut off, the tracheal cannula is straightened and rotated with an obturator and the smaller endotracheal tube is removed.

Relative contraindications to percutaneous tracheostomy include:

- difficult-to-identify anatomy;
- short neck/rigid cervical spine;
- severe coagulopathy;
- raised intracranial pressure.

The percutaneous technique has a number of potential advantages when compared to the surgical approach. The skin incision is small, disruption of deeper tissues is minimized and there is no tracheal resection. The risk of bleeding, the incidence of infection and scar formation may therefore be reduced. Percutaneous tracheostomy is quicker (average 11.7 minutes) than surgical tracheostomy (average 26.9 minutes) (Dulguerov *et al.*, 1999), is technically easier and can be performed at the bedside, thereby avoiding the hazards of transportation. Fewer personnel and less equipment are required and costs are reduced. It has also been claimed that percutaneous tracheostomy is associated with fewer operative and long-term complications, although when compared to a more recent series of surgical tracheostomies, perioperative complications are in fact more common, whereas postoperative complications are less frequent with the percutaneous approach (Dulguerov *et al.*, 1999). In particular, and perhaps not surprisingly, percutaneous tracheostomy is more frequently complicated by difficulty with tube placement, creation of a false passage and subcutaneous emphysema. Indeed, one meta-analysis has indicated that serious perioperative complications, including operative mortality and cardiorespiratory arrest, may be more common with percutaneous tracheostomy (Dulguerov *et al.*, 1999). On the other hand this review confirmed the reduced incidence of bleeding and infection with percutaneous tracheostomy, but suggested that tracheal stenosis and damage to the tracheal cartilages may be more common with this approach.

Bronchoscopic guidance increases the safety of percutaneous tracheostomy and in particular minimizes the risk of posterior tracheal wall injury. The highest complication rates are associated with techniques not involving progressive dilatation (Dulguerov *et al.*, 1999). Certainly the translaryngeal technique has been associated with a high incidence of unsolvable technical difficulties and serious complications (Cantais *et al.*, 2002). In a large series of bronchoscopically guided, percutaneous dilational tracheostomies there were no procedure-related deaths, the incidence of clinically relevant bleeding was 2.9% and insertion of the tracheostomy tube was easy, or only moderately difficult in 86.7% of cases. The incidence of tracheostomy tube-related complications (defined as hypoxaemia, cannula misplacement, accidental decannulation, cuff rupture and herniation, or posterior tracheal wall lesions) was only 0.7%. The incidence of tracheal ring fracture was higher with conic than with stepwise dilatation (Beiderlinden *et al.*, 2002). These authors also emphasized the importance of avoiding early routine tracheostomy tube changes, which can be particularly difficult following percutaneous tracheostomy, and of secure fixation of the tracheostomy tube.

The use of dilatational techniques for reformation of healed tracheostomies, where distorted anatomy increases the risk of bleeding from major vessels, is controversial. Percutaneous tracheostomy may also be a useful means of rapidly securing the airway in an emergency.

Cricothyroidotomy

The technique of cricothyroidotomy is simple and quick; it is usually reserved for emergencies. A large-bore needle and cannula (e.g. 14G) can be inserted percutaneously via the cricothyroid membrane to provide a temporary route for oxygenation, although ventilation is inefficient and a surgical tracheostomy will normally be required within 30–45 minutes to avoid hypercarbia.

Alternatively a surgical approach via a transverse skin incision allows insertion of a size 6 or 7F tracheostomy or endotracheal tube under direct vision. The percutaneous dilatational technique described above (Barrachina *et al.*, 1996) or the Penlon cricothyrotomy cannula can also be used. The latter technique involves extending the patient's head, making a small skin incision and pushing the cannula blade through the cricothyroid membrane into the trachea. The blade is then retracted and the integral metal dilators advanced and opened, allowing insertion of a tracheostomy tube.

Because the cricothyroid membrane is a relatively avascular area, serious bleeding is rarely a problem with this technique. Pneumothorax is also unusual because of the high approach. Some believe that the incidence of subglottic stenosis and vocal cord paralysis is unacceptably high with cricothyroidotomy.

Minitracheostomy (Ryan, 1990)

A small-diameter (e.g. 4.0-mm) uncuffed tube can be inserted percutaneously via the cricothyroid membrane following infiltration with local anaesthetic. A Seldinger technique, in which the minitracheostomy and a dilator are inserted over a guidewire, is probably safer and less traumatic. This provides a route for repeated tracheobronchial suction using a 10 FG catheter and for the administration of oxygen, while being comfortable and allowing the patient to speak and eat. This technique has also been used in the emergency management of upper-airway obstruction, to administer HFJV and in obstructive sleep apnoea.

Complications include haemorrhage, misplacement in the mediastinum, displacement and surgical emphysema. Minitracheostomy should not be used in patients who are unable to protect their airway or in those with coagulopathy.

TRACHEOSTOMY TUBES

During mechanical ventilation, and for protection against aspiration, a cuffed tracheostomy tube is clearly required. As with endotracheal tubes for long-term use, these should be constructed of non-irritant material and have low-pressure, high-volume cuffs. The tip is normally cut square, rather than bevelled, to decrease the risk of obstruction and mucosal injury.

When the patient's condition has improved, it is usual to deflate the cuff and later change to an uncuffed tube. Traditionally, these were made of silver, which is non-irritant and bactericidal. They had an inner tube which could be removed for cleaning at regular intervals. They could also be modified with a fenestration at the angle of the tube and a one-way flap valve to allow the patient to speak. Plastic uncuffed tubes are now available, some with disposable inner cannulae, both with and without fenestrations. In some cases a cuffed fenestrated tube with an inner cannula may be preferred as a means of protecting the airway while allowing the patient to speak intermittently. Various tracheal 'buttons' are also available to maintain patency of the tracheostomy and provide a route for endotracheal suction. In an attempt to enable mechanically ventilated patients to phonate with the cuff inflated, tracheostomy tubes are available that incorporate an additional small lumen, which allows a separate gas flow to be diverted through the larynx (**Fig. 7.14a**). One-way Passy–Muir speaking valves can also be used in ventilated patients, as well as in those breathing spontaneously (**Fig. 7.14b**). Alternatively, the patient can simply use a finger to occlude the tracheostomy temporarily (**Fig. 7.14c and d**).

MANAGEMENT

A postoperative chest X-ray should be obtained to confirm correct positioning of the tube and exclude a pneumothorax.

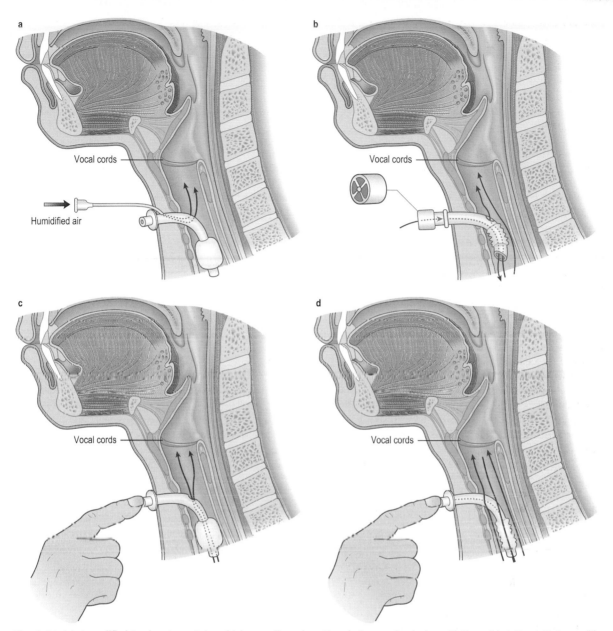

Fig. 7.14 (a) A modified tracheostomy tube which can allow phonation during mechanical ventilation. (b) A Passy–Muir speaking valve with fenestrated tube and cuff deflated. (c) The patient or member of staff can use a finger to occlude the tube during speech, in this case via a fenestrated tube with the cuff inflated. (d) Tracheostomy tube with cuff deflated.

Tracheostomy tubes must be securely fixed, a split-gauze dry dressing is used and the wound cleaned with saline. Wound swabs should be cultured regularly. The tube is left in place for 7 days and then changed every 5–6 days, depending on local policy. Emergency equipment must always be available at the bedside and should include a tracheostomy tube of the same size and one size smaller, as well as a tracheal dilator.

Decannulation

Decannulation is associated with an increase in dead space and a significant increase in the work of breathing (Chadda *et al.*, 2002). Following removal of the tracheostomy tube the stoma should be covered by a dry occlusive dressing and allowed to heal spontaneously. This usually occurs rapidly and within 1–2 days reinsertion of a similar-sized tracheostomy tube is likely to be extremely difficult.

REFERENCES

Agvald-Öhman C, Wernerman J, Nord CE, et al. (2003) Anaerobic bacteria commonly colonize the lower airways of intubated ICU patients. Clinical Microbiology and Infection 9: 397–405.

Al-Saady N, Bennett ED (1985) Decelerating inspiratory flow waveform improves lung mechanics and gas exchange in patients on intermittent positive-pressure ventilation. Intensive Care Medicine 11: 68–75.

Al-Saady NM, Fernando SS, Petros AJ, et al. (1995) External high frequency oscillation in normal subjects and in patients with acute respiratory failure. Anaesthesia 50: 1031–1035.

Antonelli M, Conti G, Rocco M, et al. (1998) A comparison of noninvasive positive-pressure ventilation and conventional mechanical ventilation in patients with acute respiratory failure. New England Journal of Medicine 339: 429–435.

Antonelli M, Pennisi MA, Pelosi P, et al. (2004) Noninvasive positive pressure ventilation using a helmet in patients with acute exacerbation of chronic obstructive pulmonary disease. A feasibility study. Anesthesiology 100: 16–24.

Ashbaugh DG, Petty TL (1973) Positive end-expiratory pressure. Physiology, indications and contraindications. Journal of Thoracic and Cardiovascular Surgery 65: 165–170.

Bach A, Boehrer H, Schmidt H, et al. (1992) Nosocomial sinusitis in ventilated patients. Nasotracheal versus orotracheal intubation. Anaesthesia 47: 335–339.

Baile EM, Albert RK, Kirk W, et al. (1984) Positive end-expiratory pressure decreases bronchial blood flow in the dog. Journal of Applied Physiology 56: 1289–1293.

Barrachina F, Guardiola JJ, Anó T, et al. (1996) Percutaneous dilatational cricothyroidotomy: outcome with 44 consecutive patients. Intensive Care Medicine 22: 937–940.

Beiderlinden M, Walz MK, Sander A, et al. (2002) Complications of bronchoscopically guided percutaneous dilational tracheostomy: beyond the learning curve. Intensive Care Medicine 28: 59–62.

Bergmans DC, Bonten MJ, Gaillard CA, et al. (2001) Prevention of ventilator-associated pneumonia by oral decontamination. A prospective, randomized double-blind, placebo-controlled study. American Journal of Respiratory and Critical Care Medicine 164: 382–388.

Bersten AD, Holt AW, Vedig AE, et al. (1991) Treatment of severe cardiogenic pulmonary edema with continuous positive airway pressure delivered by facemask. New England Journal of Medicine 325: 1825–1830.

Bjorneboe M, Ibsen B, Astrup P, et al. (1955) Active ventilation in treatment of respiratory acidosis in chronic diseases of the lungs. Lancet 269: 901–903.

Boots RJ, Howe S, George N, et al. (1997) Clinical utility of hygroscopic heat and moisture exchangers in intensive care patients. Critical Care Medicine 25: 1707–1712.

Bott J, Carroll MP, Conway JH, et al. (1993) Randomised controlled trial of nasal ventilation in acute ventilatory failure due to chronic obstructive airways disease. Lancet 341: 1555–1557.

Brimioulle S, Rocmans P, de Rood M, et al. (1990) High frequency jet ventilation in the management of tracheal laceration. Critical Care Medicine 18: 338–339.

Brochard L (2000) What is really important to make noninvasive ventilation work. Critical Care Medicine 28: 2139–2140.

Brochard L, Pluskwa F, Lemaire F (1987) Improved efficacy of spontaneous breathing with inspiratory pressure support. American Review of Respiratory Disease 136: 411–415.

Brochard L, Harf A, Lorino H, et al. (1989) Inspiratory pressure support prevents diaphragmatic fatigue during weaning from mechanical ventilation. American Review of Respiratory Disease 139: 513–521.

Brochard L, Isabey D, Piquet J, et al. (1990) Reversal of acute exacerbations of chronic obstructive lung disease by inspiratory assistance with facemask. New England Journal of Medicine 323: 1523–1530.

Brochard L, Rauss A, Benito S, et al. (1994) Comparison of three methods of gradual withdrawal from ventilatory support during weaning from mechanical ventilation. American Journal of Respiratory and Critical Care Medicine 150: 896–903.

Brochard L, Mancebo J, Wysocki M, et al. (1995) Noninvasive ventilation for acute exacerbations of chronic obstructive pulmonary disease. New England Journal of Medicine 333: 817–822.

Brun-Buisson C (2007) Preventing ventilator associated pneumonia. British Medical Journal 334: 861–862.

Canadian Critical Care Trials Group (2006) A randomized trial of diagnostic techniques for ventilator-associated pneumonia. New England Journal of Medicine 355: 2619–2630.

Cantais E, Kaiser E, Le-Goff Y, et al. (2002) Percutaneous tracheostomy: prospective comparison of the translaryngeal technique versus the forceps-dilational technique in 100 critically ill adults. Critical Care Medicine 30: 815–819.

Chadda K, Louis B, Benaisna L, et al. (2002) Physiological effects of decannulation in tracheostomized patients. Intensive Care Medicine 28: 1761–1767.

Chastre J, Wolff M, Fagon J-Y, et al. (2003) Comparison of 8 vs 15 days of antibiotic therapy for ventilator-associated pneumonia in adults. A randomized trial. Journal of the American Medical Association 290: 2588–2598.

Chatila W, Kreimer DT, Criner GJ (2001) Quality of life in survivors of prolonged mechanical ventilatory support. Critical Care Medicine 29: 737–742.

Chishti A, Batchelor AM, Bullock RE, et al. (2000) Sleep-related breathing disorders following discharge from intensive care. Intensive Care Medicine 26: 426–433.

Confalonieri M, Potena A, Carbone G, et al. (1999) Acute respiratory failure in patients with severe community-acquired pneumonia. A prospective randomized evaluation of noninvasive ventilation. American Journal of Respiratory and Critical Care Medicine 160: 1585–1591.

Cook DJ, Reeve BK, Guyatt GH, et al. (1996) Stress ulcer prophylaxis in critically ill patients. Resolving discordant meta-analyses. Journal of the American Medical Association 275: 308–314.

Cook D, Guyatt G, Marshall J, et al. (1998) A comparison of sucralfate and ranitidine for the prevention of upper gastrointestinal bleeding in patients requiring mechanical ventilation. New England Journal of Medicine 338: 791–797.

de Larminat V, Montravers P, Dureuil B, et al. (1995) Alteration in swallowing reflex after extubation in intensive care unit patients. Critical Care Medicine 23: 486–490.

de Lassence A, Alberti C, Azoulay E, et al. (2002) Impact of unplanned extubation and reintubation after weaning on nosocomial pneumonia risk in the intensive care unit. A prospective multicenter study. Anesthesiology 97: 148–156.

Delclaux C, L'Her E, Alberti C, et al. (2000) Treatment of acute hypoxemic nonhypercapnic respiratory insufficiency with continuous positive airway pressure delivered by a facemask. Journal of the American Medical Association 284: 2352–2360.

Derderian SS, Rajagopal KR, Abbrecht PH, et al. (1982) High frequency positive pressure jet ventilation in bilateral bronchopleural fistulae. Critical Care Medicine 10: 119–121.

DeRiso AJ, Ladouski JS, Dillon TA, et al. (1996) Chlorhexidine gluconate 0.12% oral rinse reduces the incidence of total nosocomial respiratory infection and nonprophylactic systemic antibiotic use in patients undergoing heart surgery. Chest 109: 1556–1561.

Dezfulian C, Shojania K, Collard HR, et al. (2005) Subglottic secretion drainage for preventing ventilator-associated pneumonia: a meta-analysis. American Journal of Medicine 118: 11–18.

Douglass JA, Tuxen DV, Horne M, et al. (1992) Myopathy in severe asthma. American Review of Respiratory Disease 146: 517–519.

Downs JB, Klein EF Jr, Desautels D, et al. (1973) Intermittent mandatory ventilation: a new approach to weaning patients from mechanical ventilators. Chest 64: 331–335.

Drakulovic MB, Torres A, Bauer TT, et al. (1999) Supine body position as a risk factor for nosocomial pneumonia in mechanically ventilated patients: a randomised trial. Lancet 354: 1851–1858.

Dreyfuss D, Soler P, Basset G, et al. (1988) High inflation pressure pulmonary edema. Respective effects of high airway pressure, high tidal volume, and positive end-expiratory pressure. American Review of Respiratory Disease 137: 1159–1164.

Dulguerov P, Gysin C, Perneger TV, et al. (1999) Percutanous or surgical tracheostomy: a meta-analysis. Critical Care Medicine 27: 1617–1625.

Ely EW, Baker AM, Dunagan DP, et al. (1996) Effect on the duration of mechanical ventilation of identifying patients capable of breathing spontaneously. New England Journal of Medicine 335: 1864–1869.

Esteban A, Frutos F, Tobin MJ, et al. (1995) A comparison of four methods of weaning patients from mechanical ventilation. New England Journal of Medicine 332: 345–350.

Esteban A, Alia I, Tobin MJ, et al. (1999) Effect of spontaneous breathing trial duration on outcome of attempts to discontinue mechanical ventilation. American Journal of Respiratory and Critical Care Medicine 159: 512–518.

Esteban A, Anzueto A, Alia I, et al. (2000) How is mechanical ventilation employed in the intensive care unit? An international utilization review. American Journal of Respiratory and Critical Care Medicine 161: 1450–1458.

Esteban A, Frutos-Vivar F, Ferguson ND, *et al.* (2004) Noninvasive positive-pressure ventilation for respiratory failure after extubation. *New England Journal of Medicine* **350**: 2452–2460.

Fabry B, Haberthur C, Zappe D, *et al.* (1997) Breathing pattern and additional work of breathing in spontaneously breathing patients with different ventilatory demands during inspiratory pressure support and automatic tube compensation. *Intensive Care Medicine* **23**: 545–552.

Farge D, de la Coussaye JE, Beloucif S, *et al.* (1995) Interactions between hemodynamic and hormonal modifications during PEEP-induced antidiuresis and antinatriuresis. *Chest* **107**: 1095–1100.

Feeley TW, Hedley-Whyte J (1975) Weaning from controlled ventilation and supplemental oxygen. *New England Journal of Medicine* **292**: 903–906.

Feeley TW, Saumarez R, Klick JM, *et al.* (1975) Positive end-expiratory pressure is weaning patients from controlled ventilation. A prospective randomised trial. *Lancet* **2**: 725–729.

Fernández MM, Villagrá A, Blanch L, *et al.* (2001) Non-invasive mechanical ventilation in status asthmaticus. *Intensive Care Medicine* **27**: 486–492.

Fernandez Mondéjar E, Vazquez Mata G, Cárdenas A, *et al.* (1996) Ventilation with positive end-expiratory pressure reduces extravascular lung water and increases lymphatic flow in hydrostatic pulmonary edema. *Critical Care Medicine* **24**: 1562–1567.

Ferrer M, Bauer TT, Torres A, *et al.* (1999) Effect of nasogastric tube size on gastroesophageal reflux and microaspiration in intubated patients. *Annals of Internal Medicine* **130**: 991–994.

Ferrer M, Esquinas A, Arancibia F, *et al.* (2003a) Noninvasive ventilation during persistent weaning failure. A randomized controlled trial. *American Journal of Respiratory and Critical Care Medicine* **168**: 70–76.

Ferrer M, Esquinas A, Leon M, *et al.* (2003b) Noninvasive ventilation in severe hypoxemic respiratory failure. A randomized clinical trial. *American Journal of Respiratory and Critical Care Medicine* **168**: 1438–1444.

Fikkers BG, Briedè IS, Verwiel JM, *et al.* (2002) Percutaneous tracheostomy with the Blue Rhino™ technique: presentation of 100 consecutive patients. *Anaesthesia* **57**: 1094–1097.

Fisher MM, Raper RF (1992) The 'cuff-leak' test for extubation. *Anaesthesia* **47**: 10–12.

Fort P, Farmer C, Westerman J, *et al.* (1997) High-frequency oscillatory ventilation for adult respiratory distress syndrome. A pilot study. *Critical Care Medicine* **25**: 937–947.

Francois B, Bellissant E, Gissot V, *et al.* (2007) 12-h pretreatment with methylprednisolone versus placebo for prevention of postextubation laryngeal oedema: a randomized double-blind trial. *Lancet* **369**: 1083–1089.

Gainnier M, Roch A, Forel J-M, *et al.* (2004) Effect of neuromuscular blocking agents on gas exchange in patients presenting with acute respiratory distress syndrome. *Critical Care Medicine* **32**: 113–119.

Gajic O, Frutos-Vivar F, Esteban A, *et al.* (2005) Ventilator settings as a risk factor for acute respiratory distress syndrome in mechanically ventilated patients. *Intensive Care Medicine* **31**: 922–926.

Gattinoni L, Agostoni, A, Pesenti A, *et al.* (1980) Treatment of acute respiratory failure with low-frequency positive-pressure ventilation and extracorporeal removal of $CO_{2\wedge}$. *Lancet* **2**: 292–294.

Gattinoni L, Pesenti A, Mascheroni D, *et al.* (1986) Low-frequency positive-pressure ventilation with extracorporeal CO_2 removal in severe acute respiratory failure. *Journal of the American Medical Association* **256**: 881–886.

Gibot S, Cravoisy A, Levy B, *et al.* (2004) Soluble triggering receptor expressed on myeloid cells and the diagnosis of pneumonia. *New England Journal of Medicine* **350**: 451–458.

Girard TD, Kress JP, Fuchs BD, *et al.* (2008) Efficacy and safety of a paired sedation and ventilator weaning protocol for mechanically ventilated patients in intensive care (Awakening and breathing controlled trial). *Lancet* **371**: 126–134.

Girault C, Daudenthun I, Chevron V, *et al.* (1999) Noninvasive ventilation as a systematic extubation and weaning technique in acute-on-chronic respiratory failure. A prospective, randomized controlled study. *American Journal of Respiratory and Critical Care Medicine* **160**: 86–92.

Girou E, Schortgen F, Delclaux C, *et al.* (2000) Association of noninvasive ventilation with nosocomial infections and survival in critically ill patients. *Journal of the American Medical Association* **284**: 2361–2367.

Gluck E, Heard S, Patel C, *et al.* (1993) Use of ultrahigh frequency ventilation in patients with ARDS. A preliminary report. *Chest* **103**: 1413–1420.

Greenbaum DM, Millen JE, Eross B, *et al.* (1976) Continuous positive airway pressure without tracheal intubation in spontaneously breathing patients. *Chest* **69**: 615–620.

Griffiths J, Barber VS, Morgan L, *et al.* (2005) Systematic review and meta-analysis of studies of the timing of tracheostomy in adult patients undergoing artificial ventilation. *British Medical Journal* **330**: 1243.

Guttmann J, Bernhard H, Mols G, *et al.* (1997) Respiratory comfort of automatic tube compensation and inspiratory pressure support in conscious humans. *Intensive Care Medicine* **23**: 1119–1124.

Hewlett AM, Platt AS, Terry VG (1977) Mandatory minute volume. A new concept in weaning from mechanical ventilation. *Anaesthesia* **32**: 163–169.

Hilbert G, Gruson D, Vargas F, *et al.* (2001) Noninvasive ventilation in immunosuppressed patients with pulmonary infiltrates, fever and acute respiratory failure. *New England Journal of Medicine* **344**: 481–487.

Hillman KM, Barber JD (1980) Asynchronous independent lung ventilation (AILV). *Critical Care Medicine* **8**: 390–395.

Ho LI, Harn HJ, Lien TC, *et al.* (1996) Postextubation laryngeal edema in adults. Risk factor evaluation and prevention by hydrocortisone. *Intensive Care Medicine* **22**: 933–936.

Holliday JE, Hyers TM (1990) The reduction of weaning time from mechanical ventilation using tidal volume and relaxation biofeedback. *American Review of Respiratory Disease* **141**: 1214–1220.

Hurst JM, Branson RD, Davis K Jr, *et al.* (1990) Comparison of conventional mechanical ventilation and high-frequency ventilation. *Annals of Surgery* **211**: 486–491.

Ibrahim EH, Mehringer L, Prentice D, *et al.* (2002a) Early versus late enteral feeding of mechanically ventilated patients: results of a clinical trial. *Journal of Parenteral and Enteral Nutrition* **26**: 174–181.

Ibrahim EH, Iregui M, Prentice D, *et al.* (2002b) Deep vein thrombosis during prolonged mechanical ventilation despite prophylaxis. *Critical Care Medicine* **30**: 771–774.

Iregui M, Ward S, Sherman S, *et al.* (2002) Clinical importance of delays in the initiation of appropriate antibiotic treatment for ventilator-associated pneumonia. *Chest* **122**: 262–268.

Jardin F, Farcot J-C, Boisante L, *et al.* (1981) Influence of positive end-expiratory pressure on left ventricular performance. *New England Journal of Medicine* **304**: 387–392.

Jenkinson C, Davies RJ, Mullins R, *et al.* (1999) Comparison of therapeutic and subtherapeutic nasal continuous positive airway pressure for obstructive sleep apnoea: a randomised prospective parallel trial. *Lancet* **353**: 2100–2105.

Jubran A, Tobin MJ (1997a) Pathophysiologic basis of acute respiratory distress in patients who fail a trial of weaning from mechanical ventilation. *American Journal of Respiratory and Critical Care Medicine* **155**: 906–915.

Jubran A, Tobin MJ (1997b) Passive mechanics of lung and chest wall in patients who failed or succeeded in trials of weaning. *American Journal of Respiratory and Critical Care Medicine* **155**: 916–921.

Katz JA, Marks JD (1985) Inspiratory work with and without continuous positive airway pressure in patients with acute respiratory failure. *Anesthesiology* **63**: 598–607.

Kollef MH (1999) The prevention of ventilator-associated pneumonia. *New England Journal of Medicine* **340**: 627–634.

Kollef MH, Rello J, Cammarata SK, *et al.* (2004) Clinical cure and survival in gram-positive ventilator-associated pneumonia: retrospective analysis of two double blind studies comparing linezolid with vancomycin. *Intensive Care Medicine* **30**: 388–394.

Krieger BP, Ershowsky PF, Becker DA, *et al.* (1989) Evaluation of conventional criteria for predicting successful weaning from mechanical ventilatory support in elderly patients. *Critical Care Medicine* **17**: 858–861.

Krishnan JA, Moore D, Robeson C, *et al.* (2004) A prospective, controlled trial of a protocol-based strategy to discontinue mechanical ventilation. *American Journal of Respiratory and Critical Care Medicine* **169**: 673–678.

Laffey JG, Tanaka M, Engelberts D, *et al.* (2000) Therapeutic hypercapnia reduces pulmonary and systemic injury following in vivo lung reperfusion. *American Journal of Respiratory and Critical Care Medicine* **162**: 2287–2294.

Lassen HC (1953) A preliminary report on the 1952 epidemic of poliomyelitis in Copenhagen with special reference to the treatment of acute respiratory insufficiency. *Lancet* **1**: 37–41.

Leithner C, Frass M, Pacher R, *et al.* (1987) Mechanical ventilation with positive end expiratory pressure decreases release of alpha-atrial natriuretic peptide. *Critical Care Medicine* **15**: 484–488.

Lellouche F, Mancebo J, Jolliet P, *et al.* (2006) A multicenter randomized trial of computer-driven protocolized weaning from mechanical ventilation. *American Journal of Respiratory and Critical Care Medicine* **174**: 894–900.

Lichtenstein D, Hulot J-S, Rabiller A, *et al.* (1999) Feasibility and safety of ultrasound-aided thoracocentesis in mechanically ventilated patients. *Intensive Care Medicine* 25: 955–958.

Lindholm CE, Grenvik A (1977) Flexible fibreoptic bronchoscopy and intubation in intensive care. In: Ledingham IMCA (ed.) *Recent Advances in Intensive Therapy 1*, pp. 47–66. Churchill Livingstone: Edinburgh.

Lorente L, Lecuona M, Martin MM, *et al.* (2005) Ventilator-associated pneumonia using a closed versus an open tracheal suction system. *Critical Care Medicine* 33: 115–119.

Luna CM, Vujacich P, Niderman MS, *et al.* (1997) Impact of BAL data on the therapy and outcome of ventilator-associated pneumonia. *Chest* 111: 676–685.

MacIntyre NR, Cook DJ, Ely EW Jr, *et al.* (2001) Evidence-based guidelines for weaning and discontinuing ventilatory support. *Chest* 120: 375S–395S.

Markowicz P, Wolff M, Djedaini K, *et al.* (2000) Multicenter prospective study of ventilator-associated pneumonia during acute respiratory distress syndrome. Incidence, prognosis and risk factors. *American Journal of Respiratory and Critical Care Medicine* 161: 1942–1948.

Martin TJ, Hovis JD, Costantino JP, *et al.* (2000) A randomized, prospective evaluation of noninvasive ventilation for acute respiratory failure. *American Journal of Respiratory and Critical Care Medicine* 161: 807–813.

Masip J, Betbesé AJ, Pàez J, *et al.* (2000) Non-invasive pressure support ventilation versus conventional oxygen therapy in acute cardiogenic pulmonary oedema: a randomised trial. *Lancet* 356: 2126–2132.

Meduri GU, Abou-Shala N, Fox RC, *et al.* (1991) Noninvasive facemask mechanical ventilation in patients with acute hypercapnic respiratory failure. *Chest* 100: 445–454.

Michard F, Chemla D, Richard C, *et al.* (1999) Clinical use of respiratory changes in arterial pulse pressure to monitor the hemodynamic effects of PEEP. *American Journal of Respiratory and Critical Care Medicine* 159: 935–939.

Montgomery AB, Holle RH, Neagley SR, *et al.* (1987) Prediction of successful ventilator weaning using airway occlusion pressure and hypercapnic challenge. *Chest* 91: 496–499.

Morris AH, Wallace CJ, Menlove RL, *et al.* (1994) Randomized clinical trial of pressure-controlled inverse ratio ventilation and extracorporeal CO_2 removal for adult respiratory distress syndrome. *American Journal of Respiratory and Critical Care Medicine* 149: 295–305.

Nava S, Ambrosino N, Clini E, *et al.* (1998) Noninvasive mechanical ventilation in the weaning of patients with respiratory failure due to chronic obstructive pulmonary disease: a randomized, controlled trial. *Annals of Internal Medicine* 128: 721–728.

Nava S, Carbone G, DiBattista N, *et al.* (2003) Noninvasive ventilation in cardiogenic pulmonary edema. A multicenter randomized trial. *American Journal of Respiratory and Critical Care Medicine* 168: 1432–1437.

Navaratnarajah M, Nunn JF, Lyons D, *et al.* (1984) Bronchiolectasis caused by positive end-expiratory pressure. *Critical Care Medicine* 12: 1036–1038.

Papazian L, Bregeon F, Thirion X, *et al.* (1996) Effect of ventilator-associated pneumonia on mortality and morbidity. *American Journal of Respiratory and Critical Care Medicine* 154: 91–97.

Park M, Sangean MC, Volpe Mde S, *et al.* (2004) Randomized, prospective trial of oxygen, continuous positive airway pressure and bilevel positive airway pressure by facemask in acute cardiogenic pulmonary edema. *Critical Care Medicine* 32: 2407–2415.

Payen DM, Farge D, Beloucif S, *et al.* (1987) Involvement of antidiuretic hormone in acute antidiuresis during PEEP ventilation in humans. *Anesthesiology* 66: 17–23.

Pepe PE, Hudson LD, Carrico CJ (1984) Early application of positive end-expiratory pressure in patients at risk for the adult respiratory distress syndrome. *New England Journal of Medicine* 311: 281–286.

Peter JV, Moran JL, Phillips-Hughes J, *et al.* (2002) Noninvasive ventilation in acute respiratory failure – a meta-analysis update. *Critical Care Medicine* 30: 555–562.

Peter JV, Moran JL, Phillips-Hughes J, *et al.* (2006) Effect of non-invasive positive pressure ventilation (NIPPV) on mortality in patients with acute cardiogenic pulmonary oedema: a meta-analysis. *Lancet* 367: 1155–1163.

Petrof BJ, Legare M, Goldberg P, *et al.* (1990) Continuous positive airway pressure reduces work of breathing and dyspnea during weaning from mechanical ventilation in severe chronic obstructive pulmonary disease. *American Review of Respiratory Disease* 141: 281–289.

Pinhu L, Whitehead T, Evans T, *et al.* (2003) Ventilator-associated lung injury. *Lancet* 361: 332–340.

Pittet D, Bonten MJ (2000) Towards invasive diagnostic techniques as standard management of ventilator-associated pneumonia. *Lancet* 356: 874.

Plant PK, Owen JL, Elliott MW (2000) Early use of non-invasive ventilation for acute exacerbations of chronic obstructive pulmonary disease on general respiratory wards: a multicentre randomised controlled trial. *Lancet* 355: 1931–1935.

Plant PK, Owen JL, Elliott MW (2001) Non-invasive ventilation in acute exacerbations of chronic obstructive pulmonary disease: long term survival and predictors of in-hospital outcome. *Thorax* 56: 708–712.

Plant PK, Owen JL, Parrott S, *et al.* (2003) Cost effectiveness of ward based non-invasive ventilation for acute exacerbations of chronic obstructive pulmonary disease: economic analysis of randomised controlled trial. *British Medical Journal* 326: 956.

Putensen C, Mutz NJ, Putensen-Himmer N, *et al.* (1999) Spontaneous breathing during ventilatory support improves ventilation–perfusion distributions in patients with acute respiratory distress syndrome. *American Journal of Respiratory and Critical Care Medicine* 159: 1241–1248.

Putensen C, Zech S, Wrigge H, *et al.* (2001) Long-term effects of spontaneous breathing during ventilatory support in patients with acute lung injury. *American Journal of Respiratory and Critical Care Medicine* 164: 43–49.

Qvist J, Pontoppidan H, Wilson RS, *et al.* (1975) Hemodynamic responses to mechanical ventilation with PEEP: the effect of hypervolemia. *Anesthesiology* 42: 45–55.

Ranieri VM, Guiliani R, Mascia L, *et al.* (1996) Patient–ventilator interaction during acute hypercapnia: pressure-support vs proportional-assist ventilation. *Journal of Applied Physiology* 81: 426–436.

Rello J, Diaz E, Roque M, *et al.* (1999a) Risk factors for developing pneumonia within 48 hours of intubation. *American Journal of Respiratory and Critical Care Medicine* 159: 1742–1746.

Rello J, Sa-Borges M, Correa H, *et al.* (1999b) Variations in etiology of ventilator-associated pneumonia across four treatment sites. Implications for antimicrobial prescribing practices. *American Journal of Respiratory and Critical Care Medicine* 160: 608–613.

Rohlfing BM, Webb WR, Schlobohm RM (1976) Ventilator-related extra-alveolar air in adults. *Radiology* 121: 25–31.

Rotondi AJ, Chelluri L, Sirio C, *et al.* (2002) Patients' recollections of stressful experiences while receiving prolonged mechanical ventilation in an intensive care unit. *Critical Care Medicine* 30: 746–752.

Ruiz M, Torres A, Ewig S, *et al.* (2000) Noninvasive versus invasive microbial investigation in ventilator-associated pneumonia. Evaluation of outcome. *American Journal of Respiratory and Critical Care Medicine* 162: 119–125.

Ryan DW (1990) Minitracheotomy. *British Medical Journal* 300: 958–959.

Sahn SA, Lakshminarayan S (1973) Bedside criteria for discontinuation of mechanical ventilation. *Chest* 63: 1002–1005.

Salam A, Tilluckdharry L, Amoateng-Adjepong Y, *et al.* (2004) Neurologic status, cough, secretions and extubation outcomes. *Intensive Care Medicine* 30: 1334–1339.

Schönhofer B, Böhrer H, Köhler D (1998) Blood transfusion facilitating difficult weaning from the ventilator. *Anaesthesia* 53: 181–184.

Schulman DS, Biondi JW, Matthay RA, *et al.* (1988) Effect of positive end-expiratory pressure on right ventricular performance. Importance of baseline right ventricular function. *American Journal of Medicine* 84: 57–67.

Segredo V, Caldwell JE, Matthay MA, *et al.* (1992) Persistent paralysis in critically ill patients after long-term administration of vecuronium. *New England Journal of Medicine* 327: 524–528.

Sha M, Saito Y, Yokoyama K, *et al.* (1987) Effects of continuous positive-pressure ventilation on hepatic blood flow and intrahepatic oxygen delivery in dogs. *Critical Care Medicine* 15: 1040–1043.

Shorr AF, Sherner JH, Jackson WL, *et al.* (2005) Invasive approaches to the diagnosis of ventilator-associated pneumonia: a meta-analysis. *Critical Care Medicine* 33: 46–53.

Simonneau G, Lemaire F, Harf A, *et al.* (1982) A comparative study of the cardiorespiratory effects of continuous positive airway pressure breathing and continuous positive pressure ventilation in acute respiratory failure. *Intensive Care Medicine* 8: 61–67.

Singer M, Bennett D (1989) Optimisation of positive end expiratory pressure for maximal delivery of oxygen to tissues using oesophageal Doppler ultrasonography. *British Medical Journal* 298: 1350–1353.

Sinclair SE, Kregenow DA, Lamm WJ, *et al.* (2002) Hypercapnic acidosis is protective in an in vivo model of ventilator-induced lung injury. *American Journal of Respiratory and Critical Care Medicine* **166**: 403–408.

Skillman JJ, Malhotra IV, Pallotta JA, *et al.* (1971) Determinants of weaning from controlled ventilation. *Surgical Forum* **22**: 198–200.

Slavin G, Nunn JF, Crow J, *et al.* (1982) Bronchiolectasis – a complication of artificial ventilation. *British Medical Journal* **285**: 931–934.

Smith TC, Marini JJ (1988) Impact of PEEP on lung mechanics and work of breathing in severe airflow obstruction. *Journal of Applied Physiology* **65**: 1488–1499.

Smulders K, van der Hoeven H, Weers-Pothoff I, *et al.* (2002) A randomized clinical trial of intermittent subglottic secretion drainage in patients receiving mechanical ventilation. *Chest* **121**: 858–862.

Stauffer JL, Olson DE, Petty TL (1981) Complications and consequences of endotracheal intubation and tracheotomy. *American Journal of Medicine* **70**: 65–76.

Straus C, Louis B, Isabey D, *et al.* (1998) Contribution of the endotracheal tube and the upper airway to breathing workload. *American Journal of Respiratory and Critical Care Medicine* **157**: 23–30.

Sydow M, Golisch W, Buscher H, *et al.* (1995) Effect of low-level PEEP on inspiratory work of breathing in intubated patients, both with healthy lungs and with COPD. *Intensive Care Medicine* **21**: 887–895.

Tanios MA, Nevins ML, Hendra KP, *et al.* (2006) A randomized, controlled trial of the role of weaning predictors in clinical decision making. *Critical Care Medicine* **34**: 2530–2535.

Teba L, Dedhia HV, Schiebel FG, *et al.* (1990) Positive-pressure ventilation with positive end-expiratory pressure and atrial natriuretic peptide release. *Critical Care Medicine* **18**: 831–835.

Tharratt RS, Allen RP, Albertson TE (1988) Pressure controlled inverse ratio ventilation in severe adult respiratory failure. *Chest* **94**: 755–762.

Thorens J-B, Kaelin RM, Jolliet P, *et al.* (1995) Influence of the quality of nursing on the duration of weaning from mechanical ventilation in patients with chronic obstructive pulmonary disease. *Critical Care Medicine* **23**: 1807–1815.

Tobin MJ (2001) Advances in mechanical ventilation. *New England Journal of Medicine* **344**: 1986–1996.

Venus B, Jacobs HK, Lim L (1979) Treatment of the adult respiratory distress syndrome with continuous positive airway pressure. *Chest* **76**: 257–261.

Weg JG, Anzueto A, Balk RA, *et al.* (1998) The relation of pneumothorax and other air leaks to mortality in acute respiratory distress syndrome. *New England Journal of Medicine* **338**: 341–346.

Yang KL, Tobin MJ (1991) A prospective study of indexes predicting the outcome of trials of weaning from mechanical ventilation. *New England Journal of Medicine* **324**: 1445–1450.

Young PJ, Ridley SA (1999) Ventilator-associated pneumonia. Diagnosis, pathogenesis and prevention. *Anaesthesia* **54**: 1183–1197.

Young PJ, Basson C, Hamilton D, *et al.* (1999) Prevention of tracheal aspiration using the pressure-limited tracheal tube cuff. *Anaesthesia* **54**: 559–563.

Zapol WM, Snider MT, Hill JD, *et al.* (1979) Extracorporeal membrane oxygenation in severe acute respiratory failure. A randomized prospective study. *Journal of the American Medical Association* **242**: 2193–2196.

8 Respiratory failure

DEFINITION

Respiratory failure occurs when pulmonary gas exchange is sufficiently impaired to cause hypoxaemia (conventionally $P_aO_2 < 8$ kPa or 60 mmHg) with or without hypercarbia (conventionally $P_aCO_2 > 7$ kPa or 55 mmHg).

TYPES, MECHANISMS AND CLINICAL FEATURES

The respiratory system consists of a gas-exchanging organ (the lungs) and a ventilatory pump (respiratory muscles/thorax), either or both of which can fail and precipitate respiratory failure.

ACUTE HYPOXAEMIC (TYPE I) RESPIRATORY FAILURE

Acute hypoxaemic (type I) respiratory failure (ARF) is caused by diseases that interfere with gas exchange by damaging lung tissue. Hypoxaemia is due to right-to-left shunts, ventilation/perfusion (V/Q) mismatch or, most often, a combination of these two. As discussed in Chapter 3, barriers to diffusion are almost never an important cause of hypoxaemia. An increase in right-to-left shunt occurs when alveoli are completely collapsed, become totally consolidated or are filled with oedema fluid. V/Q inequalities result from pulmonary parenchymal disease that causes regional variations in compliance, an increased scatter of time constants (see Chapter 3) and/or abnormalities of perfusion. Also, functional residual capacity (FRC) is reduced so that tidal exchange takes place below closing volume (i.e. airway closure is present throughout the respiratory cycle), an abnormality that is associated with an increase in the number of relatively underventilated lung units.

Initially, there is usually an increase in total ventilation, which compensates for the increased dead space (V_D) and maintains P_aCO_2 at normal levels. Indeed, relative hyperventilation, possibly in response to severe hypoxaemia and/or stimulation of irritant and mechanoreceptors within the lungs, may cause a reduction in P_aCO_2. The degree of hypoxaemia is limited by constriction of vessels supplying those alveoli with a low PO_2 – *hypoxic pulmonary vasoconstriction* – although the intensity of this response is very variable and appears to be genetically determined (see Chapter 3).

As well as the impairment of gas-exchanging properties, the lungs deteriorate mechanically with a reduction in compliance (associated with the fall in FRC; see Chapter 3) and/or an increase in resistance, so that the work and metabolic cost of breathing are increased. Under these circumstances, patients find it easier to breathe rapidly with a low tidal volume (V_T). Finally, these patients are often pyrexial, with a raised metabolic rate, and this further increases both oxygen consumption ($\dot{V}O_2$) and the volume of carbon dioxide that has to be excreted. Therefore the characteristic clinical features of ARF include:

- hypoxia;
- hypocarbia;
- tachypnoea;
- small V_T.

In contrast to the normal pattern of ventilation, there is little moment-to-moment variation in either respiratory rate or V_I.

VENTILATORY (TYPE II) RESPIRATORY FAILURE

Ventilatory failure occurs when alveolar ventilation is insufficient to excrete the volume of carbon dioxide being produced by tissue metabolism. Carbon dioxide is therefore retained, producing an increase in both arterial and alveolar PCO_2. Due to the operation of the alveolar gas equation (see Chapter 3, equation 3.16), this inevitably leads to a fall in alveolar oxygen tension (P_AO_2) and, when breathing air, hypoxaemia, even in patients with normal lungs. Inadequate alveolar ventilation may be due to:

- reduced ventilatory effort;
- inability to overcome an increased resistance to ventilation;
- failure to compensate for an increase in V_D and/or carbon dioxide production;
- a combination of these factors.

The respiratory muscles have a large reserve, however, and considerable impairment of function may be present without ventilatory failure. Characteristic clinical features of pure ventilatory failure, therefore, include:

- hypercarbia;
- hypoxia;
- a reduced rate and/or depth of breathing.

These patients may suffer from an extremely distressing sensation of breathlessness, even when ventilation is apparently adequate (e.g. judged by blood gas values).

MIXED RESPIRATORY FAILURE

Often, the two types of respiratory failure are combined to produce a mixed picture. As discussed above, acute diseases of the pulmonary parenchyma initially cause purely hypoxaemic respiratory failure. In some cases, however, exhaustion eventually supervenes; the patient is then unable to overcome the mechanical impairment of lung function and cannot compensate for the increased V_D and carbon dioxide production. At this stage, the P_aCO_2 begins to rise, leading to a picture of mixed respiratory failure.

Ventilatory failure is often complicated by the subsequent development of pulmonary abnormalities. This is because these patients are unable to cough effectively, sigh or take deep breaths, and are therefore at risk of alveolar collapse, retention of secretions and secondary infection. In those with an associated bulbar palsy, aspiration can occur and further damage the lungs.

RESPIRATORY MUSCLE DYSFUNCTION

Respiratory muscle fatigue (see Chapter 3) has been demonstrated in healthy subjects submitted to high inspiratory resistive loads and may also play a role in the development of respiratory failure, although overt respiratory muscle fatigue is probably unusual and the underlying mechanisms are not yet fully understood. Increased 'fatigability', of the sternomastoid muscle has, however, been demonstrated in patients with severe respiratory disease on admission to hospital (Efthimiou et al., 1987), and this appeared to resolve as the patient recovered. It was suggested that respiratory muscle fatigue had contributed to hypercapnia in these patients, although the exact significance of these findings remains unclear. It has also been postulated that chronic respiratory muscle fatigue, a poorly understood phenomenon, may contribute to the development of hypercapnia in chronic respiratory failure.

Predisposing factors to the development of respiratory muscle fatigue include:

- an increased load (e.g. imposed by airways obstruction, a reduction in lung compliance or chest wall abnormalities);
- muscle weakness related to neuromuscular disorders (see Chapters 3 and 15), disuse atrophy, malnutrition, generalized wasting or old age.

Muscle dysfunction may be exacerbated by:

- sepsis;
- metabolic disturbances;
- hypoxaemia;
- hypercarbia;
- hyperinflation (see later).

In addition, profound *reductions in respiratory muscle blood flow*, such as may occur in cardiogenic shock, can lead to impaired respiratory muscle contraction in the face of increased excitation, especially when combined with the increased demands imposed by compensatory hyperventilation and pulmonary oedema (Aubier et al., 1981).

Mechanisms that may mediate fatigue include:

- inhibition of neural drive;
- impaired neuromuscular transmission;
- excessive force and duration of contraction;
- impaired excitation–contraction coupling;
- depletion of muscle energy stores;
- failure of the contractile machinery.

Two types of muscle fatigue can be identified:

- *high-frequency fatigue*, which is thought to be due to impaired neuromuscular transmission and/or propagation of the action potential;
- *low-frequency fatigue*, which may reflect impaired excitation–contraction coupling.

Although high-frequency nerve stimulation generates maximum muscle tension, the force of contraction rapidly falls when it persists. If this high-frequency fatigue were allowed to develop in the respiratory muscles there would be a rapid and catastrophic loss of ventilatory capacity. Lower-frequency stimulation produces less initial force, but tension is well maintained and soon exceeds that generated by high-frequency stimulation. Low-frequency fatigue of respiratory muscles, which experimentally is long-lasting and associated with muscle fibre damage, may be an important component of ventilatory failure, but is only precipitated by massive overload and has proved difficult to demonstrate clinically. It may be that neither low-frequency fatigue, with muscle damage, nor high-frequency fatigue, with the rapid onset of extreme respiratory failure, occurs readily because the central nervous system will not (or cannot) drive the peripheral contractile apparatus sufficiently hard (Moxham, 1990). Moreover, in patients with congestive cardiac failure or severe chronic obstructive pulmonary disease (COPD) the proportion of slow-twitch fibres decreases, an adaptation which may increase the resistance of the diaphragm to fatigue and is probably a response to constant moderate exercise (Levine et al., 1997). Interestingly, in one study patients with COPD did not develop low-frequency diaphragmatic fatigue when exercised to exhaustion (Polkey et al., 1995).

The role of *central fatigue* in respiratory failure is uncertain, but it may be that respiratory drive is modified to avoid not only central, but also high-frequency and low-frequency fatigue and thereby optimize ventilation, albeit at the cost of hypercapnia. Ventilatory failure may therefore be the result of a reduction in central drive, which is intended to protect the respiratory muscles from overload and fatigue. For example, during weaning from mechanical ventilation, if the load is excessive and unsustainable, patients breathe rapidly with a low V_T. This reduces the work of breathing, but at the expense of carbon dioxide retention.

Clinical features of respiratory muscle fatigue

It has been suggested that tachypnoea, asynchronous or paradoxical respiration, respiratory alternans and eventually a rising P_aCO_2 with a reduction in respiratory rate and minute volume are indicative of respiratory muscle fatigue. In *asynchronous respiration* there is a discrepancy in the rate of movement of the thoracic and abdominal compartments, while in *paradoxical respiration* they move in opposite directions. *Respiratory alternans* is caused by recruitment and derecruitment of the accessory/intercostal muscles and the diaphragm, leading to an increase in the breath-to-breath variation in the relative contribution of the ribcage and abdomen to V_T.

At present, however, there is no convincing evidence that any particular constellation of physical signs can serve as a sensitive or specific marker of respiratory muscle fatigue. The detection of an abnormal pattern of thoracoabdominal motion does, however, suggest a significantly increased respiratory load. Objective measures of respiratory muscle strength and fatigue are discussed in Chapter 7.

CAUSES OF RESPIRATORY FAILURE

Respiratory failure is commonly precipitated by:

- surgical operations (particularly upper abdominal or thoracic);
- acute respiratory tract infections;
- the administration of depressant drugs.

The causes of respiratory failure can best be considered according to anatomical location (**Fig. 8.1**).

RESPIRATORY CENTRE

Causes of depression of the respiratory centre commonly seen in the intensive care unit (ICU) include:

- raised intracranial pressure or direct trauma (e.g. head injury);
- infections (e.g. meningoencephalitis);
- vascular lesions;
- drug overdose (e.g. narcotics, barbiturates).

Patients in traumatic coma with intracranial hypertension may also have associated pulmonary oedema, lung contusion or aspiration pneumonia. Frequently, the laryngeal reflexes are also depressed and in some cases there may be a true bulbar palsy. Both predispose the patient to aspiration

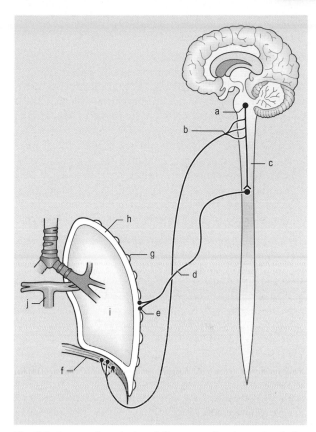

Fig. 8.1 Causes of respiratory failure according to anatomical location. a, Respiratory centre; b, phrenic nerve; c, spinal cord; d, motor nerves; e, neuromuscular junction; f, muscle; g, chest wall; h, pleura; i, lungs and airways; j, pulmonary circulation.

pneumonitis. Severe hypoxia and extreme hypercarbia can also reduce the responsiveness of the respiratory centre.

Sleep-related respiratory disturbances
CENTRAL SLEEP APNOEA

In central sleep apnoea, there is periodic cessation of spontaneous impulse formation during sleep, which leads to repeated episodes of apnoea with absent respiratory efforts.

Complaints of dyspnoea and other respiratory findings are rarely prominent. Patients may present with:

- lethargy;
- headache;
- daytime sleepiness;
- unexplained polycythaemia;
- pulmonary hypertension;
- cor pulmonale.

Patients with *primary alveolar hypoventilation*, in whom there is a blunted ventilatory response to hypoxia and hypercarbia in the absence of abnormal lung function, may present with similar signs and symptoms. An example is the *Pickwickian syndrome* in which hypoventilation occurs in very obese, somnolent men who are said to resemble the fat boy, Joe, in Charles Dickens' The Pickwick Papers.

OBSTRUCTIVE SLEEP APNOEA

Patients with obstructive sleep apnoea suffer from intermittent functional upper-airway obstruction during sleep, which is thought to be due to episodic loss of pharyngeal tone. This is associated with loud snoring, frequent apnoeic episodes, especially during rapid-eye movement (REM) sleep, with severe hypoxaemia and repeated nocturnal awakening or arousal. Although traditionally associated with obesity, many patients are not significantly overweight. The condition is also associated with COPD and a reduced size of the pharyngeal opening, even when the patient is awake.

Occasionally obstructive sleep apnoea is associated with:

- daytime hypersomnolence;
- poor concentration;
- morning headache;
- impotence;
- systemic/pulmonary hypertension;
- unexplained cor pulmonale;
- polycythaemia.

The diagnosis is made when a sleep study demonstrates frequent severe apnoeic episodes associated with marked oxygen desaturation and vigorous respiratory efforts.

Correctable factors include:

- encroachment on the pharynx (obesity, acromegaly, enlarged tonsils);
- nasal obstruction (nasal deformities, rhinitis, polyps, adenoids);
- respiratory-depressant drugs (alcohol, sedatives, strong analgesics).

SPINAL CORD

Very rarely, lesions of the high cervical cord or brainstem may interrupt the pathways involved in automatic breathing, while leaving the conscious pathways intact. Because these unfortunate patients have to remember to breathe, there are long periods of apnoea, even when the subject is awake, and serious carbon dioxide retention develops when they fall asleep. The hypercarbia increases cerebral blood flow, causing headaches, nightmares and distrubed sleep patterns. This condition has been called Ondine's curse, after a water nymph who, according to German mythology, cursed her husband by abolishing all his automatic functions. When he finally became exhausted and fell asleep, he died.

Traumatic damage to the spinal cord at or above the origin of the phrenic nerve (C3, C4, C5) causes severe ventilatory failure since only the accessory muscles are spared. Partial lesions are common, while cord damage below this level causes less severe respiratory impairment since diaphragmatic breathing remains intact (see Chapter 10).

Poliomyelitis has its major impact on the anterior horn cells in the spinal cord and/or the motor nuclei of the cranial nerves and, in some cases, the respiratory centre itself is involved. The patient may therefore have a bulbar paralysis, in which case airway protection is vital, or spinal polio, which may cause weakness of the respiratory muscles and ventilatory failure. Sometimes both bulbar and spinal motor nuclei are affected.

If the spasms of tetanus are prolonged and severe, they may interfere with ventilation, but in any case treatment of the most severe cases consists of heavy sedation, paralysis and artificial ventilation (see Chapter 15). There is also some evidence that tetanus causes respiratory depression by a direct effect on the brainstem.

Motor neurone disease is a progressive disorder affecting the cerebral cortex, brainstem and spinal cord and is manifested as muscular atrophy with spasticity and hyperreflexia. It is a disease of middle age, which usually progresses inexorably and relatively rapidly (2–5 years) until, in the absence of intervention, death supervenes from respiratory failure, often associated with aspiration pneumonia. There is no known treatment but a nihilistic approach to ventilatory support is no longer tenable. Non-invasive ventilation may improve survival and quality of life in some patients, symptoms of nocturnal hyperventilation and dyspnoea can often be controlled and the need for tracheostomy/invasive ventilation may be obviated (Simonds, 2000). Nevertheless the decision to institute respiratory support in such cases is often far from straightforward. The participation of the patient, family and carers in decision-making is therefore essential (see Chapter 2).

MOTOR NERVES

In Guillain–Barré syndrome, lower motor neurone weakness develops a few days, or even weeks, after a flu-like illness. Usually the lower limbs are affected first, but later weakness may spread to the muscles of the face and trunk. A significant proportion of patients with this syndrome then develop ventilatory failure and require ventilatory support (see Chapter 15).

NEUROMUSCULAR JUNCTION

Although myasthenia gravis may affect any voluntary muscle, ventilatory failure is unusual except during acute exacerbations (myasthenic crisis), overdosage with anticholinesterases (cholinergic crisis) or postoperatively (following thymectomy) (see Chapter 15).

Botulism is an extremely rare form of food poisoning in which botulinum toxin prevents the release of acetylcholine from motor nerve endings, causing flaccid paralysis and ventilatory failure.

Organophosphorous compounds have been developed as chemical weapons and are used as insecticides. They are long-acting anticholinesterases and produce respiratory depression, bronchospasm, salivation, bradycardia, hypertension and convulsions (see Chapter 19).

Failure to reverse the effects of neuromuscular-blocking agents used during anaesthesia is an occasional cause of admission to intensive care and high-dependency units for mechanical ventilation.

CHEST WALL

If a segment of chest wall becomes unstable (e.g. due to *multiple rib fractures*), particularly when associated with lung contusion, it may be impossible to sustain adequate ventilation (see Chapter 10). Similarly, if the thorax is deformed (e.g. due to kyphoscoliosis), lung expansion will be impaired. These patients may eventually develop ventilatory failure and are prone to recurrent chest infections. On the other hand, ventilatory failure is unusual when chest movement is restricted, but the thorax is uniform (e.g. as in ankylosing spondylitis).

Rarely, patients with *myopathies* or *myositis* may develop respiratory failure. Mechanical ventilation may be required and can allow time for the diagnosis to be established (e.g. by muscle biopsy).

PLEURA

Pneumothorax, haemothorax, pleural effusion and *empyema* may all cause or exacerbate respiratory failure.

LUNGS AND AIRWAYS

As discussed above, diseases affecting primarily the lungs and airways initially cause hypoxaemic respiratory failure, but may later progress to the mixed type. Causes of ARF include pneumonia, asthma, left ventricular failure, acute lung injury (ALI) and acute respiratory distress syndrome (ARDS) (see below). Examples of chronic type I respiratory failure include emphysema and fibrosing lung disease. The commonest cause of mixed respiratory failure is COPD. Upper-airway obstruction is usually well tolerated initially, but can rapidly progress to frank respiratory failure.

PULMONARY CIRCULATION

As well as mechanically obstructing the circulation (see Chapter 5), acute pulmonary embolism can cause *V/Q* inequalities, possibly via reflex mechanisms, with hypoxaemia and tachypnoea. Recurrent pulmonary emboli eventually produce chronic pulmonary hypertension and respiratory failure.

▮ PRINCIPLES OF MANAGEMENT

Clearly, the specific treatment of respiratory failure will vary according to the underlying cause, but the same general principles apply in all cases:

- Hypoxaemia should be corrected.
- The load on the respiratory muscles should be reduced by improving lung mechanics and controlling fever.
- Ventilatory pump capacity should be optimized.

Specific measures include:

- administration of supplemental oxygen;
- control of secretions;
- treatment of pulmonary infection;
- treatment of airways obstruction;
- measures to limit pulmonary oedema;
- mechanical respiratory support.

The importance of chest wall stiffness and decreased abdominal compliance in increasing the respiratory load is sometimes not fully appreciated. Since it seems unlikely that overt high- or low-frequency fatigue is allowed to develop in respiratory failure, specific therapy to counteract fatigue is probably of little value (Moxham, 1990).

Respiratory failure must not be considered in isolation. Not only do hypoxia and hypercarbia adversely affect cardiovascular performance, but a low cardiac output is associated with a reduction in P_{O_2}, exacerbating the adverse effect of a given degree of shunt on arterial oxygenation. Low cardiac output is also associated with a decrease in respiratory muscle blood flow, anaerobic metabolism in respiratory muscles (which exacerbates lactic acidosis) and respiratory muscle fatigue (Aubier *et al.*, 1982). Many drugs that act on the cardiovascular system, such as dopamine and glyceryl trinitrate, have been shown to increase pulmonary venous admixture, probably by reversing hypoxic pulmonary vasoconstriction. Myocardial failure often causes pulmonary congestion with increased shunting, and hypotension may lead to an increased dead space, particularly during positive-pressure ventilation. Finally, the increased work and metabolic cost of breathing increase the load on the myocardium and respiratory system.

OXYGEN THERAPY

Indications

Supplemental oxygen is always indicated in patients with *acute hypoxaemic or mixed respiratory failure*. For reasons discussed previously, oxygen therapy is most effective when the main abnormality is *V/Q* mismatch, but is less efficacious in the presence of a fixed right to left shunt (see Chapter 3).

In patients with *pure ventilatory failure*, the primary abnormality is retention of carbon dioxide; specific treatment is therefore directed towards lowering P_aCO_2 and P_ACO_2. The administration of oxygen is, however, a useful first step since it effectively reverses the hypoxia caused by the elevated P_ACO_2.

Patients with *carbon monoxide poisoning* will also benefit from oxygen administration. By increasing P_aO_2, the dissociation of carboxyhaemoglobin is accelerated and the increase in dissolved oxygen improves tissue oxygenation (see Chapters 3 and 19).

Methods of oxygen administration

In mechanically ventilated patients, the inspired oxygen concentration (F_IO_2) is easily measured (see Chapter 3) and can be maintained at the desired level by mixing air and oxygen

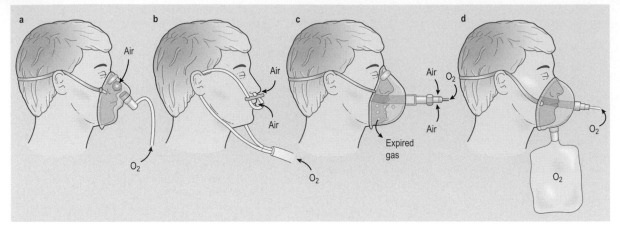

Fig. 8.2 Methods of administering supplemental oxygen to an unintubated patient. (a) Simple facemask; (b) nasal cannulae: both (a) and (b) are variable-performance devices; (c) Venturi mask (d) mask with rebreathing bag: both (c) and (d) are fixed performance devices.

in appropriate proportions. This also applies to spontaneously breathing patients with an endotracheal tube or a tracheostomy in place connected to either a T-piece or a continuous positive airway pressure (CPAP) circuit (see Chapter 7).

In the non-intubated spontaneously breathing patient, measuring F_IO_2 is not usually a practical proposition. Fortunately, in the majority of patients, the precise concentration of oxygen delivered is not crucial and a variable-performance device, such as a *simple facemask* or *nasal cannulae* (**Fig. 8.2**) will suffice. With these devices, the patient entrains a variable amount of air to supplement the flow of oxygen during inspiration, and it is not possible to predict with any degree of accuracy the concentration of oxygen being delivered to the patient's lungs. Furthermore, the F_IO_2 is dependent on the oxygen flow rate, as well as the patient's V_T and respiratory rate and therefore varies during the respiratory cycle (Goldstein *et al.*, 1982). Since the peak inspiratory flow rate may be as much as 30 L/min, considerable volumes of air may be entrained at this point in the respiratory cycle. On the other hand, if the patient hypoventilates, the inspired oxygen concentration may be higher than expected. With these devices, the F_IO_2 probably varies from about 0.35 to 0.55% with oxygen flows of 6–10 L/min. Higher concentrations of oxygen can be delivered by using a mask with a reservoir bag attached (**Fig. 8.2**).

Nasal cannulae are often preferred to facemasks because they are less claustrophobic and do not interfere with sleep, feeding or speaking. They may, however, cause ulceration of the nasal or pharyngeal mucosa, and in some cases are associated with abdominal distension caused by swallowing oxygen. Although oxygen flow rates of 0.5–15 L/min can be used through nasal cannulae, high flow rates (more than 2–4 L/min) are very uncomfortable; it may then be preferable to administer additional oxygen via a facemask. This has the added advantage that if the mask is removed (e.g. to perform mouth care), the patient continues to receive some supplemental oxygen via the nasal cannulae.

If more accurate administration of oxygen is required, a *fixed-performance device* should be used. There are three ways of delivering a known, constant F_IO_2.

Firstly, a gas mixture of the required oxygen concentration can be delivered to the patient via a tight-fitting facemask and a circuit containing a reservoir bag and a one-way valve. The reservoir bag partially collapses during inspiration and supplements the fresh gas flow; during expiration, the bag is refilled. Because there is no entrainment of air, the F_IO_2 is known and remains constant throughout the respiratory cycle. As with the use of tight-fitting facemasks for the application of CPAP, these masks are often poorly tolerated and can produce pressure necrosis of the facial skin.

The second method involves the application of the Venturi principle (**Fig. 8.2**), producing *high airflow with oxygen enrichment* (HAFOE) (Campbell, 1960a, b). If oxygen is delivered through an injector at a given flow rate, a fixed amount of air will be entrained and the F_IO_2 can be accurately predicted. Relatively low flows of oxygen entrain large volumes of air and the high flows, combined with the large volume of the mask, ensure that the patient's requirements for fresh gas are satisfied even at peak inspiration. Masks are available that will deliver 24%, 28%, 34% or 60% oxygen. For example, a 24% Ventimask uses an oxygen flow rate of only 2 L/min, but produces a total fresh gas flow of 50 L/min downstream of the injector. The design of the mask is crucial, particularly with regard to its volume, and some commercially available devices are unsatisfactory (Campbell, 1982).

Finally, *oxygen tents* can be used as fixed-performance devices and have proved to be particularly useful in children. They require a high fresh gas flow with a preset F_IO_2. Rebreathing is prevented by allowing gas to escape around the lower unsealed edges of the tent.

Physiological effects of oxygen therapy

In normal subjects, breathing oxygen causes a reduction in minute ventilation of approximately 10%, probably due to a decrease in chemoreceptor drive. The consequent rise in P_aCO_2 is exacerbated by a reduction in the buffering capacity of oxygenated haemoglobin. V_D may be increased by redistribution of pulmonary blood flow, and absorption collapse can increase venous admixture (see below). In some cases, reversal of hypoxic pulmonary vasoconstriction may be associated with a fall in pulmonary vascular resistance, while cardiac output may decrease in association with a rise in peripheral resistance. Occasionally, administration of oxygen to those with ARF leads to a transient deterioration in conscious level. This is thought to be due to an acute reduction in cerebral blood flow when the reversal of hypoxia leaves the cerebral vasoconstrictor effect of hypocarbia unopposed.

There is also increasing evidence to suggest that hyperoxia, which may occur when oxygen is administered unnecessarily or in inappropriately high concentrations, can promote reflex vasoconstriction in arteriolar smooth muscle via local regulatory mechanisms and may be harmful. For example, hyperoxia may reduce coronary blood flow, especially to ischaemic areas, and can reduce cardiac output and increase systemic vascular resistance in patients with myocardial infarction or congestive heart failure (Thomson et al., 2002).

Oxygen toxicity (Jackson, 1990)

Although oxygen is present in the air we breathe, and is essential to life, the possibility that prolonged administration of high concentrations of this gas may have toxic effects has been recognized for many years. As long ago as 1775, Joseph Priestley introduced the concept of oxygen toxicity, and a century later hyperbaric oxygen was shown to cause convulsions in birds. In 1899, Lorrain-Smith demonstrated that mice and other small animals developed pulmonary complications when exposed to high PO_2. It was not until the 1920s, however, that the therapeutic use of oxygen became common practice and the possibility of oxygen toxicity began to concern clinicians. Even now, the relevance of oxygen-induced lung damage to clinical practice remains controversial.

Experimental work has shown that continuous exposure to high concentrations of oxygen can damage mammalian lungs, but the evidence that high concentrations of oxygen cause lung injury in humans is less conclusive. Volunteers exposed to high concentrations of oxygen for more than 24 hours develop tracheobronchitis (manifested as substernal pain), with a reduction in vital capacity (VC), lung compliance and pulmonary diffusing capacity (Caldwell et al., 1966; Comroe et al., 1945). Also mucociliary clearance and macrophage function are impaired within a few hours of breathing 100% oxygen. It is more difficult to prove that oxygen damages the lungs of patients who receive high concentrations to correct hypoxaemia since clearly such patients already have underlying lung disease, the histological appearances of which are often non-specific. In addition, there are no pathognomonic chest radiographic or pathological appearances of oxygen-induced lung damage. Finally, there

are obvious difficulties in devising a study with a suitable control group.

Despite these problems, two prospective controlled studies have been performed. In one (Singer et al., 1970), postcardiac surgery patients were ventilated with either 100% oxygen or less than 50% oxygen for approximately 24 hours. There were no differences in intrapulmonary shunt, effective compliance, V_D/V_T ratio or clinical course between the two groups. The other study (Barber and Hamilton, 1970), performed in patients with irreversible brain damage, showed that after 30–40 hours, P_aO_2 was lower, while intrapulmonary shunt and the V_D/V_T ratio were greater in those ventilated with 100% oxygen than in the control group. Radiographic appearances and measurement of total lung weight supported these findings, although there were no noteworthy histological differences between the two groups. These investigations suggest that 100% oxygen can cause some deterioration in lung function, but this is probably only significant when exposure is for more than 24 hours. Pulmonary oedema is thought to develop after 72–96 hours of exposure to high concentrations of oxygen and lung fibrosis after about 96 hours.

The mechanisms by which oxygen damages the lungs are unclear, although it seems probable that, as with ARDS, the formation of reactive oxygen species is an important cause of direct cellular damage (Deneke and Fanburg, 1982) (see Chapter 5). A number of drugs, including paraquat and bleomycin, may exacerbate oxygen-induced lung injury by their effects on lung antioxidant defences and/or by increasing the rate of production of reactive oxygen species. Other factors, such as a deficiency of vitamins E and C, old age, hypermetabolic states, hyperthyroidism and catecholamines, may predispose to oxygen toxicity, while enzymes such as superoxide dismutase are generally protective (see Chapter 5).

High inspired concentrations of oxygen will also displace nitrogen from the lungs, and this may be associated with absorption collapse of underventilated lung units. The contribution of reduced surfactant production to atelectasis and lung damage in this situation is uncertain. Finally, inadequate humidification of oxygen will exacerbate pulmonary abnormalities by drying both the bronchial mucosa, which impairs the mucociliary transport mechanism, and the bronchial secretions.

Other adverse effects of high concentrations of oxygen include retrolental fibroplasia and exacerbation of barotrauma-induced bronchopulmonary dysplasia in neonates, while hyperbaric oxygen can precipitate convulsions.

Although it is clear that retrolental fibroplasia is caused by excessively high P_aO_2, it seems that lung damage is related more to P_AO_2 than to the P_aO_2. It is also worth noting that it is the normal areas of lung that are exposed to the highest PO_2 and that it is therefore these areas that may be most damaged by the use of a high F_IO_2.

In conclusion, it seems reasonable to assume that administration of oxygen can damage the lungs and that the extent of the injury depends on the duration of exposure and the concentration of oxygen. It is therefore important to use the lowest F_IO_2 compatible with adequate arterial oxygenation. Conventionally, the aim is to achieve at least 90%, and preferably 95%, saturation of haemoglobin with oxygen. It must be remembered, however, that at levels of S_aO_2 approaching 90%, the patient is close to the steep segment of the oxyhaemoglobin dissociation curve where small falls in P_aO_2 cause potentially dangerous reductions in oxygen content. Although there is only limited information on safe levels for oxygen therapy, long-term administration of an $F_IO_2 \leq 0.5$ or of 100% oxygen for less than 24 hours is traditionally considered to be acceptable. *Dangerous hypoxia should never be tolerated through a fear of oxygen toxicity.* Finally, although experimental evidence suggests that treatment with antioxidants or administration of exogenous surfactant may ameliorate oxygen toxicity, the value of such measures in clinical practice is unclear.

Monitoring the effects of oxygen therapy

In view of the risks of pulmonary oxygen toxicity and the potential dangers of hyperoxia it is important to ensure that oxygen therapy is prescribed, administered and monitored with care (Thomson *et al.*, 2002).

Some clinical improvement may be obvious following the administration of oxygen (e.g. reversal of cyanosis, slowing of the respiratory rate and a reduction in respiratory distress). Arterial blood gas analysis is, however, essential for proper assessment of the effects of treatment; ideally a baseline sample should be obtained first with the patient breathing air. In most cases, the aim is to achieve a P_aO_2 within normal limits and more than 95% saturation of haemoglobin with oxygen. It is pointless to administer oxygen in concentrations that produce a higher than normal P_aO_2 since, because of the shape of the dissociation curve, oxygen content is not significantly increased. If potentially toxic concentrations of oxygen are required to achieve a normal P_aO_2, lower values may be accepted provided that oxygen content, and by implication oxygen delivery (DO_2), remains acceptable. In particular, more than 90% saturation of haemoglobin with oxygen can sometimes be considered adequate, and this may be achieved at P_aO_2 values as low as 8 kPa (60 mmHg). Compensatory mechanisms such as polycythaemia, a shift of the dissociation curve, an increase in cardiac output and a redistribution of blood flow may preserve cellular oxygenation despite severe arterial hypoxaemia.

Clinical assessment of cellular oxygenation is difficult, although a reduction in P_vO_2 or mixed venous oxygen saturation (S_vO_2) is thought to be a reasonable indication that tissue oxygenation is impaired (see Chapters 3–6). Other indices such as the development of lactic acidosis are too insensitive to be of value in assessing oxygen therapy. It is also worth re-emphasizing that when PO_2 is low, the patient is operating on the steep segment of the oxyhaemoglobin dissociation curve and small increases in PO_2 will produce clinically useful improvements in oxygen content. This fact is utilized when administering oxygen to patients who are dependent on a hypoxic drive to respiration in whom too great an increase in P_aO_2 may cause dangerous carbon dioxide retention (see below).

CONTROL OF SECRETIONS

Many patients with respiratory failure produce large quantities of bronchial secretions, which are often infected. In order to prevent sputum retention, with its attendant dangers of pulmonary collapse and perpetuation of infection, these secretions must be cleared.

Hydration

Patients with severe respiratory failure are often unable to drink and lose large quantities of fluid due to pyrexia, hyperventilation and the excessive work of breathing. Dehydration is therefore frequent, and as a result secretions may become more tenacious. This can be avoided by humidifying inspired gases (see Chapter 7) and, more importantly, by achieving adequate systemic hydration with intravenous crystalloid solutions. On the other hand, lung water is frequently increased in patients with respiratory failure, particularly in ALI/ARDS, and some patients with COPD are unable to handle a salt or water load, perhaps at least in part due to autonomic dysfunction (Stewart *et al.*, 1995). In such patients some degree of fluid restriction is usually indicated.

Mucolytic agents

A number of mucolytic agents have been developed that can reduce sputum viscosity *in vitro*. For example, various cysteine analogues have been described that reduce the number of cross-linking disulphide bridges in polymeric mucous glycoproteins to produce less viscid thiomonomers.

Chest physiotherapy (Selsby and Jones, 1990)

Chest physiotherapy, which may be preventive or curative, conventionally uses *postural drainage*, *percussion* and *vibration* (PDPV) in an attempt to mobilize secretions and expand collapsed lung segments. In those with copious sputum production these techniques, usually in combination with *directed coughing* in those who are conscious and cooperative, may be associated with an enhanced clearance of secretions and improved lung function. Patients with acute exacerbations of COPD, but without excessive secretions, do not, however, benefit from PDPV and chest physiotherapy may even be associated with worsening airways obstruction, although this can usually be prevented by prior administration of a bronchodilator. Moreover PDPV is of no value, and may even be detrimental, in patients with acute primary pneumonia. Percussion is effective when the proximal airways are obstructed. The *forced expiratory technique* (FET), which involves expiring forcefully from mid to low lung volumes while maintaining an open glottis (*puffing exercises*) may be superior to both directed coughing and PV in enhancing sputum clearance; it may be most effective when combined with postural drainage. *Incentive spirometry* (also known as sustained maximal inspiration) uses an indicator (usually visual) to inform the patient whether or not he or she has produced sufficient flow or insufflatory volume and maintained the inspiratory effort for a sufficiently long time (at least 3 seconds). The technique is indicated for the prevention or treatment of atelectasis but is only useful in cooperative patients with an adequate VC (e.g. > 10 mL/kg). The superiority of incentive spirometry over percussion and directed cough has not been clearly demonstrated (Bellet et al., 1995). In all cases adequate analgesia is crucial.

Critically ill patients are particularly at risk during physiotherapy, not only because they often have severe lung disease, but also because of associated problems such as cardiovascular instability and raised intracranial pressure. In particular, numerous studies have demonstrated that PDPV and tracheal suctioning can precipitate dangerous hypoxaemia, which may last for an hour or more after treatment. The most likely mechanism for this hypoxaemia is atelectasis, which may be exacerbated by repetitive coughing and increased oxygen requirements in lightly sedated, unparalysed patients. Moreover, ventilator disconnection and loss of positive end-expiratory pressure (PEEP) are associated with an immediate increase in shunt, which can take as long as 60 minutes to recover. Closed suctioning systems, which obviate the need to disconnect the ventilator, and self-inflating bags incorporating a PEEP valve are now available and may be useful in selected cases.

Current evidence suggests that chest physiotherapy is indicated for critically ill patients with excessive secretions or acute atelectasis, but is likely to be of little value in those with pulmonary oedema (either cardiogenic or associated with ALI/ARDS) or pulmonary consolidation without copious secretions. In patients with acute lobar collapse, PDPV and fibreoptic bronchoscopy are usually equally effective, but success is more likely in the absence of an air bronchogram (i.e. when bronchial obstruction has led to distal collapse) than in those with an air bronchogram (indicative of peripheral collapse/consolidation). The value of prophylactic chest physiotherapy in mechanically ventilated patients is uncertain.

Tracheal intubation and tracheostomy

When chest physiotherapy with tracheal suctioning (via either the mouth or a nasopharyngeal airway) fails to clear copious secretions and the patient (who is often exhausted, confused and uncooperative) continues to deteriorate, direct access to the airway is required for effective tracheobronchial toilet. In the most urgent cases, endotracheal intubation is usually the safest technique but, when time allows, a mini-tracheostomy, which involves inserting a small-diameter tube into the trachea via the cricothyroid membrane, perhaps combined with external high-frequency oscillation (see Chapter 7) may be useful. This technique facilitates the clearance of secretions in those who are unable to cough effectively, and in some cases the need for intubation and mechanical ventilation can be averted. Glottic function is maintained. Minitracheostomy is contraindicated in those who are unable to protect their own airway. A formal tracheostomy may be required at a later stage (see Chapter 7).

Respiratory stimulants

A variety of analeptic agents have been used to increase alveolar ventilation in patients with carbon dioxide retention, as well as to arouse those who are drowsy, stimulating them to cough and cooperate with physiotherapy. The safety margin with these agents is, however, narrow and they are now rarely used. For example nikethamide, which has a short duration of action, may precipitate hypertension, tachycardia, sweating, vomiting, tremors, rigidity and convulsions, especially when administered repeatedly. Doxapram is a more potent and selective agent with a wider safety margin and is preferred. Its respiratory-stimulant effect is mediated by both peripheral and central chemoreceptors, and when given slowly it may be possible to achieve peripherally mediated stimulation while largely avoiding unwanted central effects.

Although analeptics may produce short-term improvements in ventilatory function, it appears that the central respiratory drive is usually adjusted appropriately to deal most effectively with the load (see earlier in this chapter) and there is a danger that respiratory stimulants will accelerate the onset of muscle fatigue. Since there is little evidence to suggest that doxapram reduces the need for intubation and mechanical ventilation in respiratory failure, its use is not generally recommended. There is, however, some evidence that a short-term infusion of doxapram, or even a single slow bolus intravenous dose given in the recovery area, may reduce the incidence of postoperative pulmonary complications in high-risk cases (Jansen et al., 1990). When ventilatory failure is due to drug induced central depression, therapeutic stimulation of respiratory drive, often with a specific antagonist such as naloxone, is clearly indicated.

In patients with chronic ventilatory failure, medroxyprogesterone stimulates respiration centrally and has been used to correct carbon dioxide retention during both wakefulness and sleep. Acetazolamide achieves a similar effect mediated by an increase in hydrogen ion concentration [H^+] acting at both peripheral and medullary chemoreceptors, although in some patients this response is not sustained (Skatrud and Dempsey, 1983). These two agents have been used in selected patients with chronic carbon dioxide retention and nocturnal hypoventilation. Tricyclic antidepressants are capable of suppressing REM sleep and augmenting upper-airway respiratory muscle activity. They may therefore be useful as a means of reducing the number of REM-related apnoeic episodes. The thiazide derivative almitrine bismesylate has been shown to improve P_aO_2 in hypoxic patients with cor pulmonale (Evans et al., 1990). The use of these agents has been largely superceded by CPAP and BiPAP treatments.

CONTROL OF INFECTION (British Thoracic Society Standards of Care Committee, 2001, updated 2004; COPD Guidelines Group of the Standards of Care Committee of the BTS, 1997)

When respiratory failure has been precipitated by pulmonary infection, except when this is due to a virus, appropriate antimicrobial therapy should be commenced. Ideally, the causative organism should be isolated, and its sensitivity to various antibiotics determined, before treatment is started; in practice, this is often not possible. Many patients have been receiving one or more antibiotics before admission to the ICU, and in the remainder it is not usually practicable to await the results of bacteriological investigations before starting treatment. The identification of the rarer causes of pneumonia can be difficult and time-consuming. It is, however, important to obtain a sputum sample and blood culture before initiating or changing antibiotic therapy. A Gram stain of sputum may give a valuable clue to the aetiology of the pneumonia; later, the results of culture and sensitivities may lead to appropriate modification of the antibiotic regimen. Isolation of an organism from both sputum and blood strongly suggests that this is the pathogen. In the absence of bacteriological information, a reasonable antibiotic regimen should be selected on the basis of the most likely infecting organisms (see Chapter 12).

TREATMENT OF AIRWAYS OBSTRUCTION
(British Thoracic Society; Scottish Intercollegeiate Guidelines Network, 2003; COPD Guidelines Group of the Standards of Care Committee of the BTS, 1997)
In asthma, reversal of airways obstruction is clearly fundamental, but many patients with COPD may also have an element of reversible airflow limitation.

β-Stimulants
In the past, isoprenaline was used extensively as a bronchodilator. This agent is, however, a non-selective β-stimulant and its use was often complicated by the development of tachycardia and/or arrhythmias. More selective β_2 agonists such as *salbutamol* and *terbutaline* are now therefore preferred, although even these can produce β_1 effects in high doses.

β-stimulants can be given orally, but are more effective when administered as a nebulized aerosol. The nebulizing dose of salbutamol is 2.5–5 mg every 4 hours. In resistant cases, more frequent or continuous administration may prove effective. Traditionally, small-volume nebulizers (consisting of a disposable or reusable nebulizer and a pressurized gas source) have been used to administer bronchodilator therapy to seriously ill and mechanically ventilated patients. It has been shown that using these devices bronchodilators can be delivered effectively during non-invasive respiratory support (Parkes and Bersten, 1997). Because of the inefficiency and variable performance of small-volume nebulizers, however, some prefer to use a metered-dose inhaler. It has been shown that, when delivered by metered-dose inhaler and spacer to mechanically ventilated COPD patients, four puffs of albuterol significantly reduced inspiratory resistance; no further improvement was achieved by increasing the dose. The decrease in airway resistance remained significant for 60 minutes (Dhand *et al.*, 1996). It is important to appreci-

ate, however, that deposition of bronchodilator in the lower respiratory tract may be influenced by the method of respiratory support, the tidal volume and the inspiratory time (Fink *et al.*, 1996) and in general higher doses are required in intubated patients. In spontaneously breathing patients with severe airways obstruction administration of bronchodilator via a nebulizer is still preferred, especially for anxious and uncooperative patients. Nebulizers should normally be driven by oxygen. A continuous intravenous infusion can be used when inhaled bronchodilators alone fail to reverse severe airway obstruction, although generally β_2 stimulants are more effective, and have fewer side-effects when administered into the airways (Cheong *et al.*, 1988). Salbutamol can be given as a loading dose of up to 500 μg over 1 hour, followed by an infusion at 5–20 μg/min. Side-effects include:

- tachycardia;
- tremor;
- hypokalaemia;
- hyperglycaemia;
- lactic acidosis.

Adrenaline (epinephrine) can be given subcutaneously (0.1–0.5 mg, repeated if necessary two or three times at 30-minute intervals) or intravenously, and may be effective when other agents have failed. Compared to β_2 agonists it has the additional advantage of further increasing airway diameter as a result of vasoconstriction and mucosal shrinkage.

Ipratropium bromide
Ipratropium bromide is an anticholinergic bronchodilator with no systemic atropine-like effects that does not inhibit mucociliary clearance. The rationale for the use of such anticholinergic therapy is to limit increased vagal tone in the airway which may not be overcome by high doses of inhaled β_2 agonists alone. Ipratropium bromide may be particularly useful when nebulized in combination with β_2 stimulants, since the two agents have an additive effect (COMBIVENT Inhalation Aerosol Study Group, 1994).

Theophyllines
Phosphodiesterase inhibitors increase intracellular levels of cyclic adenosine monophosphate (AMP), but there is some doubt as to whether this mediates their bronchodilator effect since at therapeutic concentrations inhibition of phosphodiesterase is minimal. These agents may also increase cardiac output and improve respiratory muscle function, although muscle fatigue may be potentiated by increased energy consumption. Theophyllines have a relatively slow onset of action.

In the UK, *aminophylline*, which contains 80% theophylline, is the most commonly used member of this group of drugs and can be given intravenously, orally or as a suppository. This agent has a low therapeutic ratio and the dose has to be carefully controlled to avoid side-effects such as:

- tachycardia;
- arrhythmias;

- sweating;
- tremor;
- nausea;
- vomiting;
- insomnia;
- seizures.

Aminophylline can also *exacerbate V/Q mismatch*, possibly by reversing hypoxic pulmonary vasoconstriction. Some therefore recommend measurement of plasma levels, which is technically difficult, or the use of nomograms to control the dose. The therapeutic range lies between 5 and 20 μg/mL; life-threatening arrhythmias and convulsions may occur at levels greater than 40 μg/mL. The intravenous loading dose of aminophylline is 5–6 mg/kg over 20–30 minutes; this can be followed by an infusion at 0.5 mg/kg per hour in patients not previously treated with theophylline. The dose should be reduced in patients with infection, cirrhosis, congestive heart failure or COPD, and in those receiving cimetidine, ciprofloxacin, erythromycin or benzodiazepines. The dose may need to be increased in younger patients, smokers without COPD, and regular alcohol consumers without liver impairment. Because it may prove difficult to find the optimal dose for an individual patient, aminophylline should only be used in those who are unresponsive to other agents.

Steroids

Mucosal inflammation is an important component of airways obstruction in asthma, as well as in many patients with acute exacerbations of COPD. Parenteral steroids (e.g. hydrocortisone 100 mg intravenously 6-hourly or as a single bolus followed by a continuous intravenous infusion at 0.5 mg/kg per hour) are therefore often used in combination with β-stimulants to suppress mucosal inflammation and help relieve airways obstruction. As well as their ability to suppress delayed hypersensitivity reactions and the inflammatory response, corticosteroids can increase cyclic AMP levels and may restore the responsiveness of the bronchial tree to catecholamines. The onset of these effects is, however, slow (3–6 hours; maximal effect in 6–12 hours), and such large doses of corticosteroids might be deleterious in the presence of active infection, as well as being implicated in the aetiology of myopathy (see Chapter 15). In less severe cases, inhaled/nebulized steroids or, in those who are able to take medication by mouth, oral administration of steroids (e.g. a once daily reducing dose of oral prednisolone) may be preferred.

β-stimulants, steroids and aminophylline can all increase urinary potassium losses.

Volatile anaesthetic agents

Halothane, enflurane and isoflurane all have bronchodilator properties and may be useful in the occasional patient when conventional treatment has failed. Isoflurane is safer than, and probably as effective as, halothane. Adequate scavenging facilities must be available if anaesthetic agents are to be used in the ICU.

Ketamine

Ketamine is an intravenous anaesthetic agent with sedative and analgesic properties that increases circulating catecholamine levels and relaxes bronchial smooth muscle. It has been suggested, therefore, that ketamine might be a useful agent for the emergency intubation of patients with severe asthma and for subsequent sedation. In one randomized, controlled trial, however, the administration of ketamine was not associated with increased bronchodilatation when compared with standard therapy (Howton *et al.*, 1996).

Heliox

Heliox is a mixture of helium and oxygen which is available as $He:O_2$ mixtures of 80:20, 70:30 and 60:40. The use of such mixtures may improve gas flow in patients with severe airways obstruction. If helium is used during mechanical ventilation, gas blenders and flow meters must be recalibrated to this low-density gas. There is evidence to suggest that the use of helium:oxygen in patients receiving non-invasive pressure support for decompensated COPD reduces dyspnoea and P_aCO_2 and might reduce the need for tracheal intubation (Jolliet *et al.*, 1999). Heliox is not currently recommended for acute asthma.

CONTROL OF LUNG WATER

In some patients with respiratory failure, alveolar–capillary permeability is increased, lowering the threshold for the development of pulmonary oedema. This is most obvious in those with ALI/ARDS (see later); it is a less-prominent feature of pneumonia and obstructive airways disease, but is an important contributory factor in many cases of postoperative respiratory failure. As discussed in Chapter 3, lung water is likely to be further increased if plasma oncotic pressure falls and/or pulmonary vascular pressures rise. The tendency to develop 'wet lungs' may also be exacerbated by the use of positive-pressure ventilation, with or without the application of PEEP (see Chapter 7).

To minimize the increase in lung water, fluids should be restricted, and it may be necessary to administer diuretics. Serum albumin should, if possible, be maintained within normal limits. This is often difficult to achieve, even with frequent administration of concentrated albumin solutions (see Chapter 5) and an aggressive approach to nutritional support, partly because these patients are often extremely catabolic, but also because of a persistent leakage of plasma proteins into the interstitial spaces (see Chapter 5 and later in this chapter). It has been recommended that in severe cases of ALI/ARDS left atrial pressure, which can be inferred from measurement of pulmonary artery occlusion pressure (PAOP), should be manipulated to produce the optimal cardiac output and DO_2, while avoiding increased hydrostatic pressures, which might contribute to the development of pulmonary oedema. In general, this means that PAOP should be maintained at 10–15 mmHg, although in ARDS, lower values (e.g. ≤8 mmHg) may be a more appropriate target. There is evidence that in patients with increased extravascular lung water, fluid restriction and diuresis are associated with a reduction in pulmonary oedema, time on the ventilator and days in intensive care (Mitchell *et al.*, 1992).

OPTIMIZING VENTILATORY PUMP CAPACITY

Respiratory muscle weakness has many causes, including:

- malnutrition;
- catabolism;
- immobility;
- metabolic disturbances;
- old age;
- steroid myopathy;
- various acquired neuromuscular disorders (see Chapter 15).

Hypophosphataemia, hypokalaemia, hypomagnesaemia, hypoxaemia and hypercapnia must all be corrected. Relief of airways obstruction will be associated with a reduction in lung volume and may restore the respiratory muscles to a more mechanically advantageous position (see later in this chapter). Adequate nutrition is clearly important, but the role of enhanced nutrition, the administration of anabolic agents/growth factors (see Chapter 11) and muscle training is uncertain. Sepsis, especially when accompanied by shock, markedly impairs respiratory muscle contractility and enhances fatigue (Hussain *et al.*, 1985).

MECHANICAL VENTILATORY SUPPORT

If the patient continues to deteriorate or fails to respond to the measures outlined above, mechanical ventilatory support should be considered (see Chapter 7).

The value of *resting the respiratory muscles* with assisted ventilation is uncertain. In those with chronic ventilatory failure, long-term nocturnal ventilation improves daytime P_aO_2 and P_aCO_2 and may improve respiratory muscle strength. The mechanism for this improvement is unclear, but may be related to improved sleep quality, control of cor pulmonale, better V/Q matching, resetting of central respiratory controllers and increases in lung and/or chest wall compliance. There is only limited evidence that rest relieves fatigue and improves muscle function in either chronic or ARF (Efthimiou *et al.*, 1987; Moxham, 1990).

Indications

Indications for instituting mechanical ventilatory support in respiratory failure vary according to the underlying disease process (see later). In *hypoxaemic and mixed respiratory failure*, the decision is made largely on clinical grounds, aided by blood gas analysis and sometimes simple bedside tests of respiratory function (e.g. V_T and maximum inspiratory force; Table 8.1). If the clinical signs of severe respiratory distress (e.g. tachypnoea > 40 breaths/min, asynchronous or paradoxical breathing, respiratory alternans, inability to

Table 8.1 Objective guidelines for instituting ventilatory support

Respiratory rate	> 40/min
Tidal volume (V_T)	< 5 mL/kg
Vital capacity (VC)	< 10–15 mL/kg
Maximum inspiratory force	< 25 cm H_2O
Arterial oxygen tension (P_aO_2)	< 8 kPa (60 mmHg)
Alveolar–arterial oxygen difference ($P_{A–a}O_2$)	> 47 kPa (350 mmHg)
Arterial carbon dioxide tension (P_aCO_2)	> 8 kPa (60 mmHg)
V_D/V_T	> 0.6

speak, sweating) persist despite maximal treatment and the patient appears exhausted, particularly if this is associated with confusion, restlessness and agitation, ventilatory support is usually required. Worsening blood gases may confirm that the situation is deteriorating: a rising P_aCO_2 (> 8 kPa) and/or extreme hypoxaemia with $P_aO_2 < 8$ kPa and alveolar–arterial oxygen difference ($P_{A–a}O_2 > 47$ kPa (350 mmHg) despite oxygen therapy are particularly significant in relation to the need for mechanical ventilation. By this stage, bedside tests of respiratory function are rarely helpful.

In contrast, the decision to institute mechanical ventilation in patients with *ventilatory failure* is influenced more by the results of blood gas analysis and bedside tests of respiratory function, in particular the VC, than by clinical assessment. Normally, mechanical ventilation should be instituted in a patient with ventilatory failure when the VC has fallen to less than 10–15 mL/kg, in order to avoid complications such as atelectasis and infection, as well as prevent respiratory arrest. V_T and respiratory rate, on the other hand, are relatively insensitive indicators of the need for mechanical ventilation in ventilatory failure because they change only late in the course of the disease. A high P_aCO_2, particularly if it is rising, is generally an indication for urgent respiratory support in these patients.

Treatment as outlined above, particularly the control of lung water, must continue once mechanical ventilation has been instituted. Additional measures that may be useful include reduction of oxygen requirements (e.g. by heavy sedation, paralysis and cooling), together with maintenance of an adequate cardiac output and haemoglobin level, the ultimate goal being to improve tissue oxygenation and prevent organ damage (see Chapter 5).

Positive end-expiratory pressure

In selected patients the application of PEEP can improve oxygenation and lung mechanics (see Chapter 7 and later in this chapter).

Continuous positive airway pressure

Patients with ARF who are not exhausted and/or hypoventilating may be allowed to continue to breathe spontaneously while a positive pressure is applied to the airway via an endotracheal tube (see Chapter 7). In those patients who can protect their own airway, and in whom retention of secretions is not a problem, CPAP may be applied using a tight-fitting facemask or hood. In selected cases, this technique is a valuable means of avoiding mechanical ventilation (see Chapter 7).

Other special techniques for respiratory support (e.g. non-invasive ventilation, high-frequency ventilation, pressure-control inverse-ratio ventilation, extracorporeal membrane oxygenation/carbon dioxide removal) may be useful in selected cases. These are considered in Chapter 7.

SOME COMMON CAUSES OF RESPIRATORY FAILURE

POSTOPERATIVE RESPIRATORY FAILURE

Pulmonary complications of surgery, including pneumonia, atelectasis, bronchospasm and exacerbations of underlying chronic lung disease. can prolong hospital stay by an average of 1–2 weeks (Lawrence *et al.*, 1996) and may precipitate respiratory failure.

Pathophysiology

Surgery and anaesthesia can be complicated by atelectasis in dependent lung regions with reductions in FRC, forced expiratory volume in 1 second (FEV$_1$), forced VC (FVC) and compliance, associated with premature small-airway closure, impaired ability to cough and muscle splinting. The pattern of breathing also alters, with a reduction in V_T and an increased respiratory rate. Diaphragmatic tone and movement are reduced, breathing becomes predominantly thoracic and the overall activity of the abdominal muscles is increased, particularly during expiration. The reduction in FRC may therefore be largely explained by a cranial shift of the diaphragm combined with loss of lung volume due to mucous plugs and alveolar collapse. There is a close relationship between the fall in FRC, the increase in pulmonary shunt and the hypoxaemia which is invariably present postoperatively and may persist for many days (Jones *et al.*, 1990). Frequent superimposed episodes of more severe hypoxaemia occur during sleep in those given opiates and are related to periods of apnoea with airways obstruction, in part due to hypotonia of the muscles of the upper airway. Hypoxia is also common later during the prolonged periods of REM sleep that are necessary to compensate for the lack of REM sleep in the early postoperative period.

These abnormalities of lung function are particularly severe following upper abdominal surgery, when FRC may fall to as little as 20% of the preoperative value, and VC and FEV$_1$ are reduced by approximately 60%. Similar, but slightly

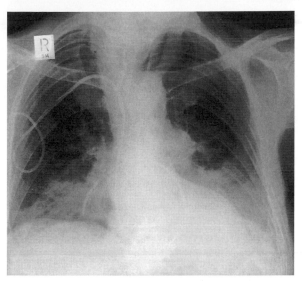

Fig. 8.3 Chest radiograph appearances of bilateral basal collapse/consolidation in a patient with postoperative respiratory failure.

less severe, changes occur after thoracic surgery. Lung function returns to normal over a period of 1–3 weeks.

Surgery and anaesthesia are also associated with depression of macrophage function and ciliary activity, while the lower respiratory tract may become colonized with bacteria. It is not surprising that in susceptible patients these changes are often associated with retention of secretions, basal lung collapse and superimposed infection (either an exacerbation of pre-existing bronchitis or secondary pneumonia), or that in some cases they precipitate respiratory failure (**Fig. 8.3**).

Predisposing factors

Suggested risk factors for postoperative pulmonary complications have included pre-existing respiratory disease (such as COPD or asthma), smoking, obesity, older age and poor general health. It also seems that pulmonary complications are more closely related to comorbidities than to chronologic age. Moreover obesity may not, in fact, be associated with a significantly increased risk and the extent of any increased risk in asthmatics is uncertain (Smetana, 1999). Clinical findings such as exercise tolerance, cough, dyspnoea, lung auscultation and chest radiography are generally more helpful in assessing risk than is spirometry, which is of variable predictive value (Lawrence *et al.*, 1996). Although an FEV$_1$ of less than 50%, an FEV$_1$/FVC ratio of less than 70% and $P_aCO_2 > 45$ mmHg have been used to define high-risk patients, it has been emphasized that neither spirometry nor blood gas analysis should be used in isolation to identify those in whom the risk of surgery is prohibitive (Smetana, 1999). There is no doubt, however, that the surgical site is an important predictor of risk, which increases as the incision approaches the diaphragm, and that surgical procedures lasting more than 3 hours are associated with a higher incidence of complications (Smetana, 1999).

Because postoperative pulmonary complications are rare in previously fit patients with normal lung function, it is logical to concentrate preventive measures on those patients known to be most at risk.

Prevention and treatment

In high-risk cases, surgery should be delayed in order to optimize respiratory function and minimize the risk of subsequent serious pulmonary complications. Thus, patients with bronchiectasis or severe COPD, particularly if associated with cor pulmonale and polycythaemia, will often benefit from a period of intensive physiotherapy, with antibiotic treatment for active infection, before surgery. In some cases, bronchodilator therapy and/or corticosteroids may be beneficial. Similarly, patients with other forms of chronic respiratory disease will require preoperative treatment of any superimposed respiratory tract infections. Patients must be persuaded to stop smoking, preferably more than 8 weeks before surgery. Educating patients about lung expansion manoeuvres should form an integral part of preoperative preparation.

In the postoperative period, simple but effective preventive measures include chest physiotherapy with deep-breathing exercises and incentive spirometry (Thomas and McIntosh, 1994). Most studies have found no difference in efficacy between these two techniques (Thomas and McIntosh, 1994). Intermittent positive-pressure breathing and CPAP are also effective, but the former is rarely used for primary prevention because of its relative expense and high incidence of complications. The application of mask or hood CPAP is particularly valuable in patients who are unable to perform deep-breathing exercises or incentive spirometry and is a useful means of achieving re-expansion of collapsed lung segments, especially in those in whom the major abnormality is a reduction in FRC (e.g. the obese patient who has recently undergone upper abdominal surgery). In patients who developed severe hypoxaemia after major elective abdominal surgery, for example, CPAP decreased the incidence of tracheal intubation, pneumonia and other serious complications (Squadrone et al., 2005). Bilevel positive airway pressure may also be an effective treatment for patients with impending, or established, postoperative respiratory failure (see Chapter 7). The provision of adequate analgesia is of paramount importance since pain seriously inhibits the patient's ability to cough and expand the lungs. Many recommend epidural analgesia after high-risk thoracic, abdominal and major vascular procedures, while intercostal nerve blocks are an alternative if an epidural is ineffective or technically difficult (see Chapter 11). If possible, the patient should be sat up at approximately 45° because in this position diaphragmatic movement is not impeded by the abdominal contents and expansion of basal lung segments is improved.

Despite these measures, some patients will need tracheal intubation, possibly combined with bronchoscopy, or a minitracheostomy to control bronchial secretions, while others will deteriorate further and require invasive or non-invasive ventilatory support. Selected cases may benefit from elective postoperative mechanical ventilation.

COMMUNITY-ACQUIRED PNEUMONIA (CAP)
(British Thoracic Society Standards of Care Committee, 2001, updated 2004)

CAP in hospitalized patients can be defined as: symptoms and signs consistent with an acute lower respiratory tract infection associated with new radiographic shadowing for which there is no other explanation (e.g. not pulmonary oedema or infarction). Further the illness should be the primary reason for admission to hospital.

The incidence of CAP in developed countries has been estimated at 2–4 cases per 1000 of the adult population, with 22–50% of cases requiring hospital admission and around 5% being admitted to ICU. Indeed CAP is the commonest infection acquired outside hospital requiring admission to the ICU. CAP is the sixth leading cause of death overall and the most common cause of death from infection, with a case fatality rate of around 5%.

Clinical presentation and assessment of severity

There is often a history of a preceding viral infection. Recent evidence has indicated that asthma is an independent risk factor for invasive pneumococcal disease (Talbot et al., 2005). In those with strep. pneumoniae infection the patient typically becomes unwell quite rapidly with high fever, dry cough and pleuritic pain. A day or two later the patient starts to produce 'rusty' coloured sputum and may develop labial herpes simplex. The patient may become tachypnoeic, with small tidal volumes and reduced movement of the affected side of the chest. There may be signs of consolidation with a pleural rub.

Complications of pneumonia can include:

- severe sepsis/septic shock;
- vital organ dysfunction;
- respiratory failure;
- ALI/ARDS;
- empyema;
- lung abscess.

Various adverse prognostic features have been identified (British Thoracic Society Standards of Care Committee, 2001, updated 2004):

- age 50 years or more;
- presence of coexisting disease.

Core clinical adverse prognostic features (CURB):

- **c**onfusion;
- **u**rea > 7 mmol/L;
- **r**espiratory rate ≥ 30 L/min;

■ **b**lood pressure low (systolic blood pressure < 90 mmHg and/or diastolic blood pressure ≤ 60 mmHg).

Additional clinical adverse prognostic features:

■ hypoxaemia (S_aO_2 < 92% or P_aO_2 < 8 kPa) regardless of F_1O_2;
■ bilateral or multilobe involvement on the chest radiograph.

These and other prediction rules for severe CAP (e.g. the American Thoracic Society Criteria and the Pneumonia Severity Index) are not, however, sufficiently discriminating to guide decision-making in individual patients (Angus et al., 2002) and should be regarded instead as useful aids to clinical judgement. Moreover the likelihood of receiving ICU care seems to be poorly predicted by most measures of severity (Angus et al., 2002). In this study ICU admission rates were higher for patients admitted from home, patients who were unemployed, patients with a history of substance abuse and patients with comorbidity. Those admitted to ICU were more likely to complain of dyspnoea and to have tachypnoea, tachycardia, hypothermia or altered mental status at presentation (Angus et al., 2002). More recently a six-point severity assessment model based on the CURB criteria and age greater or less than 65 years (CURB-65 score) at hospital admission has been shown to stratify patients according to increasing risk of mortality (score 0, 0.7%; score 1, 3.2%; score 2, 3%; score 3, 17%; score 4, 41.5%; score 5, 57%) (Lim et al., 2003).

Suggested criteria for the diagnosis of severe CAP include:

■ Clinical features:
    ■ respiratory rate ≥ 30 breaths/min;
    ■ diastolic blood pressure ≤ 60 mmHg;
    ■ confusion;
    ■ age > 65 years;
    ■ comorbidity
■ Investigations:
    ■ chest X-ray – more than one lobe involved;
    ■ P_aO_2 < 8 kPa;
    ■ low albumin (< 35 g/L);
    ■ white cell count low (< 10^9/L) or high (> 20 × 10^9/L);
    ■ raised serum urea (> 7 mmol/L);
    ■ positive blood cultures (have been associated with a worse prognosis).

Aetiology

An aetiological agent is identified in only about half of the cases of CAP in the general adult population. The organisms identified most frequently are *Streptococcus pneumoniae*, *Mycoplasma pneumoniae*, respiratory viruses and *Chlamydia pneumoniae*. *Coxiella burnetii* is prevalent in some rural areas. Other organisms such as *Legionella pneumophila*, *Haemophilus influenzae*, Gram-negative aerobic bacilli and *Staphylococcus aureus* are encountered less frequently. In those with severe CAP *Streptococcus pneumoniae* remains the most common pathogen, but *L. pneumophila*, *H. influenzae*,

enteric Gram-negatives and *Staphylococcus aureus* assume greater importance, whilst *M. pneumoniae*, *C. pneumoniae* and viruses become less common. Occasionally *Mycobacterium tuberculosis* causes severe pneumonia. When CAP is acquired in a nursing home ('*Health care associated pneumonia*'; HCAP) enteric organisms become the commonest aetiological agents. Specific organisms are more often identified in patients admitted to ICU.

Investigations and diagnosis (see Chapter 12)

A chest radiograph should always be performed on admission (**Fig. 8.4**), together with a full blood count, urea, electrolytes, liver function tests and, when available, determination of creatine phosphate or procalcitonin levels. The degree of hypoxaemia should also be assessed. Blood culture is recommended in all patients and when possible sputum samples should immediately be sent for culture and sensitivity tests, preferably before the first dose of antibiotics is given. In those with severe CAP or complications the following additional investigations are recommended:

■ immediate Gram stain of sputum;
■ pneumococcal antigen in urine, sputum and serum;
■ pleural fluid for Gram stain and culture when available;
■ invasive procedures (e.g. bronchoalveolar lavage (BAL)) in selected cases;
■ *Legionella* cultures on invasive respiratory samples (e.g. BAL); *Legionella* urinary antigen test should be rapidly available;
■ paired serological assays with complement fixation tests for atypical and common respiratory viral pathogens (also indicated in those unresponsive to β-lactam antibiotics);
■ chlamydial antigen detection tests (also when there is a strong clinical suspicion of psittacosis).

Management

Those who are hypoxic should receive *supplemental oxygen*, if necessary in high concentrations, although because hypoxia is caused predominantly by a physiological shunt, the response may be disappointing. Other general measures may include *volume repletion*, *analgesia* for pleuritic pain and administration of a *cough suppressant*.

In those admitted to hospital with severe CAP initial *empirical antibiotic therapy* should consist of intravenous co-amoxiclav or a second-generation (e.g. cefuroxime) or third-generation (e.g. cefotaxime or ceftriaxone) cephalosporin combined with a macrolide (e.g. clarithromycin or erythromycin). The patient can be transferred to an oral regime as soon as clinical improvement occurs and the temperature has been normal for 24 hours. For patients with severe CAP, in whom no organism has been identified, 10 days of treatment is recommended. In those in whom infection with *L. pneumophila*, *Staphylococcus aureus* or Gram-negative enteric bacilli is suspected or confirmed, treatment can be extended to 14–21 days. When severe CAP fails to respond to combination antibiotic treatment, changing

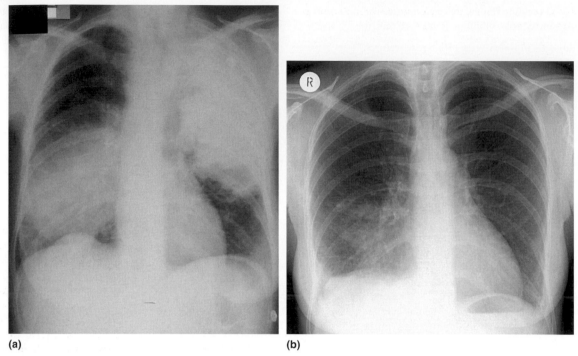

(a)   **(b)**

Fig. 8.4 Chest radiograph appearances in a patient with (a) bilateral pneumococcal pneumonia; (b) streptococcal pneumonia involving the middle lobe. (Courtesy of Dr S.P.G. Padley.)

antibiotic prescriptions empirically or adding rifampicin to the current regime are options. If a specific pathogen is identified the antibiotic regime should, if necessary, be modified appropriately (see Chapter 12).

Those with severe CAP on admission who do not respond rapidly should be considered for admission to a critical care area. Persisting hypoxia ($P_aO_2 < 8$ kPa despite supplemental oxygen), progressive hypercapnia, severe acidosis (pH < 7.26), shock or depressed consciousness are all indications for admission to the ICU. In those who require tracheal intubation fibreoptic bronchoscopy may be valuable to remove retained secretions, to obtain further samples for culture and to exclude endobronchial abnormalities such as carcinoma. Recent evidence suggests that in patients with severe CAP prolonged low-dose hydrocortisone infusion modulates the inflammatory response, hastens resolution of pneumonia and prevents the development of multiple-organ dysfunction and delayed septic shock (Confalonieri *et al.*, 2005). There was also some indication that length of hospital stay and mortality might be reduced by such treatment (Confalonieri *et al.*, 2005). *Non-invasive mechanical ventilation* may have a role in the initial management of selected cases with respiratory failure due to CAP (see Chapter 7).

Prognosis

The mortality of patients admitted to ICU with CAP remains high, at between 22 and 54%. The need for mechanical ventilation and the development of ARDS, severe sepsis/septic shock or extrapulmonary organ dysfunction are associated with a significantly worse prognosis.

SEVERE ASTHMA

The prevalence of asthma, the absolute number of hospital admissions for severe asthma and the proportion who required mechanical ventilation increased progressively from the 1960s until the late 1980s (Williams, 1989). The death rate from asthma also increased during these three decades (McFadden, 1991). Since then asthma mortality, at least in the younger age groups, seems to have declined in England and Wales, despite a continuing increase in prevalence (Campbell *et al.*, 1997), and the death rate due to asthma has also declined in Scotland (Bucknall *et al.*, 1999). Similar trends have been noted in a number of other countries. Exceptions to this decline include the USA and Japan, which continued to experience increasing asthma mortality until recently. Overall annual mortality rates from asthma in most western countries vary between 1 and 8 per 100 000 of the population. Many of these deaths are probably preventable since a high proportion of patients die before they reach hospital, most of those who die have chronically severe asthma, often inadequately treated, and a number of sudden and apparently unpredictable deaths occur after admission to hospital. Substandard hospital care is more common in fatal cases and may include incorrect diagnosis, inadequate monitoring, suboptimal treatment, administration of sedation, inadequate clinical assessment (including underestimation of severity) and failure to institute mechanical ventilation (Eason and Markowe, 1987). It has been suggested that substance abuse (especially by inhalation) may make a significant contribution to asthma morbidity and mortality. The introduction of national and international guidelines for the prevention and management of asthma may have contributed to an improvement in long-term management and possibly a reduction in the number of preventable deaths (British Thoracic Society; Scottish Intercollegiate Guidelines Network, 2003). As death rates have fallen there has been a proportionate increase in the use of inhaled steroids and it seems that relatively small doses of these agents may protect against death (Campbell *et al.*, 1997).

Aetiology

Factors precipitating severe asthma include exposure to high concentrations of allergen and respiratory infection (either bacterial or viral). The former may explain the observation that there is an increase in death rates in young people during the summer. Alterations in treatment regimens (e.g. a sudden reduction in the dose of corticosteroids), an overdose of sedatives, desensitization procedures, provocation tests and anaesthesia may all provoke intense bronchospasm. The stimuli most often associated with fatal or near-fatal airways obstruction include profound emotional upsets, serious atmospheric pollution, use of β-blockers and ingestion of non-steroidal anti-inflammatory drugs (NSAIDs) in sensitive subjects (McFadden, 1991). The overuse or abuse of β_2 agonists may provoke fatal arrhythmias or may delay seeking medical attention. There is evidence that reduced chemosensitivity to hypoxia and blunted perception of dyspnoea may predispose patients to fatal asthma attacks (Kikuchi *et al.*, 1994). Fatal attacks have also been associated with:

- underestimation of severity by patients or relatives;
- poor compliance;
- low level of education;
- poverty;
- obesity;
- alcohol or drug abuse;
- severe domestic, marital or legal stress;
- social isolation;
- psychiatric disorders.

The influence of sex differences seems to be variable. Other risk factors for death include previous intubation for asthma, hypercapnia, pneumomediastinum or pneumothorax and admission to hospital despite chronic steroid use. A history of near-fatal asthma requiring mechanical ventilation is an important predictor of subsequent death from asthma.

Aspirin-induced asthma is a common problem that affects 8–20% of adult asthmatics. The aetiology is not clear, but probably involves inhibition of cyclooxygenase, with preferential metabolism of arachidonic acid to produce bronchoconstrictor and proinflammatory leukotrienes rather than prostaglandins. An alternative explanation is that a chronic viral infection generates cytotoxic lymphocytes, which are normally suppressed by prostaglandins, but which will attack virus-infected respiratory tract cells when cyclooxygenase is inhibited (Power, 1993).

Pathophysiology

The increased airway resistance in asthma is due to oedema of the bronchial mucosa and obstruction by thick, tenacious mucous plugs, as well as an increase in bronchomotor tone. Some reports have emphasized the role of mucosal inflammation in producing airways obstruction (Djukanovic *et al.*, 1990). There is a marked increase in the number of inflammatory cells in the airways, most notably eosinophils, mast cells and lymphocytes, particularly type 2 helper CD4 T cells.

Lung elastic recoil is reduced in association with persistent activity of the inspiratory muscles throughout expiration. Alveolar pressure remains positive at the end of expiration, a phenomenon known as *intrinsic or auto-PEEP*, and this may cause a dynamic compression of the distal airways. Forced expiratory flow rates and VC are reduced, air trapping causes an increase in FRC, and total lung capacity (TLC) and the work of breathing are increased. Hyperinflation impairs respiratory muscle function (see later). Pulmonary vascular resistance increases, producing right ventricular strain and sometimes a fall in cardiac output. This will be exacerbated if, as is often the case, the patient is hypovolaemic.

Clinical features

Recognition of the severity of an attack is essential if preventable deaths are to be avoided.

An asthmatic attack can be considered severe if it is particularly prolonged (i.e. lasting several days) or if it is resistant to therapy. Such episodes are sometimes referred to as *status asthmaticus*, which has been defined as 'an acute asthmatic attack in which the degree of bronchial obstruction is either severe from the beginning or progressively increases in severity and is not relieved by conventional therapy'.

Signs that the attack is particularly severe (Table 8.2) include:

- extreme dyspnoea causing an inability to speak, eat, drink or even sleep;
- use of accessory muscles;
- tachypnoea;
- tachycardia;
- upright posture;
- mental confusion and exhaustion.

Pulsus paradoxus may be difficult to detect and is an unreliable sign, while in the most severe cases *wheezing* may be absent due to the marked reduction in airflow. Ventilatory failure with *hypercarbia* is associated with *restlessness, anxiety* and a *bounding pulse*. A *silent chest, cyanosis, feeble respiratory effort* and *bradycardia* or *hypotension* indicate a very severe attack. It is important to appreciate that the

Table 8.2 Levels of severity of acute asthma exacerbations (British Thoracic Society; Scottish Intercollegiate Guidelines Network, 2003)

Near-fatal asthma	Raised $PaCO_2$ and/or requiring mechanical ventilation with raised inflation pressures
Life-threatening asthma	Any of the following in a patient with severe asthma: PEF < 33% best or predicted S_pO_2 < 92% PaO_2 < 8 kPa Normal $PaCO_2$ (4.6–6.0 kPa) Silent chest Cyanosis Feeble respiratory effort Bradycardia Dysrhythmia Hypotension Exhaustion Confusion Coma
Acute severe asthma	Any one of: PEF 33–50% best or predicted Respiratory rate ≥ 25 breaths/min Heart rate ≥ 110 beats/min Inability to complete sentences in one breath
Moderate asthma exacerbation	Increasing symptoms PEF > 50–75% best or predicted No features of acute severe asthma
Brittle asthma	Type 1; wide PEF variability (> 40% diurnal variation for > 50% of the time over a period > 150 days) despite intense therapy Type 2; sudden severe attacks on a background of apparently well-controlled asthma

PEF, peak expiratory flow.

degree of bronchospasm often worsens appreciably in the early hours, reflected as diurnal changes in peak expiratory flow rate (*early-morning dips*), possibly because of the reduction in blood cortisol levels at this time or the diurnal variation in catecholamine levels. Extreme hypercarbia and hypoxia may be complicated by diffuse cerebral swelling and raised intracranial pressure, which in some cases may be of sufficient severity to cause pupillary changes (Dimond and Palazzo, 1997).

There is a spectrum of clinical presentations, but broadly two patterns can be defined.

■ In one, very severe airways obstruction develops extremely rapidly, sometimes leading to death within minutes or at most a few hours. This *sudden asphyxic asthma* may develop in a previously symptomless patient, is commonest in young men and is often associated with marked bronchial reactivity. Patients frequently present comatose with a silent chest, a very high P_aCO_2 and a metabolic acidosis. Respiratory arrest is relatively common. These patients do, however, respond promptly to treatment. There is probably considerable overlap between this presentation of asthma and anaphylactic reactions to specific allergens (e.g. peanuts, wasp and bee stings) (see Chapter 5).

■ At the other end of the spectrum are those whose *respiratory failure develops slowly and progressively* with muscle fatigue and exhaustion. The presentation may, however, appear precipitate because symptoms are minimized by denial, underperception of breathlessness and behaviour modification until airway obstruction is very severe. These patients tend not to seek medical help and the severity of their disease is often underestimated; they are therefore frequently undertreated and poorly controlled. Response to treatment may be slow.

The clinical presentation of *aspirin-induced asthma* is characteristic. Initially there is a sudden onset of malaise, nasal obstruction and discharge, and sneezing, frequently accompanied by a productive cough. These symptoms then evolve over a few weeks into a persistent rhinitis with nasal polyps. Over the following months the patient develops sensitivity to NSAIDS manifested as acute bronchospasm, cutaneous flushing of the head and neck, rhinorrhoea, conjunctival irritation and, in a few cases, circulatory collapse and respiratory arrest. The asthma in such cases is generally severe, protracted and difficult to control. The combination of asthma, nasal polyps and aspirin intolerance has been termed the *aspirin triad* (Power, 1993).

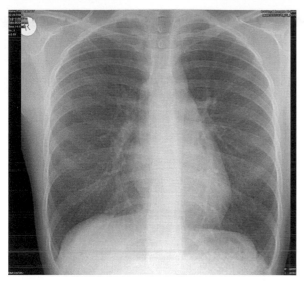

Fig. 8.5 Chest radiograph appearances in a patient with asthma. Note horizontal ribs, low flat diaphragms and vertical heart. (Courtesy of Dr S.P.G. Padley.)

Investigations

A chest radiograph should always be obtained in patients hospitalized with acute severe asthma to exclude infection and the rare possibility of a pneumothorax. Characteristically, the chest radiograph will show the features of pulmonary hyperinflation with hyperlucent lung fields, horizontal ribs, flat diaphragms and a vertical heart (**Fig. 8.5**).

Usually the patient is too breathless to perform lung function tests, but measurement of FVC, FEV_1 and PEFR may be used to assess the response to treatment. It is also important to appreciate that by performing such objective measurements in apparently less severe cases, the danger of underestimating the severity of the attack can be avoided. A PEFR < 50% of predicted or < 200 L/min suggests a severe attack.

An electrocardiogram (ECG) may reveal tachycardia, arrhythmias, ST-segment changes, P pulmonale in leads II and III and right-axis deviation.

Initially, the patient is hypoxic due to V/Q mismatch, while relative hyperventilation induces hypocarbia. A normal or high P_aCO_2 is an ominous sign that the patient is tiring, although the trend is more important that a single value. A metabolic acidosis is relatively common and may be due to circulatory failure, a reduction in hepatic metabolism of lactate and an increase in circulating catecholamines (endogenous or exogenous). Electrolyte estimation may reveal hypokalaemia secondary to the use of β_2 agonists or steroids.

Management

International and national guidelines have provided evidence-based consensus statements on the management of acute asthma in children and adults in the community and in hospital (British Thoracic Society; Scottish Intercollegiate

Table 8.3 Indications for admitting patients with severe asthma to intensive care (statement by the British Thoracic Society)

Deteriorating peak flow
Worsening or persistent hypoxia
Hypercapnia
Exhaustion
Feeble respiration
Confusion or drowsiness
Coma or respiratory arrest
Arterial blood gas analysis showing fall in pH or rising H^+ concentration

Guidelines Network, 2003). Suggested indications for admission to intensive care are shown in **Table 8.3**.

Patients with acute asthma are managed according to the principles outlined above with oxygen, rehydration, bronchodilators and steroids.

The purpose of *bronchodilator therapy* in acute asthma is to reverse any bronchial smooth-muscle spasm in order to buy time until the anti-inflammatory effect of the corticosteroid begins to work after 6–12 hours. There has been some controversy about the possible harmful effects of 'higher-efficacy' β_2 agonists such as fenoterol (a full agonist), compared with salbutamol (a weaker partial agonist) since the former was implicated as a possible cause of increased death rates from asthma in New Zealand (Sears, 1996); currently 'higher-efficacy' β_2 agonists are not considered to have a role in the routine management of severe asthma. Recent studies examining the benefit of adding nebulized ipratropium to nebulized salbutamol have been conflicting. On balance, and because there are few adverse systemic effects, this agent is advocated for patients with acute severe or life-threatening asthma and for those who do not respond to initial high-dose inhaled β_2 agonists.

It is conceivable that in acute severe asthma the considerable reduction in peripheral airway calibre might limit the delivery of nebulized drugs to the lung. This effect can be partially offset by increasing the dose and frequency of the inhaled bronchodilator or even by using continuous administration, although theoretically the intravenous route might be more predictable and effective. When the two routes of administration were compared in acute hypercapnic asthma, however, the bronchodilator response was greater when the agent was inhaled (Salmeron *et al.*, 1994), although, importantly, intravenous salbutamol does seem to improve the initial bronchodilator response when given in addition to nebulized salbutamol and systemic steroids (Cheong *et al.*, 1988). Nevertheless a meta-analysis concluded that there is no evidence to support the use of intravenous β_2 agonists in emergency department patients with severe acute asthma (Travers *et al.*, 2002). There is also conflicting evidence as to whether the addition of intravenous aminophylline is beneficial and, in view of the difficulties associated with its use (see above), this agent should be reserved for resistant cases and life-threatening situations.

The efficacy of systemic corticosteroids given to reverse the inflammatory component of airways obstruction in asthma is supported by meta-analysis (Rowe *et al.*, 1992). There is also evidence that in asthmatic patients steroids rapidly reverse the bronchodilator desensitization induced by regular treatment with inhaled formoterol (Tan *et al.*, 1997), further emphasizing the importance of early steroid administration in severe asthma. In most patients there appears to be no advantage in the intravenous as opposed to the oral route of administration and, although there is a dose–response relationship, the effect of steroids is maximal at a dose of about 50 mg prednisolone daily. Dispersible tablets can be used for those who have difficulty swallowing, while the intravenous route is reserved for patients who are vomiting or who have the features of life-threatening asthma. Provided that the patient has responded adequately to systemic steroids (PEF > 60% of predicted or best), high-dose inhaled corticosteroids can be substituted after 24–48 hours.

Magnesium sulphate has been shown to be safe and effective in acute severe asthma. A single dose of intravenous magnesium sulphate (1.2–2 g i.v. infusion over 20 minutes) has been recommended for patients with unresponsive acute severe life-threatening or near-fatal asthma (British Thoracic Society; Scottish Intercollegiate Guidelines Network, 2003), although the use of magnesium sulphate in this situation remains controversial. There is also some evidence that nebulized magnesium sulphate can provide additional bronchodilation when used in conjunction with standard measures in patients with severe asthma (Hughes *et al.*, 2003).

Antibiotics should only be given when there is strong evidence of bacterial infection. Correction of any metabolic *acidosis* with sodium bicarbonate will be associated with a transient increase in carbon dioxide production and should, if possible, be avoided. In general *oxygen* should be administered in high concentrations because respiratory drive is well maintained and there is little risk of promoting hypercarbia. There is, however, some evidence that in those with severe airways obstruction, high inspired oxygen concentrations may precipitate or worsen hypercarbia and in such cases it may be prudent to initiate oxygen therapy in a controlled fashion, adjusted according to the results of blood gas analysis (McFadden, 1991). *Humidification* is important to avoid cold-induced bronchoconstriction and minimize the risk of inspissated secretions. *Administration of sedatives, cough suppressants or β-blockers can cause rapid, and sometimes fatal, deterioration.*

MECHANICAL VENTILATION

Although ventilating patients with severe asthma is extremely hazardous, it is equally dangerous to procrastinate when the patient is exhausted. Some characteristic features of those requiring mechanical ventilation include:

- youth;
- a long history of asthma;
- previous hospital admissions in status;
- attacks lasting more than 24 hours before admission.

It can be difficult to assess which patients require ventilation, but some generally accepted criteria are:

- extreme exhaustion;
- ineffective respiratory efforts;
- increasing mental disturbance;
- coma;
- severe hypoxaemia;
- life-threatening respiratory acidosis:
- a P_aCO_2 that is rising despite aggressive therapy.

Patients who have a respiratory arrest will require immediate intubation and ventilation.

Selecting the pattern of ventilation. There are a number of important considerations when selecting an appropriate pattern of ventilation for an asthmatic patient. Because of the severe airway obstruction, a long expiratory phase is required to avoid overinflation of the lungs. On the other hand, the time constants of most lung units are markedly increased (see Chapter 3) and inspiration may have to be prolonged to allow adequate distribution of inspired gases. Therefore, a slow respiratory rate (e.g. 6–10 breaths/min), with long inspiratory and expiratory phases (e.g. to achieve an I:E ratio of at least 1:2), is usually required. V_T should be limited (e.g. to 6–8 mL/kg) to avoid high inflation pressures and the risk of barotrauma. Peak inspiratory pressures should probably not be allowed to exceed 40 cm H_2O. For a given minute volume, hyperinflation is minimized by using a lower V_T and a higher respiratory rate. The inspiratory flow rate can be increased (e.g. to > 80 L/min) to allow a longer expiratory phase, although this may adversely affect the distribution of ventilation (Tuxen and Lane, 1987). Conversely, reducing the inspiratory flow rate from 100 to 40 L/min reduces peak inspiratory pressures but also decreases expiratory time, which in turn decreases lung emptying (Tuxen, 1994). In severe cases, the minute volume is inevitably inadequate and moderate hypercarbia should be tolerated. The patient should be heavily sedated and may occasionally require muscle relaxants, particularly in the early stages (avoiding agents that might release histamine). The use of neuromuscular-blocking agents under these circumstances seems to be associated with an increased incidence of muscle weakness/myopathy and of ventilator-associated pneumonia (Adnet *et al.*, 2001). Control mode ventilation (volume or pressure) is usually used initially, but as the patient recovers and muscle relaxation is discontinued spontaneous modes (e.g. synchronized intermittent mandatory ventilation with pressure support: see Chapter 7) can be introduced. If pressure-limited ventilation is chosen, expired tidal volume must be closely monitored to avoid inadvertent underventilation.

The use of PEEP in severe asthma is controversial since an 'intrinsic PEEP' associated with airway compression and lung hyperinflation is already present. Nevertheless externally applied PEEP downstream from the compressed distal airways may overcome the obstruction to flow without increasing alveolar pressure (Marini, 1989). Although a few have recommended high levels of PEEP, most would suggest that only low levels (< 5 cm H_2O) should be used to avoid overdistension of near-normal or partially obstructed lung units. In general, however, PEEP appears to be detrimental in severe asthma since it further increases lung volume, elevates intrathoracic and airway pressures and depresses the circulation (Tuxen, 1989). Nevertheless, cautious application of low-level PEEP may be useful during spontaneous breathing. The role of CPAP and non-invasive ventilation in the management of acute severe asthma is uncertain (see Chapter 7).

Apart from increasing the risk of pneumothorax, over-inflation of the lungs compresses the heart and attenuates the pulmonary vasculature, further increasing pulmonary vascular resistance. Eventually, the right ventricle fails and cardiac output falls. This may be a terminal event. The risk of this complication can be minimized by ensuring that expiration is completed before the next inspiration begins, either by ausculation or by disconnecting the patient from the ventilator and listening at the endotracheal tube. A tape measure placed between two marks drawn on the chest is a useful means of assessing progressive hyperinflation. A rising central venous pressure (CVP) may also indicate hyperinflation. In severe cases it may be necessary to disconnect the patient from the ventilator intermittently to allow lung deflation.

Similar considerations apply when ventilating patients with chronic airflow limitation (see below). Moreover, rapidly lowering the P_aCO_2 towards normal in these patients, some of whom have a compensatory metabolic alkalosis, may cause a marked increase in pH with a reduction in ionized calcium levels, cerebral vasoconstriction and a danger of seizures. There may also be a dramatic fall in cardiac output.

BRONCHIAL LAVAGE
Obstruction by tenacious mucous plugs is an important component of the increased airway resistance in severe asthma. Some authorities therefore recommend bronchial lavage in patients who require mechanical ventilation. This procedure is almost invariably associated with severe hypoxia and hypercarbia and as a consequence is extremely hazardous. An alternative is to instil small quantities of saline into the endotracheal tube at regular intervals, although the efficacy of this technique is questionable.

EXTERNAL CHEST COMPRESSION
In severe cases expiration can be assisted by external chest compression (Fisher et al., 1989).

DISCONTINUING RESPIRATORY SUPPORT
The reported duration of mechanical ventilation in acute severe asthma varies from an average of 12 hours up to several days. Weaning and extubation of patients with reversible airway obstruction may precipitate a further episode of severe bronchospasm. In such cases the patient can be sedated with a continuous infusion of propofol or an inhalational agent during the danger period.

MORTALITY
Reported mortality rates for patients requiring mechanical ventilation for acute severe asthma vary considerably from 38% to zero, and in part depend on whether patients who have suffered brain injury as a result of cardiorespiratory arrest prior to the institution of ventilatory support are included.

ACUTE RESPIRATORY FAILURE ASSOCIATED WITH CHRONIC OBSTRUCTIVE PULMONARY DISEASE
The prevalence of, and mortality from, COPD continues to increase. COPD is now the fourth leading cause of death in the USA, where approximately 16 million people are thought to suffer from this disease. Moreover, given that chronic lung disease is probably often a contributing factor to death from other common conditions, the importance of COPD as a cause of death is likely to be underestimated. Reasons for the dramatic increase in COPD worldwide include reductions in mortality from other causes (such as cardiovascular disease in industrialized countries and infection in developing countries), together with a marked increase in cigarette smoking and environmental pollution in developing countries. It is likely that there are important interactions between these environmental factors and a genetic predisposition to COPD. Patients with COPD suffer exacerbations at regular intervals, with up to 2 or 3 episodes per annum. Furthermore exacerbations are more frequent in active smokers.

Pathophysiology
Airflow limitation in patients with COPD is not fully reversible and is due to a combination of mucosal and peribronchial inflammation and fibrosis (obliterative bronchiolitis), bronchial gland hypertrophy, mucus hypersecretion and bronchoconstriction, the latter being caused by stimulation of airway sensory receptors by inhaled irritants and the release of inflammatory mediators. Although chronic inflammation plays an important role in the pathogenesis of COPD, the mechanisms differ markedly from those seen in asthma. Inflammation is most obvious in the peripheral airways and lung parenchyma, which are infiltrated with macrophages and T lymphocytes (mainly type 1 helper T cells or CD8 T cells), whilst secretions contain increased numbers of macrophages and neutrophils. In contrast to asthma, eosinophils are not prominent, except during exacerbations or in patients with concomitant asthma. Inflammatory mediators implicated in COPD include leukotriene B_4, tumour necrosis factor and interleukin-8 (IL-8). Protease–

antiprotease imbalance (involving elastase, α_1-antitrypsin and metalloproteinases and their inhibitors) and oxidative stress are also thought to play an important role. Amplifying mechanisms (such as defective antiinflammatory responses or latent viral infection) and perpetuating mechanisms are probably important in determining susceptibility to COPD.

In those with *emphysema* there is enlargement of air spaces and destruction of lung parenchyma. The loss of lung elasticity is associated with closure of small airways and an increase in airways resistance due to reduced radial traction on the airway combined with an increase in dynamic compression during expiration. There is also a reduction in maximum expiratory flow associated with the fall in elastic recoil pressure. The combination of airflow limitation and reduced elastic recoil leads to pulmonary hyperinflation and a fall in lung compliance (see Chapter 3).

The energy cost of breathing is increased in COPD, sometimes to as much as 15% of total body $\dot{V}O_2$, and ventilatory reserve is reduced; resting ventilation may then constitute as much as 40% of maximum ventilatory capacity.

Although hyperinflation tends to minimize airway obstruction, it adversely affects *inspiratory muscle function*. The decrease in muscle fibre length reduces the force of contraction, while flattening of the diaphragm, associated with a decrease in its radius of curvature, reduces the efficiency of diaphragmatic pressure generation. Moreover, because of the orientation of the muscle fibres, diaphragmatic contraction may produce ribcage deflation rather than expansion. Similarly, the horizontal position of the ribs makes it more difficult for the respiratory muscles to expand the thorax. In patients with stable COPD, however, it seems that compensatory mechanisms may counterbalance these deleterious effects of hyperinflation on diaphragm function (Levine *et al.*, 1997; Polkey *et al.*, 1995; Rochester, 1991; Similowski *et al.*, 1991).

There is increasing evidence that the inflammatory changes associated with COPD may have deleterious systemic effects contributing, for example, to an increased metabolic rate and weight loss, with skeletal *muscle wasting and weakness*. Chronic hypoxia and immobility may also contribute to muscle weakness in these patients.

Pulmonary gas exchange is deranged in COPD due to a combination of V/Q mismatch (caused by airways obstruction, pulmonary parenchymal disease and disturbances of the pulmonary vasculature) and hypoventilation. In those with carbon dioxide retention, respiratory drive is usually increased; it is unclear whether a fall in V_T contributes to hypercarbia in stable COPD at rest. Those with ARF who develop hypercarbia do, however, breathe at smaller tidal volumes and higher respiratory rates than those who remain eucapnic, probably in an attempt to avoid fatigue and minimize respiratory distress. It seems that, as well as the deterioration in lung mechanics, other factors are likely to contribute to carbon dioxide retention (e.g. hypercarbia can itself have a depressant effect on chemoreceptors). In addition,

hypoventilation has the advantage that, as P_ACO_2 rises, a greater volume of carbon dioxide can be excreted for a given level of alveolar ventilation.

In some patients with COPD, alveolar destruction and distortion destroy the capillary bed and, combined with hypoxic pulmonary vasoconstriction, lead to *pulmonary hypertension* with secondary vascular changes. Cor pulmonale may develop and, during episodes of respiratory failure, worsening hypoxia may precipitate severe right heart failure.

Clinical presentation

ARF complicating COPD is usually precipitated by respiratory tract infection (bacterial or viral) or environmental factors such as air pollution or extremes of temperature. Airways obstruction worsens, with increased production and retention of sputum. Deterioration may also be related to the administration of sedatives or narcotic analgesics, surgery, development of a pneumothorax, rib fractures due to trauma or excessive coughing, pulmonary embolism or congestive heart failure. In some cases, respiratory failure may simply represent the final stages of irreversible lung disease.

Clinically *hyperinflation* presents as:

- intercostal and supraclavicular recession;
- decreased distance between the cricoid cartilage and the sternal notch;
- reduced cardiac dullness;
- an increased anteroposterior diameter of the chest.

Traditionally two distinct clinical types have been described;

- *pink puffers*, who present with hyperventilation, severe dyspnoea and relatively normal blood gases; they suffer predominantly from emphysema;
- *blue bloaters*, whose major abnormality is chronic bronchitis, and who are cyanosed with cor pulmonale, profuse secretions and little or no dyspnoea.

In practice the majority of patients lie somewhere between these two extremes and postmortem studies have not supported this simplistic distinction.

As well as features suggestive of a precipitating infection (fever, purulent sputum, leukocytosis, clinical evidence of pulmonary consolidation, lung infiltrates on chest radiography), patients with acute exacerbations of COPD may present with:

- worsening wheeze;
- dyspnoea;
- tachypnoea;
- use of accessory muscles;
- intercostal and supraclavicular recession;
- pulsus paradoxus;
- 'pursed-lip' breathing.

Other features include:

- cyanosis;
- rhonchi;
- prolonged expiration and expiratory wheeze.

Occasionally patients present with increasing hypercarbia and acidosis without dyspnoea (e.g. when their conscious level has been depressed by drugs or in the advanced stages of respiratory failure). Such cases are easily missed. *Cor pulmonale* may be evident as a loud pulmonary component to the second heart sound, a right ventricular heave, jugular venous distension, peripheral oedema and hepatomegaly. *Signs of acute hypercapnia* may also be present, including anxiety, dyspnoea, confusion, transient psychosis, coma and, in some cases, tremors, myoclonic jerks, asterixis and seizures. In addition, cerebral vasodilatation leads to headaches, papilloedema, and occasionally focal neurological signs, while peripheral vasodilatation is associated with warm, flushed skin and a bounding pulse. As P_ACO_2 rises P_aO_2 inevitably falls (see Chapter 3) and some believe that many of these features of carbon dioxide narcosis are mediated more by hypoxia and acidosis than by the elevated PCO_2.

Complications associated with ARF in patients with COPD include pulmonary embolism (which may occur in up to 25% of cases), pneumothorax, gastrointestinal haemorrhage and renal insufficiency. A wide variety of arrhythmias, including premature atrial beats, atrial fibrillation, premature ventricular contractions and ventricular tachycardia, may be encountered.

Investigations

A *full blood count* may reveal polycythaemia, which is not only secondary to chronic hypoxia but is also a response to persistently elevated carboxyhaemoglobin levels caused by continued heavy cigarette smoking.

A *chest radiograph* should always be obtained to diagnose or exclude pneumothorax, lobar or segmental collapse, pneumonia or obvious left ventricular failure. The chest radiograph may suggest pulmonary hypertension with prominent proximal and attenuated distal vascular markings, and an enlarged right heart. Radiological features of emphysema include hyperinflation, flattened diaphragms, a vertical heart, vascular attenuation and bullae (**Fig. 8.6**).

The *ECG* may show features of right atrial and ventricular hypertrophy, including P pulmonale, right-axis deviation, dominant R waves in V_{1-2}, right bundle branch block and ST depression, as well as T-wave flattening and inversion in V_{1-3}.

Pulmonary function tests are rarely performed in practice but characteristically show a fall in FEV_1, FVC, and the $FEV_1/$FVC ratio, a reduced diffusing capacity and an increased residual volume (RV), FRC and TLC. Hypercapnia is unlikely when the FEV_1 exceeds 35% of the predicted value, whilst patients with an FEV_1 of < 40% of predicted are likely to require hospitalization.

Sputum should be sent for microscopy and culture.

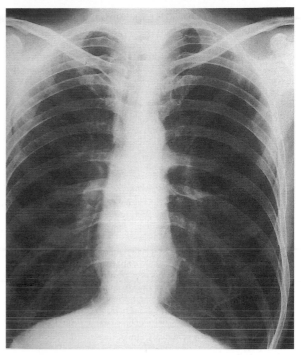

Fig. 8.6 Chest radiograph of a patient with emphysematous chronic obstructive pulmonary disease. Notice the hyperinflated lungs with low flat diaphragms and narrow cardiac silhouette.

Treatment

A number of consensus statements and guidelines for the management of acute exacerbations of COPD have been produced (COPD Guidelines Group of the Standards of Care Committee of the BTS, 1997; Pauwels *et al.*, 2001; **Table 8.4**).

Treatment consists of:

- controlled oxygen therapy;
- elimination of infection with antibiotics (usually a 5–10 day course of doxycycline, amoxicillin, co-amoxiclav, clarithromycin or a quinolone. Moxifloxacin is preferred by some: see Chapter 12);
- bronchodilators and corticosteroids;
- mechanical ventilation when indicated;
- in view of the lack of evidence, chest physiotherapy and mucolytic agents should not be routinely prescribed.

Although acute exacerbations of COPD can be non-infective or due to viral infection, current evidence supports the use of *antibiotics* for acute exacerbations of COPD when sputum is purulent (McCrory *et al.*, 2001), particularly in those with severe exacerbations (Stoller, 2002). Although antibiotics are usually recommended for patients with COPD who require mechanical ventilation, there has been little evidence to support this practice in those without pneumonia. However, a prospective, randomized, controlled trial has demonstrated that, when compared to placebo, once daily oral ofloxacin significantly reduced mortality, duration of ventilation and

Table 8.4 Recommendations for the management of acute exacerbations of chronic obstructive pulmonary disease (Pauwels *et al.*, 2001)

Investigations	Chest X-ray Electrocardiogram Arterial blood gas analysis Sputum culture and sensitivity (if no response to initial antibiotics) Electrolytes Haemoglobin/haematocrit
Bronchodilator therapy	β-adrenergic agonist as first-line treatment Anticholinergic agent in addition if poor response to β-agonist Consider methylxanthine (e.g. aminophylline) for severe exacerbations
Corticosteroids	Recommended
Antibiotics	Recommended for those with increased and/or purulent sputum
Supplemental oxygen	Recommended target $Pa_{O_2} > 8$ kPa (60 mmHg) or $S_aO_2 > 90\%$. Measure arterial blood gases 30 minutes after initiating oxygen therapy
Chest physiotherapy and clearance of secretions	Manual or mechanical chest percussion and postural drainage possibly beneficial for patients with lobar atelectasis or > 25 mL of sputum/day Facilitate sputum clearance by stimulating coughing
Mechanical ventilation	Recommended when two or more of the following present: Severe dyspnoea with accessory muscle use or paradoxical abdominal movement pH < 7.3–7.35 and $Pa_{CO_2} > 45$–60 mmHg Respiratory rate > 25 breaths/min
Other	Diet, low-molecular-weight heparin, fluids

hospital stay (Nouira *et al.*, 2001), although it has been suggested that this may have been related to a reduction in the incidence of nosocomially acquired pneumonia, rather than any impact on the precipitating infection.

Although *bronchodilators* generally cause only a small ($< 10\%$) increase in FEV_1 in patients with COPD, they can improve symptoms by reducing hyperinflation and thus dyspnoea, as well as increasing exercise tolerance. They are therefore the mainstay of current drug therapy for COPD. An additional benefit is that long-acting β_2 agonists may reduce infective exacerbations by inhibiting the adhesion of bacteria to airway epithelial cells. Some believe that, unlike asthma, COPD is more effectively treated by anticholinergic agents than by β_2 agonists. There is, however, substantial evidence that both inhaled β agonists and anticholinergic agents can improve airflow during acute exacerbations of COPD (Stoller, 2002). Specifically, the administration of a bronchodilator can increase the FEV_1 and the FVC by 15–29% over a period of 60–120 minutes (McCrory *et al.*, 2001; Stoller, 2002), although β agonists have not been shown to be superior to anticholinergic agents. As with asthma, the benefits of using aminophylline as an additional bronchodilator remain unclear, and a meta-analysis concluded that the available evidence does not support the use of methylxanthines for the treatment of exacerbations of COPD (Barr *et al.*, 2003). If used at all, these agents should be reserved for the most severe and resistant cases.

Interestingly the chronic inflammation of COPD is not suppressed by inhaled or oral *corticosteroids*, even at high doses, and there is only limited evidence that long-term treatment with high doses of corticosteroids reduces the progression of COPD (Burge *et al.*, 2000). Many believe that those who do improve probably have concomitant asthma. Nevertheless systemic glucocorticoids have been shown to produce moderate improvements in outcome in hospitalized patients with exacerbations of COPD, the maximal benefit being achieved during the first 2 weeks of treatment (Davies *et al.*, 1999; Niewoehner *et al.*, 1999). This discrepancy may be related to differences in the inflammatory response (such as increased numbers of eosinophils) or airway oedema during exacerbations as opposed to stable COPD. Steroids should probably be given for no more than 2 weeks.

In the future newer mediator antagonists, such as 5-lypoxygenase inhibitors and leukotriene B_4 antagonists, may prove useful, as may more potent and stable antioxidants. Protease inhibitors and new anti-inflammatory agents such as phosphodiesterase 4 inhibitors, are also being developed. *Diuretics* may be required in those with pulmonary hypertension and cor pulmonale or left ventricular failure.

Pulmonary rehabilitation consisting of a structured programme of education, exercise and physiotherapy has been shown to improve exercise capacity and quality of life among patients with COPD and to reduce the amount of health care needed (Griffiths *et al.*, 2000).

CONTROLLED OXYGEN THERAPY

Relief of life-threatening hypoxia is clearly the first priority; this can usually be achieved by administering supplemental oxygen and optimizing cardiac output. It is important to appreciate, however, that administration of oxygen is nearly always associated with a rise in P_aCO_2 due to:

- a fall in minute ventilation (Calverley, 2000), caused by suppression of the hypoxic drive to breathe which is mediated by the carotid chemoreceptors;
- reversal of hypoxic pulmonary vasoconstriction, with worsening V/Q mismatch and an increased physiological dead space;
- the Haldane effect (i.e. carbon dioxide dissociates from haemoglobin).

In most cases this rise in P_aCO_2 is of no consequence, but in those with severe COPD, long-standing hypercarbia and a 'hypoxic' drive to respiration, oxygen therapy may significantly decrease alveolar ventilation and precipitate severe carbon dioxide retention. Because these patients are hypoxic they are operating on the steep portion of their oxyhaemoglobin dissociation curve and small increases in P_aO_2, not sufficient to cause significant carbon dioxide retention, will lead to useful increases in arterial oxygen content (C_aO_2). Oxygen saturation values of 90–92% should be targeted. This forms the basis for controlled oxygen therapy (Campbell, 1960a) using fixed-performance masks (Ventimask) delivering 24%, 28% or 34% oxygen. Alternatively nasal cannulae can be used to administer a low flow of oxygen. Careful monitoring is essential with frequent blood gas analysis to achieve the optimal effect. Although small increases in P_aCO_2 can be tolerated, the pH should not be allowed to fall below 7.25. If significant carbon dioxide retention does occur it is important not to deprive the patient of supplemental oxygen since, because of the respiratory depression and the increase in P_aCO_2, P_aO_2 is likely to fall to a level lower than that on admission. Evidence suggests that, provided oxygen therapy is carefully controlled, hypoxaemia can be corrected with a low risk of CO_2 retention, indicating that hypercapnic ventilatory drive is preserved in most patients. Generally those who develop clinically important CO_2 retention are more severely hypercapnic on presentation (Moloney *et al.*, 2001). Inhalation of nitric oxide (see below) may worsen, rather than improve, gas exchange in COPD (Barberà *et al.*, 1996).

MECHANICAL VENTILATION

If the patient continues to deteriorate despite these measures, institution of mechanical ventilation should be considered. This decision is primarily clinical (see above) and intervention is often prompted by deteriorating mental status, ineffective cough or apnoea.

Selection of patients for mechanical ventilation. In general it is prudent to be cautious about embarking on mechanical ventilation in those with severe chronic respiratory failure because they are particularly susceptible to complications and in a proportion of cases weaning will prove to be difficult or very occasionally impossible. Selection of suitable patients is based largely on an assessment of the severity and nature of the underlying chronic pulmonary disease. The patient's previous exercise tolerance and ability to lead an independent existence are perhaps the most important considerations. Those who were severely incapacitated (e.g. able to walk only a few metres on the flat) before the acute episode will be extremely difficult to wean from the ventilator. Conversely, if the patient was previously leading a full and active life an aggressive approach to treatment should be adopted. It is also important to enquire about previous admissions to hospital with respiratory failure and whether the patient has required mechanical ventilation in the past. If possible, the duration of any previous intensive care admissions and details of the weaning process should be ascertained. Polycythaemia and cor pulmonale suggest that the patient has been hypoxic for some time, whereas an elevated bicarbonate concentration indicates that hypercarbia has been present for at least a few days. In general, success is most likely in patients with a clearly reversible component to their lung pathology (e.g. superadded infection and/or reversible airways obstruction), whereas those with end-stage lung disease associated with unresponsive airflow limitation are less likely to benefit from mechanical ventilation. Clearly if there is any doubt, as is frequently the case, the patient should be intubated and ventilated.

The principles underlying the selection of the most appropriate mode and pattern of ventilation for a patient with COPD are similar to those described earlier for patients with severe asthma. There is some evidence that the application of an external PEEP at a level close to that of the intrinsic PEEP can significantly reduce work of breathing in mechanically ventilated COPD patients (Guerin *et al.*, 2000). In one study values for static intrinsic PEEP averaged 13 ± 2.9cm H_2O in ventilator-dependent, tracheostomized COPD patients (Purro *et al.*, 1998). Non-invasive mechanical ventilation may be useful as a means of avoiding endotracheal intubation and has been associated with improved outcomes in patients with exacerbations of COPD (see Chapter 7).

GENERAL MEASURES

Mechanically ventilated patients with COPD require prophylaxis against thromboembolism and adequate nutritional support (usually via the enteral route). Hypophosphataemia, which can impair respiratory muscle function (Aubier *et al.*, 1985), is extremely common and may be related to an intracellular shift of phosphate secondary to correction of respiratory acidosis (Laaban *et al.*, 1989). Phosphate administration is indicated in those with severe hypophosphataemia, those with symptoms related to low phosphate levels, when there is pre-existing hypophosphataemia and in alcoholics. The benefits of phosphate administration in those with lesser degrees of hypophosphataemia are less clear. Hypokalaemia, hypomagnesaemia and hypocalcaemia may also adversely affect the performance of respiratory muscles and should be corrected.

Prognosis

The prognosis of patients admitted to ICU with acute exacerbations of COPD is probably considerably better than many had believed. Recent evidence suggests that, provided patients are selected appropriately, median ventilation times and length of ICU stay in ventilated patients with COPD are comparable to those of other mechanically ventilated critically ill patients, as is the total length of hospital stay. Prolonged mechanical ventilation and weaning difficulties were not a major problem in this series and the hospital survival rate was 89% (Moran *et al.*, 1998). Similarly, Nevins and Epstein (2001) reported an in-hospital mortality rate of 15%, which fell to only 12% in those without an Acute Physiology and Chronic Health Evaluation II (APACHE II)-defined comorbid illness or malignancy, with fewer than 10% of patients requiring mechanical ventilation for more than 21 days. Mortality rates are increased in those with more severe acute illness (defined by APACHE II or Acute Physiology Score), anaemia, hypoalbuminaemia, malignancy and profound weight loss. The need for mechanical ventilation for more than 72 hours and extubation failure also seem to be associated with a higher mortality (Moran *et al.*, 1998; Nevins and Epstein, 2001). Outcome does not seem to be influenced by the severity of the underlying lung disease, age, the severity of gas exchange impairment or hypophosphataemia (Nevins and Epstein, 2001). The absence of pulmonary infiltrates on the admission chest X-ray, the presence of congestive cardiac failure and an infectious aetiology have been associated with better outcomes. Interestingly, previous episodes of mechanical ventilation have also been associated with improved survival (Nevins and Epstein, 2001).

UPPER-AIRWAY OBSTRUCTION
Causes

Upper-airway obstruction is a life-threatening emergency and may be due to:

- an obstruction within the lumen of the airway;
- swelling originating from the wall of the airway;
- extrinsic compression.

Causes include:

- trauma;
- foreign bodies;
- airway burns;
- tumours (e.g. lymphoma);
- haematomas (e.g. following carotid endarterectomy or thyroid surgery);
- infections such as epiglottitis, croup, tonsillar hypertrophy or abscess, retropharyngeal abscess, diphtheria.

Instrumentation of the respiratory tract may also be complicated by obstruction; for example, endotracheal tubes can become blocked with secretions, and following extubation, laryngeal oedema or tracheal stenosis may compromise the airway (see Chapter 7).

Clinical features

Upper-airway obstruction presents acutely, insidiously or progressively as:

- dyspnoea;
- stridor;
- wheeze;
- hoarseness;
- dysphonia:
- an unusual cough.

Initially symptoms may occur only on exertion, but as the obstruction worsens respiratory difficulty becomes evident, even at rest. At first patients are usually able to compensate by increasing respiratory effort and the use of accessory muscles; V_T, respiratory rate and blood gases therefore often remain within normal limits. Once exhaustion develops or the severity of the obstruction becomes insuperable, deterioration occurs very quickly. The patient becomes extremely alarmed and agitated, inspirations are gasping, activity of the accessory muscles becomes increasingly prominent and there is nasal flaring with suprasternal and intercostal recession; these features may be combined with a persistent cough, corneal ecchymoses and subcutaneous emphysema. In the preterminal stages consciousness may be lost, the patient becomes hypoxic, hypercarbic and acidotic, cardiac arrhythmias develop and stridor usually diminishes.

In general the degree of stridor bears little relationship to the severity of the obstruction. Inspiratory stridor suggests supraglottic obstruction, while expiratory stridor is indicative of a lesion below the glottis; sometimes stridor is heard during both inspiration and expiration. In some cases the severity of symptoms is related to posture and *lying the patient supine may precipitate complete obstruction*.

Airways obstruction may be fixed or variable. *Fixed obstructions* (e.g. due to tumour or a stricture) are unaffected by dynamic changes in the cross-sectional area of the airways and airflow is equally reduced in inspiration and expiration. *Variable obstructions*, on the other hand, are influenced by the alterations in airway calibre that occur during the respiratory cycle. During inspiration the extrathoracic airway tends to collapse because the intraluminal pressure becomes negative compared to the atmosphere, whereas the intrathoracic airway has a tendency to expand because the pleural pressure becomes more negative than the intraluminal pressure. Although during normal quiet breathing these alterations are relatively small (less than 15%), during the increased respiratory effort induced by obstruction airway calibre may change by more than 50%. Therefore in a patient with a variable extrathoracic obstruction (e.g. due to vocal cord palsy or a goitre) the reduction in flow will be greater during inspiration while the reverse is true for a variable intrathoracic obstruction.

Diagnosis and investigations

The oral cavity and oropharynx should be inspected and cleared of any foreign material. Concurrent and alternative diagnoses (e.g. tension pneumothorax) must be excluded and the neck should be examined for tumours, haematomas or traumatic injury.

Anteroposterior and lateral *radiographs* of the chest and neck, *tomography* and a *computed tomography (CT) scan* may reveal the site, severity and nature of the obstruction. In some cases *endoscopy* will be required. *Blood gas analysis* should be performed. *Flow–volume loops* may differentiate extra- from intrathoracic obstruction and fixed from variable obstruction (see Chapter 6). It is important not to endanger the patient's life by delaying relief of the obstruction or by leaving the patient unaccompanied while investigations are performed.

Treatment

Because flow through the obstruction is turbulent, resistance is dependent on the density of the inspired gas and may be reduced by administering a mixture of *helium* (which is less dense than air) in oxygen. Adequate *humidification* is essential. Often, this simply allows time to prepare for endotracheal intubation and/or tracheostomy or cricothyrotomy. *Venous access* should be established.

Ideally *tracheal intubation* should only be performed by an experienced operator accompanied by a skilled assistant in an anaesthetic room or operating theatre. All the equipment that might be required to secure the airway must be immediately available, including a full range of endotracheal tubes in varying sizes, adequate suction, bougies and stylets, as well as resuscitation equipment. A surgeon should be standing by in case urgent tracheostomy is necessary. Monitoring should include ECG and pulse oximetry.

Some consider *awake intubation* using topical anaesthesia, cricoid pressure and a fibreoptic intubating laryngoscope to be the safest option, but this is often not possible in a restless and uncooperative patient. The alternative is *inhalational induction of anaesthesia* using a volatile agent in 100% oxygen or in a helium/oxygen mixture, followed by laryngoscopy and attempted intubation with the patient breathing spontaneously. This has the advantage that bubbles of saliva may form during expiration and indicate the position of the glottic opening. A transtracheal bougie, fibreoptic stylet or percutaneous retrograde cricothyroid guide wire may all prove useful.

If all else fails, *tracheostomy* should be performed, although this is extremely hazardous under these circumstances, and *cricothyrotomy* may be the preferred technique. *Transtracheal jet ventilation* should only be used when expiration is unlikely to be significantly impeded. In some instances (e.g. severe head and neck trauma), an elective tracheostomy may be performed once the airway has been secured.

SPECIFIC TREATMENT

Specific treatment of the obstruction may involve antibiotics, surgery, radiotherapy, laser or chemotherapy. Extubation can be considered when the patient is awake and cooperative, with competent laryngeal reflexes and there is a gas leak around the tube with the cuff deflated. Facilities for emergency reintubation must be immediately available. When mucosal swelling is contributing to airway narrowing, the obstruction may be relieved by administering nebulized adrenaline (1 mL of 1:1000 adrenaline diluted in 5 mL 0.9% saline); this may 'buy time' until more definitive treatment can be organized, and in some cases may circumvent the need for tracheal intubation (MacDonnell *et al.*, 1995). Over a longer time course the swelling may be reduced by dexamethasone 4 mg intravenously every 6 hours.

PULMONARY OEDEMA

Pulmonary oedema is a recognized complication of severe upper-airway obstruction (Oswalt *et al.*, 1977) and has been described most often in children with acute epiglottitis. It may be caused by the huge negative intrathoracic pressures generated to overcome the resistance to ventilation, leading to a marked reduction in the interstitial perimicrovascular pressure. A period of mechanical ventilation with PEEP is nearly always required in such cases, but resolution of the oedema is fairly rapid and weaning can usually commence within 24–48 hours. A similar mechanism may explain the pulmonary oedema that can develop when a lung that has been collapsed for some time (e.g. by a pneumothorax or pleural effusion) is re-expanded. It is thought that surfactant is inactivated during the period of lung collapse and that large negative pressures are therefore generated during reinflation.

EPIGLOTTITIS

Clinical features

Epiglottitis is caused almost exclusively by *Haemophilus influenzae* type B and usually affects children 1–6 years of age, although adult cases do occur. It has an acute onset with fever, toxaemia and noisy breathing. The child adopts a characteristic posture, sitting forward with an open mouth from which saliva dribbles, and usually does not cough. Sudden total obstruction can occur and may be precipitated by stressful procedures such as intravenous cannulation, performing lateral radiographs of the neck to confirm the diagnosis or simply lying the child supine.

Treatment

Ampicillin and chloramphenicol were until recently the antibiotics of choice, but because of the emergence of resistant strains of *Haemophilus*, cefotaxime given intravenously is being used more frequently. Airway obstruction should be relieved by nasotracheal intubation. Usually the child can be allowed to breathe spontaneously without sedation (Butt *et al.*, 1988). Criteria for extubation include resolution of fever, passage of time (12–16 hours) and improvement in the child's general appearance. Pre-extubation laryngoscopy is unnecessary. Most can be extubated within 24 hours.

CARDIOGENIC PULMONARY OEDEMA
(see Chapters 3, 5 and 9) (Fig. 8.7)
Treatment
Immediate management of acute left ventricular failure involves sitting the patient up and administering high-flow oxygen, intravenous opiates (e.g. morphine 2.5–10 mg), intravenous nitrates (e.g. glyceryl trinitrate or isosorbide dinitrite) and intravenous diuretics (e.g. furosemide 40–120 mg). Inotropic support or intra-aortic balloon counter-pulsation may be required (see Chapter 5). When pulmonary oedema is resistant to these measures, ultrafiltration or haemofiltration (see Chapter 13) should be considered. Some patients may be suitable candidates for heart transplantation.

Unless pulmonary capillary pressure falls to less than 10 mmHg, hydrostatic oedema resolves slowly by lymphatic drainage, not by the more rapid process of reversal of fluid flux.

Patients with severe respiratory distress and exhaustion due to unresponsive cardiogenic pulmonary oedema may benefit from a period of CPAP via a face mask or hood or non-invasive *mechanical ventilation* (see Chapter 7). Some may require invasive mechanical ventilation. This is particularly the case in those scheduled for corrective cardiac surgery (e.g. closure of a ventricular septal defect or replacement of a leaking mitral valve). The low cardiac output and hypotension often present in these patients need not be a deterrent to respiratory support since hypoxaemia is usually very responsive to the application of positive pressure to the airways, the net effect often being to increase DO_2. In one study, however, high-dose isosorbide dinitrate was found to be safer and more effective than biphasic positive airway pressure combined with conventional treatment (Sharon *et al.*, 2000).

ACUTE LUNG INJURY/ACUTE RESPIRATORY DISTRESS SYNDROME (Ware and Matthay, 2000; Wyncoll and Evans, 1999, Wheeler and Bernard, 2007)
In 1967, Ashbaugh *et al.* described a syndrome of acute respiratory distress in adults characterized by:

- severe dyspnoea;
- tachypnoea;
- cyanosis refractory to oxygen therapy;
- a reduction in lung compliance;
- diffuse alveolar infiltrates seen on the chest radiograph.

They remarked on the similarity between this 'adult respiratory distress syndrome' and that seen in neonates (Ashbaugh *et al.*, 1967). Before this description the same clinical syndrome had been given a variety of names, such as shock lung, Da Nang lung (during the Vietnam war), septic lung, posttraumatic pulmonary insufficiency, respiratory lung and pump lung (associated with cardiopulmonary bypass). Because it also occurs in children this condition is now known as 'acute respiratory distress syndrome'.

Definition
In order to define ARDS more precisely, as well as allow more accurate assessments and comparisons of outcome, an expanded three-part definition was proposed in 1988 in

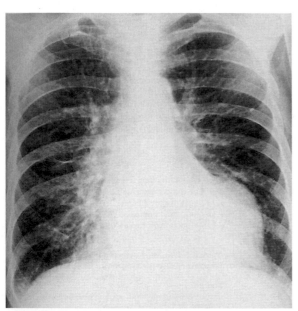
(a)

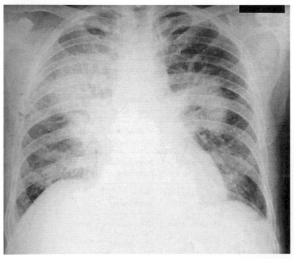
(b)

Fig. 8.7 (a) Cardiogenic pulmonary oedema in a patient with a left ventricular aneurysm. Notice the prominent upper-lobe vessels, peribronchial cuffing and Kerley B lines. (b) 'Bat's-wing' pulmonary oedema in a patient with left ventricular failure.

which the severity of the lung injury is quantified by a four-point scoring system based on: (1) chest radiographic appearances; (2) the degree of hypoxaemia; (3) the extent of the reduction in compliance; and (4) the requirement for PEEP. On the basis of this score the patient can be categorized as having no lung injury, mild to moderate lung injury or a severe ALI. Only severe ALI warrants the term ARDS. Additionally the clinical disorders responsible for, or associated with, the development of ALI are identified, the presence or absence of non-pulmonary organ dysfunction is assessed and the condition is classified as acute or chronic (Murray et al., 1988).

Six years later the American–European Consensus Conference Committee (Bernard et al., 1994) published the first widely accepted definition of ARDS. This definition is based on the following clinical criteria:

- appropriate clinical setting with one or more recognized risk factors;
- lung injury may be a consequence of a direct, pulmonary insult or an indirect, non-pulmonary insult (in many cases this distinction is not clear-cut);
- new bilateral, diffuse, patchy or homogeneous pulmonary infiltrates;
- no apparent cardiogenic cause (PAOP < 18 mmHg if measured or no clinical evidence of left atrial hypertension)*;
- oxygenation criteria:
  - ALI – arterial oxygen tension/fractional inspired oxygen (P_aO_2/F_IO_2) ratio < 40 kPa (300 mmHg);
  - ARDS – P_aO_2/F_IO_2 ratio < 26.6 kPa (200 mmHg); (in both cases despite normal P_aCO_2 and regardless of PEEP).

Although this definition is simple to use clinically and has the possible advantage of recognizing that ARDS represents the extreme end of a spectrum of lung injury, the system also has a number of disadvantages. These include:

- factors influencing outcome, such as the precipitating cause and number of other organ failures, are not assessed;
- the chest X-ray criteria may not be applied consistently, even by experienced clinicians (Rubenfeld et al., 1999) and consensus training may be required to achieve the levels of agreement necessary for conducting clinical trials (Meade et al., 2000);
- the level of P_aO_2/F_IO_2 chosen for distinguishing between ALI and ARDS is arbitrary and the level of PEEP is not specified;
- the value of distinguishing between ALI and ARDS has been questioned;

- the epidemiological significance of a diagnosis of ALI is unclear;
- it is uncertain whether ALI can be considered to be a 'pre-ARDS' state.

Moreover, because the term ALI/ARDS defined in this way can be applied to such a diverse range of disorders, it has been criticized for being too non-specific and some go so far as to question whether the condition can be considered to be a discrete entity. Most, however, accept the value of ARDS as a descriptive term, provided it is used discriminatingly, since the clinical findings, pathological features and approach to management are similar whatever the underlying cause. Indeed, some authorities (Ware and Matthay, 2000) recommend that clinicians routinely use the 1994 definitions to allow comparison of their patients with those enrolled in clinical trials. Nevertheless, most would agree that new diagnostic criteria are required which reflect the underlying pathophysiology more accurately and take into account the nature of the inciting event (Wyncoll and Evans, 1999).

Causes

ALI/ARDS can occur as a non-specific reaction of the lungs to a wide variety of direct and indirect pulmonary insults (Table 8.5), including:

- shock, sepsis, trauma, massive blood transfusion (see Chapters 5 and 10);
- fat embolism, lung contusion, inhalation of smoke and/or toxic gases (see Chapter 10);
- pancreatitis (see Chapter 16);
- amniotic fluid embolism (see Chapter 18);
- cardiopulmonary bypass (rarely);
- pneumonia;
- aspiration of gastric contents.

Hypotension alone is not an important cause of ARDS. By far the commonest predisposing factor is sepsis, and 20–40% of patients with severe sepsis will develop ARDS. The second most frequent cause of ARDS is aspiration of gastric contents (see later). Trauma patients may develop ARDS either early as a result of a direct insult or later in association with sepsis. The risk of developing ARDS increases with the number of predisposing disorders and is magnified by the presence of disseminated intravascular coagulation, alcohol abuse and chronic lung disease.

Incidence

The true incidence of ARDS has been difficult to determine, largely because of variations in the diagnostic criteria, as well as the causes and clinical manifestations of the condition. An early estimate by the US National Institutes of Health suggested that the annual incidence in the USA was 75 per 100 000 of the population. Subsequent studies from the Canary Islands (Villar and Slutsky, 1989) and the UK (Webster et al., 1988) suggested a much lower incidence of 1.5–4.5 cases/100 000 of the population. Similarly, Valta et al.

*It should be recognized that in cardiogenic pulmonary oedema, previously elevated left ventricular filling pressures may have been normalized by treatment before pulmonary artery catheterization and that radiological changes may take 24–48 hours to resolve.

Table 8.5 Disorders associated with acute respiratory distress syndrome

Direct lung injury	Indirect lung injury
Common causes	
Pneumonia	Sepsis
Aspiration of gastric contents	Severe trauma with shock and multiple transfusions
Less common causes	
Pulmonary contusion	Cardiopulmonary bypass
Blast injury	Drug overdose (heroin, barbiturates)
Fat embolism	Acute pancreatitis
Near-drowning	Transfusion-associated lung injury
Inhalational injury (smoke or corrosive gases)	Eclampsia
Reperfusion lung injury after lung transplantation or pulmonary embolectomy	High altitude
Amniotic fluid embolism	

(1999) found the frequency of ARDS to be 4.9 cases per 100 000 inhabitants per year, whilst the first epidemiological study to use the 1994 consensus definitions reported a much higher annual incidence of 17.9 per 100 000 for ALI and 13.5 per 100 000 for ARDS (Luhr *et al.*, 1999). An even higher annual incidence of ARDS (28 cases per 100 000 of the population) has been reported from Australia (Bersten *et al.*, 2002). In a recent study from the USA the incidence of ALI was found to increase with age from 16 per 100 000 person-years for those between 15 and 19 years old up to 306 per 100 000 person-years for those between 75 and 84 years old (Rubenfeld *et al.*, 2005). Within the ICU patients with ARDS may account for 16–18% of all ventilated patients and around 7% of all admissions. Interestingly, a smaller proportion of ventilated patients (4–5%) fulfil the criteria for ALI (Luhr *et al.*, 1999, Roupie *et al.*, 1999).

Pathogenesis and pathophysiology of ALI/ARDS

ALI can be considered to be the earliest manifestation of a generalized inflammatory reaction, the *non-cardiogenic pulmonary oedema* which is the cardinal feature of the early stages of the disease being the first and clinically most evident sign of a generalized increase in vascular permeability. ALI/ARDS can therefore be an early complication of the systemic inflammatory response syndrome (SIRS) and, not surprisingly, is frequently associated with the development of multiple-organ dysfunction syndrome (MODS) (Bone *et al.*, 1992). Alternatively ARDS may be precipitated by a direct insult and may or may not be complicated later by SIRS and/or MODS (see Chapter 5).

In the early exudative phase of ARDS the increased vascular permeability caused by *endothelial injury*, combined with *damage to the pulmonary epithelium* which lowers the threshold for alveolar flooding, is associated with an influx of protein-rich oedema fluid into the interstitial and air spaces of the lung. Damage to the cuboidal, type II alveolar epithelial cells (which make up only 10% of the alveolar surface area and are more resistant to injury than the flat type I cells) reduces surfactant production, thereby promoting atelectasis. The loss of epithelial integrity and injury to type II cells disrupts normal epithelial fluid transport, impeding removal of oedema fluid from the alveolar spaces, and when the injury is severe fibrosis may develop as a consequence of compromised or disorganized epithelial repair. Interestingly, it seems that in patients with bacterial pneumonia loss of the epithelial barrier may predispose to septic shock (Kurahashi *et al.*, 1999).

The early phase of pulmonary oedema in ARDS is associated with the presence of large numbers of inflammatory cells, predominantly neutrophils, in the extravascular spaces, and there is evidence that damage to the alveolar–capillary barrier is in part mediated by *granulocytes* (Heflin and Brigham, 1981) stimulated by *activated complement* (e.g. C_{5a}) (Jacob, 1981). The activated neutrophils are sequestered in the pulmonary capillaries where they attach to endothelium, migrate into the extravascular spaces and release a variety of injurious mediators including *reactive oxygen species*, *proteolytic enzymes* (trypsin, collagenase and elastase), *platelet-activating factor* and *products of arachidonic acid* (Matthay *et al.*, 1984).

There is, however, some doubt as to whether neutrophilic inflammation is the primary cause of ARDS or is a secondary event, since the condition may develop in patients with profound neutropenia (Laufe *et al.*, 1986) and some animal models are neutrophil-independent. On the other hand ALI can deteriorate during recovery of neutropenia (Azoulay *et al.*, 2002). As discussed in Chapter 5, *adhesion molecules* play a crucial role in leukocyte–endothelial interactions. Interestingly, initial plasma levels of soluble L-selectin were reduced in patients who subsequently developed ARDS and there was a significant correlation between low levels of soluble L-selectin, the severity of lung injury and mortality (Donnelly *et al.*, 1994).

Mononuclear cells such as alveolar and intravascular macrophages also contribute to pulmonary damage by triggering *coagulation/fibrinolysis* and releasing *cytokines* such as tumour necrosis factor, IL-1, IL-6 and IL-8. Proinflammatory cytokines may also be produced locally by epithelial cells or fibroblasts. Tumour necrosis factor has been found in the bronchopulmonary secretions of patients with ARDS, but not in controls (Millar *et al.*, 1989); higher levels of IL-8 in BAL fluid predict the subsequent development of ARDS in trauma victims (Donnelly *et al.*, 1993) and high concentrations of *macrophage migration-inhibitory factor* have been found in BAL fluid from patients with the syndrome (Donnelly *et al.*, 1997). As is the case with sepsis, the balance between pro- and anti-inflammatory mechanisms is thought to be a key determinant of the development and progression of this disorder.

It has been suggested that in patients with ARDS due to a direct insult the injury predominantly involves the epithelium with intra-alveolar oedema and neutrophil accumulation, whereas when the insult is indirect, endothelial damage with increased vascular permeability is the dominant feature. In practice, however, both mechanisms frequently coexist.

REACTIVE OXYGEN SPECIES (see Chapter 5)
The theory that *reactive oxygen species* derived from activated neutrophils play a key role in the pathogenesis of ARDS is supported by finding higher levels of oxidant activity in the expired breath of mechanically ventilated patients who developed ARDS than in those who did not (Baldwin *et al.*, 1986) and by the observation that elevated serum levels of superoxide dismutase and catalase are predictive of the subsequent development of ARDS (Leff *et al.*, 1993). Again an imbalance between pro- and antioxidant mechanisms appears to be important, with the antioxidant system being severely compromised and plasma levels of lipid peroxidation products being significantly elevated (Metnitz *et al.*, 1999). Similarly, BAL fluid hypoxanthine levels were found to be significantly increased in patients with ARDS, plasma hypoxanthine levels were higher in non-surviving patients than in survivors and there was a negative correlation between low protein thiols and high hypoxanthine levels (Quinlan *et al.*, 1997). In another study, however, Sznajder *et al.* (1989) found that increased hydrogen peroxide concentrations were present in the expired breath not only of patients with ARDS, but also in those with ARF associated with focal pulmonary infiltrates, suggesting that oxygen metabolites participate in the pathogenesis of other forms of ALI as well as ARDS.

PROTEOLYTIC ACTIVITY
McGuire *et al.* (1982) have found *increased proteolytic activity* attributable to neutrophil elastase in lavage fluid from the lungs of patients with ARDS, supporting the concept that proteases are involved in its pathogenesis. Numerous proteolytic enzymes may be implicated, derived not only from activated white cells, but also from the coagulation and complement cascades, and from other failing organs such as the pancreas, especially in those with sepsis and MODS. Not only may the antiproteinases then be overwhelmed by the amount of proteolytic activity, but it seems likely that neutrophils can generate both hypochlorous acid and N-chloramines, which then oxidize the surrounding α_1-proteinase inhibitor and perhaps other antiproteinases. This could then allow proteolytic enzymes, such as *neutrophil-derived elastase*, to solubilize the extracellular matrix. The ensuing loss of structural integrity and disruption of the surface anionic charge might contribute to the increase in vascular permeability. It has, however, been shown that there is a considerable excess of antiproteinase activity in patients with ARDS (Wewers *et al.*, 1988), and it has therefore been suggested that protease-induced damage may not be particularly important in the pathogenesis of ALI. Proteolytic activity may, however, be implicated in the damage to surfactant-specific proteins which has been described in ARDS.

COAGULATION DISORDERS
Thrombocytopenia and microthrombosis are frequently associated with the development of ARDS and activation of the clotting system is likely to be important in its pathogenesis. Platelet and fibrin thrombi have been found at postmortem in the lungs of patients dying with ARDS, and these can release vasoactive substances such as serotonins and prostaglandins. Fibrinolysis releases fibrin/fibrinogen degradation products, which may injure the pulmonary microvasculature, while localized vascular obstruction might be associated with episodes of ischaemia followed by reperfusion injury. These disorders do, however, also occur in patients with sepsis and major tissue injury who do not develop ARDS.

HAEMORRHAGIC INTRA-ALVEOLAR EXUDATE
This is rich in platelets, fibrin, fibrinogen and clotting factors; fibrin and fibronectin are deposited along the alveolar ducts, with the incorporation of cellular debris. This exudate may inactivate surfactant and stimulate inflammation, as well as promoting hyaline membrane formation and the migration of fibroblasts into the air spaces.

RESOLUTION, FIBROSIS AND REPAIR
Within days of the onset of ARDS, formation of a new epithelial lining is under way and activated fibroblasts accumulate in the interstitial spaces. Later type II alveolar epithelial cells proliferate to cover the denuded basement membrane and then differentiate into type I cells, restoring the normal alveolar architecture and increasing the fluid transport capacity of the alveolar epithelium. Alveolar oedema is cleared from the distal air spaces into the lung interstitium primarily by active sodium transport. Water follows passively, probably through transcellular water channels called aquaporins. Protein, both soluble and insoluble, must also be mobilized from the air spaces. Whereas soluble protein

can be removed largely by diffusion between alveolar epithelial cells, insoluble protein is probably cleared by endocytosis and transcytosis by alveolar epithelial cells and by phagocytosis by macrophages. Because hyaline membranes provide a framework for the growth of fibrous tissue it is particularly important that insoluble proteins are cleared from the air spaces. Apoptosis (see Chapter 5) is thought to be an important mechanism for the clearance of neutrophils from the injured lung.

Some patients develop an accelerated fibrosing alveolitis. Fibroblast and epithelial cell growth factors, released by macrophages and other cells in the lung, may be involved in this process. Subsequently interstitial fibrosis may progress with loss of elastic tissue and obliteration of the pulmonary vasculature, together with lung destruction and emphysema. Pulmonary hypertension may be severe and can lead to right ventricular failure. In this phase oxygenation may improve, but the increased V_D and reduced lung compliance (secondary to fibrosis and reduced surfactant) persist. The chest X-ray may show linear opacities consistent with evolving fibrosis. CT scanning shows diffuse interstitial opacities, and bullae and pneumothorax may occur. In those who recover the lungs are substantially remodelled.

PHYSIOLOGICAL CHANGES

Physiological changes include an increased shunt and $P_{A-a}O_2$, associated with a reduced FRC and compliance. Conventionally this reduction in compliance has been attributed to the lung pathology but it has been shown that, although this may be true for pulmonary ARDS (mainly due to diffuse pneumonia) in extrapulmonary cases (mainly due to intra-abdominal disease) chest wall elastance was markedly increased, probably largely due to raised intra-abdominal pressure (Gattinoni et al., 1998). As well as the reduction in compliance, airflow resistance is markedly increased in ARDS, possibly related to the reduction in lung volume, to obliteration of the conducting airways or to airway inflammation and hyperreactivity. The depletion and inactivation of surfactant may contribute to atelectasis. Pulmonary dead-space fraction is markedly elevated early in the course of ARDS and is significantly higher in non-survivors than survivors (Nuckton et al., 2002).

Pulmonary vascular resistance is often elevated in patients with ARDS. High right-sided filling pressures are then required to maintain cardiac output, and the right ventricle dilates, increasing myocardial wall tension and jeopardizing coronary perfusion. In severe cases, the interventricular septum may be distorted so that it impinges on the left ventricular cavity, causing a rise in left atrial pressure. Left ventricular end-diastolic volume and stroke index therefore remain low, while PAOP is paradoxically high (Sibbald and Driedger, 1983).

There are a number of causes of pulmonary hypertension in ARDS. Initially, mechanical obstruction of the pulmonary circulation may occur as a result of vascular compression by interstitial fluid, oedema of the vessel wall and the weight of the oedematous lung. Later, constriction of the pulmonary vasculature may occur in response to increased autonomic activity and circulating substances such as catecholamines, serotonin, prostaglandin $F_2\alpha$, thromboxane, fibrinogen degradation products and complement. Endothelial damage may impair production of endothelium-derived vasodilators such as nitric oxide (NO) and prostacyclin, and NO levels have been shown to be low in fully developed ARDS (Brett and Evans, 1998). Vessels supplying poorly oxygenated alveoli constrict (hypoxic vasoconstrictor response) in an attempt to improve V/Q matching. This response may be enhanced by local acidosis and hypercarbia, but may in some cases be inhibited by vasodilator products of arachidonic acid breakdown.

In some patients with ARDS and pulmonary hypertension, angiography will reveal beading of the arterioles and peripheral pruning of the pulmonary vasculature. This suggests fibrin deposition and is associated with a marked increase in V_D and a poor prognosis. In these cases, subpleural lung segments may be infarcted and liable to rupture. In others both pulmonary vascular resistance and angiography are normal, and the 'wet lung' is more likely to respond to dehydration and respiratory support.

CT scanning has demonstrated that in extrapulmonary ARDS ground-glass opacification is more prevalent than in pulmonary ARDS, in which consolidation is the dominant feature. In both categories of ARDS pleural effusions are common (**Fig. 8.8b**), while alveolar filling, consolidation and atelectasis are predominantly located in dependent regions (Gattinoni et al., 1991) (**Fig. 8.8a**). The likely explanation for this phenomenon is that the distribution of extravascular lung water and areas of lung collapse is influenced by gravitational increases in capillary pressure and air space compression in the lower lung regions. It has been suggested that the lung in ARDS can be considered to consist of three zones (**Fig. 8.8a**):

- apparently healthy, functioning 'baby lung' (although inflammation is present even in these non-dependent regions);
- 'recruitable';
- clearly abnormal ('non-recruitable').

This concept is consistent with the observation that the abnormality of gas exchange is largely due to true shunt, combined with areas of normal or high V/Q ratios. In the 'healthy' zone, which may represent only 20–30% of the normal lung volume, compliance and gas exchange are near-normal; with conventional techniques of ventilation this *baby lung* is exposed to high oxygen concentrations, disproportionately large tidal volumes and the potentially damaging effects of high transpulmonary pressures and alveolar overdistension (see below).

At postmortem the lungs of patients who die with ARDS are heavy and congested, with atelectasis, hyaline membranes and end-stage fibrosis.

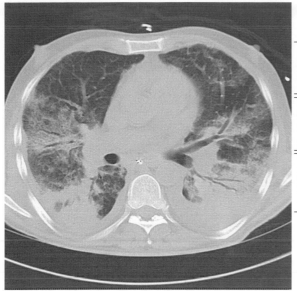

Functioning "baby lung"

"Recruitable" lung

"Non-recruitable" lung

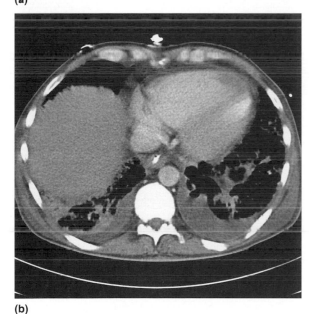

(b)

Fig. 8.8 (a) Lung computed tomography scan of patient with acute respiratory distress syndrome showing ground-glass opacification in non-dependent regions with atelectasis and consolidation in dependent regions. There are small pleural effusions. (b) Same patient as shown in (a) using soft-tissue window settings to demonstrate small bilateral effusions layering in the dependent region of both hemithoraces. (Courtesy of Dr S.P.G. Padley.)

pleural effusions are common (**Fig. 8.9**). Patchy lung densities may be more prominent when ARDS is due to a direct pulmonary insult.

The *diagnosis of ARDS* is therefore based on:

- identifying an antecedent history of a precipitating condition such as sepsis or trauma;
- refractory hypoxaemia ($P_aO_2 < 8$ kPa, $F_IO_2 > 0.4$, $P_aO_2/P_AO_2 < 0.25$);
- radiological evidence of bilateral pulmonary infiltrates;
- a PAOP < 15–18 mmHg (with normal oncotic pressure);
- a total thoracic compliance < 30 mL/cm H_2O.

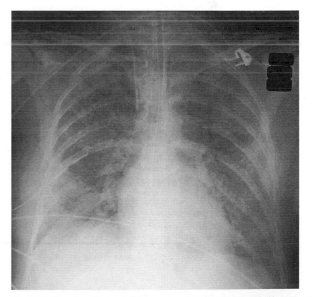

Fig. 8.9 Chest radiograph appearance in acute respiratory distress syndrome. Bilateral diffuse alveolar shadowing with air bronchograms and without cardiac enlargement.

Clinical presentation and diagnosis

ALI/ARDS usually develops insidiously 12–72 hours after the precipitating event, but in 80% of patients ALI is evident within 24 hours and many of those with sepsis develop signs and symptoms within 6 hours. The diagnosis of ALI/ARDS is mainly clinical. The first sign is often an unexplained tachypnoea, followed by increasing hypoxia with central cyanosis, dyspnoea and respiratory distress. Fine crackles are heard throughout both lung fields. Later the chest radiograph shows bilateral, patchy, asymmetrical or diffuse pulmonary infiltrates, interstitial at first, but subsequently with an alveolar pattern. Air bronchograms may be seen and

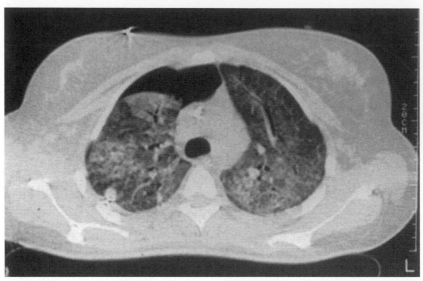

Fig. 8.10 Computed tomography scan of a patient with acute respiratory distress syndrome demonstrating a large anterior pneumothorax not visible on a plain chest radiograph (Courtesy of Dr S.P.G. Padley).

Other disorders such as fibrosing alveolitis and left ventricular failure should be excluded. As V_D rises, minute volume has to be increased to maintain a normal P_aCO_2.

Nosocomial pneumonia is a common complication of ALI/ARDS, especially during the subacute phase (see Chapter 12). The particular susceptibility of ALI/ARDS lungs to superimposed infection may be related to:

- impaired blood supply;
- poor lymphatic drainage;
- the presence of plasma/cellular debris in the air spaces;
- impaired mucociliary transport;
- retention of secretions;
- impaired immunomodulatory and antibacterial activity of surfactant.

Management *(Wyncoll and Evans, 1999)*

Management is based on treatment of the underlying condition, especially the eradication and control of sepsis, combined with the avoidance of further lung injury and complications such as ventilator-associated pneumonia (VAP), as well as supportive measures (see Chapter 11). Enteral nutrition should, if possible, be commenced early. There is some evidence that the use of a formula containing eicosapentaenoic acid, linolenic acid and antioxidants may be beneficial (Gadek *et al.*, 1999). Patients should receive stress ulcer prophylaxis and prophylactic subcutaneous heparin.

CT scanning of the lungs is increasingly used as a routine investigation in ARDS, although the cost-effectiveness of this approach has not been demonstrated. Also the patient is exposed to a significant dose of radiation and the risks of transfer to the CT scanner. Nevertheless, with experienced staff the investigation can usually be performed safely and may reveal clinically important pathology such as occult pneumothoraces (**Fig. 8.10**), lung abscesses or empyema, as well as traction bronchiectasis and evidence of barotrauma; it may also be possible to distinguish between chronic inflammation and fibrosis. CT scanning has also been useful in determining the extent and distribution of lung injury and can be used to guide drainage of pneumothoraces and loculated fluid collections. Repeat CT scanning may be helpful.

In some centres *fibreoptic bronchoscopy* with broncholalveolar lavage is performed routinely, mainly in order to obtain adequate microbiological specimens and to rule out infection if steroids are being considered in the later stages of the disease (see below).

RESPIRATORY SUPPORT *(see Chapter 7)*

Conventional methods of mechanical ventilation with large tidal volumes (10–15 mL/kg) and high levels of PEEP may exacerbate and perpetuate pulmonary damage by overdistending ventilated alveoli (in particular, overdistension of the 'baby lung' – see above) and exposing the lungs to high transpulmonary pressures. Not only do such ventilatory strategies disrupt the alveolar–capillary membrane, inactivate surfactant and promote oedema formation, but they may also stimulate a pulmonary inflammatory response which in some cases becomes systemic (Chiumello *et al.*, 1999). It seems possible that this ventilator-induced systemic inflammatory response might be associated with the development of multiple-organ failure and a worse outcome.

Cyclic opening and closing of atelectatic alveoli during mechanical ventilation are associated with damaging shear forces and may also contribute to this ventilator-associated lung injury (see Chapter 7). More recent approaches to ventilation in ARDS therefore aim to maintain a mean airway pressure just sufficient to recruit unstable alveoli and improve gas exchange whilst avoiding high inflation pressures (preferably peak inflation pressure < 35 cm H_2O, certainly < 40 cm H_2O and mean airway pressure < 20–25 cm H_2O) and alveolar overdistension (tidal volume < 8 mL/kg). Many recommend that the level of PEEP should be set just above (e.g. 2 cm H_2O) the lower inflection point of the pressure–volume curve (often around 14–16 cm H_2O) in order to minimize cyclic opening and closing of recruitable alveoli, although the best method for selecting 'ideal' PEEP continues to be debated. There is evidence to suggest that for a given applied airway pressure the transpulmonary (or distending) pressure of the lungs is higher in pulmonary than in extrapulmonary ARDS (in which chest wall compliance is low, often largely due to abdominal distension), consistent with the observation that in the former increasing PEEP mainly induced overstretching of ventilated lung units whereas in the latter there was alveolar recruitment (Gattinoni et al., 1998).

Initial results obtained with ventilatory techniques designed to limit end-inspiratory volume by using low tidal volumes whilst accepting the inevitable increase in P_aCO_2 (permissive hypercarbia) were inconsistent. Although an early, prospective, observational study suggested that outcome might be improved (Hickling et al., 1994), subsequent relatively small controlled trials failed to confirm this finding (Brochard et al., 1998; Stewart et al., 1998), neither was the incidence of barotrauma reduced (Stewart et al., 1998). More recently, however, a large, prospective, randomized controlled trial has demonstrated that mortality in ALI/ARDS can be significantly reduced (from 39.8% to 31.0%) by using low tidal volumes (6 mL/kg of predicted body weight) with plateau pressures not exceeding 30 cm H_2O, as opposed to 'traditional' high tidal volumes (12 mL/kg of predicted body weight). Interestingly, this reduction in mortality was associated with lower plasma IL-6 levels and more days without organ or systemic failure in the low-tidal-volume group (Acute Respiratory Distress Syndrome Network, 2000), a finding consistent with the observation that a lung-protective ventilatory strategy is associated with reduced plasma and BAL levels of inflammatory mediators (Ranieri et al., 1999).

The success of this trial in demonstrating a survival benefit, in contrast to previous controlled studies, may be explained by the large number of patients studied, the considerable difference in the tidal volumes (and hence plateau pressures) used (which were at the extremes of those employed in clinical practice) and the use of strict protocols for the control of pH by increasing the respiratory rate and administering sodium bicarbonate. Potentially deleterious effects of hypercarbia include impaired myocardial contractility, hypotension, arrhythmias, increased pulmonary artery pressures, raised intracranial pressure and an increased requirement for sedation/muscle relaxation. These changes can be attenuated by buffering with tromethamine (Weber et al., 2000). Some centres therefore also use tracheal gas insufflation to limit the rise in P_aCO_2. There is some evidence, however, to suggest that hypercarbia may have some beneficial effects (see Chapter 7) and that buffering of hypercapnic acidosis is unnecessary (Laffey et al., 2004).

Such low tidal volumes may be associated with alveolar derecruitment, despite PEEP set just above the lower inflection point. It has been shown that under these circumstances introducing 45 cm H_2O pressure-limited sighs leads to further lung recruitment and improvements in oxygenation (Pelosi et al., 1999). Importantly, sighs were more effective in extrapulmonary than in pulmonary ARDS, perhaps because in the latter the predominant pathology is consolidation of alveoli rather than atelectasis (i.e. the potential for recruitment is low), whereas in the former atelectasis predominates (i.e. there is considerable potential for recruitment). Moreover in extrapulmonary ARDS higher applied airway pressures are required to achieve transpulmonary pressures sufficient to recruit collapsed lung segments. Similarly transient, large increases in airway pressures (recruitment manoeuvres) (e.g. peak pressure 50 cm H_2O and PEEP above the upper inflection point of the pressure–volume curve) have been shown to produce improvements in oxygenation probably related to alveolar recruitment, in patients with ARDS.

In those undergoing protective ventilation, however, recruitment manoeuvres are often ineffective in improving oxygenation and may cause alveolar overdistension sufficient to redistribute pulmonary blood flow and increase shunt, as well as compromising haemodynamics (Grasso et al., 2002; Villagra et al., 2002). In another study of ARDS patients already ventilated with high PEEP the response to recruitment manoeuvres was only modest, although the derecruitment associated with tidal volume reduction could be reversed by increasing PEEP by 4 cm H_2O (Richard et al., 2001). On the other hand, in some patients with early ARDS oxygenation may be dramatically improved, although this improvement is often not sustained and it is suggested that in such cases PEEP should be increased following the recruitment manoeuvre. It seems that in those with extrapulmonary ARDS, and later in the evolution of lung injury (when pleural effusions are common), much of the pressure applied to the respiratory system during a recruitment manoeuvre is dissipated against the stiff pleural cavity and chest wall, thereby reducing transpulmonary pressures and limiting alveolar recruitment. Interestingly, in patients with early extrapulmonary ARDS placed in the prone position (see below) a sustained inflation at 50 cm H_2O for 30 seconds led to a further and sustained improvement in oxygenation, regardless of whether there had been a response to prone positioning (Oczenski et al., 2005).

Although constant-flow, volume-controlled ventilation was used in the successful ARDS network trial, many clinicians advocate a *descending-flow, pressure-controlled mode*. Plateau airway pressures (and thus peak alveolar pressures) are the same with both modes but peak airway pressure is less and mean airway pressure is higher with pressure-controlled ventilation. There is also some evidence that oxygenation is improved by pressure-controlled ventilation and that organ failures and in-hospital mortality may be reduced (Esteban *et al.*, 2000).

The *open-lung protective ventilation* strategy aims to prevent cyclic opening and closing of alveoli by maintaining PEEP just above the pressure at which alveoli collapse, conventionally identified clinically as the lower inflection point on the static pressure–volume curve (see Chapters 3 and 6, **Figs 3.25 and 6.4**). This approach is usually combined with low tidal volumes, permissive hypercarbia and pressure-limited ventilation. In one relatively small prospective randomized controlled trial this strategy significantly reduced 28-day mortality from 71% to 38% (Amato *et al.*, 1998), although some have expressed concern about the high control group mortality. The incidence of clinical barotrauma was also reduced.

In a more recent, larger study, however, clinical outcomes were similar whether lower or higher PEEP levels were used in patients with ARDS receiving mechanical ventilation with a tidal volume goal of 6 mL/kg (National Heart, Lung and Blood Institute ARDS Clinical Trials Network, 2004). The selection of the optimal level of PEEP can also present difficulties. In particular, the physiological correlates of the lower and upper inflection points on the static pressure–volume curve are uncertain. Thus the lower inflection point may reflect the beginning of alveolar recruitment, rather than the region in which most of the recruitment occurs, and in some cases a lower inflection point cannot be identified, although this does not necessarily indicate lack of recruitment. The upper inflection point may indicate the end of recruitment or the onset of overdistension. Moreover pressure–volume curves are representative of the whole respiratory system, including the chest wall, and may not adequately reflect a heterogeneously diseased lung. Some investigators have used CT scanning to measure recruitment and have shown that at 15 cm H_2O PEEP intratidal recruitment/derecruitment is largely avoided in the majority of patients with ARDS (Gattinoni *et al.*, 1995). More recently it has been shown that the percentage of potentially recruitable lung varies widely in patients with ALI/ARDS and correlates closely with the percentage of lung tissue in which aeration can be maintained after the application of PEEP (Gattinoni *et al.*, 2006).

Current evidence therefore supports the use of a lung-protective ventilation strategy in ARDS. This should include low tidal volumes (< 6–8 mL/kg), pressure-limited ventilation, permissive hypercarbia and an 'open-lung' technique. Importantly, the efficacy of low-tidal-volume ventilation does not appear to be influenced by the clinical risk factor (e.g. infectious versus non-infectious, pulmonary versus non-pulmonary) associated with the development of ARDS (Eisner *et al.*, 2001).

Inverse-ratio ventilation (often with pressure control) has been used to improve oxygenation by allowing ventilation of lung units with long time constants and encouraging recruitment of previously collapsed or poorly ventilated alveoli. Mean airway pressure is increased, PEEP requirements may be reduced, dead space may fall and carbon dioxide elimination may be improved. The reduction in expiratory time can, however, cause dynamic hyperinflation, with auto-PEEP, overdistension of the lungs and a reduction in cardiac output. There is a risk of pneumothorax. The value of inverse-ratio ventilation remains uncertain (McIntyre *et al.*, 2000).

High-frequency positive-pressure ventilation, jet ventilation and oscillation. These techniques are associated with effective gas exchange at lower peak airway pressures than conventional mechanical ventilation and may thereby reduce the incidence of barotrauma and ventilator-associated lung injury (see Chapter 7). Significant improvement in oxygenation can, however, only be achieved by increasing mean airway pressures. Jet ventilation at frequencies close to the natural resonant frequency of the lung (5–7 Hz) with high mean airway pressures may promote alveolar recruitment, thereby improving gas exchange when conventional ventilation has failed (Lin *et al.*, 1990). A prospective controlled trial has demonstrated that, although high-frequency jet ventilation can be used safely in ARF, outcome was no better than with standard techniques (Carlon *et al.*, 1983). There is, however, some reason to believe that newer jet ventilators may be more effective (see Chapter 7); prospective, randomized trials employing these devices are awaited. Prospective trials have suggested that high-frequency oscillation might be a safe and effective intervention for severely hypoxaemic patients with ARDS (Derdak *et al.*, 2002; Mehta *et al.*, 2001).

Non-invasive ventilation. Although the vast majority of patients with ALI/ARDS will require tracheal intubation, non-invasive ventilation via a facemask has proved effective in some studies. The place of non-invasive ventilation in the management of acute hypoxaemic respiratory failure remains unclear, however (Keenan *et al.*, 2004) (see Chapter 7).

Low-frequency positive-pressure ventilation with extracorporeal carbon dioxide removal (LFPPV-ECCO2-R) (see Chapter 7). The results of uncontrolled trials of LFPPV-ECCO2-R in ARDS were encouraging (Gattinoni *et al.*, 1986), but a randomized trial found no significant difference in survival between patients treated with ECCO2-R and those supported with pressure-controlled inverse-ratio ventilation (Morris *et al.*, 1994). Since the ability to maintain gas exchange with ECCO2-R is well established, some continue to use the technique in selected patients with intractable hypoxaemia and hypercarbia. Others feel that extracorporeal support for ARDS should be confined to controlled clinical trials (Morris et al., 1994). Although the concept of 'resting' the lung to promote recovery is theoretically attractive, these techniques are invasive, costly, can be associated with significant complications (mainly coagulopathies and haemorrhage) and have not yet been shown to improve outcome in controlled trials. It is also apparent that many fewer cases now require extracorporeal techniques merely to achieve adequate oxygenation. Even so, the role of extracorporeal gas exchange in the management of ARDS remains controversial (Peek and Firmin, 1997), especially given that improved technology with heparin-loaded circuits, non-occlusive roller pumps, improved anticoagulation and pumpless circuits (Reng et al., 2000) may reduce the incidence of complications. Many therefore believe that further controlled trials are warranted (McIntyre et al., 2000).

LIMITATION OF PULMONARY OEDEMA

Some time ago the use of diuretics and fluid restriction to minimize pulmonary oedema was shown to reduce extravascular lung water, days on the ventilator and length of stay in the ICU (Mitchell et al., 1992) and a recent large randomized, controlled trial demonstrated that, compared to a liberal strategy, a conservative strategy of fluid management improved lung function and shortened the duration of mechanical ventilation and intensive care, without increasing non-pulmonary organ failures. There was, however, no significant difference in 60-day mortality (National Heart, Lung and Blood Institute ARDS Clinical Trials Network, 2006a).

If possible, plasma oncotic pressure should be maintained by using colloidal solutions to expand the intravascular volume. In patients with ARDS, however, colloids are unlikely to be retained within the vascular compartment; once they enter the interstitial space, the intravascular oncotic gradient is lost and the main determinants of oedema formation become the microvascular hydrostatic pressure and the efficiency of lymphatic drainage. There is, therefore, some controversy about the relative merits of colloids or crystalloids for volume replacement in patients likely to develop ALI/ARDS or in whom the condition is established (see Chapter 5).

PHYSIOTHERAPY

During the acute phase of ALI/ARDS, when large volumes of pulmonary oedema are being produced continuously, chest physiotherapy, manual inflations and endotracheal suction are unlikely to be of any benefit. Later removal of secretions and re-expansion of collapsed lung segments may be helpful. Hypoxia due to discontinuation of PEEP and loss of supplemental oxygen during bronchial toilet can be avoided by using endotracheal tube adaptors with self-sealing diaphragms.

BODY POSITION CHANGES

Both lateral and prone positions have been shown to improve gas exchange. In the lateral position, with the less injured lung down, gravity increases blood flow to the good lung and V/Q matching is improved. When the patient is changed from the supine to the prone position lung densities in the dependent regions are redistributed; in some patients this is associated with improved gas exchange (Gattinoni et al., 1991). A reduced pleural pressure gradient, more uniform alveolar ventilation, caudal movement of the diaphragm, redistribution of perfusion, reduced effects of abdominal pressure on the thoracic cavity, improved postural drainage and removal of secretions and recruitment of collapsed alveoli may all contribute to this improvement in gas exchange. The triangular shape of the pleural cavity is also important because in the prone position the volume of the most dependent lung is minimized (Blanch et al., 1997). With appropriate experience, procedures and protocols, complications are infrequent but may include worsening oxygenation, skin pressure lesions, accidental extubation and removal of intravascular cannulae. Repeated position changes between prone and supine may allow reductions in airway pressures and F_IO_2, thereby attenuating ventilator-associated lung injury, especially if used early. The response to prone positioning is, however, variable (oxygenation improves in 60–70% of patients, sometimes dramatically) and can be unpredictable. Improvement is more likely in those with severe hypoxia and hypercarbia and early ARDS (Blanch et al., 1997) and the response may partly depend on whether the patient is suffering from pulmonary or extrapulmonary ARDS. Thus in extrapulmonary ARDS the redistribution of atelectasis from dorsal to ventral regions and possibly the changes in regional transpulmonary pressures may lead to rapid improvement in oxygenation whereas in pulmonary ARDS the improvement in oxygenation is less marked and more gradual; in these cases redistribution of ventilation may be a more important mechanism (Lim et al., 2001; Pelosi and Gattinoni, 2001).

The precise indications for prone positioning, the timing of position changes and the effect of this technique on outcome remain uncertain. In a recent prospective, randomized, controlled trial prone positioning failed to influence mortality from ALI/ARDS, despite improvements in oxygenation in more than 70% of the instances in which it was used (Gattinoni et al., 2001), although there was some suggestion of a short-term survival advantage for the most severe cases. Moreover the time patients spent in the prone position was relatively short (7 hours per day) and was limited to 10 days and a lung-protective ventilatory strategy was not specified. In a study of patients with hypoxaemic ARF, early systematic prone positioning for a median of 8 hours a day, for a median of 4 days, failed to improve outcome and was associated with some significant complications (e.g. endotracheal tube obstruction, pressure sores). Oxygenation was improved, however, and the incidence of VAP was reduced (Guerin et al., 2004). A more recent trial indicated that prone ventilation, when initiated early and applied for most of the day over a prolonged period (mean of 10 days), is feasible and safe and might reduce mortality (Mancebo et al., 2006).

Further, adequately powered trials of longer periods of prone positioning in patients with severe ARDS treated with lung-protective ventilation are required to determine the effects of this intervention on mortality. For the time being prone positioning cannot be recommended as routine treatment for all patients with ARDS, but should be reserved for those with severe hypoxaemia.

INHALED NITRIC OXIDE

In patients with ARDS, inhaled NO can reduce pulmonary artery pressure and increase P_aO_2 by improving V/Q matching without causing systemic vasodilatation (Rossaint et al., 1993). Inhaled NO may also reduce oedema formation and neutrophil sequestration in the lung. Although it has been shown to improve oxygenation in responders with ALI/ARDS, the response is often not sustained (Michael et al., 1998) and so far inhaled NO has not been shown to improve outcome. In one trial, for example, the clinical response was variable, with some 60% of patients showing improvements in oxygenation compared to 24% of those given placebo, and was not sustained. Mortality was unchanged (Dellinger et al., 1998) and in another trial the mortality from early ALI was unaffected (Lundin et al., 1999). Some studies have suggested an additive effect when NO administration is combined with prone positioning, especially in pulmonary ARDS (Rialp et al., 2001).

Administration of NO requires careful monitoring to avoid the production of dangerous amounts of toxic products of its combination with oxygen, such as nitrogen dioxide. There is also some concern that NO, being a reactive free radical, may be toxic to the lungs and that levels of dangerous metabolic intermediates such as peroxynitrite (see Chapter 5) may be increased. In one study, however, inhaled NO did not appear to exacerbate pulmonary inflammation or increase oxidant stress (Cuthbertson et al., 2000). Rebound pulmonary hypertension may also cause problems when inhaled NO is reduced or discontinued. NO may be useful as a short-term rescue therapy in patients with refractory hypoxaemia but cannot be recommended as standard treatment (McIntyre et al., 2000). Indeed, in one study prone positioning was more effective than inhaled NO as a means of improving hypoxaemia (Dupont et al., 2000) and a recent meta-analysis concluded that NO is associated with limited improvement in oxygenation but confers no mortality benefit and may be harmful (Adhikari et al., 2007).

ALMITRINE

Almitrine bismesylate potentiates hypoxic pulmonary vasoconstriction, thereby improving V/Q matching. Pulmonary artery pressure may increase. Not only does almitrine alone improve oxygenation but it also enhances the effects of inhaled NO (Gallart et al., 1998).

AEROSOLIZED PROSTACYCLIN

Aerosolized prostacyclin, which is easier to monitor and deliver, appears to have similar effects to inhaled NO in patients with ARDS (Walmrath et al., 1996b). Again, however, the response to inhaled prostacyclin is variable and its effects on outcome unknown.

AEROSOLIZED SURFACTANT

Because the lungs of patients with ALI/ARDS are deficient in surfactant (see above), intrapulmonary administration of exogenous surfactant might be expected to be beneficial by lowering alveolar surface tension, as well as through the immunomodulatory and antimicrobial properties of surfactant. Certainly surfactant administration reduces morbidity and mortality in neonatal respiratory distress syndrome and can improve lung function and survival in animal models of ARDS. Disappointingly, however, continuous aerosolized administration of a synthetic surfactant failed to influence outcome from sepsis-induced ARDS (Anzueto et al., 1996), perhaps because insufficient surfactant was delivered to the peripheral alveoli or because the synthetic preparation lacked the surfactant-specific proteins (Sp-A, -B, -C and -D) which contribute to the biophysical functions, anti-inflammatory and antimicrobial properties of natural surfactant. Bronchoscopically directed administration of larger doses of a natural bovine surfactant extract produced more encouraging preliminary results (Walmrath et al., 1996a), as did intratracheal instillation of a bovine preparation which improved gas exchange and was associated with a trend for increased survival (Gregory et al., 1997). Disappointingly, however, tracheal instillation of a recombinant protein C-based surfactant failed to improve overall survival in a heterogeneous population of patients with ARDS (Spragg et al., 2004).

PARTIAL LIQUID VENTILATION

Perfluorocarbons are dense, volatile liquids which ultimately evaporate from the lung with little systemic absorption. They have a low surface tension and extremely high solubility for oxygen and carbon dioxide. By filling the FRC of the lungs with perfluorocarbon liquid the alveoli are held open and gas exchange is facilitated. Lavage of cellular debris and anti-inflammatory effects may also be beneficial. In a small, prospective, uncontrolled study this technique improved gas exchange without affecting haemodynamics, but pulmonary compliance was unchanged and mortality remained near 50% (Hirschl et al., 1998). Partial liquid ventilation cannot be recommended as a treatment for ARDS at present.

CARDIOVASCULAR SUPPORT

Although patients with ALI/ARDS are usually hyperdynamic, cardiac output may be compromised by a variety of factors, including low filling pressures due to fluid restriction, high levels of PEEP, increased pulmonary vascular resistance and the myocardial effects of sepsis (see Chapter 5). Moreover, as many as 20% of patients with ARDS suffer from concomitant heart disease.

Tissue DO_2 should be optimized (see Chapter 5) by ensuring that the haemoglobin concentration is adequate, cautious expansion of the circulating volume, the use of inotropic support when required, and possibly the administration of specific agents such as inhaled NO or aerosolized prostacyclin to reduce pulmonary hypertension. Because administration of large volumes of fluid in an effort to maintain cardiac output and blood pressure is likely to exacerbate pulmonary oedema there should be no hesitation in using inotropes and vasoconstrictors to achieve an adequate cardiac output and blood pressure in the face of relative hypovolaemia. In one study early pulmonary artery catheterization did not appear to affect either morbidity or mortality in patients with shock, ARDS or both (Richard et al., 2003) and in a recent large, multicentre trial pulmonary artery catheter-guided therapy did not improve survival or organ function, and was associated with more complications when compared to central venous catheter-guided therapy. The pulmonary artery catheter should not therefore be routinely used for the management of ALI (National Heart, Lung and Blood Institute ARDS Clinical Trials Network, 2006b). It is also important to appreciate that a low PAOP does not necessarily imply hypovolaemia requiring correction and should not automatically prompt the administration of fluids. Transoesophageal echocardiography can be used to assess left ventricular filling and right ventricular impairment, whilst in some cases the oesophageal Doppler may prove useful.

Administration of prostaglandin E_1 to patients with ARDS reduces systemic and pulmonary vascular resistances; this is accompanied by increases in stroke volume, heart rate and cardiac output (Bone et al., 1989; Silverman et al., 1990). Despite these apparently beneficial physiological effects, prostaglandin E_1 failed to improve outcome in a mixed group of medical and surgical patients with ARDS (Bone et al., 1989), and in a more recent prospective randomized controlled study liposomal prostaglandin E_1 did not influence mortality (Abraham et al., 1999). Administration of prostaglandin E_1 may be complicated by hypotension (Abraham et al., 1999), a deterioration in gas exchange (Melot et al., 1989) and an increased incidence of diarrhoea (Bone et al., 1989). Prostaglandin E_1 is not recommended for patients with ARDS (McIntyre et al., 2000).

ANTI-INFLAMMATORY AGENTS

Prior administration of corticosteroids to sheep given endotoxin prevents the subsequent increase in lung vascular permeability (Brigham et al., 1981) and the early administration of high-dose corticosteroids to patients with septic ARDS may in some cases reduce alveolar–capillary permeability (Sibbald et al., 1981). High-dose corticosteroids have not, however, been shown to prevent ARDS in patients at risk or improve outcome in the acute stages of ARDS in humans (Bernard et al., 1987), although it has been suggested that they may be beneficial when administered during the late fibroproliferative phase. In a small randomized controlled trial of 24 patients, methylprednisolone 2 mg/kg daily, reducing over 32 days, improved hospital mortality in patients who had not responded to supportive techniques alone by the seventh day of respiratory failure (Meduri et al.,

1998). A recent multicentre, randomized, controlled trial, however, did not support the routine use of methylprednisolone for persistent ARDS (although such treatment was associated with some improvement in cardiopulmonary physiology and an increase in the number of ventilator-free and shock-free days). Moreover starting methylprednisolone treatment more than 14 days after the onset of ARDS was associated with significantly increased mortality rates (National Heart, Lung, and Blood Institute ARDS Clinical Trials Network, 2006c).

Ibuprofen may reduce pulmonary hypertension and improve oxygenation in ARDS but does not reduce the incidence or duration of ARDS in patients with sepsis, nor is outcome improved (see Chapter 5). The value of other agents that might limit pulmonary damage such as antioxidants/free radical scavengers (e.g. catalase, superoxide dismutase, N-acetylcysteine) and immunotherapy is uncertain (see also Chapter 5).

Outcome

There is increasing evidence to suggest that mortality from ARDS has fallen over the last two decades, from around 60% to between 30 and 40% (Abel et al., 1998; Bersten et al., 2002; Milberg et al., 1995), perhaps as a consequence of improved general care, the increasing use of management protocols and attention to infection control and nutrition, as well as the introduction of novel treatments and lung-protective strategies for respiratory support. Indeed it may now be possible to achieve hospital mortality rates as low as 25–30% (Levy, 2004; National Heart, Lung and Blood Institute ARDS Clinical Trials Network, 2004). Prognosis is, however, very dependent on aetiology. For example, when ARDS occurs in association with septic shock and persistent sepsis, mortality rates may be as high as 90%. In addition, the development of ARDS significantly worsens the prognosis in sepsis and is an independent predictor of outcome.

Patients with ARDS due to fat embolism, on the other hand, have a much better prognosis, with survival rates of around 90%. ARDS developing after cardiopulmonary bypass also has a relatively good prognosis, while medical patients tend to have a higher mortality than trauma patients. Mortality rises with increasing age (Rubenfeld et al., 2005), failure of other organs and the presence of chronic liver disease. Surprisingly, initial indices of oxygenation and ventilation do not predict outcome (Milberg et al., 1995). The failure of pulmonary function to improve during the first week of treatment is, however, a poor prognostic sign. The dead-space fraction, Simplified Acute Physiology Score II (SAPS II) and quasistatic respiratory compliance are independent risk factors for death (Nuckton et al., 2002). There is also some evidence to suggest that mortality is higher in patients with ARDS caused by direct pulmonary insults (predominantly pneumonia) than in those with extrapulmonary causes (such as cardiac surgery, abdominal pathology, sepsis and trauma) (Suntharalingam et al., 2001).

Death is rarely due to irreversible respiratory failure (Montgomery *et al.*, 1985), and more than 75% of patients who die with ARDS now do so as a result of MODS and haemodynamic instability rather than impaired gas exchange. Most early deaths are attributable to the underlying illness or injury, whereas late deaths are usually related to sepsis (Montgomery *et al.*, 1985). Acute renal failure (ARF) is common in patients with ARDS and adversely affects the prognosis, while the development of liver failure is associated with a particularly poor outlook.

Lung function of patients who recover from ARDS improves considerably over the first 3 months and typically there is little further improvement beyond 6 months. Overall lung function tests recover to about 80% of predicted values (McHugh *et al.*, 1994). When present, residual radiographic changes are normally limited to a few linear scars, isolated areas of pleural thickening and small, bullous cysts. Residual impairment of lung mechanics may include mild restriction, obstruction, impairment of carbon monoxide diffusion capacity or impaired gas exchange on exercise. In one study lung volume and spirometric measurements were normal by 6 months, but carbon monoxide diffusion capacity remained low throughout the 12-month follow-up. In only 6% of patients did oxygen saturation fall below 88% on exercise (Herridge *et al.*, 2003). These abnormalities are, however, usually asymptomatic. Those with severe disease requiring prolonged ventilation are at the highest risk for persistent abnormalities of lung function. CT scanning the lungs of ARDS survivors often reveals a reticular pattern, with a striking anterior distribution, which is most closely related to the duration of respiratory support, suggesting that alveolar overdistension in the unprotected, non-consolidated lung regions is responsible for this long-term fibrotic change (Desai *et al.*, 1999).

Long-term survivors of ARDS who report adverse experiences during intensive care often show evidence of post-traumatic stress disorders, anxiety and depression (Schelling *et al.*, 1998). Disappointingly, quality of life may be markedly impaired and there is a continuing risk of death for several months after discharge (even in previously healthy ARDS survivors) (Angus *et al.*, 2001). Persistent functional disability is common up to 1 year after discharge from ICU and is largely a result of muscle wasting and weakness and, to a lesser extent, entrapment neuropathy, heterotopic ossification and pulmonary abnormalities (Herridge *et al.*, 2003).

ASPIRATION PNEUMONITIS AND ASPIRATION PNEUMONIA (Marik, 2001)

Factors predisposing to pulmonary aspiration include obtundation, impaired laryngopharyngeal reflexes and a propensity to vomiting or regurgitation (**Table 8.6**). Nasogastric tubes, especially if wide-bore, predispose to aspiration by preventing closure of the oesophageal sphincter and interfering with coughing and clearing of the pharynx. The use of a percutaneous gastrostomy or enterostomy for enteral nutrition has not, however, been shown to reduce the incidence

Table 8.6 Factors predisposing to pulmonary aspiration

Reduced consciousness

Overdose (10% of cases)
Metabolic coma
General anaesthesia
Head injury
Cerebrovascular accident
Epilepsy

Impaired cough and gag

Motor or sensory bulbar dysfunction
Recent extubation of larynx
Elderly patients
Severe illness

Increased susceptibility to regurgitation/vomiting

Hiatus hernia
Oesophageal obstruction
Oesophagectomy
Bowel obstruction
Pregnancy
Presence of nasogastric tube

of aspiration pneumonia. Critically ill patients are at increased risk of aspiration pneumonia because of gastroparesis, the presence of a nasogastric tube and obtundation, especially when in the supine position. Although the presence of an endotracheal or tracheostomy tube protects against large-volume aspiration, the vocal cords and epiglottis are held open, allowing fluids to accumulate above the cuff. Small amounts may then trickle past the cuff into the lungs (see also ventilator associated pneumonia Chapter 7).

The consequences of pulmonary aspiration depend on the nature of the aspirate, but overall about a third of patients with clearly documented aspiration will subsequently develop ARDS.

Types of aspiration
ASPIRATION OF STERILE ACIDIC GASTRIC CONTENTS (ASPIRATION PNEUMONITIS)
Aspiration of sterile acidic gastric contents causes severe damage within minutes. The alveolar–capillary barrier loses its integrity, high-permeability oedema develops rapidly and acid denaturation of surfactant leads to atelectasis. Within a few hours there is degeneration of the bronchial epithelium, destruction of type II alveolar lining cells and an inflammatory cell infiltrate, consisting predominantly of neutrophils. This is associated with acid-mediated induction and release of proinflammatory cytokines such as tumour necrosis factor and IL-8, cyclooxygenase and lipooxygenase products,

reactive oxygen species and adhesion molecule expression. In those who survive, the inflammatory response resolves, the bronchial epithelium regenerates and the fibroproliferative phase supervenes.

Clinically there is sudden onset of severe dyspnoea, cough, cyanosis and wheeze, often associated with hypovolaemia and hypotension (Mendelson's syndrome; see Chapter 18). There may be rapid progression to ARDS. In some cases aspiration is 'silent'.

ASPIRATION OF INFECTED FLUIDS (ASPIRATION PNEUMONIA)

The stomach and oropharynx of patients who have been ill or hospitalized for some time, especially those patients with gastrointestinal pathology and those receiving antacids, are frequently colonized by pathogenic bacteria. Under these circumstances aspiration can result in severe pneumonia, often caused by Gram-negative organisms normally resident only in the lower gastrointestinal tract. Pathological changes are similar to, but generally less severe than, those of pure acid aspiration except that they may be complicated later by infection. Unlike those with aspiration pneumonitis, the episode of aspiration is often not witnessed.

ASPIRATION OF PARTICULATE MATTER

Aspiration of particulate matter (e.g. food) may cause acute large-airways obstruction or, if smaller irritant particles such as meat or vegetables are inhaled, may precipitate an inflammatory response followed by a granulomatous reaction with minimal fibrosis. Uncleared particles may lead to persistent infection, necrotizing pneumonia, abscess formation or empyema. Chest radiography may show focal collapse or consolidation.

The consequences of aspirating large quantities of fine particles in neutral gastric contents, as may occur some time after a meal, are similar, but less severe than those of pure acid aspiration.

ASPIRATION OF INERT FLUIDS

Inert fluids free of particulate matter or bacteria produce minimal pulmonary damage. The immediate clinical consequences depend solely on the volume aspirated, and resolution is usually rapid.

Diagnosing aspiration

The diagnosis of aspiration is largely clinical, but can often be confirmed by examining an endotracheal aspirate or by bronchoscopy. Chest X-ray appearances are helpful but not pathognomonic.

Management

The patient should be positioned head-down on his or her right-hand side, the airway secured, the oropharynx suctioned and oxygen given. Those with a depressed conscious level and/or impaired airway protection will require tracheal intubation. A nasogastric tube should be passed to empty the stomach.

When particulate aspiration has occurred and when focal collapse or foreign bodies are visible on the chest radiograph, *bronchoscopy* may be indicated. *Rigid bronchoscopy* is usually most effective, but a general anaesthetic is required and it may be difficult to maintain acceptable oxygenation. Also access to the upper lobes and more distal airways is limited. *Fibreoptic bronchoscopy* may therefore be preferred, especially in those with more distal airways occlusion and when attempting to remove solid foreign particles such as teeth or amalgam. Bronchial lavage is probably of no value, but *chest physiotherapy* is essential. *Bronchodilators* may be required.

The use of *antibiotics* is controversial. Recent evidence suggests that significant concentrations of bacterial pathogens are isolated in fewer than half of patients with aspiration pneumonia. In those who aspirate in the community, *Streptococcus pneumoniae*, *Staphylococcus aureus*, *Haemophilus influenzae* and *Enterobacter* predominate, whereas in patients with hospital-acquired aspiration Gram-negative organisms, including *Pseudomonas aeruginosa*, are most common. Anaerobic organisms are not usually isolated (Marik, 2001; Mier et al., 1993). Although prophylactic antibiotics are commonly administered to patients in whom aspiration has been witnessed or is suspected, this practice is not generally recommended. Empirical antibiotic therapy is, however, considered to be appropriate for patients who aspirate gastric contents and who have small-bowel obstruction or other conditions associated with gastric colonization. Antibiotic therapy should also be considered when aspiration pneumonitis fails to resolve and is clearly indicated for those with aspiration pneumonia. Sampling of the lower respiratory tract with a protected brush specimen or BAL is recommended by some to identify the causative organism(s). An appropriate broad-spectrum antibiotic should be selected (e.g. a second or third generation cephalosporin or piperacillin/tazobactam); agents with specific activity against anaerobic organisms (e.g. metronidazole) are not normally recommended but may be indicated in patients with severe periodontal disease, putrid sputum or radiographic evidence of necrotizing pneumonia or lung abscess. Because *Streptococcus pneumoniae* is frequently isolated from the lungs of patients who aspirate in the community, some have recommended routine prophylaxis with penicillin in such cases (Mier et al., 1993).

The administration of *corticosteroids* has also been controversial. The majority of studies suggest that they are of no benefit and there is a danger that they may increase the incidence of superimposed infection and impair the ability of fibroblasts to wall off aspirated foodstuffs. The administration of corticosteroids is not recommended.

SEVERE ACUTE RESPIRATORY SYNDROME (SARS)

In the last few years there have been a number of worldwide outbreaks of an acute, severe, highly infectious pneumonia caused by a novel coronavirus. This condition has been termed SARS and is characterized by high fever, with or without chills and rigors, influenza-like symptoms and new radiological infiltrates compatible with pneumonia. There may be a history of contact with infected individuals. Other possible aetiological agents should be excluded. Stringent infection control measures must be adopted to minimize droplet spread and contact with the patient's secretions, fluids or excreta. For example, patients should be isolated in cubicles with negative-pressure airflow, closed suction systems should be used for those receiving mechanical ventilation and health care workers should wear effective face-masks, protective eye wear, full-face shields, caps, gowns with full sleeve coverage, surgical gloves and shoe covers. A protocol for the management of patients with SARS which includes antibacterials (levofloxacin or co-amoxiclav with clarithromycin) and a combination of ribavirin and methylprednisolone has been described (So *et al.*, 2003). Four out of the 31 patients treated in this series received non-invasive ventilation, but none required tracheal intubation and there were no deaths (So *et al.*, 2003).

REFERENCES

Abel SJ, Finney SJ, Brett SJ, et al. (1998) Reduced mortality in association with the acute respiratory distress syndrome (ARDS). *Thorax* **53**: 292–294.

Abraham E, Baughman R, Fletcher E, et al. (1999) Liposomal prostaglandin E1 (TLC C-53) in acute respiratory distress syndrome: a controlled, randomized, double-blind, multicenter clinical trial. TLC-C-53 ARDS study group. *Critical Care Medicine* **27**: 1478–1485.

Acute Respiratory Distress Syndrome Network (2000) Ventilation with lower tidal volumes as compared with traditional tidal volumes for acute lung injury and the acute respiratory distress syndrome. *New England Journal of Medicine* **342**: 1301–1308.

Adhikari NKJ, Burns KEA, Friedrich JO, et al. (2007) Effect of nitric oxide on oxygenation and mortality in acute lung injury: systematic review and meta-analysis. *British Medical Journal* **334**: 779–781.

Adnet F, Dhissi G, Borron SW, et al. (2001) Complication profiles of adult asthmatics requiring paralysis during mechanical ventilation. *Intensive Care Medicine* **27**: 1729–1736.

Amato MBP, Barbas CS, Medeiros DM, et al. (1998) Effect of a protective ventilation strategy on mortality in the acute respiratory distress syndrome. *New England Journal of Medicine* **338**: 347–354.

Angus D, Musthafa AA, Clermont G, et al. (2001) Quality-adjusted survival in the first year after the acute respiratory distress syndrome. *American Journal of Respiratory and Critical Care Medicine* **163**: 1389–1394.

Angus D, Marrie TJ, Obrosky DS, et al. (2002) Severe community acquired pneumonia. Use of intensive care services and evaluation of American and British Thoracic society diagnostic criteria. *American Journal of Respiratory and Critical Care Medicine* **166**: 717–723.

Anzueto A, Baughman RP, Guntupalli KK, et al. (1996) Aerosolized surfactant in adults with sepsis-induced acute respiratory distress syndrome. *New England Journal of Medicine* **334**: 1417–1421.

Ashbaugh DG, Bigelow DB, Petty TL, et al. (1967) Acute respiratory distress in adults. *Lancet* **2**: 319–323.

Aubier M, Trippenbach T, Roussos C (1981) Respiratory muscle fatigue during cardiogenic shock. *Journal of Applied Physiology* **51**: 499–508.

Aubier M, Viires N, Syllie G, et al. (1982) Respiratory muscle contribution to lactic acidosis in low cardiac output. *American Review of Respiratory Disease* **126**: 648–652.

Aubier M, Murciano D, Lecocguic Y, et al. (1985) Effect of hypophosphatemia on diaphragmatic contractility in patients with acute respiratory failure. *New England Journal of Medicine* **313**: 420–424.

Azoulay E, Darmon M, Delclaux C, et al. (2002) Deterioration of previous acute lung injury during neutropenia recovery. *Critical Care Medicine* **30**: 781–786.

Baldwin SR, Simon RH, Grum CM, et al. (1986) Oxidant activity in expired breath of patients with adult respiratory distress syndrome. *Lancet* **1**: 11–14.

Barber RE, Hamilton WK (1970) Oxygen toxicity in man. A prospective study in patients with irreversible brain damage. *New England Journal of Medicine* **283**: 1478–1484.

Barberà JA, Roger N, Roca J, et al. (1996) Worsening of pulmonary gas exchange with nitric oxide inhalation in chronic obstructive pulmonary disease. *Lancet* **347**: 436–440.

Barr RG, Rowe BH, Camargo CA Jr (2003) Methylxanthines for exacerbations of chronic obstructive pulmonary disease: meta-analysis of randomised trials. *British Medical Journal* **327**: 643.

Bellet PS, Kalinyak KA, Shukla R, et al. (1995) Incentive spirometry to prevent acute pulmonary complications. *New England Journal of Medicine* **333**: 699–703.

Bernard GR, Luce JM, Sprung CL, et al. (1987) High-dose corticosteroids in patients with the adult respiratory distress syndrome. *New England Journal of Medicine* **317**: 1565–1570.

Bernard GR, Artigas A, Brigham KL, et al. (1994) The American-European Consensus Conference on ARDS: definitions, mechanisms, relevant outcomes and clinical trial coordination. *American Journal of Respiratory and Critical Care Medicine* **149**: 818–824.

Bersten AD, Edibam C, Hunt T, et al. (2002) Incidence and mortality of acute lung injury and the acute respiratory distress syndrome in three Australian states. *American Journal of Respiratory and Critical Care Medicine* **165**: 443–448.

Blanch L, Mancebo J, Perez M, et al. (1997) Short-term effects of prone position in critically ill patients with acute respiratory distress syndrome. *Intensive Care Medicine* **23**: 1033–1039.

Bone RC, Slotman G, Maunder R, et al. (1989) Randomized double-blind, multicenter study of prostaglandin E₁ in patients with the adult respiratory distress syndrome. *Chest* **96**: 114–119.

Bone RC, Balk R, Slotman G, et al. (1992) Adult respiratory distress syndrome. Sequence and importance of development of multiple organ failure. *Chest* **101**: 320–326.

Brett SJ, Evans TW (1998) Measurement of endogenous nitric oxide in the lungs of patients with the acute respiratory distress syndrome. *American Journal of Respiratory and Critical Care Medicine* **157**: 993–997.

Brigham KL, Bowers RE, McKeen CR (1981) Methylprednisolone prevention of increased lung vascular permeability following endotoxemia in sheep. *Journal of Clinical Investigation* **67**: 1103–1110.

British Thoracic Society; Scottish Intercollegiate Guidelines Network (2003) British guideline on the management of asthma. *Thorax* **58** (Suppl. 1): 1–94.

British Thoracic Society Standards of Care Committee (2001) BTS guidelines for the management of community acquired pneumonia. *Thorax* **56** (Suppl.): 41–64 (update 2004 available at www.brit-thoracic.org.uk/guidelines).

Brochard L, Roudot-Thoraval F, Roupie E, et al. (1998) Tidal volume reduction for prevention of ventilator-induced lung injury in the acute respiratory distress syndrome. *American Journal of Respiratory and Critical Care Medicine* **158**: 1831–1838.

Bucknall CE, Slack R, Godley CC, et al. (1999) Scottish confidential inquiry into asthma deaths. *Thorax* **54**: 978–984.

Burge PS, Calverley PM, Jones PW, et al. (2000) Randomised double blind, placebo controlled study of fluticasone propionate in patients with moderate to severe chronic obstructive pulmonary disease: the ISOLDE trial. *British Medical Journal* **320**: 1297–1303.

Butt W, Shann F, Walker C, et al. (1988) Acute epiglottitis: a different approach to management. *Critical Care Medicine* **16**: 43–47.

Caldwell PR, Lee WL Jr, Schildkraut HS, et al. (1966) Changes in lung volume, diffusing capacity, and blood gases in men breathing oxygen. *Journal of Applied Physiology* **21**: 1477–1483.

Calverley PM (2000) Oxygen-induced hypercapnia revisited. *Lancet* **356**: 1538–1539.

Campbell EJ (1960a) A method of controlled oxygen administration which reduces the risk of carbon-dioxide retention. *Lancet* **2**: 12–14.

Campbell EJ (1960b) Respiratory failure. The relation between oxygen concentrations of inspired air and arterial blood. *Lancet* **2**: 10–11.

Campbell EJ (1982) How to use the Venturi mask. *Lancet* **2**: 1206.

Campbell MJ, Cogman GR, Holgate ST, et al. (1997) Age specific trends in asthma mortality in England and Wales, 1983–95: results of an observational study. *British Medical Journal* **314**: 1439–1441.

Carlon GC, Howland WS, Ray C, et al. (1983) High-frequency jet ventilation. A prospective randomized evaluation. *Chest* **84**: 551–559.

Cheong B, Reynolds SR, Rajan G, et al. (1988) Intravenous β-agonist in severe acute asthma. British Medical Journal 297: 448–450.

Chiumello D, Pristine G, Slutsky AS (1999) Mechanical ventilation affects local and systemic cytokines in an animal model of acute respiratory distress syndrome. American Journal of Respiratory and Critical Care Medicine 160: 109–116.

COMBIVENT Inhalation Aerosol Study Group (1994) In chronic obstructive pulmonary disease, a combination of ipratropium and albuterol is more effective than either agent alone. An 85-day multicenter trial. Chest 105: 1411–1419.

Comroe JH Jr, Dripps RD, Dumke PR, et al. (1945) Oxygen toxicity. The effect of inhalation of high concentrations of oxygen for twenty-four hours on normal men at sea level and at a simulated altitude of 18,000 feet. Journal of the American Medical Association 128: 710–717.

Confalonieri M, Urbino R, Potena A, et al. (2005) Hydrocortisone infusion for severe community-acquired pneumonia. American Journal of Respiratory and Critical Care Medicine 171: 242–248.

COPD Guidelines Group of the Standards of Care Committee of the BTS (1997) BTS Guidelines for the management of chronic obstructive pulmonary disease. Thorax 52 (Suppl. 5): S1–28.

Cuthbertson BH, Galley HF, Webster NR (2000) Effect of inhaled nitric oxide on key mediators of the inflammatory response in patients with acute lung injury. Critical Care Medicine 28: 1736–1741.

Davies L, Angus RM, Calverley PM (1999) Oral corticosteroids in patients admitted to hospital with exacerbations of chronic obstructive pulmonary disease: a prospective randomised controlled trial. Lancet 354: 456–460.

Dellinger RP, Zimmerman JL, Taylor RW, et al. (1998) Effects of inhaled nitric oxide in patients with acute respiratory distress syndrome: results of a randomized phase II trial. Critical Care Medicine 26: 15–23.

Deneke SM, Fanburg BL (1982) Oxygen toxicity of the lung: an update. British Journal of Anaesthesia 54: 737–749.

Derdak S, Mehta S, Stewart TE, et al. (2002) High-frequency oscillatory ventilation for acute respiratory distress syndrome in adults. American Journal of Respiratory and Critical Care Medicine 166: 801–808.

Desai SR, Wells AU, Rubens MB, et al. (1999) Acute respiratory distress syndrome: CT abnormalities at long-term follow-up. Radiology 210: 29–35.

Dhand R, Duarte AG, Jubran A, et al. (1996) Dose–response to bronchodilator delivered by metered-dose inhaler in ventilator-supported patients. American Journal of Respiratory and Critical Care Medicine 154: 388–393.

Dimond JP, Palazzo MG (1997) An unconscious man with asthma and a fixed, dilated pupil. Lancet 349: 98.

Djukanovic R, Roche WR, Wilson JW, et al. (1990) Mucosal inflammation in asthma. American Review of Respiratory Disease 142: 434–457.

Donnelly SC, Strieter RM, Kunkel SL, et al. (1993) Interleukin 8 and development of adult respiratory distress syndrome in at-risk patient groups. Lancet 341: 643–647.

Donnelly SC, Haslett C, Dransfield I, et al (1994) Role of selectins in development of adult respiratory distress syndrome. Lancet 344: 215–219.

Donnelly SC, Haslett C, Reid PT, et al. (1997) Regulatory role for macrophage migration inhibitory factor in acute respiratory distress syndrome. Nature Medicine 3: 320–323.

Dupont H, Mentec H, Cheval C, et al. (2000) Short-term effect of inhaled nitric oxide and prone positioning in gas exchange in patients with severe acute respiratory distress syndrome. Critical Care Medicine 28: 304–308.

Eason J, Markowe HL (1987) Controlled investigation of deaths from asthma in hospitals in the North East Thames region. British Medical Journal 294: 1255–1258.

Efthimiou J, Fleming J, Spiro SG (1987) Sternomastoid muscle function and fatigue in breathless patients with severe respiratory disease. American Review of Respiratory Disease 136: 1099–1105.

Eisner MD, Thompson T, Hudson LD, et al. (2001) Efficacy of low tidal volume ventilation in patients with different clinical risk factors for acute lung injury and the acute respiratory distress syndrome. American Journal of Respiratory and Critical Care Medicine 164: 231–236.

Esteban A, Alia I, Gordo F, et al. (2000) Prospective randomised trial comparing pressure-controlled ventilation and volume-controlled ventilation in ARDS. Chest 117: 1690–1696.

Evans TW, Tweney J, Waterhouse JC, et al. (1990) Almitrine bismesylate and oxygen therapy in hypoxic cor pulmonale. Thorax 45: 16–21.

Fink JB, Dhand R, Duarte AG, et al. (1996) Aerosol delivery from a metered-dose inhaler during mechanical ventilation. American Journal of Respiratory and Critical Care Medicine 154: 382–387.

Fisher MM, Bowey CJ, Ladd-Hudson K (1989) External chest compression in acute asthma: a preliminary study. Critical Care Medicine 17: 686–687.

Gadek JE, DeMichele SJ, Karlstad MD, et al. (1999) Effect of enteral feeding with eicosapentaenoic acid, γ-linolenic acid and antioxidants in patients with acute respiratory distress syndrome. Critical Care Medicine 27: 1409–1420.

Gallart L, Lu Q, Puybasset L, et al. (1998) Intravenous almitrine combined with inhaled nitric oxide for acute respiratory distress syndrome. American Journal of Respiratory and Critical Care Medicine 158: 1770–1777.

Gattinoni L, Pesenti A, Mascheroni D, et al. (1986) Low-frequency positive-pressure ventilation with extracorporeal CO_2 removal in severe acute respiratory failure. Journal of the American Medical Association 256: 881–886.

Gattinoni L, Pelosi P, Vitale G, et al. (1991) Body position changes redistribute lung computed tomographic density in patients with acute respiratory failure. Anesthesiology 74: 15–23.

Gattinoni L, Pelosi P, Crotti S, et al. (1995) Effects of positive end-expiratory pressure on regional distribution of tidal volume and recruitment in adult respiratory distress syndrome. American Journal of Respiratory and Critical Care Medicine 151: 1807–1814.

Gattinoni L, Pelosi P, Suter PM, et al. (1998) Acute respiratory distress syndrome caused by pulmonary and extrapulmonary disease. American Journal of Respiratory and Critical Care Medicine 158: 3–11.

Gattinoni L, Tognoni G, Pesenti A, et al. (2001) Effect of prone positioning on the survival of patients with acute respiratory failure. New England Journal of Medicine 345: 568–573.

Gattinoni L, Caironi P, Cressoni M, et al. (2006) Lung recruitment in patients with the acute respiratory distress syndrome. New England Journal of Medicine 354: 1775–1786.

Goldstein RS, Young J, Rebuck AS (1982) Effect of breathing pattern on oxygen concentration received from standard facemasks. Lancet 2: 1188–1190.

Grasso S, Mascia L, Del Turco M, et al. (2002) Effects of recruiting maneuvers in patients with acute respiratory distress syndrome ventilated with protective ventilatory strategy. Anesthesiology 96: 795–802.

Gregory TJ, Steinberg KP, Spragg R, et al. (1997) Bovine surfactant therapy for patients with acute respiratory distress syndrome. American Journal of Respiratory and Critical Care Medicine 155: 1309–1315.

Griffiths TL, Burr ML, Campbell IA, et al. (2000) Results at 1 year of outpatient multidisciplinary pulmonary rehabilitation: a randomised controlled trial. Lancet 355: 362–368.

Guerin C, Milic-Emili J, Fournier G (2000) Effect of PEEP on work of breathing in mechanically ventilated COPD patients. Intensive Care Medicine 26: 1207–1214.

Guerin C, Gaillard S, Lemasson S, et al. (2004) Effects of systematic prone positioning in hypoxemic acute respiratory failure: a randomized controlled trial. Journal of the American Medical Association 292: 2379–2387.

Heflin AC Jr, Brigham KL (1981) Prevention by granulocyte depletion of increased vascular permeability of sheep lung following endotoxemia. Journal of Clinical Investigation 68: 1253–1260.

Herridge MS, Cheung AM, Tansey CM, et al. (2003) One-year outcomes in survivors of the acute respiratory distress syndrome. New England Journal of Medicine 348: 683–693.

Hickling KG, Walsh J, Henderson S, et al. (1994) Low mortality rate in adult respiratory distress syndrome using low-volume, pressure-limited ventilation with permissive hypercapnia: a prospective study. Critical Care Medicine 22: 1568–1578.

Hirschl RB, Conrad S, Kaiser R, et al. (1998) Partial liquid ventilation in adult patients with ARDS: a multicenter phase I-II trial. Annals of Surgery 228: 692–700.

Howton JC, Rose J, Duffy S, et al. (1996) Randomized, double-blind, placebo-controlled trial of intravenous ketamine in acute asthma. Annals of Emergency Medicine 27: 170–175.

Hughes R, Golkorn A, Masoli M, et al. (2003) Use of isotonic nebulised magnesium sulphate as an adjuvant to salbutamol in treatment of severe asthma in adults: randomised placebo-controlled trial. Lancet 361: 2114–2117.

Hussain SN, Simkus G, Roussos C (1985) Respiratory muscle fatigue: a cause of ventilatory failure in septic shock. Journal of Applied Physiology 58: 2033–2040.

Jackson RM (1990) Molecular, pharmacologic, and clinical aspects of oxygen-induced lung injury. Clinics in Chest Medicine 11: 73–86.

Jacob HS (1981) The role of activated complement and granulocytes in shock states and myocardial infarction. *Journal of Laboratory and Clinical Medicine* **98**: 645–653.

Jansen JE, Sorensen AI, Naesh O, et al. (1990) Effect of doxapram on postoperative pulmonary complications after upper abdominal surgery in high-risk patients. *Lancet* **335**: 936–938.

Jolliet P, Tassaux D, Thouret J-M, et al. (1999) Beneficial effects of helium:oxygen versus air:oxygen during noninvasive pressure support in patients with decompensated chronic obstructive pulmonary disease. *Critical Care Medicine* **27**: 2422–2429.

Jones JG, Sapsford DJ, Wheatley RG (1990) Postoperative hypoxaemia: mechanisms and time course. *Anaesthesia* **45**: 566–573.

Keenan SP, Sinuff T, Cook DJ, et al. (2004) Does non-invasive positive pressure ventilation improve outcome in acute hypoxemic respiratory failure? A systematic review. *Critical Care Medicine* **32**: 2516–2523.

Kikuchi Y, Okabe S, Tamura G, et al. (1994) Chemosensitivity and perception of dyspnea in patients with a history of near fatal asthma. *New England Journal of Medicine* **330**: 1329–1334.

Kurahashi K, Kajikawa O, Sawa J, et al. (1999) Pathogenesis of septic shock in *Pseudomonas aeruginosa* pneumonia. *Journal of Clinical Investigation* **104**: 743–750.

Laaban J-P, Grateau G, Psychoyos I, et al. (1989) Hypophosphatemia induced by mechanical ventilation in patients with chronic obstructive pulmonary disease. *Critical Care Medicine* **17**: 1115–1120.

Laffey JG, O'Croinin D, McLoughlin P, et al. (2004) Permissive hypercapnia – role in protective lung ventilatory strategies. *Intensive Care Medicine* **30**: 347–356.

Laufe MD, Simon RH, Flint A, et al. (1986) Adult respiratory distress syndrome in neutropenic patients. *American Journal of Medicine* **80**: 1022–1026.

Lawrence VA, Dhanda R, Hilsenbeck SG, et al. (1996) Risk of pulmonary complications after elective abdominal surgery. *Chest* **110**: 744–750.

Leff JA, Parsons PE, Day CE, et al. (1993) Serum antioxidants as predictors of adult respiratory distress syndrome in patients with sepsis. *Lancet* **341**: 777–780.

Levine S, Kaiser L, Leferovich J, et al. (1997) Cellular adaptations in the diaphragm in chronic obstructive pulmonary disease. *New England Journal of Medicine* **337**: 1799–1806.

Levy MM (2004) PEEP in ARDS – how much is enough? *New England Journal of Medicine* **351**: 389–391.

Lim C-M, Kim EK, Lee JS, et al. (2001) Comparison of the response to the prone position between pulmonary and extrapulmonary acute respiratory distress syndrome. *Intensive Care Medicine* **27**: 477–485.

Lim WS, van der Eerden MM, Laing R, et al. (2003) Defining community acquired pneumonia severity on presentation to hospital: an international derivation and validation study. *Thorax* **58**: 377–382.

Lin ES, Jones MJ, Mottram SD, et al. (1990) Relationship between resonance and gas exchange during high frequency jet ventilation. *British Journal of Anaesthesia* **64**: 453–459.

Luhr OR, Antonsen K, Karlsson M, et al. (1999) Incidence and mortality after acute respiratory failure and acute respiratory distress syndrome in Sweden, Denmark and Iceland. *American Journal of Respiratory and Critical Care Medicine* **159**: 1849–1861.

Lundin S, Mang H, Smithies M, et al. (1999) Inhalation of nitric oxide in acute lung injury: results of a European multicentre study. *Intensive Care Medicine* **25**: 911–919.

McCrory DC, Brown C, Gelfand SE, et al. (2001) Management of acute exacerbations of COPD: a summary and appraisal of published evidence. *Chest* **119**: 1190–1209.

MacDonnell SP, Timmins AC, Watson JD (1995) Adrenaline administered via a nebulizer in adult patients with upper airway obstruction. *Anaesthesia* **50**: 35–36.

McFadden ER Jr (1991) Fatal and near-fatal asthma. *New England Journal of Medicine* **324**: 409–411.

McGuire WW, Spragg RG, Cohen AB, et al. (1982) Studies on the pathogenesis of the adult respiratory distress syndrome. *Journal of Clinical Investigation* **69**: 543–553.

McHugh LG, Milberg JA, Whitcomb ME, et al. (1994) Recovery of function in survivors of the acute respiratory distress syndrome. *American Journal of Respiratory and Critical Care Medicine* **150**: 90–94.

McIntyre RC, Pulido EJ, Bensard DD, et al. (2000) Thirty years of clinical trials in acute respiratory distress syndrome. *Critical Care Medicine* **28**: 3314–3331.

Mancebo J, Fernández R, Blanck L, et al. (2006) A multicenter trial of prolonged prone ventilation and severe acute respiratory distress syndrome. *American Journal of Respiratory and Critical Care Medicine* **123**: 1233–1239.

Marik PE (2001) Aspiration pneumonitis and aspiration pneumonia. *New England Journal of Medicine* **344**: 665–671.

Marini JJ (1989) Should PEEP be used in airflow obstruction? *American Review of Respiratory Disease* **140**: 1–3.

Matthay MA, Eschenbacher WL, Goetzl EJ (1984) Elevated concentrations of leukotriene D4 in pulmonary edema fluid of patients with the adult respiratory distress syndrome. *Journal of Clinical Immunology* **4**: 479–483.

Meade MO, Cook RJ, Guyatt GH, et al. (2000) Interobserver variation in interpreting chest radiographs for the diagnosis of acute respiratory distress syndrome. *American Journal of Respiratory and Critical Care Medicine* **161**: 85–90.

Meduri GU, Headley AS, Golden E, et al. (1998) Effect of prolonged methylprednisolone therapy in unresolving acute respiratory distress syndrome: a randomized controlled trial. *Journal of the American Medical Association* **280**: 159–165.

Mehta S, Lapinsky SE, Hallett DC, et al. (2001) Prospective trial of high-frequency oscillation in adults with acute respiratory distress syndrome. *Critical Care Medicine* **29**: 1360–1369.

Melot C, Lejeune P, Leeman M, et al. (1989) Prostaglandin E$_1$ in the adult respiratory distress syndrome. *American Review of Respiratory Disease* **139**: 106–110.

Metnitz PG, Bartens C, Fischer M, et al. (1999) Antioxidant status in patients with acute respiratory distress syndrome. *Intensive Care Medicine* **25**: 180–185.

Michael JR, Barton RG, Saffle JR, et al. (1998) Inhaled nitric oxide versus conventional therapy. Effect on oxygenation in ARDS. *American Journal of Respiratory and Critical Care Medicine* **157**: 1372–1380.

Mier L, Dreyfuss D, Darchy B, et al. (1993) Is penicillin G an adequate initial treatment for aspiration pneumonia? A prospective evaluation using a protected specimen brush and quantitative cultures. *Intensive Care Medicine* **19**: 279–284.

Milberg JA, Davis DR, Steinberg KP, et al. (1995) Improved survival of patients with acute respiratory distress syndrome (ARDS): 1983–1993. *Journal of the American Medical Association* **273**: 306–309.

Millar AB, Foley NM, Singer M, et al. (1989) Tumour necrosis factor in bronchopulmonary secretions of patients with adult respiratory distress syndrome. *Lancet* **2**: 712–714.

Mitchell JP, Schuller D, Calandrino FS, et al. (1992) Improved outcome based on fluid management in critically ill patients requiring pulmonary artery catheterization. *American Review of Respiratory Disease* **145**: 990–998.

Moloney ED, Kiely JL, McNicholas WT (2001) Controlled oxygen therapy and carbon dioxide retention during exacerbations of chronic obstructive pulmonary disease. *Lancet* **357**: 526–528.

Montgomery AB, Stager MA, Carrico CJ, et al. (1985) Causes of mortality in patients with the adult respiratory distress syndrome. *American Review of Respiratory Disease* **132**: 485–489.

Moran JL, Green JV, Homan SD, et al. (1998) Acute exacerbations of chronic obstructive pulmonary disease and mechanical ventilation: a reevaluation. *Critical Care Medicine* **26**: 71–78.

Morris AH, Wallace CJ, Menlove RL, et al. (1994) Randomized clinical trial of pressure-controlled inverse ratio ventilation and extracorporeal CO_2 removal for adult respiratory distress syndrome. *American Journal of Respiratory and Critical Care Medicine* **149**: 295–305.

Moxham J (1990) Respiratory muscle fatigue: mechanisms, evaluation and therapy. *British Journal of Anaesthesia* **65**: 43–53.

Murray JF, Matthay MA, Luce JM, et al. (1988) An expanded definition of the adult respiratory distress syndrome. *American Review of Respiratory Disease* **138**: 720–723.

National Heart, Lung and Blood Institute ARDS Clinical Trials Network (2004) Higher versus lower positive end-expiratory pressures in patients with the acute respiratory distress syndrome. *New England Journal of Medicine* **351**: 327–336.

National Heart, Lung and Blood Institute ARDS Clinical Trials Network (2006a) Comparison of two fluid-management strategies in acute lung injury. *New England Journal of Medicine* **354**: 2564–2575.

National Heart, Lung and Blood Institute ARDS Clinical Trials Network (2006b) Pulmonary-artery versus central venous catheter to guide treatment of acute lung injury. *New England Journal of Medicine* **354**: 2213–2224.

National Heart, Lung and Blood Institute ARDS Clinical Trials Network (2006c) Efficacy and safety of corticosteroids for persistent acute respiratory distress syndrome. *New England Journal of Medicine* **354**: 1671–1684.

Nevins ML, Epstein SK (2001) Predictors of outcome for patients with COPD requiring invasive mechanical ventilation. *Chest* **119**: 1840–1849.

Niewoehner DE, Erbland ML, Deupree RH, *et al.* (1999) Effect of systemic glucocorticoids on exacerbations of chronic obstructive pulmonary disease. *New England Journal of Medicine* **340**: 1941–1947.

Nouira S, Marghli S, Belghith M, *et al.* (2001) Once daily oral ofloxacin in chronic obstructive pulmonary disease exacerbation requiring mechanical ventilation: a randomised placebo-controlled trial. *Lancet* **358**: 2020–2025.

Nuckton TJ, Alonso JA, Kallet RH, *et al.* (2002) Pulmonary dead-space fraction as a risk factor for death in the acute respiratory distress syndrome. *New England Journal of Medicine* **346**: 1281–1286.

Oczenski W, Hörman C, Keller C, *et al.* (2005) Recruitment maneuvers during prone positioning in patients with acute respiratory distress syndrome. *Critical Care Medicine* **33**: 54–61.

Oswalt CE, Gates GA, Holmstrom MG (1977) Pulmonary edema as a complication of acute airway obstruction. *Journal of the American Medical Association* **238**: 1833–1835.

Parkes SN, Bersten AD (1997) Aerosol kinetics and bronchodilator efficacy during continuous positive airway pressure delivered by facemask. *Thorax* **52**: 171–175.

Pauwels RA, Buist AS, Calverley PM, *et al.* (2001) Global strategy for the diagnosis, management and prevention of chronic obstructive pulmonary disease: NHLBI/WHO Global Initiative for Chronic Obstructive Lung Disease (GOLD). Workshop summary. *American Journal of Respiratory and Critical Care Medicine* **163**: 1256–1276 (also available at http://www. goldcopd.com).

Peek GJ, Firmin RK (1997) Extracorporeal membrane oxygenation, a favourable outcome? *British Journal of Anaesthesia* **78**: 235–237.

Pelosi P, Gattinoni L (2001) Acute respiratory distress syndrome of pulmonary and extra-pulmonary origin: fancy or reality? *Intensive Care Medicine* **27**: 457–460.

Pelosi P, Cadringher P, Bottino N, *et al.* (1999) Sigh in acute respiratory distress syndrome. *American Journal of respiratory and Critical Care Medicine* **159**: 872–880.

Polkey MI, Kyroussis D, Keilty SE, *et al.* (1995) Exhaustive treadmill exercise does not reduce twitch transdiaphragmatic pressure in patients with COPD. *American Journal of Respiratory and Critical Care Medicine* **152**: 959–964.

Power I (1993) Aspirin-induced asthma. *British Journal of Anaesthesia* **71**: 619–621.

Purro A, Appendini L, Patessio A, *et al.* (1998) Static intrinsic PEEP in COPD patients during spontaneous breathing. *American Journal of Respiratory and Critical Care Medicine* **157**: 1044–1050.

Quinlan GJ, Lamb NJ, Tilley R, *et al.* (1997) Plasma hypoxanthine levels in ARDS: implications for morbidity and mortality. *American Journal of Respiratory and Critical Care Medicine* **155**: 479–484.

Ranieri VM, Suter PM, Tortorella C, *et al.* (1999) Effect of mechanical ventilation on inflammatory mediators in patients with acute respiratory distress syndrome: a randomized controlled trial. *Journal of the American Medical Association* **282**: 54–61.

Reng M, Philipp A, Kaiser M, *et al.* (2000) Pumpless extracorporeal lung assist and adult respiratory distress syndrome. *Lancet* **356**: 219–220.

Rialp G, Betbesé AJ, Pérez-Márquez M, *et al.* (2001) Short-term effects of inhaled nitric oxide and prone position in pulmonary and extrapulmonary acute respiratory distress syndrome. *American Journal of Respiratory and Critical Care Medicine* **164**: 243–249.

Richard J-C, Maggiore SM, Jonson B, *et al.* (2001) Influence of tidal volume on alveolar recruitment. Respective role of PEEP and a recruitment maneuver. *American Journal of Respiratory and Critical Care Medicine* **163**: 1609–1613.

Richard C, Warszawski J, Anguel N, *et al.* (2003) Early use of the pulmonary artery catheter and outcomes in patients with shock and acute respiratory distress syndrome: a randomized controlled trial. *Journal of the American Medical Association* **290**: 2713–2720.

Rochester DF (1991) The diaphragm in COPD. *New England Journal of Medicine* **325**: 961–962.

Rossaint R, Falke KJ, Lopez F, *et al.* (1993) Inhaled nitric oxide for the adult respiratory distress syndrome. *New England Journal of Medicine* **328**: 399–405.

Roupie E, Lepage E, Wysocki M, *et al.* (1999) Prevalence, etiologies and outcome of the acute respiratory distress syndrome among hypoxemic ventilated patients. *Intensive Care Medicine* **25**: 920–929.

Rowe BH, Keller JL, Oxman AD (1992) Effectiveness of steroid therapy in acute exacerbations of asthma: a meta-analysis. *American Journal of Emergency Medicine* **10**: 301–310.

Rubenfeld GD, Caldwell E, Granton J, *et al.* (1999) Interobserver variability in applying a radiographic definition for ARDS. *Chest* **116**: 1347–1353.

Rubenfeld GD, Caldwell E, Peabody E, *et al.* (2005) Incidence and outcomes of acute lung injury. *New England Journal of Medicine* **353**: 1685–1693.

Salmeron S, Brochard L, Mal H, *et al.* (1994) Nebulized versus intravenous albuterol in hypercapnic acute asthma. *American Journal of Respiratory and Critical Care Medicine* **149**: 1466–1470.

Schelling G, Stoll C, Haller M, *et al.* (1998) Health-related quality of life and posttraumatic stress disorder in survivors of the acute respiratory distress syndrome. *Critical Care Medicine* **26**: 651–659.

Sears MR (1996) Epidemiological trends in asthma. *Canadian Respiratory Journal* **3**: 261–268.

Selsby D, Jones JG (1990) Some physiological and clinical aspects of chest physiotherapy. *British Journal of Anaesthesia* **64**: 621–631.

Sharon A, Shpirer I, Kaluski E, *et al.* (2000) High-dose intravenous isosorbide-dinitrate is safer and better than Bi-PAP ventilation combined with conventional treatment for severe pulmonary edema. *Journal of the American College of Cardiology* **36**: 832–837.

Sibbald WJ, Driedger AA (1983) Right ventricular function in acute disease states: pathophysiological considerations. *Critical Care Medicine* **11**: 339–345.

Sibbald WJ, Anderson RR, Reid B, *et al.* (1981) Alveolo-capillary permeability in human septic ARDS. Effect of high-dose corticosteroid therapy. *Chest* **79**: 133–142.

Silverman HJ, Slotman G, Bone RC, *et al.* (1990) Effects of prostaglandin E_1 on oxygen delivery and consumption in patients with the adult respiratory distress syndrome. *Chest* **98**: 405–410.

Similowski T, Yan S, Gauthier AP (1991) Contractile properties of the human diaphragm during chronic hyperinflation. *New England Journal of Medicine* **325**: 917–923.

Simonds AK (2000) Nasal ventilation in progressive neuromuscular disease: experience in adults and adolescents. *Monaldi Archives for Chest Disease* **55**: 237–241.

Singer MM, Wright F, Stanley LK, *et al.* (1970) Oxygen toxicity in man. A prospective study in patients after open-heart surgery. *New England Journal of Medicine* **283**: 1473–1478.

Skatrud JB, Dempsey JA (1983) Relative effectiveness of acetazolamide versus medroxyprogesterone acetate in correction of chronic carbon dioxide retention. *American Review of Respiratory Disease* **127**: 405–412.

Smetana GW (1999) Preoperative pulmonary evaluation. *New England Journal of Medicine* **340**: 937–944.

So LK, Lau AC, Yam LY, *et al.* (2003) Development of a standard treatment protocol for severe acute respiratory syndrome. *Lancet* **361**: 1615–1617.

Spragg RG, Lewis JF, Walmrath H-D, *et al.* (2004) Effect of recombinant surfactant protein C-based surfactant on the acute respiratory distress syndrome. *New England Journal of Medicine* **351**: 884–892.

Squadrone V, Coha M, Cerutti E, *et al.* (2005) Continuous positive airway pressure for treatment of postoperative hypoxemia: a randomized controlled trial. *Journal of the American Medical Association* **293**: 589–595.

Stewart AG, Waterhouse JC, Billings CG, *et al.* (1995) Hormonal, renal and autonomic nerve factors involved in the excretion of sodium and water during dynamic salt and water loading in hypoxaemic chronic obstructive pulmonary disease. *Thorax* **50**: 838–845.

Stewart TE, Meade MO, Cook DJ, *et al.* (1998) Evaluation of a ventilation strategy to prevent barotrauma in patients at high risk for acute respiratory distress syndrome. *New England Journal of Medicine* **338**: 355–361.

Stoller JK (2002) Clinical practice. Acute exacerbations of chronic obstructive pulmonary disease. *New England Journal of Medicine* **346**: 988–994.

Suntharalingam G, Regan K, Keogh BF, *et al.* (2001) Influence of direct and indirect etiology on acute outcome and 6-month functional recovery in acute respiratory distress syndrome. *Critical Care Medicine* **29**: 562–566.

Sznajder JI, Fraiman A, Hall JB, *et al.* (1989) Increased hydrogen peroxide in the expired breath of patients with acute hypoxemic respiratory failure. *Chest* **96**: 606–612.

Talbot TR, Hartert TV, Mitchel E, *et al.* (2005) Asthma as a risk factor for invasive pneumococcal disease. *New England Journal of Medicine* **352**: 2082–2090.

Tan KS, Grove A, McLean A, *et al.* (1997) Systemic corticosteroid rapidly reverses bronchodilator subsensitivity induced by formoterol in asthmatic patients. *American*

Journal of Respiratory and Critical Care Medicine **156**: 28–35.

Thomas JA, McIntosh JM (1994) Are incentive spirometry, intermittent positive pressure breathing, and deep breathing exercises effective in the prevention of postoperative pulmonary complications after upper abdominal surgery? A systematic overview and meta-analysis. *Physical Therapy* **74**: 3–16.

Thomson AJ, Webb DJ, Maxwell SR, *et al.* (2002) Oxygen therapy in acute medical care. *British Medical Journal* **324**: 1406–1407.

Travers Ah, Rowe BH, Barker S, *et al.* (2002) The effectiveness of iv β-agonists in treating patients with acute asthma in the emergency department: a meta-analysis. *Chest* **122**: 1200–1207.

Tuxen DV (1989) Detrimental effects of positive end-expiratory pressure during controlled mechanical ventilation of patients with severe airflow obstruction. *American Review of Respiratory Disease* **140**: 5–9.

Tuxen DV (1994) Permissive hypercapnic ventilation. *American Journal of Respiratory and Critical Care Medicine* **150**: 870–874.

Tuxen DV, Lane S (1987) The effects of ventilatory pattern on hyperinflation, airway pressures and circulation in mechanical ventilation of patients with severe air-flow obstruction. *American Review of Respiratory Disease* **136**: 872–879.

Valta P, Uusaro A, Nunes S, *et al.* (1999) Acute respiratory distress syndrome: frequency, clinical course, and costs of care. *Critical Care Medicine* **27**: 2367–2374.

Villagra A, Ochagavía A, Vatua S, *et al.* (2002) Recruitment maneuvers during lung protective ventilation in acute respiratory distress syndrome. *American Journal of Respiratory and Critical Care Medicine* **165**: 165–170.

Villar J, Slutsky AS (1989) The incidence of the adult respiratory distress syndrome. *American Review of Respiratory Disease* **140**: 814–816.

Walmrath D, Gunther A, Ghofrani HA, *et al.* (1996a) Bronchoscopic surfactant administration in patients with severe adult respiratory distress syndrome and sepsis. *American Journal of Respiratory and Critical Care Medicine* **154**: 57–62.

Walmrath D, Schneider T, Schermuly R, *et al.* (1996b) Direct comparison of inhaled nitric oxide and aerosolized prostacyclin in acute respiratory distress syndrome. *American Journal of Respiratory and Critical Care Medicine* **153**: 991–996.

Ware LB, Matthay MA (2000) The acute respiratory distress syndrome. *New England Journal of Medicine* **342**: 1334–1349.

Weber T, Tschernich H, Sitzwohl C, *et al.* (2000) Tromethamine buffer modifies the depressant effect of permissive hypercapnia on myocardial contractility in patients with acute respiratory distress syndrome. *American Journal of Respiratory and Critical Care Medicine* **162**: 1361–1365.

Webster NR, Cohen AT, Nunn JF (1988) Adult respiratory distress syndrome – how many cases in the UK? *Anaesthesia* **43**: 923–926.

Wewers MD, Herzyk DJ, Gadek JE (1988) Alveolar fluid neutrophil elastase activity in the adult respiratory distress syndrome is complexed to alpha-2-macroglobulin. *Journal of Clinical Investigation* **82**: 1260–1267.

Wheeler AP, Bernard GR (2007) Acute lung injury and the acute respiratory distress syndrome: a clinical review. *Lancet* **369**: 1553–1565.

Williams MH (1989) Increasing severity of asthma from 1960 to 1987 (letter). *New England Journal of Medicine* **320**: 1015–1016.

Wyncoll DLA, Evans TW (1999) Acute respiratory distress syndrome. *Lancet* **354**: 497–501.

9 Myocardial ischaemia, cardiopulmonary resuscitation and management of arrhythmias

The commonest cause of cardiac arrest and life-threatening arrhythmias is ischaemic heart disease. In the UK approximately 300 000 people annually suffer myocardial infarction (MI) and coronary artery disease is the single largest cause of death, accounting for approximately 60 deaths per 100 000 of the population each year. Recognized risk factors include increasing age, smoking, hypertension, hypercholesterolaemia, sedentary lifestyle, diabetes and familial predisposition. Men are affected more frequently than premenopausal women, but after the menopause the incidence of atheroma in women approaches that in men. Diet may also be important.

ACUTE CORONARY SYNDROMES

PATHOPHYSIOLOGY

The common mechanism underlying all acute coronary syndromes (ACS) is rupture or erosion of the fibrous surface of an atheromatous plaque. This is followed by platelet aggregation and adhesion, localized thrombus formation, distal embolization of thrombus and vasoconstriction. Persistent occlusion of a coronary artery can lead to myocardial necrosis within 15–30 minutes. Initially the vulnerable subendocardial layer is affected but if ischaemia persists the infarct zone extends through to the subepicardial myocardium, producing a transmural Q-wave MI.

DEFINITIONS

MI can be defined as death of cardiac myocytes due to myocardial ischaemia and is diagnosed on the basis of an appropriate clinical history, characteristic electrocardiogram (ECG) changes and elevated biochemical markers. The ACS were defined in an attempt to stratify patients with chest pain of cardiac origin in order to distinguish high-risk patients who require urgent intervention from those with little or no suspicion of life-threatening MI (Bertrand et al., 2002; Van der Werf et al., 2003). They comprise:

- ST-segment elevation (or new/presumed new left bundle branch block (LBBB)) MI (STEMI):
  - appropriate clinical history;
  - ST segment elevation on ECG;
  - elevated biochemical markers.
- Non-ST-segment elevation MI (NSTEMI):
  - appropriate clinical history;
  - ECG may be normal or show some evidence of acute myocardial ischaemia (usually ST-segment depression) or non-specific abnormalities (e.g. T-wave inversion);
  - elevated biochemical markers.
- Unstable angina:
  - appropriate clinical history;
  - ECG changes as for NSTEMI;
  - normal biochemical markers.

These clinical syndromes form part of a spectrum of the same disease process, although NSTEMI and unstable angina can be classified together as *non-ST-segment elevation ACS*.

DIAGNOSIS

Patients may complain of *new-onset chest pain*, *chest pain at rest* or a *deterioration in pre-existing angina*. Typically the pain radiates to the left arm, neck or jaw. Some may present with *atypical symptoms* such as pain suggestive of indigestion or pleurisy, breathlessness, fatigue, presyncope or syncope. In those with MI autonomic symptoms are common and on examination the patient may be pale, cold and sweating. Adverse clinical signs such as hypotension, bradycardia, tachycardia, basal crackles, fourth heart sound and cardiac murmurs may be detected.

The ECG may be normal or show ST depression/T-wave inversion in NSTEMI and persistent ST elevation or LBBB pattern in STEMI. The development of Q waves is indicative of transmural infarction. Characteristic ECG changes in anterior wall and inferior MI are shown in **Figure 9.1**, together with the typical evolution of ECG changes in STEMI. Lateral wall MI produces changes in leads I, AVL and V_5/V_6. In patients with a posterior MI there may be ST depression in leads V_{1-3} with a dominant R wave and ST elevation in leads V_{5-6}. The number of leads involved broadly reflects the extent of the myocardial injury, whilst the height of initial ST-segment elevation is modestly correlated with the degree of ischaemia. Other causes of ST-segment elevation or T-wave changes not related to ACS include:

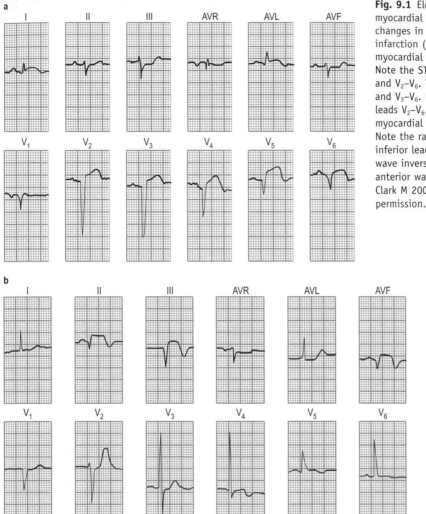

Fig. 9.1 Electrocardiogram (ECG) changes in myocardial infarction and evolution of ECG changes in ST-segment elevation myocardial infarction (STEMI). (a) An acute anterolateral myocardial infarction shown by a 12-lead ECG. Note the ST segment elevation in leads I, AVL and V_2–V_6. The T wave is inverted in leads I, AVL and V_3–V_6. Pathological Q waves are seen in leads V_2–V_6. (b) An acute inferior wall myocardial infarction shown by a 12-lead ECG. Note the raised ST segment and Q waves in the inferior leads (II, III and AVF). The additional T-wave inversion in V_4 and V_5 probably represents anterior wall ischaemia. Adapted from Kumar P, Clark M 2005 Clinical Medicine 6E Elsevier with permission.

- metabolic disturbances;
- drug toxicity;
- pericarditis;
- left ventricular hypertrophy;
- normal variant;
- Wolff–Parkinson–White syndrome and conduction defects.

Cardiac-specific troponin I and troponin T are highly sensitive and specific early markers of myocardial injury. Levels start to rise within 3–4 hours after MI and remain raised for 4–10 days. If the initial troponin assay is negative a repeat determination should be performed 9–12 hours later. Measurement of *creatinine kinase (CK)-MB* levels is less specific but may be useful for monitoring the course of established MI. It is important to appreciate that a positive cardiac troponin (> 0.1 ng/mL) does not differentiate between the various causes of myocardial injury and that troponin levels are raised in many other conditions, including sepsis, renal failure, pulmonary embolism and cerebrovascular accident (Ammann *et al.*, 2004). New markers of myocardial injury such as myeloperoxidase and glutathione peroxidase 1 are becoming available.

Echocardiography can be useful for identifying wall motion abnormalities (which support the diagnosis) and assessing the severity of left ventricular impairment, as well as for the diagnosis of specific complications such as mitral regurgitation, ventricular septal defect, pericardial effusion and myocardial rupture. Echocardiography may also detect alternative diagnoses such as aortic dissection, pericarditis or pulmonary embolism (see Chapter 4).

MANAGEMENT (Table 9.1)

The choice of treatment for ACS largely depends on an assessment of the risk of immediate extensive myocardial

c

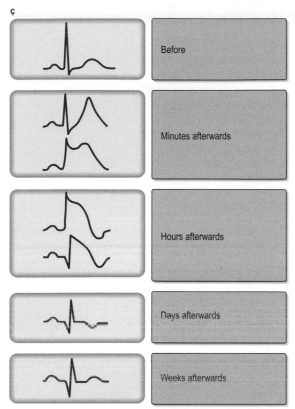

Before

Minutes afterwards

Hours afterwards

Days afterwards

Weeks afterwards

Fig. 9.1 (c) Electrocariographic evolution of myocardial infarction (STEMI). After the first few minutes the T waves become tall, pointed and upright and there is ST-segment elevation. After the first few hours the T waves invert, the R-wave voltage is decreased and Q waves develop. After a few days the ST segment returns to normal. After weeks or months the T wave may return to upright but the Q wave remains. Adapted from Kumar P, Clark M 2005 Clinical Medicine 6E Elsevier with permission.

damage or further coronary events (Bertrand *et al.*, 2002; Van der Werf *et al.*, 2003) (**Table 9.2**).

Immediate management should include general measures combined with treatment to relieve symptoms, limit myocardial damage and reduce the risk of cardiac arrest:

- oxygen in high concentrations via a facemask;
- aspirin 300 mg (chewed) as soon as possible:
  - can be combined with clopidogrel (300 mg p.o. loading dose then 75 mg p.o. daily) and low-molecular-weight heparin;
- nitroglycerine as sublingual glyceryl trinitrate (0.3–1 mg) repeated, unless the patient is hypotensive;
- continuous ECG monitoring: obtain 12-lead ECG;
- establish venous access and obtain blood for biochemical markers, full blood count, biochemistry, lipids, glucose;
- morphine or diamorphine titrated intravenously, avoiding oversedation and respiratory depression;
- consider an antiemetic if nausea is present;

- β-blockade to reduce myocardial oxygen demand (unless contraindicated);
- treat pulmonary oedema (see Chapters 7 and 8).

Treatment can be given prior to hospital admission by trained health care professionals using strict guidelines. 3-hydroxy-3-methylglutaryl coenzyme A (HMG CoA) reductase inhibitor agents (statins) are routinely administered to patients with ACS. These agents may stabilize the plaque, improve vascular and myocardial remodelling and, when given early, reduce the incidence of further cardiovascular events.

The treatment of STEMI (or MI with new/presumed new LBBB) aims to restore the blood supply to myocardium that has not been irreversibly damaged. Clinical trials have confirmed the efficacy of early reperfusion therapy in reducing infarct size, complications and mortality from MI (GUSTO Angiographic Investigators, 1993; Zijlstra *et al.*, 1993). Reperfusion should be achieved as soon as possible after the onset of chest pain. Coronary reperfusion may be achieved by percutaneous coronary intervention (PCI) or thrombolysis. In this situation coronary artery surgery is usually reserved for the complications of MI. An early invasive strategy also seems to be associated with sustained benefit in moderate- to high-risk patients with non-ST-elevation ACS (Lagerqvist *et al.*, 2006).

Percutaneous coronary intervention
PCI, performed within 90 minutes if possible, is the preferred reperfusion therapy in interventional cardiology centres with the available expertise, especially if more than 3 hours have elapsed since the onset of chest pain. Percutaneous transluminal coronary angioplasty (PTCA) performed within 12 hours of the onset of STEMI is associated with a lower risk of death or reinfarction when compared to thrombolysis (Keeley *et al.*, 2003). Rates of reintervention, hospital readmission and recurrent ischaemia may also be lower with PTCA than with thrombolysis. The superiority of PCI in this situation is largely attributable to a reduction in the incidence of recurrent MI. Stenting of the coronary arteries during primary PCI seems to reduce the need for repeat target vessel revascularization but does not appear to influence mortality. It is unclear whether the use of drug-eluting stents is advantageous in patients with acute MI (Laarman *et al.*, 2006; Spaulding *et al.*, 2006). A recent trial (Fernandez-Aviles *et al.*, 2004) suggests that PCI is safe, and improves clinical outcome at 1 year even when performed following thrombolysis. There is some evidence to suggest that atrial natriuretic peptide can reduce infarct size in patients undergoing reperfusion treatment (Kitakaze *et al.*, 2007).

Thrombolysis
Thrombolysis is most effective when administered within 6 hours of STEMI or new LBBB MI, whereas the benefits are limited when treatment is delayed for more than 12 hours (Fibrinolytic Therapy Trialists' Collaborative Group, 1994). Older patients benefit less from thrombolysis, perhaps because of their increased risk of cerebrovascular accident.

Table 9.1 Pharmacological therapy in acute coronary syndromes

Drug	Dose	Notes
Oxygen	35–50%	Check ABG in severe COPD
Antiplatelet		
Aspirin	150–300 mg chewable or soluble aspirin, then 75 mg p.o. daily	Give PPI to those with dyspepsia history
Clopidogrel	300 mg p.o. loading dose, then 75 mg p.o. daily	Caution: increased risk of bleeding; avoid if CABG planned
Analgesia		
Diamorphine	2.5–5.0 mg i.v.	Prescribe with antiemetic (e.g., metoclopramide 10 mg i.v.)
Myocardial energy consumption		
β-blockers	e.g. Atenolol 5 mg i.v. repeated after 15 min, then 25–50 mg p.o. daily or Metoprolol 5 mg i.v. repeated to a maximum of 15 mg, then 25–50 mg p.o. twice daily	Avoid in asthma, heart failure, hypotension, bradyarrhythmias
Coronary vasodilatation		
Glyceryl trinitrate	2–10 mg/h i.v./buccal or sublingual	Maintain systolic BP above 90 mmHg
Plaque stabilization/ventricular remodeling		
HMG-CoA reductase inhibitors (statins)	e.g. Simvastatin 20–40 mg p.o. daily Pravastatin 20–40 mg p.o. daily Atorvastatin 80 mg p.o. daily	Combine with dietary advice and modification
ACE inhibitors	e.g. Ramipril 2.5–10 mg p.o. daily Lisinopril 5–10 mg p.o. daily	Monitor renal function
PLUS FOR NON-ST-ELEVATION MYOCARDIAL INFARCTION (NSTEMI)		
Antithrombin		
Low-molecular-weight heparins	Enoxaparin 1 mg/kg s.c. twice daily	
Glycoprotein IIb/IIIa inhibitors		
Abciximab	250 mcg/kg i.v. bolus then 125 nanogram/kg per min up to 10 mcg/min i.v. for 12 h	If coronary intervention likely within 24 h
Eptifibatide	180 mcg/kg i.v. bolus, then 2 mcg/kg per min i.v. for 72 h	Indicated in high-risk patients managed without coronary intervention or during PCI
Tirofiban	400 nanogram/kg per min i.v. for 30 min, then 100 nanogram/kg per min for 48–108 h	Indicated in high-risk patients managed without coronary intervention or during PCI
PLUS FOR ST-ELEVATION MYOCARDIAL INFARCTION (STEMI)		
Thrombolysis		
Streptokinase	1 500 000 units i.v. over 60 min	Antibodies appear after 4 days. It should not therefore be used after this time

Drug doses are for adult patients with normal renal or hepatic function and without specific contraindications.

Table 9.1 Continued

Drug	Dose	Notes
Alteplase	15 mg i.v. bolus, then 50 mg over 30 min and 35 mg over 60 min	Dose modification if < 65 kg or 6–12 h post-MI Prescribe heparin for at least 24 h (consult product literature)
Or		
Tenecteplase	30–50 mg i.v. bolus according to weight (500–600 mcg/kg)	Prescribe heparin for at least 24 h (consult product literature)
Or		
Reteplase	10 units i.v. bolus repeated after 30 min	Prescribe heparin for 48 h (consult product literature)

ABG, arterial blood gases; ACE, angiotensin-converting enzyme; BP, blood pressure; CABG, coronary artery bypass grafting; COPD, chronic obstructive pulmonary disease; HMG-CoA, 3-hydroxy-3-methylglutaryl coenzyme A; LMW, PCI, percutaneous coronary intervention; PPI, proton pump inhibitor. Drug doses are for adult patients with normal renal or hepatic function and without specific contraindications.

Table 9.2 The thrombolysis in myocardial infarction (TIMI) risk score for acute coronary syndromes

Risk factor	Score
Age > 65	1
More than three coronary artery disease risk factors: hypertension, hyperlipidaemia, family history, diabetes, smoking	1
Known coronary artery disease (coronary angiography stenosis > 50%)	1
Aspirin use in the last 7 days	1
Severe angina (more than two episodes of rest pain in 24 hours)	1
ST deviation on ECG (horizontal ST depression or transient ST elevation > 1 mm)	1
Elevated cardiac markers (CK-MB or troponin)	1

Total score	Rate of death/MI in 14 days (%)	Rate of death/MI/urgent revascularization (%)
0–1	3	4.75
2	3	8.3
3	5	13.2
4	7	19.9
5	12	26.2
6–7	19	40.9

CK-MB, creatine kinase MB; ECG, electrocardiogram; MI, myocardial infarction.

The death rate from MI can be reduced by prompt reperfusion therapy (door to needle time < 20 minutes). Streptokinase is the agent most commonly used worldwide. Recombinant tissue-type plasminogen activator (rt-PA) achieves higher reperfusion rates but is more expensive than streptokinase and is associated with a higher risk of stroke. Some use rt-PA in preference to streptokinase in patients less than 50 years old with anterior MI, in those with hypotension and in patients who have previously received streptokinase. Recombinant t-PA appears to be considerably more effective than streptokinase if it can be given within 4 hours of the onset of chest pain. Double-bolus reteplase and single-bolus tenecteplase facilitate rapid administration of fibrinolytic therapy and can be used for pre-hospital fibrinolysis. If the patient fails to reperfuse within 60–90 minutes (as demonstrated by 50% reduction in the extent of ST-segment elevation), re-thrombolysis or referral for rescue coronary angioplasty is indicated.

Thrombolysis should be accompanied by aspirin therapy, which in STEMI should be combined with clopidogrel.

Table 9.3 Contraindications to thrombolysis

Absolute contraindications	Relative contraindications
Haemorrhagic stroke or stroke of unknown origin at any time	Transient ischaemic attack in preceding 6 months
Ischaemic stroke in preceding 6 months	Oral anticoagulant therapy
Central nervous system damage or neoplasms	Pregnancy or within 1 week postpartum
Recent major trauma/surgery/head injury (within preceding 3 weeks)	Non-compressible puncture wounds
Gastrointestinal bleeding within the last month	Traumatic resuscitation
Known bleeding disorder	Refractory hypertension (systolic blood pressure > 180 mmHg)
Aortic dissection	Advanced liver disease Infective endocarditis

Heparin is recommended adjunctive therapy with alteplase, reteplase or tenecteplase to prevent re-thrombosis but not with streptokinase. Unfractionated heparin is preferred in patients receiving tenecteplase.

The contraindications to thrombolysis are listed in **Table 9.3**.

Low-risk patients with non-ST-segment elevation ACS (no recurrence of chest pain during observation, normal ECG or minor T-wave changes only, normal troponin on the initial assay and at 6–12 hours post admission) can be managed with oral aspirin and/or clopidogrel, β-blockers and nitrates (Chen, 2005; Yusuf *et al.*, 2001). Glycoprotein (GP) IIb/IIIa platelet receptor inhibitors (e.g. abciximab, eptifibatide, tirofiban) are of most benefit in troponin-positive patients with diabetes scheduled for coronary intervention. Patients with NSTEMI should be given low-molecular-weight heparin.

Subsequent management
Delayed coronary revascularization is recommended for high-risk patients with ACS who have not been adequately revascularized acutely and low-risk patients in whom an exercise or dobutamine stress test proves positive. Those with single-vessel disease are normally treated with PCI, whereas patients with left main stem lesions or triple-vessel disease may be best managed by surgical coronary artery bypass grafting. Surgery may also be indicated in those with complex coronary lesions. Coronary stenting may stabilize the disrupted coronary plaque and reduces restenosis rates compared to PTCA alone. The incidence of complications associated with coronary intervention can be reduced by preprocedure clopidogrel and periprocedure GP IIb/IIIa inhibitors. Such an interventional approach significantly reduces mortality, as well as reducing the rate of MI, recurrent angina and hospital readmission. Patients with increased troponin levels benefit most.

Preventive strategies
Secondary prevention involves antithrombotic therapy with low-dose aspirin (75 mg daily), preservation of left ventricular function with an angiotensin-converting enzyme inhibitor, β-blockade and, for those with angina, oral nitrates. Cholesterol reduction strategies, including low-fat, high-fibre diet and regular exercise, will complement cholesterol suppression by statins. In those with diabetes blood glucose levels must be strictly controlled. Effective control of blood pressure, maintenance of optimal body weight and removal of avoidable risk factors such as smoking contribute to a reduction in the risk of future coronary events, cardiorespiratory collapse and death.

Complications
These include:

- cardiac failure/cardiogenic shock;
- myocardial rupture/aneurysmal dilatation;
- ventricular septal defect;
- mitral regurgitation;
- cardiac arrhythmias;
- conduction disturbances;
- post-MI pericarditis and Dressler's syndrome.

The Killip classification can be used to assess patients with heart failure post MI:

- Killip I – no crackles and no third heart sound
- Killip II – crackles in < 50% of the lung fields or a third heart sound
- Killip III – crackles in > 50% of the lung fields
- Killip IV – cardiogenic shock.

Prognosis
The risk of death following STEMI can be predicted using the TIMI score (**Table 9.4**) (Chesebro *et al.*, 1987).

 CARDIORESPIRATORY ARREST

Millions of people around the world have learned the fundamentals of cardiopulmonary resuscitation (CPR). Instructions are available on the internet at http://www.learncpr.org. Readers interested in refreshing their knowledge of advanced CPR can access http://www.resus.org.uk or http://www.cpr-ecc.org. For up-to-date posters of the algorithms for basic and advanced life support, go to http://www.erc.edu. Recent evidence suggests that cardiac-only resuscitation

Table 9.4 Thrombolysis in myocardial infarction (TIMI) risk score for ST-elevation myocardial infarction (STEMI)	
Risk factor	**Score**
Age > 65	2
Age > 75	3
History of angina	1
History of hypertension	1
History of diabetes	1
Systolic blood pressure < 100 mmHg	3
Heart rate > 100 beats/min	2
Killip II–IV*	2
Weight > 67 kg	1
Anterior myocardial infarction or left bundle branch block	1
Delay to treatment > 4 hours	1
Total score	**Risk of death at 30 days (%)**
0	0.8
1	1.6
2	2.2
3	4.4
4	7.3
5	12.4
6	16.1
7	23.4
8	26.8
9–16	35.9

*See text.

by bystanders should be preferred for adult patients with witnessed out-of-hospital cardiac arrest (SOS-KAMTO Study Group, 2007).

DIAGNOSIS

Cardiorespiratory arrest is diagnosed clinically. The patient rapidly loses consciousness, becoming unresponsive and lifeless with absent pulsation in the major vessels (carotid and femoral arteries). Heart sounds cannot be heard and respiratory efforts are absent or gasping. The pupils soon dilate and become unresponsive to light. It may be difficult to determine whether the primary event was respiratory or cardiac, although if a history can be obtained this may suggest the likely sequence of events. When the primary aetiology is respiratory, profound bradycardia and cyanosis often precede cardiac arrest.

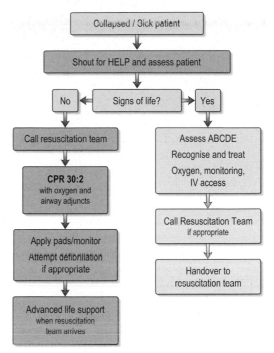

Fig. 9.2 In-hospital resuscitation guidelines. CPR, cardiopulmonary resuscitation; IV, intravenous. (Originally published at www.resus.org.uk.)

TREATMENT (www.resus.org.uk)

Having established that signs of life are absent it is vital to *call for assistance* (**Fig. 9.2**) since it is virtually impossible to perform adequate resuscitation unaided. *Basic cardiac life support* should start at once. If the patient has a monitored and witnessed collapse in hospital a single *precordial thump* (in which removal of the fist delivers the energy) can be delivered after confirmation of ventricular fibrillation (VF)/ventricular tachycardia (VT) cardiac arrest. That can be followed by defibrillation if the precordial thump is unsuccessful, provided a defibrillator is instantly available. Basic life support with chest compressions and assisted ventilation should be started immediately after the precordial thump or the direct current (dc) shock is delivered. After 2 minutes of CPR check the rhythm and give another shock (if indicated). The rationale for this recommendation is that immediately following collapse due to unheralded VF the lungs and arterial blood are likely to contain a sufficient reservoir of oxygen; the most urgent priority is therefore to try to restore the circulation.

Airway and respiration

A *clear airway* must be established as a priority. The oropharynx should be cleared of obvious obstructions such as false teeth, vomit, blood and other debris before flexing the neck, extending the head and inserting an oropharyngeal airway. The patient should then be *ventilated* with added *oxygen* at a rate of approximately 10 breaths/min using a facemask and a self-inflating bag. A pocket mask for expired air respiration (**Fig. 9.3**) may be easier to use, especially for

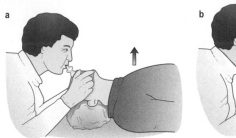
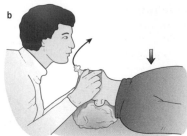

Fig. 9.3 Mask–mouth ventilation. (a) Open airway, blow into mouthpiece, observing chest inflation; (b) allow patient to exhale passively.

one-person resuscitation, but supplemental oxygen should be given as soon as possible. Alternatively, a laryngeal mask airway and bag-valve apparatus or a bag-valve-mask technique may be used according to local policy.

Whichever method is used, it is important to ensure that the chest expands with each insufflation. If it proves impossible to achieve adequate ventilation using any of these methods, then *tracheal intubation* may be required, although this should normally only be attempted by those experienced in the technique. Prolonged attempts at intubation by unskilled personnel waste valuable time, may exacerbate hypoxia and hypercarbia and can cause structural damage. Nevertheless, the trachea should be intubated as soon as skilled assistance arrives since this secures the airway, ensures effective positive-pressure ventilation and protects the lungs from aspiration of stomach contents.

Despite immediate vigorous manual ventilation, *respiratory acidosis* is common during CPR. This impairs cerebral autoregulation and may exacerbate ischaemic brain injury. *Hypoxia* is also common during CPR and is probably largely a result of collapsed distal lung units caused by chest compression and inefficient ventilation, combined with reduced lung perfusion. Arterial hypoxaemia is further exacerbated by the fall in mixed venous oxygen tension (PO_2) caused by poor tissue perfusion (Weil *et al.*, 1986). Finally, lung function may be further compromised during CPR by pre-existing cardiac failure or lung disease and by aspiration of gastric contents. In some circumstances, the application of positive end-expiratory pressure (PEEP) during CPR can improve oxygenation, and, although often associated with a reduction in cardiac output (see Chapter 7), may actually enhance forward flow by further augmenting the overall rise in intrathoracic pressure.

Cardiac massage
EXTERNAL CARDIAC MASSAGE
Effective external cardiac massage (ECM) can only be performed on a *hard surface*. This may be provided by an intensive care or coronary care unit bed, a board placed under the mattress or, failing either of these, by placing the patient on the floor. *Chest compression* must be achieved using a vertical force in the midline. A downward pressure should be delivered with a rhythmic rather than a jerky action using straight arms, with the heel of the hand placed in the middle of the chest. The sternum should be depressed to a depth of 4–5 cm. keeping

the fingers away from the chest wall. With an unprotected airway compressions and breaths should be delivered in a ratio of 30:2 but following definitive airway management lung inflation and external cardiac compression need no longer be synchronized. Chest compressions at a rate of approximately 100 per minute should continue uninterrupted (except for defibrillation and pulse checks when indicated) and ventilation should be continued at roughly 10 breaths/min.

Once effective cardiac massage and artificial ventilation have been established, the patient's colour should improve, the pupils may return to normal size, there should be a palpable pulse (although this does not necessarily indicate adequate flow, merely that the pressure wave has been transmitted along a patent fluid-filled vessel) and the conscious level may improve (head shaking, grimacing). At this stage, *ECG monitoring* should be attached to the patient if not already in place, and more specific treatment should be instituted.

Although clinical assessment of the efficacy of CPR is extremely difficult it has been suggested that measurement of the *end-tidal carbon dioxide concentration* may be a suitable means of monitoring blood flow generated by precordial compression (Higgins *et al.*, 1990; Levine *et al.*, 1997).

Complications of ECM include:

- traumatic injury to the abdominal viscera (in particular, rupture of the liver and spleen);
- damage to the myocardium;
- chest wall injury;
- pulmonary aspiration;
- impaired lung function.

Injury to thoracic or abdominal structures may follow prolonged energetic CPR in as many as 60% of cases.

The *mechanisms by which ECM produces forward flow* have been the subject of debate. It was originally suggested that forward flow through the aortic and pulmonary valves was produced by direct compression of the heart between sternum and spine, which elevated intraventricular pressures above those in the great vessels. Cyclical release of sternal pressure allowed chest recoil, reducing intrathoracic pressure and encouraging venous return, while reflux of blood from the aorta and pulmonary artery was prevented by the one-way valves. Measurement of intravascular pressures in experimental situations has demonstrated, however, that ECM produces simultaneous and equal pressure increases in both central venous and arterial vessels (Rudikoff *et al.*, 1980). Moreover, the increases in intrathoracic pressure were transmitted fully to the carotid artery, but only minimally to the jugular vein, creating a peripheral arteriovenous pressure gradient and antegrade flow. Therefore, the whole thorax appears to perform as a pump during ECM with flow from intra- to extrathoracic vessels, the heart and lungs acting as a single one-way reservoir of blood.

During chest compression, blood is expelled from the thorax into patent arteries and during this phase retrograde venous flow is minimized by the presence of valves and by venous collapse at high intrathoracic pressures (Mair *et al.*, 1993). Venous return occurs during chest recoil and may be augmented by methods of CPR that provide active decompression of the chest wall, e.g. using a hand-held suction device or active compression of the chest and abdomen in an alternating fashion (Cohen *et al.*, 1993; Stiell *et al.*, 1996). Other developments have included the use of pneumatic vests to achieve circumferential chest compression (Halperin *et al.*, 1993) or inspiratory impedence valves (Lurie *et al.*, 2000). The latter occlude the airway during active decompression with a suction cup device and therefore may augment venous return by achieving a greater intrathoracic vacuum. It remains to be seen, however, whether these techniques will impact significantly on the survival of patients with cardiac arrest.

INTERNAL CARDIAC MASSAGE

Open-chest cardiac compression produces a radically different haemodynamic response to ECM since antegrade blood flow is achieved by direct ventricular compression. Between 1950 and 1960, open chest cardiac compression became a routine procedure, access to the heart being gained through a left thoracotomy, by a subdiaphragmatic approach or via a median sternotomy. Following the description of closed-chest cardiac compression, internal cardiac massage was rapidly and almost completely abandoned (except following cardiac surgery), even though a number of studies (Bircher and Safar, 1984; Sanders *et al.*, 1984) have demonstrated that the open technique is associated with better forward flow, improved coronary perfusion and well-maintained cerebral blood flow. Moreover in cases of suspected intrathoracic trauma, thoracotomy can facilitate the diagnosis and treatment of some of the common reversible causes for cardiac arrest such as pericardial tamponade, tension pneumothorax or occult intrathoracic bleeding.

Despite these advantages, open-chest cardiac compression is currently rarely used outside the operating theatre and intensive care unit. It may, however, still be preferred in those with profound hypothermia following drowning or in the younger patient with cardiac arrest complicating status asthmaticus. It may also be useful when ECM is ineffective.

Intravenous access

Expansion of the circulating volume is generally not required during CPR, but powerful pressor agents must be given into

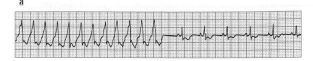

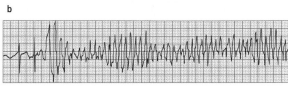

Fig. 9.4 (a) Ventricular tachycardia terminating spontaneously. (b) Ventricular fibrillation.

a large vein to ensure rapid delivery to the myocardium and the peripheral vasculature. The peripheral veins may be collapsed and difficult to cannulate and it may be necessary to use the *internal jugular vein*. *Intratracheal instillation* of drugs has been recommended as an alternative when venous cannulation proves difficult, and even as an immediate measure before intravascular access is established. Some, however, have considered this route to be unreliable (McCrirrick and Monk, 1994). In children an *intraosseus infusion device* inserted into the tibia may also prove life-saving (Glaeser *et al.*, 1993).

Management of life-threatening arrhythmias and pulseless electrical activity
VENTRICULAR FIBRILLATION AND OTHER PULSELESS RHYTHMS

VF and pulseless VT (Fig. 9.4) are most easily terminated by delivering a dc *shock* with minimal delay. The paddles of the defibrillator should be positioned so as to enclose as much ventricular muscle as possible, but should avoid contact with monitoring electrodes, the nipples, glyceryl trinitrate patches and permanent pacemaker generators. One shock should be delivered as quickly as possible followed by immediate resumption of CPR (30 compressions to 2 ventilations) without reassessing the rhythm or feeling for a pulse. After 2 minutes of CPR check the rhythm and give another dc shock (if indicated). The recommended energy when using a *monophasic defibrillator* is 360 J for both the initial and subsequent shocks. By reversing the current flow during defibrillation, *biphasic defibrillators* appear to be effective at lower energy levels than conventional devices. The recommended initial energy for biphasic defibrillators is 150–200 J, with second and subsequent shocks being delivered at 150–360 J. These devices use small batteries and, when combined with analysis software, have enabled the manufacture of portable automatic defibrillators that use voice prompts to guide the rescuer. Automated external defibrillators (AEDs) are now available in many public places (Fromm *et al.*, 2002; Liddle *et al.*, 2003), as well as in the hospital environment. Moreover, training and equipping volunteers to attempt early defibrillation with AEDs within a structured response system can increase the number of survivors to hospital

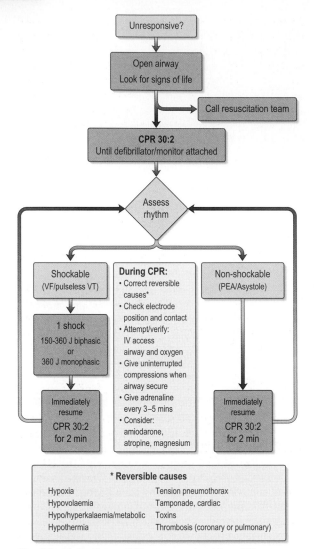

```
┌─────────────────────┐
│    Unresponsive?    │
└─────────────────────┘
           │
           ▼
┌─────────────────────┐
│    Open airway      │
│ Look for signs of life│
└─────────────────────┘
           │        └──────────┐
           │                   ▼
           │         ┌─────────────────────────┐
           │         │ Call resuscitation team │
           │         └─────────────────────────┘
           ▼
┌─────────────────────────────┐
│         CPR 30:2            │
│ Until defibrillator/monitor │
│        attached            │
└─────────────────────────────┘
           │
           ▼
        ◇ Assess ◇
        ◇ rhythm ◇
```

Shockable
(VF/pulseless VT)

1 shock
150–360 J biphasic
or
360 J monophasic

Immediately resume
CPR 30:2
for 2 min

During CPR:
• Correct reversible causes*
• Check electrode position and contact
• Attempt/verify: IV access airway and oxygen
• Give uninterrupted compressions when airway secure
• Give adrenaline every 3–5 mins
• Consider: amiodarone, atropine, magnesium

Non-shockable
(PEA/Asystole)

Immediately resume
CPR 30:2
for 2 min

* Reversible causes

Hypoxia	Tension pneumothorax
Hypovolaemia	Tamponade, cardiac
Hypo/hyperkalaemia/metabolic	Toxins
Hypothermia	Thrombosis (coronary or pulmonary)

Fig. 9.5 Adult advanced life support algorithm. CPR, cardiopulmonary resuscitation; IV, intravenous; PEA, pulseless electrical activity; VF, ventricular fibrillation; VT, ventricular tachycardia. (Originally published at www.resus.org.uk.)

discharge after cardiac arrest in out-of-hospital public places (Hallstrom *et al.*, 2004). On the other hand the addition of advanced life support interventions seems not to improve survival rates further (Stiell *et al.*, 2004).

If a promptly administered dc shock fails to restore a coordinated rhythm, prolonged CPR is likely to be required (**Fig. 9.5**). At this stage the patient's trachea should be intubated, positive-pressure ventilation should commence, intravenous access should be secured and emergency drugs should be prepared.

The drug of first choice is *adrenaline* (epinephrine) 1 : 10 000 1 mg given into the central circulation if possible. Chest compressions continue for 2 minutes, uninterrupted for ventilation, before the heart rhythm is reassessed and a

further dc shock at 360 J (or biphasic equivalent) is delivered if indicated. If VF/pulseless VT remains refractory, the loop is repeated again, including intravenous adrenaline 1 mg or, alternatively, adrenaline 3 mg via the endotracheal tube every 3–5 minutes (and ideally just before shock delivery). The administration of high-dose adrenaline (5 mg) is no longer advocated as there is no evidence that long-term survival is improved (Vandycke and Martens, 2000). There is also no clear advantage to the use of vasopressin rather than adrenaline for the treatment of cardiac arrest (Aung and Htay, 2005).

An intravenous bolus of amiodarone 300 mg should be considered when VF or pulseless VT does not respond to three dc shocks. A further dose of 150 mg may be given for refractory VF/pulseless VT. When VF/VT is recurrent a continuous intravenous infusion of amiodarone (900 mg over 24 hours) can be given. In patients with out-of-hospital cardiac arrest, treatment of refractory ventricular arrhythmias with amiodarone has been shown to improve the rate of survival to hospital admission (Kudenchuk *et al.*, 1999). Magnesium sulphate (4–8 mmol intravenously) has also been recommended for refractory VF and polymorphic VT. Lidocaine 1 mg/kg intravenously can be considered if amiodarone is not available but should not be given if amiodarone has already been administered. A total dose of 3 mg/kg should not be exceeded during the first hour. The administration of an alkalinizing agent (e.g. 8.4% sodium bicarbonate 50 mL intravenously) should be considered after 3–5 minutes of resuscitation and when the pH ≤ 7.1 and/or the patient is hyperkalaemic. If the patient's rhythm changes to asystole or pulseless electrical activity (PEA), the non-shockable rhythm algorithm should be followed (**Fig. 9.5**) (see below).

Persistent ventricular arrhythmias may be related to:

- hypoxia;
- hypovolaemia;
- hyperkalaemia/hypokalaemia and metabolic disorders;
- alterations in plasma levels of calcium or magnesium;
- acidosis or alkalosis;
- hypothermia;
- tension pneumothorax;
- cardiac tamponade;
- toxic/therapeutic disturbances;
- myocardial failure;
- thromboembolic/mechanical obstruction.

ASYSTOLE AND PULSELESS ELECTRICAL ACTIVITY

In *asystole* electrical activity is absent in association with clinical cardiac arrest. Although malfunction of the ECG monitor must be excluded, it is also important to consider whether the apparent asystole is in fact VF. If this possibility cannot be excluded, do not defibrillate but continue chest compression and ventilation for 2 minutes and reassess the rhythm.

For confirmed asystole drug therapy comprises, first, *adrenaline* 1 mg intravenously (or 3 mg via the endotracheal tube) and then a single dose of *atropine* 3 mg intravenously (or 6 mg via the endotracheal tube). *Transthoracic external pacing* is very occasionally effective in those with some residual electrical activity and can be used while a transvenous pacing system is established. If absence of electrical activity persists, further adrenaline 1 mg intravenously every 3–5 minutes and continued CPR are recommended whilst potentially reversible contributing factors are excluded. If VF/VT is subsequently identified, change to the shockable rhythm algorithm (**Fig. 9.5**).

PEA, including *electrical mechanical dissociation* (EMD) is a clinical condition in which there is no cardiac output in spite of ordered ventricular electrical activity. This may be *primary*, when the myocardium fails to contract adequately in response to electrical stimulation, or *secondary*, when the loss of forward flow is due to mechanical problems such as:

- hypovolaemia;
- pneumothorax;
- cardiac tamponade or acute rupture of the heart;
- pulmonary embolism.

Hypothermia, hypoxia, profound electrolyte disturbances and drug overdose may also be associated with EMD.

Specific therapies must be considered from the outset, especially volume replacement for hypovolaemia, pericardial aspiration for tamponade and urgent drainage of a tension pneumothorax.

When there is no immediately obvious remediable cause, the drug of first choice is *adrenaline*. The dose is 1 mg given centrally if possible. *Atropine* 3 mg is also indicated for PEA with a ventricular rate of less than 60 beats/min. *Calcium chloride* administration should be considered for the treatment of PEA due to hyperkalaemia, hypocalcaemia or an overdose of calcium channel-blocking drugs (Vincent, 1987). If VF/VT is subsequently identified, change to the shockable rhythm algorithm (Fig. 9.5).

CORRECTION OF ELECTROLYTE DISTURBANCES

Hyperkalaemia is relatively common during CPR, partly due to the release of potassium into the circulation from injured and/or hypoxic tissues. It should be treated with *calcium chloride, glucose and insulin mixtures*, and diuretics such as *furosemide*. In the presence of acidosis hyperkalaemia may temporarily respond to sodium bicarbonate administration (see below).

In some cases (e.g. following cardiac surgery) VF or VT may have been precipitated by *hypokalaemia or hypomagnesaemia* and urgent treatment with intravenous potassium or magnesium will be required.

CORRECTION OF ACIDOSIS

Anaerobic metabolism during the period of poor tissue perfusion is associated with increased lactic acid production. Furthermore, metabolism of lactic acid by the liver is impaired by a reduction in hepatic blood flow, and during extreme ischaemia the liver itself contributes to lactate pro-

duction. Nevertheless, since metabolic acidosis is only deleterious when severe, the routine administration of large quantities of sodium bicarbonate during CPR is unnecessary, particularly following short periods of cardiorespiratory arrest, and may be dangerous. The only exception may be when the patient is known to have had a pre-existing severe acidosis, for example due to cardiogenic shock. Potential adverse effects of excessive sodium bicarbonate administration include:

- hypernatraemia with an increased plasma osmolality;
- hypokalaemia;
- increased cardiac irritability;
- impaired myocardial performance;
- exacerbation of respiratory and intracellular acidosis;
- increased affinity of haemoglobin for oxygen.

In addition, sympathomimetic agents may be inactivated when mixed with sodium bicarbonate.

As an approximation, about 0.5 mmol of sodium bicarbonate per litre of extracellular fluid (ECF) is required for each minute of CPR in order to neutralize acidosis. Ideally, subsequent administration of alkali should be guided by frequent acid–base determinations.

POSTRESUSCITATION MANAGEMENT

A minority of patients will be resuscitated easily and quickly. They rapidly regain consciousness and resume spontaneous ventilation. They may be extubated immediately and further treatment should be aimed at preventing a recurrence. Many of those who are successfully resuscitated, however, will initially remain unconscious, often with absent or inadequate spontaneous respiratory efforts and hypotension. In these cases, subsequent management is aimed at restoring cardiovascular and respiratory function and minimizing cerebral damage.

RESPIRATORY FUNCTION

The tracheal tube must be left in place until the patient is conscious and has effective cough, gag and swallowing reflexes. Some patients may later require a tracheostomy. Mechanical ventilation is clearly indicated when respiratory function is impaired (e.g. in those with pulmonary oedema, aspiration pneumonitis or a significant chest wall injury). Furthermore, a modest degree of hyperventilation may improve cerebral autoregulation, as well as reducing cerebral acidosis (see Chapter 15). Nevertheless, although it is accepted that *hypoxaemia and hypercarbia must be avoided*, there is no evidence to support the use of deliberate hyperventilation or prolonged (> 48 hours) elective controlled ventilation when respiratory function is adequate. A reasonable approach is to initiate controlled ventilation in all patients who have suffered a global ischaemic insult and to reassess the situation 4–6 hours later. Selected patients may then be allowed to breathe spontaneously.

CARDIOVASCULAR FUNCTION

It is vital to ensure that cerebral and coronary blood flow are adequate following resuscitation and it is therefore essential to *restore systemic blood pressure*. Even mild hypotension must be avoided at all costs and a few hours of controlled slight hypertension may be beneficial (see below). This may require manipulation of the circulating volume and, if necessary, the administration of inotropic or vasopressor agents. Metabolic derangements, including metabolic acidosis and fluid and electrolyte disturbances, must also be corrected. Intra-aortic balloon counterpulsation (IABCP) may be indicated in selected patients with cardiogenic shock or persistent myocardial ischaemia (see Chapter 5).

CEREBRAL FUNCTION

Provided there is no pre-existing intracranial pathology (e.g. cerebrovascular disease) and cardiac arrest was not preceded by hypoxia, ischaemic brain damage during CPR may be prevented by maintaining a cerebral blood flow as low as one-seventh of normal values. This can usually be achieved if CPR is correctly performed. Nevertheless, cerebral perfusion is not usually sufficient to sustain normal brain activity during CPR and patients may remain unconscious, sometimes with fixed dilated pupils, and yet recover normal cerebral function. Sometimes, signs of cerebral activity such as frowning, head shaking, struggling and an eyelash reflex may be present during CPR and these may suggest that the brain is being adequately oxygenated.

If, however, resuscitation is protracted, cerebral function usually deteriorates progressively due to a gradual reduction in cerebral blood flow and persistent relative ischaemia. Furthermore, cerebral lactic acidosis, which is not corrected by the systemic administration of sodium bicarbonate, impairs cerebral autoregulation (the mean perfusion pressure during CPR is generally less than 50 mmHg and is therefore below the lower limit for autoregulation) and depresses cerebral function.

The ultimate outcome for those patients who are successfully resuscitated could be considerably improved if it were possible to ameliorate the cerebral damage caused by cardiorespiratory arrest and protracted CPR. Clearly, this could be achieved if improved techniques of CPR were developed that maintained normal cerebral perfusion. It is also evident that events occurring during or after reperfusion may initiate or exacerbate cell damage and that appropriate interventions might therefore limit the degree of brain damage.

Control of seizures

Seizure discharges can exacerbate postischaemic cerebral damage by increasing metabolic demands and precipitating neuronal hypoxia in areas of marginally perfused brain. Moreover, sympathetic nervous activity is increased, placing an extra demand on the patient's limited cardiorespiratory reserve. It is therefore accepted that prophylactic administration of anticonvulsants and aggressive treatment of seizures (e.g. with diazepam/phenytoin), both of which are associ-

ated with minimal risks, are normally justified (see Chapter 15).

Cerebral perfusion

There is evidence that the degree of cerebral damage is influenced by the adequacy of cerebral perfusion following restoration of cardiac activity. Thus, it appears that the brain can recover from quite prolonged periods of normothermic relative ischaemia (up to 20 minutes) provided that cerebral blood flow is subsequently adequate.

Initially, systemic hypertension combined with the loss of autoregulation may cause cerebral hyperperfusion with oedema formation and disruption of the blood–brain barrier, although a spontaneous or induced episode of hypertension during or immediately after restoration of a circulation seems to be associated with better outcomes. Subsequently hypoperfusion is nearly always the dominant abnormality. This is associated with prolonged severe depression of cerebral cortical blood flow and an increased cerebrovascular resistance. Possible explanations have included cellular swelling with raised intracranial pressure, intravascular coagulation, increases in viscosity, microvascular endothelial swelling and release of vasoactive metabolites of arachidonic acid such as thromboxane. It has also been suggested that cerebrovascular spasm may be caused by an influx of calcium ions into anoxic vascular smooth muscle.

Based on these observations, suggested therapeutic interventions have included:

- anticoagulation;
- haemodilution with dextrans or oxygen-carrying blood substitutes;
- calcium antagonists (see below);
- prostacyclin;
- diuretics;
- steroids;
- manipulation of the arachidonic acid cascade.

There is little evidence to support the use of steroids, diuretics or anticoagulants in this situation, and it appears that cerebral oedema is unusual following global brain ischaemia, except in those who have sustained extensive neuronal damage incompatible with survival. The value of other measures remains uncertain. The aim should be to achieve normotension or slight hypertension during the postarrest period; but because autoregulation is impaired, extreme hypertension, which might exacerbate oedema formation and intracranial hypertension, should be avoided. Haemodilution to a haematocrit of about 30% has been recommended.

Metabolic factors

It has also been suggested that elevated brain glucose levels predispose to cerebral oedema and enhance lactic acid production by increasing the supply of substrate, thereby exacerbating neuronal damage. A number of experimental studies have demonstrated that high blood glucose levels prior to cardiac arrest are associated with a worse neurological outcome (Pulsinelli et al., 1982). The clinical implications of these findings are unclear, although it would seem sensible to avoid significant hyperglycaemia (see Chapter 17: tight glycaemic control).

Hyperthermia must be avoided. Moreover, two prospective randomized controlled trials have indicated that mild therapeutic hypothermia may improve neurological outcome in selected patients after out-of-hospital VF cardiac arrest (Bernard et al., 2002; Hypothermia After Cardiac Arrest Study, 2002) and new guidance now recommends early induction of mild hypothermia (32–34°C), sustained for at least 12 hours (Safar and Kochanek, 2002), in such patients when they remain unconscious in the absence of circulatory shock. Methods for inducing hypothermia include surface cooling with cold air or the application of ice packs to the head and torso, nasopharyngeal cold irrigation, gastric and intravenous cold loads and invasive brain cooling (e.g. using cardiopulmonary bypass). Shivering must be prevented. The feasibility and efficacy of external cooling in routine clinical practice have recently been confirmed (Oddo et al., 2006). Further studies are required to confirm these findings following in-hospital collapse, as well as to determine the optimum target temperature, duration of hypothermia and preferred rates of rewarming to normothermia.

Biochemical abnormalities
The rapid depletion of cellular energy stores that follows sudden complete ischaemia leads to failure of the ionic pump, membrane depolarization and cellular swelling. There is also an accumulation of calcium ions within the cells. This may initiate a number of harmful reactions, including the release of free fatty acids, particularly arachidonic acid, and the production of reactive oxygen species, and could be the final common pathway leading to cell death. The potential of calcium entry-blocking drugs as cerebral-protective agents has therefore been investigated. It was postulated that these agents might prevent cerebrovascular spasm and maintain cerebral blood flow as well as reducing the calcium-induced liberation of free fatty acids and reactive oxygen species. In a randomized clinical trial, however, the calcium channel blocker lidoflazine was ineffective in reducing either mortality or brain damage after cardiac arrest (Brain Resuscitation Clinical Trial II Study Group, 1991).

It was also suggested that barbiturates might protect the brain from ischaemic damage by virtue of their free radical scavenging activity. These agents also suppress brain metabolism, as well as reducing cerebral blood flow and intracranial pressure, and may improve the cerebral oxygen supply/demand ratio. A number of experimental studies suggested that pretreatment, and possibly early postinsult therapy might be beneficial in focal ischaemia. The results in experimental global ischaemia were, however, conflicting and in a randomized clinical trial of thiopental loading in

comatose survivors of cardiac arrest, there were no significant differences in outcome between treatment and control groups (Brain Resuscitation Clinical Trial 1 Study Group, 1986).

In view of the multifactorial nature of postischaemic/hypoxic cerebral injury it seems likely that multiple therapeutic interventions may ultimately be required to achieve a significant beneficial effect. Furthermore, the timing of each intervention in relation to the episode of cardiorespiratory arrest will probably prove to be crucial. Current management of patients following CPR is therefore based on supporting cardiorespiratory function to ensure optimum conditions for brain recovery (Saltuari and Marosi, 1994), and the only undisputed therapeutic principles are to:

- restore systemic blood pressure;
- ensure adequate oxygenation;
- avoid hypercapnia;
- avoid hyperthermia/induce hypothermia;
- abolish seizures.

THROMBOLYTIC THERAPY
Thrombolysis should be considered for those in whom cardiac arrest was precipitated by MI provided there are no contraindications (Table 9.3).

The safety of thrombolysis following CPR seems to depend on the duration of the resuscitation attempt, and successful resuscitation immediately following early defibrillation should not normally preclude thrombolytic therapy. Although conventionally thrombolysis was thought to be contraindicated if vigorous resuscitation had taken place, particularly when prolonged energetic ECM had been performed, a prospective trial of thrombolytic therapy using recombinant t-PA combined with heparin after initially unsuccessful out-of-hospital resuscitation has suggested improved patient outcome, without increased bleeding complications related to CPR (Böttiger et al., 2001).

■ CARDIORESPIRATORY ARREST ASSOCIATED WITH SPECIAL CIRCUMSTANCES

A number of conditions other than major cardiac arrhythmias can present with life-threatening disturbances of circulatory or respiratory function. The diagnosis can often be suspected from the patient's immediate history or surroundings, but sometimes the underlying pathology is obscure. Airway protection, ventilation and circulatory support, as previously described, remain central to their treatment.

PRIMARY RESPIRATORY ARREST
In adults primary respiratory arrest is uncommon but is usually the result of:

- an acute severe intracerebral event (e.g. intracranial haemorrhage);

- the effect of depressant drugs (e.g. opioids or tricyclic antidepressants);
- profound metabolic derangements;
- acute upper-airway obstruction (e.g. asphyxiation in an eating place –'*café coronary*').

Initially cardiac output is maintained, but in the face of progressive hypoxaemia heart rate falls and myocardial contractility is impaired, culminating in asystole.

The diagnosis usually rests on the observation of an apnoeic and cyanosed patient with a palpable pulse. The essential requirement is to establish an unobstructed airway and restore oxygenation, if necessary with tracheal intubation or tracheostomy and assisted ventilation. If the patient is treated promptly, recovery of a satisfactory circulation may follow restoration of the airway and ventilatory support alone; in such cases the eventual outcome is usually determined by the underlying diagnosis. Chest compressions and adrenaline administration will be required for the patient who remains pulseless.

ASTHMA AND SEVERE BRONCHOSPASM
(see Chapter 8)

Asthmatic patients are vulnerable to episodes of severe lower-airway narrowing and in the most serious cases profound hypoxia can lead to marked bradycardia followed by asystole. Immediate support of ventilatory function is essential. Patients should be intubated and ventilated with 100% oxygen. Bilateral air entry should be confirmed clinically and the possibility of a complicating tension pneumothorax excluded. Profound bronchospasm and air trapping may necessitate external chest compression to reduce hyperinflation. Internal cardiac massage should be considered for prolonged cardiac arrest complicating life-threatening asthma.

PULMONARY EMBOLISM (see Chapter 5)

Massive pulmonary embolism characteristically causes circulatory arrest with a markedly elevated jugular venous pressure, deep cyanosis and an initial tachypnoea before spontaneous respiration ceases. Adrenaline should be administered early to reverse bradycardia, maintain systemic venous return and coronary perfusion, and augment right ventricular contraction. When pulmonary obstruction is severe, cardiac compression is ineffective and the patient remains suffused, pulseless and deeply cyanosed. In successful cases the embolus may be dispersed into distal vessels and as oxygenation improves pulmonary arterial pressure may fall. If resuscitation fails to restore the circulation within a few minutes, continued CPR is likely to prove futile.

ANAPHYLAXIS (see Chapter 5)

The airway should be opened, cleared and maintained. One hundred percent oxygen should be administered using assisted ventilation if necessary. If an effective airway cannot be established and laryngeal oedema prevents orotracheal intubation, emergency cricothyroidotomy may prove necessary. If there is no detectable cardiac output, chest compressions should commence together with rapid volume expansion and administration of *adrenaline* (an intramuscular or a slow intravenous injection of 500 µg repeated as necessary, the dose titrated against the response). *Antihistamines* (H_1-receptor antagonists) given by slow intravenous injection (e.g. chlorpheniramine 10–20 mg) are a useful adjunctive treatment. *Hydrocortisone*, 100–500 mg, can also be administered intravenously. Intravenous aminophylline or a β_2-agonist such as salbutamol are useful additional measures if bronchospasm is a major feature and does not respond rapidly to other treatment.

ELECTROCUTION

Casualties may be struck by lightning or injured by domestic or industrial electricity. Lightning consists of direct current of an extremely high voltage. It may cause immediate asystole or VF, as well as inflicting a severe primary injury on the central nervous system.

VF is the commonest initial arrhythmia and should be treated by defibrillation as soon as possible. For other arrhythmias, standard protocols should be followed. After successful resuscitation, myoglobinuria may result from muscle damage. Intravenous fluid therapy and mannitol administration may help to maintain an adequate urinary output (see Chapter 13). Electrical burns, compartment syndromes and other traumatic lesions may require specialist surgical attention.

RESUSCITATION IN LATE PREGNANCY
(see Chapter 18)

Circulatory arrest from a variety of acute conditions remains an important cause of maternal mortality. The causes of maternal cardiac arrest include:

- pulmonary embolism;
- massive haemorrhage;
- amniotic fluid embolism;
- placental abruption;
- eclampsia;
- sepsis;
- drug toxicity.

An obstetrician and a paediatrician should be involved at an early stage.

After clearing and opening the airway, early tracheal intubation is recommended since gastric emptying is prolonged in pregnant women and there is an increased risk of regurgitation and pulmonary aspiration. In the later stages of pregnancy the diaphragm will be splinted by the large uterus and high inflation pressures may be required. To improve venous return and cardiac output it is vital that pressure on the inferior vena cava from the gravid uterus is relieved by placing sandbags, pillows or a purpose-made wedge under the patient's right side. Alternatively, the uterus can be moved to the left by manual displacement or the patient's right hip can be raised. Arrhythmias should be treated according to standard protocols. During epidural anaesthesia high levels of local anaesthetic agents may be present in the blood and lidocaine administration should therefore be avoided.

In the pregnant woman emergency Caesarean section is indicated after 5 minutes of unsuccessful in-hospital resuscitation in an attempt to save the fetus and improve the mother's chances of survival. Surgery must be accompanied by uninterrupted CPR.

MISCELLANEOUS CAUSES OF CARDIAC ARREST

Collapse following drug overdose and poisoning is dealt with in Chapter 19. Cardiopulmonary arrest following near-drowning is discussed in Chapter 10 and hypothermia in Chapter 20.

PROGNOSIS OF CARDIORESPIRATORY ARREST

It is perhaps not surprising that the results of CPR initiated in the community are inferior to those achieved within the hospital environment, probably largely because of delays in initiating resuscitation combined with lack of skill and interruptions in CPR while the patient is moved. In particular, coma is more frequent in those who suffer a cardiorespiratory arrest outside hospital (Bur et al., 2001).

Even within hospitals, organizational deficiencies and absent or malfunctioning equipment may significantly delay the institution of effective CPR, and the outcome for those who arrest on general wards is poor. The outlook for those who arrest in the coronary or intensive care unit, operating theatre or emergency department is, however, considerably better (Goldhill et al., 1999; Tunstall-Pedoe et al., 1992). This disparity between survival rates in the different locations appears not to be attributable to differences in the immediate response to CPR. Rather, it seems to reflect the severity of the underlying illness in those receiving CPR on general wards, for some of whom attempted resuscitation may be inappropriate. Importantly, it seems that earlier recognition of those at risk may reduce the incidence of, and improve the outcome from, 'unexpected cardiac arrest' (Buist et al., 2002) (see Chapter 1).

Good prognostic features include a previously normal heart, prompt initiation of effective CPR and cardiac arrest due to primary VF. Conversely, when cardiac arrest occurs in a patient with progressive myocardial failure, often in asystole, the outlook is grave. Outcome is also poor when the cardiac collapse is not witnessed, the initial cardiac rhythm is not VT/VF and when resuscitation does not lead to restoration of a pulse within the first 10 minutes (van Walraven et al., 2001). Finally the prognosis for cerebral recovery is closely related to the duration of unconsciousness.

ASSESSMENT OF NEUROLOGICAL PROGNOSIS IN COMATOSE SURVIVORS OF CARDIAC ARREST

Early, accurate prediction of neurological outcome in comatose survivors of cardiac arrest would encourage the clinician to continue aggressive supportive treatment in those with a favourable prognosis while avoiding the futile prolongation of costly therapy when the situation is hopeless. A recent systematic review concluded that findings on simple physical examination strongly predict death or poor neurological outcome in comatose survivors of cardiac arrest. In particular the chance of meaningful neurological recovery seems to be extremely small in patients who lack pupillary and corneal reflexes at 24 hours and have no motor response at 72 hours. In the first few hours after cardiac arrest clinical signs are unreliable and none strongly predict a good neurological outcome (Booth et al., 2004). Although persistent unresponsiveness at 3–7 days after cardiac arrest and CPR has been predictably followed by permanent severe brain damage, the suggestion that in patients with hypoxic/ischaemic coma a permanent vegetative state can be accurately predicted after 3 days of intensive care is contentious. Some have even suggested that in view of the uncertainty, unlimited care should be maintained in such cases, particularly since recovery from persistent vegetative state has apparently been observed after 4 or more months (Andrews, 1993). As is always the case, decisions to withdraw or limit therapy in comatose survivors of cardiac arrest must be made on an individual basis, informed by an objective assessment of the prognosis, and only after discussion with the next of kin and all those involved in the patient's care (see Chapter 2).

ABANDONING CPR AND 'DO NOT ATTEMPT RESUSCITATION' ORDERS (British Medical Association (BMA), The Resuscitation Council (UK) and the Royal College of Nursing (RCN), 2001)

It is not possible to diagnose brainstem death with confidence during CPR and therefore attempts at resuscitation should only be abandoned when it proves impossible to restore effective myocardial activity. Time should not be a major factor in reaching this decision, which is the responsibility of the leader of the resuscitation team. The size of the pupils or their lack of response to light should not be taken as a guide to the activity of the central nervous system or the likelihood of recovery. CPR should continue for longer in those who are hypothermic or the victims of near-drowning and when cardiac arrest is associated with drug overdose (see Chapters 10, 19 and 20).

In some patients with terminal disease, CPR is started inappropriately and should then be abandoned as soon as the circumstances become clear. This situation can usually be avoided by establishing beforehand that, because of the nature and extent of the underlying disease, resuscitation would be inappropriate. Most hospitals have instituted formal 'do not attempt resuscitation' policies. Once a decision not to resuscitate has been made, it must be reviewed regularly and changed if circumstances alter. All such decisions should be discussed with the next of kin and must be communicated to the medical and nursing staff involved in the patient's care, as well as being clearly recorded in the patient's notes and dated and signed by the most senior available medical member of the team caring for that patient. Each case must be considered on its own merits, in particular the patient's quality of life and perception of the situation are important. Age alone should not be a bar to resuscitation. It is appropriate to endeavour to discuss such decisions with patients who are both conscious and mentally competent (see also Chapter 2).

MANAGEMENT OF ARRHYTHMIAS

Arrhythmias occurring in critically ill patients are frequently secondary to associated abnormalities such as:

- hypoxia;
- electrolyte disturbances (particularly hypokalaemia or hypomagnesaemia);
- sudden alterations in arterial carbon dioxide tension (P_aCO_2);
- increased circulating catecholamine levels;
- sepsis;
- drug effects.

In some cases, pre-existing *cardiac disease*, *myocardial contusion* (see Chapter 10) or *pulmonary disease* may contribute to the development of rhythm disturbances.

Because of the dangers associated with the use of antiarrhythmic agents (see below), these precipitating factors must be identified and if possible corrected before resorting to specific therapy. Subsequent definitive treatment is then only indicated when the arrhythmia persists and is associated with a significant haemodynamic disturbance. Specific therapy may also be required when persistence of the abnormality is likely to impair cardiac performance (e.g. when the ventricular rate is very rapid) or if the arrhythmia is of a type conventionally considered to predispose to more serious rhythm disturbances (e.g. 'R on T' ventricular premature contractions: VPCs). Furthermore, if it is not possible to correct the underlying abnormality immediately (e.g. a patient with atrial fibrillation (AF) secondary to pneumonia and sepsis), it may prove difficult to restore, and subsequently maintain, sinus rhythm (Mayr *et al.*, 1999). Under these circumstances, treatment should be directed at controlling the ventricular rate and minimizing any haemodynamic disturbance (Sanai *et al.*, 1993).

Critically ill patients are generally intolerant of antiarrhythmics, almost all of which are negatively inotropic, and in general these agents should be avoided. If this is not possible, they should be administered cautiously, usually in reduced dosage. *dc cardioversion* does not impair myocardial function unless high-energy shocks are used and adminis-

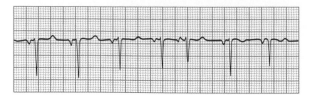

Fig. 9.6 Atrial premature contraction associated with an inferior myocardial infarction.

tered repeatedly, and this is therefore often the most appropriate initial treatment when restoration of sinus rhythm is essential. Similarly, *digoxin*, which does not depress the myocardium and may have a modest positive inotropic effect, remains a valuable agent in seriously ill patients.

The choice of the most appropriate antiarrhythmic for a particular patient is often difficult and the various classifications of the available agents are unlikely to be of much practical help to the intensive care clinician (Aronson, 1985).

When complex arrhythmias are encountered and/or the abnormality fails to respond to simple measures, a cardiologist should be consulted.

MANAGEMENT OF SPECIFIC ARRHYTHMIAS

Treatment of asystole, VF and pulseless VT has been discussed earlier in this chapter.

Atrial premature contractions (APCs)

APCs (**Fig. 9.6**) are *usually benign* and do not therefore normally warrant intervention. Treatment may be indicated:

- in a patient who has reverted to sinus rhythm following an episode of AF because in this situation closely coupled APCs may precipitate recurrence;
- when APCs are not conducted (this may lead to a very slow effective ventricular rate);
- in those in whom APCs are known to precipitate a re-entry tachycardia.

APCs can be treated with *β-blockers* or *disopyramide*.

Ventricular premature contractions

The significance of VPCs (**Fig. 9.7**) is uncertain, particularly in the absence of ischaemic heart disease. They may be idiopathic and benign or related to associated abnormalities, most commonly hypokalaemia or hypomagnesaemia. Ventricular 'escape' beats are also sometimes seen in association with bradycardia and may respond to atropine administration.

Specific treatment is usually instituted because of concern that VPCs may precipitate VF/VT. Traditionally, 'warning arrhythmias', which may degenerate into VF/VT and therefore require treatment, are considered to include:

- a bigeminal rhythm;
- VPCs occurring more frequently than 5 per minute or in runs of 2 or more;

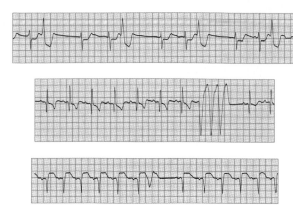

Fig. 9.7 Ventricular premature contractions (VPCs): (top) unifocal trigeminy; (middle) salvo of VPCs; (bottom) R on T VPC.

- multifocal VPCs;
- those in which the R wave is superimposed on the T wave.

The value of prophylactic treatment has, however, been questioned since, although it is possible to reduce the incidence of these warning arrhythmias and possibly the occurrence of VF/VT, it is uncertain whether this influences the ultimate outcome. Nevertheless most would recommend prophylactic treatment in those with sinister VPCs that persist after correction of associated abnormalities, and certainly it is usual to institute such therapy after a recurrence of VF/VT.

Lidocaine is relatively safe when used by slow intravenous injection and can be considered first for emergency use. Side-effects include dizziness, drowsiness, speech disturbances, tremor and agitation. Lidocaine is metabolized by the liver and the dose should therefore be reduced in those with hepatic failure or a low cardiac output. In overdose, lidocaine can produce hypotension, fits and conduction disturbances. Alternatives to lidocaine include *amiodarone* (see VT). β-blockers can also sometimes be effective.

Broad-complex tachycardias

Although broad-complex tachycardias (QRS complexes ≥ 0.12 second) may result from supraventricular rhythms with aberrant conduction, in a periarrest context they should be assumed to be ventricular in origin.

VT usually originates in a small group of abnormal myocardial cells and may be associated with an area of infarction or ischaemia. It may also arise in ventricular muscle that is hypertrophied or myopathic. Hypokalaemia, reduced tissue magnesium concentrations, raised catecholamine levels and a slow sinus rate all predispose to the development of VT. Established VT may be preceded by warning arrhythmias such as R on T or multiform ectopics and brief runs of VT.

Therapy for VT is directed at conversion to sinus rhythm and the prevention of recurrence. The priorities for treat-

ment (Fig. 9.8) depend on the rate and the haemodynamic consequences of the arrhythmia. VT with poor or deteriorating haemodynamics or sustained VT in symptomatic patients require DC *cardioversion*. Normally this should be synchronized to the R wave to avoid a 'shock on T' phenomenon, although if VT is truly pulseless or is very rapid the ventricles may be 'fluttering', in which case synchronization is unnecessary. dc cardioversion is always performed under sedation/general anaesthesia. For VT at rates less than 150/min with acceptable haemodynamics or when VT is paroxysmal and recurrent rather than sustained, pharmacological treatment is indicated once other predisposing conditions such as slow atrial rate or hypokalaemia have been corrected. Hypokalaemia may be associated with hypomagnesaemia, especially in those who were receiving diuretic treatment before admission; an intravenous magnesium infusion can be considered in such cases, as well as in those with underlying conduction defects.

Many antitachycardia drugs exacerbate *torsades de pointes* (a special form of VT characterized by changing wave fronts of ventricular activation, which is often related to a long Q-T interval). This disorder should if possible be treated by correcting electrolyte disorders, especially hypokalaemia and hypomagnesaemia, and by attempting to increase the underlying heart rate if it is slow with atrial (or ventricular) pacing. Alternatively β-blockers may be considered. Where possible, expert help should be sought with the assessment and treatment of irregular broad-complex tachyarrhythmias.

In the absence of adverse signs and in situations in which broad-complex regular tachycardia may be supraventricular in origin, *amiodarone* (300 mg) should be given by slow intravenous injection over 20–60 minutes (preferably via a central venous catheter) followed by an infusion up to a total of 1.2 g in 24 hours.

Agents that can be considered if amiodarone fails to stabilize the cardiac rhythm include:

- *Mexiletine*, 100–250 mg intravenously at a rate of 25 mg/min followed by an infusion of 250 mg over 1 hour, 125 mg/hour for 2 hours and then 500 μg/min.
- *Propranolol*, 0.5–1 mg intravenously and repeated if necessary; should only be used when the underlying pathology is MI or ischaemia.
- *Sotalol*, 20–120 mg intravenously over 10 minutes. This agent has been shown to be superior to lidocaine for the acute termination of sustained VT (Ho *et al.*, 1994).

Single- or dual-chamber pacing can also suppress VT by increasing the heart rate.

The presence of an implanted automatic defibrillator should not influence the conduct of the recommended emergency measures for treating VT/VF.

Narrow-complex tachycardia

The term supraventricular tachycardia (SVT) encompasses all tachycardias originating above the division of the His bundle and includes atrial flutter and fibrillation, atrial

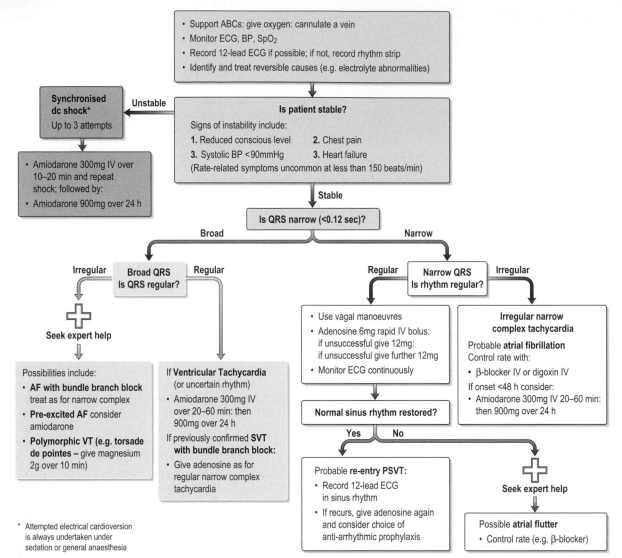

Fig. 9.8 Tachycardia algorithm (doses based on adult of average body weight). AF, atrial fibrillation; BP, blood pressure; dc, direct current; ECG, electrocardiogram; IV, intravenous. (Originally published at www.resus.org.uk.)

ectopic tachycardia, multifocal atrial tachycardia and ectopic junctional rhythms (Delacretaz, 2006).

In all forms of SVT the QRS complexes are narrow (≤ 0.12 second duration) unless there is a pre-existing antegradely conducting accessory pathway, bundle branch block or the increased heart rate precipitates aberrant conduction. It must be emphasized, however, that it can sometimes be extremely difficult to distinguish between an SVT with abnormal conduction and VT on the ECG (**Table 9.5**); *broad-complex tachycardias must therefore be treated as sustained VT unless proved to be otherwise.*

It is uncommon for a narrow-complex tachycardia to cause profound circulatory collapse, but the circulation may

Table 9.5 Electrocardiogram distinction between supraventricular tachycardia with bundle branch block and ventricular tachycardia

VT is the more likely diagnosis when there is:

A very broad QRS (> 0.14 seconds)

Atrioventricular dissociation

A bifid upright QRS with a taller first peak in V_1

A deep S wave in V_6

A concordant (same polarity) QRS direction in all chest leads (V_1–V_6)

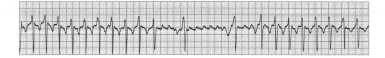

Fig. 9.9 Carotid sinus massage reveals atrial flutter.

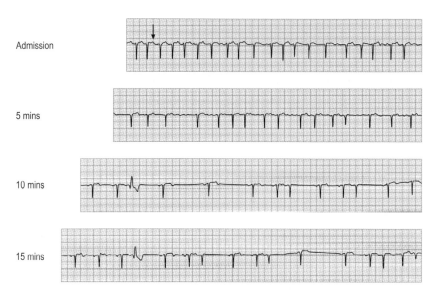

Admission

5 mins

10 mins

15 mins

Fig. 9.10 Atrial fibrillation. The ventricular rate is slowed by the administration of a beta-blocker.

be compromised if the attack is prolonged, if the patient is hypovolaemic and if unusually high ventricular rates are superimposed on underlying coronary, valvular or myocardial disease. Particularly high ventricular rates may be seen when the speed of atrioventricular (AV) conduction is enhanced by an abnormal pathway that bypasses the AV node, e.g. AV nodal re-entry tachycardia or AV re-entry tachycardia due to Wolff–Parkinson–White syndrome.

Patients with circulatory collapse require immediate *synchronized dc cardioversion* following intravenous sedation/general anaesthesia. Occasionally *carotid sinus massage* restores AV block enabling atrial and junctional tachycardias to be distinguished from each other and from atrial flutter (**Fig. 9.9**).

Adenosine has also become popular for the management of narrow-complex tachycardias (Garratt *et al.*, 1992). This agent is a naturally occurring compound that has profound short-lived electrophysiological actions when administered intravenously. It depresses AV nodal conduction with a half-life of 2–10 seconds and often converts paroxysmal SVT to sinus rhythm, particularly where AV nodal re-entry is the underlying mechanism. Adenosine is administered as a rapid intravenous bolus injection over 2 seconds followed by a saline flush. An initial 3–6-mg injection may be followed if required by two doses each of 12 mg at 1–2-minute intervals (**Fig. 9.8**). Further increments should not be given if high-level AV block develops. (This dosing schedule is currently outside the UK licence). Care should be taken with asthmatic patients, since adenosine is a bronchoconstrictor and in patients with known Wolff–Parkinson–White syndrome.

Also patients receiving dipyridamole or carbamazepine and those with a denervated heart may experience a markedly exaggerated effect. Other side-effects include flushing and headache.

If adenosine is not successful in establishing a satisfactory rhythm or if fast irregular narrow-complex tachycardia persists at a rate greater than 130 beats/min, subsequent management will depend upon the perceived urgency. If adverse signs (hypotension, chest pain or heart failure) are present treatment should consist of synchronized DC countershock under sedation/general anaesthesia. If this is unsuccessful an intravenous infusion of 300 mg *amiodarone* given over 10–20 minutes can be followed by synchronized dc shock, with another 900 mg of amiodarone given intravenously over 24 hours. If adverse signs are not evident and amiodarone proves ineffective, other drug strategies should be considered.

β-blocking agents are sometimes used to slow the ventricular rate in narrow-complex tachycardia (**Fig. 9.10**) and may occasionally restore sinus rhythm in those with a junctional tachycardia. They must be given cautiously when myocardial function is impaired. β-blockade may also be used to prevent recurrence and *esmolol* 40 mg intravenously over 60 seconds, followed by an infusion of 4–12 mg/min, has proved particularly effective in this respect.

Verapamil, a calcium channel blocker predominantly affecting the AV node, is also likely to slow the ventricular rate and may restore sinus rhythm in paroxysmal narrow-complex tachycardia (**Fig. 9.11**). It should be administered slowly intravenously in a dose of 2.5–5 mg repeated if necessary after approximately 5–10 minutes. Verapamil can

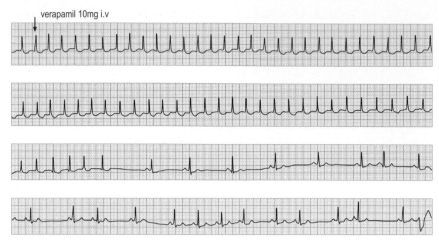

Fig. 9.11 Supraventricular tachycardia terminated by intravenous verapamil.

however, produce marked myocardial depression with profound hypotension and should be used extremely cautiously in the critically ill. In addition, it should never be given with intravenous β-blockade since the combination is known to cause extreme bradycardia, hypotension (Packer *et al.*, 1982) and even asystole. Provided the patient is not digitalized, and there is no possibility of digitalis toxicity, *digoxin* (500 µg orally or intravenously over 30 minutes) can be used as a safer alternative to verapamil to slow the ventricular rate. In cases of paroxysmal SVT with block, digitalis toxicity should be suspected. As well as correcting any electrolyte abnormality, intravenous administration of a β-blocker may be useful. Specific digoxin antibody is available for known or strongly suspected life-threatening overdosage (see Chapter 19).

If it proves impossible to restore sinus rhythm or if the above measures fail to prevent a recurrence, *atrial 'overdrive' pacing* may sometimes effectively terminate the arrhythmia.

ATRIAL FLUTTER

Synchronized direct current cardioversion is nearly always the treatment of choice, particularly since this arrhythmia usually responds poorly to drug therapy. Intravenous *amiodarone* may be used in an attempt to restore sinus rhythm. *Atrial 'overdrive' pacing* is also sometimes effective. Digoxin is not generally recommended since very large, potentially toxic doses are often required to control the ventricular rate.

ATRIAL FIBRILLATION

This arrhythmia may present with a wide range of ventricular rates; treatment depends on the likely underlying cause, as well as the degree of any haemodynamic disturbance (Sanai *et al.*, 1993) (**Fig. 9.8**).

Patients who develop AF with a heart rate less than 100 beats/min with mild or no symptoms and well-maintained perfusion are considered to be at low clinical risk. If the onset of AF was more than 24 hours previously, anticoagula-tion should be considered, followed by attempted cardioversion 3–4 weeks later. An anteroposterior electrode position is more effective than the anterolateral position for external cardioversion of persistent AF (Kirchhof *et al.*, 2002). If the onset of AF is known to have been within 24 hours the patient can be heparinized before attempting to restore sinus rhythm with *amiodarone* 300 mg given over 20–60 minutes or *flecainide* 100–150 mg intravenously over 30 minutes, followed by attempted cardioversion.

Patients at intermediate clinical risk from the arrhythmia may have higher heart rates, symptoms of breathlessness and/or signs of poor perfusion. If there is no evidence of structural heart disease or impaired haemodynamics and the onset of AF was likely to have been more than 24 hours previously, the heart rate should be controlled with *β-blockers, verapamil, diltiazem* (unlicensed indication) or *digoxin*. Verapamil and diltazem should not be used in patients receiving β-blockers (see above). The addition of intravenous *magnesium sulphate* (20 mmol/L over 20 minutes followed by 20 mmol/L over 2 hours) to these standard measures has been shown to enhance rate reduction and conversion to sinus rhythm (Davey and Teubner, 2005). Cardioversion should not be attempted until the patient has been anticoagulated for several weeks. If the onset of the AF is known to have been within the last 24 hours patients at intermediate risk from the arrhythmia should be heparinized and receive amiodarone or flecainide. If sinus rhythm is not restored attempted cardioversion can subsequently be undertaken with a synchronized dc shock.

In the presence of structural heart disease or impaired haemodynamics and prolonged AF the heart rate should be controlled with digoxin or amiodarone. dc cardioversion should not be attempted for several weeks until the patient has been fully anticoagulated.

In compromised patients with recent-onset AF (less than 24 hours) heparinization and attempts at dc cardioversion should be undertaken. If attempted cardioversion fails, or the AF recurs, a bolus of amiodarone can be given before a further attempt at dc cardioversion and should be followed by an amiodarone infusion. *Paroxysmal AF associated with critical illness can also often be controlled with amiodarone.*

It should be remembered that if AF or atrial flutter have been present for more than a few hours, restoration of sinus rhythm occasionally results in arterial embolization.

SINUS TACHYCARDIA

Sinus tachycardia is nearly always a secondary phenomenon related to one or more of the following:

- hypovolaemia;
- pyrexia;
- hypoxaemia;
- hypercarbia;
- anaemia;
- pain;
- anxiety.

These abnormalities must be identified and, when possible, corrected. Specific treatment is therefore not usually required, and because a reduction in heart rate may be associated with a fall in cardiac output, it can actually be deleterious.

Bradycardia

Bradycardia is defined as a heart rate of less than 60 beats/min, although it may be more helpful to classify bradycardias as absolute or relative. The former can be defined as a heart rate less than 40 beats/min and the latter as a heart rate which is inappropriately slow for the individual patient's clinical condition.

A pathological bradycardia may be the result of conducting system disease, inferior MI or both. Bradycardia may be exacerbated by β-blockade, calcium channel blockers and other depressant agents. In acute ischaemic syndromes a modest bradycardia is advantageous in reducing myocardial oxygen consumption, but more serious slowing predisposes to arrhythmias and reduces cardiac output. The management of bradycardia is outlined in **Figure 9.12.** *Therapeutic cardiac pacing* will be required in any patient with sustained symptomatic or haemodynamically compromising bradycardia (**Table 9.6**).

Profound bradycardia and asystole may also follow severe hypoxia or hypothermia or the massive parasympathetic outflow of facial injury or near-drowning. Treatment in these cases should initially be directed at the underlying pathology.

SINUS BRADYCARDIA

As heart rate falls, cardiac output is maintained by an increase in stroke volume, due largely to a rise in end-diastolic volume. If this compensatory mechanism fails, blood pressure falls, ventricular filling pressures rise and coronary perfusion is jeopardized. Sometimes nodal or ventricular 'escape' rhythms are seen. The heart rate should be increased, initially by administering *atropine* intravenously.

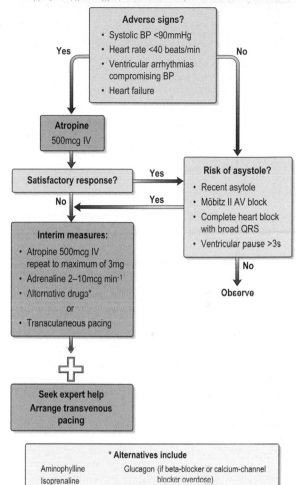

Fig. 9.12 Bradycardia algorithm (doses based on adult of average body weight). AV, atrioventricular; BP, blood pressure. (Originally published at www.resus.org.uk.)

In persistent cases, repeated administration of atropine up to a maximum of 3 mg may be required. Supplies of isoprenaline are limited by difficulties in obtaining the raw material. An alternative in those resistant to atropine is to give a continuous intravenous infusion of adrenaline in a dose of 2–10 μg/min. Other alternatives include dobutamine, dopamine and aminophylline. Intravenous glucagon should be considered if beta-blockers or calcium channel blockers are a possible cause of bradycardia. *Transcutaneous (external) pacing* may also sometimes be required until transvenous pacing can be established. Provided there is no abnormality of AV conduction, transvenous *atrial pacing* is occasionally effective, but a temporary ventricular electrode should also be inserted in case the atrial system fails or an AV conduction abnormality supervenes. As well as pro-

Table 9.6 Common pacing modes

AOO	Fixed-rate atrial pacing (useful in atrial standstill)
VOO	Fixed-rate ventricular pacing (useful in emergencies if ventricular sensing proves unreliable)
AAI	Senses low atrial rates and triggers atrial pacing (useful in sick sinus syndrome)
VVI	Ventricular sensing over a set rate inhibits ventricular pacing
VDD	'Atrial tracking' where atrial sensing triggers a ventricular pacing spike (used in complete heart block with normal sinus node activity)
DVI	Physical atrioventricular sequential pacing if ventricular rate slows below a threshold. Lack of atrial sensing makes it useful only if the pacing rate is greater than the atrial rate; therefore DDD or AAI modes may be more appropriate
DDD	Atrioventricular sequential pacing if intrinsic rate slows below a set threshold

The various combinations of chamber sensing and pacing interactions have been coded using five symbols.
Chambers paced and sensed (0, none; A, atrium; V, ventricle; D, atrium and ventricle).
Response to sensing (0, none; T, triggered; I, inhibited; D, triggered and inhibited).

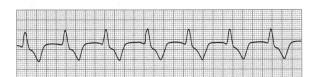

Fig. 9.13 Idioventricular rhythm associated with inferior myocardial infarction.

ducing haemodynamic improvement, increasing the heart rate may abolish escape rhythms.

IDIOVENTRICULAR RHYTHM

A reduction in the sinus rate, sinus arrest or sinoatrial block may be associated with an idioventricular escape rhythm (**Fig. 9.13**). Often, the ventricular rate is increased above the expected 40–60 beats/min by the effects of the underlying disease (e.g. an MI). This rhythm can be benign, but if associated with a haemodynamic disturbance, can usually be abolished by increasing the sinus rate.

DISTURBANCES OF CONDUCTION

First-degree AV block (Fig. 9.14). This is generally benign, but may progress to second-degree block, in which case the Wenckebach phenomenon (Mobitz type I) usually develops.

Second-degree AV block – Mobitz type I (Wenckebach) (Fig. 9.15). This is commonly associated with an inferior MI and is almost always self-limiting. The Wenckebach phenome-

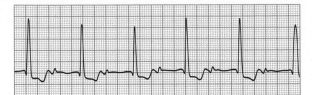

Fig. 9.14 First-degree atrioventricular block.

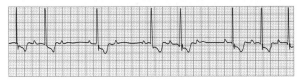

Fig. 9.15 Second-degree atrioventricular block: Mobitz type I.

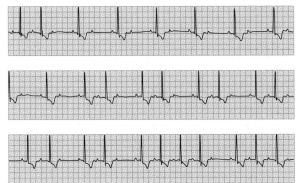

Fig. 9.16 Second-degree atrioventricular block: Mobitz type II.

non does not usually therefore require treatment, although if a 2:1 cycle develops it may be associated with haemodynamic deterioration.

Mobitz type II (Fig. 9.16). This infranodal conduction disorder often progresses to complete heart block; some authorities therefore recommend prophylactic insertion of a temporary transvenous pacing wire.

Third-degree AV block (Fig. 9.17). When associated with inferior MI, this is caused by ischaemia of the AV node and the conduction disturbance is usually transient. When complete heart block accompanies anterior MI, however, it is indicative of a large infarct sufficient to damage the His–Purkinje system. This implies a poor prognosis.

Treatment involves the administration of drugs to increase the ventricular rate (e.g. *atropine*, if the ventricular complexes are narrow, or *adrenaline*), followed by insertion of a temporary transvenous wire. β-stimulants should only be used if the patient is hypotensive since they may increase infarct size and precipitate arrhythmias.

Fascicular block. Prophylactic pacemaker insertion has been recommended for patients with right bundle branch block

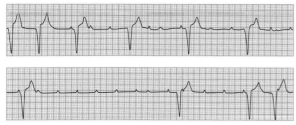

Fig. 9.17 Third-degree atrioventricular block.

and left anterior or posterior hemiblock, as well as for those with bifascicular block and a prolonged P-R interval. This is most often indicated in the context of evolving acute MI.

In patients with impaired ventricular function, the loss of atrial transport may be poorly tolerated and in these cases *AV sequential pacing* may produce haemodynamic improvement.

REFERENCES

Ammann P, Pfisterer M, Fehr T, *et al.* (2004) Raised cardiac troponins. *British Medical Journal* **328**: 1028–1029.

Andrews K (1993) Recovery of patients after four months or more in the persistent vegetative state. *British Medical Journal* **306**: 1597–1600.

Aronson JK (1985) Cardiac arrhythmias: theory and practice. *British Medical Journal* **290**: 487–488.

Aung K, Htay T (2005) Vasopressin for cardiac arrest. A systematic review and meta-analysis *Archives of Internal Medicine* **165**: 17–24.

Bernard SA, Gray TW, Buist MD, *et al.* (2002) Treatment of comatose survivors of out-of-hospital cardiac arrest with induced hypothermia *New England Journal of Medicine* **346**: 557–563.

Bertrand ME, Simoons ML, Fox K, *et al.* (2002) Management of acute coronary syndromes in patients presenting without persistent ST-segment elevation. *European Heart Journal* **23**: 1809–1840.

Bircher N, Safar P (1984) Manual open-chest cardiopulmonary resuscitation. *Annals of Emergency Medicine* **13**: 770–773.

Booth CM, Boone RH, Tomlinson G, *et al.* (2004) Is this patient dead, vegetative or severely neurologically impaired? Assessing outcome for comatose survivors of cardiac arrest. *Journal of the American Medical Association* **291**: 870–879.

Böttiger BW, Bode C, Kern S, *et al.* (2001) Efficacy and safety of thrombolytic therapy after initially unsuccessful cardiopulmonary resuscitation: a prospective clinical trial. *Lancet* **357**: 1583–1585.

Brain Resuscitation Clinical Trial I Study Group (1986) Randomized clinical study of thiopental loading in comatose survivors of cardiac arrest. *New England Journal of Medicine* **314**: 397–403.

Brain Resuscitation Clinical Trial II Study Group (1991) A randomized clinical study of a calcium-entry blocker (lidoflazine) in the treatment of comatosed survivors of cardiac arrest. *New England Journal of Medicine* **324**: 1225–1231.

British Medical Association (BMA), The Resuscitation Council (UK) and the Royal College of Nursing (RCN) (2001) Decisions relating to cardiopulmonary resuscitation: a joint statement. Available online at: http://www.bma.org.uk/publications/nsf.

Buist MD, Moore GE, Bernard SA, *et al.* (2002) Effects of a medical emergency team on reduction of incidence of an mortality from unexpected cardiac arrests in hospital: preliminary study. *British Medical Journal* **324**: 387–390.

Bur A, Kittler H, Sterz F, *et al.* (2001) Effect of bystander first aid, defibrillation and advanced life support on neurologic outcome and hospital costs in patients after ventricular fibrillation cardiac arrest. *Intensive Care Medicine* **27**: 1474–1480.

Chen Z (2005) COMMIT/CCS-2: Clopidogrel and metoprolol in myocardial infarction trial/ second Chinese cardiac study – the clopidogrel arm. Available online at: http://www.medscape.com/viewarticle/501637.

Chesebro JH, Knatterud G, Roberts R, *et al.* (1987) Thrombolysis in myocardial infarction (TIMI) Trial phase I: a comparison between intravenous tissue plasminogen activator and intravenous streptokinase. Clinical findings through hospital discharge. *Circulation* **76**: 142–154.

Cohen TJ, Goldner BG, Maccaro PC, *et al.* (1993) A comparison of active compression–decompression cardiopulmonary resuscitation with standard cardiopulmonary resuscitation for cardiac arrests occurring in the hospital. *New England Journal of Medicine* **329**: 1918–1921.

Davey MJ, Teubner D (2005) A randomized controlled trial of magnesium sulfate, in addition to usual care, for rate control in atrial fibrillation. *Annals of Emergency Medicine* **45**: 347–353.

Delacretaz E (2006) Supraventricular tachycardia. *New England Journal of Medicine* **354**: 1039–1051.

Fernandez-Aviles F, Alonso JJ, Castro-Beiras A, *et al.* (2004) Routine invasive strategy within 24 hours of thrombolysis versus ischaemia-guided conservative approach for acute myocardial infarction with ST-segment elevation (GRACIA-1): a randomised controlled trial. *Lancet* **364**: 1045–1053.

Fibrinolytic Therapy Trialists' Collaborative Group (1994) Indications for fibrinolytic therapy in suspected acute myocardial infarction: collaborative overview of early mortality and major morbidity results from all randomised trials of more than 1000 patients. *Lancet* **343**: 311–322.

Fromm RE Jr, Weltge A, Varon J (2002) Public use of automatic defibrillators: a bolt from the blue. *Lancet* **360**: 1712.

Garratt CJ, Malcolm AD, Camm AJ (1992) Adenosine and cardiac arrhythmias. The preferred treatment for supraventricular tachycardia. *British Medical Journal* **305**: 3–4.

Glaeser PW, Hellmich TR, Szewczuga D, et al. (1993) Five year experience in prehospital intraosseous infusions in children and adults. *Annals of Emergency Medicine* **22**: 1119–1124.

Goldhill DR, Worthington L, Mulcahy A, *et al.* (1999) The patient-at-risk team: identifying

and managing seriously ill ward patients. *Anaesthesia* **54**: 853–860.

GUSTO Angiographic Investigators (1993) The effects of tissue plasminogen activator, streptokinase or both on coronary-artery patency, ventricular function and survival after acute myocardial infarction. *New England Journal of Medicine* **329**: 1615–1622.

Hallstrom AP, Ornato JP, Weisfeldt M, *et al.* (2004) Public-access defibrillation and survival after out-of-hospital cardiac arrest. *New England Journal of Medicine* **351**: 637–646.

Halperin HR, Tsitlik JE, Gelfand M, *et al.* (1993) A preliminary study of cardiopulmonary resuscitation by circumferential compression of the chest with use of a pneumatic vest. *New England Journal of Medicine* **329**: 762–768.

Higgins D, Hayes M, Denman W, *et al.* (1990) Effectiveness of using end tidal carbon dioxide concentration to monitor cardiopulmonary resuscitation. *British Medical Journal* **300**: 581.

Ho DS, Zecchin RP, Richards DA, *et al.* (1994) Double-blind trial of lignocaine versus sotalol for acute termination of spontaneous sustained ventricular tachycardia. *Lancet* **344**: 18–23.

Hypothermia After Cardiac Arrest Study Group (2002) Mild therapeutic hypothermia to improve the neurologic outcome after cardiac arrest. *New England Journal of Medicine* **346**: 549–556.

Keeley EC, Boura JA, Grines CL (2003) Primary angioplasty versus intravenous thrombolytic therapy for acute myocardial infarction: a quantitative review of 23 randomised trials. *Lancet* **361**: 13–20.

Kirchhof P, Eckardt L, Loh P, *et al.* (2002) Anterior-posterior versus anterior-lateral electrode positions for external cardioversion of atrial fibrillation: a randomised trial. *Lancet* **360**: 1275–1279.

Kitakaze M, Asakura M, Kim J, *et al.* and the J-WIND investigators (2007) Human atrial natriuretic peptide and nicorandil as adjuncts to reperfusion treatment for acute myocardial infarction (J-WIND): two randomised trials. *Lancet* **370**: 1483–1493.

Kudenchuk PJ, Cobb LA, Copass MK, *et al.* (1999) Amiodarone for resuscitation after out-of-hospital cardiac arrest due to ventricular fibrillation. *New England Journal of Medicine* **341**: 871–878.

Laarman GJ, Suttorp MJ, Dirksen MT, *et al.* (2006) Paclitaxel-eluting versus uncoated stents in primary percutaneous coronary intervention. *New England Journal of Medicine* **355**: 1105–1113.

Lagerqvist B, Husted S, Kontny F, *et al.* (2006) 5-year outcomes in the FRISC-II randomised trial of an invasive versus a non-invasive strategy in non-ST-elevation acute coronary syndrome: a follow-up study. *Lancet* **368**: 998–1004.

Levine RL, Wayne MA, Miller CC (1997) End-tidal carbon dioxide and outcome of out-of-hospital cardiac arrest. *New England Journal of Medicine* **337**: 301–306.

Liddle R, Davies CS, Colquhoun M, et al. (2003) The automated external defibrillator. *British Medical Journal* **327**: 1216–1218.

Lurie K, Voelckel W, Plaisance P, et al. (2000) Use of an inspiratory impedance threshold valve during cardiopulmonary resuscitation: a progress report. *Resuscitation* **44**: 219–230.

McCrirrick A, Monk CR (1994) Comparison of i.v. and intra-tracheal administration of adrenaline. *British Journal of Anaesthesia* **72**: 529–532.

Mair P, Furtwaengler W, Baubin M (1993) Aortic valve function during cardiopulmonary resuscitation. *New England Journal of Medicine* **329**: 1965–1966.

Mayr A, Knotzer H, Mutz N, et al. (1999) Atrial tachyarrhythmia after cardiac surgery. *Intensive Care Medicine* **25**: 242–243.

Oddo M, Schaller M-D, Feihl F, et al. (2006) From evidence to clinical practice: effective implementation of therapeutic hypothermia to improve patient outcome after cardiac arrest. *Critical Care Medicine* **34**: 1865–1873.

Packer M, Meller J, Medina N, et al. (1982) Hemodynamic consequences of combined beta-adrenergic and slow calcium channel blockade in man. *Circulation* **65**: 660–668.

Pulsinelli WA, Waldman S, Rawlinson D, et al. (1982) Moderate hyperglycemia augments ischemic brain damage: a neuropathologic study in the rat. *Neurology* **32**: 1239–1246.

Rudikoff MT, Maughan WL, Effron M, et al. (1980) Mechanisms of blood flow during cardiopulmonary resuscitation. *Circulation* **61**: 345–352.

Safar PJ, Kochanek PM (2002) Therapeutic hypothermia after cardiac arrest. *New England Journal of Medicine* **346**: 612–613.

Saltuari L, Marosi M (1994) Coma after cardiac arrest: will he recover all right? *Lancet* **343**: 1052–1053.

Sanai L, Armstrong IR, Grant IS (1993) Supraventricular tachy-dysrhythmias in the critically ill: a review of antidysrhythmic therapy in patients with SVT. *British Journal of Intensive Care* **3**: 358–364.

Sanders AB, Kern KB, Ewy GA, et al. (1984) Improved resuscitation from cardiac arrest with open-chest massage. *Annals of Emergency Medicine* **13**: 672–675.

SOS-KAMTO Study Group (2007) Cardiopulmonary resuscitation by bystanders with chest compression only (SOS-KAMTO): an observational study. *Lancet* **369**: 920–926.

Spaulding C, Henry P, Teiger E, et al. (2006) Sirolimus-eluting versus uncoated stents in acute myocardial infarction. *New England Journal of Medicine* **355**: 1093–1104.

Stiell IG, Hebert PC, Wells GA, et al. (1996) The Ontario trial of active compression-decompression cardiopulmonary resuscitation for in-hospital and prehospital cardiac arrest. *Journal of the American Medical Association* **275**: 1417–1423.

Stiell IG, Wells GA, Field B, et al. for the Ontario Prehospital Advanced Life Support Study Group (2004) Advanced cardiac life support in out-of-hospital cardiac arrest. *New England Journal of Medicine* **351**: 647–656.

Tunstall-Pedoe H, Bailey L, Chamberlain DA, et al. (1992) Survey of 3765 cardiopulmonary resuscitations in British hospitals (the BRESUS study): methods and overall results. *British Medical Journal* **304**: 1347–1351.

Van der Werf F, Ardissino D, Betriu A, et al. (2003) Management of acute myocardial infarction in patients presenting with ST segment elevation. *European Heart Journal* **24**: 28–66.

Vandycke C, Martens P (2000) High dose versus standard dose epinephrine in cardiac arrest – a meta-analysis. *Resuscitation* **45**: 161–166.

van Walraven C, Forster AJ, Parish DC, et al. (2001) Validation of a clinical decision aid to discontinue in-hospital cardiac arrest resuscitations. *Journal of the American Medical Association* **285**: 1602–1606.

Vincent JL (1987) Should we still administer calcium during cardiopulmonary resuscitation? *Intensive Care Medicine* **13**: 369–370.

Weil MH, Rackow EC, Trevino R, et al. (1986) Difference in acid–base state between venous and arterial blood during cardiopulmonary resuscitation. *New England Journal of Medicine* **315**: 153–156.

Yusuf S, Zhao F, Mehta SR, et al. (2001) Effects of clopidogrel in addition to aspirin in patients with acute coronary syndromes without ST-segment elevation. *New England Journal of Medicine* **345**: 494–502.

Zijlstra F, de Boer MJ, Hoorntje JC, et al. (1993) A comparison of immediate coronary angioplasty with intravenous streptokinase in acute myocardial infarction. *New England Journal of Medicine* **328**: 680–684.

10 Trauma

Trauma is the leading cause of death in people aged between 1 and 35 years in the developed world. Road traffic crashes (RTCs) still account for the majority of these trauma deaths. Death following civilian trauma has been described as having a trimodal distribution (Trunkey, 1983):

- The *first peak* comprises individuals who die within 30 minutes of the event, in these cases death being due to injuries which are so complex and severe that survival is almost certainly impossible within the constraints of current knowledge and expertise. Typical examples would be deaths resulting from major cerebral or brainstem lacerations or massive vascular disruption within the thorax.
- The *second peak*, occurs within 4 hours of injury. These deaths are characterized by major losses of circulating blood volume, are often associated with severe head injuries and are frequently compounded by a failure to provide and maintain an adequate airway and ventilation.
- The *third peak*, accounting for the remaining 20% of trauma deaths, includes those patients who die days or weeks following trauma. This is commonly a result of multiple-organ failure and sepsis, or pulmonary embolism (see Chapter 5). There is evidence that with rapid resuscitation and competent early surgical intervention this third peak of mortality can be significantly reduced.

The principles of respiratory support are discussed in Chapter 7, the management of shock in Chapter 5, and head trauma in Chapter 15.

ADVANCED TRAUMA LIFE SUPPORT AND TRAUMA RESUSCITATION

Three fundamental principles underpinned the development of the Advanced Trauma Life Support (ATLS) programme by the American College of Surgeons.

1. The greatest threat to life should be treated first.
2. The lack of a definitive diagnosis should not hinder the application of an indicated treatment.

3. A detailed history is not an essential prerequisite for the evaluation of an acutely injured patient.

The result was the development of the ABCs (airway, breathing and circulation) approach to the assessment and treatment of trauma victims.

The ATLS programme emphasizes that life-threatening injuries kill and maim in certain reproducible timeframes. Obstruction of the airway kills more quickly than impaired respiration, and the latter is more rapidly lethal than loss of the circulating volume. An expanding intracranial mass lesion is the next most dangerous problem. The letters 'ABCDE' define a specific, ordered, prioritized sequence of evaluations and treatments, which should be followed in injured patients. Judgement is required, however, to determine which procedures are necessary in a particular patient (Pepe, 2003). ATLS provides one acceptable method for the safe, immediate management of trauma (Coats and Davies, 2002; Driscoll and Skinner, 2000a, b; Trunkey, 1991) (**Table 10.1**).

A: AIRWAY WITH CERVICAL SPINE CONTROL
(Watson, 2000)

All severely injured patients are to a greater or lesser extent hypoxaemic. Immediate administration of supplementary *oxygen* to the *unobstructed airway* is of paramount importance. Simultaneously the *neck* must at all times be kept *immobilized* without traction (for example, using a spine board, sandbags and a hard collar or manual in-line immobilization) until the possibility of neck injury is excluded. The only exception is the restless and thrashing patient where suboptimal immobilization with a semirigid collar is preferred to risking spinal cord damage caused by excessive and unrestrained body movement with the head and neck immobile.

In an unconscious patient, foreign bodies obstructing the airway must be removed under direct vision. The laryngeal and pharyngeal reflexes should then be assessed and respiratory performance evaluated. If protective reflexes are adequate, retracting the tongue forward by employing the chin lift/jaw thrust manoeuvre or by inserting an *oropharyngeal* or *nasopharyngeal airway* may suffice. The role of the laryngeal mask airway (LMA) in the resuscitation of the injured patient has not been clearly defined. When a patient arrives in the emergency department with an LMA in place it must be decided whether removal or replacement with a definitive airway is indicated. If the reflexes are depressed or absent (i.e. there is no gag reflex when oropharyngeal suction is attempted) the airway must be secured at the earliest opportunity by intubation with an appropriately sized *endotracheal tube*. Many patients will require bag-mask ventilation with oxygen before intubation is attempted. During these manoeuvres the neck should be kept immobilized (**Fig. 10.1**) (Criswell *et al.*, 1994).

A large-bore *gastric tube* should also be passed. Nasal passage of a gastric tube is contraindicated in patients with suspected basal skull fractures or injury to the soft palate.

Tracheostomy is rarely necessary as an emergency procedure. Severe distorting injury to the structures above or at the level of the larynx can render endotracheal intubation impossible, but *cricothyroidotomy* is preferred to emergency tracheostomy in such circumstances (see Chapter 7).

B: BREATHING (Rooney *et al.*, 2000)

Hypoxic patients can often decompensate rapidly and unpredictably. Once a secure airway has been established adequate ventilation must be ensured, although it is important to remember that positive-pressure ventilation may precipitate circulatory collapse, especially if the patient is hypovolaemic. Moreover raised intrathoracic pressure during positive-pressure ventilation is associated with an increased risk of pneumothorax in patients with chest injuries and may induce tension in existing pneumothoraces. This complication must be anticipated and chest drains should be inserted in all patients with a pneumothorax who require positive-pressure ventilation (see Chapter 7). Because hypercapnia and hypoxia from asphyxia or inadequate ventilation can cause considerable deterioration in cerebral function, especially when combined with fluctuations in arterial blood pressure, mechanical ventilation must always be considered when there is coincidental head injury, even in those without overt respiratory failure (see Chapter 15).

Six life-threatening injuries may be identified in relation to the airway and breathing.

1. airway obstruction;
2. tension pneumothorax;
3. open pneumothorax (sucking chest wound) caused by a large defect of the chest wall;
4. massive haemothorax;
5. flail chest;
6. cardiac tamponade.

A further *six 'hidden' potentially lethal chest injuries* may be identified in a secondary examination after primary resuscitation.

1. pulmonary contusion;
2. myocardial contusion;
3. aortic disruption;
4. traumatic diaphragmatic rupture;
5. tracheobronchial disruption;
6. oesophageal disruption.

C: CIRCULATION

The classical sign of shock, namely hypotension, is not observed in previously fit young patients until they have lost 30% or more of their circulating volume (**Tables 10.2 and 10.3**). Intravenous *volume replacement* should ideally be instituted before blood pressure falls to minimize the duration of tissue ischaemia and reduce the risk of subsequent multiple-organ dysfunction (see Chapter 5). If the signs of shock do not rapidly improve, blood transfusion will be required and a surgical opinion must be obtained. The possibility of concealed intra-abdominal bleeding should be considered (Cope and Stebbings, 2000), while major thoracic injuries may require immediate thoracotomy.

In contrast to traditional teaching there is some controversial evidence to suggest that in hypotensive patients with penetrating torso injuries outcome is improved if aggressive

Table 10.1 Immediate management of trauma	
A	Airway with cervical spine control
B	Breathing
C	Circulation with haemorrhage control
D	Disability or neurological status
E	Exposure (undress) with temperature control

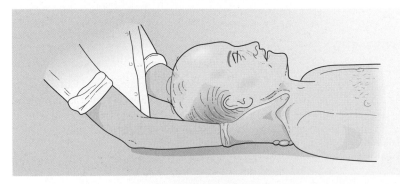

Fig. 10.1 Manual immobilization of the neck.

Table 10.2 Classification of severity of haemorrhage in previously fit young patients	
Class 1	Loss of up to 15% of the circulating volume (up to 750 mL in a 70-kg patient) No change in vital signs
Class 2	Loss of 15–30% (up to 1500 mL) of circulating volume Fall in pulse pressure Sweating, restless patient with moderate tachycardia, tachypnoea
Class 3	Loss of 30–40% (up to 2000 mL) of circulating volume Marked tachycardia (> 120 beats/min) and tachypnoea (> 20 breaths/min) Systolic blood pressure falls to 90 mmHg Patient very restless, agitated, sweating
Class 4	Loss of greater than 40% (> 2000 mL) of circulating volume Patient is drowsy, the pulse is thready and tachycardia (> 140 beats/min) or preterminal, bradycardia may be present Tachypnoea (> 35 breaths/min) The blood pressure is less than 90 mmHg and may be unrecordable by non-invasive means

fluid resuscitation is delayed until operative intervention (Bickell *et al.*, 1994). It is suggested that fluids given before surgery may accentuate ongoing bleeding or disrupt effective blood clots, leading to fatal secondary haemorrhage. Bleeding may be further exacerbated by dilution of coagulation factors and a reduction in viscosity. The application of this approach to patients with polytrauma is, however, difficult and contentious; a selective approach to treatment based on the judgement of an experienced, discerning and knowledgeable clinician has been advocated (Pepe, 2003).

Although coagulopathy following major trauma is conventionally considered to be due to activation and consumption of coagulation factors, there is evidence to suggest that early coagulopathy is triggered by tissue hypoperfusion, which in turn activates protein C, causing systemic anticoagulation (Brohi *et al.*, 2007). In patients with severe, uncontrollable bleeding unresponsive to conventional measures, consideration should be given to the administration of factor VIIa (Spahn *et al.*, 2005).

D: DISABILITY OR NEUROLOGICAL STATUS
(Bullock *et al.*, 2000)
The patient's *conscious level* should be recorded using the Glasgow Coma Scale. The *pupillary response to light* must also be examined. Any deterioration in consciousness should prompt re-evaluation of airway control, adequacy of ventilation, oxygenation and volume replacement.

F: EXPOSURE AND CONTROL OF THE ENVIRONMENT
The patient should be completely undressed to allow a thorough examination and assessment, but it is imperative to *prevent hypothermia*. Warm blankets are useful, intravenous fluids should be warmed and a warm environment should be maintained.

Although *limb injuries* are not generally immediately lethal in themselves (Rossiter *et al.*, 2000b), except when associated with life-threatening haemorrhage, it is particularly important to identify those injuries that may threaten the survival of a limb, as well as fractures, the acute management of which may influence overall mortality and morbidity. *Compartment syndrome*, *crush syndrome* and *fat embolism syndrome (FES)* can all cause multiple-organ dysfunction in the early postinjury phase.

At the earliest opportunity following the immediate resuscitative procedures the patient's *back and perineum must be carefully inspected*. This will usually involve logrolling the patient, during which it is important to maintain in-line cervical spine immobilization. While the patient is on his or her side the spine should be palpated along its entire length for tenderness and any 'gaps' indicating spinal injury. The anal reflex should be observed and sensation in the perineum tested and recorded (see Spinal injuries, below). In males, *rectal examination* will identify the position of the prostate, which may be displaced upwards or feel *boggy* in those with urethral injury. Rectal examination will also detect blood in the rectum, indicating bowel injury.

RE-EVALUATION
The secondary survey, a head-to-toe examination, should not begin until the primary survey has been completed and the adequacy of initial resuscitation has been re-evaluated by repeated assessments of the patient's vital signs.

RADIOLOGICAL ASSESSMENT
Although radiological investigations have an important role in the initial management of trauma patients, it is important not to allow these procedures to compromise treatment and continued monitoring of the patient. In those with a head injury, however, a computed tomography (CT) head scan may be performed in spite of unstable vital signs to confirm the need for neurosurgical intervention, since under these circumstances stabilization is often impossible until the intracranial haematoma has been evacuated.

Three radiographs are of prime importance in patients who have been subjected to blunt trauma:

1. *The chest radiograph*: it is important to appreciate that pneumo- or haemothorax and widening of the mediastinum are less easily detected on supine, anteroposterior chest radiographs.
2. *A lateral cervical spine* film: this must include the base of the skull and all vertebrae from C1 to T1.

3. *Pelvic radiograph*: in particular the sacroiliac regions must be closely inspected as major disruptions can lead to significant concealed haemorrhage.

Further radiographs, particularly of the limbs, should not be performed until cardiovascular stability has been achieved. A *lateral skull film* and a *lateral view of the thoracolumbar spine* may then be obtained (Rankine *et al.*, 2000).

OTHER INVESTIGATIONS

Once intravenous access has been established, blood should be taken immediately for cross-matching, full blood count, haematocrit, and urea and electrolyte estimation. Regular and repeated estimations of blood lactate values, coagulation, arterial blood gas tensions and acid–base state should be performed, particularly if the admission values are abnormal and following any intervention involving the airway or ventilation.

Imaging techniques such as focused assessment sonography in trauma (FAST) scanning and CT should be used after initial stabilization and when there is no indication for immediate surgery. The position of diagnostic peritoneal lavage may be downgraded in centres with rapid access to spiral CT.

Diagnostic peritoneal lavage

Peritoneal lavage may help decide which patients subsequently require surgical assessment by laparotomy. The technique should be considered in the following categories of patient:

- patients in whom blunt or penetrating intra-abdominal injury is suspected and in whom clinical examination is difficult or impossible because of altered consciousness (e.g. due to head injury or substance abuse);
- multiple-trauma patients who require general anaesthesia for other injuries, or those already intubated and sedated/paralysed;
- trauma patients with unexplained hypotension or those with equivocal findings on clinical examination of the abdomen, lower chest or pelvis.

Peritoneal lavage involves the aseptic insertion of a dialysis catheter into the peritoneal cavity at a point one-third of the distance from the umbilicus to the symphysis pubis in the midline. If gross blood or enteric contents are not aspirated then 10 mL/kg body weight of warmed Ringer's lactate/0.9% saline (up to 1 litre) is instilled into the peritoneum through intravenous tubing attached to the dialysis catheter. If peritoneal lavage fluid drains via a chest tube or an indwelling urinary catheter, or if the fluid is heavily blood-stained, urgent laparotomy is indicated. Otherwise lavage fluid should be drained off by gravity and after 5 minutes a sample should be sent to the laboratory for an erythrocyte count. More than 100 000 erythrocytes/mL indicate a positive result and the need for exploratory laparotomy. Diagnostic peritoneal lavage, if undertaken, should be performed by the general surgeon who will be responsible for any subsequent laparotomy.

CHEST INJURIES (Tai and Boffard, 2003)

In Europe and Australasia, most cases of chest trauma involve *non-penetrating* injuries, usually as a result of RTCs. *Penetrating* injuries caused by knife or gunshot wounds are also seen, but are more common in the USA and South Africa.

Fewer than 15% of patients with chest injuries require surgical intervention. Multiple rib fractures with pulmonary contusion, haemothorax or pneumothorax can usually be dealt with simply and effectively by insertion of a chest drain, administration of analgesics, judicious fluid resuscitation and physiotherapy. When ignored, underestimated or inadequately treated, however, such injuries may ultimately prove fatal. The necessity for surgical intervention is based on the rate of bleeding or leakage of air from the intercostal drain. If 1500 mL of blood is immediately evacuated or the hourly drainage exceeds 200 mL for 4 hours or more, then it is highly likely the patient will require early thoracotomy, as will those with continued haemodynamic instability. It is important to appreciate that if the drain is incorrectly sited or becomes blocked, the severity of haemorrhage may not be appreciated. Chest drains should never be clamped in an attempt to tamponade bleeding. Other indications for thoracotomy include:

- cardiac tamponade;
- transmediastinal missile track;
- injury to the major airways or oesophagus.

Patients who have suffered traversing wounds of the mediastinum must be evaluated to exclude the possibility of tracheobronchial, oesophageal or vascular injury even if there are no clinical or chest X-ray signs of damage to mediastinal structures and the patient is haemodynamically stable. Chest drain insertion is performed as required and if no immediate surgical intervention is indicated, contrast-enhanced helical CT or angiography should be performed. If these investigations are negative, water-soluble contrast oesophagography can be undertaken, with consideration to subsequent oesophagoscopy and bronchoscopy.

SPECIFIC INJURIES
Lungs and airways

Tears or *punctures* of lung tissue, often involving small airways, are relatively common following penetrating injuries and chest wall trauma with rib fractures. They are associated with pneumo- or haemopneumothoraces, and the presence of surgical emphysema will often alert the clinician to the diagnosis. *Rupture of a large bronchus* may cause:

- haemoptysis;
- complete atelectasis of the affected lung;

Table 10.3 Immediate effects of blasts and explosions

Primary – direct effects (e.g. overpressurization and underpressurization)

Pulmonary damage

Rupture of tympanic membranes

Rupture of hollow viscera

Secondary

Penetrating trauma

Fragmentation injuries

Tertiary – effects of structure collapse and of persons being thrown by the blast wind

Crush injuries and blunt trauma

Penetrating trauma

Fractures and traumatic amputations

Open or closed brain injuries

Quaternary – burns, asphyxia and exposure to toxic substances

- mediastinal emphysema,
- persisting pneumothorax and air leak.

Less commonly, the *trachea* itself may be either partially or totally *disrupted*. If there is a wide separation of the two ends, the patient usually dies rapidly from asphyxia. Lesser degrees of separation are, however, compatible with survival. Stridor, hoarseness, persistent cough with or without haemoptysis and subcutaneous emphysema suggest injury to the proximal trachea. More distal injuries are associated with subcutaneous emphysema and pneumomediastinum. In such cases respiratory distress may be insignificant unless the tear is large. In some cases the injury is not recognized until some time later when the patient may present with recurrent pneumonia or atelectasis.

Lung contusion may be diffuse and bilateral (e.g. following a blast injury: **Table 10.3**) (DePalma *et al.*, 2005; Rossiter *et al.*, 2000a), or relatively localized (e.g. underlying a limited area of blunt chest wall trauma). Pulmonary contusion may also follow a high-energy transfer missile injury. Occasionally, an *isolated intrapulmonary haematoma* is seen. Severe respiratory failure usually ensues in those with extensive contusion, especially when associated with chest wall instability, and in those who develop acute respiratory distress syndrome, but oedema formation and chest radiograph changes are often delayed for about 24 hours. Patients with pulmonary contusion are also prone to the later development of pneumonia.

MANAGEMENT

Although, in those breathing spontaneously, a small *pneumothorax* can be allowed to resolve spontaneously (provided it is not enlarging and not compromising respiratory func-

tion), larger collections of air, haemopneumothoraces, sucking chest wounds and those under tension will require insertion of an underwater seal drain. If a patient with a tension pneumothorax is haemodynamically unstable, immediate needle decompression via the second intercostal space in the midclavicular line is indicated. A conventional chest drain can be inserted later. A chest drain should always be inserted when a patient with a pneumothorax requires mechanical ventilation. Some authorities recommend prophylactic insertion of chest drains in those with multiple rib fractures who need mechanical ventilation, even in the absence of a pneumothorax. This practice is, however, associated with a risk of damaging the underlying lung. It may be preferable simply to be alert to the possibility of this complication and to have the facilities for immediate chest drain insertion available at the bedside.

In order to ensure satisfactory drainage of blood and fluid, the drain should be inserted through the fourth or fifth intercostal space just anterior to the mid-axillary line (see Chapter 7). If the pneumothorax fails to re-expand, and the air leak persists, it may be necessary to apply a negative pressure (e.g. −5 cm H_2O) using a high-volume, low-pressure suction device. Chest drains can be removed when:

- there is no air leak;
- there is only a small 'swing' of the tubing air–fluid level;
- there is less than 100 mL drainage in 24 hours;
- the lung has re-expanded.

Patients with a persistent pneumothorax associated with a large air leak may require surgical repair or resection of the damaged lung. Broad-spectrum antibiotics should be administered for 24 hours following chest drain insertion (Tai and Boffard, 2003).

Intubation of patients with suspected tracheal disruption should be performed using fibreoptic bronchoscopic guidance, with a competent surgeon standing by to perform emergency tracheostomy if needed. Once the airway has been secured, the patient has been stabilized and other injuries have been addressed, the tracheal injury can be repaired surgically. Distal injuries also require bronchoscopy to define the lesion. Smaller injuries can be managed conservatively whereas larger lesions will require operative repair.

As with other causes of non-cardiogenic pulmonary oedema, treatment of *lung contusion* consists of:

- supplemental oxygen;
- continuous positive airway pressure (CPAP), non-invasive ventilation or controlled ventilation with positive end-expiratory pressure (PEEP) (see Chapter 7);
- judicious fluid therapy;
- diuretics for overhydration.

Prophylactic antibiotics should not be used, except possibly in those with pre-existing chronic obstructive pulmonary disease (COPD). In the past some authorities suggested that corticosteroids might limit the degree of pulmonary

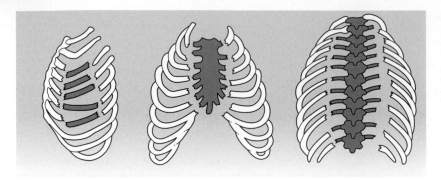

Fig. 10.2 Types of flail chest. A lateral injury is the most common. Anterior injuries are caused by frontal impact and may be associated with damage to the heart. Posterior injuries are unusual and strong muscular support prevents serious paradoxical movement. From Webb (1978), with permission.

abnormality (Trinkle *et al.*, 1975), particularly in those with blast injuries, but this is not currently recommended.

Chest wall

Major chest wall injuries produce instability of the thoracic cage and lung contusion.

If several ribs are fractured in more than one place, or if broken ribs are combined with fracture dislocations of the costochondral junctions or sternum, the negative intrapleural pressure generated on inspiration causes the isolated segment of chest wall to collapse inwards (*flail segment*), compromising ventilation. There is usually an associated haemopneumothorax. These mechanical problems, exacerbated by severe pain, can cause significant hypoventilation, as well as impairing the patient's ability to cough and maintain lung expansion. There is, then, a risk of atelectasis, sputum retention and secondary infection.

Flail segments can be classified according to their anatomical location (**Fig. 10.2**). An associated fractured clavicle exacerbates chest wall instability, and raises the possibility that ventilation may be further compromised by phrenic nerve injury. Sternal fractures can be particularly unstable.

Associated *pulmonary contusion* (see above) causes hypoxaemia and a progressive fall in lung compliance. The latter exacerbates chest wall instability; as lung compliance falls, increasingly negative intrapleural pressures are generated in order to sustain ventilation and the flail segment becomes progressively more obvious. Indeed, in some cases *paradoxical chest wall movement* is only noticed when lung mechanics have deteriorated 12–24 hours after the injury.

MANAGEMENT

The most appropriate management for a particular patient not only depends on the severity and nature of the chest injury, but is also influenced by the presence of pre-existing obesity or lung disease, the nature of any associated injuries and the patient's age.

Associated injuries to the head, face, abdomen or extremities can significantly complicate the management of chest trauma. In particular, comatose patients should always be intubated and ventilated, while painful laparotomy wounds can further embarrass ventilation. The prognosis following chest wall injury is significantly worse in:

- the obese;
- the elderly;
- those with pre-existing chronic lung disease;
- patients with pre-existing hypertension;
- those with myocardial ischaemia.

Patients with diseases such as ankylosing spondylitis that interfere with normal chest wall expansion will be particularly seriously compromised by chest wall injuries.

Following initial assessment and treatment, the patient must be closely observed for several days, since deterioration is almost inevitable over the first 24–48 hours. As well as *clinical evaluation* and *blood gas analyses*, serial measurements of *vital capacity* provide a useful means of assessing the patient's progress.

As a guide to the most appropriate management for a particular patient, chest injuries can be categorized into one of *three grades of severity*: minor, intermediate or severe.

Minor. These patients are able to maintain adequate alveolar ventilation and can cough. They may have a small flail segment, underlying pulmonary damage is minimal and there is no pre-existing lung disease. Associated trauma is limited to moderate peripheral injuries and there is no head or intra-abdominal injury.

Minor injuries can be treated with:

- oxygen;
- analgesia;
- careful fluid management to maintain euvolaemia;
- physiotherapy;
- early mobilization.

The success of this regimen depends on the provision of adequate analgesia. In some cases, *non-steroidal anti-inflammatory drugs (NSAIDs)* may be sufficient. Others will require *opiates* by continuous intravenous infusion or patient-controlled analgesia, perhaps combined with transcutaneous electrical nerve stimulation. *Intercostal blocks* may be useful, but they usually have to be repeated at approximately 12-hourly intervals. This may be facilitated by using a catheter technique. Premixed 50% nitrous oxide in oxygen (*Entonox*) can be used to provide supplementary analgesia during painful procedures.

Although this regimen is often referred to as 'conservative management', this is a misleading term since, to be successful, it requires a particularly active approach to all aspects of patient care and is very demanding of both the patient and staff. If possible, therefore, even patients with minor injuries should be admitted to a high-dependency or intensive care facility.

Intermediate. Although these patients can ventilate adequately, their ability to cough is seriously impaired. They may have an obvious flail segment and associated lung contusion. As compliance falls and intrapulmonary shunt increases, these patients can deteriorate significantly during the first 24–48 hours following injury. Patients with associated extensive limb injuries, a mild head injury, pre-existing lung disease, obesity or old age are also at risk.

Treatment consists of:

- supplemental oxygen;
- analgesia;
- physiotherapy;
- careful fluid management to maintain euvolaemia;
- early mobilization.

Some patients may also require *endotracheal intubation* or *tracheostomy* to protect their airway and control secretions. Pulmonary contusion should be treated as outlined above with avoidance of over-vigorous fluid resuscitation and diuretics if there is evidence of overhydration (see also Chapter 8).

It is especially important to control pain in this category of patient in order to permit coughing and effective physiotherapy (Karmakar and Ho, 2003). *Thoracic epidurals* are particularly effective and can increase functional residual capacity (FRC), compliance, vital capacity and P_aO_2, as well as decreasing paradoxical movement of the chest wall. *Intercostal blocks* are generally less satisfactory, but *opiates* can be effective if administered as a continuous intravenous infusion or as patient-controlled analgesia (PCA), and when combined with NSAIDs or paracetamol. Pleural analgesia via a chest drain or thoracic paravertebral blocks may also be effective.

Some have recommended the application of *CPAP by facemask* (see Chapter 7) for 20–30 minutes each hour in order to increase FRC (Dittmann *et al.*, 1982), although the efficacy of non-invasive ventilation in this situation has not been established. With this regimen, it may be possible to avoid mechanical ventilation, even in those with a large flail segment. This may, however, be at the expense of a degree of permanent chest wall deformity.

Severe. These patients have serious chest wall instability with extensive pulmonary contusion. They are extremely hypoxaemic, cannot cough and are often unable to sustain adequate alveolar ventilation. They rapidly become exhausted and require mechanical ventilation. Patients with associated visceral injuries requiring laparotomy and/or a severe head injury, as well as those with moderate chest injury, but who are elderly, obese or who have pre-existing lung disease, may also require ventilation. PEEP can be used to improve oxygenation (see Chapter 7). Although traditionally patients have been prevented from making spontaneous respiratory efforts because of concern that this could perpetuate chest wall instability, most now recommend the use of synchronized intermittent mandatory ventilation or one of the other spontaneously breathing modes of respiratory support, with the addition of PEEP. Patients with severe unilateral pulmonary abnormalities may occasionally require independent lung ventilation (see Chapter 7). An alternative is to nurse the patient in the lateral position with the damaged lung uppermost. This diverts pulmonary blood flow away from the damaged lung and limits preferential ventilation of the good lung. In those with a large and persistent air leak, high-frequency ventilation may prove useful (Chapter 7). Weaning should commence as soon as the lung lesion has resolved and can be facilitated by thoracic epidural analgesia. There is some evidence that internal fixation and stabilization of the chest wall reduce the length of stay in these patients. A selective approach, restricting, but not ignoring, surgical stabilization has been recommended (Galan *et al.*, 1992).

Although secondary chest infection is common, especially in the presence of lung contusion, *antibiotics* should be withheld until infection is obvious and preferably until the responsible organism has been identified, although some administer prophylactic antibiotics to those with pre-existing COPD.

Early mobilization is recommended, even for these severely injured patients.

Heart (Pretre and Chilcott, 1997)
PENETRATING INJURY

Surprisingly, a number of patients with penetrating cardiac injuries make a complete recovery, although high velocity gunshot wounds of the heart are invariably fatal.

In those who remain shocked despite apparently adequate volume replacement, with signs of cardiac tamponade (see Chapter 5), subxyphoid *pericardiocentesis* (**Fig. 10.3**) may help to stabilize the patient haemodynamically until the patient can undergo thoracotomy, pericardiotomy and attempted surgical repair. The pericardial sac can be aspirated using an intravenous cannula or continuously drained with a soft, flexible catheter. Improvement is often dramatic following removal of relatively small amounts of blood. Relief of tamponade may, however, simply encourage further haemorrhage and some patients may be more stable if a degree of cardiac compression is allowed to persist. In the more stable patient cardiac tamponade may be suspected when the chest X-ray reveals a globular cardiac shadow, the electrocardiogram (ECG) complexes are of low voltage and central venous pressure (CVP) measurements are high. The diagnosis may be confirmed by echocardiography, ultrasound of the pericardial sac as part of the FAST examination or direct examination via a pericardial window.

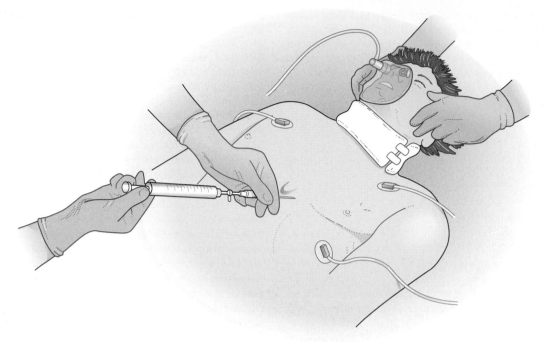

Fig. 10.3 Needle pericardiocentesis. With the patient supine, the skin is punctured slightly to the left of the xiphisternum and the cannula is directed upwards, backwards and to the left until the pericardial sac is entered. Electrocardiogram monitoring is essential in order to detect arrhythmias or myocardial injury.

If possible, emergency thoractomy or sternotomy should be performed by a competent cardiothoracic surgeon, because once the pericardium is opened, haemorrhage can be catastrophic and is most likely to be controlled quickly by those with experience of cardiac surgery. Ideally, the facilities for cardiopulmonary bypass should be available.

BLUNT INJURY

Myocardial contusion is a common, but often unrecognized, complication of non-penetrating chest injury. It is characterized by patchy areas of muscle necrosis and haemorrhagic infiltrate, usually predominantly involving the right ventricle. The diagnosis is suggested by ST-segment and T-wave changes or transient prolongation of the QT interval on serial ECGs, sinus tachycardia and arrhythmias. Elevated serum levels of creatine kinase-MB do not predict the likelihood of complications following blunt cardiac injury. Cardiac troponins may also be elevated although this finding is nonspecific. Clinically significant cardiac injury is unlikely when troponin levels are normal. *Echocardiography* is a useful technique for identifying or excluding structural cardiac damage and for assessing myocardial function in such cases (see Chapter 4).

Management is as for myocardial infarction. When contusion is severe, myocardial function may be significantly impaired, in which case cardiac output monitoring or, in selected patients, catheterization of the pulmonary artery may be indicated to guide volume replacement. Some patients will require inotropic support or, rarely, intra-aortic balloon counterpulsation.

Complications are common and may include sudden unexpected cardiac arrest, as well as supraventricular and ventricular arrhythmias. The prophylactic use of antiarrhythmics, however, remains controversial. *Cardiac rupture* may occur either at the time of impact or later as a delayed consequence of myocardial contusions. Intracardiac lesions, such as *disruption of a valve* or *rupture of the interventricular septum*, may also occur and are often fatal. These complications are, however, uncommon. Cardiac failure due to traumatic aortic or mitral insufficiency may develop within a few weeks, whereas tricuspid regurgitation may not present until several years have elapsed. *Intrapericardial haemorrhage* following blunt injuries originates from torn pericardial and epicardial vessels or, occasionally, small myocardial tears. If cardiac tamponade develops it should be relieved by pericardiocentesis. In some cases, bleeding will stop spontaneously while others will require surgical intervention.

PERICARDIUM

The pericardium may be torn by a blunt injury, usually in association with rupture of the diaphragm (see later in this chapter). More often, however, pericardial damage is the result of a penetrating injury. The main danger of a pericardial tear is that the heart may herniate through the defect, severely compromising cardiac function. If this happens, immediate surgery is indicated.

Aorta (Pretre and Chilcott, 1997)

The aorta can be disrupted, usually as a result of a rapid deceleration injury, at the junction between the fixed and mobile portions of the aortic arch (i.e. most frequently just distal to the origin of the left subclavian artery at the level of the ligamentum ateriosum). This is usually rapidly fatal in the elderly in whom the aorta is rigid, but young patients may suffer partial rupture and survive for long enough to be investigated and undergo definitive surgery. Disruption of the aorta just above the aortic valve may also occur, but is usually fatal.

DIAGNOSIS

The possibility of traumatic aortic disruption must be actively excluded in all patients with a history of a fall from a height or high-speed motor vehicle crash. Aortic rupture should be suspected when widening of the superior mediastinum, sometimes in association with some fluid in the pleural cavity, is seen on the chest radiograph of a patient who has suffered an injury compatible with this complication (Fig. 10.4). Other features suggestive of aortic rupture include depression of the left main bronchus, blurred outline of the arch or descending aorta, enlarged paratracheal stripe, fractured first rib or left apical haematoma and displacement of the mid-oesophagus to the right. The patient may complain of retrosternal or intrascapular pain, whilst pressure from a mediastinal haematoma may cause dysphagia, stridor or a hoarse voice. On examination, there may be a discrepancy between the blood pressure in each arm and femoral pulses may be diminished or absent, with upper-extremity hypertension. A harsh systolic murmur may be audible over the anterior or posterior chest wall.

The significance of mediastinal widening is, however, notoriously difficult to assess in trauma patients and *helical contrast-enhanced CT scanning* of the chest has now been shown to be an accurate diagnostic method for mediastinal haematoma and aortic rupture in haemodynamically stable patients with suspected blunt aortic injury. Should blunt aortic injury be detected, the extent of the injury can be defined by *aortography* (Fig. 10.4). Transoesophageal echocardiography can be performed rapidly and is a highly sensitive and specific method for detecting injury to the thoracic aorta (Smith *et al.*, 1995). Surgical treatment is by either primary repair of the aorta or resection of the injured segment and grafting. Surgical repair of aortic rupture should not be delayed beyond the time required to evaluate and treat other emergency conditions. The role of novel endovascular therapies in the treatment of traumatic aortic disruption has yet to be established.

Diaphragmatic rupture

Diaphragmatic rupture is rare and usually follows significant trauma to the truncal region. It may also be associated with acetabular fractures, when the force of the impact is transmitted along the length of the femur and through the abdomen. It is a relatively benign injury and may not be recognized until many years after the accident when the patient presents with abdominal contents within the left hemithorax, sometimes associated with bowel obstruction or strangulation. If the right hemidiaphragm is ruptured, the liver usually prevents herniation. Large ruptures may cause collapse of the ipsilateral lung with dyspnoea and reduced breath sounds. Imaging is often unhelpful and the diagnosis can only be established by laparascopy, video-assisted thoracoscopy or at laparotomy.

Oesophageal trauma

Oesophageal injuries are rare but should be considered in any patient who has a left pleural effusion or pneumothorax without a rib fracture and when there is particulate matter in the chest drain. The presence of mediastinal air also suggests oesophageal rupture. Patients may complain of pleuritic retrosternal pain radiating to the neck. There may be haematemesis, surgical emphysema in the neck or a characteristic crunching sound on auscultation of the heart, caused by air tracking around the pericardium (*Hamman's sign*). The diagnosis can be confirmed by contrast studies and endoscopy, but may only become apparent later when the patient develops mediastinitis.

Drainage of the pleural space and mediastinum with direct repair of the injury is the definitive surgical option. Occasionally more extensive procedures have to be undertaken to prevent continued soiling of the mediastinum and pleura by gastric and oesophageal contents.

PROGNOSIS

Reported overall mortality rates for those with chest injuries vary considerably depending on the patient population studied. Thoracic trauma is, however, a significant cause of mortality in trauma victims, particularly when associated with extrathoracic injuries, or pre-existing morbidity, such as COPD and old age (Galan *et al.*, 1992).

BURNS (Robertson and Fenton, 2000)

The majority of burn injuries occur in the home and frequently involve children aged 1–5 years who are scalded by hot liquids or whose clothing is ignited. Among teenagers and adults, men aged 17–30 years are the most frequent victims, usually as a result of accidents with inflammable liquids. Bedding and house fires most frequently affect the elderly and infirm, while about 25% of burns admissions are due to industrial accidents. Major structural fires account for only a small proportion of those admitted to hospital with thermal injury.

Although improved fire-fighting techniques and emergency medical services, as well as the increased use of smoke detectors, may have made some contribution to a reduction in burn-related deaths, in general preventive measures have had only limited success. In contrast, major advances in the resuscitation and subsequent care of burns patients have been responsible for a dramatic improvement in overall survival rates and a reduction in hospital stay among those admitted to specialized burn centres. Therefore, high-risk

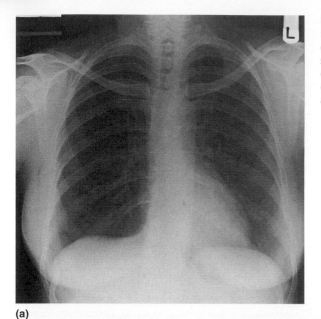

(a)

Fig. 10.4 Traumatic disruption of the aorta. (a) Normal chest radiograph 10 days before the accident. (b) Obvious widening of the mediastinum with displacement of the right paratracheal stripe. There is a left-sided pleural effusion overlying the apex of the lung in this supine film. (c) Aortogram showing a complete tear of the aorta at the level of the isthmus, with an aneurysm extending to the origin of the left subclavian artery.

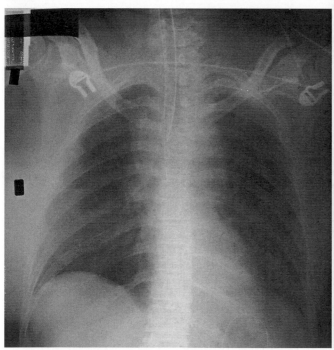

(b)

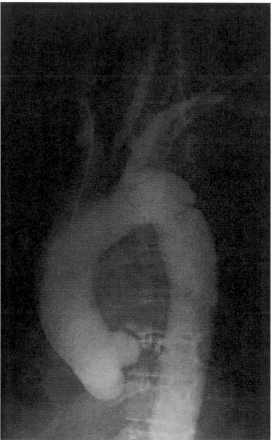

(c)

patients should always be referred to such units following initial resuscitation (**Table 10.4**).

ASSESSMENT

The severity of a thermal injury depends on the area damaged and the depth of the burn. The percentage surface area burned can be estimated using the 'rule of nine' (**Fig. 10.5**), modified in children to take into account the greater proportion of the body represented by the head and neck and the lesser contri-

bution of the legs. In those with extensive burns, it may be easier to assess the area of undamaged skin and subtract this from 100. The depth of the burn can be classified as:

- erythema only;
- partial-thickness;
- full-thickness.

Erythematous changes, without blistering, will usually resolve spontaneously within a few days and should not be

Table 10.4 Guidelines to aid in the selection of patients for referral to a burn centre
Burns greater than 10% of total body surface area (TBSA)
Burns of special areas: face, hands, feet, genitalia, perineum, over major joints
Full-thickness burns greater than 5% of TBSA in adults and 2% of TBSA in children
Electrical burns
Chemical burns
Burns with an associated inhalation injury
Circumferential burns of the limbs and chest
Burns at the extremes of age
Burn injury in patients with pre-existing medical disorders that could complicate management, prolong recovery or affect mortality rate
Any burn patient with associated trauma
Burns associated with self-harm or assault

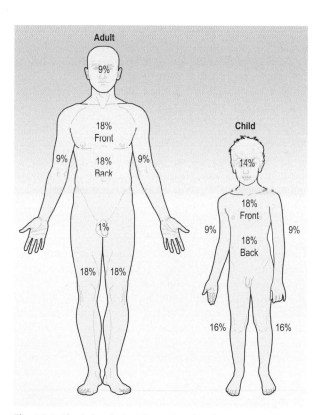

Fig. 10.5 The 'rule of nine' for estimating the percentage surface area burned in an adult and a child. The palmar surface (including the fingers) of the patient's hand represents approximately 1% of the patient's total body surface area (TBSA).

included in the calculation of the surface area burned. In areas of partial-thickness involvement, some viable deep epithelial elements remain, from which regeneration of skin is possible. This occurs beneath the eschar of dead dermis within 1–4 weeks. Because nerve endings are exposed and remain intact, partial-thickness burns are extremely painful. In contrast, epithelial structures and nerve endings are virtually completely destroyed following a full-thickness burn. Healing can therefore only occur by ingrowth of skin from surrounding structures or by contraction, but the conventional view that pain sensation is absent is a misconception; patients may in fact suffer from a severe, dull, pressure-like pain. Full-thickness burns may also involve underlying structures. In some cases, the distribution of the burn suggests the possibility of child abuse.

It is also important to identify *associated trauma* to other organs and vital structures.

MANAGEMENT
Volume replacement and cardiovascular support
Thermal injury increases microvascular permeability, in part because of the release of vasoactive substances (Demling and LaLonde, 1990) both locally and systemically, and plasma is lost not only externally (into blisters and as an exudate on the surface of the burn) but also into the interstitial spaces. The increase in regional blood flow is accompanied by an early rise in capillary pressure, which may enhance oedema formation. There is also intracellular swelling due to a generalized cell membrane defect. Increases in the osmotic pressure within the interstitium of both burned and adjacent non-burned tissue also appear to be important in the genesis of oedema and may be related to the release of osmotically active cellular elements. Oedema formation is most rapid during the first 6–8 hours after injury but continues for 18–24 hours. These changes, combined with evaporation of salt and water from the exposed surfaces, cause a considerable reduction in circulating volume and haemoconcentration. Without aggressive volume replacement, hypovolaemic shock supervenes (Monafo, 1996) and, if this is allowed to persist, acute renal failure may follow.

Because survival after near-total burns is no longer uncommon provided that early organ failure is avoided, vigorous resuscitation is always indicated in previously healthy patients with injuries that inexperienced observers might judge to be lethal (Monafo, 1996).

ASSESSING FLUID REQUIREMENTS
Because fluid losses are not obvious, and the patient may at first appear well, the extent of the volume deficit is often underestimated. Significant reductions in plasma volume follow burns involving more than 15% body surface area (BSA) in adults and more than 10% BSA in children. Although the magnitude of the losses is variable (e.g. partial-thickness scalds may be associated with massive reductions in plasma volume whereas deep flame burns are often charred and relatively dry), the volume of intravenous fluid

required can be estimated using one of a number of formulae. For example, *the Mount Vernon formula* (Muir, 1981) recommends:

Volume of plasma to be given in each period = % area burned × weight (kg)/2

Provided the patient's condition remains satisfactory, the calculated volume of plasma is infused in successive periods of 4, 4, 4, 6, 6 and 12 hours.

Most now favour resuscitation with crystalloid, usually Ringer's lactate solution, for example 2–4 mL/kg of body weight multiplied by the percentage of second- and third-degree BSA burned in the first 24 hours. Half of the calculated fluid requirements is administered during the first 8 hours after injury, coincident with the period of most rapid oedema formation (Monafo, 1996). Crystalloid requirements during the second day of treatment are about half of those required in the first 24 hours. It must be emphasized, however, that frequent clinical assessment of the adequacy of volume replacement is essential and that the rate of transfusion should be adjusted as indicated. This should be guided by the urine output (which should be maintained at more than 1.0 mL/kg per hour), in conjunction with vital signs, peripheral perfusion (temperature gradient), lactate levels and the haematocrit. Haematocrit is influenced by red cell destruction and extravascular extravasation, as well as plasma losses. Retrospectively collected evidence has demonstrated that those with smoke inhalation may require a higher than expected fluid input to maintain adequate cardiovascular performance (Navar *et al.*, 1985) and in these patients aggressive volume replacement reduces the incidence of organ dysfunction. Fluid requirements are also increased when resuscitation has been delayed and in children with large burns.

Some consider that CVP is an unreliable guide to volume requirements in burns patients and, in view of the high risk of infection and often limited availability of suitable access sites, avoid cannulating central veins. Others have recommended CVP monitoring in all patients with serious burns; occasionally more invasive haemodynamic monitoring may be required (see Chapter 4).

CHOICE OF FLUID FOR VOLUME REPLACEMENT

Severely burned patients require replacement of their circulating volume with large quantities of salt-containing solutions, but the type of fluid used for resuscitation is perhaps less important than the volume given and the experience of those responsible for its administration. Most authorities now suggest that crystalloids alone should be administered during the first 24 hours, in part because accumulated extravascular water can later be mobilized relatively easily (see Chapter 5). Subsequently, colloids and blood can be given as required to maintain the circulating volume and the packed cell volume respectively. For reasons discussed in Chapter 5, a few continue to use colloids even during the early phase of resuscitation, while others add colloid to a background crystalloid regimen in an attempt to maintain intravascular

volume and the plasma albumin concentration. There is, however, some evidence that colloids such as 5% albumin may be harmful in this situation. The role of hypertonic saline in the resuscitation of burns victims remains unclear.

Despite this aggressive approach to the restoration and maintenance of an adequate circulating volume, *acute renal failure* or transient episodes of *renal impairment* may complicate thermal injury. These may follow periods of hypoperfusion and hypoxia, and can be exacerbated by haemoglobinuria or myoglobinuria in those with electrical or crush injuries. Delayed renal failure is usually a consequence of sepsis, often in the context of multiple-organ dysfunction syndrome. Established acute renal failure is associated with a particularly high mortality in burns patients and must be avoided if at all possble (see Chapter 13).

Myocardial dysfunction may occur during the acute phase, and has been attributed to a circulating myocardial-depressant factor, primarily causing diastolic dysfunction. Myocardial oedema may also be a contributing factor. *Myocardial infarction* is a rare complication.

Surgery

Urgent surgical intervention may be required for patients with circumferential burns of the trunk or the limbs, which can impair respiration, or constrict blood vessels and cause ischaemic damage, respectively. Decompression is achieved by incising the skin and, sometimes, the deep fascia.

Elective surgery is performed to repair areas of full-thickness skin loss, and to prevent infection, by excision of eschar and autologous skin grafting. This should be performed as soon after resuscitation as is feasible and is usually first undertaken 2–4 days after burning. Wound excisions can be staged in those with deep burns that are too extensive to be closed in one procedure. Alternatively the burns can be completely excised within the first days after the injury and covered with a temporary skin substitute (allogenic cadaver skin or an artificial skin substitute), once the supply of autologous skin has been exhausted. Some deep partial-thickness burns may also be treated surgically since some believe (Monafo, 1996) that this approach results in better joint function and less severe scarring than more conservative treatment. These procedures can be associated with considerable blood loss. Grafting skin on to established, granulating wounds from which the eschar has sloughed may occasionally be necessary in those who are severely ill or have systemic complications, but is generally a poor surgical option.

Analgesia (Gallagher et al., 2000) (see Chapter 11)

Initially, analgesia is best achieved by administering small incremental doses of an opiate intravenously (e.g. 1 mg increments of morphine up to a total of 10 mg over 10 minutes). Cooling the burn and inhalation of Entonox may also be used to provide immediate pain relief. Subsequently, a continuous intravenous infusion of morphine can be given at a rate of 1–4 mg/h; alternatively patient-controlled analgesia can be used for alert patients. As is usually the case, combinations of drugs are often more effective than single agents. More severe procedural pain may require the addition of local blocks and/or general anaesthesia.

Control of infection (Ansermino and Hemsley, 2004)

A number of factors contribute to the susceptibility of burns patients to infective complications. These include:

- destruction of the skin or mucosal surface barrier;
- necrotic tissue and serosanguineous exudate provides a medium to support the growth of microorganisms;
- impaired immune function;
- use of invasive monitoring.

It is not surprising, therefore, that the commonest causes of death in those successfully resuscitated after thermal injury are *sepsis* and *multiple-organ failure*. Most often, this is related to infection of the lungs, or less often the burn wound, but in some cases urinary tract infections or contamination of intravascular catheters are implicated. As with other infections occurring in the critically ill, the most common pathogens causing burn wound sepsis have changed from the Gram-positive cocci (e.g. the β-haemolytic streptococcus) to resistant Gram-negative rods, such as *Pseudomonas aeruginosa*. Recently, however, methicillin-resistant strains of *Staphylococcus aureus* have been responsible for a number of epidemics of infection in burns units and there has been an increase in the incidence of Gram-positive infections. Invasive fungal infection may occur later.

The burn wound usually becomes colonized within a few days of admission, as a result of either autogenous infection or cross-contamination from another patient. The topical application of antimicrobial agents (most often silver sulfadiazine) for prophylaxis may delay colonization and reduce the concentration of bacteria before definitive surgery. Systemic antibiotics should only be used to treat documented infection. Distinguishing between infection, colonization and the systemic inflammatory response to the burn injury can be difficult, however. Interpretation of surface wound cultures is also difficult. Blood cultures and wound biopsy with histological examination and quantitative culture can help to differentiate invasive infection from burn wound colonization, although the latter is time-consuming and costly. The risk of cross-contamination can be minimized by barrier nursing in a single cubicle. Antitetanus prophylaxis is routine in most units.

Metabolic response and nutritional support

Serious burns are associated with:

- increased basal metabolic rate (resting energy expenditure may increase by more than 100% of basal metabolic rate);

- raised core temperature;
- hyperdynamic circulation;
- protein catabolism;
- lipolysis;
- increased susceptibility to infection;
- poor wound healing.

Previously established means of controlling hypermetabolism include a warm ambient environment (32°C) and effective pain relief (Wilmore *et al.*, 1974, 1975). Excision and closure of the burn wound and the recognition and treatment of infection are also important.

Provision of adequate nutritional support is vital. Enteral feeding is preferred because it maintains intestinal mucosal integrity and may diminish translocation of bacteria from the gut lumen (Herndon and Ziegler, 1993); enteral nutrition may also reduce the incidence of gastric ulceration. Total parenteral nutrition has been associated with reduced survival (see Chapter 11).

Pulmonary embolism is an unusual complication of thermal injury, but some centres use *prophylactic subcutaneous heparin* (see Chapter 11).

PROGNOSIS

The mortality of thermal injury is related to the depth of the burn, the percentage of BSA involved and the age of the patient. Survival rates have significantly improved over the last decade or so. For example, in 1964, 50% of patients between 10 and 30 years of age with second- and third-degree burns involving 50% of their BSA would have died. In-hospital mortality rates of less than 5% are now being reported for major burn injuries treated in specialized burn units.

INHALATION INJURY (Ansermino and Hemsley, 2004; Monafo, 1996)

Burns sustained within an enclosed space should suggest the potential for inhalation injury. Not only does this increase the mortality for a given surface area burn, but inhalation injury is also associated with an increased risk of death at the scene of the accident. The incidence of inhalation injury increases with the extent of the burn.

Patients with inhalation burns may develop *pharyngeal* and *laryngeal oedema*, with *upper-airways obstruction*, due to thermal and/or chemical damage. There may also be *pulmonary parenchymal damage*, which can cause acute hypoxaemic respiratory failure.

Pathophysiology

Few gases, except superheated steam, have sufficient thermal capacity to carry heat beyond the trachea. Pulmonary parenchymal damage is therefore usually chemical and due to water-soluble gaseous products of combustion such as ammonia, chlorine and sulphur dioxide. These react with the water in mucous membranes to produce strong acids and alkalis, which can induce bronchospasm, ulceration of the mucous membranes and oedema. Lipid-soluble compounds such as phosgene, nitrous oxide, hydrogen chloride and aldehydes can reach the distal airways on carbon particles that adhere to the mucosa. These damage the cell membrane directly and impair ciliary clearance. Moreover, the inflammation is aggravated by activation of alveolar macrophages. Smoke inhalation promotes tracheobronchitis and formation of casts (destroyed epithelium and fibrin), and also enhances leukocyte margination in pulmonary capillaries and the release of inflammatory mediators.

Presentation and diagnosis

Airway burns should be suspected in any patient with:

- facial burns;
- stridor, hoarseness or cough;
- dysphagia;
- erythema of the nasopharyngeal mucosa;
- singed nasal vibrissae;
- soot in expectorated secretions, nose or mouth;
- hypoxaemia;
- dyspnoea, decreased level of consciousness or confusion.

Such an injury is most likely following facial flame burns or when the victim has been confined within a small, smoke-filled room. *Elevated carboxyhaemoglobin (COHb) levels* on admission also suggest that there has been significant respiratory involvement, provided allowance is made for the time interval between smoke inhalation and admission (**Fig. 10.6**) (Clarke *et al.*, 1981). Although there is a significant correlation between carbon monoxide levels and blood cyanide concentrations (Baud *et al.*, 1991), it is not possible to predict with confidence the presence or absence of cyanide poisoning from COHb levels. One study suggested that in fire victims with minor or no cutaneous burns, a *high plasma lactate concentration* strongly suggests that the patient is suffering from cyanide poisoning (Baud *et al.*, 1991).

The *chest radiograph* and *blood gas analysis* may be within normal limits initially, but should be repeated at intervals in order to detect subsequent deterioration. In some centres, *indirect laryngoscopy* or *fibreoptic bronchoscopy* is performed early to assess airway obstruction, confirm the diagnosis, define the extent and severity of the airway burn and to perform tracheobronchial toilet.

Early increases in extravascular lung water are rare, but may result from the direct chemical toxicity of inhaled gases in the most severe cases of inhalation injury. More often the increase in microvascular permeability leads to *pulmonary oedema* some 1–3 days after injury and to pneumonia, which is often severe and recurrent, some days later. Delayed increases in lung water may be related to systemic or pulmonary sepsis. *Pulmonary fibrosis* is commonly encountered among survivors. *Bronchorrhoea*, which is usually a response to the inhaled irritants rather than a sign of infection, is common after smoke inhalation.

Presentation is frequently delayed, but *early diagnosis* may be possible using fibreoptic bronchoscopy.

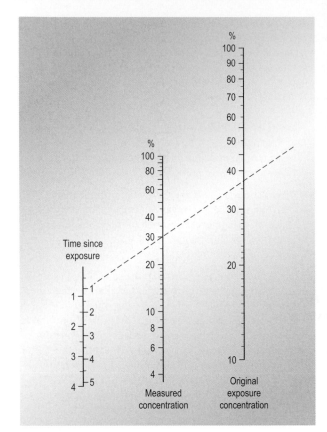

Fig. 10.6 Nomogram for calculating carboxyhaemoglobin concentration at time of exposure. Time since exposure is given in two scales to allow for the effects of previous oxygen administration on the half-life of carboxyhaemoglobin. (Left scale assumes a half-life of 3 hours, that on the right assumes a half-life of 4 hours.) Reproduced from Clarke CJ, Campbell D, Reid WH (1981) Blood carboxy haemoglobin and cyanide levels in fire survivors *Lancet* **i** 1332–1335. © by the Lancet Ltd with permission.

Monitoring

The value of pulse oximetry is limited because current instruments do not distinguish between oxyhaemoglobin and COHb. Importantly, carbon monoxide toxicity may result in falsely elevated pulse oximetry readings. The difficulties of adequately measuring arterial blood pressure indirectly in extensively burned patients and the need to measure arterial blood gases frequently justify arterial cannulation. Invasive monitoring may also be required to guide fluid administration (see volume replacement and cardiovascular support p. 275).

Management of inhalation injury

Management should begin as soon as possible with the administration of *supplemental oxygen*. All those with suspected airway burns must be closely observed for the signs of impending airway obstruction and/or respiratory failure. Early *intubation* is preferable to a late *tracheostomy* under unfavourable circumstances. Indeed, tracheostomy should be avoided if possible because it is associated with an increased risk of pulmonary infection in burns injury. Supplemental oxygen should be continued at least until the COHb concentration has fallen to less than 10%. If hypoxia persists despite oxygen the application of *CPAP* may be beneficial, although mask CPAP can be difficult to achieve in those with facial burns and tracheal intubation may then be required. Mechanical ventilation with PEEP is often necessary, but patients with inhalation injury are particularly prone to barotrauma, probably due to air-trapping in small airways obstructed by casts. Aggressive airway toilet is essential. Diluted heparin and acetyl cystine nebulization may be helpful (Desai *et al.*, 1998). Prophylactic corticosteroids and antibiotics have no role in treatment. There is no specific treatment for airway burns other than ensuring adequate oxygenation and minimizing further alveolar injury.

The value of *hyperbaric oxygen therapy* in carbon monoxide poisoning remains uncertain (see Chapter 19). Similarly, the use of *cyanide antidotes* is controversial and, in view of their potential toxicity, their use is difficult to justify as blind therapy for an already ill patient (see Chapter 19).

■ SPINAL INJURIES (Swain *et al.*, 2000)

Spinal injuries are a feature of modern mechanized societies, the majority of cases being the result of RTCs. Other causes include falls at work or in the home, sports injuries (mainly diving accidents) and battlefield casualties. The cervical spine is injured in 2–12% of patients following blunt polytrauma and injuries to the head and neck are associated in up to one-third of cases. It is estimated that there are approximately 15–50 new cases of spinal injury/million population per year, although this is probably an underestimate since many immediately fatal cases are unrecognized and many others are inadequately documented. Spinal injuries are most frequent in young adults, with a male-to-female ratio of about 4:1.

PATHOPHYSIOLOGY

Traumatic injury to the spinal cord produces a variable degree of irreversible neuronal destruction and haemorrhage caused by traction and compression forces, often compounded by direct compression of neural elements by fractured and displaced bone fragments, disc material and ligaments. Within minutes of the injury the spinal cord swells to occupy the entire diameter of the spinal canal at the level of the injury, compromising local blood flow. Cord ischaemia is exacerbated by the systemic hypotension caused by spinal neurogenic shock, often compounded by hypovolaemia. Thus, as is the case in head injuries (see Chapter 15), the ultimate neurological deficit is worsened by secondary ischaemia as well as ensuing cellular and molecular events, including apoptosis.

IMMEDIATE MANAGEMENT

Patients with isolated spinal injury should be *resuscitated* and, if possible, transferred immediately to a specialized unit. Those with serious associated injuries or respiratory failure are usually admitted directly to an intensive care unit. (Chest trauma is common in those with thoracolumbar fracture dislocations, and damage to the cervical spine is frequently associated with head injury. Many patients will have multiple injuries.)

High thoracic or cervical lesions may produce immediately life-threatening respiratory failure and cardiovascular disturbances (see later in this section). Some patients may therefore require *emergency tracheal intubation* and *controlled ventilation*, as well as measures to *restore haemodynamic stability*.

Further damage to the spinal cord must be avoided when moving the patient from the site of the accident and during transfer. Patients must therefore be lifted on a spine immobilization device and extricated from wreckage with extreme care; this will usually require several people. Flexion, extension and lateral movements of the spinal column should be prevented by using in-line manual immobilization, a cervical collar or sandbags placed on either side of the head, and by positioning pillows to maintain the natural curvatures of the spine. Slight hyperextension at the site of the fracture is preferred and slight traction should be applied to the patient's head and legs.

DIAGNOSIS AND ASSESSMENT

Spinal injury is easily overlooked in the absence of significant cord damage and in those who are unconscious. If the patient is comatose, a cord lesion should be suspected if deep tendon *reflexes are absent* and in the presence of *urinary retention* or *priapism*. Lesions above T11 produce intercostal paralysis and an *abnormal respiratory pattern*, while cervical cord damage may be associated with *Horner's syndrome*. Nevertheless, all comatose patients should be handled as if a cord injury is present until this possibility has been excluded. Every effort should be made to remove the rigid spine board as early as possible to reduce the risk of decubitus ulcer formation. The spine board is often removed as part of the secondary survey when the patient is log-rolled for inspection and palpation of the back.

On admission to hospital, a full neurological examination should be performed to determine the level and completeness of the lesion. Damage to the lower motor neurones in the central grey matter at the site of injury, and in several segments above and below the lesion, results in flaccid paralysis at the level of the injury. Variable damage to the surrounding white matter affects the long tracts, producing upper motor neurone signs below the level of the injury. It is also worth remembering that multilevel cord injury is a possibility. Subsequently, neurological assessment should be repeated at frequent intervals in order to detect extension of the deficit as cord oedema progresses upwards. It is particularly important to recognize increasing paralysis of respiratory muscles so that controlled ventilation can be instituted without delay. *Neck movements should only be examined in conscious patients and by an expert.*

Investigations *(Morris et al., 2004)*

Clinically trauma patients can be regarded as having a stable cervical spine if:

- the Glasgow Coma Scale is 15 and the patient is alert and oriented;
- the patient has not consumed any intoxicants or drugs;
- there are no serious distracting injuries;
- no signs or symptoms are found on cervical examination:
  - no midline tenderness or pain;
  - no impairment to full range of active movement;
  - no referable neurological deficit.

When these criteria are not fulfilled, as will be the case in most patients with multiple injuries, a lateral cervical spine film should be obtained, soon after life-threatening problems are identified and controlled. The base of the skull, all seven cervical vertebrae and the first thoracic vertebra must be visualized. Anteroposterior and odontoid peg views should also be obtained. Fractures, especially those involving the facet joints, may, however, be missed on plain radiographs. A *CT scan* better defines bony structures and can further demonstrate the nature and extent of any spinal injury. Helical CT scanning has been shown to allow rapid, effective and safe evaluation of the cervical spine in unconscious, intubated trauma patients (Brohi *et al.*, 2005) and significantly outperforms plain radiography as a screening test for patients at high risk of cervical spine injury (Holmes and Akkinepalli, 2005). A *magnetic resonance imaging (MRI) scan* allows detailed visualization of neural tissue but is impractical for screening injuries of the cervical spine in critically ill patients. Most now recommend that cervical injury should be routinely screened and excluded in unconscious patients with multiple injuries by plain radiography combined with directed CT. Further, in trauma units with access to a helical, multiplane, CT scanner the entire cervical spine should be imaged at high resolution (Morris *et al.*, 2004). *Somatosensory evoked responses* (Chapter 15) can be used to assess the completeness of the cord lesion and to document subsequent recovery or deterioration.

MANAGEMENT
Respiratory system

Lesions above T11 interrupt the innervation of respiratory muscles. *Intercostal paralysis* may be partial or complete, and may be asymmetrical. Diaphragmatic breathing in the presence of intercostal paralysis produces a *paradoxical pattern of respiration* with abdominal distension and indrawing of the affected segments of the chest wall during inspiration. Lesions at or above C4 deprive the diaphragm of its major segmental nerve supply and ventilation is grossly impaired. Immediate intubation and ventilation may be life-saving in such cases.

Associated *chest injuries* are common, particularly in those with thoracolumbar injuries, and can further impair respiratory function. These abnormalities may be exacerbated by *aspiration* of gastric contents (the patient is usually nursed supine and often has an impaired ability to cough, a reduced conscious level and paralytic ileus) and *pulmonary oedema* (see later in this section).

It is recommended that *controlled ventilation* is instituted early on the basis of a clinical assessment, assisted by blood gas analysis, in order to avoid a progressive deterioration in respiratory function. Because of the sympathetic denervation, many of these patients are unable to compensate for the increased intrathoracic pressure during positive-pressure ventilation and become markedly hypotensive. Cautious volume replacement, with or without inotropes/vasopressors support, may then be required to restore perfusion of vital organs.

The management of these respiratory abnormalities is complicated by the positioning and immobilization required to treat the spinal injury, which hampers effective physiotherapy. Moreover, vital capacity is reduced and the ability to cough impaired. Importantly, diaphragmatic breathing in the presence of intercostal paralysis is most efficient in the supine position. *Intensive physiotherapy* is essential.

Cardiovascular support

There is some experimental evidence to suggest that spinal cord injury can produce *immediate hypertension and bradycardia* lasting for approximately 3–4 minutes (Rawe and Perot, 1979). This may be associated with a *transient rise in intracranial pressure* and an increase in *pulmonary artery pressure*. These changes can be compared with those described in neurogenic pulmonary oedema (see Chapter 15).

Subsequently, *spinal shock* supervenes, vasomotor tone is lost and both resistance and capacitance vessels dilate. The sympathetic innervation of the heart, which arises from spinal segments T1–T5, is interrupted by lesions above this level, while parasympathetic fibres remain intact. Patients with high thoracic or cervical injuries are therefore *hypotensive* (systolic blood pressure, commonly 80–90 mmHg), but *without an associated tachycardia*. Furthermore, vagal stimulation, for example in response to hypoxia or endotracheal suction, is unopposed and can produce a profound *bradycardia*, or even *asystole* (Welply *et al.*, 1975). This can be prevented by administering atropine regularly or, in resistant cases, by isoprenaline. Hypoxaemic episodes must be avoided.

Despite the hypotension and relative hypovolaemia, which may or may not be combined with significant blood loss from associated injuries, the circulating volume must be replaced cautiously. The CVP may be an unreliable guide to volume requirements and cardiovascular function in these patients, necessitating more invasive monitoring in difficult cases. Patients with high spinal injuries are unable to respond to a volume challenge by increasing heart rate and contractility, and there is therefore a considerable risk of overtransfusion. In some cases, a vasopressor agent will be required to restore the systemic blood pressure to an acceptable level. Furthermore, these patients are particularly prone to pulmonary oedema, possibly because pulmonary capillaries are disrupted during the initial hypertensive episode.

Following the period of spinal shock, reflex activity gradually returns and there is some recovery of sympathetic tone. Nevertheless, although the tendency to bradycardia diminishes, a degree of postural hypotension generally persists. Furthermore continued autonomic dysreflexia may be encountered in quadriplegia complicating spinal cord injury above T6. This life-threatening syndrome characterised by hypertension, bradycardia and vasodilation above the level of the cord injury can be triggered by visceral or somatic stimuli such as distension of the bladder or bowel, faecal impaction and cold or pressure on the skin. Treatment entails finding and removing the cause whilst treating the accompanying hypertension.

Management of the spinal fracture or fracture dislocation

The stability of the spinal column is dependent on the integrity of the posterior ligamentous complex. This consists of the supraspinous and interspinous ligaments, the ligamentum flavum and the capsules of the facet joints. If these are disrupted, the spinal injury will be unstable. Conventionally many clinicians have believed that occult ligamentous injury could only be reliably excluded once the patient had recovered consciousness sufficiently to undergo clinical evaluation. As a result many patients have been subjected to the risks of prolonged immobilisation with the application of a cervical collar. Complications of this approach include (Morris *et al.*, 2004):

- cutaneous pressure ulceration;
- venous obstruction and raised intracranial pressure;
- delayed tracheostomy;
- difficulty in obtaining central venous access;
- inability to adequately maintain oral hygiene;
- failed enteral nutrition;
- gastrostasis, reflux and pulmonary aspiration;
- restricted physiotherapy;
- thromboembolism;
- increased risk of cross infection.

In view of the considerable morbidity and mortality associated with prolonged immobilisation in a cervical collar many now recommend the combined use of plain radiographs and CT (which may have a false negative rate as low as 0.1%) to 'clear' the cervical spine in patients who fail to regain consciousness within 48–72 hrs. The patient can then be mobilised cautiously under close supervision (Morris *et al.*, 2004).

The role of early surgery to decompress the spinal cord by removing bone, disc and ligamentous fragments remains controversial, unless canal integrity is severely compromised. In general, however, early internal stabilisation has distinct practical advantages during rehabilitation when compared to external ('halo') devices.

CERVICAL SPINE INJURIES

In the absence of facet joint dislocation, cervical spine injuries can be managed with a *cervical collar* or *skull traction* to maintain the position and immobilize the site of injury. If one, or both, posterior facet joints are dislocated, *early reduction* is indicated. This can be achieved either by manipulation under a relaxant general anaesthetic, guided by an image intensifier, or by graded traction using skull tongs. An MRI scan should be obtained before reduction of the cervical spine using traction if the patient is uncooperative or will require reduction under general anaesthesia. Some centres perform *open reduction* in all cases, whereas others only resort to this method when more conservative measures have failed. Subsequently, the position must be maintained with traction. Patients can be nursed in a *Stryker frame*, although this is unsuitable for those with limb fractures requiring traction and the prone position is poorly tolerated by those with associated chest injuries. In most situations, therefore, *tilting and turning beds*, e.g. a Rotorest or an Egerton Stoke Mandeville bed are more satisfactory.

Specific types of cervical spine injury. The atlas may be fractured where the arch meets the lateral masses. Displacement occurs if the transverse ligament is torn (**Fig. 10.7**). Such an injury is usually caused by a vertical force, such as a fall on the head. Neurological damage is generally minimal and the injury may be treated with a cervical collar worn for three months.

The *odontoid process* may be fractured, usually through the base, most often as a result of an RTC or a severe fall (**Fig. 10.8**). Cord damage is usually mild or absent, but skull traction is generally indicated and surgery may be necessary if the fracture fails to unite.

Posterior dislocation of the *axis* may occur without a fracture. This causes few neurological signs and is treated with traction followed, if necessary, by fusion

Burst fractures (**Fig. 10.9**) are very painful, but stable. Unless there is marked bony displacement, cord damage is unusual, but they require support in a collar until fusion is seen radiologically.

Lateral radiographs of the cervical spine may appear normal in patients with *hyperextension injury*, although

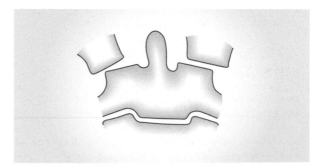

Fig. 10.7 Displaced lateral masses of the atlas. From Johnson PG (1978) The management of spinal injuries. In: Hanson GC, Wright PL (eds) *The Medical Management of the Critically Ill*, pp. 412–429. Academic Press: London, with permission.

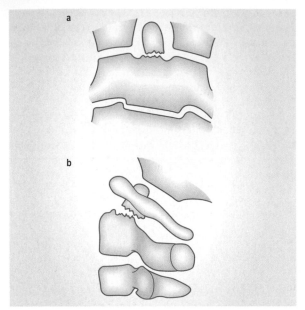

Fig. 10.8 Fractured odontoid process. (a) Anteroposterior view through the mouth of a basal fracture. (b) Lateral view in extension. From Johnson PG (1978) The management of spinal injuries. In: Hanson GC, Wright PL (eds) *The Medical Management of the Critically Ill,* pp. 412–429. Academic Press: London, with permission.

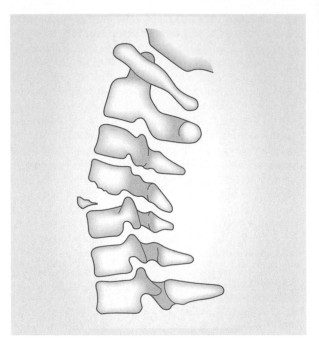

Fig. 10.10 Hyperextension injury of C4/C5: avulsion of fragment from C4. From Johnson PG (1978) The management of spinal injuries. In: Hanson GC, Wright PL (eds) *The Medical Management of the Critically Ill,* pp. 412–429. Academic Press: London, with permission.

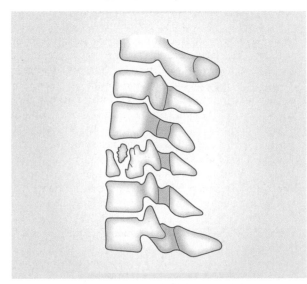

Fig. 10.9 Burst fracture of C5. From Johnson PG (1978) The management of spinal injuries. In: Hanson GC, Wright PL (eds) *The Medical Management of the Critically Ill,* pp. 412–429. Academic Press: London, with permission.

instability is demonstrable if films are obtained with the neck extended. In some cases, a small fragment of bone may be avulsed from the lower anterior edge of a vertebral body (**Fig. 10.10**). Because the posterior ligaments remain intact, these injuries are stable in the neutral position and can be treated with a cervical collar. The degree of neurological damage is variable.

Anterior dislocations (**Fig. 10.11**) disrupt the posterior ligaments and are therefore unstable unless the facet joints lock. Tetraplegia may occur as a result of this type of injury, but often neurological damage is minimal. Treatment consists of immediate reduction (e.g. using graded skull traction under radiographic control), followed by fusion.

The great majority of serious neck injuries involve *fracture dislocations* (**Fig. 10.12**), most often at C5/6 or C6/7. These injuries are unstable and are associated with the highest incidence of severe neurological damage. The safest treatment is probably continuous skull traction under radiographic control, although some surgeons will manipulate the injury under general anaesthesia. Traction may be followed by operative fusion.

THORACIC SPINE INJURIES
Anterior wedge fractures often occur in association with osteoporosis or malignant deposits. They are stable and should be treated symptomatically. On the other hand, traumatic fracture dislocations in this region are irreducible and almost invariably cause paraplegia.

THORACOLUMBAR INJURIES
Anterior wedge and burst fractures are stable and require only symptomatic treatment. The integrity of the posterior ligaments in this region can be assessed by palpating the midline. If there is a palpable gap between the spinous pro-

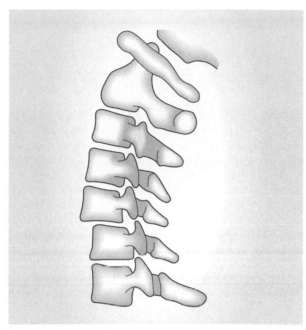

Fig. 10.11 Anterior dislocation: unifacet dislocation of C5 on C6. From Johnson PG (1978) The management of spinal injuries. In: Hanson GC, Wright PL (eds) *The Medical Management of the Critically Ill*, pp. 412–429. Academic Press: London, with permission.

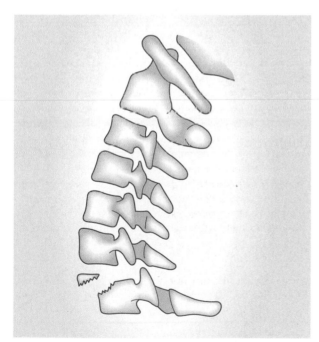

Fig. 10.12 Fracture dislocation of C6/C7: avulsion of fragment of C7. From Johnson PG (1978) The management of spinal injuries. In: Hanson GC, Wright PL (eds) *The Medical Management of the Critically Ill*, pp. 412–429. Academic Press: London, with permission.

cesses, into which the finger sinks, then the fracture is unstable. These injuries can be treated by postural reduction with the patient extended over a foam bolster positioned at the level of the injury. Some cases will require open reduction and fixation.

Treatment of spinal cord injury

It is generally accepted that *early immobilization and reduction of fracture dislocations*, together with *prompt resuscitation* to restore oxygen delivery, can minimize neurological damage.

A number of additional measures aimed at preventing or minimizing secondary cord damage have been evaluated, but in general the results have been either inconclusive or discouraging. Nevertheless evidence suggests that *high-dose methylprednisolone* may be of value in certain patients following non-penetrating trauma with incomplete spinal cord injuries (Bracken *et al.*, 1997). There is, however, some concern that such treatment may be associated with an increased risk of gastric bleeding and wound infection. The use of steroids should be determined in consultation with a neurosurgeon or the local spinal injury centre. One accepted regimen is to administer methylprednisolone (30 mg/kg bolus) within 8 hrs after the injury. Treatment started within the first 3 hrs is continued (5.4 mg/kg/hr) for 24 hrs. Treatment initiated between 3 and 8 hrs is continued for 48 hrs.

Gastrointestinal tract, fluid and electrolyte balance, nutrition

In the acute phase, it can be difficult to exclude significant intra-abdominal trauma since patients with spinal injury are unable to appreciate abdominal pain and a proportion develop a neurogenic paralytic ileus. *Peritoneal lavage* is rarely performed and interpretation may be complicated by blood leaking into the abdominal cavity from a paravertebral haematoma. *CT scanning* is now normally undertaken in these circumstances.

Some patients develop discoordinated bowel activity with progressive *abdominal distension* and *vomiting*, despite the presence of bowel sounds. This is associated with an increased risk of aspiration, fluid and electrolyte disturbances and impaired ventilation. Usually, these abnormalities resolve within 4–7 days and in most cases it is possible to establish enteral nutrition. Occasionally, parenteral nutrition is indicated.

The rectum must be emptied on about the fourth day after injury and this should be followed by regular bowel evacuation. This is achieved with oral aperients, rectal suppositories and, if necessary, manual evacuation. Provided this regimen is started soon after the injury, so that overdistension of the bowel is avoided, a pattern of reflex evacuation can be established and faecal incontinence prevented.

Urinary tract

Initially, patients admitted to the intensive care unit will require urethral or suprapubic catheterization with continuous drainage. Later, a regimen of intermittent catheterization may be instituted to encourage the return of reflex bladder function.

Body temperature

The ability to adjust skin blood flow and sweating is lost below the level of a complete spinal cord lesion. This is a particular problem for tetraplegics who are therefore prone to hypothermia and may require air conditioning during hot weather.

General measures

Finally, prophylactic measures to minimize the risk of gastrointestinal haemorrhage and thromboembolic complications are essential (see Chapter 11), as are first-class nursing care and physiotherapy to prevent decubitus ulceration and fixed deformities.

Anaesthetic considerations

Tracheal intubation can be difficult and hazardous in those with unstable cervical spines. In such cases, the *head and neck should be immobilized* with sandbags or by an assistant before intubation. The usual flexion–extension manoeuvres must be avoided. Because of the dangers of vagal stimulation, the patient should be *preoxygenated* and given *atropine* (Welply et al., 1975). Suxamethonium can precipitate *hyperkalaemia* between 3 days and 6 months after the injury (Snow et al., 1973) and should therefore be avoided. In the acute situation, however, patients are at risk of aspiration and some recommend *rapid-sequence induction* with a fast-acting non-depolarizing muscle relaxant and the application of cricoid pressure. Many authorities recommend *awake intubation*, if necessary using a fibreoptic laryngoscope, as the safest technique. Emergency *cricothyrotomy* or *tracheostomy* is occasionally necessary. Adequate monitoring of cardiovascular and respiratory function is essential throughout.

PROGNOSIS

The outlook for patients with spinal injury has markedly improved since the First World War, when approximately 90% of all cases died within 1 year; currently the mortality is only 2–5% in the first 12 months. Furthermore, although the life expectancy of a tetraplegic is undoubtedly reduced, on average by about 15 years, paraplegics can generally anticipate a normal lifespan. However, these figures only apply to young patients; the prognosis is considerably worse in the elderly. Nevertheless, since the majority of spinally injured patients are less than 25 years old, they represent a considerable long-term financial commitment. Effective preventive measures are therefore of the utmost importance and should include improvements in safety standards on the roads, at work and in the home.

◼ NEAR-DROWNING (Golden et al., 1997)

In the UK, 1000–1500 people die each year as a result of accidental drowning. The incidence is higher in North America and Australia because of the large number of domestic swimming pools and the popularity of water sports. Almost half of those who drown are less than 20 years old, the highest incidence being in the second decade, and approximately 75% of the victims are male. Blood alcohol levels are often high. About one-third are competent swimmers and a number of these individuals drown during an attempt at prolonged underwater swimming. In these cases, it is thought that the swimmer hyperventilates before diving in order to lower the arterial carbon dioxide tension and extend the length of time he or she can remain under water. The swimmer may then lose consciousness due to severe hypoxia before the arterial carbon dioxide tension has reached a level sufficient to stimulate respiration. Subsequently, P_aCO_2 rises and the ensuing inspiratory effort is accompanied by pulmonary aspiration.

Competent, healthy young swimmers may also drown following immersion in cold water. Under these circumstances the initial respiratory responses to the cold, which include an immediate gasp followed by uncontrollable hyperventilation and an extreme sense of dyspnoea, cause swim-stroke/respiration asynchrony and make effective swimming difficult or impossible. Moreover in turbulent or choppy water the inability to breath-hold for more than 10–20 seconds makes aspiration more likely.

Deciding whether and when to stop resuscitation of a drowning victim is notoriously difficult. No single factor predicts prognosis accurately (Soar et al., 2005).

PATHOPHYSIOLOGY

Drowning can be defined as suffocation by submersion/immersion in a liquid medium, especially water (Modell, 1993). In fact, drowning occurs without aspiration in only approximately 10% of victims; the remaining 90% aspirate liquid, predominantly water (Modell et al., 1976). Although the composition of the water influences the ultimate physiological response, all victims of submersion are hypoxaemic. In those who have not aspirated, hypoxaemia is simply related to a period of apnoea, whereas in those who have inhaled water, there is often primary lung injury. In addition to hypoxaemia, metabolic acidosis is also present in the majority of patients and occasionally there are significant fluid and electrolyte abnormalities. Disseminated intravascular coagulation and rhabdomyolysis have also been described. Cerebral damage and renal dysfunction may complicate the most serious cases. Delayed deaths following near-drowning are usually associated with unrecognized pulmonary insufficiency, secondary chest infection, hypoxic cerebral damage or raised intracranial pressure.

Respiratory abnormalities

Aspiration of large volumes of fresh water alters the alveolar surface tension by interfering with surfactant and, even though the water is rapidly absorbed into the circulation, this produces hypoxaemia due to *ventilation/perfusion mismatch* and *alveolar collapse*. Salt water, on the other hand, remains within the alveoli and draws fluid into the lungs from the intravascular space. Although the total amount of surfactant is reduced, that which remains continues to function normally. This produces predominantly a large, fixed *right-to-left shunt*. In both instances, a severe *permeability pulmonary oedema* can develop and lung compliance is reduced. Development of non-cardiogenic pulmonary oedema may be delayed for many hours – so-called *secondary drowning*.

Overexpansion of the lungs with areas resembling *acute emphysema* can frequently be demonstrated at postmortem in those who have drowned, and is probably the result of violent fluctuations in intrathoracic pressure occurring during the period of airway obstruction. In many, there is also evidence of *aspiration of particulate matter*, such as gastric contents, mud or sand. In those who die later, there may be *bronchopneumonia*, sometimes with multiple *abscess formation* but, in those who survive, recovery of lung function is usually complete.

Cardiovascular abnormalities

The initial cardiovascular responses to cold immersion include an immediate intense peripheral vasoconstriction, tachycardia and an increase in cardiac output, with an increase in arterial and venous pressures. Vasoconstriction may divert blood flow to the brain and myocardium and, together with the protective effect of hypothermia, may account for survival following prolonged submersion in cold water. (A 5-year-old Norwegian boy survived without neurological sequelae after 40 minutes' submersion in iced water (Siebke *et al.*, 1975).) In those with pre-existing cardiovascular disease these responses may, however, precipitate myocardial ischaemia or a cerebrovascular accident. *Bradycardia*, often associated with intense *vasoconstriction* and apnoea, can be elicited by submerging the face in water at less than 20°C, when it is known as the *diving reflex* (Ramey *et al.*, 1987). Bradycardia and vasoconstriction can also occur as a response to hypoxaemia and acidosis, whereas catecholamine release and hypothermia may further contribute to the increased vascular tone.

Theoretically, salt-water drowning would be expected to cause hypovolaemia, while aspiration of fresh water should expand the circulating volume. In clinical practice, however, victims of near-drowning rarely inhale sufficient quantities to cause significant changes in blood volume. Nevertheless, *hypovolaemia* may be present because of the diuresis and natriuresis that follow the increase in venous return and cardiac output caused by the hydrostatic pressure of the water on the body. Moreover peripheral vasoconstriction can further increase right atrial pressure and may enhance urine output by as much as one-third. Losses of circulating volume (e.g. as pulmonary oedema) can further exacerbate hypovolaemia.

A wide variety of *ECG changes* have been described in association with near-drowning. These have included:

- absent P waves;
- ST-segment elevation;
- increased PR interval;
- atrioventricular dissociation;
- ventricular tachycardia/fibrillation.

Generally, these are secondary changes that revert to normal following correction of hypoxaemia, acidosis, hypothermia and hypovolaemia.

Electrolyte disturbances

Although plasma levels of sodium and chloride may be elevated following experimental salt-water drowning (sea water contains 509 mmol/L of sodium), and low plasma sodium levels have been demonstrated in animal studies of fresh-water aspiration, serious electrolyte disturbances are clinically unusual and it is doubtful that they play a significant role in determining survival. Occasionally, *hyperkalaemia* occurs in association with metabolic acidosis or acute renal failure, and rarely complicates haemolysis caused by absorption of very large volumes of fresh water. *Magnesium* levels may be elevated following sea-water drowning.

Body temperature (see Chapter 20)
Hypothermia is a common complication of near-drowning and may protect vital organs from hypoxic/ischaemic damage. As body temperature falls below 30°C, however, ventricular fibrillation becomes increasingly likely, and at less than 28°C, established ventricular fibrillation is usually resistant to cardioversion. Rapid rewarming may then be necessary. Unlike other causes of hypothermia, near-drowning is often associated with aspiration of cold water into the lungs, stomach or both; this may accelerate the reduction in deep body temperature.

Renal dysfunction

Renal dysfunction is unusual, but may occur in association with hypoxia, metabolic acidosis, severe haemoglobinuria or hypothermia. Established acute renal failure is even more unusual and usually follows an extended period of hypotension.

Neurological damage
Ischaemic cerebral damage can follow prolonged asphyxia, hypoxaemia or cardiac arrest, while some patients develop *cerebral oedema* and *intracranial hypertension*.

MANAGEMENT
Immediate care
Once the victim has been removed from the water, the first priority is to relieve hypoxia by establishing a *clear airway* followed, if necessary, by *mouth-to-mouth resuscitation* and *external cardiac massage*. If it is impossible to reach dry land immediately, expired air ventilation should be attempted in the water since a few breaths may be sufficient to restart spontaneous respiration and cardiac activity. Where possible casualties wearing a life jacket whose airway is clear of the water should be recovered in the horizontal position. Time

should not be wasted in attempting to remove water from the patient's lungs, since the amount recovered, if any, is usually too small to be significant. The Heimlich manoeuvre is not recommended. It is, however, essential to *prevent further heat loss* by wrapping the victim in blankets or warm clothing.

Once experienced personnel arrive at the scene, comatose patients and those requiring continued artificial ventilation should be *intubated* (there is a significant risk of regurgitation and aspiration) and an *intravenous infusion* should be established. An ECG will allow the detection and treatment of arrhythmias. The patient should be evacuated to hospital as soon as possible. Some recommend that all severely hypothermic and clinically lifeless patients should be transferred to an institution with the facilities for cardiopulmonary bypass.

Hospital care

On admission to hospital it is important to determine the circumstances of the accident (duration of immersion, salt or fresh water, warm or cold, history of alcohol or drug ingestion) as well as the results of any attempts at resuscitation. The patient should be fully examined, including a search for associated injuries, which may significantly complicate the management of near-drowning. In particular, cervical spine and head injuries are frequently associated with diving accidents, water slide use and alcohol intoxication and are easily missed in comatose patients (see earlier in this chapter). Analysis of serum electrolyte concentrations should be performed as necessary. Body temperature should be measured. Predisposing injuries or medical conditions should be excluded.

RESPIRATORY MANAGEMENT

Hypoxaemia is almost invariable following immersion, even in those who appear to have recovered fully. All patients should therefore receive *supplemental oxygen* and should be admitted to hospital for observation because of the risk of delayed respiratory failure, e.g. secondary drowning – see earlier in this chapter. The single most effective means of reversing hypoxaemia is the application of *CPAP* in patients breathing spontaneously or *PEEP* in those receiving controlled ventilation. Some patients develop irritative bronchospasm requiring *bronchodilator therapy*. The principles of treatment for acute respiratory failure are discussed in Chapter 8.

CARDIOVASCULAR SUPPORT

This will involve the *restoration of sinus rhythm, volume replacement* and, occasionally, *inotropic support*. In complicated cases, invasive monitoring may provide useful information, particularly in those with pulmonary oedema. The principles of cardiovascular support are discussed in Chapter 5.

NEUROLOGICAL MANAGEMENT

With improvements in emergency services, bystander resuscitation and intensive care during the last few decades, the prevention and treatment of brain injury have become the main therapeutic challenge in the increasing proportion of victims who survive near-drowning. Unfortunately, the value of aggressive measures aimed at minimizing cerebral damage and controlling intracranial hypertension in comatose victims of near-drowning is uncertain; for example, pentobarbital therapy failed to improve outcome in nearly drowned, flaccid and comatose children (Nussbaum and Maggi, 1988). Although many advocate monitoring intracranial pressure, significant intracranial hypertension is unusual after near-drowning and when cerebral swelling does occur it does so late, often after irreversible brain damage has occurred. The value of such monitoring is therefore questionable.

EXPOSURE AND ENVIRONMENT

Victims of near-drowning are frequently hypothermic and their body temperature must be closely monitored. The degree of hypothermia depends not only on the temperature of the water from which patients are retrieved, but also on the amount of insulation provided by their clothing. Several methods of rewarming patients with hypothermia have been advocated (see Chapter 20). It is important to choose a technique that does not produce shivering and increase oxygen demand before the circulation has been restored.

ADDITIONAL MEASURES

Administration of *steroids* is not recommended in near-drowning since they do not appear to limit the pulmonary abnormality (Calderwood *et al.*, 1975) and may inhibit lung healing.

Although the use of *prophylactic antibiotics* has been advocated by some authorities, it is generally considered preferable to perform frequent bacteriological investigations and treat only established infections.

PROGNOSIS

The proportion of victims who survive with normal cerebral function following near-drowning varies considerably in retrospective studies. Factors associated with a good outcome are listed in **Table 10.5**.

Conversely, factors reported to influence outcome adversely include:

- prolonged submersion;
- delay in initiating effective cardiopulmonary resuscitation;
- severe metabolic acidosis (pH < 7.1);
- asystole on arrival in hospital;
- fixed, dilated pupils;
- a low Glasgow Coma Score (< 5).

None of these predictors is infallible, however, and survival with normal cerebral function has been reported even in apparently hopeless cases. For children who are comatose on arrival at the hospital, up to 40% can be expected to survive with normal cerebral function, 30% will die, and the remainder will survive with moderate to severe brain damage. For

Table 10.5 Factors associated with a good outcome from near-drowning
Children
Females
Water temperature < 10°C
Duration of submersion < 10 minutes
No aspiration
Time to effective basic life support < 10 minutes
Rapid return of spontaneous cardiac output on arrival in the Emergency Department
Core temperature < 33°C
Minimum blood pH > 7.1
Blood glucose < 11.2 mmol/L
Glasgow Coma Scale > 6
Pupillary responses present

comatose adults, the mortality is broadly comparable, although survival with impaired brain function is less likely. Since outcome appears to be largely dependent on the extent of irreversible brain damage, prevention of drowning accidents must remain the highest priority.

CRUSH INJURIES

TRAUMATIC RHABDOMYOLYSIS AND COMPARTMENT SYNDROME

Crush syndrome or traumatic rhabdomyolysis refers to the clinical effects caused by a significant mass of injured muscle that may precipitate acute renal failure if untreated. The syndrome is caused by a combination of direct muscle injury, muscle ischaemia and muscle cell death with release of myoglobin, most often as a result of prolonged continuous pressure on the limbs or torso. Acute renal failure following crush injuries was reported during the London blitz during the Second World War (Bywaters and Beall, 1941) although the incidence of rhabdomyolysis after the attacks on the New York World Trade Center in 2001 was low (Goldfarb and Chung, 2002), perhaps reflecting the high fatality rate. Similarly, no cases of acute renal failure were reported after the South-east Asian tsunami in 2004, probably because all victims who were crushed subsequently drowned. Mass disasters such as earthquakes may, however, involve numerous casualties with crush injuries and crush-related acute renal failure (Sever et al., 2006). Rhabdomyolysis can also be induced by ischaemia/reperfusion, overuse of skeletal muscle (e.g. marathon running, prolonged seizures), hyperthermia, poisoning, alcohol, infections (e.g. viral) or drugs (e.g. theophyllines, statins) and the risk is increased by

metabolic disturbances (e.g. hypokalaemia, hypophosphataemia) (Lane and Phillips, 2003).

PATHOGENESIS

Crush syndrome is a consequence of the destruction of muscle tissue, leading to an efflux of myoglobin, potassium, calcium and phosphate into the circulation. Systemic release of muscle constituents is normally delayed until the limbs have been extricated, decompressed or revascularized. Direct compression of muscle is aetiologically important in many patients with rhabdomyolysis, although a similar situation may arise following temporary interruption of the vascular supply to a limb.

The microvascular damage induced by ischaemia and reperfusion, and the resulting interstitial oedema, is thought to have an important role in the pathogenesis of skeletal muscle crush injury (Odeh, 1991). Since many muscles are enclosed by a sheath of tight fascia, the development of oedema and swelling is associated with a marked increase in intracompartmental pressure. This may in turn lead to ischaemic necrosis, nerve compression and rhabdomyolysis (compartment syndrome).

Acute renal failure in rhabdomyolysis results from renal vasoconstricton, intraluminal myoglobin cast formation, tubular obstruction by uric acid crystals and haem protein nephrotoxicity.

CLINICAL FEATURES

Typically the patient has suffered some form of entrapment or compression injury. Following extrication and decompression, the crush syndrome is characterized by hypovolaemic shock and hyperkalaemia, and, unless preventive measures are instituted early, usually precipitates acute renal failure. Massive rhabdomyolysis may also be associated with disseminated intravascular coagulation, life-threatening haemorrhage, acute cardiomyopathy and multiple-organ failure. Hyperkalaemia may precipitate fatal cardiac arrhythmias.

Compartment syndromes usually develop over a period of several hours. They may be initiated by crush injuries, closed or open fractures or sustained compression of an extremity in a comatose patient, or may follow restoration of blood flow to a previously ischaemic extremity.

The signs and symptoms of compartment syndrome are:

- pain, which is typically increased by passively stretching involved muscles;
- decreased sensation within the area of the involved compartment;
- tense swelling of the limb;
- weakness or paralysis of involved muscles.

DIAGNOSIS

The serum creatine phosphokinase level is elevated to more than five times the upper-normal limit (in the absence of myocardial infarction). There may be visible myoglobinuria (tea or cola-coloured urine). Myoglobinuria can also be inferred by a positive urine dipstick for haem in the absence of red cells on microscopic examination. The serum potassium can be markedly elevated. Hypocalcaemia may also occur as a consequence of calcium binding by damaged muscle proteins and phosphate. Intracompartmental pressure can be measured by inserting a hypodermic needle connected to a transduced manometer line. Pressures greater than 35 mmHg are considered to be abnormal.

MANAGEMENT

Aggressive fluid resuscitation is essential (Better and Stein, 1990). In extensive traumatic rhabdomyolysis, it is quite common to sequester huge volumes of fluid in the damaged muscle. Inadequate replacement of these losses, which are often compounded by haemorrhage, will increase the risk of acute renal failure. Sometimes, bleeding can only be controlled by amputating the affected limb.

The management and prevention of renal insufficiency in patients with rhabdomyolysis are discussed elsewhere (Chapter 13). Administration of *mannitol* and *alkalinization of the urine* are the mainstays of treatment. When renal failure ensues despite these measures, dialysis will be required.

Prompt recognition of the compartment syndrome is essential. If there are symptoms or a suspicion of a compartment syndrome all potentially constricting circumferential dressings or casts must be removed. If there is not a prompt symptomatic improvement, *fasciotomy* must be performed to release tight muscle compartments before necrosis ensues. Decompressive fasciotomy may have to be combined with excision of necrotic tissue and may not avert amputation of the affected limb.

OUTCOME

Provided the cause of the rhabdomyolysis is identified, and is reversible, outcome may be good. Indeed, one of the most effective tools for decreasing the death toll after disasters is successful treatment of the crush syndrome and related acute renal failure.

 FAT EMBOLISM SYNDROME (Mellor and Soni, 2001)

FES is a collection of respiratory, haematological and cutaneous symptoms and signs associated with trauma as well as other unrelated conditions. No single theory satisfactorily explains all the pathophysiological features of FES. Embolism of fat may occur during orthopaedic procedures, as identified by transoesophageal echocardiography without clinical sequelae. The reported incidence of the clinical syndrome is low (< 1%) (Bulger *et al.*, 1997).

CLINICAL FEATURES

Presentation may be fulminating with pulmonary and systemic embolization, right ventricular insufficiency and car-

Table 10.6 Features of fat embolism syndrome
Major criteria
Petechial rash
Respiratory symptoms and signs – tachypnoea, dyspnoea, bilateral inspiratory crepitations, haemoptysis
Neurological signs – confusion, drowsiness, coma
Minor criteria
Tachycardia (> 120 beats/min)
Pyrexia (> 39.4°C)
Retinal changes – fat or petechiae
Jaundice
Anuria or oliguria
Laboratory features
Thrombocytopenia (> 50% decrease)
Sudden decrease in haemoglobin level (> 20% decrease)
High erythrocyte sedimentation rate (> 71 mm/h)
Fat macroglobulinaemia

diorespiratory collapse. More usually the onset is gradual with hypoxaemia, neurological symptoms, fever and a petechial rash.

DIAGNOSIS

It has been suggested that the use of major and minor features would provide a consistent and reliable standard for diagnosis of FES (**Table 10.6**). The presence of any one major plus four minor criteria in addition to fat macroglobulinaemia consitutes the syndrome (Gurd and Wilson, 1974).

MANAGEMENT

Treatment is non-specific and supportive, and aims to minimize hypovolaemia, hypoxaemia and repetitive embolization (e.g. by early operative stabilization of fractures). No adjunctive medical treatments have been demonstrated to be effective in this self-limiting condition.

RELATIONSHIP OF FAT EMBOLISM SYNDROME AND BONE MARROW NECROSIS TO MULTIPLE-ORGAN FAILURE FROM OTHER CAUSES

FES shares many of the features of the systemic inflammatory response syndrome (see Chapter 5), as well as multiple-organ failure associated with other conditions, such as soft-tissue injury, burns not involving bone marrow, trauma, hepatic necrosis and fatty liver (where fat embolization from damaged hepatocytes may be involved). Acute pancreatitis and altitude sickness have also been associated with FES. Both propofol and total parenteral nutrition involving lipid infusions have been reported to be associated with respiratory failure, but without all the features of FES. FES is, however, recognized as part of sickle-cell crisis when complicated by *acute chest syndrome*.

Bone marrow necrosis also occurs in a wide variety of other conditions such as bacterial infections (Bulvik *et al.*, 1995) and can be associated with coagulopathy. Fat and bone marrow necrosis might, therefore, be implicated in the genesis of acute lung injury, shock and multiple organ dysfunction complicating general critical illness (Rae *et al.*, 1994).

COMPLICATIONS OF TRAUMA

Systemic inflammation accompanies extensive tissue injury, surgical excision of necrotic tissue and fat embolism, as well as the process of wound repair. Complications serve to amplify the original inflammatory injury and its consequences. The goal of trauma management is to limit the extent of these systemic insults by rapid resuscitation and timely, effective surgical intervention. There is some evidence to suggest that the risk of death is significantly reduced when care is provided in a trauma centre (MacKenzie *et al.*, 2006) (see Chapter 21).

Intensive care management of the trauma patient should be viewed as a continuation of measures initiated by the emergency services for patients at high risk of organ failure. Monitoring, interpretation and treatment of acute physiological changes accompanying haemorrhagic shock, reperfusion injury and compartment syndrome may influence the subsequent development of multiple-organ dysfunction. Controversially there is some retrospective evidence to suggest that for severely injured patients who arrive in severe shock, and in the elderly, the use of a pulmonary artery catheter may improve survival (Friese *et al.*, 2006) (see Chapter 4). Causes of death following trauma include not only hypovolaemic shock but also acute lung injury, disseminated intravascular coagulation, tachyarrhythmias, cardiac failure, acute renal failure, electrolyte disturbances and sepsis. Survivors may experience significant psychological trauma, whilst limb compartment syndromes may be complicated by permanent paralysis or necrosis, which can lead to a form of Volkmann's ischaemic contracture or gangrene.

REFERENCES

Ansorrimo M, Hemsley C (2004) ABC of burns: intensive care management and control of infection. *British Medical Journal* 329: 220–223.

Baud FJ, Barriot P, Toffis V, et al. (1991) Elevated blood cyanide concentrations in victims of smoke inhalation. *New England Journal of Medicine* 325: 1761–1766.

Better OS, Stein JH (1990) Early management of shock and prophylaxis of acute renal failure in traumatic rhabdomyolysis. *New England Journal of Medicine* 322: 825–829.

Bickell WH, Wall MJ Jr, Pepe PE, et al. (1994) Immediate versus delayed fluid resuscitation for hypotensive patients with penetrating torso injuries. *New England Journal of Medicine* 331: 1105–1109.

Bracken MB, Shepard MJ, Holford TR, et al. (1997) Administration of methylprednisolone for 24 or 48 hours or tirilazad mesylate for 48 hours in the treatment of acute spinal cord injury. Results of the Third National Acute Spinal Cord Randomised Controlled Trial. National Acute Spinal Cord Injury Study. *Journal of the American Medical Association* 277: 1597–1604.

Brohi K, Healy M, Fotheringham T, et al. (2005) Helical computed tomographic scanning for the evaluation of the cervical spine in the unconscious intubated trauma patient. *Journal of Trauma Injury, Infection and Critical Care* 58: 897–901.

Brohi K, Cohen MJ, Ganter MT, et al. (2007) Acute traumatic coagulopathy: initiated by hypoperfusion. Modulated through the protein C pathway? *Annals of Surgery* 245: 812–818.

Bulger EM, Smith DG, Maier RV, et al. (1997) Fat embolism syndrome: a 10-year review. *Archives of Surgery* 132: 435–439.

Bullock R, Teasdale G, Swann I (2000) Head injuries. In: Driscoll P, Skinner D, Earlam R (eds) *ABC of Major Trauma*, 3rd edn. BMJ Publications: London, p. 4.

Bulvik SAI, Ross S, Jacobs D (1995) Extensive bone marrow necrosis associated with antiphospholipid antibodies. *American Journal of Medicine* 98: 572–574.

Bywaters EGL, Beall D (1941) Crush injuries with impairment of renal function. *British Medical Journal* I: 427–432.

Calderwood HW, Modell JH, Ruiz BC (1975) The ineffectiveness of steroid therapy for treatment of fresh-water near-drowning. *Anesthesiology* 43: 642–650.

Clarke CJ, Campbell D, Reid WH (1981) Blood carboxyhaemoglobin and cyanide levels in fire survivors. *Lancet* i: 1332–1335.

Coats TJ, Davies G (2002) Prehospital care for road traffic casualties. *British Medical Journal* 324: 1135–1138.

Cope A, Stebbings W (2000) Abdominal trauma. In: Driscoll P, Skinner D, Earlam R (eds) *ABC of Major Trauma*, 3rd edn. BMJ Publications: London, p. 4.

Criswell JC, Parr MJA, Nolan JP (1994) Emergency airway management in patients with cervical spine injuries. *Anaesthesia* 49: 900–903.

Demling RH, LaLonde C (1990) Identification and modification of the pulmonary and systemic inflammatory and biochemical changes caused by a skin burn. *Journal of Trauma* 30: 557–562.

DePalma RG, Burris DG, Champion HR, et al. (2005) Blast injuries. *New England Journal of Medicine* 352: 1335–1342.

Desai MH, Micak R, Richardson J, et al. (1998) Reduction in mortality in pediatric patients with inhalation injury with aerosolised heparin/acetylcystine therapy. *Journal of Burn Care and Rehabilitation* 19: 210–212.

Dittmann M, Steenblock U, Kränzlin M, et al. (1982) Epidural analgesia or mechanical ventilation for multiple rib fractures? *Intensive Care Medicine* 8: 89–92.

Driscoll P, Skinner D (2000a) Initial assessment and management-I: primary survey and resuscitation. In: Driscoll P, Skinner D, Earlam R (eds) *ABC of Major Trauma*, 3rd edn. BMJ Publications: London, p. 2.

Driscoll P, Skinner D (2000b) Initial assessment and management-II: the secondary survey. In: Driscoll P, Skinner D, Earlam R (eds) *ABC of Major Trauma*, 3rd edn. BMJ Publications: London, p. 2.

Friese RS, Shafi S, Gentilello LM (2006) Pulmonary artery catheter use is associated with reduced mortality in severely injured patients: A national Trauma Data Bank analysis of 53,312 patients. *Critical Care Medicine* 34: 1597–1601.

Galan G, Penalver JC, Paris F, et al. (1992) Blunt chest injuries in 1696 patients. *European Journal of Cardiothoracic Surgery* 6: 284–287.

Gallagher G, Rae CP, Kinsella J (2000) Treatment of pain in severe burns. *American Journal of Clinical Dermatology* 1: 329–335.

Golden F St C, Tipton MJ, Scott RC (1997) Immersion, near-drowning and drowning. *British Journal of Anaesthesia* 79: 214–225.

Goldfarb DS, Chung S (2002) The absence of rhabdomyolysis-induced renal failure following the World Trade Center collapse. *American Journal of Medicine* 113: 260.

Gurd AR, Wilson RI (1974) The fat embolism syndrome. *British Journal of Bone and Joint Surgery* 56B: 408–416.

Herndon DN, Ziegler ST (1993) Bacterial translocation after thermal injury. *Critical Care Medicine* 21: S50–S54.

Holmes JF, Akkinepalli R (2005) Computed tomography versus plain radiography to screen for cervical spine injury: a meta-analysis. *Journal of Trauma Injury, Infection and Critical Care* 58: 902–905.

Johnson PG (1978) The management of spinal injuries. In: Hanson GC, Wright PL (eds) *The Medical Management of the Critically Ill*, pp. 412–429. Academic Press: London.

Karmakar MK, Ho AM-H (2003) Acute pain management in patients with multiple fractured ribs. *Journal of Trauma-Injury, Infection and Critical Care* **54**: 615–625.

Lane R, Phillips M (2003) Rhabdomyolysis. *British Medical Journal* **327**: 115–116.

MacKenzie EJ, Rivara FP, Jurkovich GJ, et al. (2006) A national evaluation of the effect of trauma-center care on mortality. *New England Journal of Medicine* **354**: 366–378.

Mellor A, Soni N (2001) Fat embolism. *Anaesthesia* **56**: 145–154.

Modell JH (1993) Drowning. *New England Journal of Medicine* **328**: 253–256.

Modell JH, Graves SA, Ketover A (1976) Clinical course of 91 consecutive near-drowning victims. *Chest* **70**: 231–238.

Monafo WW (1996) Initial management of burns. *New England Journal of Medicine* **335**: 1581–1586.

Morris CG, McCoy W, Lavery GG (2004) Spinal immobilisation for unconscious patients with multiple injuries. *British Medical Journal* **329**: 495–499.

Muir I (1981) The use of the Mount Vernon formula in the treatment of burn shock. *Intensive Care Medicine* **7**: 49–53.

Navar PD, Saffle JR, Warden GD (1985) Effect of inhalational injury on fluid resuscitation requirements after thermal injury. *American Journal of Surgery* **150**: 716–720.

Nussbaum E, Maggi JC (1988) Pentobarbital therapy does not improve neurological outcome in nearly drowning, flaccid-comatose children. *Paediatrics* **81**: 630–634.

Odeh M (1991) The role of reperfusion-induced injury in the pathogenesis of the crush syndrome. *New England Journal of Medicine* **324**: 1417–1422.

Pepe PE (2003) Shock in polytrauma. *British Medical Journal* **327**: 1119–1120.

Pretre R, Chilcott M (1997) Blunt trauma to the heart and great vessels. *New England Journal of Medicine* **336**: 626–632.

Rae D, Porter J, Beechey-Newman N, et al. (1994) Type I prophoospholipase AZ propeptide in acute lung injury. *Lancet* **344**: 1472–1473.

Ramey CA, Ramey DN, Hayward JS (1987) Dive response of children in relation to cold-water near-drowning. *Journal of Applied Physiology* **63**: 665–668.

Rankine J, Nicholson D, Driscoll P (2000) Radiological assessment. In: Driscoll P, Skinner D, Earlam R (eds) *ABC of Major Trauma,* 3rd edn. BMJ Publications: London, p. 6.

Rawe SE, Perot PL Jr (1979) Pressor response resulting from experimental contusion injury to the spinal cord. *Journal of Neurosurgery* **50**: 58–63.

Robertson C, Fenton O (2000) Management of severe burns. In: Driscoll P, Skinner D, Earlam R (eds) *ABC of Major Trauma,* 3rd edn. BMJ Publications: London, p. 17.

Rooney SJ, Hyde JAJ, Graham TR (2000) Chest injuries. In: Driscoll P, Skinner D, Earlam R (eds) *ABC of Major Trauma,* 3rd edn. BMJ Publications: London, p. 3.

Rossiter ND, Hodgetts T, Ryan J, et al. (2000a) Blast and gunshot/missile injuries. In: Driscoll P, Skinner D, Earlam R (eds) *ABC of Major Trauma,* 3rd edn. BMJ Publications: London.

Rossiter NJ, Willett KM, Ross R, et al. (2000b) Limb injuries. In: Driscoll P, Skinner D, Earlam R (eds) *ABC of Major Trauma,* 3rd edn. BMJ Publications: London, p. 8.

Sever MS, Vanholder R, Lameire N (2006) Management of crush-related injuries after disasters. *New England Journal of Medicine* **327**: 115–116.

Siebke H, Breivik H, Rod T, et al. (1975) Survival after 40 minutes' submersion without cerebral sequelae. *Lancet* **i**: 1275–1277.

Smith MD, Cassidy JM, Souther S, et al. (1995) Transesophageal echocardiography in the diagnosis of traumatic rupture of the aorta. *New England Journal of Medicine* **332**: 356–362.

Snow JC, Kripke BJ, Sessions GP, et al. (1973) Cardiovascular collapse following succinylcholine in a paraplegic patient. *Paraplegia* **11**: 199–204.

Soar J, Deakin CD, Nolan JP, et al. (2005) European Resuscitation Council Guidelines for Resuscitation 2005, section 7: cardiac arrest in special circumstances. *Resuscitation* **67** (Suppl. 1): S135-S170.

Spahn DR, Tucci MA, Makris M (2005) Is recombinant FVIIa the magic bullet in the treatment of major bleeding? *British Journal of Anaesthesia* **94**: 553–555.

Swain A, Dove J, Baker H (2000) The spine and spinal cord. In: Driscoll P, Skinner D, Earlam R (eds) *ABC of Major Trauma,* 3rd edn. BMJ Publications: London, p. 25.

Tai NRM, Boffard KD (2003) Thoracic trauma: principles of early management. *Trauma* **5**: 123–136.

Trinkle JK, Richardson JD, Franz JL, et al. (1975) Management of flail chest without mechanical ventilation. *Annals of Thoracic Surgery* **19**: 355–363.

Trunkey DD (1983) Trauma. *Scientific American* **249**: 28–35.

Trunkey DD (1991) Initial treatment of patients with extensive trauma. *New England Journal of Medicine* **324**: 1259–1263.

Watson D (2000) The upper airway. In: Driscoll P, Skinner D, Earlam R (eds) *ABC of Major Trauma,* 3rd edn. BMJ Publications: London, p. 2.

Webb AK (1978) Flail chest: management and complications. *British Journal of Hospital Medicine* **20**: 406–412.

Welply NC, Mathias CJ, Frankel HL (1975) Circulatory reflexes in tetraplegics during artificial ventilation and general anaesthesia. *Paraplegia* **13**: 172–182.

Wilmore DW, Long JM, Mason AD Jr, et al. (1974) Catecholamines: mediator of the hypermetabolic response to thermal injury. *Annals of Surgery* **180**: 653–669.

Wilmore DW, Mason AD Jr, Johnson DW, et al. (1975) Effect of ambient temperature on heat production and heat loss in burn patients. *Journal of Applied Physiology* **38**: 593–597.

11 General aspects of managing critically ill patients

FLUID AND ELECTROLYTE BALANCE
(Lobo, 2004)

PHYSIOLOGICAL BACKGROUND

In normal individuals water constitutes 45–60% of lean body weight, depending on age, sex and body build, the proportion being greater in men and infants and less in the obese. Approximately two-thirds of body water is contained within the *intracellular* compartment, the remainder being extracellular fluid (ECF) distributed between the *interstitial* space (two-thirds) and the *vascular* space (one-third). There is also a fourth *transcellular* compartment, which includes water in the gut as well as cerebrospinal, synovial, pericardial and pleural fluid (**Fig. 11.1**). Although in health this compartment is small, it may become important in disease (e.g. in those with bowel obstruction in whom as much as 6 litres of water may be pooled in the gut and therefore lost from the ECF). In addition small amounts of water are contained in bone and dense connective tissue.

Each of these spaces has a unique function and composition, the distribution of water between the compartments depending on the osmotic equilibrium between them, the osmotic pressure exerted by non-diffusible plasma proteins (the colloid osmotic pressure: see Chapter 3) and the Gibbs–Donnan equilibrium (which requires that the products of diffusible ions on each side of a semipermeable membrane must be equal). The latter explains the unequal distribution of diffusible ions on either side of a semipermeable membrane when one side contains poorly diffusible ions such as the electrical charge on protein molecules. Allowing for the Gibbs–Donnan distribution and the plasma colloid osmotic pressure, the electrolyte content of plasma and interstitial fluid is essentially the same, whereas the composition of the intracellular fluid (ICF) differs considerably from the other two. Due to the operation of cellular pumps (e.g. Na^+/K^+ ATPase), sodium and chloride ions are largely extracellular, whereas potassium is the dominant intracellular cation, balanced by phosphate, sulphate and bicarbonate anions, as well as protein (**Table 11.1a**). The equilibrium between the intravascular and interstitial compartments is determined by the pore size in the capillary membrane, the relative concentration of proteins on either side of the membrane and the capillary hydrostatic pressure.

REGULATION OF EXTRACELLULAR VOLUME

The extracellular volume is controlled by the sodium concentration, which is regulated primarily by the kidneys. Renal conservation of sodium is very efficient but the kidneys have a limited capacity to excrete excess sodium (perhaps because evolving mammals have rarely been exposed to high sodium concentrations). It is believed that the effective arterial blood volume (EABV) is the most important determinant of renal sodium and water excretion; when EABV is expanded urinary sodium excretion is increased and may exceed 100 mmol/L, whilst sodium losses can be almost eliminated when EABV is severely depleted, provided kidney function is normal. These alterations in sodium excretion can result from changes in both the filtered load (determined largely by the glomerular filtration rate (GFR)) and tubular reabsorption. Neurohumoral regulation of extracellular volume is mediated by volume receptors which sense changes in the EABV, rather than changes in sodium concentration:

- *Extrarenal receptors* (located in the left atrium, major thoracic veins, carotid sinus and aortic arch) respond to slight reductions in effective circulating volume by increasing sympathetic nervous activity and circulating catecholamine levels, whilst volume receptors in the cardiac atria control the release of atrial natriuretic peptide (ANP) from granules in the atrial walls.
- *Intrarenal receptors* in the walls of the afferent glomerular arterioles respond, via the juxtaglomerular apparatus, to changes in renal perfusion and control the activity of the renin–angiotensin–aldosterone system. Renin release from the juxtaglomerular cells is also influenced by the sodium concentration in the distal tubule and sympathetic nervous activity. Prostaglandins I_2 and E_2 are also produced within the kidney in response to angiotensin II, thereby modulating the degree of sodium retention by maintaining GFR and sodium and water excretion.

Normal day-to-day adjustments in sodium excretion are mediated by aldosterone, and possibly ANP, with high-pressure arterial receptors (carotid, aortic arch, juxtaglomerular apparatus) being more important than low-pressure volume receptors (cardiac atria, right ventricle, thoracic veins, pulmonary vasculature). When there is more significant hypovolaemia, increased sympathetic activity causes a reduction in GFR and enhances proximal and thin ascending limb sodium reabsorption, both directly and by stimulating the secretion of renin–angiotensin II and the non-osmotic release of antidiuretic hormone (ADH). Marked, persistent hypovolaemia associated with hypotension leads to increased salt and water absorption in the proximal tubules and ascending limb of Henle, perhaps mediated by changes in renal interstitial hydrostatic pressure and local production of nitric oxide and prostaglandins.

In *oedematous conditions* such as cardiac failure, liver cirrhosis and hypoalbuminaemia salt and water are retained despite the increased extracellular volume, probably as a consequence of arterial underfilling due to a reduction in cardiac output or peripheral vasodilatation. The unloading of arterial volume receptors leads to activation of the sympathetic nervous and serum–angiotensin–aldosterone systems, as well as the release of ADH. Whereas normally the increased delivery of sodium to the site of action of aldosterone in the collecting ducts limits the degree of sodium retention, this mechanism fails in those with oedematous states, probably largely because sodium delivery to the collecting duct remains markedly reduced. Such patients therefore respond to spironolactone with a large natriuresis.

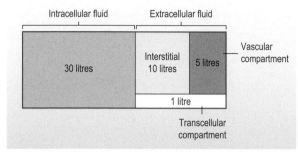

Fig. 11.1 Distribution of body water in a 75-kg man.

Table 11.1a Electrolyte composition of intracellular and extracellular fluids			
	Plasma (mmol/L)	Interstitial fluid (mmol/L)	Intracellular fluid (mmol/L)
Na^+	142	144	10
K^+	4	4	160
Ca^{2+}	2.5	2.5	1.5
Mg^{2+}	1	0.5	13
Cl^-	102	114	2
HCO_3^-	26	30	8
PO_4^{2-}	1	1	57
SO_4^{2-}	0.5	0.5	10
Organic acid	3	4	3
Protein	16	0	55

Table 11.1b Composition of commonly prescribed crystalloids				
	NaCl (9 g/L)	Hartmann's	NaCl (1.8 g/L)-dextrose (40 g/L)	Dextrose (50 g/L)
Na^+ (mmol/L)	154	131	31	0
Cl (mmol/L)	154	111	31	0
$Na^+:Cl^-$	1:1	1.18:1	1:1	–
K^+ (mmol/L)	0	5	0	0
HCO_3^- (mmol/L)	0	29	0	0
Ca^{2+} (mmol/L)	0	4	0	0
Glucose (mmol/L)	0	0	222.2 (40 g)	277.8 (50 g)
pH	5.0	6.5	4.5	4.0
Osmolality (mOsm/L)	308	274	286	280

REGULATION OF WATER EXCRETION

Total body water is regulated by *thirst* and by *intracellular osmoreceptors* (mainly located in the hypothalamus), the *renin–angiotensin* system and, to some extent, *volume receptors* in capacitance vessels close to the heart. The osmoreceptors sense changes in the plasma sodium concentration and osmolality and influence both thirst and the release of ADH from the supraoptic and paraventricular nuclei. ADH acts on V_2 (vasopressin) receptors causing preformed cytoplasmic vesicles that contain unique water channels (*aquaporins*) to move to and be inserted into the luminal membrane. These aquaporins span the luminal membrane and permit movement of water across the cells down a favourable osmotic gradient. As the effect of ADH diminishes the aquaporins aggregate within clathrin-coated pits, from which they are removed from the luminal membrane by endocytosis and returned to the cytoplasm. Defects in this mechanism can lead to *nephrogenic diabetes insipidus*.

It is important to appreciate that volume regulation and osmoregulation operate independently (for example, in response to a saline load or in the syndrome of inappropriate ADH secretion), although both systems may be activated simultaneously. In general maintenance of volume always takes precedence over maintenance of osmolality. Also ADH secretion may occur in response to non osmotic stimuli such as stress and a marked reduction in circulating volume. Under these circumstances ADH may cause vasoconstriction through stimulation of V_1 (vasopressin) receptors.

GENERAL PRINCIPLES OF FLUID AND ELECTROLYTE MANAGEMENT

The average water requirement for a normal adult is 20–60 mL/kg per day. In most intensive care patients, however, the stress response promotes sodium and water retention, a tendency that is exacerbated by mechanical ventilation (see Chapter 7), while in those breathing humidified gases, insensible losses are approximately half the estimated normal 500–900 mL/day. In many patients there is also a degree of renal dysfunction, which further impairs their ability to excrete a salt and water load. It must also be remembered that normal oxidation of food produces significant volumes of water (0.41, 0.60 and 1.07 mL of water/g of protein, carbohydrate and fat, respectively). Critically ill patients are therefore particularly susceptible to salt and water overload and, especially when combined with an increase in vascular permeability and hypoproteinaemia (see Chapter 3), they are at considerable risk of developing pulmonary and peripheral oedema. The latter may compromise tissue oxygenation and impede microcirculatory flow, as well as reducing lymphatic drainage, thereby further exacerbating accumulation of oedema fluid. Salt and water excess may also delay both gastric emptying and small intestinal transit, whereas oedema of the limbs can inhibit mobilization and compromise neuromuscular function.

Potassium excretion is usually increased in the critically ill as a consequence of muscle breakdown and the actions of mineralocorticoids, so that total body potassium is reduced, often in the presence of a normal serum potassium concentration. On refeeding serum potassium levels fall as potassium re-enters the cells (see later in this chapter).

Some degree of fluid restriction with reduced sodium intake is therefore usually necessary, and potassium supplements are normally required. As a guide the daily requirements for an adult critically ill patient who is not eating can be calculated as:

Water = 40 mL/kg per day (e.g. for an 80-kg patient = 2.5 litres/day)

Sodium = 1 mmol/kg per day (e.g. for a 70-kg patient = 70 mmol/day)

Potassium = 1–1.5 mmol/kg per day (e.g. for a 70-kg patient = 70–105 mmol/day)

In order to avoid ketosis the patient will also require:

Glucose (dextrose) = 2–4 g/kg per day (e.g. for a 70-kg patient = 140–280 g/day).

For an 80-kg patient a suitable regime for routine maintenance might, therefore, consist of 3 litres of 0.18% NaCl (30 mmol/litre) in 4% glucose (40 g/litre) and 0.2% KCl (27 mmol/litre).

Additional sources of fluid and electrolytes, such as the saline used to flush intravascular catheters, as well as the high sodium content of colloid replacement fluids and the solutions used as vehicles for intravenous drugs, must also be taken into account. Conversely, some patients will be losing abnormally large volumes of fluid and electrolytes (e.g. as diarrhoea or drainage from fistulae). If the patient is pyrexial, sweating or hyperventilating with inadequate humidification, insensible losses will be increased. Urine output may be increased by diuretic therapy or by an osmotic diuresis, as may occur with hyperglycaemia. Sometimes polyuria may be the result of diabetes insipidus (e.g. complicating a head injury; see Chapters 15 and 17).

In some cases, therefore, ill-advised fluid restriction or inadequate replacement of large losses can cause significant dehydration with intravascular volume depletion and a risk of renal impairment, whereas in others excessive administration of fluid and electrolytes may lead to overhydration with 'wet lungs' and peripheral oedema.

An appropriate intravenous fluid regimen must be devised for each individual patient based on clinical assessment and experience, guided by the results of laboratory investigations. Most of the variables routinely monitored in intensive care patients, such as blood pressure, heart rate, central venous pressure (CVP) and even to some extent urine output, are largely a reflection of the volume of the intravascular space. Assessment of the interstitial and intracellular volumes is more difficult and is usually based on chest radiograph appearances and the detection of peripheral oedema on clinical examination, although invasive techniques are now available for the estimation of extravascular lung water (see Chapter 6). In some units, patients are weighed daily to assist assessment of fluid balance, although this is practically difficult and requires a meticulous technique to be accurate. Plasma urea, creatinine, electrolyte and blood sugar levels should be measured at least once a day, and sometimes more frequently. The total output of fluid as urine, gastric aspirate and from any drains, together with the total intravenous and oral input, should be calculated 12-hourly and the overall fluid balance recorded. In difficult cases it may be helpful to measure urinary urea and electrolyte concentrations, as well as plasma and urinary osmolalities and the electrolyte content of the gastric aspirate and any drainage fluid. The total input and output of each individual constituent can then be calculated.

The differential distribution of body water between the four compartments, and of sodium and chloride between the intracellular and extracellular spaces, has important implications when selecting an appropriate intravenous fluid regime. Intravenous infusion of the inappropriately called 'normal', 'physiological' or 'isotonic' (0.9%) saline primarily expands the extracellular compartment and, because this solution contains 154 mmol sodium/litre there is a small increase in the osmolality of the ECF, which causes a slight shift of fluid into the vascular space. In practice isotonic sodium containing fluids expand the circulating volume by only about 20–25%, the remainder being sequestered in the interstitial space. Administration of Hartmann's solution, which is more physiological than the slightly hyperosmolar 0.9% saline (**Table 11.1**), is associated with a larger diuresis, perhaps because, being of lower osmolality, the ADH response to the administration of this crystalloid is less pronounced. Despite its lower sodium content excretion of sodium is also greater following the administration of Hartmann's solution, an observation that may be partly explained by the higher concentration of chloride ions, and ratio of chloride to sodium ions, in 0.9% saline which can cause renal vasoconstriction and a reduction in GFR. Moreover the kidneys are slow to excrete a chloride load and the hyperchloraemia caused by the administration of large volumes of 0.9% saline can precipitate a persistent metabolic acidosis (see Chapter 6). Also 0.9% saline does not contain a number of other important mineral and organic constituents of plasma and cannot, therefore, be considered to be a 'physiological' solution. For these reasons most now recommend the use of Hartmann's solution in preference to 0.9% saline for re-expansion of the ECF and vascular space.

Administration of 0.18% saline in glucose 4% reduces the osmolality of the ECF, water moves into the cells until a new osmolar equilibrium is established and the increase in ECF volume is considerably less than that achieved with 0.9% saline or Hartmann's solution. When dextrose solutions are administered they are distributed throughout the total body water according to the relative volumes of the various compartments; consequently only about one-tenth of the infused volume remains in the intravascular space.

Finally colloidal solutions are normally confined to the intravascular space, at least initially, and have traditionally been considered to be the most effective solutions for expanding the circulating volume, although their distribution varies depending on the colloid used and can be profoundly influenced by changes in vascular permeability (see Chapters 3 and 5).

Fortunately, patients are generally surprisingly tolerant of what are inevitably rather crude attempts to control their fluid and electrolyte balance, particularly when the kidneys are functioning normally. Nevertheless, if the basic principles of management are not understood, or careless mistakes are made, serious abnormalities will result.

The important constituents to be considered are water, sodium, potassium and magnesium. There may be an excess or deficit of each, either singly or in combination.

WATER DEPLETION
Causes
Water depletion rarely occurs in isolation since it is usually combined with some degree of sodium loss. Predominant water depletion may occur if:

- intake is inadequate;
- there are excessive losses of hypotonic fluid (diabetes insipidus, diarrhoea, sweating, hyperventilation).

Diagnosis
Losses of water are initially distributed evenly throughout the body compartments. Once the deficit is severe enough to cause a decreased circulating volume, aldosterone is released, causing renal retention of sodium. Because of the osmotic effect of the increase in plasma sodium concentration, water then leaves the cells and there is a reduction in tissue turgor. The patient is oliguric with a concentrated urine. Plasma sodium is increased, plasma urea is slightly increased and plasma osmolality is normal or increased. The haematocrit rises only in the later stages of water depletion.

Treatment
5% dextrose or, if, as is more usual, sodium has been lost as well, 0.18% saline in dextrose 4% should be administered intravenously. The management of diabetes insipidus is discussed in Chapter 17 (see also section on treatment of hypernatraemia, below).

WATER INTOXICATION
Causes
Water intoxication is *usually iatrogenic* and caused by excessive intravenous administration of hypotonic solutions (e.g. 5% dextrose) in the presence of a reduced ability to excrete water, often caused by *increased levels of ADH* in response to stress (e.g. perioperatively) or in association with an 'inappropriate' secretion of ADH. It may also complicate *absorption of irrigation fluid* during urological surgery.

Diagnosis
Plasma sodium is low, often less than 120 mmol/L. Acute severe water intoxication can cause confusion which may

progress to convulsions and coma (see also Hyponatraemia, below).

Treatment

Mild water intoxication can be treated simply by restriction of intake (to 1000 mL or even 500 mL per day); in more severe cases 0.9% saline or occasionally hypertonic saline may be required (see section on treatment of hyponatraemia, below). If renal function is impaired, hypertonic saline may be dangerous and dialysis will be required. In some patients with inappropriate ADH secretion, fluid restriction alone may be insufficient and in such cases drugs that antagonize ADH (e.g. *demeclocycline*) may be used to induce nephrogenic diabetes insipidus.

HYPONATRAEMIA
Causes and clinical features

A low plasma sodium (< 135 mmol/L) can be caused by *water intoxication*, or by *depletion of total body sodium*, although changes in plasma sodium are usually a reflection of changes in water rather than sodium balance. Some commonly encountered causes and contributing factors are:

- diuretic therapy;
- psychogenic polydipsia (a common cause of hyponatraemia, but a rare cause of admission to the intensive care unit (ICU));
- renal disease;
- cardiac failure;
- end-stage liver disease;
- fluid losses from the alimentary tract or intra-abdominal drains;
- syndrome of inappropriate ADH.

Hyponatraemia is often precipitated by the use of *hypotonic intravenous fluids* (e.g. 5% dextrose, 0.18% saline in dextrose 4%) to replace isotonic losses (e.g. from the alimentary tract) or to maintain blood sugar levels in hepatic insufficiency.

Despite repeated warnings (Lane and Allen, 1999) *postoperative hyponatraemia* remains common, perhaps especially in women undergoing orthopaedic surgery, and is usually attributable to the routine administration of large volumes of isotonic dextrose to patients whose ADH levels have risen in response to the stress of surgery. The risk of hyponatraemia is further increased in the elderly, in whom the ability to handle a water load is impaired, and by long-term preoperative treatment with thiazide diuretics.

Early symptoms of hyponatraemia include progressive headache, nausea, vomiting and weakness. Often the significance of these symptoms is not recognized and if not treated the patient may progress to obtundation, hallucinations, decorticate posturing, myoclonic jerks, seizures, respiratory arrest, coma and brain damage or death. Premenopausal women with hyponatraemic encephalopathy are at particular risk of developing brain damage, whereas men and postmenopausal women are far less likely to develop encephalopathy. Thus premenopausal women and children are at

risk of brain damage at sodium concentrations as high as 128 mmol/L, whereas postmenopausal women do not usually become symptomatic until sodium concentrations have fallen below 120 mmol/L, although symptoms can occur at higher levels if the rate of change is rapid.

The true nature of a cause of hyponatraemia in the critically ill, the '*sick-cell syndrome*' (Flear and Singh, 1973), is still controversial. This syndrome was thought to occur only in the most severely ill patients and was said to account for the close association between a low plasma sodium and a poor prognosis. It was postulated that a defect at cellular level, possibly a failure of the sodium pump due to an inadequate supply of energy in the form of adenosine triphosphate (ATP), causes sodium to enter the cell in exchange for potassium ions, which are then lost in the urine. An alternative explanation has been that this abnormality is simply a response to total body potassium depletion that causes intracellular hypotonia and a redistribution of body water. More recently it has been suggested that in critically ill patients intracellular solutes may leak out of the cell because of an increase in membrane permeability and that this could lead to intracellular redistribution of sodium, with an increased osmolar gap. Simultaneous correction of hyponatraemia and the osmolar gap supports this concept of the sick-cell syndrome (Guglielminotti *et al.*, 2002).

Diagnosis

In hyperlipidaemia the plasma sodium concentration may be *spuriously low* because the sodium is confined to the aqueous phase, whereas its concentration is expressed in terms of the total plasma volume. Significant sodium depletion will cause a fall in intravascular volume and stimulate the release of aldosterone. In true hyponatraemia, therefore, urinary potassium excretion increases while sodium ions are retained. In hyperlipidaemia (or 'pseudohyponatraemia') the concentration of other plasma electrolytes (potassium, chloride and bicarbonate) will also be reduced. Failure to recognize pseudohyponatraemia can have dangerous consequences (Editorial, 1980).

When the cause of hyponatraemia is not obvious it is important to exclude:

- Addison's disease;
- hypothyroidism;
- the syndrome of inappropriate ADH.

Treatment

The brain oedema and raised intracranial pressure associated with hyponatraemia can result in a number of devastating consequences, including central diabetes insipidus, cerebral infarction, cortical blindness and a permanent vegetative state. Hypoxia plays an important role in the genesis of the cerebral damage associated with hyponatraemia and neurological sequelae are almost inevitable in those who suffer a respiratory arrest. Prompt treatment, including securing the airway, ensuring adequate oxygenation and mechanical ventilation when indicated, is therefore essential.

When there are no symptoms conservative treatment, consisting of eliminating the precipitating cause, including correction of any hormone deficiency (e.g. cortisol, aldosterone, thyroid hormone), and simple water deprivation is the preferred course of action. Normal saline should be given to those who are volume-depleted. Symptomatic hyponatraemia can be treated with intravenous hypertonic sodium chloride (3%, 514 mmol/L) sometimes combined with administration of a loop diuretic such as furosemide.

Although conventionally too rapid correction of profound, chronic (> 2 days) hyponatraemia is thought to increase the risk of precipitating severe shrinkage of brain cells and *central pontine myelinolysis* (Sterns *et al.*, 1986), it seems that prompt judicious therapy with intravenous sodium chloride before the development of respiratory insufficiency is associated with better outcomes than fluid restriction alone (Ayus and Arieff, 1999). Certainly chronic symptomatic hyponatraemia in postmenopausal women can be associated with serious morbidity and mortality (Ayus and Arieff, 1999) and the risk of not correcting cerebral oedema exceeds the small risk of osmotic demyelination as a result of treatment. Nevertheless, in cases of symptomatic hyponatraemia the rise in plasma sodium should not usually exceed 1–2 mmol/h. The plasma sodium concentration should be monitored frequently (e.g. every 2 hours) and should not be allowed to increase to above about 133 mmol/L. In those with seizures and/or respiratory distress the sodium concentration should be increased more rapidly, for example by about 8–10 mmol/L over the first 4 hours in profound hyponatraemia or until cessation of seizure activity. This rate of correction can only be accomplished using hypertonic saline. Treatment with hypertonic saline should be discontinued when either the patient becomes asymptomatic or the plasma sodium reaches a concentration of between 124 and 132 mmol/L. The plasma sodium should not normally be increased by more than about 20 mmol during the initial 48 hours of treatment and as a general principle should not be rapidly increased to normal or high levels. As a guide, and assuming that water comprises 50% of total bodyweight, 1 mL/kg of 3% sodium chloride will raise the plasma sodium by 1 mmol/L.

A recent multicentre trial demonstrated that in patients with euvolaemic or hypervolaemic hyponatraemia caused by chronic heart failure, cirrhosis or the syndrome of inappropriate ADH an oral vasopressin V_2-receptor antagonist was effective in increasing serum sodium concentrations (Schrier *et al.*, 2006).

HYPERNATRAEMIA (Pavlevsky *et al.*, 1996)
Causes
Hypernatraemia (a plasma sodium > 145 mmol/L) is one of the most commonly encountered electrolyte abnormalities in the hospital population and is seen most often in situa-

tions of predominant *water depletion* (e.g. diabetic coma, diabetes insipidus, fever, elevated ambient temperature, infirmity). It may also occur in association with *salt retention* in acute renal failure and can be exacerbated by the excessive administration of sodium ions, often as isotonic saline, artificial colloids or 8.4% sodium bicarbonate.

Clinical features
Conscious level is frequently impaired and seizures are common. Associated laboratory abnormalities may include metabolic acidosis, azotaemia, hypophosphataemia and hyperglycaemia. Most patients have severe concomitant disease and hypernatraemia is associated with substantial long-term morbidity and mortality.

Treatment
Associated medical conditions must be treated as a matter of urgency. Pure water depletion should be treated with hypotonic intravenous fluids or dialysis, but rapid falls in plasma sodium greater than 2 mmol/h may precipitate cerebral oedema and must be avoided. Too rapid correction of hypernatraemia has been implicated in the morbidity and mortality of diabetic ketoacidosis (see Chapter 17). When required (e.g. following excessive administration of isotonic saline) solute removal should be accomplished by diuretic therapy or dialysis.

HYPOKALAEMIA
Causes
The normal daily intake of potassium is 50–150 mmol (1–1.5 mmol/kg per day). Hypokalaemia is usually related to *inadequate replacement of excessive urinary or gastrointestinal losses* (e.g. diarrhoea). For a number of reasons, critically ill patients are particularly prone to the development of hypokalaemia. Elevated levels of *aldosterone* are found in both cardiac and liver failure, as well as in response to stress, while *steroids* and *diuretics* also increase urinary potassium losses. Movement of potassium into cells is promoted by β_2 agonists, insulin, mineralocorticoids and theophyllines. Also potassium may be lost in the urine during the recovery phases of *acute renal failure*, and severe hypokalaemia may itself lead to tubular dysfunction. Severe vomiting may be accompanied by a hypochloraemic alkalosis which leads to a shift of potassium into the cells and increased potassium losses from the kidney. Conversely, acidosis favours the movement of potassium out of cells in exchange for hydrogen ions. These changes in plasma potassium are more marked with metabolic than with respiratory acid–base disturbances.

Clinical features and diagnosis
Plasma potassium levels are not always a good guide to total body potassium, which may be significantly depleted even when the patient is normokalaemic. In this situation the diagnosis is suggested by finding a *metabolic alkalosis* with a paradoxically acid urine, caused by renal conservation of

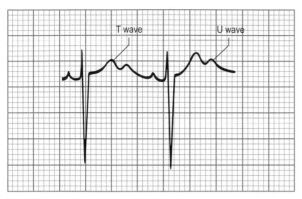

Fig. 11.2 Electrocardiographic changes in hypokalaemia: lead V₃, showing U waves. These are best seen in the anterior chest leads. Because of T-wave flattening and ST depression, the U wave may sometimes be mistaken for a T wave.

potassium ions in exchange for hydrogen ions, with renal retention of sodium and bicarbonate.

Hypokalaemia may also be detected by recognizing the associated *electrocardiographic (ECG) changes* of ST-segment depression, decreased T-wave amplitude and prominent U waves (**Fig. 11.2**). Subsequently there may be widening of the QRS complex and atrioventricular block. Hypokalaemia can also cause supraventricular tachycardias, particularly in the presence of digoxin, as well as more serious ventricular arrhythmias.

Profound potassium depletion may be associated with *skeletal muscle dysfunction*, severe weakness, hyporeflexia and, in extreme cases, paralysis (e.g. hypokalaemic periodic paralysis). Muscle weakness may be exacerbated by accompanying hypophosphataemia as potassium depletion leads to renal tubular phosphate wasting. Weaning from mechanical ventilation may be prevented, while gut motility and vascular responsiveness to pressor agents may be reduced. Acute respiratory failure due to severe hypokalaemia in the presence of a hyperchloraemic acidosis has been reported (Dunn *et al*, 1999).

Metabolic effects of hypokalaemia include reduced protein and carbohydrate synthesis and glucose intolerance.

Treatment

Underlying causes should be corrected when possible. Treatment is with potassium chloride by infusion. Concentrated solutions of potassium are extremely irritant and must therefore be administered via a centrally placed catheter. If potassium is given too rapidly, plasma concentrations may reach dangerous levels before equilibration between extra- and intracellular compartments has occurred. Except in exceptional circumstances, intravenous administration of potassium should not exceed 40 mmol/h. When there is a coexisting metabolic acidosis potassium should be replaced before correcting the acidosis in order to avoid further dangerous reductions in plasma potassium levels. Resolution of metabolic alkalosis can be a useful guide to correction of the whole-body potassium deficit. Magnesium is required for

cellular potassium uptake and to prevent continued renal potassium losses.

HYPERKALAEMIA
Causes

Hyperkalaemia can be defined as a plasma potassium level of more than 5 mmol/L and may be associated with a high, normal or low total body potassium. Regulation of the distribution of potassium between compartments has to be extremely efficient since the extracellular movement of as little as 2% of the intracellular potassium could result in potentially fatal hyperkalaemia.

Hyperkalaemia is most often caused by renal insufficiency but is also frequently *iatrogenic* as a consequence of excessive potassium administration. Administration of *suxamethonium* to patients with diffuse tissue damage (e.g. muscle trauma, burns, tetanus or paralysis) can release large quantities of potassium into the circulation. There is a risk of this complication 5–15 days after the injury and the danger persists for 2–3 months in those who have sustained burns or trauma, and for perhaps 3–6 months in those with upper motor neurone lesions (Gronert and Theye, 1975). Other causes of hyperkalaemia include *hypercatabolism, diabetic ketoacidosis, rhabdomyolysis, tumour lysis syndrome, severe burns, haemolysis and reperfusion of ischaemic tissues.* *Metabolic acidosis* may be associated with, or exacerbate hyperkalaemia. It is important to exclude causes of *pseudohyperkalaemia* such as faulty venesection technique, *in vitro* haemolysis, extreme leukocytosis or thrombocytosis.

Diagnosis and treatment

Signs and symptoms may be absent. The *ECG changes* associated with hyperkalaemia are peaked T waves and widening of the QRS complexes, followed by bradycardia and asystole (**Fig. 11.3**).

Treatment is therefore urgent. Obviously potassium administration, and drugs that promote potassium retention, should be stopped. In extreme emergencies *10 mL 10% calcium gluconate* injected intravenously will temporarily antagonize the cardiac effects of hyperkalaemia. An intravenous injection of *50 mL 50% dextrose containing 15 units soluble insulin* given over 15–20 minutes will drive potassium into the cells. The effect may last for up to 6 hours, after which the treatment may be repeated. Alkalinization with *sodium bicarbonate* and, if possible, *hyperventilation* will also shift potassium into the intracellular compartment, as well as enhancing potassium excretion via the kidneys. The former has by far the greater effect on plasma potassium levels. Sodium bicarbonate should be avoided in patients prone to sodium overload (e.g. those with renal failure). *Promotion of a diuresis* with loop diuretics or a thiazide will increase potassium excretion, in part by increasing sodium delivery to the distal tubule. In cell lysis syndromes an osmotic diuretic may be more appropriate. Potassium levels may be further reduced by the slow intravenous administration of a β_2 *adrenoreceptor agonist* (e.g. salbutamol 500 µg), which will promote cellular

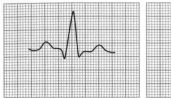

a Normal

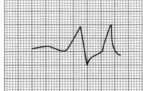

c Reduced P wave with broadend QRS complex

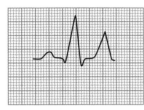

b Tented T wave

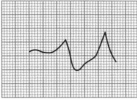

d 'Sine wave' pattern (pre-cardiac arrest)

Fig. 11.3 Progressive electrocardiographic changes with increasing hyperkalaemia. Apapted from Kumar P, Clark M 2005 Clinical Medicine 6E Elsevier with permission.

uptake of potassium by a cyclic adenosine monophosphate (AMP)-dependent activation of the Na$^+$/K$^+$ pump. Nebulized salbutamol (10 mg) has also been recommended. In practice, however, β_2 agonists are rarely prescribed for this indication, in part because of their chronotrophic and arrhythmogenic actions. Rectally, or orally, administered sodium or calcium *exchange resins*, which physically remove potassium cations, have an onset of action within about 30 minutes that should last for up to 6 hours. In many cases, however, and particularly in those with renal insufficiency, these measures only defer the dangerous consequences of hyperkalaemia while arrangements are made for definitive treatment with *haemofiltration* or *dialysis*.

Coexisting metabolic disturbances should be corrected and the underlying cause treated if possible.

HYPOMAGNESAEMIA (Noronha and Matuschak, 2002)

Magnesium (Mg) is the fourth commonest cation in the body and the second most abundant intracellular cation. Approximately 53% of total Mg stores are in bone, 27% in muscle and 19% in soft tissues, with only 0.3% in serum and 0.5% in red blood cells. Measurements of serum total Mg concentration (normal 0.8–1.2 mmol/L) are therefore a poor reflection of total body stores, and even red cell or mononuclear cell Mg concentrations are not a reliable guide to tissue levels. Moreover the relationship between circulating total Mg concentration and biologically active ionized magnesium (Mg^{2+}) is not straightforward, especially in the critically ill. Measurement of serum, rather than plasma, Mg concentrations is often recommended because additives (such as anticoagulants) may be contaminated with Mg or may interfere with the assay. More complex methods for assessing total body Mg, such as 24-hour excretion rates or

a Mg loading test, are not readily applicable in the routine management of critically ill patients.

Causes

Magnesium homeostasis is regulated by the kidneys and by alterations in absorption from the bowel, whilst extracellular levels are maintained by the exchangeable stores in bone. In critically ill patients Mg deficiency can be caused by:

- reduced intestinal absorption;
- increased renal losses;
- compartmental redistribution;
- a combination of these.

Consequences of magnesium deficiency

Hypomagnesaemia is common in the critically ill and is associated with increased mortality and prolonged hospital stay. Magnesium plays an important role in the storage, transfer and utilization of high-energy phosphates and is therefore essential for the metabolism of protein, fat, carbohydrate and nucleic acid and for energy-dependent cellular functions, including membrane stability and action potential generation. In addition intracellular Mg^{2+} maintains low resting levels of intracellular Ca^{2+} and may modulate calcium balance by influencing parathormone secretion. Whether Mg deficiency also increases skeletal muscle resistance to parathormone is currently uncertain.

Mg^{2+} also plays a crucial role in the maintenance of intracellular K$^+$ concentrations, so that decreases in Mg^{2+} concentrations are associated with efflux of K$^+$ from myocardial cells, thereby inducing depolarization. In the nervous system Mg has a depressant effect at synapses (see Chapter 15), for example through presynaptic inhibition of acetylcholine release at the neuromuscular junction and, centrally, non-competitive blockade of N-methyl-D-aspartic acid (NMDA) receptors. Thus Mg deficiency has the potential to impair oxidative phosphorylation, protein metabolism and transmembrane electrolyte flux in cardiac and neural tissues. Potentially important effects of hypomagnesaemia on immune function, the inflammatory response, calcium-induced cell injury and mitochondrial function have also been described. It is perhaps not surprising, therefore, that magnesium deficiency has been shown to be associated with a worse outcome from endotoxin challenge (Salem *et al.,* 1995), supporting the practice of correcting magnesium deficiency in the critically ill.

Clinical features of magnesium deficiency

Most patients with hypomagnesaemia remain asymptomatic and in general signs and symptoms correlate poorly with circulating magnesium levels. It seems that overt manifestations may depend more on the rate at which depletion develops, on tissue rather than circulating levels and on serum ionized rather than total levels of Mg.

The *neuromuscular manifestations* of magnesium deficiency (irritability and weakness) seem to be related to the combined effects of ionized hypomagnesaemia and the associated hypocalcaemia. The extent to which these abnormalities contribute to delayed weaning from mechanical ventilation is, however, uncertain. Similarly, it seems that alterations in serum total Mg concentrations are unlikely to precipitate *arrhythmias* unless accompanied by changes in other cations, especially potassium. Importantly, associated hypokalaemia and hypocalcaemia are refractory to treatment unless Mg is first repleted. The *ECG changes* associated with severe hypomagnesaemia are indistinguishable from those seen in hypokalaemia (ST-segment depression, flattened T waves, prolongation of PR and Q-T intervals). Associated arrhythmias include premature atrial contractions, atrial fibrillation, multifocal atrial tachycardia, premature ventricular contractions, ventricular tachycardia and ventricular fibrillation. Digitalis-induced arrhythmias are promoted. Magnesium therapy is also recommended for *torsades de pointes*. Hypomagnesaemia is associated *with increased vasomotor tone, hypertension and coronary artery spasm* and has been implicated in sudden death related to ischaemic heart disease. Indeed, magnesium replacement has been shown to prevent arrhythmias and improve survival after myocardial infarction. Hypomagnesaemia is also common after cardiopulmonary bypass surgery and is implicated in postoperative arrhythmias in such patients. The role of magnesium in the pathogenesis and treatment of neurological disorders is discussed further in Chapter 15.

Treatment

Renal function must be assessed prior to the initiation of therapy. Treatment is with oral magnesium hydroxide, intramuscular magnesium chloride or the slow intravenous infusion of magnesium sulphate repeated as necessary according to plasma estimations. In an emergency 8–12 mmol Mg can be given over 1–2 minutes intravenously followed by 40 mmol over the next 5 hours. In the severely ill 40 mmol Mg can be given on day 1, with 16–24 mmol on days 2–5, either intravenously or intramuscularly. Intravenous magnesium can precipitate hypotension and prolong conduction times. Oral maintenance is with 12–24 mmol Mg hydroxide per day.

HYPERMAGNESAEMIA
Causes

Hypermagnesaemia occurs most commonly as a result of *excessive magnesium administration* (e.g. magnesium-containing laxatives or antacids) usually in the context of *acute or chronic renal impairment*.

Diagnosis and treatment

The main adverse effects of hypermagnesaemia are on *cardiac conduction*, with prolongation of the PR interval and QRS complexes and peaked T waves. At even higher levels, *weakness, hyporeflexia, respiratory paralysis* and *coma* may occur, with *cardiac arrest* as the terminal event.

Magnesium therapy should be discontinued. Intravenous *calcium gluconate* may be used as emergency treatment for the cardiac conduction defects. *Dextrose and insulin* can be given as for the treatment of hyperkalaemia. *Haemofiltration/dialysis* may be required in the most severe cases, especially in those with renal failure.

HYPOPHOSPHATAEMIA (Bugg and Jones, 1998)

The majority of the total body phosphate (85%) is stored in bone as hydroxyapatite crystals within the organic matrix. Of the remainder, 14% is contained in soft tissues as phosphate and only 1% is found in the blood. The latter is present in both organic (mainly phospholipid) and inorganic (HPO_4^{2-}, $H_2PO_4^-$ and PO_4^{3-}) forms. Standard laboratory tests measure only inorganic phosphate (normal range 0.8–1.3 mmol/L). Once again the exact relationship between plasma phosphate concentrations (which have a diurnal variation), total body levels and the onset of symptoms is unclear. Certainly low plasma phosphate levels may be due to a transcellular shift from the extracellular to the intracellular compartment. Also spuriously low phosphate levels may be found in patients treated with mannitol. Moderate hypophosphataemia has been arbitrarily defined as a serum level of 0.32–0.65 mmol/L, whilst levels less than 0.32 mmol/L are considered to be severe.

Phosphate homeostasis is regulated by parathormone, 1–25 dihydroxycholecalciferol, and calcitonin and is closely linked to calcium. Intestinal absorption is inhibited by calcitonin (and can be blocked by diphosphonates) and enhanced by the vitamin D metabolite, 1–25 dihydroxycholecalciferol, whilst calcium ions can bind intraluminal phosphate to form insoluble complexes, thereby reducing the bioavailability of both ions. In the kidney parathormone decreases tubular reabsorption whilst hyperphosphateaemia and respiratory or metabolic acidosis increase urinary losses of phosphate. As well as affecting intestinal phosphate absorption, 1–25 dihydroxycholecalciferol enhances mobilization of phosphate from bone.

Phosphates fulfil a large number of important physiological and biochemical functions, including:

- as high-energy phosphate bonds in adenosine diphosphate (ADP)/adenosine triphosphate (ATP);
- as intracellular messengers (e.g. cyclic AMP);
- as a component of 2, 3 diphosphoglycerate in red blood cells;
- as a component of other intracellular compounds such as phospholipids, nucleic acids, nucleoproteins and enzyme cofactors;
- as a regulator of enzymes in the glycolytic pathway;
- as a pH buffer.

Phosphates are also involved in the immune system and the coagulation cascade.

Causes of hypophosphataemia

Moderate hypophosphataemia is common in critically ill patients (25–30%) and has been reported particularly in

Table 11.2 Causes of hypophosphataemia

Inadequate intake

Chronic malnourishment/starvation

Phosphate-depleted feed (especially total parenteral nutrition)

Reduced absorption (e.g. binding to iron, magnesium or aluminium, small-bowel disease such as Crohn's disease, vitamin D deficiency)

Vomiting or nasogastric suctioning

Redistribution of phosphate into cells

Catabolism is associated with muscle breakdown and phosphate depletion. Subsequent nutritional support can lead to redistribution of phosphate back into the cells and hypophosphataemia ('refeeding syndrome')

Catecholamines (endogenous or exogenous), β-adrenergic receptor agonists, steroids and insulin enhance phosphate uptake

Metabolic or respiratory alkalosis can promote an intracellular shift of phosphate

Recovery from hypothermia

Increased losses

Drugs (e.g. acetazolamide, theophyllines, glucocorticoids, dopamine, paracetamol)

Massive diuresis

Primary or secondary hyperparathyroidism

Dialysis

Respiratory or metabolic acidosis

Multiple mechanisms

Burns

Diabetic ketoacidosis

Chronic alcoholism

---

patients with *respiratory failure* and *trauma victims*. Hypophosphataemia may be caused by inadequate intake, redistribution of phosphate into cells, increased losses of phosphate or a combination of these (**Table 11.2**). In *chronic alcoholism*, for example, hypophosphataemia may be related to malnutrition, diarrhoea, vomiting and the use of antacids, as well as the effect of coexistent hypomagnesaemia and hypocalcaemia. Morever, episodes of ketoacidosis caused by starvation can damage intracellular components leading to increased losses of phosphate. Similar mechanisms, exacerbated by glycosuria, ketonuria, polyuria and exogenous insulin administration, probably account for the hypophosphataemia which can complicate *diabetic ketoacidosis*. Hypophosphataemia is also common during the recovery phase from *burns*, when it is caused by a combination of increased

urinary losses as salt and water are mobilized and excreted by the kidney and rapid cellular uptake as the patient becomes anabolic. Other circumstances in which hypophosphataemia is commonly encountered on the ICU include *refeeding syndrome* (see later in this chapter), *salcylate poisoning, paracetamol overdose, haemodialysis, recovery from hypothermia* and *sepsis*.

Consequences of phosphate deficiency

These may include:

- muscle weakness (can cause diaphragmatic weakness and respiratory failure and prevent weaning from mechanical ventilation – see also Chapters 7 and 8);
- reduction in red cell 2,3-diphosphoglycerate with a left shift of the oxyhaemoglobin dissociation curve (see Chapter 3);
- reversible myocardial dysfunction;
- impaired response to vasopressors;
- ventricular arrhythmias;
- paraesthesia, tremor, neuropathy, myopathy, seizures, coma;
- leukocyte and platelet dysfunction;
- increased red cell fragility, haemolytic anaemia;
- osteomalacia.

Treatment

Phosphate replacement is relatively safe and effective, although rapid infusion of high doses can precipitate hypotension, hypocalcaemia, hyperphosphataemia, metastatic calcification and renal failure. Particular care is required in those with renal impairment. It is important to remember that many phosphate preparations contain potassium. Treatment of moderate hypophosphataemia is with 0.16–0.32 mmol/kg of phosphate over 4–6 hours and of severe cases is with 0.64 mmol/kg over 8–12 hours.

HYPERPHOSPHATAEMIA

Hyperphosphataemia is defined as a fasting plasma concentration of more than 1.5 mmol/L. *Pseudohyperphosphataemia* may occur in paraproteinaemias, hyperlipidaemia, haemolysis and hyperbilirubinaemia.

Causes (Table 11.3)

The most common cause of hyperphosphataemia in the critically ill is end-stage renal failure; hyperphosphataemia is rare in those with normal or only mildly impaired renal function. Other causes encountered on the ICU include rhabdomyolysis, malignant hyperpyrexia, transcellular shifts caused by acidosis and exogenous administration in the form of laxatives or enemas.

Consequencies of hyperphosphataemia

Hyperphosphataemia is usually asymptomatic but if severe can result in precipitation of calcium phosphate, particularly in the presence of a normal or raised calcium or of alkalosis.

Table 11.3 Causes of hyperphosphataemia

Decreased excretion

Chronic renal failure

Hyperparathyroidism

Hyperthyroidism

Acromegaly

Hypermagnesaemia

Biphosphonates

Increased intake

Laxatives/enemas

Injudicious phosphate administration

Transcellular shift

Metabolic or respiratory acidosis

Sepsis

Tumour lysis syndrome

Malignant hyperpyrexia

Rhabdomyolysis

Acute haemolysis

Tetany, hypotension and even convulsions may occur when calcium levels fall precipitously.

Treatment

In mild hyperphosphataemia identification and treatment of the cause are usually sufficient. Severe acute hyperphosphataemia can often be successfully managed by promoting renal excretion with intravenous saline and diuretics. Correction of acidosis and administration of glucose and insulin may correct transcellular shifts. Rarely haemodialysis may be required.

HYPER- AND HYPOCALCAEMIA (see Chapter 17)

NUTRITIONAL SUPPORT (Souba, 1997)

The indications for the provision of nutritional support are not well defined but it has been recommended that such support should be initiated when it is anticipated that a critically ill patient will be unable to meet his or her nutritional needs orally for a period of 5–10 days (ASPEN Board of Directors and the Clinical Guidelines Task Force, 2002). In normal individuals short periods of starvation are of little consequence and the same is true for previously well-nourished intensive care patients who resume eating within a few days (e.g. those admitted electively following cardiac surgery). In the majority of critically ill patients, however, most would suggest that nutritional support should be insti-

tuted as soon as practicable (usually within 1–2 days of the acute episode) in an attempt to prevent serious reductions in body cell mass as well as to ensure adequate supplies of protein and energy for tissue repair and resisting infection. Many patients are malnourished when admitted (15–40% of patients admitted to UK hospitals are malnourished at the time of their admission) and if loss of muscle bulk is allowed to progress, muscle weakness may delay mobilization and compromise the patient's ability to breathe spontaneously (see Chapters 7 and 8). In addition, malnutrition may be associated with abnormalities of the lung parenchyma, as well as an increased susceptibility to pulmonary infection (Askanazi et al., 1982), whilst immune function and wound healing may be compromised. There is also an association between malnutrition and mortality, although a cause-and-effect relationship has not been established and the ability of nutritional support to improve outcome in many clinical situations remains unproven.

Objective measures of the patient's nutritional state might help the clinician to assess the need for nutritional support. Unfortunately, although the parameters that can be assessed reasonably easily (e.g. weight loss, serum albumin and transferin levels, anthropometric measurements such as mid-arm muscle circumference, triceps skinfold thickness, hand grip strength and cutaneous responses to recall antigens) can define the nutritional status of a population of patients, they are generally relatively insensitive and lack specificity in critically ill patients. In practice it seems that malnourished patients can be accurately identified on the basis of a subjective clinical assessment of their nutritional status without reference to a rigid scoring system (Detsky, 1991).

The efficacy and safety of nutritional support are improved when supervised by a *multidisciplinary nutrition team*. The exact composition of such teams will vary according to local circumstances, but most will include at least one clinician (physician, surgeon, intensive care specialist), a dietitian, a pharmacist, a clinical biochemist and a nurse specialist. The roles of team members must be clearly defined.

ENTERAL NUTRITION

In the very early days of intensive care many, if not the majority, of critically ill patients were fed intravenously, but because of the risk of complications and the increased costs associated with parenteral nutrition (PN) (Gramlich et al., 2004) the enteral route, which seems to be associated with certain specific benefits, is now preferred (ASPEN Board of Directors and the Clinical Guidelines Task Force, 2002). In particular, in contrast to PN, enteral nutrition improves autoregulation of blood flow to the gut and is thought to:

- encourage gastrointestinal motility;
- maintain intestinal mucosal integrity;
- support the mucosal immune system;
- reduce bacterial translocation (Alexander, 1990) (see Chapter 5).

Moreover, when delivered enterally nutrients enter the bloodstream via the normal route, are presented directly to the liver for processing and may therefore be better utilized.

In 1989 a prospective study was published indicating that, following major abdominal trauma, postoperative enteral nutrition significantly reduced septic complications when compared with total PN (TPN) (Moore *et al.*, 1989). This finding was later confirmed by a meta-analysis of prospective trials comparing enteral and PN (Moore *et al.*, 1992) and the authors of a more recent systematic review also concluded that in critically ill patients the use of enteral nutrition as opposed to PN results in an important reduction in the incidence of infectious complications, although mortality seems not to be affected (Gramlich *et al.*, 2004). In patients with gastrointestinal cancer it has been shown that enteral nutrition, when instituted early, can significantly reduce the complication rate and duration of postoperative stay when compared with PN (Bozzetti *et al.*, 2001). Similarly, after liver tranplantation early jejunal feeding was found to be practicable and was thought to have potential benefits compared to PN in terms of reduced complications and costs (Wicks *et al.*, 1994). Certainly, in comparison to a 'nil by mouth' policy after major gastrointestinal surgery, early enteral feeding reduces infection rates and length of stay in hospital and may also reduce the risk of anastomotic breakdown, wound infection, pneumonia, intra-abdominal abscess and mortality (Lewis *et al.*, 2001). In one such study immediate postoperative enteral feeding via a nasojejunal tube (see below) was found to be safe, prevented an increase in gut mucosal permeability, produced a positive nitrogen balance and reduced complications (Carr *et al.*, 1996). A recent systematic review of randomized, controlled studies that compared early with delayed enteral nutrition in various categories of critically ill surgical and trauma patients confirmed that early institution of feeding is associated with a lower incidence of infections and a reduced length of hospital stay, although the incidence of non-infectious complications and mortality rates seem to be unaffected (Marik and Zaloga, 2001). This finding should, however, be interpreted with some caution given the heterogeneity of the patient populations and in particular the absence of trials conducted in medical intensive care patients. Nevertheless current evidence supports the now generally accepted practice of instituting enteral feeding as early as possible in all critically ill patients. When enteral nutrition cannot be initiated within 24 hours of admission there is evidence to suggest that the early use of PN may be associated with improved outcomes, despite an increased risk of infectious complications (Simpson and Doig, 2005).

Administration

Enteral feeding is normally administered via a *nasogastric tube* and can be commenced provided that the gastric aspirate is not excessive (e.g. not more than 40 mL/h). Bowel sounds are a poor indicator of small-bowel activity; their absence should not delay institution of enteral feeding. In patients who require long-term nutritional support, especially those with impaired consciousness or dysphagia, the feed may be delivered via a *gastrostomy* and it has been shown that endoscopically guided *percutaneous gastrostomy* (percutaneous endoscopic gastrostomy – PEG) is a simple, safe and well-tolerated procedure. In some patients, for example those with impaired gastric emptying, it may be advantageous to position a *fine tube in the jejunum* (usually this is most easily achieved endoscopically: Davies *et al.*, 2002). Alternatively a *jejunostomy* can be fashioned at the time of surgery (Moore and Moore, 1991) or positioned percutaneously. Self-propelled feeding tubes that migrate spontaneously into the jejunum have also been described (Berger *et al.*, 2002).

The benefits of *routinely* using the transpyloric route for enteral feeding in critically ill patients remain uncertain. In one randomized prospective study the use of a nasojejunal tube to deliver enteral nutrition was associated with a significant reduction in gastric residual volume, a strong trend toward improved tolerance of enteral nutrition and an extremely low requirement for PN (Davies *et al.*, 2002), while in another the incidence of gastrointestinal complications was reduced (Montejo *et al.*, 2002). Other studies, however, have found no benefit from routine transpyloric feeding (Neumann and Delegge, 2002). It is also unclear whether jejunal feeding reduces the risk of aspiration. Although in one randomized trial postpyloric feeding was associated with a significant reduction in gastric oesophageal regurgitation and a trend towards less microaspiration (Heyland *et al.*, 2001a), in others there was no difference in pulmonary aspiration rates between those fed via the gastric or transpyloric routes (Esparzel *et al.*, 2001; Neumann and Delegge, 2002), neither was there a reduction in the incidence of nosocomial pneumonia (Montejo *et al.*, 2002). Finally, the authors of a systematic review were unable to demonstrate a clinical benefit from postpyloric compared to gastric tube feeding in a mixed group of critically ill patients (Marik and Zaloga, 2003). Moreover, it is now recognized that the more invasive routes of enteral feeding are associated with an increased risk of complications, including the rare but fatal *non-occlusive bowel necrosis*. On balance, therefore, most believe that the routine use of jejunal feeding is unnecessary and that transplyoric feeding should be confined to those who are intolerant of gastric feeds. Jejunal feeding, may, however be beneficial in those with severe pancreatitis (Pupelis *et al.*, 2001).

Fine-bore nasogastric and nasojejunal tubes are more comfortable, as well as less likely to cause oesophageal ulceration and stricture than traditional tubes; they are ideal for long-term use. Most fine-bore tubes are supplied with a wire introducer, some can be stiffened by placing them in a refrigerator and others have mercury-weighted tips. Whichever is used it is possible to push these fine-bore tubes past the low-pressure cuff of an endotracheal or tracheostomy tube and into the lungs. Unconscious, sedated or debilitated patients and those with bulbar palsy may not react to the presence of such a tube in their major airways, and it is therefore essential to check for correct placement before starting the feed. Although it can be more difficult to aspirate gastric contents through some fine-bore tubes, testing the pH of the aspirate can be an unreliable means of confirming correct tube placement. A radiograph should therefore always be taken to verify that the tube is correctly positioned. The position of the tube should also be checked after procedures which may have caused the tube to be dislodged (e.g. tracheostomy, transoesophageal echocardiography, endoscopy).

The majority of intensive care patients are unable to protect their own airways. Some patients are supine and the presence of a nasogastric tube renders the gastro-oesophageal sphincter incompetent, allowing reflux of gastric contents. The presence of a cuffed endotracheal or tracheostomy tube is not a certain barrier to inhalation since liquids may find their way past a low-pressure cuff. In such patients, therefore, fluid must not be allowed to accumulate in the stomach and the nasogastric tube must be of a sufficient size to allow aspiration. Some fine-bore tubes are sufficiently rigid and have a large enough lumen to allow aspiration of gastric contents and can therefore be used in those who are tolerating a gastric feed even when they are unable to protect their airways. In the early stages of critical illness, in patients at high risk of aspiration and for short-term use, however, larger-bore nasogastric tubes are sometimes preferred. It is also easier to be certain of the position of these larger tubes. A variety of double- and triple-lumen nasogastric and nasojejunal tubes are now available to facilitate gastric decompression, thereby reducing the risk of aspiration. Patients should be nursed with at least a 30° head-up tilt (see Chapter 7, prevention of ventilator-associated pneumonia).

The administration sets used for enteral feeding should be sterile and have connections incompatible with intravenous infusion giving sets. In most units the feed is administered at a constant rate using an infusion pump, to reduce the incidence of diarrhoea (Jones et al., 1980). To avoid the risk of regurgitation, the feed can be discontinued every 5 hours and the stomach aspirated after a 1-hour 'rest period'. In addition, feeding can be discontinued during the night to simulate a more normal dietary pattern. When using 'tight glycaemic control' (see Chapter 17), however, it is probably easier and safer to feed patients throughout the 24-hour period.

Although bolus feeding may have a more positive effect on nitrogen balance it does not appear to reduce the incidence of ventilator-associated pneumonia or mortality. There seems to be no advantage in commencing enteral nutrition with one-quarter- or one-half-strength feeds, although it is sensible to use reduced volumes initially (e.g. 30–50 mL rather than 100 mL/h) until it is clear that there is no problem with gastric emptying. Volumes of aspirate up to 150 mL can be returned and the feed continued. If larger quantities are obtained, indicating gastric stasis, up to 150 mL can be returned, but the excess should be discarded and the volume of feed administered should be reduced.

Some recommend continuing the enteral feed at a rate of 10 mL/h in all cases in the belief that this may help to preserve gastrointestinal mucosal integrity. Prokinetic agents are often given to encourage gastric emptying. These include:

- metoclopramide – inhibits the actions of dopamine in the gut, increases lower oesophageal sphincter tone, sensitizes the gut to acetylocholine;
- erythromycin – activates motilin receptors on enteric nerves and smooth muscle.

These promotility drugs have been shown to have beneficial effects on gastrointestinal transient times, gastric residual volumes and feeding tolerance but do not appear to influence clinically important outcomes, such as pneumonia and mortality (Booth et al., 2002). Cisapride has been withdrawn from the market because of its association with lethal cardiac arrhythmias and there is some concern that the use of erythromycin may encourage microbial resistance, as well as being known to provoke *torsades de pointes* in some patients. Metoclopramide is therefore the agent of choice for this indication and there is some evidence that a dose of 20 mg may be more effective than the usual 10 mg. Conversely it seems that very low doses of erythromycin (e.g. 40 mg p.o.) can improve motility, although this does not circumvent the potential for encouraging the emergence of resistant microbial strains. A new generation of promotility agents, including macrolide derivatives with prokinetic but no antimicrobial activity, are currently being evaluated. A single dose of intravenous erythromycin (500 mg) can be used to facilitate bedside placement of postpyloric feeding tubes (Griffith et al., 2003).

Choice of feed

In general, one of the proprietary low-residue whole protein and fat polymeric diets should be used. These provide approximately 75 g of protein and 2000 kcal in 2 litres of feed, with a non-protein calorie:nitrogen ratio that is usually less than 200:1. The majority are lactose-free and contain most of the daily requirements of electrolytes, trace elements and vitamins. Low-sodium feeds may be useful in hypernatraemic patients, potassium and magnesium content may need to be reduced in those with renal impairment and feeds containing 2 kcal/mL can be used to limit fluid intake. Although it has been suggested that hyperosmolar feeds may be more likely to produce diarrhoea, this was not the case in one study (Keohane et al., 1984). Elemental diets are occasionally required for those with severely impaired gastrointestinal function. The use of an acidified enteral feed has been shown to reduce gastric microbial colonization (Heyland et al., 1999) and might, therefore reduce the incidence of ventilator-associated pneumonia.

IMMUNONUTRITION

In recent years there has been considerable interest in the potential of modified enteral formulations containing

Table 11.4 Potential (beneficial) effects of pharmaconutrients

Arginine

Improved immune function

Improved wound healing

Reduced nitrogen losses

Stimulates secretion of insulin, glucagon, prolactin and growth hormone

Precursor of nitric oxide

Glutamine

Augments lymphocyte and macrophage proliferation

Maintains gastrointestinal barrier function

Precursor of glutathione, an antioxidant

Precursor of nucleotides

Interorgan transporter of nitrogen

ω3 fatty acids

Inhibit a variety of cellular and humoral immune mechanisms

Increase production of prostaglandin E_3

Influence release of thromboxane A_2 and prostaglandin I_2

RNA* or synthetic polynucleotides

Essential for cell-mediated immunity and T-lymphocyte function

Enhance host defences (at least in patients with cancer)

*There is little evidence to support the use of dietary RNA supplementation.

pharmacological doses of specific nutrients to influence favourably host defences, the inflammatory response, nutritional status and gastrointestinal mucosal barrier function. The *pharmaconutrients* most often employed have been arginine, nucleotides, ω3 fatty acids, glutamine and branched-chain amino acids. Some of the potentially beneficial effects of these compounds are shown in **Table 11.4**. The most commonly used commercial preparation (Impact) contains a combination of arginine, ω3 fatty acids and RNA. Although the experimental evidence to support the administration of these various substrates to seriously ill humans is limited and the rationale for the dose and relative proportions of these additives is not clear, the use of such formulations has been shown to restore or enhance immune function in critically ill or septic patients (Cerra *et al.*, 1991) and in postoperative cancer patients (Kemen *et al.*, 1995). In addition a number of prospective, randomized controlled trials have indicated that early administration of enteral immunonutrition may reduce the frequency of acquired infections and length of hospital stay in critically ill patients (Bower *et al.*, 1995), the severity of postoperative infections and length of postoperative stay in patients undergoing surgery for gastric or pancreatic cancer (Braga *et al.*, 1995) and the requirement

for mechanical ventilation and length of hospital stay in a mixed group of critically ill patients (Atkinson *et al.*, 1998). Moreover enteral nutrition with a preparation containing eicosapentaenoic acid, gamma-linolenic acid and antioxidants improved gas exchange and reduced the requirement for mechanical ventilation, the developments of new organ failures and the length of ICU stay in patients with acute respiratory distress syndrome (Gadek *et al.*, 1999), whilst in another study of septic patients admitted to the ICU immunonutrition not only reduced the infection rate but also improved survival rates amongst the less severely ill patients (Galbán *et al.*, 2000). The addition of glutamine alone to enteral feeds may also reduce the incidence of acquired infections and seems to be safe, but does not appear to influence either length of stay or mortality (Conejero *et al.*, 2002; Houdijk *et al.*, 1998), possibly because of the limited systemic availability of enterally administered glutamine (see below). Conversely, a formulation enriched with glutamine, arginine, ω3 fatty acids, antioxidants and a mixture of fibres failed to improve clinical outcome in a heterogeneous population of intensive care patients (Kieft *et al.*, 2005).

Whilst acknowledging the heterogeneity of these and other published studies, recent meta-analyses and systematic reviews have concluded that in the overall population of seriously ill patients, immunonutrition may reduce the risk of developing major infectious complications, the duration of mechanical ventilation and the length of ICU and hospital stay but does not appear to influence mortality (Heyland *et al.*, 2001b; Heys *et al.*, 1999, Montejo *et al.*, 2003). Indeed, some have raised concerns that the non-glutamine formulations may actually increase mortality in certain subsets of critically ill patients, and that in some studies this may account for the observed lower incidence of complications and reduced length of hospital stay (Griffiths, 2003; Heyland *et al.*, 2001b; Heys *et al.*, 1999; Kennedy and Hall, 2000), although others have rejected this suggestion (Montejo *et al.*, 2003; Wyncoll and Beale, 2001). The role of immunonutrition in the management of critically ill patients therefore remains controversial. Current evidence suggests that, although immune-modulating enteral feeds may have a number of beneficial clinical effects, especially when used perioperatively in elective surgical and cancer patients, these may not translate into reductions in mortality and doubts remain about the efficacy and safety of this approach in the general population of critically ill patients, particularly those who are more severely ill (Calder, 2003; Griffiths, 2003; Heyland *et al.*, 2001b; Heys *et al.*, 1999). Disturbingly, a more recent randomized, multicentre trial of enteral immunonutrition in patients with severe sepsis was discontinued because of excess mortality in the treatment group (Bertolini *et al.*, 2003). In view of this uncertainty it has been suggested that for now the use of fixed-formula, commercial, immunonutrient preparations should be reserved for trauma patients undergoing surgery and for pre- and peri-operative administration to elective surgical patients (Griffiths, 2003). Moreover a recent consensus group concluded that arginine-enriched formulations should not be used in the critically ill, but that there is increasing evidence to support the use of antioxidants, such as selenium (Macfie, 2004). Further studies are required to establish the role of immunonutrition in the management of specific, more homogeneous subgroups of critically ill patients and to determine the most effective combination of pharmaconutrients.

Complications

It is well recognized that enteral feeding targets are rarely achieved (De Jonghe *et al.*, 2001). Inadequate calorie intake may be attributable to underprescription or failure to deliver the prescribed quantity of feed, but is often due to upper gastrointestinal intolerance, which in one study was associated with pneumonia, a longer ICU stay and increased mortality (Mentec *et al.*, 2001). Failure to tolerate enteral feeding seems to be associated with the administration of sedatives and catecholamines.

Abdominal distension and *diarrhoea* are also common problems in the critically ill and appear to be closely related to concomitant antibiotic therapy (Keohane *et al.*, 1983, 1984). Occasionally, but more often in recent years, *Clostridium difficile* infection may be responsible. Lactase deficiency is probably a rare cause of diarrhoea (Keohane *et al.*, 1983). If diarrhoea does occur, some form of fibre may be added to the feed, for example partially hydrolysed guar (Spapen *et al.*, 2001). In fact most newer formulations contain a source of fibre. Agents such as codeine phosphate (30–60 mg orally or nasogastrically 4-hourly) or loperamide (4 mg initially, followed by 2 mg after each loose stool up to a maximum of 16 mg daily orally or nasogastrically) can be used to reduce gastrointestinal motility. Currently it is not clear whether adding specific bacteria, such as lactobacilli, to the feed is beneficial. Other complications of enteral nutrition include:

- bacterial colonization of the feed (do not leave hanging at the bedside for more than 12–24 hours);
- regurgitation and aspiration;
- oesophageal ulceration with bleeding and stricture formation (particularly with large-bore tubes);
- hyperglycaemia;
- deficiencies of potassium, phosphate, magnesium and zinc;
- mild abnormalities of liver function.

Finally *refeeding syndrome* (Hearing, 2004) may occur when feeding follows a prolonged period of starvation (e.g. anorexia nervosa, cancer, alcoholism). During starvation insulin secretion is decreased in response to the reduced carbohydrate intake and fat and protein stores are catabolized to produce energy. During this process intracellular electrolytes, and in particular phosphate, are lost. On refeeding increased insulin secretion stimulates cellular uptake of phosphate, leading to profound hypophosphataemia (see above). The clinical features of refeeding syndrome include:

- rhabdomyolysis;
- leukocyte dysfunction;
- respiratory failure;
- cardiac failure;
- oedema;
- hypotension;
- arrhythmias;
- seizures;
- coma and death.

Treatment is with intravenous phosphate 50 mmol over 24 hours. Severe hypophosphataemia requiring further phosphate administration may recur after initial correction. The risk of refeeding syndrome can be reduced by starting feeds at a reduced calorific rate in vulnerable patients.

TOTAL PARENTERAL NUTRITION (Dominguez Cherit *et al.*, 2002)
Indications

PN will be required for those patients in whom enteral feeding is contraindicated (e.g. small-bowel anastomoses, intrinsic small-bowel disease) or fails due to gastric stasis, ileus, intractable diarrhoea or malabsorption. Supplementary PN may also be required when it proves impossible to provide sufficient energy via the enteral route alone, although the authors of a systematic review could find no evidence that starting PN at the same time as enteral nutrition improved clinical outcomes when compared to using enteral nutrition alone (Dhaliwal *et al.*, 2004).

PERIOPERATIVE TPN

It has been recognized for many years that there is an increased risk of complications in surgical patients with pre-existing protein/energy malnutrition (Studley, 1936) and that this is largely related to sepsis, presumably associated with inadequate immune responses and impaired tissue repair. While it is undoubtedly possible to provide adequate nutritional support for an indefinite period using home TPN in otherwise healthy patients with severe irreversible malabsorption (e.g. a short-bowel syndrome), there is little evidence that perioperative TPN improves outcome in surgical patients (Detsky, 1991). An early meta-analysis of 11 studies concluded that any possible benefit of preoperative TPN in well-nourished patients was small and clinically unimportant, although it was suggested that it might be of greater value in malnourished patients (Detsky *et al.*, 1987). A later multicentre study, however, not only confirmed the lack of efficacy of TPN in borderline malnourished patients, who had more infectious complications when given TPN, but also failed to prove unequivocal benefit, despite some encouraging trends, even in severely malnourished patients (Veterans Affairs Total Parenteral Nutrition Cooperative Study Group, 1991). A subsequent meta-analysis (Heyland *et al.*, 1998) confirmed that TPN had no effect on mortality overall, although major complications were reduced in malnourished compared with nourished patients and in surgical rather than critically ill patients. It would seem that in the absence of severe malnutrition most patients are probably best served by prompt surgery.

TPN IN THE ACUTE PHASE OF CRITICAL ILLNESS

It has also proved difficult to establish the value of PN during the acute phase of a non-surgical critical illness, although it is known that patients who lose more than 30% of their initial body weight in the course of an acute illness have only a remote chance of survival (Detsky, 1991). Certainly during the first 48–72 hours of an acute episode, PN may seriously complicate management and even with aggressive nutritional support it is often impossible to achieve a positive nitrogen balance in critically ill patients. This reflects the use of amino acids as oxidative fuels (Cerra *et al.*, 1987) with reduced protein synthesis and increased protein catabolism, combined with impaired fat and glucose tolerance. In practice, the ability to meet the national nutritional requirements of critically ill patients may also be limited by the need for fluid restriction, often in the presence of impaired renal function. Nevertheless the provision of adequate nutritional support should always be given a high priority; diuretics or haemofiltration should be used to prevent fluid overload, early haemofiltration/dialysis should be instituted to prevent azotaemia and supplemental PN should be given when enteral feeding alone is insufficient.

Administration

INSERTION AND CARE OF CENTRAL INTRAVENOUS CATHETERS FOR PN (see Chapter 4)

The *infraclavicular approach to the subclavian vein* is often preferred for the insertion of a long-term intravascular catheter since it allows the patient unrestricted movement of the upper limb, head and neck, and minimizes movement of the catheter at the skin puncture site.

Intravenous feeding is never an emergency and catheter placement should be performed as a planned procedure with full aseptic precautions. A *silicone catheter* should be used as these are the least thrombogenic, and some authorities recommend the use of a *subcutaneous 'tunnel'* to reduce the incidence of catheter-related sepsis. For long-term PN large-bore *Hickman silicone catheters* inserted surgically or percutaneously seem to be associated with a lower risk of obstruction, as well as allowing greater patient mobility, and are being used increasingly frequently. Although it is preferable to use dedicated vascular access for PN, in critically ill patients it may be acceptable to use one lumen of a *multi-lumen catheter* inserted via either the subclavian or internal jugular vein, particularly when venous access is difficult. An alternative is to use a dedicated *peripherally inserted central catheter* (PICC) introduced via a vein in the anticubital fossa. These catheters are also made of materials which have a low potential for thrombogenesis and can be used for several weeks.

The puncture sites should be sprayed with an antiseptic such as chlorhexidene and a porous dressing applied. The dressing should not be disturbed unless there is a suggestion of catheter-related infection. Central lines should be removed if signs of infection (unexplained fever, pus or erythema at puncture sites) or thrombophlebitis develop (see Chapter 12).

Correct positioning of the catheter must be confirmed before intravenous feeding is started. It should be possible to aspirate venous blood freely and a chest radiograph should be performed to confirm that the catheter tip is in the superior vena cava. An infusion pump should be used to ensure that the solution is administered constantly at the required rate throughout the 24-hour period.

Once inserted, the catheter port should be used only for intravenous feeding and never for administering drugs, blood or blood products, or for sampling blood. Except under exceptional circumstances, the use of two- or three-way taps and Y-connectors must be avoided. Recently, *double-lumen Hickman catheters* have been introduced; these can be used to ensure that one lumen is dedicated solely to the administration of PN, even in those in whom venous access is restricted.

PERIPHERAL PARENTERAL NUTRITION

The central venous route for the administration of PN was originally developed in order to avoid the thrombophlebitis that complicated peripheral infusion of hyperosmolar nutrient solutions. It is now recognized that thrombophlebitis associated with peripheral administration of nutritional support is related not only to the osmotic load of the infusion mixture, but also to the irritant effect of the cannula and infection. Admixtures consisting of a 3.5% solution of amino acids, with a lower concentration of glucose (5–10%), the majority of calories provided as fat emulsion and an osmolarity of less than 900 mosm/L minimize the risk of chemical phlebitis and have been shown to be suitable for peripheral administration. Since most courses of PN rarely exceed 14 days, preservation of a peripheral vein for around 5 days allows peripheral PN to be given to most patients with just two or three cannula changes. Peripheral PN therefore has a role for patients in whom adequate nutritional support cannot be provided by the enteral route and when there are difficulties with central venous access. It is also useful when it is anticipated that PN will be required for only a relatively short period (e.g. < 1 week).

Paediatric silicon feeding lines are used in some centres to minimize thrombophlebitic complications (Madan *et al.*, 1992). A number of other techniques have been used in an attempt to reduce the incidence of peripheral venous thrombophlebitis and prolong catheter life. These have included:

- in-line filters;
- heparin and steroid additives;
- buffering;
- transdermal administration of glyceryl trinitrate.

Selection of an appropriate intravenous feeding regimen

Intravenous feeds must provide the patient with protein, energy (carbohydrate and fats), electrolytes, water, vitamins and trace elements. It is important to avoid overfeeding (see below).

Protein is administered in the form of solutions containing a balanced mixture of essential and semi-essential amino acids. The body can only use L-amino acids and approximately 25% of the total nitrogen content should consist of essential amino acids, while a mixture of non-essential amino acids is also required for efficient protein synthesis. High concentrations of a single non-essential amino acid such as glycine should be avoided.

Depending on the degree of catabolism, patients will require in the order of 1.2–1.5 g of protein/kg per day (Bistrian and Babineau, 1998; Ishibashi *et al.*, 1998) (i.e. about 0.2–0.35 g/kg per day of nitrogen). In malnourished individuals, restoration of body cell mass is very slow and appears to be directly related to the total energy intake, provided adequate quantities of protein are also given. Increasing the protein intake to more than 1.5–2 g/kg per day will not, however, accelerate weight gain (Shizgal and Forse, 1980), whilst others have shown that protein losses are unlikely to be significantly reduced by increasing protein intake to more than 1.5 g/kg fat free mass per day (Ishibashi *et al.*, 1998). Surprisingly, it is possible to achieve protein sparing in a previously well nourished patient following moderately severe trauma (e.g. elective surgery) by administering only amino acids via a peripheral vein, aiming to achieve the optimal intake of 1.5 g protein/kg per day. In this way, body cell mass may be preserved until full nutritional support is established either enterally or parenterally. In practice, however, this technique is rarely used.

Glucose is the *carbohydrate* of choice, the only disadvantages being the tendency to develop hyperglycaemia and, when excessive amounts of glucose are given, fatty liver. Critically ill patients are usually intolerant of glucose, whilst exogenously administered steroids and other drugs, such as thiazide diuretics, are diabetogenic. The recommended daily glucose intake of 4–6 g/kg (about 300–400 g/day) is, however, safe and generally well tolerated. Exogenous insulin should be given in doses sufficient to control blood sugar levels close to the normal range (see Chapter 17).

Fat solutions are an excellent source of calories and are usually given as the soya bean preparation Intralipid (10 or 20%). They also prevent the development of essential fatty acid deficiency and are a source of cholesterol and phosphate (as phospholipids), although the latter may not be readily available. Recently, there has been some interest in supplementation with ω3 and ω6 fatty acids (see earlier in this chapter). The recommended daily dose is 0.7–1.4 g lipid/kg per day (about 50–100 g/day). Fat solutions are non-irritant and can be administered via a peripheral vein (see earlier in this chapter) because they are iso-osmolar, with a neutral pH.

Although in the past it was considered sufficient to administer Intralipid peripherally once or twice a week, currently fat solutions are usually administered daily. Some patients, especially those with hepatic disease, acute pancreatitis or extensive sepsis who are not being given insulin, may show intolerance of fat. Before obtaining blood samples it is therefore important to check that the plasma is not lipaemic. If fat globules are seen, there is a risk of contaminating autoanalysers. There is some evidence that fat emulsions may worsen ventilation/perfusion mismatch, embolize to the lungs and increase pulmonary vascular resistance (Moore, 2001), although when conventional formulations are used these theoretical risks do not seem to be clinically significant (Askanazi *et al.*, 1982; Radermacher *et al.*, 1992). Although the potentially deleterious pulmonary effects of lipid emulsions might be expected to be more relevant, in patients with acute lung injury in one study adverse effects were only seen in those who had received rapid infusions. When infused continuously over the recommended 24 hours as an all-in-one formulation, no deleterious effects were apparent (Suchner *et al.*, 2001).

Energy requirements can be estimated assuming that minimally stressed patients require about 25–30 kcal/kg per day, which may be increased by around 10% in the critically ill and by up to 50% in those with severe burns or major trauma. Current evidence suggests, however, that hypermetabolic and septic critically ill patients should be given energy intakes close to their basal requirements. The optimum combination of carbohydrate and lipid as non-protein energy substrates remains to be clarified. In general it is usual to give 30–40% of the total calorie intake as lipid and to provide 100–200 kcal of non-protein energy for each gram of nitrogen. In the hypercatabolic patient the optimal calorie:nitrogen ratio may fall to less than 140:1, whereas in those who are less catabolic the ratio may be closer to 200:1; typically the ratio is 150:1. While inadequate provision of energy substrates results in depletion of body stores, the administration of excessive quantities of non-protein energy may lead to the development of generalized fat deposition and a *fatty liver*. Moreover, such overprovision, even when accompanied by large quantities of protein, often fails to reverse the negative nitrogen balance in catabolic patients. It is recommended that the exogenous glucose load should not exceed approximately 500 g/day.

Appropriate solutions should be included in the regimen to provide adequate quantities of sodium, potassium, magnesium, calcium and phosphate. Phosphate deficiency is associated with a reduced red cell 2,3-diphosphoglycerate concentration and an increase in the oxygen affinity of haemoglobin, as well as respiratory muscle weakness (see earlier in this chapter and Chapters 7 and 8). Extra iron may also be required, and in long-term intravenous feeding, replacement of trace elements such as copper, manganese, chromium, selenium and zinc will become important. Zinc deficiency may be associated with impaired wound healing. All water- and fat-soluble vitamins must also be provided.

Glutamine is a precursor for nucleotide synthesis, an important fuel source for rapidly dividing cells, the principal interorgan transporter of nitrogen and a precursor for the formation of the important antioxidant glutathione (**Table 11.4**). In catabolic states mobilization of glutamine from muscle may fail to maintain plasma concentrations of glutamine, which becomes a 'conditionally essential' amino acid. Due to problems of solubility and stability, traditional amino acid solutions have omitted glutamine. The recent development of glutamine dipeptides (with alanine or

Table 11.5 Examples of total parenteral nutrition regimens

Central	All mixed in 3-litre bags and infused over 24 hours	
Nitrogen	L-Amino acids 14 g/L	1 litre
Energy	Glucose 50%	0.5 litre
	Glucose 20%	0.5 litre
	Plus:	
	Lipid 10%	0.5 litre
	as either intralipid	Fractionated soya oil 100 g/L
	or lipofundin	Soya oil 50 g, medium-chain
		triglycerides 50 g/L
	Electrolytes, water-soluble vitamins, fat-soluble vitamins, trace elements and heparin may be added if required.	
	Nitrogen 14 g, non-protein calories 9305 kJ (2250 kcal)	
Peripheral	All mixed in 3-litre bags and infused over 24 hours	
Nitrogen	L-Amino acids 9 g/L	1 litre
Energy	Glucose 20%	1 litre
	Lipid 20%	0.5 litre
	Trace elements, electrolytes and water-soluble and fat-soluble vitamins, heparin 1000 IU and hydrocortisone 100 mg are added if required.	
	Nitrogen 9 g, non-protein calories 7206 kJ (1700 kcal)	

glycine) have solved this pharmaceutical problem. There is evidence to suggest that glutamine supplementation can prevent or ameliorate the gastrointestinal mucosal atrophy seen during prolonged TPN (van der Hulst *et al.*, 1993) and supplementing PN solutions with glutamine in dipeptide form has been shown to improve nitrogen balance and immune function and shorten hospital stay in surgical patients (Morlion *et al.*, 1998), as well as to reduce the incidence of Gram-negative bacteraemia in severely burned patients (Wischmeyer *et al.*, 2001).

In a study of critically ill patients unable to receive enteral nutrition, glutamine-supplemented PN improved survival at 6 months and reduced the hospital cost per survivor (Griffiths *et al.*, 1997). This difference in survival was almost entirely explained by a reduced death rate in the ICU from multiple-organ failure, associated with a reduction in the incidence of catheter-related sepsis and *Candida* infections. In keeping with the concept that the benefits of exogenous glutamine in this situation are explained by correction or prevention of a deficiency of this amino acid, the excess mortality was seen predominantly in those patients who were dependent on standard TPN for a prolonged period (Griffiths *et al.*, 2002). Similarly, Goeters *et al.* (2002) found that parenteral glutamine improved 6-month survival, but only in those fed for more than 9 days. A systematic review of studies investigating both enteral and parenteral glutamine administration supported the suggestion that parenteral glutamine reduces mortality and indicated that glutamine supplementation is associated with lower rates of infection and shorter hospital stays. Importantly, there was no evidence of harm resulting from this intervention (Novak *et al.*, 2002).

Arginine plays an important role in nitrogen and ammonia metabolism and in the generation of nitric oxide, and may improve immune function, encourage wound healing and reduce nitrogen losses (**Table 11.4**). Administration of TPN enriched with arginine and glutamate has been shown to generate glutamine and limit protein catabolism in surgical intensive care patients (Bérard *et al.*, 2000). There is little evidence, however, that more arginine is required than is already provided in standard PN formulations. Moreover administration of excess arginine may be deleterious and, in any case, additional arginine can be safely generated from glutamine if required.

The various constituents of the appropriate 24-hour feeding regimen, including fat, are preferably premixed by the pharmacy in a *single bag* (normally containing 1.5–3 litres of solution) using an aseptic technique. Subsequently no further additives should be introduced to this bag. The composition of typical PN solutions is shown in **Table 11.5**. The giving set should be changed with each new feeding bag or at the end of each 24-hour cycle. If facilities for making up a feeding bag are not available, the various constituents of the regimen should be administered simultaneously using three-way taps or Y-connectors, although this carries an increased risk of infective complications.

Complications (Table 11.6)

Some authorities believe that modern all-in-one PN formulations, when administered by experienced clinicians to patients in whom enteral nutrition is difficult or impossible using the latest techniques and taking care to avoid overfeeding, are not associated with significantly more complications

Table 11.6 Complications of parenteral nutrition

Catheter-related

Complications related to insertion (see Chapter 4)

Displacement

Fracture and embolism

Occlusion

Venous thrombosis

Infection and bacteraemia

Metabolic

Hyperglycaemia

Hypoglycaemia (sudden cessation of feeding)

Hypo/hyperkalaemia

Hypophosphataemia

Metabolic acidosis

Sepsis

Fluid overload

Deficiencies of vitamins and trace elements

Hepatobiliary

Abnormal liver function tests

Jaundice

Intestinal

Villous atrophy

Bacterial translocation/endotoxaemia

Table 11.7 Monitoring parenteral nutrition

At least daily	Frequent bedside estimation of blood sugar Body weight (if practicable) Urea, electrolytes and blood sugar
At least twice weekly	Liver function tests Calcium and phosphates Full blood count
At least weekly	Mg^{2+} Nitrogen balance
Monthly	Vitamin B_{12} Folate Iron and total iron-binding capacity Zinc

than enteral nutrition (Dominguez Cherit *et al.*, 2002; Griffiths, 2003). Moreover recent meta-analyses have indicated that, despite an increased risk of infectious complications, mortality rates are not increased by the use of PN rather than enteral nutrition (Peter *et al.*, 2005; Simpson and Doig, 2005).

Probably the most serious complication of intravenous feeding is the development of *infection* and *bacteraemia*. Experimental studies suggest that conventional TPN fails to prevent the intestinal mucosal atrophy normally associated with starvation and has been associated with an increase in mucosal permeability and bacterial translocation from the gut lumen (Alverdy *et al.*, 1988) (see Chapter 5), although this phenomenon may not be important during short-term TPN in humans. The incidence of pneumonia and sepsis may also be increased in patients receiving PN.

PN can also be complicated by displacement of the catheter, mechanical problems, fluid overload, metabolic acidosis, electrolyte imbalance, deficiencies of vitamins and trace elements and metabolic derangements. Intravenous fat emulsions have been used to supplement glucose as an energy source because they are a more concentrated source

of calories and because of the problems caused by overfeeding with glucose such as hyperglycaemia (which should now be controlled with high doses of insulin — see Chapter 17) and fatty liver (Driscoll and Blackburn, 1990). Overfeeding with carbohydrate can also lead to increased CO_2 production which might precipitate respiratory failure in those with poor respiratory reserve.

PN may also be associated with *abnormalities of liver function*. Most commonly there is an increase in alkaline phosphatase, but in some cases bilirubin levels are also elevated, sometimes to the extent that the patient becomes jaundiced. Transaminase levels may also rise. These abnormalities of liver function are probably most often due to the provision of energy (either as fat or carbohydrate) in excess of requirements, which leads to *fatty infiltration of the liver*. Another contributory factor may be *intrahepatic cholestasis*, possibly due to changes in the composition of bile. Of course, in critically ill patients, many other factors, including shock, sepsis and drug therapy, can precipitate liver dysfunction. In adults, changes in liver function induced by PN are almost always reversible (e.g. by reducing the energy input or by changing to enteral nutrition), but in children, for reasons that are not entirely clear, they can persist and lead to chronic liver disease.

Monitoring patients receiving TPN

Careful monitoring of patients receiving TPN is therefore required if these complications are to be avoided (**Table 11.7**). Most importantly, overfeeding must be avoided. It is clearly essential to keep an accurate *daily record of fluid balance* and the patient should be *weighed* daily if this is practicable. Urea, creatinine, electrolytes and blood sugar should also be measured daily. In particular, if, as is usual, the patient is receiving an insulin infusion, blood sugar levels should be determined frequently by the nursing staff at the bedside. Initially, this may be performed hourly, but once a stable regimen is established, the frequency of blood sugar estimations can be progressively reduced to 4-hourly. Liver function tests (including estimation of calcium and phosphate) and a full blood count should be performed at least twice weekly. Plasma magnesium should be measured once a week, and blood levels of vitamin B_{12}, folate, iron, total iron-binding capacity and zinc should be estimated monthly. Normally, all these investigations should also be performed before feeding begins. A 24-hour collection of urine for determination of urea, electrolyte and creatinine concentrations allows calculation of creatinine clearance and nitrogen balance. Estimating total urinary nitrogen excretion from urinary urea excretion is, however, of dubious value, especially in unstable critically ill patients (Konstantinides et al., 1991).

MODIFYING THE CATABOLIC RESPONSE (Hadley and Hinds, 2002)

The metabolic response to critical illness is associated with hypermetabolism, insulin resistance, alterations in substrate utilization and a negative nitrogen balance. Initially protein is lost predominantly from skeletal muscle but later the viscera becomes a major site for proteolysis, although cardiac muscle seems to be relatively spared. During the acute phase of critical illness at least some aspects of this catabolic response are likely to be beneficial, for example the increased availability of amino acids for gluconeogenesis, increased immune cell replication, synthesis of acute-phase proteins and wound healing. In the context of modern intensive care, however, where critically ill and injured patients can often be supported for prolonged periods, persistence of the catabolic response has a number of important detrimental effects, including:

- immune dysfunction;
- impaired wound healing;
- loss of integrity of the gastrointestinal mucosal barrier;
- skeletal muscle wasting and weakness:
  - difficulty weaning from mechanical ventilation;
  - delayed mobilization;
  - prolonged rehabilitation.

Unfortunately conventional nutritional support only partially ameliorates this process and muscle protein catabolism cannot be prevented. The role of *glutamine supplementation* and *immunonutrition* in modifying the catabolic response and reducing morbidity and mortality has been discussed earlier in this chapter, while the benefits of *tight glycaemic control* are reviewed in Chapter 17. The value of *gonadal steroids, adrenergic agents* (in particular β_2 agonists), *muscle stimulation, elevated ambient temperature* and *afferent blockade* in this context remains unclear. For many years there was also considerable interest in the potential of treatment with *growth hormone* (GH) and other growth factors, to limit protein catabolism and reduce muscle wasting in the critically ill.

In health, GH secretion is pulsatile, with large nocturnal peaks superimposed on a barely detectable baseline. This pattern of secretion is controlled by the balance between a hypothalamic releasing hormone (GH-releasing hormone: GHRH) and the inhibitory effects of somatostatin. The actions of GH are mediated both directly via peripheral GH receptors and indirectly via the enhanced hepatic synthesis of insulin-like growth factor-I (IGF-I). Although basal circulating levels of GH are increased in critical illness, normal pulsatility is lost and serum concentrations of IGF-I and its GH-dependent binding protein (IGFBP-3) are reduced (Timmins et al., 1996). Initially a number of relatively small studies suggested that administration of recombinant human (rh) GH to catabolic patients could increase circulating levels of IGF-I, improve nitrogen balance, attenuate the fall in muscle glutamine levels, improve protein synthetic rates and preserve lean body mass. Some studies also suggested that rhGH could increase muscle strength, reduce weaning time, improve wound healing, reduce hospital length of stay and, in burns victims, improve survival. Disappointingly, however, two parallel prospective randomized controlled trials subsequently demonstrated that high-dose rhGH significantly increased mortality when given to heterogeneous groups of long-stay critically ill adults. Weaning times were prolonged and duration of hospital and ICU length of stay were also increased (Takala et al., 1999). Possible explanations for this unexpected finding include the immune-modulating effects of growth factors, inhibition of glutamine mobilization from muscle and the adverse effects of increased insulin resistance, perhaps compounded by an increased metabolic rate and suboptimal nutritional support. Importantly, recent evidence suggests that the neuroendocrine response to critical illness is biphasic and that during the chronic phase there is complete loss of GH pulsatility and mean circulating levels are lower than during the acute phase (Van den Berghe, 2000). It seems that GH resistance may not be a feature of this chronic phase and under these circumstances exogenous high-dose GH could be harmful. Interestingly, the administration of GH secretagogues during prolonged critical illness can stimulate GH secretion and restore pulsatility, and the combination of GH-releasing peptide and thyrotrophin-releasing hormone (TRH) has been shown to restore pulsatile secretion of GH and TSH, with associated increases in circulating levels of IGF-I and IGFBP-3 and reduced protein breakdown (Van den Berghe et al., 1999). Whether this more physiological approach to modifying the metabolic response to prolonged critical illness will be safer and more effective than growth factor administration remains to be seen.

SEDATION, ANALGESIA AND MUSCLE RELAXATION (Gehlbach and Kress, 2002)

Most patients admitted to intensive care will require analgesia and, in the majority, administration of a sedative will be indicated to achieve some or all of the following:

- allay anxiety;
- relieve discomfort;
- encourage sleep;
- modulate the physiological response to stress and decrease oxygen consumption;
- promote synchronous breathing with the ventilator and tolerance of the endotracheal tube;
- alleviate dyspnoea;
- prevent self-extubation and removal of invasive catheters.

Sedatives may also be used to manage acute confusional states (see later in this chapter) and during diagnostic or invasive procedures. The combination of an opiate and a sedative or intravenous anaesthetic agent is generally used to facilitate mechanical ventilation and to obtund the physiological response to stress. Morphine and the benzodiazepines are the most common agents used to provide analgesia and sedation in intensive care and are often administered in combination although, given the large variety of recommended agents and drug combinations, it is clear that no regime is ideal. In selected cases, neuromuscular blockade may be indicated and, in some, heavy sedation or even anaesthesia may be required to control intracranial hypertension, seizures or the spasms of tetanus (see Chapter 15). Heavy sedation may also be indicated in patients with severe respiratory failure, especially since current lung-protective ventilatory strategies are inherently uncomfortable.

The properties that should be considered when choosing the most appropriate sedative for an individual patient include:

- sedation potential;
- anxiolysis;
- analgesia;
- amnesia (may predispose to delirium);
- rate of onset and duration of action;
- predictability of effect;
- speed of reversal on cessation;
- degree of respiratory depression;
- degree of cardiovascular depression;
- gastrointestinal effects;
- venous irritation;
- addictive potential;
- cost;
- interaction with other drugs;
- tolerance.

An ideal agent would be effective, safe, easily titratable, cheap and rapidly acting. It would also provide sedation, analgesia and anxiolysis. As the goals of sedation vary between patients it is unlikely, however, that any one agent will be suitable in all circumstances. For example, in a patient receiving controlled ventilation, the respiratory depression and cough reflex suppression caused by an opiate are of little consequence and may be advantageous, whereas a patient with Guillain–Barré syndrome may have less need for analgesia,

Table 11.8 Adverse effects of inadequate or excessive sedation/analgesia

Inadequate	Excessive
Hypertension	Hypotension
Tachycardia	Bradycardia
Increased oxygen consumption	Respiratory depression
Myocardial ischaemia	Constipation, ileus
Cerebrovascular accident	Nausea, vomiting
Tracheal tube intolerance	Immune suppression
	Prolonged time on the ventilator and intensive care unit stay
	Tolerance

but the establishment of adequate sleeping patterns and normal gastrointestinal function will be an important goal. In the early phase after surgery or trauma, on the other hand, provision of effective analgesia must be a priority.

Tolerance to opioids and benzodiazepines may develop quite rapidly, especially when given by continuous infusion, and may necessitate progressive escalation of the dose. Withdrawal symptoms can complicate weaning from long-term mechanical ventilation as the dose of sedatives/analgesics is reduced (Cammarano et al., 1998).

ASSESSING THE LEVEL OF SEDATION

Inadequate sedation and analgesia are not only distressing for the patient but may also be associated with specific complications and increased morbidity (Table 11.8). In particular increased sympathetic activity may be associated with hypertension and tachycardia, as well as a risk of myocardial ischaemia or cerebrovascular accident. Moreover oxygen consumption is increased and failure to synchronize with the ventilator may lead to pulmonary atelectasis and hypoxaemia. Conversely, oversedation may precipitate bradycardia, hypotension, respiratory depression and ileus, as well as prolonging time on the ventilator and ICU stay. Also sedatives compromise host immunity by inhibiting leukocyte function. Indeed, in one observational study sedation was identified as an independent risk factor for the development of ventilator-associated pneumonia (see Chapter 7) (Rello et al., 1999).

In most cases the aim is for the patient to appear drowsy and comfortable, but easily rousable and cooperative. Deep sedation is normally reserved for specific indications such as severe head injury or tetanus. The ideal level of sedation is, however, often difficult to achieve in critically ill patients in whom the volumes of distribution, availability and elimination of drugs are profoundly altered by, for example, alterations in protein binding, renal or liver dysfunction and drug interactions. Importantly, it has been shown that daily interruption of sedative infusions until the patient is awake decreases the duration of mechanical ventilation and the length of stay in the ICU (Kress *et al.*, 2000), without increasing the risk of self-extubation/catheter removal or adverse psychological effects (Kress *et al.*, 2003). The number of diagnostic tests (e.g. computed tomography scanning) performed to exclude cerebral pathology may also be reduced (Kress *et al.*, 2000), as may the incidence of other complications associated with critical illness and mechanical ventilation such as ventilator-associated pneumonia, upper gastrointestinal haemorrhage and bacteraemia (Schweickert *et al.*, 2004). Similarly, the introduction of sedation scoring, written guidelines and an educational programme with continuous feedback has been shown to reduce time on the ventilator and length of stay (Brattebo *et al.*, 2002).

The level of sedation can be assessed as described by Ramsay *et al.* (1974) for patients sedated with an infusion of the anaesthetic induction agent althesin (alphaxalone-alphadolone). Six levels of sedation were proposed:

1. anxious and agitated or restless, or both;
2. cooperative, oriented and tranquil;
3. responds to commands only;
4. asleep, but with a brisk response to light glabellar tap or loud auditory stimulus;
5. asleep, sluggish response to light glabellar tap or loud auditory stimulus;
6. asleep, no response.

It is suggested that levels 2–5 can be considered suitable for patients requiring sedation in the ICU. The use of this *Ramsay* scale allows sedation to be tailored to individual patients' needs and also facilitates comparative clinical studies between different agents or techniques.

More recently a simplified five-point scale (*the Brussels sedation scale*) has been shown to be reproducible, objective and reliable (Detriche *et al.*, 1999). In addition the use of this scale was found to be better than clinical assessment, especially as a means of avoiding oversedation (Detriche *et al.*, 1999). Similarly the *Richmond Agitation-Sedation Scale* (RASS), which is a 10-point scale with four levels of anxiety or agitation (+1 to +4 (combative)), one level to denote a calm and alert state (0) and five levels of sedation (−1 to −5 (unrousable)) has been shown to be easy to administer, valid and reliable (Sessler *et al.*, 2002).

Physical methods for assessing sedation have also been developed, but are not yet used routinely. For example, the level of cortical electrical activity can be assessed using the *cerebral function monitor* (CFM) or *cerebral function-analysing monitor* (CFAM) (see Chapter 15), and *auditory evoked potentials* have been used to assess the depth of sedation or anaesthesia (Thornton *et al.*, 1989). More recently a new processed electroencephalographic signal, the *bispectral index* (BIS), has been used to monitor the level of sedation on a relative scale, continuously and non-invasively (Triltsch

Table 11.9 Guidelines for adult doses for some of the opioids commonly administered to mechanically ventilated patients

Drug	Intravenous bolus dose	Intravenous infusion rate
Morphine	2–6 mg	2–8 mg/h
Pethidine	10–50 mg	10–50 mg/h
Fentanyl	50–200 μg	100–200 μg/h
Alfentanil	1–5 mg	1–6 mg/h
Sufentanil	10–70 μg	10–70 μg/h

Table 11.10 Guidelines for bolus doses and lock-out intervals for opioids in patient-controlled analgesia systems (the use of a background infusion has been shown to increase opioid use and side-effects)

Opioid	Bolus dose (mg)	Lock-out time interval (minutes)
Morphine	0.5–3	5–20
Pethidine	5–30	5–15
Fentanyl	0.01	3–10

et al., 2002). This technique requires further validation in the ICU setting.

ANALGESIA

Achieving adequate analgesia and sedation can be considered to be independent goals of treatment, priority being given to pain control. It is particularly important to recognize when agitation and sympathetic hyperactivity are due to unrelieved pain and therefore indicate the need for effective analgesia rather than increased sedation. In alert patients a visual or numerical analogue pain scale, or a verbal descriptor scale, can be used to guide analgesic requirements. In difficult cases the assistance of the pain management team should be requested.

Opiates

These agents are the mainstay of effective pain relief during the early phase of intensive care. Because intramuscular administration of opiates is associated with irregular absorption, fluctuating blood levels and periods of pain between doses, analgesics are best administered to critically ill patients by continuous intravenous infusion (**Table 11.9**). The dose can be adjusted according to the individual's requirements, guided, for example, by the clinical response to nursing or medical interventions (*nurse-directed analgesia*). *Patient-controlled analgesia* (PCA, **Table 11.10**) may be preferred for patients who are sufficiently alert and cooperative.

Morphine remains the most commonly used opiate and may be less deleriogenic than the alternatives. *Fentanyl*, which is a potent lipid-soluble synthetic opioid, is rapidly redistributed to the tissues and has a shorter duration of action, although long-term administration leads to accumulation and prolongation of its elimination half-life; fentanyl's duration of action then approaches that of morphine. Similarly the duration of action of the ultra-short-acting agent *alfentanil* increases considerably after prolonged administration, especially in patients with liver failure. After a few days the analgesic efficacy of alfentanil diminishes. In contrast the duration of action of *sufentanil* increases only slightly after prolonged administration and development of tolerance seems to be less pronounced, perhaps because of its high receptor affinity and lipophilicity. *Remifentanil* has a rapid onset of action (about 1 minute) and a steady state is quickly achieved. It has a *context-sensitive half-life* (the time required for the central compartment drug concentration to decrease by 50%) of 2–3 minutes which is independent of the duration of infusion. Unlike other opioids, remifentanil is rapidly and predictably metabolized by non-specific esterases in the blood and tissues, principally to a carboxylic acid derivative, remifentanil acid. Thus remifentanil can be administered in higher doses and for long periods without the risk of significant accumulation. In view of this organ-independent elimination remifentanil should be particularly useful in critically ill patients, although its routine use is currently limited by cost. In one study remifentanil facilitated more rapid emergence from analgesia and sedation than did sufentanil, one disadvantage being that patients complained of considerable pain within 20 minutes of stopping the infusion (Soltész *et al.*, 2001). Although remifentanil acid does accumulate in patients with renal impairment current evidence suggests that prolongation of μ-opioid effects is unlikely (Pitsiu *et al.*, 2004). *Tramadol* is an atypical opioid which is an agonist for μ receptors. It inhibits serotonin and causes less sedation and respiratory depression than other opiates.

The side-effects of the opioids are dose-related and include:

- nausea and vomiting;
- dysphoria;
- decreased gut motility;
- ventilatory depression;
- cardiovascular depression.

High doses of meperidine (pethidine) may produce muscle twitching and convulsions due to the accumulation of the neurotoxic metabolite normeperidine. It is also important to remember that morphine elimination is reduced in renal failure (Ball *et al.*, 1985) and that there may be accumulation of the pharmacologically active metabolite morphine-6-glucuronide (Osborne *et al.*, 1986). *Naloxone* (0.1–0.4 mg intravenously) can be used to antagonize opioid side-effects (see Chapter 19).

Non-opiate analgesics

Although the opioids are the most commonly used analgesics in critically ill patients, discomfort from bones, joints or muscles following prolonged immobilization, inflammatory disorders (e.g. pleuritic chest pain) and less severe pain may not require, and may respond poorly to, opioid administration. Non-steroidal anti-inflammatory drugs (NSAIDs), which block prostaglandin biosynthesis by inhibiting cyclooxygenase (COX), may be useful in such cases and are widely used perioperatively as an alternative or as a supplement to opioid analgesics (Dahl and Kehlet, 1991).

Aspirin is contraindicated in children under 12 years of age because of an association with Reye's syndrome, otherwise a dose of 300–900 mg may be given orally every 4–6 hours to a maximum of 4 g in 24 hours. *Paracetamol* 500 mg–1 g can be given orally, intravenously or rectally every 4–6 hours to adults, and is most effective when given regularly. Since these less-powerful analgesics are also available in many different combinations (e.g. co-codamol contains paracetamol combined with codeine phosphate), it is essential that the precise contents of these commercial preparations are known. *Diclofenac* is available not only as an oral sustained-release preparation and a suppository, but also as a parenteral preparation. *Ketorolac* may also be given orally, intramuscularly or intravenously, initially 10 mg four times a day. The dose should be reduced in the elderly.

The use of NSAIDs in critical illness is, however, significantly limited by *side-effects* related to inhibition of prostaglandin biosynthesis such as:

- gastrointestinal haemorrhage;
- renal impairment (see Chapter 13);
- bronchospasm;
- platelet dysfunction.

COX-2-selective inhibitors (e.g. celecoxib, parecoxib) are as effective as conventional NSAIDs but are less likely to cause gastric ulceration and have little effect on platelet function. Whether these agents are less likely to cause renal dysfunction is as yet unclear and, disturbingly, recent evidence suggests that the long-term use of these agents can be associated with an increased risk of myocardial infarction and other cardiovascular events (Hippisley-Cox and Coupland, 2005; Solomon *et al.*, 2005).

Sometimes severe muscular pain or chronic pain syndromes similar to sympathetic dystrophy are encountered in patients recovering from critical illness neuropathy. Such neuropathic pain may not respond to conventional analgesics, but requires involvement of a specialist pain team to coordinate the use of membrane-stabilizing agents such as carbamazepine, tricyclic antidepressants, gabapentin or α-adrenoreceptor modulation.

α₂-adrenoreceptor agonists

α₂-adrenoreceptors are located in the central and peripheral nervous systems and in autonomic ganglia, both pre- and postsynaptically. Stimulation of postsynaptic receptors in the central nervous system leads to a reduction in sympathetic activity, while stimulation of presynaptic receptors in sympathetic nerve endings inhibits noradrenaline release, the overall effect being to induce sedation with a decrease in blood pressure and heart rate. Stimulation of α_2-adrenore-ceptors in the spinal cord produces analgesia. Because peripheral α_2-receptors in blood vessels mediate vascular smooth-muscle contraction, rapid injection of a potent α_2-agonist can cause transient hypotension.

The prototype α_2-agonist *clonidine* has been used in the management of withdrawal from alcohol, benzodiazepines and opiates and as an adjuvant to facilitate analgesia and sedation and prevent tolerance during long-term respiratory support. It has also been used in the treatment of tetanus (see Chapter 15). Clonidine can cause hypotension, particularly in the presence of hypovolaemia, and arrhythmias, whilst withdrawal has been associated with rebound hypertension. High doses can cause constipation.

Dexmedetomidine is a lipophilic, imidazole derivative with a higher affinity and selectivity for the α_2-receptor than clonidine. Dexmedetomidine has potent sedative, analgesic and anxiolytic effects and can blunt the stress response to surgery and intensive care procedures. It does not affect respiratory rate or carbon dioxide clearance but can cause hypotension and bradycardia. In one study, however, dexmedetomidine seemed to improve haemodynamic stability, particularly during weaning and after extubation (Triltsch et al., 2002). Importantly, the quality of sedation produced by dexmedetomidine differs from that associated with the use of conventional sedatives. Whereas gamma-aminobutyric acid (GABA) inhibitors such as the benzodiazepines produce a clouding of consciousness, which at higher doses progresses into unconsciousness, α_2-agonists reduce sympathetic activity and the level of arousal; although calm when undisturbed, patients are therefore easily roused to full consciousness, without showing signs of stress (Venn and Grounds, 2001). Consequently sedation with an α_2-agonist alone is not recommended for patients receiving muscle relaxants. In clinical practice dexmedetomidine is well tolerated, provides effective sedation and reduces the requirement for other (respiratory-depressant) analgesics and sedatives (Triltsch et al., 2002; Venn and Grounds, 2001; Venn et al., 1999). It is reassuring that in one study patients who had received dexmedetomidine described their stay in intensive care as 'pleasant' and were not disturbed by any increased awareness, neither did lack of sleep seem to be as frequent a complaint as in those sedated with propofol (Venn and Grounds, 2001). A recent randomised controlled trial in mechanically ventilated patients demonstrated that the use of a dexmedetomidine infusion was associated with more days alive without delirium or coma than sedation with lorazepam (Pandharipande et al., 2007).

Regional blockade

Regional techniques have a number of potential advantages over intravenous analgesia for the relief of postoperative pain and may be useful in the management of pain following traumatic injury, especially in those with chest injuries (see Chapter 10).

EPIDURAL ANALGESIA

Epidural analgesia can improve the quality of postoperative pain relief and attenuates the stress response to surgery, as well as allowing the patient to cough and deep-breathe more effectively and change position more easily, while remaining more alert. Diaphragmatic dysfunction, a consequence of reflex muscle spasm after surgery, may also be ameliorated.

A number of clinical studies and meta-analyses have suggested that epidural techniques can promote earlier recovery and improve outcome by decreasing the incidence of thromboembolic and pulmonary complications, as well as hastening recovery of gut function, in the postoperative period (Buggy and Smith, 1999). More recently, however, a large prospective randomized trial in high-risk patients undergoing major abdominal surgery or oesophagectomy found no overall difference in mortality or major morbidity between those receiving epidural analgesia and a control group, although there was a modest reduction in the incidence of respiratory failure (Rigg et al., 2002).

In many critically ill patients, placement of an extradural catheter is contraindicated (e.g. because of general or local infection, coagulopathy or anticoagulant administration). It has been suggested that an epidural should not be attempted if the partial thromboplastin time or the international normalized ratio is prolonged or if the platelet count is less than $100\,000 \times 10^9$/L. Epidural placement should be delayed for at least 4 hours after the last dose of unfractionated heparin and for at least 12 hours after administering a dose of fractionated or low-molecular-weight heparin. Similar considerations apply to the removal of epidural catheters.

For the control of lower-limb, pelvic and abdominal pain, the epidural catheter can be inserted in the lumbar region at L1–2 or L2–3; an initial dose of 10–15 mL of 0.5% bupivacaine can be followed by an infusion of 0.125% bupivacaine at 5–20 mL/h (the use of a continuous infusion rather than repeated bolus doses is less likely to be associated with acute episodes of hypotension). In those with upper abdominal or thoracic pain the epidural catheter is best inserted in the mid-thoracic region between T7 and T10. Here an initial dose of 4–6 mL of 0.5% bupivacaine can be followed by an infusion of 6–10 mL/h of 0.125% bupivacaine.

Epidural administration of opiates may be associated with less hypotension and produces longer-lasting, although less dense, analgesia. Opiates act synergistically with local anaesthetic agents and the combination may reduce the potential for side-effects, as well as minimizing the tendency for local anaesthetic agents to exhibit tachyphylaxis (**Table 11.11**).

As well as determining the sensory level of the block, careful observation of cardiorespiratory function is necessary for all epidural techniques, but particularly when local anaesthetics and opiates are used in combination, when there is a significant risk of delayed, insidious, opiate-induced respiratory depression as well as the sudden cardiovascular collapse that may follow local anaesthetic-induced sympathetic blockade. Opiate-induced respiratory depression fol-

Table 11.11 Suggested adult doses of opioid drugs given extradurally

Opioid	Extradural bolus dose
Diamorphine	2.5–5 mg
Fentanyl	100–200 µg
Extradural infusion	
Bupivacaine	0.125% plus
Diamorphine	5 mg
or Morphine	10 mg
or Fentanyl	100 µg

diluted in a total volume of 50 mL infused at 4–10 mL/h initially and adjusted according to patient response

Table 11.12 Guidelines for bolus doses and infusion rates for sedative and anaesthetic agents in mechanically ventilated patients

Sedative or analgesic agent	Bolus dose	Infusion rate
Diazepam	2.5–5 mg	1–4 mg/h
Lorazepam	1–2 mg	Not suitable
Midazolam	2.5–5 mg	0.5–6 mg/h
Propofol	1–2.5 mg/kg	1–4 mg/kg per h
Thiopental	250–500 mg	100–200 mg/h

Age, obesity, concomitant medication, hepatic and renal dysfunction may change dose requirements.

lowing epidural injection is least likely to occur with the more lipid-soluble agents such as fentanyl and diamorphine. Other side-effects of epidural opiates include nausea and vomiting, urinary retention and pruritus. It may be possible to antagonize these side-effects with naloxone without reducing analgesia. Other potential complications of epidural analgesia include:

- subarachnoid injection of local anaesthetic leading to coma, bradycardia, hypotension and respiratory arrest;
- intravascular injection;
- high block leading to respiratory muscle paralysis;
- epidural haematoma or abscess (rare: presents as triad of back pain, progressive motor weakness and incontinence. Diagnosis can be confirmed by magnetic resonance imaging. Treatment is immediate surgical exploration).

It is suggested that in critically ill patients epidural catheters should not remain in place for more than 3 days.

INTERPLEURAL BLOCKADE
Local anaesthetic agents can be infused continuously into the interpleural space. Alternatively, their administration can be patient-controlled. This technique has been used for the management of multiple rib fractures, as well as following upper abdominal surgery (Murphy, 1993) and thoracic procedures (Ferrante et al., 1991).

PERIPHERAL NERVE BLOCKS
Intercostal (or *paravertebral*) nerve blocks can provide good analgesia in the relevant dermatomes and may be useful to allow patients with, for example, thoracotomy wounds or rib fractures (not more than three or four) to cough without pain. Unfortunately there is a risk of pneumothorax and multiple injections may be required. Paravertebral blocks can, however, be maintained with a catheter and the action of bupivacaine can be prolonged by the addition of adrenaline (epinephrine). *Femoral nerve* infusions have been used for lower-limb pain.

SEDATIVES
Benzodiazepines
Benzodiazepines interact with specific receptors in the central nervous system to augment or facilitate the inhibitory effect of GABA on synaptic transmission, thereby producing sedation, hypnosis and anxiolysis. Other properties of the benzodiazepines include amnesia, a reduction in vagal tone, some cardiorespiratory depression in larger doses, potent anticonvulsant activity and a minor degree of muscle relaxation. Importantly, in some cases there may be paradoxical confusion and agitation and it seems that benzodiazepines may increase the risk of developing delirium (Panharipande et al., 2006) (see later in this chapter). Withdrawal symptoms may be seen following long-term use and include:

- anxiety;
- insomnia;
- dysphoria;
- unpleasant dreams;
- sweating.

The effects of benzodiazepines can be reversed by the specific antagonist *flumazenil*, but because the effect lasts for only about 60 minutes repeated bolus injections or a continuous infusion may be required. Also there is a danger of precipitating seizures.

Diazepam or *diazepam emulsion* (a soya bean oil/water emulsion, which is less irritant and painful on intravenous injection) has been a popular benzodiazepine for bolus intravenous administration. Although blood levels initially fall rapidly due to redistribution, the elimination half-life is long (20–50 hours) and accumulation is a significant problem. Moreover diazepam is metabolized in the liver to produce active metabolites such as desmethyldiazepam and oxazepam. Consequently *midazolam*, which is more potent and rapidly acting, with a shorter elimination half-life, has been preferred (**Table 11.12**). In critically ill patients, midazolam is frequently administered as a continuous intravenous infusion. The active metabolite of midazolam (α-hydroxy-midazolam) makes an important contribution to the effects of this agent during long-term sedation and may accumulate in those with renal impairment. Also the unpredictable pharmacokinetics of midazolam, especially in hepatic insufficiency and when liver blood flow is reduced, mean that in the long term, cumulative effects may present a significant problem (Dirksen *et al.*, 1987; Shelley *et al.*, 1987). The elimination half-life of midazolam is also sensitive to drug interactions involving the cytochrome P450 3A4 isoenzyme.

Lorazepam is directly glucuronidated and this metabolite has not yet been shown to be pharmacologically active, so that although its elimination half-life is much longer than that of midazolam, recovery times are not prolonged following long-term use. There is also some evidence to suggest that attaining the desired level of sedation is easier with lorazepam than with midazolam, and that the former can offer significant cost savings (Swart *et al.*, 1999). Lorazepam is, however, dissolved in propylene glycol and a number of cases of propylene glycol toxicity with hyperosmolarity, lactic acidosis and renal dysfunction have been reported following high-dose continuous intravenous infusions. It is important to recognize that other symptoms of propylene glycol toxicity, such as decline in mental status, seizures and arrhythmias, can mimic alcohol withdrawal, for which lorazepam may have been prescribed (Tuohy *et al.*, 2003). Although this syndrome usually resolves promptly on discontinuing the infusion, in patients with multiple-organ dysfunction haemodialysis may be a useful method for reducing serum concentrations of propylene glycol and correcting the increased osmolar gap (Parker *et al.*, 2002).

Intravenous anaesthetic agents

The barbiturate *thiopental* is occasionally administered as a continuous intravenous infusion to control raised intracranial pressure or to treat convulsions refractory to more conventional measures (see Chapter 15). Its use may be complicated by cardiovascular and respiratory depression. The effects of thiopental are cumulative and prolonged recovery must be anticipated.

Propofol (an alkylphenol which is chemically unrelated to any other sedative) is rapidly metabolized, principally in the liver, and its effects are not cumulative. The pharmacokinetics of propofol are essentially unchanged by hepatic or renal impairment, although concomitant use of fentanyl may decrease the volume of distribution and clearance of propofol and thereby reduce the dose required. Sedation with this agent is easily controllable and has been associated with more rapid weaning from ventilation and extubation than midazolam (Aitkenhead *et al.*, 1989; Barrientos-Vega *et al.*, 1997; Hall *et al.*, 2001), although this may not influence time to discharge from intensive care (Hall *et al.*, 2001). As a consequence of the shorter weaning times, overall costs may be less with propofol than with midazolam (Barrientos-Vega *et al.*, 2001). Propofol causes dose-related falls in blood pressure, largely due to a reduction in systemic vascular resistance. Severe bradycardia and conduction disturbances are occasionally seen. Propofol is a respiratory depressant.

Although originally used in intensive care to provide sedation after cardiac surgery (Grounds *et al.*, 1987), propofol is now widely used in general intensive care patients.

There have been a number of reports linking propofol infusion in children to a frequently fatal syndrome characterized by lipaemia, acidosis, bradyarrhythmia and rhabdomyolysis of cardiac and skeletal muscle, with myocardial and renal failure (Parke *et al.*, 1992). It has been suggested that the cause may be related to mitochondrial dysfunction with impaired fatty acid oxidation (Wolf *et al.*, 2001). This syndrome has also been reported in adults, albeit extremely rarely (Perrier *et al.*, 2000), although it is important to appreciate that a direct causal relationship has not been conclusively established.

Inhalational anaesthetic agents

It has been suggested that inhalational anaesthetic agents such as *isoflurane* (Kong *et al.*, 1989; Willatts and Spencer, 1994) may be used as alternatives to intravenous agents, the main advantages being dependable and rapid pulmonary uptake and excretion. The low blood/gas solubility of isoflurane allows rapid titration to the desired level of sedation. Also the elimination of inhalational agents is not compromised by renal or hepatic failure. The main concerns relate to the potential adverse cardiovascular effects of isoflurane, fluoride ion nephrotoxicity with prolonged administration and practical issues regarding the special equipment required for its administration and scavenging. A vaporizer developed specifically for use in the ICU is now available, however, and an absorber, which contains activated charcoal, is a convenient means of scavenging anaesthetic vapour; exposure of staff can be further reduced by the use of closed suction systems.

Of the newer inhalational anaesthetic agents, *enflurane* and *sevoflurane* are also potentially nephotoxic and the long-term use of *desflurane* has been inhibited by the cost. Nevertheless desflurane is even less toxic than isoflurane and has been shown to allow shorter and more predictable emergence times, and quicker mental recovery after short-term postoperative sedation than propofol. Moreover, by using a low fresh gas flow pure drug costs were lower than for propofol (Meiser *et al.*, 2003).

The use of *nitrous oxide* is limited by myocardial depression, the risk of pulmonary hypertension and inhibition of methionine synthase activity which can cause bone marrow depression and peripheral neuropathy with prolonged use. *Entonox* (50% nitrous oxide in 50% oxygen) can sometimes be useful in intensive care patients to provide analgesia in situations where pain is predictable and of short duration (e.g. physiotherapy, drain removal, change of dressing).

The readily controlled level of sedation and rapid recovery associated with the use of inhalational agents is particularly advantageous for the short-term sedation of postoperative patients but the safety and efficacy of these agents for the long-term sedation of critically ill patients have not been established. Inhalational agents may also be useful to facilitate procedures such as bronchoscopy. Because inhalational anaesthetic agents cause bronchial relaxation they may be particularly useful in patients with asthma or chronic obstructive pulmonary disease (see Chapter 8).

Major tranquillizers

Butyrophenones (e.g. haloperidol, 5–10 mg orally, intravenously or intramuscularly, as required) can be particularly useful in severe agitation resistant to other sedatives, delirium or psychosis (see later in this chapter). They may also be useful for withdrawal symptoms. Butyrophenones produce a detached, tranquil state, have an antiemetic effect and are not usually associated with cardiovascular depression, even in high doses. Haloperidol may cause Q-T prolongation, as well as extrapyramidal side-effects. Interestingly, haloperidol, which is known to inhibit the secretion of pro-inflammatory cytokines, has been associated with a reduction in hospital mortality in mechanically ventilated patients (Milbrandt *et al.*, 2005). *Neuroleptic malignant syndrome* (see Chapter 20) is a rare complication. These agents have largely replaced the phenothiazines.

Ketamine

Ketamine is a phencyclidine derivative widely used in emergency situations to produce dissociative anaesthesia with cardiovascular stability, maintained muscle tone and profound analgesia. It has also proved useful in mechanically ventilated patients with severe asthma (Park *et al.*, 1987) (see Chapter 8). In subanaesthetic concentrations ketamine has analgesic and sedative properties. Ketamine is an NMDA receptor antagonist and thereby prevents or limits the hyperalgesia which can develop in response to prolonged nociceptive stimuli. When tolerance to opioids has developed ketamine may therefore restore analgesia and allow a reduction in the opiate dose. The initial intravenous dose is 1–4.5 mg/kg, followed by an infusion of 10–45 µg/kg per min adjusted according to response. Although useful in hypotensive patients and those with bronchospasm, ketamine's catecholamine-releasing properties may precipitate tachycardia and hypertension. Emergence delirium, vivid dreams and occasionally hallucinations have also limited its usefulness during routine anaesthesia, but these can be ameliorated by concomitant benzodiazepine administration.

MUSCLE RELAXATION

In the critically ill, muscle relaxants are used:

- to allow tracheal intubation;
- to facilitate mechanical ventilation, especially in those with critical gas exchange or severe airways obstruction;
- to enable procedures to be performed (e.g. bronchoscopy, percutaneous tracheostomy);
- occasionally to decrease metabolic requirements in ventilated patients with reduced cardiorespiratory reserves (see Chapters 7 and 8);
- to facilitate control of intracranial hypertension (see Chapter 15);

Table 11.13 Suggested adult doses of neuromuscular blocking agents given to critically ill mechanically ventilated patients

Neuromuscular-blocking drug	Bolus dose	Infusion rate
Suxamethonium	0.5–1.5 mg/kg	Not suitable
Pancuronium	0.5–4 mg	Not suitable
Vecuronium	40–100 µg/kg	50–80 µg/kg per h
Atracurium	600 µg/kg	300–600 µg/kg per h
Rocuronium	600 µg/kg	300–600 µg/kg per h

- to control abnormal movements refractory to the administration of sedative or hypnotic agents alone;
- in the management of tetanus (see Chapter 15).

The use of muscle relaxants in the ICU is more complicated than in the operating theatre because treatment is prolonged, and their activity may be influenced by associated therapies, as well as the severity of the patient's condition and organ failures, including critical illness polyneuropmyopathy. There have also been difficulties because their administration has usually not been monitored using peripheral nerve stimulators. In practice train of four following stimulation of the ulnar nerve with a hand-held stimulator is the most convenient method for monitoring the degree of neuromuscular blockade.

If precise control of the degree of muscle relaxation is not required, on-demand repeat injections are acceptable, otherwise a continuous intravenous infusion is preferred (**Table 11.13**). Nevertheless it must be remembered that, even with *atracurium*, a muscle relaxant with little interpatient pharmacodynamic variation, the individual dose requirements for continuous infusion may vary as much as fivefold (Yate *et al.*, 1987).

The *side-effects* of neuromuscular-blocking drugs include various histaminic reactions as well as severe or even life-threatening bronchospasm. Although cardiovascular changes are generally negligible, bolus injection of muscle relaxants may be accompanied by brady- or tachyarrhythmias, and even cardiac arrest. In particular, succinylcholine can cause extreme bradycardia or asystole and is contraindicated in a variety of conditions in which muscle fasciculations might precipitate hypertonia or systemic hyperkalaemia. Succinylcholine may be indicated when the airway must be secured rapidly, especially when a full stomach is suspected, although one of the newer, rapid-onset non-depolarizing muscle relaxants such as *rocuronium* may also be used in this situation. *Pancuronium* and *vecuronium* do not release histamine, whilst with *atracurium* histamine is released only at high doses. Pancuronium is associated with a tachycardia and a well-maintained blood pressure, whilst with vecuronium and atracurium cardiovascular stability is usually well maintained.

The duration of action of all non-depolarizing muscle relaxants can be prolonged in critically ill patients. This may be attributable to immobilization, metabolic disorders, malnutrition and concomitant steroid or aminoglycoside antibiotic therapy. It may be more likely to follow the uncontrolled administration of *vecuronium*, active metabolites of which may accumulate, especially in the presence of renal impairment (Segredo *et al.*, 1990). *Atracurium besilate* is the only agent whose action is not dramatically increased in cases of multiple-organ failure because of its rapid spontaneous degradation by the Hofmann elimination reaction in all clinical situations except deep hypothermia.

Perhaps understandably, muscle relaxant administration has been implicated as a cause of the neuromuscular weakness sometimes encountered in patients who survive life-threatening illness. It would seem, however, that in many cases the development of acquired neuromuscular disorders in intensive care patients is unrelated to the use of these agents, although disuse atrophy is likely with prolonged use (see Chapter 15). Other disadvantages of the use of muscle relaxants include the risk of awareness, the danger of disconnection from the ventilator, the inability to perform a full neurological assessment and an increased risk of infection and thromboembolism.

ANTIEMETICS

As well as the prokinetics (see earlier in this chapter), such as metoclopramide and domperidone, the following agents may prove useful from time to time as antiemetics in critically ill patients:

- Phenothiazines – these agents block dopamine D_2 receptors in the chemoreceptor trigger zone and have variable anticholinergic effects. Prochlorpherazine is the most commonly used phenothiazine for this indication in a dose of 5–12.5 mg i.v. Side-effects, including hypotension, sedation and extrapyramidal reactions, are common. Neuroleptic malignant syndrome is rare.
- Butyrophenones – droperidol (0.25–5 mg i.v.) is most often used. Side-effects are similar to those of the phenothiazines.
- Antihistamines – these agents act principally on vestibular efferents. Cyclizine, which has additional anticholinergic effects, is currently a popular antiemetic in a dose of 50 mg i.m.
- Dexamethasone – effective when used prophylactically. Probably acts by reducing the inflammatory response to surgery.
- 5-HT receptor antagonists (ondansetron, granisetron) – these agents block vagal afferent pathways and 5-HT receptors in the area postrema. They can be effective for otherwise unresponsive nausea and vomiting. Ondansetron can be given in a dose of 4–8 mg i.v. Side-effects are few.

A recent trial of antiemetics for the prevention of postoperative nausea and vomiting concluded that since the various interventions were equally effective, the safest and least expensive should be used first (Apfel *et al.*, 2004).

PREVENTION OF DEEP VENOUS THROMBOSIS AND PULMONARY THROMBOEMBOLISM (Weinmann and Salzman, 1994)

The pathophysiological processes involved in the causation of deep venous thrombosis (DVT) and pulmonary embolism (PE) were first studied by Rudolf Virchow. He proposed three main predisposing factors:

1. damage to the vessel wall;
2. diminution of blood flow;
3. increased coagulability of the blood.

These three factors (Virchow's triad) are still thought to account for most cases of thromboembolism occurring in the critically ill, in whom coexistent risk factors such as prolonged immobility, surgery and indwelling vascular catheters are common. In many cases thromboembolic disease is silent and difficult to diagnose with certainty. DVT is common in critically ill patients, with rates varying from 22% to almost 80% depending on patient characteristics (Attia *et al.*, 2001). Venous thromboembolism is a particularly common complication of major trauma (Geerts *et al.*, 1994), acute spinal cord injury (Attia *et al.*, 2001), infectious polyneuritis (see Chapter 15) and pregnancy (see Chapter 18). In such patients some form of screening practice, such as repeat duplex scanning studies, may be advantageous. Even in a group of critically ill patients receiving universal, protocol-directed thromboprophylaxis the incidence of DVT was 9.6% (Cook *et al.*, 2005). In this prospective cohort study (from which those with a diagnosis of trauma, orthopaedic surgery and pregnancy were excluded) risk factors for ICU-acquired DVT were:

- personal or family history of venous thromboembolism;
- end-stage renal failure;
- platelet transfusion;
- vasopressor use.

Duration of mechanical ventilation, ICU stay and hospitalization were longer in those with DVT than in those without (Cook *et al.*, 2005).

In most intensive care patients, passive leg exercises combined with subcutaneous *low-dose heparin* and early mobilization offer sufficient protection. Heparin prophylaxis may be contraindicated in neurosurgical patients, as well as in some trauma patients (e.g. those with head or ophthalmic injuries) and those with documented haemostatic failure. In such cases *intermittent pneumatic compression* of the legs may be effective. *Elastic graduated-compression stockings* may also be beneficial, especially when combined with other measures. There is little information on the risks and benefits of the various thromboembolic prophylactic regimes in critically ill patients and methods of prophylaxis proven in one group are not necessarily as effective in another (Attia et al., 2001). High-risk patients may benefit from the use of prophylactic regimes which combine mechanical and pharmacological interventions. Clearly the risk-to-benefit ratio will vary from patient to patient and should be assessed individually.

Low-molecular-weight heparins (e.g. enoxaparin) (Weitz, 1997) are fragments of unfractionated heparin produced by controlled enzymatic or chemical depolymerization processes that yield chains with a mean molecular weight of about 5000. Unlike unfractionated heparin (molecular weight 3000–30 000), which has equivalent activity against factor Xa and thrombin, low-molecular-weight heparins are predominantly active against factor Xa. They also cause less inhibition of platelet function and do not increase microvascular permeability. Low-molecular-weight heparins produce a more predictable anticoagulant response than unfractionated heparin, reflecting their greater bioavailability, longer (two to four times) half-life and dose-independent clearance. These differences are largely explained by the reduced binding affinity of low-molecular-weight heparins for plasma proteins, endothelial cells and macrophages. Consequently, unlike therapeutic unfractionated heparin, treatment with low-molecular-weight heparin does not normally require laboratory monitoring.

The risk of bleeding seems to be reduced compared to unfractionated heparin, as does the incidence of heparin-induced thrombocytopenia. Nevertheless low-molecular-weight heparins should not be used in patients wih established heparin-induced thrombocytopenia because of the considerable cross-reactivity of the responsible antibody. An alternative in this situation is to use danaparoid sodium, which exhibits minimal cross-reactivity in vitro, or a direct thrombin inhibitor such as hirudin. In patients with major trauma, low-molecular-weight heparin has been shown to be more efficacious than low-dose heparin (Geerts et al., 1996), consistent with findings in orthopaedic patients and following spinal cord injury. Disadvantages of low-molecular-weight heparins in the critically ill include the need for subcutaneous absorption when peripheral perfusion may be poor and the lack of a means of reversing their anticoagulant effects. In some cases, therefore, a low-dose intravenous infusion of unfractionated heparin (e.g. 500 iu/hour initially), which can be discontinued and reversed with protamine if necessary, may be preferred.

PREVENTION OF STRESS ULCERATION

Stress-related gastric mucosal injury may lead to superficial erosions that are usually diffuse and associated with a low risk of serious bleeding, or to 'stress ulcers', that are deeper, more focal lesions and are more likely to be complicated by significant haemorrhage. Occasionally mucosal lesions may penetrate more deeply and erode larger blood vessels. Mucosal injury associated with NSAIDs often consists of multiple erosions combined with some deeper ulcers. The pathogenesis of stress-related mucosal disease is complex but is thought to be largely related to reductions in mucosal blood flow and ischaemia–reperfusion injury, rather than excess acid production. Bleeding from the injured mucosa may be:

- occult (guaiac-positive nasogastric aspirate or stools; can be caused by nasogastric trauma);
- overt (haematemesis, gross blood or 'coffee grounds' in the gastric aspirate, melaena);
- clinically significant (overt bleeding complicated by hypotension, tachycardia, an orthostatic change, a fall in haemoglobin of > 2 g/dl or the need for transfusion of 2 units of blood within 24 hours).

Acute gastrointestinal haemorrhage associated with stress-related mucosal injury was at one time a very common, serious and life-threatening complication of critical illness (see Chapter 16). Those with burns (Curling's ulcers – may be single and deep), head injuries (Cushing's ulcers), multiple trauma, renal failure, respiratory failure, jaundice, hypotension and severe sepsis were conventionally considered to be at greatest risk. The incidence of gastrointestinal haemorrhage from stress ulceration has, however, decreased dramatically since the early days of intensive care (Cook et al., 1994), perhaps in part due to the widespread use of prophylactic measures, but also as a result of more effective treatment of acute hypoxaemia and hypotension, as well as improved respiratory care (Tryba, 1994). The use of early enteral alimentation has also been associated with a significant decrease in the risk of gastrointestinal haemorrhage (Pingleton and Hadzima, 1983). Nevertheless, in the absence of prophylactic measures the frequency of acute upper gastrointestinal mucosal injury may approach 90% within 3 days of admission to intensive care (Eddleston et al., 1994) and currently overt bleeding is thought to occur in around 5% of heterogeneous groups of intensive care patients, while clinically important bleeding occurs in only approximately 1–4% of critically ill patients. The mortality in those who do develop clinically important bleeding may be as high as 50%, although most die with, rather than as a direct consequence of, haemorrhage. Clinically significant bleeding is also associated with considerable morbidity and increased costs.

Antacids, H_2 receptor antagonists, and sucralfate all appear to decrease the rate of bleeding compared to placebo (Cook et al., 1991, 1996), as do proton pump inhibitors.

Antacid therapy is directed at maintaining the gastric pH consistently higher than 3.5, the value at which the incidence of bleeding diminishes significantly. This regimen has proved effective in many studies, but is inconvenient to administer and can result in diarrhoea and metabolic abnormalities.

H_2-receptor blockers can be administered orally or intravenously, by either bolus or continuous infusion, the intention being to maintain the gastric pH above 3.5. These agents also increase mucosal blood flow, as well as stimulating mucus production and prostaglandin synthesis (Friedman *et al.*, 1982; Shuman *et al.*, 1987). Development of tolerance over a period of 2–3 days may, however, lead to a significant reduction in acid suppression. Moreover a number of observational studies have suggested that the higher gastric pH consequent on treatment with H_2-receptor antagonists (and antacids) may be associated with bacterial overgrowth in the stomach, tracheobronchial colonization and an increased risk of ventilator-associated pneumonia.

Sucralfate is an aluminium hydroxide salt of sucrose octasulphate that can be administered orally or nasogastrically. It is only a weak antacid, but has antipepsin activity, stimulates prostaglandin synthesis and forms a protective coating over inflamed areas of mucosa (Tryba *et al.*, 1985). It has been associated with a lower incidence of nosocomial pneumonia, and a lower mortality than agents that cause marked reductions in gastric acidity (Driks *et al.*, 1987). Aluminium absorption may, however, lead to toxicity (osteomalacia, microcytic hypochromic anaemia, encephalopathy) in patients with renal failure, and rapid increases in plasma aluminium to toxic levels have been described in critically ill patients on continuous renal replacement therapy (Mulla *et al.*, 2001). In such patients alternative prophylactic agents should be used.

Proton pump inhibitors block H_2-receptor gastrin- and cholinergic-mediated acid production and inhibit gastric secretion at the final common pathway of the H^+/K^+ ATP proton pump. Tolerance does not develop to these agents and the reduction in gastric acidity can be maintained over prolonged periods. Continuous infusion of proton pump inhibitors is superior to bolus administration.

Prostaglandin E_2 derivatives have been used as stress ulcer prophylaxis in several studies, but have not proved to be effective. Misoprostol has been specifically recommended for protection against gastric injury induced by NSAIDs.

It is difficult to provide definitive recommendations for prophylactic therapy. Most now accept that prophylaxis against stress ulcers can be safely withheld from critically ill patients unless they have a coagulopathy or require mechanical ventilation for 48 hours or more (Cook *et al.*, 1994), the risk of bleeding in such patients being around 3–5% compared to less than 0.1% in other categories of intensive care patients. Many also believe that those who are tolerating large-volume enteral feeds do not require prophylaxis against gastrointestinal haemorrhage. In general the risk of bleeding appears to increase with the duration of mechanical ventilation, time in ICU and the severity of illness. In contrast to previous evidence indicating that H_2-receptor antagonists and sucralfate were more or less equally effective in preventing stress ulceration, but that the use of sucralfate was associated with a lower risk of pneumonia and mortality (Cook *et al.*, 1996; Driks *et al.*, 1987), a more recent prospective randomized controlled trial demonstrated that patients receiving ranitidine have a significantly lower risk of gastrointestinal bleeding than those given sucralfate. Importantly,

in keeping with the results of other more recent trials, there was no significant difference in the incidence of ventilator-associated pneumonia, nor was there any difference in mortality or length of ICU stay, between the groups (Cook *et al.*, 1998). On this basis most now recommend the use of H_2-receptor antagonists in at-risk patients. The debate continues, however, and a recent meta-analysis controversially concluded that ranitidine is ineffective as a means of preventing gastrointestinal bleeding in ICU patients and might increase the risk of pneumonia (Messori *et al.*, 2000). It should also not be forgotten that, although prophylaxis for gastrointestinal bleeding reduces morbidity (Cook *et al.*, 1991) and possibly the duration of intubation and length of ICU stay (Eddleston *et al.*, 1994), it has not been shown to influence mortality.

PSYCHOLOGICAL AND BEHAVIOURAL DISORDERS

Patients treated in the ICU can develop various acute psychological disturbances or alterations in mental state, which may become manifest either in the unit or following discharge. In many cases the disorder has an organic cause, whereas in others it is a result of the emotional impact of the critical illness and its treatment, or a combination of these. A number of patients, especially those admitted after accidents or self-harm, have a pre-existing psychiatric disorder or other predisposing factors.

DELIRIUM

Delirium is the most commonly encountered serious mental disturbance in critically ill patients and is now being increasingly recognized, with a prevalence, depending on case-mix, that ranges from 15 to 18% of patients at some time during their stay. This syndrome is characterized by an acute and often reversible fluctuation or clouding of consciousness with reduced awareness of the environment, agitation and confusion. Many patients present with decreased psychomotor activity, reduced awareness, apathy and drowsiness (*hypoactive subtype*) and are not easily recognized unless formally examined. Others are agitated and may become restless, and even violent, with illusions, hallucinations and delusions of persecution (*hyperactive subtype*). In some cases there are features of both hyper- and hypoactivity. Characteristically, the severity of the mental disturbance fluctuates, with lucid intervals during the day and deterioration at night. Attention deficits can be regarded as the hallmark of confusional states. Patients are easily distracted and cannot maintain their focus of attention during a task. Memory and orientation for time and place are also typically impaired. Patients are often disorganized, irrational and manifest impaired reasoning.

An underlying cause can be identified in more than 85% of cases of delirium. It is important to recognize the following predisposing factors and causes:

- hypoxia (including carbon monoxide poisoning);
- hypotension;
- hypo- or hyperglycaemia;
- hypertensive encephalopathy;
- Wernicke's encephalopathy;
- withdrawal from drugs (alcohol, opiates, sedatives – see below);
- meningitis/encephalitis;
- cerebrovascular accident/intracranial haematoma, abscess or tumour;
- seizures (especially when complex/partial);
- poisoning/medications (e.g. benzodiazepines);
- metabolic disturbances (acidosis, alkalosis, dehydration, electrolyte disturbance, uraemia, hepatic encephalopathy);
- trauma (heat stroke, severe burn, postoperative).

Delirium is commoner in surgical patients (especially post cardiac surgery and burns) and in the older age groups: children appear to be particularly resistant. The risk of developing delirium is increased by sleep deprivation.

The majority of delirious patients recover without observable sequelae, although some progress to stupor or coma and die. Delirium and agitation increase the risk of complications such as retention of pulmonary secretions, lung collapse and aspiration pneumonia; length of stay is prolonged and mortality rates are high. In one study of mechanically ventilated patients delirium was common and appeared to be an independent predictor of higher 6-month mortality and longer duration of hospital stay (Ely et al., 2004). Delirium is also associated with increased costs (Milbrandt et al., 2004). In another study severe agitation was seen in 16% of mechanically ventilated patients and was associated with prolonged ICU stay and duration of mechanical ventilation, as well as a higher rate of self-extubation. Mortality was not, however, increased (Woods et al., 2004).

Agitation (defined as a state of increased psychomotor activity, often accompanied by an increased rate and volume of speech, as well as labile and inappropriate affect) can also occur in critically ill patients in the absence of altered consciousness (i.e. they are not considered to be delirious). Predisposing factors include:

- poor comprehension (language barrier, intellectual impairment);
- sensory impairment (e.g. visual or auditory);
- anxiety/fear;
- pain;
- personality disorder.

Confusion (defined as lack of certainty, orderly thought or power to distinguish, choose or act decisively) is also not specific to delirium. In those with clear consciousness the differential diagnosis should include:

- dementia;
- functional psychosis (may resemble delirium when disorganized, agitated and confused);
- mood disorder;
- seizure;
- conversion disorder;
- malingering; ⎫ rarely seen in intensive care
- dissociative disorder. ⎭

ACUTE FUNCTIONAL PSYCHOSES

Some patients in ICU experience extreme stress, anxiety and fear of impending death, although others have little real experience of, and often have complete amnesia for, the acute phase of their critical illness. Some authors have implicated the restrictions that critically ill patients suffer, such as being unable to speak, unable to communicate and being restrained in the development of psychosis. In addition, they are severely deprived of sleep, and stages 3 and 4 and rapid-eye movement sleep are severely or completely suppressed (Aurell and Elmqvist, 1985). They also suffer from reduced stimulation, social isolation and physical confinement. Such sensory deprivation is known to induce hallucinations of sound, vision, touch and movement as well as reduced vigilance and an underestimation of time. Patients may also be subjected to significant noise and light pollution, repetitive stimulation (e.g. flashing lights on monitors and infusion pumps, the sound of alarms) and occasional severe discomfort or pain. However convincing evidence that any of these extrinsic features is sufficient on its own to induce psychosis is lacking. Impairment of cerebral function (e.g. caused by drugs or metabolic derangement, particularly in sepsis) may exaggerate the psychological response of the patient to these environmental stresses and predispose to the development of an acute functional psychosis. These may present as thought disorder, delusions or hallucinations in a patient who is fully conscious and oriented with an intact memory. Unlike delirium, which always has an organic cause, acute functional psychoses resolve when the patient is removed from the intimidating environment that triggered the acute syndrome (Lloyd, 1993). It is now also recognized, however, that patients who have no recollection of intensive care but have suffered delusional, often paranoid experiences are prone to the subsequent development of acute stress reactions (Jones et al., 2001a).

Cardiopulmonary bypass has been particularly associated with delirium and psychosis, although the incidence of serious mental disturbance in this category of patient is now relatively low. This is probably due to a number of factors, including shorter bypass times, careful preoperative preparation and attention to environmental factors within the ICU.

ANXIETY AND DEPRESSION

Intensive care patients may also exhibit a variety of less severe psychological reactions to their predicament. These range from overwhelming fear, tension and sustained anxiety to severe, often agitated, depression and negativism. Patients may exhibit obsessive-compulsive behaviour in which they analyse every aspect of their situation and illness in minute detail; alternatively, they may display repression by rejecting their problem and allowing staff a 'free hand'. Some patients become totally dependent, while others are wholeheartedly involved in their own treatment, denying any feelings of fear or hopelessness. Because many critically ill patients are unable to speak it is, however, difficult to diagnose anxiety or depression confidently. Indeed many of the non-verbal symptoms of these disorders can be explained by delirium, which is probably much more common.

PRE-EXISTING DISORDERS

Many patients admitted to ICU will have pre-existing psychological problems. These will then manifest themselves, sometimes in exaggerated form, as the patient recovers. It has been suggested that certain abnormal personality traits or mental diseases may predispose to particular types of physical illness; cases of self-poisoning, drug addiction and alcohol abuse are among the more obvious examples.

The features of *narcotic addiction* include pinpoint pupils and transitory elation, which is followed by marked anxiety and restlessness. Anorexia, constipation and extreme weight loss are common, as is loss of libido. Examination may reveal multiple injection sites, sometimes with bruising, abscesses and septic thrombophlebitis. *Signs and symptoms of withdrawal* include:

- running eyes and nose;
- sneezing;
- perspiration;
- gooseflesh;
- vague aches and pains;
- anxiety, restlessness, aggression;
- dilated pupils.

Nausea, vomiting, abdominal pain, diarrhoea, limb cramps, sleeplessness and agitation may also occur.

Alcohol withdrawal is characterized by nervous system excitation, which varies from mild sleeplessness and irritability to *delirium tremens*. In mild cases there is:

- tremor;
- perspiration;
- nervousness;
- dyspepsia;
- weakness;
- anorexia;
- hyperreflexia;
- labile affect;
- increased arousal;
- insomnia.

Severe cases exhibit:

- hypertension;
- tachycardia;
- fever;
- hallucinations (visual, tactile or auditory);

- disorientation;
- convulsions.

Delirium tremens is characterized by:

- delirium;
- clouding of consciousness;
- convulsions.

In addition, alcohol can exacerbate pre-existing psychiatric disorders such as aggressive psychopathy, manic-depressive psychoses and paranoid schizophrenia.

PREVENTION

Prevention of these psychological disturbances involves maintaining the patient's contact with reality, together with frequent explanation and reassurance, control of metabolic disturbances and the provision of adequate analgesia and anxiolysis. This presents a considerable challenge in the ventilated patient.

For those who are conscious and alert, some form of occupational therapy is required; this may take the form of radio, television or 'talking' books. Maintaining effective communication between staff and the patient is crucial and may involve the use of writing boards, cards displaying letters of the alphabet or illustrations or speaking valves. As normal an environment as possible should be maintained (e.g. darkness, silence and, if possible, uninterrupted sleep at night with natural daylight and wakefulness during the day). Assessment and treatment can also disturb the patient's sleep and should be kept to a minimum. Staff should consider clustering their activities to provide adequate rest periods (at least 90 minutes). Night sedation (e.g. with temazepam 10–20 mg or lorazepam 1–2 mg orally) is often useful to initiate sleep. Even when conditions are optimal, however, normal sleep patterns are disrupted and do not return to normal until the patient recovers. Although sleep is abnormal, whether patients are deprived of sleep remains unclear. Even though sleep deprivation alone is not a cause of delirium or psychosis, lack of sleep may predispose critically ill patients to develop disorientation, hallucinations, delusions and mood changes.

It is also important that ICUs are provided with windows (see Chapter 1), preferably with a view, although this is probably more important to staff and visitors than to patients. Frequent information regarding the time, day of the week and season of the year should be provided. It has been suggested that a digital clock/radio and possibly a calendar can therefore be very useful. The patient should be allowed as much privacy as possible, while monitoring and other equipment should be unobtrusively sited, preferably behind the patient's head. Finally, all procedures must be fully explained before they are performed and frequent encouragement must be provided about the progress of the illness. It is important to remember that some patients who appear to be unconscious may not be; they will require local anaesthesia or intravenous sedation to avoid awareness before painful therapeutic interventions, procedures to establish invasive monitoring or elective direct current cardioversion. Although conventional wisdom has been that amnesia for their time in intensive care helps to protect patients from psychological sequelae, evidence has suggested that amnesia and oversedation are associated with an increased incidence of the delusions which predispose to the subsequent development of posttraumatic stress disorder (PTSD) (Jones *et al.*, 2001b).

These psychological aspects of patient care are particularly dependent on the nurses who spend many hours at the bedside of one individual patient and have the opportunity to establish a close and understanding relationship.

TREATMENT

In the intensive care unit setting delirium can be diagnosed reliably and rapidly using the Confusion Assessment Method for the Intensive Care Unit (CAM-ICU) (Ely *et al.*, 2001).

When present, underlying causes such as encephalitis, encephalopathy and cerebrovascular accident (see above) will require specific treatment, while hypotension, hypoxia, electrolyte and acid–base disorders should be corrected as rapidly as possible. Pain and discomfort must be controlled. In those with drug-induced delirium the offending drug should be stopped and an alternative agent substituted if necessary. In some cases administration of an antidote may be indicated (e.g. naloxone, flumazenil – see Chapter 19). Drug withdrawal should be actively managed. Those with inadequate coping skills will require sensitive support from the medical and nursing staff, family and friends and, in some cases, a psychiatrist.

Although the patient's inevitable anxiety can usually be safely controlled using benzodiazepines, severe depression is less easily treated. *Tricyclic antidepressants* are often ineffective and may be associated with dangerous cardiovascular side-effects; a *selective serotonin reuptake inhibitor* may therefore be preferred. Acute agitation/confusion may require treatment with either benzodiazepines or butyrophenones to avoid self-harm. *Haloperidol*, which has minimal autonomic effects, is probably the agent of choice in the critically ill; intravenous and/or intramuscular injection of this agent in a dose of 2–10 mg, repeated as necessary (up to a total of 18 mg per day), is effective in most cases, although larger doses may occasionally be required. Smaller doses (as low as 0.5 mg) may be appropriate in the elderly. Continuous infusions of haloperidol have been shown to be effective in controlling severe agitation in critically ill patients. This approach may also reduce the requirement for bolus administration of sedatives, reduce nursing workload and facilitate weaning from mechanical ventilation (Riker *et al.*, 1994). Side-effects include prolonged QT_c interval, arrhythmias (including *torsades de pointes*), hypotension and extrapyramidal effects. Alternatively *diazepam* 2.5–5 mg or *lorazepam* 0.5–1 mg in repeated intravenous doses may be preferred. A continuous infusion of *midazolam* can be effective in severely agitated patients. Some patients benefit from combined administration of a neuroleptic and a benzodiazepine, whilst

in others an α_2-agonist may successfully control confusional agitation and in view of recent evidence (Panharipande *et al.*, 2007) may be preferred. In extreme cases patient safety may only be guaranteed by heavy sedation and tracheal intubation, sometimes with mechanical ventilation and administration of muscle relaxants. The use of high doses of sedatives, analgesics and muscle relaxants to control agitation is, however, likely to be associated with delayed weaning and prolongation of ICU stay. If necessary, symptoms of narcotic withdrawal can be controlled with *methadone*, 10–20 mg, which can be repeated 1–2 hours later and should be effective for about 12 hours.

Mechanical restraint may be indicated to protect severely agitated patients from self-harm (e.g. by removal of intravascular cannulae or endotracheal tubes, falling out of bed) and may in some cases be preferable to (and safer than) heavy sedation (pharmacological restraint) (Nirmalan *et al.*, 2004).

RELATIVES AND FRIENDS

The morale of relatives and close friends is also most important; they should receive every possible care and attention. In particular, they should be given frequent detailed explanations about the patient's treatment and progress; because of their high levels of stress and anxiety repetition is essential to ensure understanding and retention of important facts. As far as possible, free visiting should be allowed since this is beneficial not only to the visitor, but also to the patients, helping them to maintain contact with reality. Visitors should be encouraged to talk to and touch the patient. Some derive comfort and support from participating in the patient's care. Some relatives develop clinical levels of anxiety and acute stress disorders that may need support.

LONG-TERM OUTCOME

Until recently little was known about the long-term psychological effects of hospitalization following critical illness on either the patients or their relatives and close friends. It is now well recognized that those who have been in exceptionally threatening or catastrophic accidents are prone to prolonged psychological reactions, particularly *PTSD* and other phobic anxiety syndromes. Characteristic features of PTSD include:

- flashback memories of the original incident;
- recurrent nightmares;
- emotional numbing;
- autonomic hyperarousal;
- avoidance behaviour.

Certainly memories of dreams, nightmares, hallucinations and paranoid delusions are common in survivors of prolonged critical illness (Rundshagen *et al.*, 2002). In some cases the persistent recollection of unpleasant experiences, sometimes accompanied by other features of PTSD (Perry *et al.*, 1992; Roca *et al.*, 1992), can interfere with normal psychosocial function and quality of life may be significantly impaired. PTSD-related symptoms are also common in relatives of patients who have undergone intensive care (Jones *et al.*, 2004) and are more frequent amongst those who feel they have received incomplete information, those whose relative died in the ICU, those whose relative died after end-of-life decisions and those who shared in such decision making (Azoulay *et al.*, 2005). Severe posttraumatic stress reaction in family members is associated with increased rates of anxiety and depression and a decreased quality of life (Azoulay *et al.*, 2005).

Those working in follow-up clinics are best placed to evaluate, in collaboration with the general practitioner, psychological symptoms following hospital discharge (Jones and Griffiths, 2002). They can also arrange treatment with antidepressant drugs or psychotherapy when indicated, as well as counselling for the patient and relatives or close friends. A self-help rehabilitation manual has been shown to be effective in assisting physical recovery and reducing depression but was less effective for treating anxiety and PTSD (Jones *et al.*, 2003)

REFERENCES

Aitkenhead AR, Pepperman ML, Willatts SM, *et al.* (1989) Comparison of propofol and midazolam for sedation in critically ill patients. *Lancet* **2**: 704–709.

Alexander JW (1990) Nutrition and translocation. *Journal of Parenteral and Enteral Nutrition* **14** (Suppl): 170S–174S.

Alverdy JC, Aoys E, Moss GS (1988) Total parenteral nutrition promotes bacterial translocation from the gut. *Surgery* **104**: 185–190.

Apfel CC, Korttila K, Abdalla M, *et al.* (2004) A factorial trial of six interventions for the prevention of postoperative nausea and vomiting. *New England Journal of Medicine* **350**: 2441–2451.

Askanazi J, Weissman C, Rosenbaum SH, *et al.* (1982) Nutrition and the respiratory system. *Critical Care Medicine* **10**: 163–172.

ASPEN Board of Directors and the Clinical Guidelines Task Force (2002) Guidelines for the use of parenteral and enteral nutrition in adult and pediatric patients *Journal of Parenteral and Enteral Nutrition* **26** (suppl.): 1SA–138SA.

Atkinson S, Sieffert E, Bihari D, *et al.* (1998) A prospective, randomized, double-blind, controlled clinical trial of enteral immunonutrition in the critically ill. *Critical Care Medicine* **26**: 1164–1172.

Attia J, Ray JG, Cook DJ, *et al.* (2001) Deep vein thrombosis and its prevention in critically ill adults. *Archives of Internal Medicine* **161**: 1268–1279.

Aurell J, Elmqvist D (1985) Sleep in the surgical intensive care unit: continuous polygraphic recording of sleep in nine patients receiving postoperative care. *British Medical Journal* **290**: 1029–1032.

Ayus JC, Arieff AI (1999) Chronic hyponatremic encephalopathy in postmenopausal women: association of therapies with morbidity and mortality. *Journal of the American Medical Association* **281**: 2299–2304.

Azoulay E, Pochard F, Kentish-Barnes N, *et al.* (2005) Risk of post-traumatic stress symptoms in family members of intensive care unit patients. *American Journal of Respiratory and Critical Care Medicine* **171**: 987–994.

Ball M, McQuay HJ, Moore RA, *et al.* (1985) Renal failure and the use of morphine in intensive care. *Lancet* **1**: 784–786.

Barrientos-Vega R, Sánchez-Soria MM, Morales-Garcia C, *et al.* (1997) Prolonged sedation of critically ill patients with midazolam or propofol: impact on weaning and costs. *Critical Care Medicine* **25**: 33–40.

Barrientos-Vega R, Sánchez-Soria MM, Morales-Garcia C, *et al.* (2001) Pharmacoeconomic assessment of propofol 2% used for prolonged sedation. *Critical Care Medicine* **29**: 317–322.

Bérard M-P, Zazzo J-F, Condat P, *et al.* (2000) Total parenteral nutrition enriched with arginine and glutamate generates glutamine and limits protein catabolism in surgical patients hospitalized in intensive care units. *Critical Care Medicine* **28**: 3637–3644.

Berger MM, Bollmann MD, Revelly J-P, *et al.* (2002) Progression rate of self-propelled feeding tubes in critically ill patients. *Intensive Care Medicine* **28**: 1768–1774.

Bertolini G, Iapichino G, Radrizzani D, *et al.* (2003) Early enteral immunonutrition in patients with severe sepsis: results of an interim analysis of a randomized multicentre clinical trial. *Intensive Care Medicine* **29**: 834–840.

Bistrian BR, Babineau T (1998) Optimal protein intake in critical illness. *Critical Care Medicine* **26**: 1476–1477.

Booth CM, Heyland DK, Paterson WG (2002) Gastrointestinal promotility drugs in the critical care setting: a systematic review of the evidence. *Critical Care Medicine* **30**: 1429–1435.

Bower RH, Cerra FB, Bershadsky B, *et al.* (1995) Early enteral administration of a formula (impact) supplemented with arginine, nucleotides, and fish oil in intensive care unit patients: results of a multicenter, prospective, randomized, clinical trial. *Critical Care Medicine* **23**: 436–449.

Bozzetti F, Braga M, Gianotti L, *et al.* (2001) Postoperative enteral versus parenteral nutrition in malnourished patients with gastrointestinal cancer: a randomised multicentre trial. *Lancet* **358**: 1487–1492.

Braga M, Vignali A, Gianotti L, *et al.* (1995) Benefits of early postoperative enteral feeding in cancer patients. *Infusionsther Transfusionsmed* **22**: 280–284.

Brattebo G, Hofoss D, Flaatten H, *et al.* (2002) Effect of a scoring system and protocol for sedation on duration of patients' need for ventilator support in a surgical intensive care unit. *British Medical Journal* **324**: 1386–1389.

Bugg NC, Jones JA (1998) Hypophosphataemia: pathophysiology, effects and management on the intensive care unit. *Anaesthesia* **53**: 895–902.

Buggy DJ, Smith G (1999) Epidural anaesthesia and analgesia: better outcome after major surgery? *British Medical Journal* **319**: 530–531.

Calder PC (2003) Immunonutrition. *British Medical Journal* **327**: 117–118.

Cammarano WB, Pittet J-F, Weitz S, *et al.* (1998) Acute withdrawal syndrome related to the administration of analgesic and sedative medications in adult intensive care unit patients. *Critical Care Medicine* **26**: 676–684.

Carr CS, Ling KD, Boulos P, *et al.* (1996) Randomised trial of safety and efficacy of immediate postoperative enteral feeding in patients undergoing gastrointestinal resection. *British Medical Journal* **312**: 869–871.

Cerra F, Blackburn G, Hirsch J, *et al.* (1987) The effect of stress level, amino acid formula, and nitrogen dose on nitrogen retention in traumatic and septic stress. *Annals of Surgery* **205**: 282–287.

Cerra FB, Lehmann S, Konstantinides FN, *et al.* (1991) Improvement in immune function in ICU patients with enteral nutrition supplemented with arginine, RNA and menhaden oil is independent of nitrogen balance. *Nutrition* **7**: 193–199.

Conejero R, Bonet A, Grau T, *et al.* (2002) Effect of a glutamine-enriched enteral diet on intestinal permeability and infectious morbidity at 28 days in critically ill patients with systemic inflammatory response syndrome: a randomized, single-blind, prospective, multicenter study. *Nutrition* **18**: 716–721.

Cook DJ, Witt LG, Cook RJ, *et al.* (1991) Stress ulcer prophylaxis in the critically ill: a meta-analysis. *American Journal of Medicine* **91**: 519–527.

Cook DJ, Fuller HD, Guyatt GH, *et al.* (1994) Risk factors for gastrointestinal bleeding in critically ill patients. *New England Journal of Medicine* **330**: 377–381.

Cook DJ, Reeve BK, Guyatt GH, *et al.* (1996) Stress ulcer prophylaxis in critically ill patients. Resolving discordant meta-analyses. *Journal of the American Medical Association* **275**: 308–314.

Cook D, Guyatt G, Marshall J, *et al.* (1998) A comparison of sucralfate and ranitidine for the prevention of upper gastrointestinal bleeding in patients requiring mechanical ventilation. *New England Journal of Medicine* **338**: 791–797.

Cook D, Crowther M, Meade M, *et al.* (2005) Deep venous thrombosis in medical-surgical critically ill patients: prevalence, incidence, and risk factors. *Critical Care Medicine* **33**: 1565–1571.

Dahl JB, Kehlet H (1991) Non-steroidal anti-inflammatory drugs: rationale for use in severe postoperative pain. *British Journal of Anaesthesia* **66**: 703–712.

Davies AR, Froomes PR, French CJ, *et al.* (2002) Randomized comparison of nasojejunal and nasogastric feeding in critically ill patients. *Critical Care Medicine* **30**: 586–590.

De Jonghe B, Appere-De-Vechi C, Fournier M, et al. (2001) A prospective survey of nutritional support practices in intensive care unit patients: what is prescribed? What is delivered? *Critical Care Medicine* 29: 8–12.

Detriche O, Berré J, Massaut J, et al. (1999) The Brussels sedation scale: use of a simple clinical sedation scale can avoid excessive sedation in patients undergoing mechanical ventilation in the intensive care unit. *British Journal of Anaesthesia* 83: 698–701.

Detsky AS (1991) Parenteral nutrition – is it helpful? *New England Journal of Medicine* 325: 573–575.

Detsky AS, Baker JP, O'Rourke K, Goel V (1987) Perioperative parenteral nutrition: a meta-analysis. *Annals of Internal Medicine* 107: 195–203.

Dhaliwal R, Jurewitsch B, Harrietha D, et al. (2004) Combination enteral and parenteral nutrition in critically ill patients: harmful or beneficial? A systematic review of the evidence. *Intensive Care Medicine* 30: 1666–1671.

Dirksen MS, Vree TB, Driessen JJ (1987) Clinical pharmacokinetics of long term infusion of midazolam in critically ill patients. *Anaesthesia and Intensive Care* 15: 440–444.

Dominguez Cherit G, Borunda D, Rivero-Sigarroa E (2002) Total parenteral nutrition. *Current Opinion in Critical Care* 8: 285–289.

Driks MR, Craven DE, Celli BR, et al. (1987) Nosocomial pneumonia in intubated patients given sucralfate as compared with antacids or histamine type 2 blockers. The role of gastric colonization. *New England Journal of Medicine* 317: 1376–1382.

Driscoll DF, Blackburn GL (1990) Total parenteral nutrition 1990. A review of its current status in hospitalised patients and the need for patient-specific feeding. *Drugs* 40: 346–363.

Dunn SR, Farnsworth TA, Karunaratne WU (1999) Hypokalaemic, hyperchloraemic metabolic acidosis requiring ventilation. *Anaesthesia* 54: 566–568.

Eddleston JM, Pearson RC, Holland J, et al. (1994) Prospective endoscopic study of stress erosions and ulcers in critically ill adult patients treated with either sucralfate or placebo. *Critical Care Medicine* 22: 1949–1954.

Editorial (1980) Dangerous pseudohyponatraemia. *Lancet* 2: 1121.

Ely EW, Inouye SK, Bernard GR (2001) Delirium in mechanically ventilated patients. Validity and reliability of the Confusion Assessment Method for the Intensive Care Unit (CAM-ICU). Journal of the American Medical Association 286:2703–2710.

Ely EW, Shintani A, Truman B, et al. (2004) Delirium as a predictor of mortality in mechanically ventilated patients in the intensive care unit. *Journal of the American Medical Association* 291: 1753–1762.

Esparzel J, Boivin MA, Hartshorne MF, et al. (2001) Equal aspiration rates in gastrically and transpylorically fed critically ill patients. *Intensive Care Medicine* 27: 660–664.

Ferrante FM, Chan VW, Arthur GR, et al. (1991) Interpleural analgesia after thoracotomy. *Anaesthesia and Analgesia* 72: 105–109.

Flear CT, Singh CM (1973) Hyponatraemia and sick cells. *British Journal of Anaesthesia* 45: 976–994.

Friedman CJ, Oblinger MJ, Suratt PM, et al. (1982) Prophylaxis of upper gastrointestinal hemorrhage in patients requiring mechanical ventilation. *Critical Care Medicine* 10: 316–319.

Gadek JE, DeMichele SJ, Karlstad MD, et al. (1999) Effect of enteral feeding with eicosapentaenoic acid, γ linolenic acid, and antioxidants in patients with acute respiratory distress syndrome. *Critical Care Medicine* 27: 1409–1420.

Galbán C, Montejo JC, Mesejo A, et al. (2000) An immune-enhancing enteral diet reduces mortality rate and episodes of bacteremia in septic intensive care unit patients. *Critical Care Medicine* 28: 643–648.

Geerts WH, Code KI, Jay RM, et al. (1994) A prospective study of venous thromboembolism after major trauma. *New England Journal of Medicine* 331: 1601–1606.

Geerts WH, Jay RM, Code KI, et al. (1996) A comparison of low-dose heparin with low-molecular-weight heparin as prophylaxis against venous thromboembolism after major trauma. *New England Journal of Medicine* 335: 701–707.

Gehlbach BK, Kress JP (2002) Sedation in the intensive care unit. *Current Opinion in Critical Care* 8: 290–298.

Goeters C, Wenn A, Mertes N, et al. (2002) Parenteral L-alanyl-L-glutamine improves 6-month outcome in critically ill patients. *Critical Care Medicine* 30: 2032–2037.

Gramlich L, Kichian K, Pinilla J, et al. (2004) Does enteral nutrition compared to parenteral nutrition result in better outcomes in critically ill adult patients? A systematic review of the literature. *Nutrition* 20: 843–848.

Griffith DP, McNally AT, Battey CH, et al. (2003) Intravenous erythromycin facilitates bedside placement of postpyloric feeding tubes in critically ill adults: a double-blind, randomized, placebo-controlled study. *Critical Care Medicine* 31: 39–44.

Griffiths RD (2003) Specialized nutrition support in critically ill patients. *Current Opinion in Critical Care* 9: 249–259.

Griffiths RD, Jones C, Palmer TE (1997) Six-month outcome of critically ill patients given glutamine-supplemented parenteral nutrition. *Nutrition* 13: 295–302.

Griffiths RD, Allen KD, Andrews FJ, Jones C (2002) Infection, multiple organ failure, and survival in the intensive care unit: influence of glutamine-supplemented parenteral nutrition on acquired infection. *Nutrition* 18: 546–552.

Gronert GA, Theye RA (1975) Pathophysiology of hyperkalemia induced by succinylcholine. *Anesthesiology* 43: 89–99.

Grounds RM, Lalor JM, Lumley J, et al. (1987) Propofol infusion for sedation in the intensive care unit: preliminary report. *British Medical Journal* 294: 397–400.

Guglielminotti J, Pernet P, Maury E, et al. (2002) Osmolar gap hyponatremia in critically ill patients: evidence for the sick cell syndrome. *Critical Care Medicine* 30: 1051–1055.

Hadley JS, Hinds CJ (2002) Anabolic strategies in critical illness. *Current Opinion in Pharmacology* 2: 700–707.

Hall RI, Sandham D, Cardinal P, et al. (2001) Propofol vs midazolam for ICU sedation: a Canadian multicenter randomized trial. *Chest* 119: 1151–1159.

Hearing SD (2004) Refeeding syndrome. *British Medical Journal* 328: 908–909.

Heyland DK, MacDonald S, Keefe L, et al. (1998) Total parenteral nutrition in the critically ill patient: a meta-analysis. *Journal of the American Medical Association* 280: 2013–2019.

Heyland DK, Cook DJ, Schoenfeld PS, et al. (1999) The effect of acidified enteral feeds on gastric colonization in critically ill patients: results of a multicenter randomized trial. *Critical Care Medicine* 27: 2399–2406.

Heyland DK, Drover JW, MacDonald S, et al. (2001a) Effect of postpyloric feeding on gastroesophageal regurgitation and pulmonary microaspiration: results of a randomised controlled trial. *Critical Care Medicine* 29: 1495–1501.

Heyland DK, Novak F, Drover JW, et al. (2001b) Should immunonutrition become routine in critically ill patients? A systematic review of the evidence. *Journal of the American Medical Association* 286: 944–953.

Heys SD, Walker LG, Smith I, Eremin O (1999) Enteral nutritional supplementation with key nutrients in patients with critical illness and cancer: a meta-analysis of randomized controlled clinical trials. *Annals of Surgery* 229: 467–477.

Hippisley-Cox J, Coupland C (2005) Risk of myocardial infarction in patients taking cyclo-oxygenase-2 inhibitors or conventional non-steroidal anti-inflammatory drugs: population based nested case-control analysis. *British Medical Journal* 330: 1366.

Houdijk AP, Rijnsberger ER, Jansen J, et al. (1998) Randomised trial of glutamine enriched enteral nutrition on infectious morbidity in patients with multiple trauma. *Lancet* 352: 772–776.

Ishibashi N, Plank LD, Sando K, et al. (1998) Optimal protein requirements during the first 2 weeks after the onset of critical illness. *Critical Care Medicine* 26: 1529–1535.

Jones C, Griffiths RD (2002) Physical and psychological recovery. In: Griffiths RD, Jones C (eds) *Intensive Care Aftercare*, pp 53–75. Oxford: Butterworth Heinemann.

Jones BJ, Payne S, Silk DB (1980) Indications for pump-assisted enteral feeding. *Lancet* 1: 1057–1058.

Jones C, Griffiths RD, Humphris G, et al. (2001a) Memory, delusions, and the development of acute posttraumatic stress disorder-related symptoms after intensive care. *Critical Care Medicine* 29: 573–580.

Jones C, Griffiths RD, Humphris G (2001b) Acute post traumatic stress disorder: a new theory for its development after intensive care. *Critical Care Medicine* 29: 573–580.

Jones C, Skirrow P, Griffiths RD, et al. (2003) Rehabilitation after critical illness: a randomized, controlled trial. *Critical Care Medicine* 31: 2456–2461.

Jones C, Skirrow F, Griffiths RD, et al. (2004) Post-traumatic stress disorder-related symptoms in relatives of patients following intensive care. *Intensive Care Medicine* 30: 456–460.

Kemen M, Senkal M, Homann H-H, et al. (1995) Early postoperative enteral nutrition with arginine-ω-3 fatty acids and ribonucleic acid-supplemented diet verses placebo in cancer patients: an immunologic evaluation of impact. *Critical Care Medicine* 23: 652–659.

Kennedy BC, Hall GM (2000) Metabolic support of critically ill patients: parenteral nutrition to immunonutrition. *British Journal of Anaesthesia* 85: 185–188.

Keohane PP, Attrill H, Jones BJ, et al. (1983) The roles of lactose and *Clostridium difficile* in the pathogenesis of enteral feeding associated diarrhoea. *Clinical Nutrition* 1: 259–264.

Keohane PP, Attrill H, Love M, *et al.* (1984) Relation between osmolality of diet and gastrointestinal side effects in enteral nutrition. *British Medical Journal* 288: 678–680.

Kieft H, Roos AN, van Drunen JD, *et al.* (2005) Clinical outcome of immunonutrition in a heterogeneous intensive care population. *Intensive Care Medicine* 31: 524–532.

Kong KL, Willatts SM, Prys-Roberts C (1989) Isoflurane compared with midazolam for sedation in the intensive care unit. *British Medical Journal* 298: 1277–1280.

Konstantinides FN, Konstantinides NN, Li JC, *et al.* (1991) Urinary urea nitrogen: too insensitive for calculating nitrogen balance studies in surgical clinical nutrition. *Journal of Parenteral and Enteral Nutrition* 15: 189–193.

Kress JP, Pohlman AS, O'Connor MF, *et al.* (2000) Daily interruption of sedative infusions in critically ill patients undergoing mechanical ventilation. *New England Journal of Medicine* 342: 1471–1477.

Kress JP, Gehlbach B, Lacy M, *et al.* (2003) The long-term psychological effects of daily sedative interruption on critically ill patients. *American Journal of Respiratory and Critical Care Medicine* 168: 1457–1461.

Lane N, Allen K (1999) Hyponatraemia after orthopaedic surgery. *British Medical Journal* 318: 1363–1364.

Lewis SJ, Egger M, Sylvester PA, *et al.* (2001) Early enteral feeding versus 'nil by mouth' after gastrointestinal surgery: systematic review and meta-analysis of controlled trials. *British Medical Journal* 323: 773–776.

Lloyd GG (1993) Psychological problems and the intensive care unit. *British Medical Journal* 307: 458–459.

Lobo DN (2004) Fluid, electrolytes and nutrition: physiological and clinical aspects. *Proceedings of the Nutrition Society* 63: 453–466.

MacFie J (2004) European round table: the use of immunonutrients in the critically ill. *Clinical Nutrition* 23: 1426–1429.

Madan M, Alexander DJ, McMahon MJ (1992) Influence of catheter type on occurrence of thrombophlebitis during peripheral intravenous nutrition. *Lancet* 339: 101–103.

Marik PE, Zaloga GP (2001) Early enteral nutrition in acutely ill patients: a systematic review. *Critical Care Medicine* 29: 2264–2270.

Marik PE, Zaloga GP (2003) Gastric versus post-pyloric feeding: a systematic review. *Critical Care* 7: R46–R51.

Meiser A, Sirtl C, Bellgardt M, *et al.* (2003) Desflurane compared with propofol for postoperative sedation in the intensive care unit. *British Journal of Anaesthesia* 90: 273–280.

Mentec H, Dupont H, Bocchotti M, *et al.* (2001) Upper digestive intolerance during enteral nutrition in critically ill patients: frequency, risk factors and complications. *Critical Care Medicine* 29: 1955–1961.

Messori A, Trippoli S, Vaiani M, *et al.* (2000) Bleeding and pneumonia in intensive care patients given ranitidine and sucralfate for prevention of stress ulcer: meta-analysis of randomised controlled trials. *British Medical Journal* 321: 1103–1106.

Milbrandt EB, Deppen S, Harrision PL, *et al.* (2004) Costs associated with delirium in

mechanically ventilated patients. *Critical Care Medicine* 32: 955–962.

Milbrandt EB, Kersten A, Kong L, *et al.* (2005) Haloperidol use is associated with lower hospital mortality in mechanically ventilated patients. *Critical Care Medicine* 33: 226–229.

Montejo JC, Grau T, Acosta J, *et al.* (2002) Multicenter, prospective, randomized, single-blind study comparing the efficacy and gastrointestinal complications of early jejunal feeding with early gastric feeding in critically ill patients. *Critical Care Medicine* 30: 796–800.

Montejo JC, Zarazaga A, Lopez-Martinez J, *et al.* (2003) Immunonutrition in the intensive care unit. A systematic review and consensus statement. *Clinical Nutrition* 22: 221–233.

Moore F (2001) Caution: use fat emulsions judiciously in intensive care patients. *Critical Care Medicine* 29: 1644–1645.

Moore EE, Moore FA (1991) Immediate enteral nutrition following multisystem trauma: a decade perspective. *Journal of the American College of Nutrition* 10: 633–648.

Moore FA, Moore EE, Jones TN, *et al.* (1989) TEN versus TPN following major abdominal trauma-reduced septic morbidity. *Journal of Trauma* 29: 916–923.

Moore FA, Feliciano DV, Andrassy RJ, *et al.* (1992) Early enteral feeding compared with parenteral reduces postoperative septic complications. The results of a meta-analysis. *Annals of Surgery* 216: 172–183.

Morlion B, Stehle P, Wachtler P, *et al.* (1998) Total parenteral nutrition with glutamine dipeptide after major abdominal surgery. *Annals of Surgery* 227: 302–308.

Mulla H, Peek G, Upton D, *et al.* (2001) Plasma aluminum levels during sucralfate prophylaxis for stress ulceration in critically ill patients on continuous venovenous hemofiltration: a randomised, controlled trial. *Critical Care Medicine* 29: 267–271.

Murphy DF (1993) Interpleural analgesia. *British Journal of Anaesthesia* 71: 426–434.

Neumann DA, Delegge MH (2002) Gastric verses small-bowel tube feeding in the intensive care unit: a prospective comparision of efficacy. *Intensive Care Medicine* 30: 1436–1438.

Nirmalan M, Dark PM, Nightingale P, *et al.* (2004) Physical and pharmacological restraint of critically ill patients: clinical facts and ethical considerations. *British Journal of Anaesthesia* 92: 789–792.

Noronha JL, Matuschak GM (2002) Magnesium in critical illness: metabolism, assessment and treatment. *Intensive Care Medicine* 28: 667–679.

Novak F, Heyland DK, Avenell A, *et al.* (2002) Glutamine supplementation in serious illness: a systematic review of the evidence. *Critical Care Medicine* 30: 2022–2029.

Osborne RJ, Joel SP, Slevin ML (1986) Morphine intoxication in renal failure: the role of morphine-6-glucuronide. *British Medical Journal* 292: 1548–1549.

Panharipande PP, Pun BT, Herr DL, *et al.* (2007) Effect of sedation with dexmedetomidine vs lorazepam on acute brain dysfunction in mechanically ventilated patients. The MENDS randomized controlled trial. *Journal of American Medical Association* 298:2644–2653.

Panharipande PP, Shintani A, Peterson J, *et al.* (2006) Lorazepam is an independent risk

factor for transitioning to delirium in intensive care unit patients. *Anesthesiology* 104:21–26.

Park GR, Manara AR, Mendel L, *et al.* (1987) Ketamine infusion. *Anaesthesia* 42: 980–983.

Parke TJ, Stevens JE, Rice AS, *et al.* (1992) Metabolic acidosis and fatal myocardial failure after propofol infusion in children: five case reports. *British Medical Journal* 305: 613–616.

Parker MG, Fraser GL, Watson DM, *et al.* (2002) Removal of propylene glycol and correction of increased osmolar gap by hemodialysis in a patient on high dose lorazepam infusion therapy. *Intensive Care Medicine* 28: 81–84.

Pavlevsky PM, Bhagrath R, Greenberg A (1996) Hypernatremia in hospitalized patients. *Annals of Internal Medicine* 124: 197–203.

Perrier ND, Baerga-Varela Y, Murray MJ (2000) Death related to propofol use in an adult patient. *Critical Care Medicine* 28: 3071–3074.

Perry S, Difede J, Musngi G, *et al.* (1992) Predictors of posttraumatic stress disorder after burn injury. *American Journal of Psychiatry* 149: 931–935.

Peter JV, Moran JL, Phillips-Hughes J (2005) A metaanalysis of treatment outcomes of early enteral versus early parenteral nutrition in hospitalized patients. *Critical Care Medicine* 33: 213–220.

Pingleton SK, Hadzima S (1983) Enteral alimentation and gastrointestinal bleeding in mechanically ventilated patients. *Critical Care Medicine* 11: 13–16.

Pitsiu M, Wilmer A, Bodenham A, *et al.* (2004) Pharmacokinetics of remifentanil and its major metabolite, remifentanil acid, in ICU patients with renal impairment. *British Journal of Anaestheisa* 92: 493–503.

Pupelis G, Selga G, Austrums E, *et al.* (2001) Jejunal feeding, even when instituted late, improves outcome in patients with severe pancreatitis and peritonitis. *Nutrition* 17: 91–94.

Radermacher P, Santak B, Strobach H, *et al.* (1992) Fat emulsions containing medium chain triglycerides in patients with sepsis syndrome: effects on pulmonary hemodynamics and gas exchange. *Intensive Care Medicine* 18: 231–234.

Ramsay MA, Savege TM, Simpson BR, *et al.* (1974) Controlled sedation with alphaxalone alphadolone. *British Medical Journal* 2: 656–659.

Rello J, Diaz E, Roque M, *et al.* (1999) Risk factors for developing pneumonia within 48 hours of intubation. *American Journal of Respiratory and Critical Care Medicine* 159: 1742–1746.

Rigg JRA, Jamrozik K, Myles PS, *et al.* (2002) Epidural anaesthesia and analgesia and outcome of major surgery: a randomised trial. *Lancet* 359: 1276–1282.

Riker RR, Fraser GL, Cox PM (1994) Continuous infusion of haloperidol controls agitation in critically ill patients. *Critical Care Medicine* 22: 433–440.

Roca RP, Spence RJ, Munster AM (1992) Posttraumatic adaptation and distress among adult burn survivors. *American Journal of Psychiatry* 149: 1234–1238.

Rundshagen I, Schnabel K, Wegner C, *et al.* (2002) Incidence of recall, nightmares and hallucinations during analgosedation in intensive care. *Intensive Care Medicine* 28: 38–43.

Salem M, Kasinski N, Munoz R, *et al.* (1995) Progressive magnesium deficiency increases mortality from endotoxin challenge: protective effects of acute magnesium replacement therapy. *Critical Care Medicine* 23: 108–118.

Schrier RW, Gross P, Gheorghiade M, *et al.* (2006) Tolvaptan, a selective oral vasopressin V_2 receptor antagonist, for hyponatremia. *New England Journal of Medicine* 355: 2099–2112.

Schweickert WD, Gehlbach BK, Pohlman AS, *et al.* (2004) Daily interruption of sedative infusions and complications of critical illness in mechanically ventilated patients. *Critical Care Medicine* 32: 1272–1276.

Segredo V, Matthay MA, Sharma ML, *et al.* (1990) Prolonged neuromuscular blockade after long-term administration of vecuronium in two critically ill patients. *Anesthesiology* 72: 566–570.

Sessler CN, Gosnell MS, Grap MJ, *et al.* (2002) The Richmond Agitation-Sedation scale: validity and reliability in adult intensive care unit patients. *American Journal of Respiratory and Critical Care Medicine* 166: 1338–1344.

Shelley MP, Mendel L, Park GR (1987) Failure of critically ill patients to metabolise midazolam. *Anaesthesia* 42: 619–626.

Shizgal HM, Forse RA (1980) Protein and calorie requirements with total parenteral nutrition. *Annals of Surgery* 192: 562–569.

Shuman RB, Schuster DP, Zuckerman GR (1987) Prophylactic therapy for stress ulcer bleeding: a reappraisal. *Annals of Internal Medicine* 106: 562–567.

Simpson F, Doig GS (2005) Parenteral vs enteral nutrition in the critically ill patient: a meta-analysis of trials using the intention to treat principle. *Intensive Care Medicine* 31: 12–23.

Solomon SD, McMurray JJV, Pfeffer MA, *et al.* (2005) Cardiovascular risk associated with celecoxib in a clinical trial for colorectal adenoma prevention. *New England Journal of Medicine* 352: 1071–1080.

Soltész S, Biedler A, Silomon M, *et al.* (2001) Recovery after remifentanil and sufentanil for analgesia and sedation of mechanically ventilated patients after trauma or major surgery. *British Journal of Anaesthesia* 86: 763–768.

Souba WW (1997) Nutritional support. *New England Journal of Medicine* 336: 41–48.

Spapen H, Diltoer M, Van Malderen C, *et al.* (2001) Soluble fiber reduces the incidence of diarrhea in septic patients receiving total enteral nutrition: a prospective, double-blind, randomized and controlled trial. *Clinical Nutrition* 20: 301–305.

Sterns RH, Riggs JE, Schochet SS Jr (1986) Osmotic demyelination syndrome following correction of hyponatremia. *New England Journal of Medicine* 314: 1535–1542.

Studley HO (1936) Percentage of weight loss: a basic indicator of surgical risk in patients with chronic peptic ulcer. *Journal of the American Medical Association* 106: 458–460.

Suchner U, Katz DP, Furst P, *et al.* (2001) Effects of intravenous fat emulsions on lung function in patients with acute respiratory distress syndrome or sepsis. *Critical Care Medicine* 29: 1569–1574.

Swart EL, van Schijndel RJ, van Loenen AC, *et al.* (1999) Continuous infusion of lorazepam versus midazolam in patients in the intensive care unit: sedation with lorazepam is easier to manage and is more cost-effective. *Critical Care Medicine* 27: 1461–1465.

Takala J, Ruokonen E, Webster NR, *et al.* (1999) Increased mortality associated with growth hormone treatment in critically ill adults. *New England Journal of Medicine* 341: 785–792.

Thornton C, Barrowcliffe MP, Konieczko KM, *et al.* (1989) The auditory evoked response as an indicator of awareness. *British Journal of Anaesthesia* 63: 113–115.

Timmins AC, Cotterill AM, Hughes SC, *et al.* (1996) Critical illness is associated with low circulating concentrations of insulin-like growth factors-I and -II, alterations in insulin-like growth factor binding proteins and induction of an insulin-like growth factor binding protein -3 protease. *Critical Care Medicine* 24: 1460–1466.

Triltsch AE, Welte M, von Homeyer P, *et al.* (2002) Bispectral index guided sedation with dexmedetomidine in intensive care: a prospective, randomized, double-blind, placebo-controlled phase II study. *Critical Care Medicine* 30: 1007–1014.

Tryba M (1994) Stress ulcer prophylaxis. *Intensive Care Medicine* 20: 311–313.

Tryba M, Zevounou F, Torok M, *et al.* (1985) Prevention of acute stress bleeding with sucralfate, antacids or cimetidine. A controlled study with pirenzepine as a basic medication. *American Journal of Medicine* 79: 55–61.

Tuohy KA, Nicholson WJ, Schiffman F (2003) Agitation by sedation. *Lancet* 361: 308.

Van den Berghe G (2000) Novel insights into the neuroendocrinology of critical illness. *European Journal of Endocrinology* 143: 1–13.

Van den Berghe G, Wouters P, Weekers F, *et al.* (1999) Reactivation of pituitary hormone release and metabolic improvement by infusion of growth hormone-releasing peptide and thyrotropin-releasing hormone in patients with protracted critical illness. *Journal of Clinical Endocrinology and Metabolism* 84: 1311–1323.

Van der Hulst RR, Van Kreel BK, Von Meyenfeldt MF, *et al.* (1993) Glutamine and the preservation of gut integrity. *Lancet* 341: 1363–1365.

Venn RM, Grounds RM (2001) Comparison between dexmedetomidine and propofol for sedation in the intensive care unit: patient and clinician perceptions. *British Journal of Anaesthesia* 87: 684–690.

Venn RM, Bradshaw CJ, Spencer R, *et al.* (1999) Preliminary UK experience of dexmedetomidine, a novel agent for postoperative sedation in the intensive care unit. *Anaesthesia* 54: 1136–1142.

Veterans Affairs Total Parenteral Nutrition Cooperative Study Group (1991) Perioperative total parenteral nutrition in surgical patients. *New England Journal of Medicine* 325: 525–532.

Weinmann EE, Salzman EW (1994) Deep vein thrombosis. *New England Journal of Medicine* 331: 1630–1641.

Weitz JI (1997) Low-molecular-weight heparins. *New England Journal of Medicine* 337: 688–698.

Wicks C, Somasundaram S, Bjarnason I, *et al.* (1994) Comparison of enteral feeding and total parenteral nutrition after liver transplantation. *Lancet* 344: 837–840.

Willatts SM, Spencer EM (1994) Sedation for ventilation in the critically ill. A role for isoflurane? *Anaesthesia* 49: 422–428.

Wischmeyer PE, Lynch J, Liedel J, *et al.* (2001) Glutamine administration reduces gram-negative bacteremia in severely burned patients: a prospective, randomized, double-blind trial versus isonitrogenous control. *Critical Care Medicine* 29: 2075–2080.

Wolf A, Weir P, Segar P, *et al.* (2001) Impaired fatty acid oxidation in propofol infusion syndrome. *Lancet* 357: 606–607.

Woods JC, Mion LC, Connor JT, *et al.* (2004) Severe agitation among ventilated medical intensive care unit patients: frequency, characteristics and outcomes. *Intensive Care Medicine* 30: 1066–1072.

Wyncoll D, Beale R (2001) Immunologically enhanced enteral nutrition: current status. *Current Opinion in Critical Care* 7: 128–132.

Yate PM, Flynn PJ, Arnold RW, *et al.* (1987) Clinical experience and plasma concentrations during the infusion of atracurium in the intensive therapy unit. *British Journal of Anaesthesia* 59: 211–217.

12 Infection in the critically ill

The incidence of hospital-acquired (nosocomial) infection has increased dramatically over the last half-century and the costs related to the treatment, prevention and surveillance of these infections are now considerable. Currently approximately 5–10% of hospitalized patients develop a nosocomial infection, a significant proportion require admission to an intensive care unit (ICU) and overall around 3% die as a result of their infection. In ICUs the prevalence of nosocomial infections has been estimated to be in the region of 18–36%.

The organisms predominantly responsible for hospital-acquired infections have altered since antibiotics were introduced into clinical practice. In the 1940s, the majority of fatal infections were caused by streptococci (*Streptococcus pyogenes* and *S. pneumoniae*) or staphylococci. Later, the emergence of resistant strains of *Staphylococcus aureus* caused concern, but during the late 1950s and the 1960s there was a progressive increase in the number of cases of sepsis and the streptococci and staphylococci were largely superseded as a cause of life-threatening infection in hospitalized patients by aerobic Gram-negative bacilli (Altemeier *et al.*, 1967). Initially, the dominant organism was *Escherichia coli*, but subsequently other Gram-negative bacteria, such as *Klebsiella* spp., *Proteus* spp., *Pseudomonas* spp., *Enterobacter* and *Citrobacter* spp., assumed greater importance. An increasing number of these organisms have since developed antibiotic resistance, probably encouraged by the wide-spread use of broad-spectrum antimicrobial agents, many of which were intrinsically more active against Gram-positive bacteria.

The most common mechanism of bacterial resistance is the introduction of β-lactamases which hydrolyse the β-lactam ring of penicillins, cephalosporins, monobactams and carbapenems. These enzymes are numerous, and they mutate continuously in response to the pressure of widespread antibiotic use, leading to the development of extended-spectrum β-lactamases. The synthesis of β-lactamases is either chromosomal or plasmid-mediated. *Plasmids* are an important cause of the spread of bacterial resistance as they can be transferred between Gram-negative bacteria by conjugation, for example in the gut, and between Gram-positive organisms by bacterial viruses called *phages*. There are in addition many other mechanisms by which bacteria can develop resistance to the non-β-lactam antimicrobials (**Table 12.1**).

More recently Gram-positive infections have again assumed greater prominence. During the 1980s Gram positive cocci resistant to multiple antibiotics (e.g. methicillin-resistant *Staphylococcus aureus* (MRSA), vancomycin-resistant enterococci (VRE)) first emerged as important pathogens and disturbingly in recent years strains of MRSA resistant to vancomycin have been identified (Chang *et al.*, 2003). Moreover, new strains of MRSA have emerged that are now an important cause of community-acquired infection worldwide. Many of these strains produce Panton-Valentine leucocidin (PVL), a toxin that destroys leucocytes and causes extensive tissue necrosis (Ferry and Étienne, 2007).

Unusual pathogens are encountered increasingly frequently in immunocompromised hosts, and fungal infection is always a danger in such patients, especially when they have received broad-spectrum antibiotics. It is important to appreciate, however, that ICUs develop their own resistant bacterial flora, which reflects the predominant case mix and pattern of antibiotic usage.

FACTORS PREDISPOSING TO INFECTION IN HOSPITALIZED PATIENTS

The changing pattern of infection and the increasing incidence of nosocomial infections are not, of course, solely attributable to the effects of antibiotic therapy; alterations in both the susceptibility of the hospital population and the procedures to which they are subjected have also contributed to this phenomenon.

An increasing number of hospitalized patients survive with impaired immune responses. This immune compromise may be a consequence of their disease, for example:

- renal failure;
- diabetes mellitus;
- malignancy;
- human immunodeficiency virus (HIV) infection;
- severe trauma;
- burns.

Alternatively impaired immune responses may be caused by therapy with:

- immunosuppressants;
- cytotoxics;

Table 12.1 Antimicrobial agents, their modes of action and the corresponding mechanisms of bacterial resistance

Antimicrobial agents	Mode of action	Resistance mechanisms
β-lactams	Cell wall synthesis, cell division	β-lactamase, altered penicillin-binding proteins
Glycopeptides (azoles, cycloserine)	Cell wall division	Blocking of drug access to pentapeptide
Aminoglycosides (spectinomycin)	Inhibit protein synthesis (bind to 30S ribosome)	Enzymatic inactivation, altered target, impermeability
Macrolides	Inhibit protein synthesis (bind to 50S ribosome)	Altered target, enzymatic inactivation
Tetracyclines	Inhibit protein synthesis (affect t-RNA binding to 30S ribosome)	Efflux, altered target, impermeability, enzymatic inactivation
Chloramphenicol (lincosamides, streptogramin)	Inhibit protein synthesis (bind to 50S ribosome)	Enzymatic inactivation, impermeability
Quinolones	Replication: inhibit DNA gyrase	Altered target enzymes, impermeability
Rifampin	Transcription: inhibit DNA-dependent RNA polymerase	Altered target enzymes, impermeability
Sulfonamides	Folic acid synthesis	Altered target
Trimethoprim	Folic acid synthesis	Altered target, impermeability
Polyones (nystatin, amphotericin B)	Cell membrane permeability	Ergosterol-deficient mutants

- steroids;
- radiotherapy.

Furthermore, the risk of infection increases:

- at the extremes of age;
- in the presence of malnutrition (see Chapter 11);
- with the severity of the underlying disease.

Risk of infection may also be influenced by genetic variation (Roy *et al.*, 2002) (see Chapter 5).

Critical illness is associated with impaired immunity, the aetiology of which is complex and probably multifactorial (see Chapter 5). There are widespread abnormalities of macrophage, T and B-cell function, neutrophil chemotaxis and intracellular killing.

Cell-mediated immunity (CMI), as measured by the delayed-type hypersensitivity skin reaction to recall antigens, has been shown to be impaired in the critically ill and persistent anergy is associated with a poor prognosis (Bradley *et al.*, 1984). The lymphocyte response to mitogens may be impaired by a number of factors, including surgery, trauma, burns, infection, malignancy, malnutrition, the effects of anaesthesia, hypoxia and blood transfusion. Circulating depressant factors, increased suppressor cell (mainly T-cell), activity and defective T-helper cell function may also be involved (Wolfe *et al.*, 1981), as may impaired natural killer cell function.

Activated *macrophages* elaborate immunosuppressive factors and have been implicated in the impaired immunity associated with critical illness. Moreover antigen presentation by macrophages may be depressed.

Neutrophil chemotaxis and *intracellular killing* may also be impaired. Chemotaxis may be impaired by an intrinsic intracellular defect, or defective production of chemotactic factors, but inhibition is most likely to be mediated by circulating depressant factors. There may also be a reduction in bactericidal activity. Neutrophil function can also be depressed by phosphate deficiency and the administration of volatile anaesthetic agents. Some of the most seriously ill patients become *leukopenic* and this is recognized as a bad prognostic sign in the presence of infection.

Depletion of *complement*, reduced *fibronectin* levels (O'Connell *et al.*, 1984) and *defective phagocytosis* due to reduced opsonic activity may also predispose to infective complications. Not uncommonly, *immunoglobulin levels* are reduced as a result of extravascular leakage, reduced synthesis and increased consumption. Moreover B-cell numbers are decreased, and the percentage of resting B cells available to be activated to produce antibodies is reduced so that inadequate levels of secretory antibodies are available at mucosal sites (Abraham and Chang, 1990). Presumably this contributes to the increased incidence of bacterial colonization at these surfaces and the increased susceptibility to bloodstream invasion.

Table 12.2 Potentially pathogenic microorganisms (PPM) causing infections in intensive care unit patients

Previously healthy (community PPM)

Streptococcus pneumoniae

Haemophilus influenzae

Moraxella catarrhalis

Escherichia coli

Staphylococcus aureus

Candida albicans

With underlying disease (hospital PPM)

Klebsiella spp.

Proteus spp.

Morganella spp.

Enterobacter spp.

Citrobacter spp.

Serratia spp.

Acinetobacter spp.

Pseudomonas spp.

These highly susceptible patients are now more frequently subjected to:

- extensive surgery;
- invasive procedures – intravascular and urethral catheterization, insertion of intercostal drains, tracheal intubation or tracheostomy;
- parenteral nutrition.

It is not surprising, therefore, that persistent or recurrent sepsis is such an intractable problem in the critically ill.

SOURCES AND PREVENTION OF INFECTION

ENDOGENOUS (AUTOGENOUS) INFECTION

Very often, the source of infection is the patient's own skin or, most importantly, oropharyngeal cavity and gastrointestinal tract. Potentially pathogenic microorganisms (PPM) involved in infection in the ICU can be conveniently divided into those present in otherwise healthy people (the so-called community PPM) and those commonly present in the hospital environment (i.e. in individuals with underlying disease – the so-called hospital PPM) (**Table 12.2**). This classification also implies that individuals with a chronic illness, but resident in the community, may carry hospital PPM. There are three basic patterns of infection in the ICU:

1. primary endogenous;
2. secondary endogenous;
3. exogenous.

In *exogenous infection*, there is no preceding microbial carriage in the throat and/or gut. In *endogenous (autogenous)* infection, oropharyngeal and/or intestinal carriage precedes infection. A *primary endogenous infection* is caused by a PPM carried by the patient on admission to the ICU, whereas a *secondary endogenous infection* is caused by PPMs acquired in the ICU. Endemic infection in the ICU is more often primary endogenous (Van Saene *et al.*, 1994).

In health, *colonization of the alimentary tract* by aerobic bacteria is resisted by:

- the integrity of the mucosal lining;
- normal gastrointestinal motility, including swallowing and peristalsis;
- the desquamation of mucosal cells;
- mucus production;
- secretory immunoglobulin A (IgA).

Normal flora, mainly the resident anaerobes, also inhibit the proliferation of aerobic organisms. These protective mechanisms are frequently impaired in the critically ill, leading to colonization of the oropharynx and gastrointestinal tract by large numbers of aerobic Gram-negative bacteria such as *E. coli*, *Klebsiella* spp., *Proteus* spp. and *Pseudomonas aeruginosa*, as well as by *Staphylococcus aureus* and yeasts, especially *Candida* spp.

An important factor promoting colonization and subsequent overgrowth of abnormal flora in the critically ill appears to be increased adherence of bacteria to the mucosa due to alteration of the epithelial surface. *Oropharyngeal colonization* is more likely in those with a tracheal or nasogastric tube in place, pre-existing pulmonary disease or uraemia, and in patients receiving antibiotics. It becomes increasingly likely the longer patients stay in hospital and the more severely ill they are, and in older age groups.

Colonization of the stomach with Gram-negative organisms is also common in critically ill patients, perhaps particularly when gastric pH is elevated by antacid prophylaxis (see Chapter 11), and in those with gastroduodenal reflux (Inglis *et al.*, 1992). It has been suggested that under these circumstances regurgitation and aspiration of gastric contents may contribute to colonization or infection of the oropharynx and respiratory tract (Du Moulin *et al.*, 1982). In a later study, however, the frequency of gastric colonization was confirmed, but there was no evidence that microorganisms migrated to the nasopharynx or that there was a relationship between such colonization and clinically important infection. Neither was there any relationship between gastric pH and colonization (Cade *et al.*, 1992) (see Chapter 7, ventilated-associated pneumonia).

The vector in many cases of autogenous infection is the patient's own hands, or those of the attendants. The patient must therefore be prevented from handling infected areas and transferring organisms to vulnerable sites elsewhere (e.g. a tracheostomy stoma). Meticulous hygiene is essential to protect the patient from endogenous infection, necessitating frequent changes of bed linen, cleaning of contaminated areas and handwashing.

Selective decontamination of the digestive tract

Decontamination of the digestive tract is designed to prevent autogenous or endogenous infection by reducing the numbers of PPM in the oropharynx and gastrointestinal tract (Stoutenbeek *et al.*, 1994). The technique was originally introduced to reduce infective complications in neutropenic oncology patients; at first unselective decontamination was often used, but this was associated with a risk of overgrowth of Gram-negative bacteria acquired from the hospital environment, probably because of a decrease in the numbers of anaerobic bacilli. *Selective decontamination of the digestive tract* (SDD) aims to avoid this problem by eliminating carriage of aerobic bacilli and yeasts while preserving the normal anaerobic flora and thereby maintaining *colonization resistance*. As well as minimizing the risk of nosocomial infection, SDD might potentially reduce the incidence of multiple-organ failure by decreasing the load of bacteria and endotoxin within the gut lumen and limiting the extent of translocation of PPM and absorption of faecal bacterial cell wall components (see Chapter 5). Successful decontamination of individual patients might also reduce the general level of contamination within the critical care area, thereby contributing to an overall reduction in infection rates.

Various regimens have been used to achieve SDD. Most use a combination of non-absorbable antibacterial and antifungal agents instilled via the nasogastric tube, together with a topical preparation applied to the oropharynx; many have also included a variable period of intravenous antimicrobial prophylaxis. It is suggested that with this combined approach the parenteral antibiotic component might prevent primary endogenous infection (caused by PPM carried on admission) and, together with the topical antimicrobials, might lower the incidence of secondary endogenous infection (caused by newly acquired microorganisms colonizing the digestive tract).

The use of SDD in critically ill patients was first described by Stoutenbeek *et al.* in 1984. They administered tobramycin, polymyxin (which binds endotoxin) and amphotericin B via the nasogastric tube, combined with systemic cefotaxime for at least 4 days, to a group of multiple trauma patients; they also emphasized the importance of decontaminating the oropharyngeal cavity using a sticky paste containing 2% tobramycin, polymyxin and amphotericin B. The infection rate fell from 81% in historical controls to 16% in treated patients, although the effect on mortality was not reported.

A subsequent prospective double-blind randomized placebo-controlled study in mechanically ventilated ICU patients confirmed that SDD can dramatically reduce the incidence of nosocomial infections, but failed to demonstrate any improvement in survival, or any reduction in the incidence of multiple-organ failure. There was also a substantial increase in the cost of antimicrobial drugs (Gastinne *et al.*, 1992). Another prospective, randomized, double-blind study reached a similar conclusion (Hammond *et al.*, 1992).

More recently, however a randomized, controlled trial conducted in two physically separate units within the same institution demonstrated a reduction in mortality, length of ICU stay, the frequency of colonization with resistant bacteria and the total costs of antibiotic treatment (de Jonge *et al.*, 2003). It is worth noting, however, that in this study additional measures were used to control colonization with PPM (persistent tracheal colonization with Gram-negative bacteria was treated with aerosolized polymyxin E and patients with blind bowel loops were given additional SDD by suppository).

A number of meta-analyses have been performed in an attempt to resolve some of the controversy surrounding the use of SDD in the critically ill. One of the first included 4142 patients in 22 studies. Although the incidence of respiratory tract infections was significantly reduced (by about 60%), the authors concluded that in long-stay (> 5 days), mechanically ventilated (> 48 hours) general intensive care patients, the effect on mortality remained uncertain, being at best only a moderate improvement in survival. Moreover, there appeared to be only a weak association between the reduction in infection rates and improved survival. A beneficial effect on mortality seemed most likely when combined topical and systemic treatment was used since in these cases there was a significant 20% reduction in the odds of death. The authors also pointed out that in no trial has there been any suggestion that SDD worsens outcome (Selective Decontamination of the Digestive Tract Trialists' Collaborative Group, 1993).

Two further meta-analyses of 2270 patients in 16 studies (Kollef, 1994) and of 3395 patients in 25 randomized studies (Heyland *et al.*, 1994) concluded that SDD reduces the incidence of acquired pneumonia, but indicated that its effect on mortality was small or non-existent. There was, however, a suggestion that when topical antibiotics were combined with a short course of intravenous antibiotics the reduction in mortality was significant, and more recent meta-analysis/ systematic reviews have also indicated that in some ICU populations SDD can reduce rates of nosocomial pneumonia, bacteraemia and nosocomial infections at remote sites and may significantly improve outcome (D'Amico *et al.*, 1998; Nathens and Marshall, 1999; van Nieuwenhoven *et al.*, 2001). It seems that critically ill surgical patients are more likely to benefit than medical patients (Nathens and Marshall, 1999) but the value of SDD in patients undergoing liver transplantation or major elective surgery and in those with burns or acute pancreatitis remains uncertain (Nathens and Marshall, 1999). A more recent randomized controlled trial, however, demonstrated a reduction in the incidence of pneumonia and mortality in patients with severe burns receiving SDD (de La Cal *et al.*, 2005).

There has been considerable concern that SDD, which contradicts traditional microbiological advice to use narrow-spectrum antibiotics only to treat clearly established infection and not colonization, might contribute to the emergence of antibiotic resistance. In general these fears do not seem to have been justified, but there is limited information on the long-term microbial consequences of SDD and some remain concerned that the widespread use of these regimens could lead to the emergence of antibiotic-resistant bacilli. In particular the safety of SDD in centres where resistant Gram-positive organisms are common has not been established and several studies have documented an increase in rates of isolation of Gram-positive organisms, especially *S. aureus*, coagulase-negative staphylococcus and enterococcus, when SDD is implemented (Gastinne *et al.*, 1992). On the other hand de Jonge *et al.* (2003) found no increase in microbial resistance associated with the use of SDD in a unit where the prevalence of VRE and MRSA was low. It also remains unclear whether combined systemic and topical regimens are superior to the use of topical or systemic antimicrobials alone. Although this seemed to be the case in one meta-analysis (Nathens and Marshall, 1999), others have found that topical administration alone can at least reduce the incidence of ventilator-associated pneumonia (see Chapter 7). Finally it is unclear whether SDD is a cost-effective infection prevention strategy, although in one trial antibiotic costs were reduced (de Jonge *et al.*, 2003).

Several factors have complicated interpretation of the large number of published trials of SDD. These include the variety of antimicrobial regimens used (e.g. some have omitted the systemic component), the different patient groups studied, the variable quality of microbiological surveillance (it is important to confirm decontamination microbiologically) and the different criteria used for the diagnosis of pneumonia. Moreover, not all studies have been prospective, randomized and double-blind, co-interventions have rarely been reported and the use of concurrent controls may influence the results by acting as a source of acquired infection for the treatment group. Indeed the reduction in the relative risk for pneumonia demonstrated with SDD seems to be inversely related to the methodological quality of the trial (van Nieuwenhoven *et al.*, 2001). Finally the discrepancy between the dramatic reduction in nosocomial infection produced by SDD and the less impressive improvement in survival suggests that many of those who die in ICUs, especially medical patients, do so with, but not because of, infection.

Nevertheless, some are now convinced that SDD does have a role in intensive care since it undoubtedly reduces colonization rates and the incidence of nosocomial infection, and because there is evidence to suggest that, at least in certain subgroups, mortality may also be reduced. The use of SDD has been advocated in units that have a low prevalence of resistant Gram-positive organisms, for patients expected to be on mechanical ventilation for at least 2 days or to be in the ICU for at least 3 days (de Jonge *et al.*, 2003). In general surgical and trauma patients are more likely to benefit than medical cases. If a decision is made to use SDD, regular surveillance samples must be taken to monitor the long-term effects of this intervention on microbial ecology and resistance patterns. Others remain unconvinced and believe that further adequately powered trials are required to determine whether SDD has a clinically significant effect on survival in selected homogeneous subgroups of patients, whether the emergence of microbial resistance is in fact a serious problem and whether SDD is cost-effective.

An alternative approach to colonization resistance is the administration of a *probiotic* in an attempt to restore a more normal gastrointestinal flora. *Prebiotics* (food for the microbes) may also be required. The value of these interventions remains unclear (Bengmark, 2002), indeed a recent randomised controlled trial found that probiotic prophylaxis was associated with increased mortality in patients with severe acute pancreatitis (Besselink *et al.*, 2008).

EXOGENOUS INFECTION

Exogenous nosocomial infection is relatively unusual, but hospitals, patients, staff and contaminated equipment such as ventilators can act as a reservoir of PPM. Critically ill patients are therefore at risk of acquiring an exogenous infection from:

- the environment;
- their attendants;
- their fellow patients.

The precautions taken to prevent exogenous infection vary from one unit to another, reflecting the lack of evidence as to the efficacy of many of the measures that can be adopted. For example, in some, clean gowns and overshoes are worn by all staff and visitors who enter the unit. Although this has not been shown to reduce the incidence of infection conclusively, it has the advantage of limiting the number of casual visitors and emphasizing the need for personal cleanliness.

The greatest risk to the patient, however, is from PPM transmitted from other patients or from contaminated areas of the unit such as the sinks, usually on the hands of the staff. The most important preventive measure is therefore *thorough handwashing* between patients (Daschner, 1985); the use of an antimicrobial agent (chlorhexidine) may be more effective than soap and alcohol (Doebbeling *et al.*, 1992) but soap is required to combat *Clostridium difficile*. Although this is the cheapest and most effective infection control measure, compliance is frequently inadequate; all units should implement measures to improve the reliability with which handwashing is performed and promote the correct use of gloves. Provision of alcohol hand rubs by patients' beds and at the entrance to cubicles can encourage more frequent hand disinfection. *Fomites*, such as stethoscopes, may also be responsible for transmitting organisms between patients. In some units, disposable aprons, and gloves, are worn at all times and are changed when moving from one patient to another. In others, such precautions are only employed when a patient is known to harbour resistant organisms. Caps and masks are generally considered to be unnecessary, except when performing aseptic procedures, while environmental monitoring is expensive, tedious and probably of little value (Daschner, 1985).

Unit design (see Chapter 1) is an important element in minimizing transmission of PPM. There must be adequate space around each bed and single cubicles should be available for barrier or reverse barrier nursing. These cubicles can be equipped with unidirectional plenum ventilation. Adequate handwashing facilities are essential and a basin should be provided adjacent to each bed area. The environment must be kept clean and all surfaces should be damp-wiped at least daily. Cleaning of isolation rooms when vacated may require disinfection. Clinical equipment must be clean or sterile.

Staff must be trained in the correct procedures for reducing transmission, and must be motivated to perform them to a high standard at all times. If staffing levels are inadequate, these procedures may be overlooked and movement between patients will increase, particularly in times of stress; as a consequence, the contact rate is increased and the incidence of transmission and subsequent secondary endogenous and/or exogenous infection may rise. Because medical staff make contact with many different patients they are more likely than nurses to transmit infection.

Isolation of colonized or infected patients may also reduce the risk of transmission of PPMs, although these patients may receive less attention than those in an open unit and may suffer more frequent preventable adverse events (Stelfox *et al.*, 2003). Moreover, in a recent study, performed in units where MRSA is endemic, there was no evidence that moving MRSA-positive patients into single rooms or into bays for cohort nursing was associated with a reduction in cross-infection (Cepeda *et al.*, 2005). Although the role of *active surveillance* to identify colonized patients also remains uncertain, some northern European countries seem to have successfully controlled MRSA by adopting 'search and destroy' and 'cordon sanitaire' policies which have included routine surveillance cultures, strict isolation procedures and identification and decolonization of patients and staff carrying MRSA. Nevertheless such aggressive control measures remain controversial, not least because of the cost and associated logistical difficulties, especially when MRSA is already endemic (Huskins and Goldmann, 2005).

INFECTION CONTROL TEAMS

Preventive measures are most likely to be successful when supervised by an infection control team. This group can assume responsibility for monitoring rates of infection, antibiotic usage and sensitivity patterns and reporting these to clinicians. They can also establish procedures for sterilization and disinfection, develop and enforce policies to contain infection, including isolation procedures, and promote effective preventive measures, such as handwashing. In conjunction with the occupational health department, the team should also be concerned with staff health and safety and should, for example, develop procedures for the management of needlestick injuries and supervise vaccinations.

ENHANCING HOST DEFENCES

Measures that may improve host defences include:

- nutritional support (see Chapter 11);
- active and passive immunization;

- granulocyte colony stimulating factor;
- granulocyte transfusions;
- immune stimulation (e.g. bacillus Calmette-Guérin (BCG) and levamisole);
- fibronectin, fresh frozen plasma, cryoprecipitate, γ-globulin.

NOSOCOMIAL INFECTIONS IN THE CRITICALLY ILL

The acquisition of a nosocomial infection significantly increases the risk of death in intensive care patients (Bueno-Cavanillas *et al.*, 1994). In a 1-day, point prevalence study conducted in European ICUs 45% of patients were infected, 14% had become infected in the community, 10% had hospital-acquired infection and 21% had an ICU-acquired infection; of these infections nearly 50% were pneumonia and 12% were bloodstream infections. The most frequently reported microorganisms were enteric Gram-negative bacilli (34%), *Staphylococcus aureus* (30%), *Pseudomonas aeruginosa* (29%), coagulase-negative staphylococci (19%) and fungi (17%) (Vincent *et al.*, 1995).

NOSOCOMIAL PNEUMONIA (see Chapter 7: ventilator-associated pneumonia)
Nosocomial pneumonia represents 10–30% of all nosocomial infections in the critically ill and is associated with a high mortality of 20–50%. Most (around 60%) are caused by Gram-negative bacteria, but more recently there has been an increase in pneumonia due to Gram-positive organisms, including MRSA.

Predisposing factors
The risk of nosocomial pneumonia is increased in:

- patients with endotracheal tubes or tracheostomies in place/those mechanically ventilated (ventilator-associated pneumonia: see Chapter 7);
- those with laryngeal dysfunction (neurological disorders, drugs, nasogastric tube);
- the elderly;
- the immunosuppressed;
- smokers;
- those with chronic lung disease;
- following surgery (particularly thoracoabdominal);
- after large-volume aspiration;
- when consciousness is depressed;
- the more seriously ill.

Diagnosis
Diagnosis can be difficult, especially in those with pre-existing lung pathology such as pulmonary oedema. The diagnosis should be suspected when:

- the patient develops a fever;
- there is leukocytosis or leukopenia;

- there are new and persistent infiltrates on the chest radiograph;
- there is a change in the quantity or appearance of the sputum;
- lung function deteriorates;
- there is an otherwise unexplained deterioration in the patient's general condition.

Unfortunately in most critically ill patients there are several potential sources of fever, the significance of purulent sputum is often uncertain, and the appearance of new infiltrates on the chest radiograph may represent not only infection, but also acute lung injury (ALI)/acute respiratory distress syndrome (ARDS), pulmonary oedema or atelectasis. Not surprisingly, therefore, the clinical diagnosis of nosocomial pneumonia has been shown to be incorrect in about one-third of cases when compared to histological findings (Andrews *et al.*, 1981).

Investigations (see Chapter 7: ventilator-associated pneumonia)

Sputum, either expectorated or obtained by endotracheal suction, should be sent for culture and determination of antibiotic sensitivities. In some cases it may not be possible to obtain an adequate quantity of sputum from the lower airways and expectorated samples are often contaminated with bacteria or fungi during their passage through the upper airways. Although aspirates obtained via an endotracheal or tracheostomy tube are less likely to be contaminated than expectorated sputum, they can still produce false-positive cultures. *Blood cultures* are rarely positive (10–20% of cases), but when an organism is isolated it is very likely to be the cause of the pneumonia.

Because clinical criteria for the diagnosis of nosocomial pneumonia are unreliable, and the results obtained from standard microbiological studies of central tracheobronchial secretions are frequently misleading (Berger and Arango, 1985), some have recommended that both the diagnosis and the causative organism should be pursued more aggressively using *invasive techniques*. More recently, however, the value of these techniques in clinical practice has been increasingly questioned (see Chapter 7: ventilator-associated pneumonia). It is often particularly difficult to identify the causative organism in immunocompromised patients with an opportunistic infection and some of the more invasive procedures may be particularly useful in such cases (see later).

TRANSTRACHEAL NEEDLE ASPIRATION (TTA)

In unintubated patients oropharyngeal contamination can be avoided by sampling via the cricothyroid membrane. The risk of complications with this technique is low, haemorrhage being the main concern, and the diagnostic yield is excellent in bacterial pneumonia, provided antibiotics have not already been given. There is, however, a significant incidence of false-positive results. In practice this technique is rarely used.

FIBREOPTIC BRONCHOSCOPY

Diagnostic material can be obtained during fibreoptic bronchoscopy by:

- aspiration;
- bronchial brushings;
- bronchoalveolar lavage (BAL);
- transbronchial lung biopsy.

Complications include:

- hypoxaemia;
- bronchospasm;
- cardiac arrhythmias;
- pneumothorax;
- haemorrhage;
- infection.

Because directly aspirated material and samples obtained by conventional bronchial brushings are likely to be contaminated by organisms colonizing the large airways, *protected specimen brushing* (PSB) has been advocated for the diagnosis of bacterial pneumonia. This technique involves passing a double-lumen catheter with a protected brush through the fibreoptic bronchoscope to collect uncontaminated specimens from suspected areas of infection. The sample can then be cultured quantitatively; growth of more than 10^3 colony-forming units/mL is generally considered significant. The overall sensitivity of PSB may be as high as 93% and the incidence of false-positives is low. The number of false-negative results can be minimized by sampling from several areas of lung. Bronchial brushings can also be useful for the detection of *Pneumocystis carinii* and fungi. Complications of brush biopsy include pneumothorax, haemorrhage and infection.

BAL has also been advocated for the diagnosis of nosocomial bacterial pneumonia, although contamination with upper-airway organisms is again a problem and some therefore consider this technique to be most suitable for demonstrating parasites and fungi. Immediate microscopic analysis of BAL fluid may allow rapid identification of the causative organism in patients with pneumonia. In general BAL is rather more sensitive than PSB since a wider area of the lung is sampled, but the most accurate diagnostic information in bacterial pneumonia may be obtained when BAL is combined with PSB. BAL has also been used successfully to diagnose opportunistic pulmonary infections in immunocompromised hosts. Complications of BAL include worsening hypoxaemia and infection.

It is almost always possible to obtain lung tissue using *transbronchial biopsy* and an aetiological diagnosis is made in 40–80% of cases. However, the incidence of complications, particularly pneumothorax, is highest with this technique, especially in those undergoing mechanical ventilation, and its use is therefore normally restricted to establishing the cause of pulmonary infiltrates in spontaneously breathing patients, especially those who are immunocompromised. In patients with malignant disease, sampling errors and false-negatives may occur: in particular the biopsy may show only non-specific interstitial pneumonitis in nearly half the cases, many of whom may in fact have active infection. The incidence of haemorrhage is low provided thrombocytopenic patients are given a platelet transfusion before the procedure. Uraemic patients are more likely to bleed. Supplemental oxygen must be given during the procedure.

PERCUTANEOUS TRANSTHORACIC NEEDLE BIOPSY
Percutaneous transthoracic needle biopsy produces a reasonable diagnostic yield, but the incidence of pneumothorax is around 25%, although significant haemoptysis is unusual. Its use is confined to spontaneously breathing patients who are sufficiently alert and cooperative to be able to stop breathing for 5-second periods while the needle is advanced.

OPEN-LUNG BIOPSY
A small segment of lung can be excised through a minithoracotomy; this usually allows a histological and microbiological diagnosis to be made. Pneumothorax, haemothorax and infection may all occur, but in experienced hands the morbidity and mortality of this procedure are acceptably low. Open-lung biopsy is indicated when transbronchial techniques fail to establish the diagnosis and when a definitive diagnosis must be established with the first procedure. It is probably safer than transbronchial biopsy in mechanically ventilated patients and those with uncorrectable hypoxaemia or a bleeding disorder. In immunosuppressed patients with pulmonary infiltrates a specific diagnosis can be established in about 70% of cases, while a non-specific interstitial pneumonitis is found in the remainder.

CHOOSING THE MOST SUITABLE INVESTIGATION
The choice of the most suitable technique in an individual patient depends on a number of factors, including:

- the presumed diagnosis (bacterial, fungal or viral);
- the presence of coagulation disorders;
- the severity of respiratory failure;
- the experience of available personnel.

URINARY TRACT INFECTIONS
Urinary tract infections account for about 40% of all nosocomial infections, but mortality rates are generally low. Most are related to the presence of a urinary catheter, which provides a route for infection with faecal organisms colonizing the perineal region. Bacteria gain access to the bladder by intra- or extraluminal migration. It is therefore important to catheterize the bladder only when clearly indicated, not simply for convenience. Urethral catheterization must be performed aseptically. The catheter must be carefully secured and connected to a closed drainage system, and continuous, unobstructed drainage must be ensured.

INFECTION RELATED TO INTRAVASCULAR DEVICES
Bloodstream infection is the most common life-threatening complication of obtaining percutaneous vascular access.

Approximately 11–16% of central venous and pulmonary artery catheters may become contaminated with PPMs and the incidence of catheter-related bloodstream infections (CRBSIs) is around 2–5% (Cobb et al., 1992; Pinilla et al., 1983). Indeed, central venous catheter-related infections may be responsible for up to 90% of all nosocomial bloodstream infection, with infection rates of 3–20 per 1000 days of catheterization. Pulmonary artery catheters have a similar incidence of CRBSIs, whilst the rate is higher for dialysis catheters and more than 70% of infections in haemodialysis patients are associated with the vascular access site. The attributable mortality of central venous CRBSIs is uncertain but seems to be between 3 and 25%, although it is clear that for those who survive, length of hospital stay is significantly prolonged and costs are substantially increased. The risk of CRBSIs associated with intra-arterial cannulae may approach that of central venous cannulae (Mermel et al., 2001).

Infection related to intravascular devices may be due to poor aseptic technique during cannulation or inadequate care of the catheter, the infusion lines or the skin puncture site. Immediately after insertion central venous catheters become coated with proteins, particularly fibrin. Colonization of the catheter occurs when bacteria migrate, either from the skin via the insertion track or from the hub through the catheter lumen to become embedded in this protein sheath. In up to one-third of cases adherent thrombus, which acts as a culture medium, forms on the catheter; this blood clot may become secondarily contaminated during a bacteraemic episode or via a contaminated infusion set and thrombus formation increases the risk of CRBSI. This is particularly likely to occur in patients receiving parenteral nutrition. Immunocompromised patients are also at increased risk of CRBSI. Infection related to intravascular devices may be complicated not only by bacteraemia and septic shock but also by septic thrombophlebitis, septic arthritis or infective endocarditis. The organisms most often implicated are coagulase-negative staphylococci and S. aureus, although Gram-negative bacilli, enterococci, streptococci, Pseudomonas or yeasts may also be responsible.

Prevention (Table 12.3)
The risk of bacterial colonization increases dramatically with the duration of catheterization. All intravascular catheters must be inserted with full aseptic precautions after adequate skin disinfection (see Chapter 4). Current evidence indicates that chlorhexidine alcoholic solution is a more effective skin disinfectant than povidone-iodine for the prevention of vascular catheter-related infections, although it is important to allow the alcohol to dry on the skin before inserting the catheter (this may take up to 2–3 minutes) (Chaiyakunapruk et al., 2002). Explanations include the superior bactericidal activity of chlorhexidine against Gram-positive cocci, as well as its prolonged antimicrobial suppressive activity and resistance to deactivation by blood serum and other protein-rich biomaterials. Chlorhexidine is, however, more expensive than povidone-iodine and it seems

Table 12.3 Prevention of infection related to central venous catheters (CVCs)

Selection of catheter type

Use a single-lumen catheter unless multiple ports are essential

For parenteral nutrition, a dedicated CVC or lumen should be used exclusively

Use an implantable or tunnelled catheter for long-term (> 30 days) use

Consider the use of an antimicrobial-impregnated catheter for patients at high risk of CRBSI

Selection of catheter insertion site

Balance risks of infection against mechanical risks of insertion

Consider the use of peripherally inserted catheters as an alternative to CVCs

Aseptic technique during insertion

Use full aseptic precautions

Clean the insertion site with alcoholic chlorhexidene gluconate solution and allow to dry

Catheter and catheter site care

Before accessing the CVC, disinfect the external surfaces of the catheter hub and connection ports with an aqueous solution of chlorhexidene gluconate (unless against manufacturer's recommendations)

Use sterile gauze or transparent dressing over the insertion site

Catheter flush solutions should contain anticoagulant

Replacement strategies

Do not routinely replace non-tunnelled CVCs as a method of CRBSI infection control

Guidewire exchange is acceptable for malfunctioning catheters if there is no evidence of infection

that alcoholic povidone-iodine may be more effective than the aqueous 10% solution for skin disinfection (Parienti *et al.*, 2004). Intravenous infusion sets should be changed regularly (e.g. every 48 hours), although the use of in-line bacterial filters may allow less frequent replacement. Routine scheduled replacement of central venous catheters may actually increase the risk of infection and is no longer recommended (Cobb *et al.*, 1992).

It is important to fix intravascular cannulae firmly, to use closed systems and to avoid contamination of three-way taps. The puncture site should be covered with a highly permeable dressing and inspected at least daily. Parenteral nutrition must be administered via a dedicated catheter or lumen (see Chapter 11). The use of occlusive antimicrobial

dressings, in-line filters, regular flushing, antiseptic cream or spray applied to the puncture site and subcutaneous tunnelling have not been conclusively shown to reduce the incidence of infection. Unfortunately compliance with guidelines for central venous catheter insertion techniques and site care is often poor. Moreover rates of infection may be higher when there is a shortage of nurses and with multiple-lumen than with single-lumen catheters (Hilton *et al.*, 1988).

Antimicrobial-impregnated catheters (e.g. coated with chlorhexidine/silver sulphadiazine or minocycline/rifampin) can reduce colonization and CRBSI, and may be cost-effective, but there are concerns about the induction of bacterial resistance and immunological reactions to the catheter coatings. They are likely to be of most value when catheters are left in place for prolonged periods (e.g. more than 7 days) and should probably be considered for high-risk cases. In patients with acute renal failure, for example, the use of haemodialysis catheters impregnated with minocycline and rifampin decreased the risk of catheter-related infections by at least sevenfold (Chatzinikolaou *et al.*, 2003).

Recently an evidence-based intervention designed to prevent CRBSIs (involving hand washing, full barrier precautions during insertion procedures, skin cleaning with chlorhexidine, avoiding the femoral site, removal of unnecessary catheters) was found to result in a large and sustained reduction in rates of CRBSI (Pronovost *et al.*, 2006).

Diagnosis

Diagnosing CRBSI without removing the catheter is difficult. Catheter-related infection should be suspected if the patient develops clinical symptoms and signs of bacateraemia in the absence of an obvious source or if they persist after apparent eradication of a septic focus. The diagnosis is more likely if there are signs of infection at the puncture site (e.g. purulent discharge or lymphangitis) and if the symptoms and signs of bacteraemia resolve after removal of the suspect catheter.

Clinical findings are, however, non-specific and conventionally CRBSI is confirmed by the combination of a positive blood culture and the same organism isolated from the catheter. Either the catheter tip or a subcutaneous segment should be submitted for culture (Mermel *et al.*, 2001). When pulmonary artery catheter infection is suspected the introducer should be cultured because this provides a higher yield (Mermel *et al.*, 2001). A recent meta-analysis concluded that simple qualitative cultures of catheter segments lack specificity, but that quantitative, or semiquantitative, culture of the catheter, combined with blood cultures drawn through the suspect catheter and from a peripheral vein, do allow accurate diagnosis of CRBSI. With long-term catheters paired quantitative blood cultures seemed to be the most accurate diagnostic method. Paired qualitative conventional blood culture using *differential time to positivity* (when blood from the catheter demonstrates microbial growth at least 2 hours earlier than the peripheral blood culture) may also be adequate (Safdar et al., 2005). With these techniques it is essential that the blood samples are drawn concomitantly (< 10 minutes apart), that similar volumes of blood are cultured and that blood is obtained before antibiotics are given. Routine culture of all central venous catheter tips following removal is unhelpful and may prompt unnecessary treatment with antibiotics. Newer techniques such as *acridine orange leukocyte cytospin* of blood taken from the central venous catheter and *endoluminal brush sampling* are not yet widely available and their role in clinical practice is uncertain.

Treatment

Conventionally intravascular catheters are removed if CRBSI is suspected. If the fever subsides it is then assumed that one or other of the catheters was responsible. Ideally replacement of central venous catheters should be delayed to allow elimination of residual organisms and in some cases it may subsequently be possible to use only peripheral venous access.

As we have seen establishing a diagnosis of CRBSI can be extremely difficult and many of the catheters removed for suspected CRBSI are subsequently found not to have been the source of infection. Moreover unnecessary catheter replacement is costly and time-consuming and increases the risk of iatrogenic complications. Some have therefore advocated postponing catheter removal in stable, low-risk patients and observing the subsequent evolution of their clinical condition while awaiting culture results. If signs of sepsis persist and/or cultures are positive then the catheter is removed. In one study such an approach led to a 62% reduction in the incidence of unnecessary catheter removal (Rijnders et al., 2004) without affecting time to defervescence, the total amount of antibiotics used, the length of hospital stay or mortality. It also seems that catheters need not be removed routinely when there is only modest inflammation at the insertion site and there are no other signs of catheter-related infection (Safdar and Maki, 2002). In those with *S. aureus* CRBSI a transoesophageal echo is recommended to exclude endocarditis.

Because long-term, cuffed, large-bore silicone catheters are more difficult to insert and remove it may be reasonable to attempt to clear the infection by injecting antibiotics through the catheter. When venous access is limited it may be acceptable to change the catheter over a guidewire, although this can be associated with an increased risk of bloodstream infection in the following 3 days. Replacement at a new site, on the other hand, increases the risk of mechanical complications (Cobb et al., 1992). It has been recommended that *antibiotic lock therapy* (instillation of antibiotic into the dead space of the catheter) should be combined with standard systemic therapy for 2 weeks when attempting to salvage venous catheters (Mermel et al., 2001).

WOUND INFECTIONS

Wound infections account for 20–25% of all nosocomial infections and are usually caused by autogenous infection at the time of surgery. A wound infection is diagnosed when there is a purulent discharge and a PPM is isolated in high concentrations. Commonly implicated organisms include *E. coli*, enterococci, *P. aeruginosa*, *Enterobacter* spp. and *Citrobacter* spp.

Wound infections are more common in the elderly, the poorly nourished, in those with renal failure or diabetes mellitus and in patients receiving steroids. The risks are greater following prolonged surgery and contaminated or dirty procedures. Importantly, administration of supplemental oxygen in high concentrations during the perioperative period can significantly reduce the incidence of wound infection (Belda et al., 2005).

THE RATIONAL USE OF ANTIBIOTICS

The successful treatment of septic, critically ill patients is critically dependent on early, empirical treatment with antibiotics to which the infecting organism is sensitive. Inadequate antimicrobial therapy (not given, delayed administration or organism-resistant) has been associated with increased mortality in various categories of patient with life-threatening infections (Kollef et al., 1999), including those with bloodstream infections (Ibrahim et al., 2000; Vallés et al., 2003), bacteraemic pneumococal pneumonia (Lujan et al., 2004) and severe sepsis (Harbarth et al., 2003). It is also clear that antimicrobial therapy is inadequate in a significant proportion (up to 19%) of such cases. Moreover the likelihood of receiving inadequate antimicrobial treatment seems to be increased when the patient has received prior antibiotic therapy during the same hospitalization, when central venous catheterization is prolonged, in those with bloodstream infection caused by *Candida* species or antibiotic-resistant pathogens (Ibrahim et al., 2000) and when the source of a bloodstream infection is unknown (Vallés et al., 2003).

Nevertheless, because critically ill patients often receive prolonged courses of the most expensive broad-spectrum antibiotics there is considerable potential for their abuse. In order to limit the emergence and spread of resistant organisms, and to control costs, antibiotics must be used rationally and sparingly:

- Antibiotics should be prescribed only when clearly indicated.
- Narrow-spectrum agents should be used whenever possible.
- Normally only short courses of antibiotics should be given (e.g. 5 days).
- Prophylactic administration should be carefully controlled.
- Unit antibiotic policies must be developed and continually reviewed.
- There is evidence that scheduled, empirical rotation of antibiotic regimes on the ICU reduces hospital-acquired and resistant hospital-acquired infection rates, not only in the unit but also on the wards to which ICU patients are transferred (Hughes et al., 2004). This approach may,

however, encourage resistance to multiple agents and was not supported in a recent systematic review (Brown and Nathwani, 2005).

■ Unnecessary treatment of non-infectious inflammatory conditions and colonization must be avoided (but see SDD above).

In practice it can be extremely difficult to distinguish between infectious and non-infectious causes of systemic inflammation, as well as to differentiate between microbial colonization and infection, in critically ill patients. Conventional clinical criteria (fever, leukocytosis, visibly purulent sputum, haemodynamic changes) are unreliable, whilst the results of microbiological investigations are usually delayed and may be inconclusive. A reliable, early laboratory-based marker of sepsis might, when used to complement clinical signs and routine laboratory investigations, help to restrict the overuse of antibiotics and encourage prompt administration when indicated. Although some investigators have concluded that C-reactive protein can be used as an early indicator of infection in patients with systemic inflammatory response syndrome (Sierra et al., 2004), this acute-phase protein has limited diagnostic specificity and a protracted response with delayed peak concentrations. Procalcitonin (circulating levels of which increase within 2–6 hours of bacterial or endotoxin challenge) may be a more reliable indicator of sepsis in critically ill patients (Chirouze et al., 2002; Harbarth et al., 2001; Müller et al., 2000), although findings have sometimes been inconsistent and procalcitonin assays, which can be performed easily and rapidly, are significantly more expensive than measurement of C-reactive protein. It is possible that specificity might be improved by combining measurement of both these markers (see Chapter 5).

Usually antimicrobial agents have to be given before the organism has been identified. Under these circumstances, material from all possible sites of infection and blood should be obtained and sent for culture and antimicrobial sensitivities before the first dose of antibiotics is administered. If the specimen is frank pus or is from a site that is usually sterile, an immediate Gram stain will sometimes provide a valuable clue as to the probable pathogen. Otherwise, a rational choice of antibiotic should be made on the basis of the organisms most likely to arise from the presumed site of sepsis and knowledge of the local prevalent organisms (hospital or unit-specific) and their resistance patterns. Many hospitals produce policies that guide the choice of antibiotic regimen in particular clinical situations (Table 12.4) and these help to rationalize the use of antimicrobial agents within the hospital environment. Close cooperation with the microbiology department is essential at all times, particularly in view of the increasing prevalence of antibiotic-resistant pathogens; infection with such an organism is more likely to prolong hospitalization, to increase the risk of death and to require treatment with more toxic or more expensive antibiotics (Holmberg et al., 1987).

In some units, sputum, urine and other available material are regularly cultured (e.g. twice a week). The results may then guide the initial choice of antibiotic. Surveillance cultures including nose, throat and perineal swabs, as well as sputum and urine can be obtained routinely on admission, and weekly thereafter.

It is recommended that initial antimicrobial therapy should be broad-spectrum, often involving a combination of agents, but that if possible treatment should subsequently be 'de-escalated'. In general, if the pathogen has been identified and its drug sensitivities are known, administration of a single antibiotic, if possible with a narrow spectrum of activity, is preferred to the use of combinations. The latter may, however, be required for empirical therapy, to prevent the emergence of resistant strains (e.g. in the treatment of tuberculosis) and for the treatment of polymicrobial infections. Furthermore, certain antibiotic combinations are synergistic (e.g. ampicillin and gentamicin against *Enterococcus faecalis*) and may therefore be particularly useful for the treatment of life-threatening infections. On the other hand, the combination of some bacteriostatic and bactericidal agents might be expected to be antagonistic, although this is no longer generally considered to be clinically important. Bactericidal antibiotics are probably superior in the treatment of endocarditis, and for neutropenic patients, but there is no evidence that they offer any advantages in other situations.

In a proportion of patients, failure of organism-sensitive antibiotic treatment to prevent death from sepsis may be related to antibiotic-mediated endotoxin liberation (Editorial, 1985). It might be possible to prevent some of these deaths by developing treatments to neutralize endotoxin and its mediators (see Chapter 5) or by developing antibiotics with a reduced propensity to liberate endotoxin.

PNEUMONIA

The appropriate initial regimen for a patient with pneumonia depends largely on whether the infection was acquired in hospital or in the community (see Chapter 8).

Pneumonias contracted outside the hospital environment (community-acquired pneumonia) can be treated initially with a combination of amoxicillin and erythromycin or clarithromycin. The former will cover the common respiratory pathogens, such as *Haemophilus influenzae* and *Streptococcus pneumoniae*, while the latter may be effective against *Mycoplasma pneumoniae* and *Legionella pneumophila*. Co-axomiclav (amoxicillin combined with clavulanic acid – a powerful inhibitor of many bacterial β-lactamases) or a second- or third-generation cephalosporin may be substituted for amoxicillin in patients with severe community-acquired pneumonia and to broaden the spectrum of activity for pneumonias acquired in hospital. In those allergic to penicillin a glycopeptide and a macrolide can be used, whilst levofloxacin may be useful in those intolerant of both penicillins and macrolides. Because an increasing number of community-acquired *H. influenzae* are resistant to amoxicillin, some have recommended using cefuroxime, ceftriaxone or cefotaxime in combination with teicoplanin for severe cases (www.brit.thoracic.org.uk). Alternatively a fluoroquinolone with enhanced

Table 12.4 Suggested antibiotic regimens in the UK

Nature of infection	Possible causative organisms	Suggested antibiotic regimen
Pneumonia		
Acquired in the community	*Streptococcus pneumoniae* *Haemophilus influenzae* *Mycoplasma pneumoniae* *Legionella pneumophila* *Chlamydiophora pneumoniae* or *psittaci* *Coxiella burnetii*.	Amoxicillin and a macrolide (can substitute a second- or third-generation cephalosporin or co-amoxiclav for amoxicillin in patients with severe community-acquired pneumonia). For those allergic to penicillin use a glycopeptide and a macrolide. Levofloxacin for those intolerant of both penicillins and macrolides
Confirmed	Staphylococcal pneumonia Pneumococcal pneumonia Staphylococcal pneumonia not responding to flucloxacillin Methicillin-resistant *Staphylococcus aureus* (MRSA) pneumonia *M. pneumoniae* *Chlamydiophora pneumoniae* *Chlamydiophora psittaci* *Coxiella burnetii* *Legionella* spp.	Flucloxacillin ± rifampicin Penicillin Add sodium fusidate to flucloxacillin Vancomycin, Teicoplanin or linezolid Clarithromycin or tetracycline Clarithromycin or tetracycline Tetracycline, clarithromycin or erythromycin Clarithromycin or tetracycline. Rifampicin in severe cases Clarithromycin ± rifampicin; levofloxacin is an alternative
Acquired in hospital	As above plus aerobic Gram-negative bacilli *Pseudomonas* pneumonia and/or bacteraemia a possibility	A second or third generation cephalosporin or piperacillin/tazobactam which may be combined with an aminoglycoside. If patient has received a cephalosporin in previous 7–10 days can use a quinolone or a carbapenem Piperacillin/tazobactam, ceftazidime or ciprofloxacin usually combined with gentamicin
Aspiration pneumonia		A second or third generation cephalosporin or piperacillin/tazobactam, sometimes combined with metronidazole Penicillin can be used for aspiration outside hospital
Exacerbation of chronic obstructive pulmonary disease	*Haemophilus influenzae* *Streptococcus pneumoniae* *Moraxella catarrhalis* Pseudomonas aeruginos a possibility	Doxycycline, amoxicillin (or co-amoxiclav), clarithromycin or moxifloxacin Quinolone
Intra-abdominal infection	Gram-negative bacilli, staphylococci and anaerobes (e.g. *Bacteroides fragilis*)	Piperacillin/tazobactam or a carbapenem with or without metronidazole. Can be combined with an aminoglycoside in severely ill patients
Ascending cholangitis		Co-amoxiclav and metronidazole. If patient has received antibiotics recently or has been instrumented, use pipercillin/ tazobactam or a carbapenem
Pelvic infections	Anaerobes Gram-negative bacilli	Metronidazole plus co-amoxiclav, a quinolone or a second- or third-generation cephalosporin

Table 12.4 Continued

Nature of infection	Possible causative organisms	Suggested antibiotic regimen
Urinary tract infections	*Escherichia coli; Proteus* spp. *Klebsiella* spp.	Co-amoxiclav or trimethoprim. A cephalosporin or nitrofurantoin are alternatives. Add an aminoglycoside if severe sepsis and/or indwelling urinary catheter
Pyelonephritis		Co-amoxiclav or piperacillin/tazobactam with gentamicin (discuss with Microbiologist for those with penicillin allergy)
Catheter-related bloodstream infections	Coagulase-negative staphycococci, *Staphylococcus aureus, Enterococcus* or *Streptococcus* spp., coliforms, *Pseudomonas aeruginosa, Corynebacterium* spp., yeasts	Glycopeptide Flucloxacillin for sensitive *Staphylococcus aureus*
Septic shock Acquired in the community	*Staphylococcus aureus Escherichia coli Streptococcus pneumoniae* Group A streptococcus *Neisseria meningitidis*	Second- or third-generation cephalosporin or piperacillin/tazobactam, perhaps combined with an aminoglycoside (discuss with Microbiologist for those with penicillin allergy)
Acquired in hospital	As above but may also include MRSA, Gram-negatives such as *Pseudomonas* spp.	Add gentamicin and a glycopeptide
Meningococcal sepsis (with or without meningitis)	*Neisseria meningitidis*	Cefotaxime or ceftriaxone
Neurological infections		
Meningitis	*Neisseria meningitidis Streptococcus pneumoniae Haemophilus influenzae Listeria monocytogenes*	Ceftriaxone in high doses Add ampicillin
Suspected viral encephalitis		Aciclovir
Brain abscess		Seek microbiological advice
Wound infections	*Staphylococcus aureus, Streptococcus* spp.	Flucloxacillin (or cefuroxime following contaminated surgery) Add metronidazole for traumatic wounds or when mucosal surface has been breached A glycopeptide if MRSA suspected
Cellulitis		Flucloxacillin Clindamycin if allergic to penicillin A glycopeptide if MRSA suspected
Necrotizing fasciitis	Mixed aerobic and anaerobic organisms Group A streptococcus	Second- or third-generation cephalosporin or piperacillin/tazobactam combined with an aminoglycoside and metronidazole. Clindamycin for group A streptococcus Penicillin for streptococcal infection Some recommend clindamycin and gentamicin for those allergic to penicillin
Gas gangrene	*Clostridium* spp.	Benzylpenicillin, gentamicin, metronidazole and clindamycin
Unusual pathogens	*Pneumocystis jirovecii* Fungi	High-dose co-trimoxazole Amphotericin B

pneumococcal activity such as levofloxacin can be used. It is, however, important to appreciate that broad spectrum antibiotics such as cephalosporins and quinolones are major risk factors for *Clostridium difficile* infection.

If *staphylococcal pneumonia* is a possibility (e.g. during an influenza epidemic), flucloxacillin combined with rifampicin should be used. If this diagnosis is subsequently confirmed and the patient is not responding, the addition of sodium fusidate may prove to be more effective. Penicillin remains the drug of first choice in patients with documented *pneumococcal pneumonia*.

If *Pseudomonas pneumonia* (or bacteraemia) is a possibility (for example, community-acquired pneumonia in patients with bronchiectasis or immune compromise, nosocomial pneumonia following prolonged antibiotic therapy), it is usually preferable to administer an antipseudomonal penicillin such as piperacillin/tazobactam, usually in combination with an aminoglycoside. Alternatively, ceftazidime or ciprofloxacin, which have good antipseudomonal activity, can be considered.

Aspiration pneumonia can be treated with piperacillin/tazobactam or a second- or third-generation cephalosporin, perhaps combined with metronidazole. Some recommend penicillin for aspiration in the community (see Chapter 8).

In patients with *ventilator-associated pneumonia* due to MRSA, initial therapy with linezolid (which penetrates more effectively into the lungs) has been associated with significantly greater survival and clinical cure rates than treatment with vancomycin (Wunderink *et al.*, 2003).

In general, aminoglycosides penetrate poorly into lungs and sputum and are therefore rarely used for pulmonary infections, except when bloodstream invasion is suspected.

EXACERBATIONS OF CHRONIC OBSTRUCTIVE PULMONARY DISEASE (see Chapter 8)

Doxycycline or amoxicillin can be given first and are nearly always effective in those cases due to pneumococcus. Because 10–14% of sputum isolates of *H. influenzae* are resistant to ampicillin, co-amoxiclav may be used as an alternative. Recent evidence suggests that moxifloxacin is more effective in terms of eradicating bacteria and is associated with a reduction in the frequency of exacerbations (Wilson *et al.*, 2004).

INTRA-ABDOMINAL INFECTION

Infections arising from sites within the abdomen usually require combination therapy to provide an adequate spectrum of activity, at least until the results of cultures and drug sensitivities are available. In this situation, an aminoglycoside is usually administered in combination with piperacillin/tazobactam or a carbapenem can be used and metronidazole. There is little to choose between gentamicin and tobramycin, both of which are active against the majority of aerobic Gram-negative bacilli, as well as staphylococci. In order to achieve effective therapy, without the risk of oto- or nephrotoxicity, it is important to monitor the blood levels of both these agents. Once-daily administration is associated with a reduction in toxicity and increased efficacy. (There is some evi-

dence that netilmicin is a less toxic alternative to the older aminoglycosides.) Amikacin should be reserved for the treatment of documented infection with gentamicin-resistant organisms.

Metronidazole is given to control infection caused by anaerobic organisms such as *Bacteroides fragilis*, and has superseded clindamycin and lincomycin, both of which were particularly implicated in the causation of pseudomembranous colitis (see later). This combination will not cover *Enterococcus faecalis* and may be ineffective against some strains of *Pseudomonas aeruginosa*. The use of an antipseudomonal penicillin will cover both these organisms.

Patients in whom ascending cholangitis is suspected should receive co-amoxiclav and metronidazole to cover mixed gut flora, including coliforms and anaerobes. Piperacillin/tazobactam can be used in those who have recently received antibiotics or been instrumented. Patients with severe acute pancreatitis complicated by necrosis, in whom secondary infection is a possibility, should be given imipenem or an agent with a narrower spectrum active against *Enterobacteriaciae* (see Chapter 16).

PELVIC INFECTIONS

Pelvic sepsis arising from the female genital tract is frequently associated with anaerobic infection and will always require treatment with metronidazole, initially in combination with co-amoxiclav or a second- or a third-generation cephalosporin. An aminoglycoside can be added in the most seriously ill or in those who fail to respond.

If clostridial infection is suspected (e.g. following a criminal abortion), penicillin should be used, whereas if staphylococcal infection is a possibility (e.g. in tampon-associated toxic shock syndrome), flucloxacillin and clindamycin (which decreases toxin production) can be used. In this situation the benefits of clindamycin are considered to outweigh the risks.

URINARY TRACT INFECTIONS

Urinary tract infections often respond well to co-amoxiclav which is active against most strains of *Escherichia coli*, *Proteus* and *Klebsiella* and has the advantage of excellent diffusion into the urinary tract. Trimethoprim, a cephalosporin or nitrofurantoin can be used as an alternative. An aminoglycoside should be considered in severe sepsis and/or the presence of an indwelling urinary catheter.

INTRAVASCULAR DEVICE INFECTION

Localized entry-site infections can be treated with the topical application of a disinfecting agent such as taurolin 2%, sometimes combined with a systemic antibiotic. Empirical therapy, when indicated, must cover *Staphylococcus aureus*; a glycopeptide is usually suitable. Flucoxacillin should be used for sensitive *S. aureus*. In those with tunnelled lines or who are immune compromised the possiblility of gram negative infection should be considered. The antibiotic regime should be modified subsequently in the light of any positive cultures. A 7-day course may be appropriate when the catheter has been removed but 14 days is recommended for infections caused by *S. aureus* or fungi. More deep-seated infection (e.g. endocarditis) may require prolonged antibiotic therapy.

NEUROLOGICAL INFECTIONS (see Chapter 15)

The three most common pathogens in adult acute bacterial meningitis are *Neisseria meningitidis, Streptococcus pneumoniae* and *H. influenzae* (now rare in western countries), although in neonates group B streptococci and *E. coli* predominate. Less common causes of meningitis in adults include group B streptococci, *Listeria monocytogenes, Staphylococcus aureus* and Gram-negative bacilli. Ceftriaxone, in high doses, is now the empirical antibiotic of choice. Ampicillin should be added when infection with Listeria is suspected. Acilovir should be given when viral encephalitis is a possibility. A blood sample should be sent for meningococcal polymerase chain reaction (PCR), blood and a throat swab should be sent for culture and serum should be sent for meningococcal serology.

WOUND INFECTIONS

In the absence of a systemic response, localized infection is treated by the topical application of disinfecting agents such as taurolin 2% at least twice a day. Local collections of pus and abscesses must be drained. Systemic antibiotics are only indicated when there are signs of generalized inflammation. Organisms commonly implicated include *S. aureus,* and haemolytic *Streptococcus* spp. Coliforms, enterococci and coagulase-negative staphylococci are usually considered to be contaminants unless they are isolated in pure culture or when the wound contains prosthetic material. Empirical therapy can be with flucloxacillin (or cefuroxime following contaminated surgery) combined with metronidazole if the wound is traumatic or a mucosal surface has been breached. When MRSA is prevalent, vancomycin and teicoplanin are suitable agents.

Cellulitis can be treated with flucloxacillin, or, if the patient is allergic to penicillin, cefuroxime or clindamycin. *Gas gangrene* is caused by deep-tissue infection with *Clostridium* spp., especially *C. perfringens,* and usually complicates penetrating traumatic injury, although it may also be seen following surgery and in intravenous drug abusers. Treatment includes urgent surgical removal of necrotic tissue and the administration of benzylpenicillin, gentamicin, metronidazole and clindamycin.

NECROTIZING FASCIITIS (Hasham *et al.,* 2005)

Necrotizing soft-tissue infections range from mild pyodermas to necrotizing fasciitis. The latter is a life-threatening, but uncommon, condition (around 500 cases per annum in the UK) in which the organisms spread rapidly along fascial planes, causing necrosis of subcutaneous tissue and fascia and, in some cases, the epidermis, but with relative sparing of the underlying muscle. Gas production is frequently prominent. Necrosis is usually limited in depth to the plane of the muscle fascia. Necrotizing fasciitis is most often caused by a synergistic infection with a mixture of enteric Gram-negative rods and anaerobes (e.g. *Bacteroides* spp., *Clostridium* spp. and anaerobic streptococci). Staphylococci may also be isolated, but overall *Streptococcus* is the most common causative organism. In particular, group A β-haemolytic streptococci have been associated with a toxic shock-like syndrome with profound discoloration and sloughing of the skin. Worryingly, necrotizing fasciitis caused by community-associated MRSA has recently been reported as an emerging clinical entity (Miller *et al.,* 2005). Organisms often gain access to the subcutaneous tissues through a trivial skin wound such as an insect bite, scratch or abrasion. Necrotizing fasciitis is more common in diabetics, the elderly, the immune-compromised and drug abusers. The condition occurs slightly more frequently in males.

Clinical presentation and diagnosis

Necrotizing fasciitis can affect any part of the body but the extremities, the perineum and the truncal areas are most commonly involved. The patient is usually extremely toxic and may be shocked, often with disproportionately severe pain and, in the early stages, only minor skin changes (erythema and swelling). The skin then becomes increasingly tense and erythematous, with indistinct margins. Later the colour may change from a red-purple to a dusky blue, before progressing to necrosis, blistering and formation of bullae, which may be haemorrhagic or may discharge 'dishwater fluid'. Crepitus of the area may be felt and air in the soft tissues can sometimes be seen on a plain radiograph. When the male genitals (usually the scrotum) are involved the condition is called *Fournier's gangrene*; in these cases infection may spread rapidly to the perineum, pelvis and abdominal wall.

Microscopy and culture of a fine-needle aspirate or incisional biopsy (which can be performed on the ward) may reveal the organisms. Computed tomographic (CT) scanning and magnetic resonance imaging may be useful when the signs are equivocal or the diagnosis is in doubt. Characteristic findings at surgery include grey, oedematous fat, which strips off the underlying fascia with a sweep of the finger.

Treatment

Prompt diagnosis and treatment are key to a successful outcome. *Radical surgical excision* until normal tissue is exposed improves survival, albeit at the cost of greater deformity. The aim is to perform definitive surgery, no matter how radical, at the first operation. Extensive cleansing with taurolin 2% is generally recommended. *Re-exploration* should be performed 24–48 hours later. Repeated debridements may be required. These procedures can be complicated by considerable blood loss.

Systemic broad-spectrum antibiotics should include a second- or third-generation cephalosporin, a carbapenem or piperacillin/tazobactam combined with an aminoglycoside and metronidazole. In those with suspected invasive streptococcal disease benzylpenicillin should be administered intravenously. Clindamycin has been recommended for group A streptococcal infection. Some recommend clindamycin and gentamicin for those allergic to penicillin. If readily available, *hyperbaric oxygen* treatment, the efficacy of which remains unproven, should be considered. *High-dose intravenous polyspecific immunoglobulin G* may limit the need to perform immediate extensive debridement or amputations in unstable patients (Norrby-Teglund *et al.*, 2005).

Prognosis

When aggressive surgery is performed early at an experienced centre, mortality rates as low as 10% or less can be achieved. Otherwise more than 70% of patients may die. Overall mortality rates have been reported to be in the region of 25%. Many of those who do survive are left with considerable scarring and deformity.

COMMUNITY ACQUIRED MRSA
(Ferry and Etienne, 2007)

Community acquired MRSA can infect even young healthy individuals without risk factors and usually causes skin or soft tissue infections. Life-threatening invasive infections such as necrotising pneumonia, necrotising fasciitis and severe sepsis have also been reported.

PROPHYLACTIC ANTIBIOTICS

The use of prophylactic antibiotics should be carefully controlled because their indiscriminate use encourages the emergence of resistant strains with which the patient, whose normal bacterial flora is destroyed, then becomes colonized. Situations in which the use of prophylactic antibiotics is generally accepted include:

- asplenia/sickle-cell disease (amoxicillin or penicillin V);
- prevention of endocarditis (see *British National Formulary* for details);
- manipulation of urinary catheters where there is a risk of endocarditis, the patient is neutropenic or the patient has a prosthesis (generally an aminoglycoside, but see *British National Formulary* for details);
- cardiac surgery (gentamicin and flucloxacillin);
- selected cases undergoing general, orthopaedic, urological or gynaecological/obstetric surgery (cefuroxime with or without metronidazole as indicated);
- insertion of prosthetic vascular grafts (flucloxacillin);
- the prevention of gas gangrene following major trauma or amputation of an ischaemic limb (penicillin).

ANTIBIOTIC-ASSOCIATED DIARRHOEA

Antibiotic-associated diarrhoea is a common complication of antibiotic therapy and can significantly complicate the management of critically ill patients. Mild forms may simply be a consequence of alterations in the bacterial flora, but in some instances there may be a low-grade *clostridium difficile* infection. Particularly severe diarrhoea with abdominal pain

or discomfort occurs in patients who develop *pseudomembranous colitis*, which is caused by the toxins produced by C. *difficile* and is more common in the elderly and debilitated. This condition is usually encountered in patients receiving broad-spectrum antibiotics and was originally described in association with the administration of lincomycin and clindamycin. Since then most other antibiotics, except parenteral aminoglycosides, have also been incriminated. The onset of diarrhoea may be delayed for up to 6 weeks after taking antibiotics. An emerging strain of C. *difficile* which produces much higher levels of toxins A and B has recently been described in association with particularly severe epidemic disease (Warny *et al.*, 2005). *Toxic megacolon* is an unusual complication of pseudomembranous colitis. This life-threatening complication should be suspected when there is increasing abdominal pain, abdominal distension, fever and tachycardia.

There is evidence that C. *difficile* is frequently transmitted between hospitalized patients and that the organism is often present on the hands of hospital personnel (McFarland *et al.*, 1989). A significant proportion of those who acquire the organism during their hospitalization remain asymptomatic and a few patients are already carrying C. *difficile* when they are admitted. The diagnosis of C. *difficile* colitis is made by growing the organism from the stools and by identifying toxins. Three negative samples are required to exclude the diagnosis. In those with pseudomembranous colitis, typical pseudomembranes may be seen on flexible procto/sigmoidoscopy.

C. *difficile* is always sensitive to vancomycin, which should be administered orally, but oral metronidazole may also be effective and is cheaper. Severe colitis may respond to high-dose oral vancomycin (up to 500 mg every 6 hours) combined with intravenous metronidazole (250 mg every 6 hours). Causative antibiotics should be discontinued if possible. Resistant cases may respond to treatment with *Saccharomyces boulardii* given as a probiotic. Patients with toxic megacolon who continue to deteriorate despite medical treatment need surgical review. Worsening abdominal pain and increasing colonic diameter are indications for subtotal colectomy. Sometimes patients relapse or develop a persistent carrier state. There is also evidence that C. *perfringens* may be responsible for some cases of antibiotic-associated diarrhoea, but this requires demonstration of cytotoxicity in cell culture as the toxin cannot be identified by routine techniques.

There is some evidence to suggest that administration of probiotics can reduce the incidence of antibiotic and C. *difficile*-associated diarrhoea (McFarland, 2007).

UNUSUAL PATHOGENS – DIAGNOSIS AND TREATMENT

Clearly, not all the infections seen on the ICU are caused by common PPM. This applies particularly to pulmonary infections, which are sometimes caused by unusual pathogens such as:

- *Mycobacterium tuberculosis;*
- viruses;
- *M. pneumoniae;*
- *Chlamydia psittaci* (psittacosis);
- *Legionella pneumophila* (legionnaires' disease);
- *Coxiella burnetii* (Q fever);
- fungi (e.g. *Pneumocystis jirovecii, Candida* spp.).

MYCOPLASMA PNEUMONIAE

M. pneumoniae is a relatively common cause of pneumonia which is often seen in teenagers or young adults. It presents as pneumonia with flu-like symptoms, sometimes associated with extrapulmonary complications such as:

- myocarditis and pericarditis;
- rashes and erythema multiforme;
- haemolytic anaemia and thrombocytopenia;
- myalgia and arthralgia;
- meningoencephalitis and other neurological abnormalities;
- gastrointestinal symptoms (e.g. vomiting, diarrhoea).

Cough may not be obvious initially and physical signs in the chest are often minimal or absent. The chest radiograph usually shows involvement of only one lower lobe, although sometimes there is dramatic shadowing in both lungs.

The white blood count is not raised, cold agglutinins occur in half the cases and the diagnosis is confirmed by a rising antibody titre.

Treatment is with clarithromycin, although tetracycline is also effective. Most patients recover in 10–14 days but in some the condition is protracted and in others there may be relapses. Lung abscesses and pleural effusions are rare.

CHLAMYDIA PSITTACI

Characteristically psittacosis presents as a low-grade illness developing over several months in a patient who has been in contact with infected birds, especially parrots. Symptoms include malaise, high fever, cough and muscular pains. The liver and spleen are sometimes enlarged and scanty 'rose spots' may be seen on the abdomen. Sometimes there is no history of contact with infected birds and occasionally the patient presents with a high swinging fever and dramatic prostration with photophobia and neck stiffness that can be confused with meningitis.

The chest radiograph shows a diffuse or segmental pneumonia and the diagnosis is confirmed by a rising titre of complement-fixing antibody. It may be possible to isolate the causative organism in psittacosis, but this is dangerous and only performed in specialist centres.

Treatment is with a macrolide or, alternatively, tetracycline.

COXIELLA BURNETII

Q fever presents as a pneumonia, which sometimes runs a chronic course and is occasionally associated with endocarditis.

The chest radiograph often shows multiple lesions. The diagnosis is confirmed by a rising titre of complement-fixing antibody.

Treatment is with clarithromycin or tetracycline. Severe cases may require rifampicin.

LEGIONELLA PNEUMOPHILA

Infection with *L. pneumophila* may occur as outbreaks in previously fit individuals when institutional shower facilities or cooling systems have been contaminated, as well as in immunocompromised patients or older male smokers. Sporadic cases, where the source is unknown, may also be seen. Characteristically the patient presents with malaise, headache, myalgia and a fever of up to 40°C with rigors. Gastrointestinal symptoms such as nausea, vomiting, diarrhoea and abdominal pain are common. Some patients have mental confusion and other neurological signs; some have haematuria and occasionally renal failure develops. The diagnosis of legionnaires' disease is extremely likely if the patient has three of the four following features:

- a prodromal flu-like illness;
- a dry cough, confusion or diarrhoea;
- lymphopenia without marked leukocytosis;
- hyponatraemia.

The chest radiograph usually shows unilateral lobar and then multilobar shadowing, sometimes with a small pleural effusion. Cavitation is rare.

It is possible to visualize *L. pneumophila* using direct immunofluorescent staining of pleural fluid, sputum or BAL fluid. The diagnosis is confirmed by rising serum IgG antibody titres and the organism can be cultured, although this takes up to 3 weeks. Urinary antigen detection may allow rapid diagnosis.

Although most consider erythromycin or clarithromycin to be the antibiotic of choice, some now recommend fluoroquinolones such as ciprofloxacin which are more active against intracellular *L. pneumophila*. In one study administration of a fluoroquinolone within 8 hours of admission to intensive care was associated with improved outcomes (Gacouin *et al.*, 2002) and many would now consider levofloxacin to be the antibiotic of choice (Sabria *et al.*, 2005). It is unclear whether the high mortality associated with severe *L. pneumophila* pneumonia can be reduced by combined treatment with erythromycin and a fluoroquinolone. Similarly the role of rifampicin either alone or in combination with clarithromycin is uncertain.

VIRAL PNEUMONIA

Viral pneumonia is unusual in adults, although *influenza A* or *adenovirus* infection are occasionally implicated. Infection with *cytomegalovirus* (CMV) is most commonly encountered in the immunocompromised, particularly those infected with HIV and recipients of bone marrow or solid-organ transplants. The virus may be transmitted by transfusion with infected blood. Whereas in healthy adults CMV causes an illness similar to infectious mononucleosis, in immunocompromised patients infection may be disseminated, with encephalitis, retinitis, diffuse involvement of the gastrointestinal tract and pneumonitis.

Serological tests can be used to detect latent (IgG) or primary (IgM) infection and the virus can be identified in tissue culture as well as by PCR. Lung biopsy can be useful to establish the diagnosis of CMV pneumonitis.

In immunosuppressed patients treatment with ganciclovir (5 mg/kg daily for 14–21 days) and immunoglobulin (Report from the British Society for Antimicrobial Chemotherapy Working Party on Antiviral Therapy, 2000) reduces retinitis and gastrointestinal damage and can eliminate CMV from blood, urine and respiratory secretions. It is less effective against pneumonitis and encephalitis. Drug resistance has been reported. Alternatives are foscarnet and cidofovir.

PNEUMOCYSTIS JIROVECII (Thomas and Limper, 2004)

This is by far the most prevalent opportunistic infection in patients infected with HIV. Although at one time reactivation of latent infection was considered to be an important cause of *Pneumocystis carinii* pneumonia (PCP), it now seems that person-to-person transmission is the most likely means by which new infections are acquired. Environmental sources may also be implicated. Nevertheless respiratory isolation is not currently recommended for patients with PCP.

In PCP the alveoli are filled with microorganisms and there is alveolar epithelial damage with increased pulmonary microvascular permeability. The alveoli are flooded with proteinaceous fluid and depleted of surfactant. The number of *Pneumocystis* organisms is greater and the number of neutrophils is lower in patients with, than in those without, acquired immunodeficiency syndrome (AIDS).

Clinical features of PCP include malaise, a low-grade fever, the subtle onset of progressive breathlessness, tachypnoea, tachycardia and a dry cough developing over a period of several weeks. Lung auscultation may be normal but diffuse crackles can be heard throughout both lung fields in severe cases. Marked hypoxaemia is characteristic. Acute dyspnoea with pleuritic chest pain may indicate the development of a pneumothorax. In patients with AIDS the onset may be more insidious with less severe hypoxaemia, and is sometimes associated with diarrhoea and weight loss.

Chest radiography typically reveals diffuse bilateral alveolar and interstitial shadowing spreading out from the perihilar region in a butterfly pattern. Less commonly there may be solitary or multiple nodules, upper-lobe infiltrates or pneumatoceles. If the chest radiograph is normal a high-resolution CT scan may reveal extensive ground-glass attenuation or cystic lesions.

Because *Pneumocystis* cannot be cultured, and the immunocompromised host may be simultaneously infected with multiple organisms (such as CMV), the diagnosis of PCP requires microscopical identification of the organism from a clinically relevant source such as sputum, BAL fluid or lung tissue. Sputum induction with hypertonic saline has a diagnostic yield of 50–90% but if this specimen is negative, bronchoscopy with BAL should be performed. Lung biopsy is rarely required. Monoclonal antibodies may have higher sensitivity and specificity than conventional staining for the detection of *Pneumocystis*. Another advantage of monoclonal antibodies is their ability to identify trophic forms and cysts, which is important because the trophic forms generally predominate in PCP. PCR can also be used to detect *Pneumocystis* nucleic acids. Because of the greater organism burden in AIDS-related PCP the diagnostic yield of sputum and BAL fluid is higher in these cases than in those with other causes of immune suppression.

Treatment is with high-dose co-trimoxazole (75–100 mg/kg daily in divided doses) normally given intravenously for 2 weeks and continued for a further week orally. Side-effects occur in up to 80% of patients and include nausea, skin rashes, megaloblastic bone marrow change and agranulocytosis. There is also some concern about the possible emergence of strains of *Pneumocystis* resistant to co-trimoxazole. Intravenous pentamidine, oral primaquine plus clindamycin or oral atovaquone are alternatives. Nebulized pentamidine (600 mg once a day for 21 days) rarely produces unwanted effects and has been shown to be effective in milder cases.

Primary prophylaxis against PCP is indicated in HIV-infected adults when the CD4 count is less than 200 cells/mm^3 or if there is a history of oropharyngeal candidiasis. Primary, and secondary, prophylaxis against PCP can be safely discontinued after the CD4 cell count has increased to above 200 cells/mm^3 for more than 3 months (Lopez Bernaldo de Quiros et al., 2001). Low-dose co-trimoxazole, dapsone, nebulized pentamidine or atovaquone can be used for prophylaxis.

The mortality rate among patients without AIDS who develop PCP is around 30–60%, although the risk of death is greater in those with cancer. Perhaps in part because of the smaller number of inflammatory cells in the lungs of AIDS patients with PCP, mortality rates are lower in such cases, at around 10–20%. Mortality is higher in those who require mechanical ventilation.

FUNGAL INFECTIONS

The incidence of nosocomial bloodstream infections caused by *Candida* species has increased 5–10-fold over the last 20 years or so and fungal infections now account for nearly 8% of all nosocomial infections. Mortality rates are high (20–57%), and although in the immune-competent host septic shock attributable to candidaemia is unusual, fewer than half of such patients will survive (Hadley et al., 2002). Risk factors for invasive fungal infection in critically ill patients include:

- broad-spectrum antibiotic therapy;
- renal or hepatic failure (Hadley et al., 2002);
- high Acute Physiology and Chronic Health Evaluation (APACHE) II score;

- indwelling central venous catheters;
- mechanical ventilation;
- recurrent perforated viscous or anastomotic leaks;
- colonization with *Candida* spp.;
- steroid therapy;
- immunocompromised patients are especially vulnerable.

Colonization of the throat, tracheostomy wounds, stomach and gut is relatively common in the critically ill and rarely requires systemic treatment. Because yeast cells adhere firmly to plastic, oropharyngeal and rectal carriage of yeasts frequently leads to contamination of tubes and catheters. Treatment of colonization should therefore include removal or replacement of endotracheal tubes, nasogastric tubes and urinary catheters, for example, and the application of topical antifungals. This will usually lead to clearance of yeasts from the lower airways and bladder.

When fungi are obtained in significant quantities from diagnostic samples such as sputum or urine, however, it can be difficult to make the important distinction between colonization and invasive infection. Invasive fungal disease may present as either localized organ involvement or generalized sepsis. Positive blood cultures may indicate significant infection but are often negative, even in autopsy-proven disease. Biopsy of infected tissue may provide the highest diagnostic yield and serology may be helpful.

In patients with *candidiasis* endophthalmitis (hard, greyish-white exudates seen on retinoscopy) is occasionally present and confirms invasive fungal disease. Haematogenous spread to the skin can also occur, in which case lesions present as small maculopapular eruptions. Other complications include meningitis, endocarditis, lung involvement and osteomyelitis. *Candida* pneumonia following aspiration of contaminated oropharyngeal secretions is extremely unusual, except in immunocompromised patients in whom fungaemia may also be due to translocation from the gut. Nevertheless if a heavy growth of fungus with pus cells is obtained repeatedly from the sputum of a ventilated patient in the presence of chest radiographic signs of consolidation, treatment for systemic fungal infection may be indicated, although more invasive techniques will normally be required to establish the diagnosis with certainty.

Invasive aspergillosis can occur in immunosuppressed patients and may present as acute pneumonia, meningitis, intracerebral abscess, lytic bone lesions or granulomatous lesions in the liver. *Pulmonary aspergillosis* may produce a mycetoma with a characteristic, mobile crescentic translucency seen on the chest radiograph and CT scan. The serum from such patients may contain *Aspergillus* precipitins.

Successful treatment of invasive disease depends on removing all possible sources of continuing infection such as intravascular catheters and prosthetic heart valves, as well as administering specific antifungal agents. *Amphotericin* remains an effective, and is certainly the longest established, antifungal agent, sometimes effecting a cure in disseminated candidiasis and producing a beneficial effect in some cases

of aspergillosis. Some degree of renal impairment usually develops soon after commencing amphotericin, but if treatment is continued the glomerular filtration rate usually stabilizes at 20–60% of normal. Renal function almost always improves rapidly once treatment is discontinued. Other adverse effects of amphotericin include anaemia, hypokalaemia, thrombocytopenia, pulmonary toxicity and hepatic dysfunction. Anaphylaxis and ventricular fibrillation have also been reported.

Liposomal amphotericin is less toxic in terms of nephrotoxicity and infusion-related reactions. Moreover, liposomal amphotericin is equivalent or superior to conventional amphotericin B for use as empirical antifungal therapy in neutropenic patients with persistent fever (Walsh *et al.*, 1999), although it is more expensive. *Fluconazole,* which can be given orally or intravenously, is a useful agent for the treatment of *C. albicans* and cryptococcal infections in immunocompromised patients but it has a narrow antifungal spectrum confined to yeasts. Adverse reactions include nausea, headache and skin rashes. The usefulness of orally administered *itraconazole* is limited by erratic bioavailability and gastrointestinal side-effects. The second generation of antifungal triazoles, such as *voriconazole,* have a broad *in vitro* spectrum, potent *in vivo* activity, a favourable safety profile and excellent bioavailability. In one study, voriconazole was found to be a suitable alternative to liposomal amphotericin which preserved renal function and was associated with a reduced frequency of acute infusion-related toxicity (Walsh *et al.*, 2002). Voriconazole has also been shown to be more effective and better tolerated than amphotericin B in immunosuppressed patients with invasive aspergillosis (Herbrecht *et al.*, 2002) and in non-neutropenic patients with candidaemia was as effective as, and less toxic than, amphotericin B followed by fluconazole (Kullberg *et al.*, 2005).

Another alternative antifungal agent is *caspofungin,* an echinocandin, which has activity against *Candida* and *Aspergillus* spp. and has been shown to be more effective, and less toxic, than amphotericin B for the treatment of invasive candidiasis (Mora-Duarte *et al.*, 2002). Caspofungin also seems to be as efficacious as liposomal amphotericin B, with the advantages of greater safety and improved survival and response rates in neutropenc patients with invasive fungal disease (Walsh *et al.*, 2004).

The role of prophylactic or pre-emptive antifungal strategies in critically ill patients remains uncertain. Current evidence suggests that, although the incidence of fungal infection can be reduced, length of stay and mortality are unchanged.

THE IMMUNOCOMPROMISED PATIENT

ACQUIRED IMMUNODEFICIENCY SYNDROME

AIDS is a consequence of infection with HIV, which infects, enters and destroys CD4 lymphocytes and impairs the function of those that remain, leading to a progressive impairment of CMI. Antibody-mediated immune responses are also defective and some patients, especially children, are particularly prone to recurrent infection with encapsulated bacteria. HIV-1 and the related HIV-2 are both retroviruses, which can be further classified as lentiviruses ('slow' viruses) because of their slowly progressive clinical effects.

Although HIV can be isolated from a wide range of tissues and body fluids, the majority of infections are transmitted by semen, cervical secretions and blood. Individuals who have an increased risk for infection with HIV are:

- individuals who have multiple sexual partners (it is particularly common among homosexuals or bisexuals in North America, western Europe and Australasia, while in much of sub-Saharan Africa, Asia and Latin America, heterosexuals and prostitutes are at considerable risk; heterosexual spread is increasingly common in Europe);
- intravenous drug users who share needles;
- children born to infected women;
- recipients of blood and blood products (e.g. haemophiliacs and transfusion recipients, especially in countries where blood donation is not screened) and donor organs.

AIDS is now the fourth commonest cause of death worldwide. Approximately 16 000 new HIV infections occur daily (the majority in young adults) and in high-prevalence countries in Africa 33% of 15-year-olds will die of HIV. Although in many of the more wealthy countries deaths due to HIV are falling, new cases continue to be diagnosed (2500 per year in the UK) and as a consequence the prevalence is rising.

Clinical features

Some weeks after infection with the virus there may be an *acute febrile illness*, which is easily mistaken for influenza or infectious mononucleosis. The patient may develop lymphopenia, thrombocytopenia and raised liver enzymes. CD4 lymphocytes may be markedly depleted and the CD4 : CD8 ratio reversed. Occasionally this initial illness may lead to transient severe immunosuppression sufficient to cause oesophageal candidiasis, or, rarely, PCP. There is then a *symptom-free period*, which may last for months or many years (median 10 years). Some symptomless individuals show *persistent generalized lymphadenopathy*, but this does not signify increased risk of progression.

Early symptomatic HIV disease includes:

- progressive weight loss;
- fatigue;
- mild chronic diarrhoea;
- minor opportunistic infections, e.g. oral candidiasis, herpes zoster, viral (hairy) leukoplakia.

A high proportion of individuals infected with HIV will eventually develop AIDS; the proportion increases with time – about 50% develop symptomatic disease within 10 years

and about 65% at 14 years. Some, however, remain well for many years. AIDS is characterized by major opportunistic infections (patients with a CD4 count greater than 200/mm^3 are at low risk of developing such infections) and tumours, which include the following:

- bacterial infections, which are often disseminated – *Listeria monocytogenes*, *Salmonella* (non-*typhi*), *Mycobacterium avium-intracellulare*, *M. kansasii*, *M. tuberculosis*. *Streptococcus pneumoniae*, *Haemophilus*, *Staphylococcus aureus*. Nosocomially acquired bacterial infection (e.g. *Pseudomonas aeruginosa*);
- viral infections – herpes simplex (ulcerating), CMV (retinitis, colitis, oesophageal ulcers, pneumonitis, encephalitis), herpes zoster, JC virus (progressive multifocal leukoencephalopathy), Epstein–Barr virus (fever, lymphoproliferative syndromes);
- fungal infections – *Candida* oesophagitis; *Cryptococcus neoformans* (meningitis or disseminated), *Histoplasma* spp.;
- protozoal infections – PCP; *Cryptosporidium* spp., *Isospora belli*, *Strongyloides stercoralis* (hyperinfection), *Toxoplasma gondii*;
- malignancies – Kaposi's sarcoma, primary brain lymphomas, Burkitt's or other B-cell lymphomas and squamous cell carcinoma of anus.

Multiple pathogens may coexist and *neurological manifestations* (e.g. dementia, subacute encephalitis, peripheral neuropathy, atypical aseptic meningitis) rarely occur in isolation. The US Centers for Disease Control classification of HIV infection is shown in **Table 12.5**.

Diagnosis

The diagnosis should be suspected in individuals presenting with any of the clinical features outlined above in the absence of other causes for immunodeficiency, especially if they have been involved in high-risk behaviour. PCP remains a common index diagnosis, although primary prophylaxis in those with CD4 counts < 200/mm^3 has reduced the incidence of this infection. The incidence of Kaposi's sarcoma has also fallen since the introduction of potent antiretroviral therapy.

Acute clinical management is concerned primarily with the opportunistic diseases and attention must be focused on prompt identification and treatment of these. The diagnosis of infection can, however, be made more difficult by the paucity of clinical features (e.g. neck stiffness in meningitis) caused by the impaired inflammatory response.

Before confirming a suspected diagnosis of HIV infection by testing for the presence of antibody to HIV, competent patients must be carefully counselled, preferably by someone experienced in the implications of a positive test. In some acutely ill patients of unknown HIV status, it may be wise to defer consideration of HIV testing until the wider issues can be discussed and the patient can be more adequately informed and counselled. Up to 40% of patients with HIV

Table 12.5 Summary of Centers for Disease Control classification of human immunodeficiency virus (HIV) infection

Absolute CD4 count (/mm³)	A: Asymptomatic or persistent generalized lymphadenopathy or acute seroconversion illness	B: HIV-related conditions*, not A or C	C: Clinical conditions listed in AIDS surveillance case definition
> 500	A1	B1	C1
200–499	A2	B2	C2
< 200	A3	B3	C4

AIDS, acquired immunodeficiency syndrome.
*Examples of category B conditions include: bacillary angiomatosis, candidiasis (oropharyngeal), constitutional symptoms, oral hairy leukoplakia, herpes zoster involving more than one dermatome, idiopathic thrombocytopenic purpura, listeriosis, pelvic inflammatory disease, especially if complicated by tubo-ovarian abscess, peripheral neuropathy.

infection are unaware of their status at the time of ICU admission; knowledge of their HIV status might influence the differential diagnosis, as well as affecting diagnostic and treatment decisions, including the use of antiretroviral therapy. Moreover the availability of a rapid HIV test that can provide a result within hours has increased the potential usefulness of a diagnosis of HIV in the treatment of patients. Nevertheless most continue to recommend that only in exceptional circumstances should tests be performed without full discussion with the patient and in the absence of the patient's express consent. In the USA some states require informed consent whereas others permit a surrogate to consent on behalf of the patient. In some cases it may be appropriate to consult the hospital ethics committee or legal representative. It is important to appreciate that the CD4 count may be low in critically ill patients without HIV and is not therefore diagnostic. Normally disclosure of a patient's HIV status requires patient consent, although in certain circumstances it may be appropriate to disclose the diagnosis to a spouse or legal surrogate.

Because the enzyme-linked immunosorbent assay (ELISA) used to test for antibody to HIV may produce both false-positive and false-negative results, confirmatory tests are required (e.g. by Western blot) and expert advice should be sought if there are unexpected findings. False-positives with some methods may occur in patients with autoimmune disease, chronic liver disease or myeloma, while the test may be falsely negative in those who have not yet seroconverted (this is common during the first 2 months after infection) or in patients with defects of antibody production. Occasionally detection of viral antigen, PCR or isolation of the virus in culture may be used to confirm the diagnosis.

Multiple immunological abnormalities may be detected in patients with AIDS, including:

- lymphopenia, especially of CD4 (T helper) cells (CD4 count < 100/mm³ is associated with severe immune compromise and infection with organisms of low virulence);
- defects in the function of CD4 cells;
- B-cell abnormalities with polyclonal activation of B cells and hypergammaglobulinaemia;

- macrophage defects;
- neutropenia (retroviral infection of haematopoietic progenitors, secondary infections, antiretroviral therapy).

Intensive care for HIV-infected patients (Huang et al., 2006)

The spectrum of diseases responsible for the admission of HIV-positive patients to hospital and critical care areas is changing. Approximately half of such patients are admitted with respiratory failure, the commonest cause of which is still PCP, although the number of patients admitted to ICU with PCP has fallen in recent years (Morris et al., 2002), probably as a consequence of improved prophylaxis, the use of adjunctive steroids and the increasing use of highly active antiretroviral therapy (HAART). Conversely the incidence of bacterial sepsis as a cause of ICU admission seems to be increasing (Rosenberg et al., 2001), especially in those who fail to respond to HAART, have low CD4 counts or become neutropenic. Other complications that may require intensive care include:

- dehydration due to diarrhoea and vomiting;
- cardiomyopathy;
- acute renal failure/end-stage renal disease (due to HIV-associated nephropathy, hepatitis B or C co-infection, diabetes or hypertension);
- pancreatitis;
- severe central nervous system disease (cryptococcal meningitis, toxoplasmosis, listeriosis);
- seizures;
- cardiac tamponade (usually due to tuberculosis);
- gastrointestinal haemorrhage;
- complications of antiretroviral therapy (e.g. mitochondrial toxicity with lactic acidosis, hepatic steatosis and, rarely, liver failure; immune reconstitution with manifestations of a more effective inflammatory response to a variety of pathogens; hypersensitivity reactions; Stevens–Johnson syndrome; pancreatitis);
- complications of a diagnostic procedure (e.g. pneumothorax following transbronchial biopsy or respiratory decompensation following BAL).

Importantly, adrenal insufficiency is common in HIV-positive patients who become critically ill. It has been recommended, therefore, that adrenal function should be assessed using an adrenocorticotrophic hormone stimulation test in all such patients (Marik *et al.*, 2002). End-stage liver disease secondary to viral hepatitis is now a frequent cause of morbidity and mortality in HIV-infected patients.

RESPIRATORY FAILURE ASSOCIATED WITH HIV INFECTION

Although PCP continues to be the most common cause of respiratory failure in HIV-infected patients (see above), mycobacteria (especially tuberculosis), pyogenic bacteria, fungi or CMV are sometimes responsible. In some cases respiratory failure is due to lymphocytic pneumonitis or pulmonary infiltration with Kaposi's sarcoma (often complicating bacterial infection). Respiratory failure due to non-HIV causes such as asthma and emphysema is increasingly common as patients infected with HIV live longer. Immune reconstitution syndromes to PCP, tuberculosis or other mycobacterial infections, occurring days to weeks after the initiation of antiretroviral therapy, can also precipitate respiratory failure.

Except in those with bacterial pneumonia, the chest radiograph usually shows diffuse shadowing. Mediastinal adenopathy is uncommon and when present suggests mycobacterial infection or lymphoma. Pleural effusions may be seen in association with pulmonary Kaposi's sarcoma (when they are usually haemorrhagic), and should also raise the possibility of tuberculosis.

Diagnostic methods have been discussed elsewhere in this chapter.

Treatment. Patients with severe respiratory failure may benefit from continuous positive airways pressure (CPAP), non-invasive ventilation (NIV) (Confalonieri *et al.*, 2002) or mechanical ventilation with positive end-expiratory pressure (PEEP) (see Chapter 7), although in those with PCP any increase in P_aO_2 is often relatively modest. The risk of pneumothorax or barotrauma is high and adherence to a lung-protective ventilatory strategy is particularly important (see Chapter 8).

The treatment of specific infections has been considered earlier in this chapter, but of particular importance in patients with severe AIDS-related PCP is the observation that the early addition of short intensive courses of corticosteroids (e.g. 40 mg methylprednisolone 8-hourly for 3–6 days) to standard therapy improves survival and reduces the incidence of respiratory failure (Bozzette *et al.*, 1990; Gagnon *et al.*, 1990). Steroids may also improve outcome in those who require ventilatory support (Montaner *et al.*, 1989). Treatment of the immune reconstitution syndrome also includes the administration of corticosteroids.

USE OF ANTIRETROVIRAL THERAPY IN CRITICALLY ILL PATIENTS

Critical illness may compromise the effective delivery and absorption of oral antiretroviral medications and only zid-

ovudine is available in an intravenous formulation. Renal insufficiency reduces the clearance of all nucleoside reverse transcriptase inhibitors (except abacavir), whilst hepatic impairment interferes with the metabolism of many protease inhibitors and non-nucleoside reverse transcriptase inhibitors. Moreover there are a number of important interactions between antiretroviral medications and drugs commonly used in critically ill patients. For example, H_2 blockers and proton pump inhibitors are contraindicated with atazanavir, and benzodiazepine levels may be markedly increased in those receiving non-nucleoside reverse transcriptase inhibitors or protease inhibitors.

It remains unclear whether antiretroviral therapy can improve the outcome of critically ill HIV-infected patients. Theoretically, improved immune function could be beneficial, whereas immune reconstitution syndromes might worsen outcome. It has been suggested (Huang *et al.*, 2006) that:

- patients who are receiving antiretroviral therapy, with evidence of viral suppression before submission to the ICU, should continue their antiretroviral drugs;
- patients who are admitted with an AIDS-defining diagnosis, especially PCP, are likely to benefit from instituting antiretroviral therapy (Morris *et al.*, 2003), especially when their condition is worsening despite treatment;
- initiation of antiretroviral therapy should be deferred when patients are admitted to the ICU with a condition that is not associated with AIDS, although when the CD4 count is < 200/mm^3 and ICU stay is prolonged, antiretroviral therapy should be considered;
- antiretroviral therapy should be given to those with HIV-associated nephropathy, since this may reduce the rate of disease progression;
- antiretroviral therapy should be discontinued immediately in those with lactic acidosis, hepatic steatosis or acute liver failure.

Prognosis

In many developed countries the mortality and morbidity (particularly the incidence of opportunistic infections) associated with HIV infection have declined dramatically since the introduction of HAART. On the other hand individual responsiveness to these medications varies (only about 50–70% of patients have significant virological responses), loss of response is common (30–50%), some are intolerant of these agents, some are non-compliant and many more do not have access to HAART. Furthermore there is increasing evidence that HAART may substantially increase the risk of cardiovascular mortality. Factors other than HAART which may have contributed to this reduction in morbidity and mortality include:

- earlier presentation, diagnosis and treatment;
- more effective therapy and prophylaxis for opportunistic infections;
- the use of corticosteroids in severe PCP.

In the early 1980s hospital mortality rates for HIV-infected patients admitted to ICU were high (in the region of 70%) and long-term survival was poor (median of around 7 months). Later in that decade mortality rates fell dramatically, largely as a result of the introduction of adjunctive corticosteroids for those with PCP. During the 1990s survival rates decreased slightly, perhaps reflecting an increasing reluctance to withdraw or withhold supportive treatment from such patients, and mortality rates stabilized at around 30–40%. In one UK study, for example, ICU mortality was 33% although, as in other studies, hospital mortality was considerably higher, at 56% (Gill *et al.*, 1999). More recently it was reported that 71% of HIV-infected patients admitted to intensive care survived to hospital discharge and that median survival times had also improved to 11 months, with survival in some subgroups as long as 2.5 years (Morris *et al.*, 2002). Most survival gains were, however, realized in those admitted with a non-AIDS-associated diagnosis whilst those with an AIDS-associated diagnosis survived, on average, for less than 1 month. Interestingly, patients receiving HAART at the time of ICU admission were 1.8 times more likely to survive than those not receiving such treatment, perhaps because CD4 counts were higher, viral loads were lower and albumin levels were higher in HAART-treated patients. Moreover admission for a non-AIDS-associated diagnosis (which carries a better prognosis) was more frequent in those receiving HAART. Low serum albumin, a high APACHE II score, the need for tracheal intubation and PCP (particularly in the setting of mechanical ventilation or pneumothorax) were all associated with a worse outcome (Morris *et al.*, 2002). Mortality rates are particularly high when HIV-positive patients develop septic shock (Gill *et al.*, 1999; Thyrault *et al.*, 1997).

ICU staff may have a variety of concerns about the provision of intensive care for these patients, including their relative youth, the generally poor long-term prognosis and the risks of occupational infection. Many of these anxieties can be ameliorated by allowing informed patients to participate in treatment decisions and by educating staff in basic infection control procedures and the nature of the disease.

Measures to minimize the risk of cross-infection

Although the risk of acquiring HIV infection during occupational exposure to HIV-positive patients in the ICU is low (approximately 0.3% following a single needlestick injury with HIV-infected blood), the importance of minimizing sharp injuries and accidental exposure to potentially infected body fluids and of adhering to universal precautions cannot be overemphasized (see Chapter 14). Appropriate measures should be taken for isolating patients with suspected tuberculosis, which is especially common in African patients.

There is no evidence that reverse isolation can reduce the incidence of nosocomial infection in patients with AIDS, as most are not acquired acutely from the environment (see earlier in this chapter).

INTENSIVE CARE FOR PATIENTS WITH MALIGNANT DISEASE

During the latter half of the twentieth century enormous progress was made in improving the once-dismal prognosis of malignant disease. More recently new, improved and more intensive chemotherapeutic regimes, with or without bone marrow transplantation (BMT) or peripheral blood stem cell transplantation (PBSCT), combined with advances in supportive care, have led to further significant increases in disease-free and overall survival times, particularly for those with haematological and lymphoreticular malignancies.

Patients with malignant disease are, however, prone to a wide variety of acute life-threatening disturbances related either to the effects of the malignancy itself or to complications of its treatment. It has been estimated that around 26% of all new referrals to a haemato-oncology unit may become critically ill at some time, a figure which may rise to over 30% in those undergoing haematopoietic stem cell support (Bach *et al.*, 2001; Gordon *et al.*, 2005). The majority of these disorders are, at least theoretically, potentially reversible and in view of the much improved prognosis it is now generally considered to be appropriate to offer intensive care to selected cases, provided there is a reasonable prospect of cure or at least worthwhile palliation (Hinds *et al.*, 1998).

Dangerous complications directly or indirectly caused by the malignancy include:

- infection;
- pleural or pericardial effusions;
- renal failure due to ureteric compression;
- pancytopenia due to marrow invasion;
- airway obstruction;
- metabolic disturbances (uraemia, ectopic hormone production);
- hypercalcaemia;
- hyperosmolar coma;
- neurological syndromes;
- massive haemorrhage from an ulcerated lesion;
- superior vena cava obstruction;
- cardiac tamponade;
- gastrointestinal disorders (obstruction, perforation, haemorrhage);
- renal failure (many causes):
- constrictive pericarditis;
- hyperviscosity syndrome (e.g. myeloma).

Life-threatening complications of treatment are most often the result of immunosuppression associated with chemotherapy, radiotherapy, steroids or, increasingly, high-dose chemotherapy and haematopoietic stem cell transplantation (HSCT). Such patients are very susceptible to overwhelming infection, particularly during the period of profound neutropenia induced by aggressive chemotherapy. In the majority of those with haematological malignancy, admission to ICU is precipitated by *pneumonia* and/or *severe sepsis/septic shock*, often complicated by *acute respiratory failure*

(Kroschinsky *et al.*, 2002; Lloyd-Thomas *et al.*, 1988; Staudinger *et al.*, 2000).

Sometimes *bleeding*, which is usually a result of marrow suppression with thrombocytopenia or less often disseminated intravascular coagulation, liver failure or the effects of drugs, is of sufficient severity to warrant admission. Other dangerous, but less frequent, complications of anticancer treatment include:

- cardiac arrhythmias;
- cardiomyopathy induced by irradiation or cytotoxic agents;
- pulmonary fibrosis related to chemotherapy or radiotherapy;
- graft-versus-host disease (GvHD);
- tumour lysis syndrome;
- gastrointestinal disorders (neutropenic enterocolitis, perforation, haemorrhage, diarrhoea, paralytic ileus).

Patients with malignant disease may also benefit from *elective admission* to the ICU following extensive surgical procedures, particularly if they have coexistent medical disorders. Intensive care may also be required for *postoperative complications*.

Infectious complications of malignant disease
(Pizzo, 1999)

Infection is a frequent complication of malignant disease and an important cause of death in patients with cancer, particularly those with haematological malignancy, in whom it is the commonest factor precipitating admission to the ICU (Lloyd-Thomas *et al.*, 1988).

IMPAIRED RESISTANCE TO INFECTION IN PATIENTS WITH MALIGNANT DISEASE (Table 12.6)

The increased susceptibility of patients with malignancy to infection may be related to:

- neutropenia;
- alterations in phagocytic function;
- lymphopenia;
- hypogammaglobulinaemia;
- impaired cellular immunity;
- disruption of mucocutaneous barriers (oral and gastrointestinal mucositis);
- obstruction of drainage tracts;
- invasive procedures.

In general immune competence is relatively intact before treatment and the majority of those with impaired cellular and humoral immunity are receiving chemotherapy, radiotherapy or steroids. Neutropenia is by far the most important cause of the increased susceptibility to infection and there is an inverse correlation between the granulocyte count and both the incidence and the severity of infection. The most pronounced immune suppression is seen in patients in relapse, probably largely as a result of previous courses of chemotherapy.

Table 12.6 Immune defects in patients with malignant disease

Carcinomas and sarcomas	Cell-mediated immunity more compromised than humoral response (degree depends on extent of metastatic spread) Effects of chemotherapy
Acute leukaemia	Abnormal neutrophil function Deficiency in the maturation of macrophages Defects in humoral immunity Neutropenia (most profound in those receiving intensive remission induction chemotherapy)
Haematopoietic stem cell transplantation	Profound marrow aplasia until transplanted marrow starts to function Prolonged cellular immune dysfunction Prolonged impaired humoral immunity
Chronic leukaemia	Defective cellular and humoral immunity Neutropenia
Lymphoproliferative disorders	Markedly impaired cell-mediated immunity Impaired humoral immunity in some cases

ORGANISMS CAUSING INFECTION

Virtually any organism can become invasive if host defences are severely impaired. The degree and duration of immune suppression, the type of immune defect, the treatment given and the patient's location may all provide a clue to the most likely infecting organism.

Bacteria still account for the majority of infections and pose the most immediate threat to the immunocompromised host. Most often aerobic Gram-negative bacilli (such as *Escherichia coli*, *Klebsiella* spp., *Pseudomonas* spp., *Proteus* spp. or *Enterobacter* spp.) are implicated, although there has been a recent resurgence in infections due to Gram-positive cocci, including coagulase-negative staphylococci. Multiple infections are relatively common. In general anaerobic infections are unusual in leukaemic patients, but are common in those with gastrointestinal and genitourinary malignancies. Less frequently, especially in those with impaired cellular immunity, infection may be due to unusual bacteria such as *Legionella pneumophila* and *Nocardia asteroides*. *Mycobacteria* are occasionally implicated. Humoral immune dysfunction renders the patient susceptible to infection with encapsulated bacteria (*Streptococcus pneumoniae*, *Haemophilus influenzae* and *Neisseria meningitidis*), as well as aerobic Gram-negative bacilli and *Pseudomonas* spp. Following haematological reconstitution, particularly during the late posttransplantation period (more than 100 days post-procedure) those who have received HSCT are particularly susceptible to infection with encapsulated bacteria, especially *Streptococcus pneumoniae*. Similarly, patients with chronic lymphoproliferative malignancies, which are often treated with steroids, are at increased risk of pneumococcal sepsis (Gowda *et al.*, 1995). Patients at high risk (those who have been neutropenic for more than 10 days and patients who have recently received a HSCT) are vulnerable not only to isolated acute bacterial infection but also to a second or even multiple infectious complications caused by bacteria, fungi, viruses or parasites.

The incidence of *fungal* infections in patients with leukaemia has increased and is usually related to a prolonged period of neutropenia combined with suppression of the normal bacterial flora by broad-spectrum antibiotics. Fungi are also an important cause of infection in BMT recipients. The majority of fungal infections in cancer patients are caused by organisms such as *Candida* and *Aspergillus* spp., which seldom cause infection unless host defence mechanisms are compromised. When cellular immunity is impaired the risk of infection with fungi such as *Cryptococcus neoformans* and *Histoplasma capsulatum* is increased.

Infection with *viruses* such as CMV, herpes simplex and varicella-zoster is seen particularly in those with impaired cellular immunity. Certain viruses, such as respiratory syncytial virus, adenovirus, parainfluenza virus and CMV, can cause acute fever. Adenovirus can also cause necrotizing hepatitis, pneumonitis or haemorrhagic cystitis, whilst CMV can cause an interstitial pneumonitis, especially in patients who have received an allogeneic HSCT. Conversely CMV is relatively uncommon following autologous HSCT. In haematologically reconstituted HSCT recipients herpes simplex infections tend to occur early (2–6 weeks after transplantation), CMV infections after 1–3 months and varicella-zoster infections after 6–12 months. Infections due to *protozoa* (*Pneumocystis jirovecii* and *Toxoplasma gondii*) and the helminth *Strongyloides stercoralis* are also seen most often in the context of compromised CMI.

SITES OF INFECTION

Common sites of infection include:

- the lung (commonest);
- mucosal surfaces (oral and perirectal);
- disseminated;
- central nervous system (unusual, except cryptococcal meningitis in those with impaired CMI and secondary to bacteraemia or fungaemia);
- genitourinary (unusual except in the elderly and those with urinary catheters or pelvic tumours);
- skin and soft tissues.

PREVENTION OF INFECTION

Once the patient has been admitted to the ICU measures to prevent infection that have been instituted on the ward (e.g. selective decontamination of the digestive tract) should in general be continued. Patients at high risk of fungal infection, such as those undergoing stem cell or BMT may be receiving prophylactic antifungal therapy with, for example, fluconazole. Careful attention to handwashing and other routine infection control measures (see earlier in this chapter) is essential. Invasive procedures should only be used when clearly indicated; strict attention to an aseptic technique and meticulous care of all intravascular cannulae, skin puncture sites and infusion lines are essential.

DIAGNOSIS OF INFECTION

In neutropenic patients the usual signs and symptoms of infection (except fever) are often absent because the patient is unable to mount an adequate inflammatory response and in nearly two-thirds of cases a focus of infection cannot be identified on initial evaluation. Sputum may not be purulent, cough may be minimal or absent, the appearance of physical signs is delayed and the chest radiograph often appears normal initially. Similarly urinary tract infection may not be accompanied by pyuria, and meningitis may be clinically silent. Finally it is important to appreciate that in these patients an apparently minor infection such as mild perianal cellulitis may cause bacteraemia with fever and chills. The diagnosis of infection in such patients is therefore often based solely on the presence of fever. (The observation that even profoundly neutropenic patients can develop a high fever in response to infection indicates that polymorphonuclear leukocytes are not the only source of endogenous pyrogens.)

Immediately infection is suspected a thorough clinical examination should be performed in an attempt to identify the source. Attention should be directed to the most common sites of infection, including the oral cavity, lungs, gastrointestinal tract (including the perineal area), skin and soft tissues. Diagnostic investigations should include:

- three blood cultures (three sets in each case);
- culture of sputum;
- bronchoscopy and BAL (in selected cases);
- aspiration or biopsy specimens from suspicious mucosal or skin lesions;
- culture of urine;
- lumbar puncture (when indicated);
- removal and culture of indwelling cannulae (except sometimes long-term intravenous catheters. Blood cultures should be obtained through the catheter);
- blood gas analysis (in those who are tachypnoeic or showing signs of respiratory distress);
- special investigations to establish the identity of the infecting organism (unusual bacteria, fungi, viruses, protozoa).

The appearance of *new pulmonary infiltrates* on the chest radiograph of a patient with malignant disease is not necessarily indicative of infection since there are also a large number of non-infectious causes (**Table 12.7**). Standard diagnostic procedures, including TTA, often fail to establish

Table 12.7 Causes of new pulmonary infiltrates in patients with malignant disease

Infectious	Bacterial pneumonia
	Fungal pneumonia
	Pneumocystis pneumonia
	Viral pneumonia (e.g. interstitial pneumonitis, especially with cytomegalovirus, 30–60 days after allogeneic haematopoietic stem cell transplantation)
Non-infectious	Radiation pneumonitis
	Cytotoxic drug-induced lung disease (e.g. bleomycin, methotrexate, busulphan and procarbazine)
	Malignant infiltration
	Pulmonary leukostasis (in uncontrolled leukaemia with very high blood counts)
	Diffuse alveolar haemorrhage
	Pulmonary oedema
	Non-specific interstitial pneumonitis

the aetiology of lung disease in these immunosuppressed patients, particularly when there is diffuse, bilateral involvement. Invasive procedures (see earlier in this chapter) are therefore often required to establish the diagnosis, although the risks of these techniques are increased in many patients with malignant disease because of associated problems such as thrombocytopenia, coagulopathy, respiratory failure and impaired tissue healing.

PRINCIPLES OF TREATMENT

Unless there is an obvious non-infectious cause, empirical antibiotic therapy must be instituted promptly whenever a neutropenic patient develops a fever. This approach dramatically reduces morbidity and mortality. A combination of two or three agents is usually required to cover the range of potential pathogens, the choice depending on the organisms known to be prevalent at a particular institution and their sensitivity patterns. Most often an aminoglycoside is combined with a cephalosporin or an antipseudomonal penicillin. If the patient remains febrile and unwell after 48 hours empirical antifungal therapy may be initiated and a glycopeptide, teicoplanin or vancomycin substituted for the aminoglycoside. Some centres use monotherapy with a third-generation cephalosporin or carbapenem as initial treatment. The chosen combination should be administered intravenously.

Subsequently it may be possible to modify the antibiotic regimen according to the results of cultures and sensitivities to a more specific, less toxic and less expensive combination. Often, however, clinicians are reluctant to alter a combination that has produced resolution of fever and clinical improvement, regardless of the culture results.

If the patient remains pyrexial and unwell, and there is no microbiological confirmation of the responsible organ-

ism, the antibiotic regimen may be changed empirically. In some cases antifungal and/or antiviral therapy or treatment for *Pneumocystis jirovecii* may also be instituted empirically. Current practice is to administer antifungal agents to neutropenic patients in whom fever persists or relapses despite antibiotic treatment (see above).

SEVERE SEPSIS/SEPTIC SHOCK

Severe sepsis/septic shock is a common cause of admission to the ICU, especially in those with haematological malignancy in whom it often occurs in association with respiratory failure (Lloyd-Thomas et al., 1988). The commonest source of infection in these patients is the lungs.

The principles governing the management of septic shock complicating malignant disease are the same as those for patients without cancer and should include early administration of appropriate antibiotics and prompt adequate resuscitation. Effective treatment is similarly dependent on the percutaneous insertion of intravascular cannulae (see Chapters 4 and 5). The risks of these invasive techniques, particularly infection and haemorrhage, are especially high in patients with malignancy. The danger of serious haemorrhage can be minimized by prior administration of fresh frozen plasma and/or platelet concentrates as indicated and by puncturing the smaller peripheral arteries and veins where bleeding is more easily controlled. It may be possible to insert central venous and pulmonary artery catheters via a vein in the antecubital fossa. Failing this the internal jugular vein should be used for central venous access since direct pressure can be applied to control venous bleeding or if the carotid artery is accidentally punctured. The subclavian approach should be avoided if possible, except for long-term catheters. Although cannulation of femoral vessels is thought by some to be associated with an increased risk of infection, this route can be used when others have failed. In practice serious complications related to vascular cannulation are rare.

PROGNOSIS

Mortality rates are high when patients with malignant disease develop an acute illness severe enough to warrant admission to ICU, particularly in those with respiratory failure who require mechanical ventilation, in whom hospital mortality rates of 60–70% or more can be expected (Azoulay et al., 1999; Depuydt et al., 2004; Gordon et al., 2005; Kroschinsky et al., 2002; Lloyd-Thomas et al., 1988; Staudinger et al., 2000). Reported survival rates for critically ill patients with haematological malignancy have varied widely from just a few percent to around 50%, depending on the patient population studied. Not surprisingly, mortality rates are lower when patients with all types of malignancy, including solid tumours, as well as surgical patients and those with metabolic disturbances are considered. In a recent prospective study of all hospitalized patients with haematological malignancy who were treated for critical illness either on the ward or in the ICU, 53% survived to leave hospital and 34% were still alive after 6 months (Gordon *et al.*, 2005).

A number of factors have been associated with a poor prognosis in such patients, including:

- mechanical ventilation;
- hypotension and need for vasopressors;
- increasing number of failed organs (mortality 90–100% when 4 or more organs fail);
- renal or hepatic dysfunction;
- central nervous system failure;
- cardiopulmonary resuscitation;
- older age;
- unresponsive or recurrent malignancy; } relationship to poor outcome has been less consistent
- persistent neutropenia;
- increasing time on the ventilator or in the ICU.

In some studies a diagnosis of acute myeloid leukaemia has been associated with a worse prognosis and female sex with a better outcome (Depuydt *et al.*, 2004). Mortality is also related to the severity of the acute illness, as assessed by the APACHE and Simplified Acute Physiology Score (SAPS) scores (Gordon *et al.*, 2005; Kroschinsky *et al.*, 2002; Lloyd-Thomas *et al.*, 1988; Staudinger *et al.*, 2000) and to the presence or absence of comorbidities (Soares *et al.*, 2005).

Outcomes are particularly poor in those who require mechanical ventilation following BMT and mortality is extremely high when such patients also suffer from shock and acute renal failure (Staudinger *et al.*, 2000). In one study only 18% of BMT recipients requiring mechanical ventilation survived to ICU discharge and only 5% were alive at 6 months (Huaringa *et al.*, 2000). A systematic review of the literature supported by a validation cohort concluded that patients requiring mechanical ventilation after HSCT have a baseline probability of death of 82–96%, which rises to 98–100% in the setting of combined hepatic and renal dysfunction (Bach *et al.*, 2001). In those who recover from respiratory failure the proportion surviving for 6 months or longer ranges from 27% to 88% (Bach *et al.*, 2001).

It has been reported that the prognosis is relatively good for those who require mechanical ventilation during the first month after BMT when respiratory failure is often due to regimen-related toxicity or cardiogenic pulmonary oedema. Conversely, late-onset respiratory failure (more than 100 days after BMT) was typically due to infection or diffuse alveolar haemorrhage and in these cases the prognosis was extremely poor (Huaringa *et al.*, 2000). The development of GvHD is associated with an extremely poor outcome following allogeneic transplants, whereas outcomes may be better in those who have undergone PBSCT, possibly because they receive less intensive preparatory regimes, they are less immunosuppressed after transplantation, marrow engraftment is quicker and they do not develop GvHD (Khassawneh *et al.*, 2002).

There is some evidence that the outcome of critically ill patients with malignant disease, including HSCT recipients with acute respiratory failure, has improved in recent years and that some of the conventional predictors of a poor outcome, such as neutropenia and BMT, have become less discriminatory (Azoulay *et al.*, 1999; Depuydt *et al.*, 2004; Khassawneh *et al.*, 2002; Kress *et al.*, 1999; Kroschinsky *et al.*, 2002; Larché *et al.*, 2003). In those with respiratory failure the use of non-invasive mechanical ventilation has been associated with improved outcomes in some, but not all, studies (perhaps because this approach is only effective when instituted early) (Depuydt *et al.*, 2004) (see Chapter 7), whilst increased survival rates in those with septic shock (56% mortality in one recent cohort) have been associated with early administration of appropriate antibiotics and prompt admission to ICU (Larché *et al.*, 2003). This reduction in reported mortality rates may also be attributable to changes in case selection, improved management of multiple organ dysfunction and new treatments for the underlying malignancy, including the use of haematopoietic growth factors.

Clearly the hospital mortality of critically ill patients with haematological malignancy is disappointingly high and the long-term prognosis for those who do survive is often poor and depends largely on the nature and progress of the underlying malignancy. Moreover the overall cost of intensive care per life-year gained and resource consumption are extremely high. Nevertheless, for some patients, intensive care is life-saving, the prospects for long-term survival can be good and the quality of life for those with haematological malignancy who do survive long-term seems to be good (Yau *et al.*, 1991).

Despite these high mortality rates, most believe that intensive care is justified for patients with acute life-threatening complications of malignancy unless or until it is clear that there is no prospect of recovery from the acute illness or that the underlying malignancy cannot be controlled. Often these patients are young and were previously fit and well; for such individuals aggressive support can be justified even when the chances of survival are slim. Nevertheless both for a humane approach to the management of critically ill patients with haematological malignancy and to ensure that finite resources are used appropriately, it is important to avoid admitting patients who cannot hope to benefit from intensive care and to limit further aggressive treatment when the outlook is obviously hopeless. Equally it is important to identify those cases with a relatively good prognosis.

Withholding or limiting treatment can be extraordinarily difficult, especially because these patients are often relatively young, but our decisions, and our advice to the patient and their next of kin, must always be based on the best possible understanding of the factors which determine both the immediate and the long-term outcome in the various categories of patient (see Chapter 2). Clearly each patient must be treated as an individual but in those with a combination of features associated with a poor outcome it will often be appropriate to limit or withdraw aggressive supportive treatment.

Once a patient has been admitted to intensive care the prognosis and treatment strategy should be reassessed at least daily. Certainly to continue to support a mechanically ventilated BMT recipient with diffuse pulmonary infiltrates who requires vasopressors or has developed hepatic and renal insufficiency could reasonably be considered to be futile and inappropriate. When making such decisions a consensus must be reached as to the most appropriate plan of management based on an accurate assessment of the prognosis. This will involve close liaison with the oncologists, nursing and support staff, as well as effective and honest communication with the patient and family and friends.

REFERENCES

Abraham E, Chang YH (1990) Hemorrhage in mice produces alterations in intestinal B cell repertoires. *Cellular Immunology* 128: 165–174.

Altemeier WA, Todd JC, Inge WW (1967) Gram-negative septicemia: a growing threat. *Annals of Surgery* 166: 530–542.

Andrews CP, Coalson JJ, Smith JD, et al. (1981) Diagnosis of nosocomial bacterial pneumonia in acute, diffuse lung injury. *Chest* 80: 254–258.

Azoulay E, Recher C, Alberti C, et al. (1999) Changing use of intensive care for hematological patients: the example of multiple myeloma. *Intensive Care Medicine* 25: 1395–1401.

Bach PB, Schrag D, Nierman DM, et al. (2001) Identification of poor prognostic features among patients requiring mechanical ventilation after hematopoietic stem cell transplantation. *Blood* 98: 3234–3240.

Belda FJ, Aguilera L, Garcia de la Asuncion J, et al. (2005) Supplemental perioperative oxygen and the risk of surgical wound infection: a randomized controlled trial. *Journal of the American Medical Association* 294: 2035–2042.

Bengmark S (2002) Gut microbial ecology in critical illness: is there a role for prebiotics, probiotics and synbiotics? *Current Opinion in Critical Care* 8: 145–151.

Berger R, Arango L (1985) Etiologic diagnosis of bacterial nosocomial pneumonia in seriously ill patients. *Critical Care Medicine* 13: 833–836.

Besselink MGH, van Santvoort HC, Baskens E, et al. for the Dutch Acute Pancreatitis Study Group (2008) Probiotic prophylaxis in predicted severe acute pancreatitis: a randomised, double-blind, placebo-controlled trial. *Lancet* 371: 651–659.

Bozzette SA, Sattler FR, Chiu J, et al. (1990) A controlled trial of early adjunctive treatment with corticosteroids for *Pneumocystis carinii* pneumonia in the acquired immunodeficiency syndrome. California Collaborative Treatment Group. *New England Journal of Medicine* 323: 1451–1457.

Bradley JA, Hamilton DN, Brown MW, et al. (1984) Cellular defense in critically ill surgical patients. *Critical Care Medicine* 12: 565–570.

British National Formulary BMJ Publishing Group/RPS Publishing, London.

Brown EM, Nathwani D (2005) Antibiotic cycling or rotation: a systematic review of the evidence of efficacy. *Journal of Antimicrobial Chemotherapy* 55: 6–9.

Bueno-Cavanillas A, Delgado-Rodriguez M, Lopez-Luque A, et al. (1994) Influence of nosocomial infection on mortality rate in an intensive care unit. *Critical Care Medicine* 22: 55–60.

Cade JF, McOwat E, Siganporia R, et al. (1992) Uncertain relevance of gastric colonization in the seriously ill. *Intensive Care Medicine* 18: 210–217.

Cepeda JA, Whitehouse T, Cooper B, et al. (2005) Isolation of patients in single rooms or cohorts to reduce spread of MRSA in intensive care units: prospective two-centre study. *Lancet* 365: 295–304.

Chaiyakunapruk N, Veenstra DL, Lipsky BA, et al. (2002) Chlorhexidine compared with povidone-iodine solution for vascular catheter-site care: a meta-analysis. *Annals of Medicine* 136: 792–801.

Chang S, Sievert DM, Hageman JC, et al. (2003) Infection with vancomycin-resistant *Staphylococcus aureus* containing the vanA resistance gene. *New England Journal of Medicine* 348: 1342–1347.

Chatzinikolaou I, Finkel K, Hanna H, et al. (2003) Antibiotic coated hemodialysis catheters for the prevention of vascular catheter-related infections: a prospective, randomized study. *American Journal of Medicine* 115: 352–357.

Chirouze C, Schuhmacker H, Rabaud C, et al. (2002) Low serum procalcitonin level accurately predicts the absence of bacteremia in adult patients with acute fever. *Clinical Infectious Diseases* 35: 156–161.

Cobb DK, High KP, Sawyer RG, et al. (1992) A controlled trial of scheduled replacement of central venous and pulmonary-artery catheters. *New England Journal of Medicine* 327: 1062–1068.

Confalonieri M, Calderini E, Terraciano S, et al. (2002) Noninvasive ventilation for treating acute respiratory failure in AIDS patients with *Pneumocystis carinii* pneumonia. *Intensive Care Medicine* 28: 1233–1238.

Daschner FD (1985) Useful and useless hygienic techniques in intensive care units. *Intensive Care Medicine* 11: 280–283.

D'Amico R, Pifferi S, Leonetti C, et al. (1998) Effectiveness of antibiotic prophylaxis in critically ill adult patients: systematic review of randomised controlled trials. *British Medical Journal* 316: 1275–1285.

de Jonge E, Schultz MJ, Spanjaard L, et al. (2003) Effects of selective decontamination of digestive tract on mortality and acquisition of resistant bacteria in intensive care: a randomised controlled trial. *Lancet* 362: 1011–1016.

de La Cal MA, Cerda E, Garcia-Hierro P, et al. (2005) Survival benefit in critically ill burned patients receiving selective decontamination of the digestive tract. *Annals of Surgery* 241: 424–430.

Depuydt PO, Benoit DD, Vandewoude KH, et al. (2004) Outcome in noninvasively and invasively ventilated hematologic patients with acute respiratory failure. *Chest* 126: 1299–1306.

Doebbeling BN, Stanley GL, Sheetz CT, et al. (1992) Comparative efficacy of alternative handwashing agents in reducing nosocomial infections in intensive care units. *New England Journal of Medicine* 327: 88–93.

Du Moulin GC, Paterson DG, Hedley-Whyte J, et al. (1982) Aspiration of gastric bacteria in antacid-treated patients: a frequent cause of postoperative colonisation of the airway. *Lancet* 1: 242–245.

Editorial (1985) A nasty shock from antibiotics? *Lancet* 2: 594.

Ferry J, Etienne J (2007) Community acquired MRSA in Europe. British Medical Journal 335: 947–948.

Gacouin A, Le Tulzo Y, Lavoue S, et al. (2002) Severe pneumonia due to *Legionella pneumophila*: prognostic factors, impact of delayed appropriate antimicrobial therapy. *Intensive Care Medicine* 28: 686–691.

Gagnon S, Boota AM, Fischl MA, et al. (1990) Corticosteroids as adjunctive therapy for severe *Pneumocystis carinii* pneumonia in the acquired immunodeficiency syndrome. A double-blind placebo-controlled trial. *New England Journal of Medicine* 323: 1444–1450.

Gastinne H, Wolff M, Delatour F, et al. (1992) A controlled trial in intensive care units of selective decontamination of the digestive tract with nonabsorbable antibiotics. The French Study Group on Selective Decontamination of the Digestive Tract. *New England Journal of Medicine* 326: 594–599.

Gill JK, Greene L, Miller R, et al. (1999) ICU admission in patients infected with the human immunodeficiency virus – a multicentre survey. *Anaesthesia* 54: 727–732.

Gordon AC, Oakervee HE, Kaya B, et al. (2005) Incidence and outcome of critical illness amongst hospitalised patients with haematological malignancy: a prospective observational study of ward and intensive care unit based care. *Anaesthesia* 60: 340–347.

Gowda R, Razvi FM, Summerfield GP (1995) Risk of pneumococcal septicaemia in patients with chronic lymphoproliferative malignancies. *British Medical Journal* 311: 26–27.

Hadley S, Lee WW, Ruthazer R, et al. (2002) Candidemia as a cause of septic shock and multiple organ failure in nonimmunocompromised patients. *Critical Care Medicine* 30: 1808–1814.

Hammond JM, Potgieter PD, Saunders GL, et al. (1992) Double-blind study of selective decontamination of the digestive tract in intensive care. *Lancet* 340: 5–9.

Harbarth S, Holeckova K, Froidevaux C, et al. (2001) Diagnostic value of procalcitonin, interleukin-6 and interleukin-8 in critically ill patients admitted with suspected sepsis. *American Journal of Respiratory and Critical Care Medicine* 164: 396–402.

Harbarth S, Garbino J, Pugin J, et al. (2003) Inappropriate initial antimicrobial therapy and its effect on survival in a clinical trial of immunomodulating therapy for severe sepsis. *American Journal of Medicine* 115: 529–535.

Hasham S, Matteucci P, Stanley PR, et al. (2005) Necrotizing fasciitis. *British Medical Journal* **330**: 830–833.

Herbrecht R, Denning DW, Patterson TF et al. (2002) Voriconazole versus amphotericin B for primary therapy of invasive aspergillosis. *New England Journal of Medicine* **347**: 408–415.

Heyland DK, Cook DJ, Jaeschke R, et al. (1994) Selective decontamination of the digestive tract. An overview. *Chest* **105**: 1221–1229.

Hilton E, Haslett TM, Borenstein MT, et al. (1988) Central catheter infections: single versus triple-lumen catheters. Influence of guide wires on infection rates when used for replacement of catheters. *American Journal of Medicine* **84**: 667–672.

Hinds CJ, Martin R, Quinton P (1998) Intensive care for patients with medical complications of haematological malignancy: is it worth it? *Schweizerische medizinische Wochenschrift* **128**: 1467–1473.

Holmberg SD, Solomon SL, Blake PA (1987) Health and economic impacts of antimicrobial resistance. *Reviews of Infectious Diseases* **9**: 1065–1078.

Huang L, Quartin A, Jones D, et al. (2006) Intensive care of patients with HIV infection. *New England Journal of Medicine* **355**: 173–181.

Huaringa AJ, Leyva FJ, Giralt SA, et al. (2000) Outcome of bone marrow transplantation patients requiring mechanical ventilation. *Critical Care Medicine* **28**: 1014–1017.

Hughes MG, Evans HL, Chong TW, et al. (2004) Effect of an intensive care unit rotating empiric antibiotic schedule on the development of hospital-acquired infections on the non-intensive care unit ward. *Critical Care Medicine* **32**: 53–60.

Huskins WC, Goldmann DA (2005) Controlling methicillin-resistant *Staphylococcus aureus* aka 'superbug'. *Lancet* **365**: 273–275.

Ibrahim EH, Sherman G, Ward S, et al. (2000) The influence of inadequate antimicrobial treatment of bloodstream infections on patient outcomes in the ICU setting. *Chest* **118**: 146–155.

Inglis TJ, Sproat LJ, Sherratt MJ, et al. (1992) Gastroduodenal dysfunction as a cause of gastric bacterial overgrowth in patients undergoing mechanical ventilation of the lungs. *British Journal of Anaesthesia* **68**: 499–502.

Khassawneh BY, White P Jr, Anaissie EJ, et al. (2002) Outcome from mechanical ventilation after autologous peripheral blood stem cell transplantation. *Chest* **121**: 185–188.

Kollef MH (1994) The role of selective digestive tract decontamination on mortality and respiratory tract infections. A meta-analysis. *Chest* **105**: 1101–1108.

Kollef MH, Sherman G, Ward S, et al. (1999) Inadequate antimicrobial treatment of infections: a risk factor for hospital mortality among critically ill patients. *Chest* **115**: 462–474.

Kress JP, Christenson J, Pohlman AS, et al. (1999) Outcomes of critically ill cancer patients in a university hospital setting. *American Journal of Respiratory and Critical Care Medicine* **160**: 1957–1961.

Kroschinsky F, Weise M, Illmer T, et al. (2002) Outcome and prognostic features of intensive care unit treatment in patients with hematological malignancies. *Intensive Care Medicine* **28**: 1294–1300.

Kullberg BJ, Sobel JD, Ruhnke M, et al. (2005) Voriconazole versus a regimen of amphotericin B followed by fluconazole for candidaemia in non-neutropenic patients: a randomised non-inferiority trial. *Lancet* **366**: 1435–1442.

Larché J, Azoulay E, Fieux F, et al. (2003) Improved survival of critically ill cancer patients with septic shock. *Intensive Care Medicine* **29**: 1688–1695.

Lloyd-Thomas AR, Wright I, Lister TA, et al. (1988) Prognosis of patients receiving intensive care for lifethreatening medical complications of haematological malignancy. *British Medical Journal* **296**: 1025–1029.

Lopez Bernaldo de Quiros JC, Miro JM, Peña JM, et al. (2001) A randomized trial of the discontinuation of primary and secondary prophylaxis against *Pneumocystis carinii* pneumonia after highly active antiretroviral therapy in patients with HIV infection. *New England Journal of Medicine* **344**: 159–167.

Lujan M, Gallego M, Fontanals D, et al. (2004) Prospective observational study of bacteremic pneumococcal pneumonia: effect of discordant therapy on mortality. *Critical Care Medicine* **32**: 625–631.

McFarland LV, Mulligan ME, Kwok RY, et al. (1989) Nosocomial acquisition of *Clostridium difficile* infection. *New England Journal of Medicine* **320**: 204–210.

McFarland LV (2007) Diarrhoea associated with antibiotic use. *British Medical Journal* **335**: 54–55.

Marik PE, Kiminyo LK, Zaloga GP (2002) Adrenal insufficiency in critically ill patients with human immunodeficiency virus. *Critical Care Medicine* **30**: 1267–1273.

Mermel LA, Farr BM, Sherertz RJ, et al. (2001) Guidelines for the management of intravascular catheter-related infections. *Clinical Infectious Diseases* **32**: 1249–1272.

Miller LG, Perdreau-Remington F, Reig G, et al. (2005) Necrotizing fasciitis caused by community-associated methicillin-resistant *Staphylococcus aureus* in Los Angeles. *New England Journal of Medicine* **352**: 1445–1453.

Montaner JSG, Russell JA, Lawson L, et al. (1989) Acute respiratory failure secondary to *Pneumocystis carinii* pneumonia in the acquired immunodeficiency syndrome. A potential role for systemic corticosteroids. *Chest* **95**: 881–884.

Mora-Duarte J, Betts R, Rotstein C, et al. (2002) Comparison of caspofungin and amphotericin B for invasive candidiasis. *New England Journal of Medicine* **347**: 2020–2029.

Morris A, Creasman J, Turner J, Luce JM, et al. (2002) Intensive care of human immunodeficiency virus-infected patients during the era of highly active antiretroviral therapy. *American Journal of Respiratory and Critical Care Medicine* **166**: 262–267.

Morris A, Wachter RM, Luce J, et al. (2003) Improved survival with highly active antiretroviral therapy in HIV-infected patients with severe *Pneumocystis carinii* pneumonia. *AIDS* **17**: 73–80.

Müller B, Becker KL, Schächinger H, et al. (2000) Calcitonin precursors are reliable markers of sepsis in a medical intensive care unit. *Critical Care Medicine* **28**: 977–983.

Nathens AB, Marshall JC (1999) Selective decontamination of the digestive tract in surgical patients: a systematic review of the evidence. *Archives of Surgery* **134**: 170–176.

Norrby-Teglund A, Muller MP, McGeer A, et al. (2005) Successful management of severe group A streptococcal soft tissue infections using an aggressive medical regimen including intravenous polyspecific immunoglobulin together with a conservative surgical approach. *Scandinavian Journal of Infectious Diseases* **37**: 166–172.

O'Connell MT, Becker DM, Steele BW, et al. (1984) Plasma fibronectin in medical ICU patients. *Critical Care Medicine* **12**: 479–482.

Parienti J-J, du Cheyron D, Ramakers M, et al. (2004) Alcoholic povidone-iodine to prevent central venous catheter colonization: a randomized unit-crossover study. *Critical Care Medicine* **32**: 708–713.

Pinilla JC, Ross DF, Martin T, et al. (1983) Study of the incidence of intravascular catheter infection and associated septicemia in critically ill patients. *Critical Care Medicine* **11**: 21–25.

Pizzo PA (1999) Fever in immunocompromised patients. *New England Journal of Medicine* **341**: 893–900.

Pronovost P, Needham D, Berenholtz S (2006) An intervention to decrease catheter-related bloodstream infections in the ICU. *New England Journal of Medicine* **355**: 2725–2732.

Report from the British Society for Antimicrobial Chemotherapy Working Party on Antiviral Therapy (2000) Management of herpes virus infections following transplantation. *Journal of Antimicrobial Chemotherapy* **45**: 729–748.

Rijnders BJ, Peetermans WE, Verwaest C, et al. (2004) Watchful waiting versus immediate catheter removal in ICU patients with suspected catheter-related infection: a randomized trial. *Intensive Care Medicine* **30**: 1073–1080.

Rosenberg AL, Seneff MG, Atiyeh L, et al. (2001) The importance of bacterial sepsis in intensive care unit patients with acquired immunodeficiency syndrome: implications for future care in the age of increasing antiretroviral resistance. *Critical Care Medicine* **29**: 548–556.

Roy S, Knox K, Segal S, et al. (2002) MBL genotype and risk of invasive pneumococcal disease: a case control study. *Lancet* **359**: 1569–1573.

Sabria M, Pedro Botet ML, Gomez J, et al. (2005) Fluoroquinolones vs macrolides in the treatment of legionnaires disease. *Chest* **128**: 1401–1405.

Safdar N, Maki DG (2002) Inflammation at the insertion site is not predictive of catheter-related bloodstream infection with short-term, noncuffed central venous catheters. *Critical Care Medicine* **30**: 2632–2635.

Safdar N, Fine JP, Maki DG (2005) Meta-analysis: methods for diagnosing intravascular device-related bloodstream infection. *Annals of Internal Medicine* **142**: 451–466.

Selective Decontamination of the Digestive Tract Trialists' Collaborative Group (1993) Meta-analysis of randomised controlled trials of selective decontamination of the digestive tract. *British Medical Journal* **307**: 525–532.

Sierra R, Rello J, Bailen MA, et al. (2004) C-reactive protein used as an early indicator of infection in patients with systemic inflammatory response syndrome. *Intensive Care Medicine* **30**: 2038–2045.

Soares M, Salluh JI, Ferreira CG, et al. (2005) Impact of two different comorbidity measures on the 6-month mortality of critically ill cancer patients. *Intensive Care Medicine* **31**: 408–415.

Staudinger T, Stoiser B, Müllner M, *et al.* (2000) Outcome and prognostic factors in critically ill cancer patients admitted to the intensive care unit. *Critical Care Medicine* **28**: 1322–1328.

Stelfox HT, Bates DW, Redelmeier DA (2003) Safety of patients isolated for infection control. *Journal of the American Medical Association* **290**: 1899–1905.

Stoutenbeek CP, Van Saene HK, Miranda DR, *et al.* (1984) The effect of selective decontamination of the digestive tract on colonisation and infection rate in multiple trauma patients. *Intensive Care Medicine* **10**: 185–192.

Stoutenbeek CP, van Saene HKF, Liberati A (1994) Prevention of respiratory tract infections in intensive care by selective decontamination of the digestive tract. In: Niederman MS, Sarosi GA, Glassroth J (eds) *Respiratory Infections: A Scientific Basis for Management*, pp 579–594. WB Saunders: Philadelphia.

Thomas CF, Limper AH (2004) *Pneumocystis* pneumonia. *New England Journal of Medicine* **350**: 2487–2498.

Thyrault M, Gachot B, Chastang C, *et al.* (1997) Septic shock in patients with the acquired immunodeficiency syndrome. *Intensive Care Medicine* **23**: 1018–1023.

Vallés J, Rello J, Ochagavía A, *et al.* (2003) Community-acquired bloodstream infection in critically ill adult patients: impact of shock and inappropriate antibiotic therapy on survival. *Chest* **123**: 1615–1624.

van Nieuwenhoven CA, Buskens E, van Tiel FH, *et al.* (2001) Relationship between methodological trial quality and the effects of selective digestive decontamination on pneumonia and mortality in critically ill patients. *Journal of the American Medical Association* **286**: 335–340.

Van Saene HKF, Nunn AJ, Petros AJ (1994) Viewpoint: survival benefit by selective decontamination of the digestive tract (SDD). *Infection Control and Hospital Epidemiology* **15**: 443–446.

Vincent J-L, Bihari DJ, Suter PM, *et al.* (1995) The prevalence of nosocomial infection in intensive care units in Europe: results of the European Prevalence of Infection in Intensive Care (EPIC) study. *Journal of the American Medical Association* **274**: 639–644.

Walsh TJ, Finberg RW, Arndt C *et al.* (1999) Liposomal amphotericin B for empirical therapy in patients with persistent fever and neutropenia. *New England Journal of Medicine* **340**: 764–771.

Walsh TJ, Pappas P, Winston DJ, *et al.* (2002) Voriconazole compared with liposomal amphotericin B for empirical antifungal therapy in patients with neutropenia and persistent fever. *New England Journal of Medicine* **346**: 225–234.

Walsh TJ, Teppler H, Donowitz GR, *et al.* (2004) Caspofungin versus liposomal amphotericin B for empirical antifungal therapy in patients with persistent fever and neutropenia. *New England Journal of Medicine* **351**: 1391–1402.

Warny M, Pepin J, Fang A, *et al.* (2005) Toxin production by an emerging strain of *Clostridium difficile* associated with outbreaks of severe disease in North America and Europe. *Lancet* **366**: 1079–1084.

Wilson R, Allegra L, Huchon G, *et al.* (2004) Short-term and long-term outcomes of moxifloxacin compared to standard antibiotic treatment in acute exacerbations of chronic bronchitis. *Chest* **125**: 953–964.

Wolfe JHN, Saporoschetz I, Young AE, *et al.* (1981) Suppressive serum, suppressor lymphocytes, and death from burns. *Annals of Surgery* **193**: 513–520.

Wunderink RG, Rello J, Cammarata SK, *et al.* (2003) Linezolid vs vancomycin. Analysis of two double-blind studies of patients with methicillin-resistant *Staphylococcus aureus* nosocomial pneumonia. *Chest* **124**: 1789–1797.

Yau E, Rohatiner AZ, Lister TA, *et al.* (1991) Long term prognosis and quality of life following intensive care for life-threatening complications of haematological malignancy. *British Journal of Cancer* **64**: 938–942.

13 Acute renal failure

DEFINITION, INCIDENCE AND CAUSES
(Table 13.1)

Acute renal failure (ARF) can be defined as a sudden (and usually reversible) failure of the kidneys to excrete the waste products of metabolism leading to an abrupt and sustained rise in serum urea and creatinine. Recently the terms *acute renal dysfunction,* or *acute kidney injury* have been suggested to encompass the entire range of acute abnormalities in kidney function. ARF may be broadly categorized as prerenal (about 70% of cases), postrenal (≤ 5% of cases) or intrarenal (intrinsic: about 25% of cases).

The incidence of ARF depends on the definition used and the population studied. When defined as a temporary increase in serum creatinine to at least 300 μmol/L or clinical features indicating acute deterioration of previously normal renal function, the annual incidence of ARF in the UK ranged from 486 to 620 per million of the population. Advanced ARF (defined as a first measured serum creatinine concentration of at least 500 μmol/L) was found in 102 individuals per million of the population per annum (Khan et al., 1997; Stevens et al., 2001). ARF occurs in approximately 23% of patients with severe sepsis and 51% of those with septic shock when blood cultures are positive (Schrier and Wang, 2004).

Prerenal failure, in which function is impaired, but there is no parenchymal damage, is due to reduced renal perfusion below the autoregulatory limit with a reduction in glomerular filtration rate (GFR), usually related to an episode of shock, hypovolaemia or dehydration. Prerenal uraemia can also result from excessive production of waste products, which may then accumulate in those with pre-existing mild renal impairment.

Postrenal ARF is caused by an obstruction to urine flow. This may be due to a lesion at the urethra or bladder neck, bilateral upper urinary tract obstruction or unilateral ureteric obstruction in patients with one functioning kidney or chronic renal insufficiency. Severe ureteric obstruction may also occur in association with small inflammatory aortic aneurysms.

Intrinsic ARF, in which the structure of the nephron is affected, is most often related to ischaemic (50%) or nephrotoxic (35%) injury to the kidney, frequently in the context of a multisystem disorder such as severe trauma or sepsis. Most cases of ARF in hospital are associated with *acute tubular necrosis* (ATN), a histological diagnosis describing the necrosis of kidney tubule cells which is common to ARF of various aetiologies, including ischaemia (vasomotor nephropathy) and exposure to nephrotoxins (direct injury to the tubule epithelial cell).

Nephrotoxins that can precipitate ATN include:

■ organic solvents (e.g. carbon tetrachloride);
■ antimicrobials (e.g. gentamicin, amphotericin);
■ heavy metals (e.g. mercuric chloride);
■ radiological contrast media;
■ myoglobin (in the presence of hypovolaemia) released from damaged muscle in patients with severe crush injuries, compartment syndrome (see Chapter 10) or non-traumatic rhabdomyolysis (e.g. alcohol withdrawal, barbiturate poisoning or uncontrolled seizure activity);
■ free haemoglobin from mismatched blood transfusions or severe haemolytic anaemia.

Extensive burns can be complicated by hypovolaemia, infection, rhabdomyolysis, ventricular dysfunction or disseminated intravascular coagulation (DIC) and are therefore frequently associated with ARF. Other situations in which ARF is commonly encountered include *severe sepsis, major gastrointestinal or postpartum haemorrhage, septic abortion, acute pancreatitis, biliary tract infection* and *postoperatively*, especially after *aortic aneurysm repair* and in the *elderly* or *jaundiced. Raised intra-abdominal pressure* to above about 30 cm H_2O also causes renal dysfunction, perhaps due to direct pressure effects on the kidney or compression of the renal veins, which can be relieved by decompressing the abdomen. Intra-abdominal pressure can be measured using a water manometer or transducer attached to a urinary catheter filled with sterile water; an increase to above 25 mmHg has been suggested as a criterion for abdominal re-exploration (Kron et al., 1984) (see Chapter 16).

Severe, acute *hyperuricaemia* is a relatively uncommon cause of ARF, the basis of which is uric acid deposition in the distal tubules and collecting ducts. Hyperuricaemic ARF is now seen most frequently as a complication of

Table 13.1 Causes of acute renal failure
Acute tubular necrosis (ATN)
Bilateral cortical necrosis
Acute glomerulonephritis
Rapidly progressive glomerulonephritis (RPGN)
Systemic lupus erythematosus (SLE)
Necrotizing vasculitis (e.g. polyarteritis nodosa, Wegener's granulomatosis, Goodpasture's syndrome)
Malignant hypertension
Acute interstitial nephritis
Severe pyelonephritis (papillary necrosis)
Occlusive renovascular disease
Acute exacerbations of chronic renal impairment
Acute obstructive uropathy

Table 13.2 Pathogenesis of acute renal failure
Renal ischaemia
Decreased glomerular filtration
Tubular injury
Tubular backleak of filtrate
Tubular obstruction
Inflammation

chemotherapy for lymphomas or leukaemias. Finally, ARF is a common complication of *liver disease*, including fulminant hepatic failure, decompensated cirrhosis and obstructive jaundice, but the term 'hepatorenal syndrome' is non-specific and is generally unhelpful (see Chapter 14).

ARF may also, but less commonly, be due to a variety of *glomerular lesions* (e.g. a rapidly progressive glomerulonephritis (RPGN) related to a systemic illness such as systemic lupus erythematosus (SLE), polyarteritis nodosa (PAN) or Goodpasture's syndrome). The diagnosis of RPGN must not be missed, since early treatment may prevent the development of end-stage renal failure (see below).

Acute tubulointerstitial nephritis (TIN) is now recognized as an unusual, but important, cause of intrinsic ARF and is usually the result of an acute or subacute 'allergic' reaction to drugs. While classically described in association with methicillin or other penicillins, sulphonamides, rifampicin and diuretics may also be implicated, whilst non-steroidal anti-inflammatory drugs (NSAIDs) are becoming an increasingly important cause of this condition. Severe infections, allograft rejection and, rarely, infiltrative disorders such as sarcoid, lymphoma or leukaemia may also cause TIN.

Myeloma is a relatively common cause of ARF presenting from the community, particularly in older patients. In such cases ARF may have been precipitated by hypercalcaemia, hyperuricaemia, cast nephropathy, hyperviscosity syndrome, light-chain deposition, amyloid or any combination of these.

Renal failure due to *vascular lesions* is uncommon but the incidence may be increasing. Vascular obstruction may be embolic (e.g. atheroemboli or from a mural thrombus) or thrombotic (e.g. following trauma or major vascular surgery) or may occur as a complication of aortic dissection. Renal vein thrombosis may cause a sudden deterioration in renal function, for example in patients with nephrotic syndrome. Microvascular occlusion may complicate pre-eclampsia,

haemolytic–uraemic syndrome, vasculitis and malignant hypertension. In patients with bilateral renal artery stenosis, in whom high levels of angiotensin help to maintain GFR, ARF is classically precipitated by administration of an angiotensin-converting enzyme (ACE) inhibitor.

PATHOGENESIS AND PATHOPHYSIOLOGY OF ACUTE RENAL FAILURE (Lameire et al., 2005; Schrier and Wang, 2004) (Table 13.2)

The production of urine by ultrafiltration of plasma is largely dependent on the glomerular capillary hydrostatic pressure, which in turn is determined by the cardiac output, aortorenal blood flow and the balance between afferent and efferent renal arteriolar tone. Afferent arterioles constrict in response to α_1-agonists such as noradrenaline (norepinephrine), and vasoconstrictor prostaglandins such as thromboxane, as well as vasopressin, endothelin and inhibition of nitric oxide (NO) synthase (MacAllister and Vallance, 1994): they are dilated by β_2 and dopaminergic stimulation, as well as by vasodilator prostaglandins (PG) such as prostacyclin, PGE_1 and PGE_2. Efferent vasoconstriction is mediated principally by angiotensin II, while larger doses of NO synthase inhibitors constrict both the afferent and efferent arteriole and reduce both renal blood flow and GFR (MacAllister and Vallance, 1994).

Total blood flow to the kidneys is extremely high – nearly one-quarter of the cardiac output – the majority being directed to the renal cortex where the cortical tubules therefore consume only a small proportion of their profuse supply of oxygen. By contrast, blood flow to the outer medulla is limited in order to avoid disrupting the gradient of osmolality generated by the countercurrent mechanism within the vasa recta. Moreover the thick ascending limb of Henle's loop and the terminal portion of the proximal tubule (S_3 segment, pars recta) avidly consume oxygen for sodium transport and oxygen diffuses directly from the descending (arterial) to the ascending (venous) branches of the vasa recta; in this region the balance between oxygen supply and demand is therefore much more precarious. The medulla is, however, protected from hypoxic injury by various mechanisms. These include the release of adenosine from the breakdown of cellular adenosine triphosphate (ATP), which enhances medullary blood flow while decreasing tubular transport and GFR, and PGE_2 (Brezis *et al.*, 1986), which is a medullary vasodilator and an inhibitor of active transport by medullary thick limbs. The reduction in cortical flow that occurs in response to hypotension may also be considered as an appropriate protective mechanism since GFR falls and blood is redistributed to the medulla, thereby helping to restore the balance between tubular oxygen supply and demand.

Except for those cases caused by nephrotoxins, the onset of ATN is almost always related to an episode of reduced renal blood flow and is precipitated by the vasomotor response to hypovolaemia, hypotension, a reduced cardiac output or sepsis (see Chapter 5). Initially renal perfusion and glomerular filtration are maintained by preglomerular arteriolar vasodilatation (triggered by a local myenteric reflex within the vessel wall as well as intrarenal production of vasodilator prostaglandins, kallikrein kinins and NO), combined with efferent vasoconstriction induced by angiotensin II. This autoregulation of renal blood flow is, however, overwhelmed when mean arterial blood pressure (MAP) falls to below 60–80 mmHg and prolonged, severe ischaemia damages renal parenchymal cells.

It is important to appreciate that the GFR is particularly sensitive to reductions in perfusion pressure in those with diseases of the microvasculature (e.g. hypertension, diabetes), the elderly and those with localized renal arterial pathology. Although extreme ischaemia can induce bilateral renal cortical necrosis and irreversible renal failure, renal injury is normally largely confined to the vulnerable outer medullary tubule segments where there is tubular epithelial damage with loss of cell polarity, dissolution of integrin-dependent cell matrix adhesion and shedding of viable, necrotic and apoptotic tubule cells (ATN). The reduction in GFR caused by impaired renal blood flow and reduced ultrafiltration pressure is then compounded by backleak of glomerular filtrate through the disrupted tubular epithelium and obstruction of urine flow due to intratubular formation of casts consisting of detached tubular epithelial cells and cellular debris. Inflammatory mechanisms, including neutrophil infiltration into the renal interstitium with release of reactive oxygen species and activation of inflammatory processes in the renal vasculature, are also thought to play an important role in the pathogenesis of ARF. Inflammation becomes prominent following reperfusion (ischaemia–reperfusion injury; see Chapter 5).

Renal blood flow usually remains low (30–50% reduction) throughout the oliguric, maintenance phase of ARF, even when volume deficits have been replaced and blood pressure restored, but then returns to normal during recovery of renal function. The continued reduction in GFR may be related to persistent afferent arteriolar constriction, possibly combined with efferent arteriolar dilatation, or to occlusion of small blood vessels and decreased capillary permeability caused by ischaemic cell swelling. Glomerular cap-

illary loops may 'shut down', thereby reducing the surface area available for filtration. Medullary ischaemia due to dysregulated release of vasoactive mediators from injured endothelial cells (e.g. decreased NO and increased endothelin production) and other mediators derived from leukocytes or renal parenchymal cells, as well as continued tubular obstruction with backdiffusion and reabsorption of filtrate, may also contribute to persistent oliguria.

Histological features of ATN typically include vacuolation, loss of brush border in proximal tubular cells and sloughing of tubular cells into the lumen, leading to cast obstruction. Interstitial oedema with leukocyte infiltration can produce widely spaced tubules. Frankly necrotic cells are not common and *histological evidence of injury is often limited despite striking functional impairment.*

The kidney is especially vulnerable to *nephrotoxic injury* because of its rich blood supply and capacity to concentrate toxins within tubule epithelial cells and the interstitium via the actions of epithelial cell transporters and renal countercurrent exchange. As with ischaemic ATN nephrotoxins impair GFR by causing intrarenal vasoconstriction; they also cause direct injury to the tubular epithelium and tubule obstruction. In contrast to ischaemic injury, however, the basement membrane remains intact and epithelial regeneration can occur after only a few days. The extent to which each of these mechanisms contributes to the development of ARF varies according to the toxic agent. For example, intrarenal vasoconstriction is the dominant mechanism in ARF induced by ciclosporin, radiocontrast media, haemoglobinuria and myoglobinuria, whereas direct tubular injury is the primary event in ATN caused by many antimicrobials (e.g. aminoglycosides, amphotericin B) and anticancer agents (e.g. cisplatin, ifosfamide). Intratubular obstruction is prominent in ARF triggered by myeloma light chains, uric acid and aciclovir crystalluria.

Simultaneous renal ischaemic and toxic insults act synergistically to increase the probability of ARF, which in most cases seems to be the result of a combination of risk factors (Shusterman *et al.*, 1987). For example, NSAIDs interfere with the intrarenal biosynthesis of vasodilator prostaglandins whilst ACE inhibitors and angiotensin II receptor blockers limit angiotensin-induced increases in systemic blood pressure and maintenance of GFR by selective efferent arteriolar constriction. Also underperfused kidneys produce more concentrated urine containing increased levels of toxins, nephrotoxic agents such as ciclosporin and radiocontrast media. Similarly, increased concentrations of myoglobin (which avidly binds NO) will exacerbate renal vasoconstriction. Common associations include:

- hypoperfusion and pre-existing renal disease, diabetes mellitus or hypertension;
- hypovolaemia and rhabdomyolysis;
- the administration of ciclosporin, amphotericin or radiocontrast media in the presence of salt and water depletion;

■ the administration of NSAIDs, an ACE inhibitor or an angiotensin II receptor blocker during an episode of renal underperfusion.

Dangerous hyperkalaemia, out of proportion to the degree of renal impairment, can occur in those treated with a combination of potassium-sparing diuretics and ACE inhibitors or angiotensin II receptor blockers.

Obstructive jaundice may be incriminated in the development of ARF when there is no other obvious cause, but the precise mechanism is unclear. Although the toxic effects of circulating endotoxin or bile have been held responsible for the renal haemodynamic disturbances observed in these patients, others have suggested that jaundice renders the kidneys more sensitive to ischaemia.

ARF is also common in *hepatic failure*. Although most cases are due to identifiable prerenal factors or to vasomotor nephropathy associated with hypotension, gastrointestinal haemorrhage or sepsis, in a few the mechanism is unclear. In decompensated cirrhosis, ARF is probably caused by a redistribution of renal blood flow, with a reduction in total flow and GFR occurring only as late events. This redistribution of flow may largely account for the intense sodium retention that occurs in cirrhosis, with hyperaldosteronism playing a less important role. The ability to handle a water load, concentrate urine and excrete hydrogen ions is also impaired in cirrhotics. ARF may then be precipitated by an episode of gastrointestinal bleeding, a sudden increase in ascites or overvigorous diuretic administration.

In *critically ill patients*, ARF commonly occurs in association with sepsis, severe sepsis, septic shock and multiple-organ dysfunction syndrome (MODS) (see Chapter 5). *Perioperative* ATN accounts for 20–25% of all cases of ARF occurring in hospital. Patients at risk include those with pre-existing renal impairment, hypertension, cardiac disease, peripheral vascular disease, diabetes mellitus, jaundice and advanced age.

In summary, therefore, although it has been suggested that renal cortical ischaemia is the main pathogenic event in ARF, it seems likely that in most cases more than one mechanism is involved and that the factors initiating the damage are not necessarily the same as those that perpetuate renal dysfunction. In the recovery phase renal function is restored by repair, regeneration and proliferation of renal parenchymal cells. Growth factors play an important role in this process.

DIAGNOSIS AND INVESTIGATIONS
(Table 13.3)

In critically ill patients, *oliguria* (urine output < 0.5 mL/kg per hour) is usually the first indication that renal function is impaired. The diagnosis is then confirmed by:

■ a progressive rise in blood urea and creatinine levels;
■ a metabolic acidosis;

Table 13.3 Investigations in acute renal failure

Urea, creatinine
Sodium, potassium
Blood gases/acid–base
Plasma and urine osmolality
Urine sodium and protein content
Urine microscopy
Cultures of urine and blood
Ultrasound scan of kidney
Renography
Renal arteriography
High-dose intravenous urography
Ureterography
Renal biopsy

■ hyperkalaemia;
■ salt and water retention.

Occasionally, an unexpected increase in plasma potassium concentration is the earliest sign of impaired renal function, particularly in the presence of extensive tissue injury.

Oligo/anuria is not, however, an essential prerequisite for the diagnosis of ARF, since when renal concentrating ability is reduced even a urine production of 2–3 L/day may not reflect a sufficiently high GFR to excrete the nitrogenous metabolic waste products, particularly if the patient is hypercatabolic. It is also important to appreciate that, in critically ill patients, alterations in circulating levels of antidiuretic hormone (ADH), aldosterone and atrial natriuretic factor (ANF) play an important role in the development of oliguria, as do the effects of positive-pressure ventilation, positive end-expiratory pressure (PEEP), fluid restriction and diuretics in those with respiratory failure (see Chapters 7 and 8). Anuria is suggestive of renal tract obstruction, although rarely it may be due to renal cortical necrosis, necrotizing glomerulonephritis or loss of vascular supply to the kidneys.

In all cases, and particularly if the patient is anuric or has intermittent complete anuria, *bladder outflow obstruction* must be excluded. This possibility should be suspected in patients with previous symptoms of prostatic enlargement and in those who have suffered recent trauma or surgery to the pelvic area. Examination may reveal an enlarged bladder. If there is any doubt, aseptic bladder catheterization should be performed or, if a urinary catheter is already in place, obstruction of the catheter should be excluded (bladder washout). It is usually advisable to obtain the assistance of a urologist and in those with trauma an ultrasound scan should be performed before catheterizing the bladder. Rectal and vaginal examinations should be performed and the external genitalia must be inspected.

Anuria is an ominous sign in patients who have recently undergone surgery to the aorta in close proximity to the renal arteries. If loss of vascular supply to the kidneys is a serious possibility, then the implications for management are profound. An early *contrast-enhanced computed tomography (CT)* scan, perhaps followed by direct *renal arteriography* if no perfusion is shown, is indicated.

Once bladder outflow obstruction has been excluded, it is important to determine whether the patient has prerenal, intrarenal or postrenal failure.

The *history* can provide a clue to the aetiology and may establish whether there was any pre-existing renal impairment (e.g. long-standing diabetes, hypertension). Patients with markedly elevated plasma urea and creatinine concentrations who are not overtly symptomatic are more likely to have slowly progressive renal failure. Many critically ill patients will be unable to communicate, but relatives or close friends can be interviewed and documented case histories will often be available from the admitting team or referring hospital. It is important to establish whether there is any evidence of previous renal disorders (childhood nephrotic syndrome, haematuria, nocturia, renal colic, hypertension, failed medical examinations for insurance purposes or for entry into the armed forces) as well as to ask about recognized aetiological factors such as ingestion of NSAIDs (particularly in patients with arthritis or migraine), 'mainlining' of drugs, diabetes mellitus, and recent infections, surgery or trauma. The family history may suggest the possibility of polycystic disease. Finally, it is important to enquire about exposure to unusual chemicals or solvents at work or in the home and recent travel abroad.

Old case notes should be scrutinized for the results of previous urine testing (proteinuria, haematuria), urea and creatinine determinations and blood pressure recordings. Plain abdominal films, intravenous urograms or ultrasound examinations may also be available and can give an indication of previous kidney size and the presence of stones.

Recent notes may reveal an episode of hypotension (e.g. on the anaesthetic chart) or sepsis, as well as providing a record of drugs administered (look particularly for gentamicin, NSAIDs and contrast media).

PRERENAL FAILURE

In prerenal failure the excretory function of the kidneys is impaired by shock, hypovolaemia or dehydration; this causes an appropriate oliguria and a reduction in GFR, with maximal tubular reabsorption of salt and water. Usually proteinuria is absent and the urinary sediment unremarkable. In general, blood urea rises more than creatinine and the urine is concentrated (osmolality > 500 mmol/L) with a high urea and low sodium content (< 20 mmol/L), and a low fractional excretion of sodium (FENa < 1%). In some cases, however, there may be a renal leak of sodium, in which case urinary sodium content may be higher than 30 mmol/L and oliguria is less marked or absent. In the absence of hypovolaemia, low urine sodium concentrations may also be seen

with radiocontrast nephropathy, haemoglobinuria and vasculitis, as well as in those with hepatorenal syndrome or cardiac failure. Classically, in prerenal oliguria the urine: plasma ratios of osmolality, urea and creatinine are greater than 2, 30 and 15 respectively.

Unfortunately, in many intensive care patients, values for these biochemical indices are borderline or misleading, especially in non-oliguric renal failure, when diuretics, or osmotically active agents such as radiocontrast media, have been administered, and in those with pre-existing renal or hepatic disease, cardiac failure or electrolyte disturbances (particularly hypokalaemia). Also a raised urea/creatinine ratio may be a consequence of a high-protein diet, catabolism, gastrointestinal bleeding, steroid therapy and a reduced body mass. Importantly, ARF secondary to rhabdomyolysis is associated with a low urea-to-creatinine ratio because creatine released from injured muscle leads to a disproportionate increase in plasma creatinine concentration. A low urea-to-creatinine ratio may also be the result of reduced urea synthesis due to malnutrition or liver disease, or a consequence of increased elimination of urea due to an increased GFR, as occurs in pregnancy. Biochemical indices are, therefore, rarely of value and the diagnosis can only be made on the basis of a clinical assessment of the state of hydration (oedema, neck veins, blood pressure, postural hypotension) and the response to a volume challenge, guided as necessary by measurements of central venous pressure (CVP) and, in some cases, more complex haemodynamic monitoring.

URINARY TRACT OBSTRUCTION

Once prerenal failure has been excluded, the most immediate priority is the exclusion or identification of urinary tract obstruction. In most patients, *ultrasound scanning* can reliably identify obstruction, as well as providing a reasonable estimate of kidney size, and is the most practical and useful imaging technique in intensive care patients. Enlarged kidneys in a patient with ARF suggest obstruction, amyloidosis, renal infiltration (e.g. lymphoma) or TIN. In some cases of obstructive uropathy, however, dilatation of the urinary tract does not occur, for example when malignancy is the cause of the obstruction, when the patient is severely dehydrated, in those with retroperitoneal fibrosis and in acute obstructon. If ultrasound is inconclusive, *contrast-enhanced CT scanning* or *high-dose intravenous urography* provides the same information and very occasionally may define the site of the obstruction. Usually, however, when obstruction is detected, *antegrade or retrograde ureterography* is necessary to define the site. Obstruction requires skilled urological assessment with a view to urgently re-establishing free drainage of urine.

ACUTE RENAL FAILURE

The diagnosis of *intrinsic ARF* is suggested by demonstrating that urine osmolality is similar to that of plasma (< 350 mmol/l), that the urinary sodium concentration is high (> 20 50 mmol/l), the FENa is above 2% and that the urinary potassium concentration is low (< 10 mmol/l). There is some evidence to suggest that serum cystatin may be an early and reliable marker of the development of ARF in critically ill patients (Herget-Rosenthal *et al.,* 2004). Other biomarkers which may prove to be useful for the early diagnosis of ARF include urinary interleukin-18 and tubular enzymes, such as the intestinal form of alkaline phosphatase, *N*-acetyl-β-glucasaminidase, alanine aminopeptidase and neutrophil gelatinase-associated lipocalin (NGAL) (Mishra *et al.,* 2005). Proteinuria is usually present and the urine contains casts composed of tubule epithelial cells and/or cellular debris. The differential diagnosis then includes:

- ATN;
- glomerular lesions (acute glomerulonephritis, vasculitis);
- cortical necrosis;
- TIN;
- renal vascular lesions;
- an acute exacerbation of chronic renal disease.

Renal size must be determined since small kidneys are indicative of underlying chronic renal disease, although renal size may be maintained in some chronic disease such as diabetes. An ultrasound scan may reveal the size of the kidneys or even suggest polycystic disease. The diagnosis of *rhabdomyolysis* is supported by an elevated serum creatine phosphokinase level and by detecting myoglobin in the urine. The serum potassium is usually markedly elevated and there may be hypocalcaemia due to a shift of calcium into injured muscle (see Chapter 10).

Glomerular disease

The possibility that ARF is due to a glomerular lesion should be considered, particularly when there are extrarenal signs such as:

- skin lesions indicative of systemic vasculitis;
- arthritis;
- neurological manifestations (e.g. mononeuritis);
- pulmonary involvement.

Hypertension is usual in these cases. Serum complement levels may be reduced and, in some, circulating immune complexes are identified. Examination of the urine may reveal red cell casts and proteinuria, whereas in vasomotor nephropathy the urinary sediment will contain only tubular cells with a few granular casts. Urine and blood cultures are essential to exclude infection. *Ultrasound examination* may reveal increased cortical echogenicity, although this is a nonspecific finding. If the presentation suggests the possibility of a treatable lesion, *renal biopsy* may be indicated. There is, however, a significant incidence of complications with this procedure, particularly haemorrhage, and the risks should be weighed against the likely benefits.

When glomerular disease presents as ARF, it is usually due to an acute process such as RPGN or a systemic disease such as Wegener's granulomatosis, PAN, SLE or Goodpasture's syndrome. Goodpasture's syndrome should be suspected when there is pulmonary involvement with haemorrhage; the diagnosis can be confirmed by demonstrating linear deposits of immunoglobulin G (IgG) along the glomerular basement membrane and by identifying circulating antiglomerular basement membrane antibody. Pulmonary involvement, sometimes with haemorrhage, is also a feature of Wegener's disease and SLE but is very uncommon in PAN. Antineutrophil cytoplasmic antibodies (ANCA) are present in more than 90% of patients with Wegener's granulomatosis.

Renal cortical necrosis

Renal cortical necrosis is extremely rare in adults, but usually presents as ARF and cannot normally be distinguished from vasomotor nephropathy in the acute stage. The aetiological factors are often the same and include:

- severe shock;
- major surgery;
- transfusion reactions;
- infections;
- burns.

Cortical necrosis occurs particularly in association with *obstetric disasters*, especially later in pregnancy. It has been suggested, therefore, that cortical necrosis occurs most often in those with a hypercoagulable state in whom development of DIC may cause particularly severe renal ischaemia. Cortical necrosis may simply be a more severe form of ATN with less chance of recovery, and should be suspected if oliguria is prolonged. The diagnosis is likely if the kidney size is found to be decreasing: cortical calcification, which appears in approximately half the patients after about 6 weeks, is virtually diagnostic. In such cases, a renal biopsy may be performed to confirm the diagnosis.

Acute interstitial nephritis

Acute interstitial nephritis is suggested by:

- a rash;
- fever;
- joint involvement;
- eosinophilia (not invariable);
- raised serum IgE levels.

Large numbers of eosinophils may be identified in the urine. Renal biopsy confirms the diagnosis.

Renal vascular lesions

Renal vascular lesions present as *sudden oliguria*, or often *complete anuria*, accompanied by hypertension, macroscopic haematuria and *loin pain*. The diagnosis can be confirmed by *radioisotope scan, renal vascular Doppler studies, CT scan* or *renal arteriography*. The latter will be required to define the site of the lesion.

Table 13.4 The RIFLE classification of acute renal dysfunction

	GFR criteria	Urine output criteria
Risk	Serum creatinine increased 1.5 times	< 0.5 mL/kg per h for 6 h
Injury	Serum creatinine increased 2.0 times	< 0.5 mL/kg per h for 12 h
Failure	Serum creatinine increased 3.0 times or creatinine = 355 µmol/L when there was an acute rise of > 44 µmol/L	< 0.3 mL/kg per h for 24 h or anuria for 12 h
Loss	Persistent acute renal failure, complete loss of kidney function for longer than 4 weeks	
End-stage renal disease	End-stage renal disease for longer than 3 months	

GFR, glomerular filtration rate.

CONSENSUS DEFINITIONS

It has been suggested that the absence of consensus defini tions for ARF, as have been applied to acute lung injury, for example, has hampered research and progress in this field (Bellomo *et al.*, 2001). These investigators have therefore proposed definitions to cover the spectrum of renal injury, the concept being similar to that applied to sepsis (see Chapter 5). Recently the Acute Dialysis Quality Initiative group proposed the RIFLE system in which ARF is classified into three categories of severity (*risk*, *injury* and *failure*) and two clinical outcome categories (*loss* and *end-stage renal disease*) (Table 13.4). This system seems to be a valid predictor of clinical outcomes (Herget-Rosenthal *et al.*, 2004).

CLINICAL COURSE AND MANAGEMENT
(Tables 13.5 and 13.6)

Outside hospital ARF typically presents as isolated, single-organ disease, which, provided that the cause is readily identified and treated, can have a good prognosis. Most cases occur in hospital, however, and ARF complicates around 5% of all hospital admissions and up to 25% of admissions to intensive care depending on the patient population and criteria for definition. Although the development of ARF in hospitalized patients may occasionally be attributable to a single identifiable event such as hypotension or drug toxicity, it is usually associated with multiple insults, especially hypovolaemia, hypotension and nephrotoxic drugs, frequently in the context of multiple-organ failure and sepsis. The outcome in this latter category of patient is often poor, particularly in those with respiratory failure. Moreover there is now good evidence that the development of ARF is strongly associated with an increased risk of death, independent of the underlying condition and comorbidities (Levy *et al.*, 1996).

Prevention of ARF is therefore a fundamental aspect of intensive care practice. This entails:

- early identification of those at risk, including:
  - the elderly;
  - diabetics;
  - hypertensives;
  - patients with atherosclerosis, chronic heart failure or hepatic cirrhosis;
  - patients receiving NSAIDs, cyclooxygenase-2 inhibitors, ACE inhibitors, angiotensin II receptor antagonists, amphotericin, gentamicin;
  - patients given radiocontrast agents;
  - patients with pre-existing renal impairment (Fig. 13.1) or renal artery stenosis;
- optimization of renal perfusion (Chapter 5);
  - restore intravascular volume;
  - maintain MAP > 70 mmHg (or > 80–90 mmHg in those with impaired autoregulation)
  - maintain cardiac output with vasopressors/inotropes as indicated;
  - avoid vasoconstriction;
- careful maintenance of crystalloid balance (Chapter 11);
- aggressive treatment of sepsis (Chapter 5);
- the avoidance of nephrotoxic drugs (gentamicin is less toxic when administered as a single daily dose);
- the avoidance of drugs that impair autoregulation of renal blood flow (NSAIDs, ACE inhibitors, angiotensin II receptor blockers);
- allopurinol to decrease uric acid synthesis in patients with leukaemia or lymphoma who are prone to uric acid nephropathy, particularly following chemotherapy;
- constant vigilance for the early signs of impaired renal function, followed by immediate corrective measures when required, is also essential. In some circumstances, the use of specific preventive therapy is warranted (see later in this chapter).

PRERENAL FAILURE

Prerenal failure should be treated by optimizing the circulating volume, replacing fluid and electrolyte deficits, and restoring the blood pressure. If cardiac output and blood pressure remain low despite volume expansion, inotropes and vasopressors should be administered as indicated, the objective being to avoid afferent arteriolar constriction and efferent vasodilation while maintaining an adequate renal

Table 13.5 Management of acute renal failure

Prerenal oliguria

Optimize the circulating volume

Correct fluid and electrolyte deficits

Restore blood pressure and cardiac output

Avoid nephrotoxins

Incipient renal failure

Mannitol

Furosemide

Dopamine
(Calcium entry blockers)

Specific measures:
  Immunosuppression
  Steroids
  Plasma exchange

Early oliguric phase

Fluid-restrict

Modify drug doses

Control hyperkalaemia (stop K$^+$ supplements, calcium
  exchange resins, dextrose and insulin, sodium
  bicarbonate)

Consider correcting acidosis (with sodium bicarbonate)

Consider controlling hypertension

Established acute renal failure

Blood purification: peritoneal dialysis, haemodialysis,
  haemofiltration

Nutritional support

Antacid prophylaxis

Prevent infection

Adjust drug doses

Careful fluid balance

Treat underlying cause

Diuretic phase

Extreme care with fluid and electrolyte balance

Table 13.6 Complications of acute renal failure

Hypervolaemia

Hyperkalaemia

Hyponatraemia

Hyperphosphataemia

Hypocalcaemia

Hypermagnesaemia

Metabolic acidosis

Uraemic syndrome

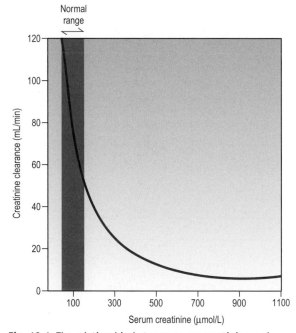

Fig. 13.1 The relationship between serum creatinine and glomerular filtration rate (creatinine clearance). Note: it is important to appreciate that renal function may be significantly impaired with little or no change in serum creatinine concentration. For example, a reduction in glomerular filtration rate from the normal 120 mL/min to 60 mL/min may result in only a small increase in serum creatinine levels, whereas a further fall to 30 mL/min can lead to a doubling of the serum creatinine concentration. It is also important to recognize that serum creatinine levels are influenced by the patient's size, sex and age, as well as by diet and drugs that compete for tubular secretion of creatinine (e.g. trimethoprim, cimetidine, amiloride and spironolactone). Thus a serum creatinine of 100 μmol/L in a 45-year-old man weighing 80 kg corresponds to a creatinine clearance of about 85 mL/min, whereas in an 80-year-old woman weighing 45 kg the same serum creatinine indicates a creatinine clearance of only around 25 mL/min. Adapted from Kumar P, Clark M 2005 Clinical Medicine 6E Elsevier with permission.

perfusion pressure (this will be higher in those with pre-existing hypertension). In septic shock noradrenaline has not only been shown to increase blood pressure but may also increase renal blood flow (Bellomo *et al.*, 1999) and creatinine clearance (Redl-Wenzl *et al.*, 1993). Arginine vasopressin constricts the efferent arteriole in the glomerulus, thereby maintaining renal perfusion (see Chapter 5). Hypoxaemia, hypercarbia and metabolic acidosis may require correction. Diuretics, including low-dose dopamine, should generally be avoided in patients with prerenal oliguria; in this respect it is important to appreciate that there may be a delay of several hours between institution of corrective measures and restoration of the urine output. Nephrotoxic agents must, of course, be avoided.

INCIPIENT RENAL FAILURE

Although the treatment of ARF is largely supportive, a number of active measures have been employed based on the premise that there may be an incipient phase of ATN that can be reversed by prompt intervention. While this is a popular concept, the evidence that such a phase exists is largely anecdotal and the efficacy of measures designed to attenuate the severity of renal injury or hasten renal recovery is still debated. Nevertheless, because non-oliguric ARF is easier to manage and may be associated with a more favourable prognosis, conversion of oliguric to non-oliguric ARF is an important objective of treatment. The potential benefits include less stringent restrictions on salt and water intake and a decreased requirement for dialysis.

Patients with *glomerulonephritis* and vasculitis may respond to immunosuppressive therapy, whilst allergic interstitial nephritis typically resolves spontaneously once the offending agent is discontinued, although steroids may hasten recovery. Plasma exchange can be useful in the management of haemolytic–uraemic syndrome and thrombotic thrombocytopenic purpura.

Mannitol

Many years ago it was suggested that this osmotic diuretic, which is also a weak antioxidant and stimulates prostaglandin production, might have a protective effect when used prophylactically in those with obstructive jaundice (Dawson, 1964), during surgery on the abdominal aorta (Barry et al., 1961), and during renal transplantation. Although there is some experimental evidence that mannitol can produce potentially beneficial effects in ARF, including prevention of cellular swelling, improved renal haemodynamics, and attenuation or prevention of tubular obstruction by increasing proximal intratubular pressures and urine flow rates, there is no clinical evidence to support the use of this agent to prevent or abort ARF. Furthermore, administration of mannitol may be complicated by circulatory overload and pulmonary oedema, particularly if there is no ensuing diuresis, as well as intracellular dehydration. Nevertheless, a few continue to administer intravenous mannitol (e.g. 20 g of a 20% solution) within up to 48 hours after the renal insult.

Furosemide

Experimental studies have suggested that this loop diuretic and vasodilator can increase renal cortical blood flow, stimulate production of vasodilator prostaglandins and specifically improve GFR. It has also been suggested that furosemide may protect the kidneys from hypoxic/ischaemic insults by decreasing reabsorptive activity, thereby limiting metabolic requirements in the vulnerable thick ascending limb of the tubules (Brezis and Rosen, 1995).

Nevertheless, the clinical value of furosemide in ARF remains uncertain. Minuth et al. (1976) performed a retrospective non-randomized study and claimed that a response to furosemide decreased the need for dialysis, although it did not appear to affect mortality. Some authorities therefore believe that furosemide may be valuable because it converts oliguric renal failure to non-oliguric renal failure, thereby minimizing the risks of hyperkalaemia and fluid overload, facilitating nutritional support and decreasing dialysis requirements. Others have suggested that furosemide only produces a diuresis in those in whom ARF would in any case have been rapidly reversible. Indeed, a number of controlled studies have shown furosemide to be ineffective in ARF (Kleinknecht et al., 1976). In a more recent prospective, double-blind, placebo-controlled, randomized study the use of bolus doses of loop diuretics in patients with ARF was associated with an increased urine output but there was no evidence that these drugs altered the time to renal recovery, dialysis requirements or mortality (Shilliday et al., 1997).

There are also theoretical objections to the use of furosemide since it may increase the nephrotoxicity of some antibiotics and could actually precipitate ARF when used in the presence of hypovolaemia. Moreover, in a controlled trial of patients with chronic renal insufficiency undergoing cardiac angiography, hydration with 0.45% saline provided better protection against acute decreases in renal function induced by radiocontrast agents than did hydration with 0.45% saline combined with mannitol or furosemide (Solomon et al., 1994). Indeed there was some evidence that furosemide might exacerbate renal dysfunction (Solomon et al., 1994). A more recent study, on the other hand, suggested that forced diuresis with intravenous crystalloid combined with furosemide and mannitol (if haemodynamics permit), beginning at the start of angiography, provides modest protection as long as a high urine flow can be achieved (Stevens et al., 1999). There is also some evidence to suggest that hydration with sodium bicarbonate is more effective than saline loading for the prevention of contrast induced renal failure (Merten et al., 2004).

Finally, although a recent observational study suggested that the use of diuretics in critically ill patients with ARF might be associated with an increased risk of death and non-recovery of renal function (Mehta et al., 2002), a subsequent large multinational study concluded that this was not the case (Uchino et al., 2004). Importantly a recent meta-analysis concluded that furosemide was not associated with any significant clinical benefits in relation to the prevention and treatment of ARF (Ho and Sheridan, 2006).

Despite these generally negative findings furosemide is still recommended by some clinicians as a means of stimulating and maintaining a diuresis, traditionally as an initial bolus dose of 100 mg followed, if ineffective, by repeated high doses (e.g. 200–500 mg in 100 mL 5% dextrose infused over 20 minutes) or, increasingly often, as a continuous intravenous infusion (2–40 mg/h). Some suggest that plasma levels should be measured to reduce the risk of ototoxicity, especially if the patient is also receiving aminoglycosides, but this is not usually possible. If there is no response within 4–8 hours, furosemide should be discontinued.

Dopamine (see Chapter 5)

In healthy subjects it has been shown that low to moderate doses of dopamine not only increase cardiac output and reduce peripheral vascular resistance, but also increase GFR, estimated renal plasma flow and sodium excretion (McDonald et al., 1964). Such observations suggested that dopamine, which often increases urine output and may also reduce tubular work through its direct tubular actions, could be a useful agent for the prevention of ARF in at-risk patients and to abort incipient renal failure.

In an early study (Parker et al., 1981), administration of dopamine 1.5–2.5 µg/kg per min to oliguric critically ill patients with a falling creatinine clearance increased urine output, creatinine clearance, osmolar clearance and the excreted fraction of filtered sodium without affecting haemodynamics or free water clearance. Dialysis requirements were reduced. In a more recent study in critically ill patients with mild, non-oliguric renal impairment dopamine increased creatinine clearance, diuresis and the fractional excretion of sodium, whereas dobutamine had no effect on those variables (Ichai et al., 2000). There is also some experimental evidence to suggest that the combination of furosemide and dopamine may act synergistically in oliguric ARF (Lindner, 1983), and that dopamine may preserve renal blood flow when noradrenaline is used to restore blood pressure. On the other hand low-dose dopamine appeared to be of no value when given prophylactically to patients undergoing elective major vascular surgery (Baldwin et al., 1994) and dopamine failed to increase gastric intramucosal pH or improve creatinine clearance in non-oliguric patients with sepsis syndrome (Olson et al., 1996).

Based on these theoretical considerations, experimental findings and some uncontrolled clinical studies, and despite the often conflicting evidence, many considered that the administration of low-dose dopamine could be justified for prophylaxis in high-risk cases and when oliguria persisted following exclusion and correction of prerenal causes. If a diuresis ensued the infusion was usually continued to simplify management. Others believed that until the efficacy and safety of this agent had been clearly demonstrated in prospective controlled trials its use for this indication could not be recommended (Thompson and Cockrill, 1994).

A prospective randomized controlled trial has resolved much of the uncertainty. In this study administration of low-dose dopamine to patients with systemic inflammatory response syndrome and clinical evidence of early renal dysfunction failed to influence creatinine levels, the requirement for renal replacement therapy or the duration of hospital or intensive care unit stay: mortality was similar in the two groups (Bellomo et al., 2000). Moreover the authors of a recent meta-analysis concluded that, although low-dose dopamine can increase urine output, there is no convincing evidence that renal dysfunction is improved or prevented, or that death rates are reduced (Friedrich et al., 2005). Clinicians have also become increasingly aware of the potential adverse effects of dopamine, which may include increased myocardial oxygen consumption, arrhythmias, inappropriate vasoconstriction, pulmonary hypertension, increased intrapulmonary shunt, decreased respiratory drive, hypokalaemia, hypophosphataemia, inappropriate diuresis in the presence of volume depletion, metabolic and immune dysfunction and predisposition to gut ischaemia (Segal et al., 1992) (see Chapter 5).

Administration of low-dose dopamine in an attempt to produce specific renal effects which might abort or limit the severity or duration of ARF in at-risk patients can therefore no longer be recommended. Nevertheless dopamine remains a useful vasopressor agent which, by virtue of its haemodynamic effects, may prove effective in the management of patients with incipient ARF. In this context it is important to appreciate that, in critically ill patients, especially those with renal impairment, clearance of dopamine is reduced, resulting in higher than expected plasma levels and significant haemodynamic effects, even when given in doses that would conventionally be considered to be 'low' or 'renal' (Juste et al., 1998) (see Chapter 5).

N-acetyl-L-cysteine

This agent is an antioxidant and vasodilator which has been shown to ameliorate ischaemic renal failure in animal models and has been reported to block the expression of vascular cell adhesion molecule-1 (VCAM-1) and NF-κB in glomerular mesangial cells. Acetylcysteine may also protect the kidneys in patients with paracetamol-induced liver failure and may improve renal function in the hepatorenal syndrome (see Chapter 14). Acetylcysteine has been shown to prevent radiographic contrast agent-induced reductions in renal function (Tepel et al., 2000), a finding confirmed by a meta-analysis (Birck et al., 2003). This agent is not effective, however, in the absence of adequate hydration and there is some evidence to suggest that acetylcysteine may reduce serum creatinine without increasing GFR.

Insulin-like growth factor-1 (IGF-1)

The rationale for the use of growth factors (epidermal growth factor (EGF), hepatocyte growth factor (HGF) and IGF-1) in ARF is as follows:

- They bind to specific receptors on proximal tubular cells where they regulate metabolism and transport.
- EGF and HGF are mitogens for proximal tubular cells in vitro.
- Expression of IGF-1 and HGF and the receptors for EGF, HGF and IGF-1 in the kidney is increased in experimental ARF.
- They may facilitate the regeneration of tubular cells.

Clinical trials indicate that, although IGF-1 may be beneficial when used to prevent the postoperative decline in renal function (Franklin *et al.*, 1997), this growth factor is of no value when administered to patients with established ARF (Hirschberg *et al.*, 1999; Kopple *et al.*, 1996).

Atrial natriuretic peptide (ANP)

ANP inhibits sodium and water reabsorption in the collecting ducts, redistributes renal medullary blood flow, reverses endothelin-induced vasoconstriction, vasodilates the afferent arterioles and vasoconstricts the efferent arterioles. GFR is increased while renal blood flow is unchanged. Although anaritide (a synthetic form of ANP) significantly reduced the need for dialysis and mortality rate in a subgroup of oliguric patients, dialysis-free survival was worsened in the non-oliguric group and was unaffected overall (Allgren *et al.*, 1997). A follow-up study was discontinued early because of lack of benefit. There is no evidence to support the use of ANP for the prevention of ARF.

Other therapeutic interventions

The preventive role of a number of other agents such as theophylline, adhesion molecule antibodies, free radical scavengers, amino acid infusions, calcium channel blockers and prostaglandins remains unclear. There is some evidence that erythropoietin may protect against renal ischaemia–reperfusion injury.

EARLY OLIGURIC PHASE

In the early oliguric phase, many patients are fluid-overloaded due to delayed recognition of the onset of ARF, often exacerbated by volume challenges administered in an attempt to restore urine output. Although the plasma sodium concentration may be low, total body sodium is usually normal or increased. In extreme cases, the combination of *salt and water overload* can produce peripheral and pulmonary oedema, sometimes with hypertension, and these constitute an indication for early dialysis. It is therefore often necessary to *fluid-restrict* patients as soon as the diagnosis of established intrinsic ARF is certain. Intravenous fluids should be limited to the volume required to replace insensible losses. In general, administration of sodium and potassium should be avoided except to replace specific identified losses. *Drug doses* must be modified appropriately at this time, with monitoring of drug levels where appropriate.

Although the rising blood urea and creatinine levels seldom create a problem at this stage, dangerous *hyperkalaemia* (see Chapter 11) can occur early, particularly if potassium supplements continue to be administered after the onset of renal impairment. A combination of factors contribute to hyperkalaemia, including reduced renal excretion and increased cellular release of potassium. The latter may be attributable to direct tissue trauma, haemolysis, protein catabolism, infection, steroids and the effects of acidosis. The rate of increase in plasma potassium, as well as the rise in urea and creatinine levels, therefore depends largely on the degree of catabolism and the extent of any tissue damage, so it is particularly rapid in those with severe trauma, sepsis or

rhabdomyolysis. Hyperkalaemia may also be compounded by metabolic acidosis which encourages potassium efflux from cells.

Hyperkalaemia produces characteristic electrocardiogram (ECG) abnormalities (elevated and pointed T waves, flattened or absent P waves followed by widened QRS complexes: see **Fig. 11.3** in Chapter 11) and if unchecked can culminate in cardiac arrest in diastole. Although the rise in potassium levels may be attenuated by the use of *calcium exchange resins* (15–30 g orally or rectally and repeated as necessary), these are difficult to use and slow to act. Dangerous hyperkalaemia should be treated with *dextrose and insulin* (e.g. 50 mL 50% dextrose with 20 units soluble insulin) and/or correction of the acidosis with 8.4% *sodium bicarbonate* (to encourage cellular uptake of potassium). In more urgent cases, 10–20 mL 10% *calcium gluconate* can be used to counteract the effects of hyperkalaemia on the myocardium. These measures will only alleviate the situation temporarily and preparations for dialysis should begin immediately. In extreme cases with marked bradycardia or asystole, isoprenaline or cardiac massage may sustain the patient until hyperkalaemia can be corrected by dialysis.

Because metabolic acidosis develops relatively slowly, and is compensated by hypocarbia, it is not usually a problem at this stage unless it is a significant component of the precipitating illness (e.g. septic shock, low cardiac output or diabetic ketoacidosis). Administration of bicarbonate (which will exacerbate salt and water overload, may precipitate hypocalcaemia and causes a left shift of the oxyhaemoglobin dissociation curve) is therefore rarely indicated, except to counteract hyperkalaemia and when acidosis is extreme.

Occasionally, severe malignant *hypertension* complicates the early oliguric phase of ARF and this should be controlled (e.g. by administering hydralazine or an infusion of glyceryl trinitrate).

ESTABLISHED ARF

In the phase of established ARF, the measures outlined above must be combined with the *removal of uraemic toxins* and with *nutritional support*.

Derangement of other functions of the kidney such as erythropoietin production, the formation of 1,25-dihydroxycholecalciferol and the metabolism of parathyroid hormone, are of limited clinical relevance in ARF. Mild *hyperphosphataemia* (1.6–3.2 mmol/L) is relatively common, however, and can be severe (3.2–6.4 mmol/L) in catabolic patients and those with rhabdomyolysis or tumour lysis syndrome. Rarely deposition of calcium phosphate can precipitate *hypocalcaemia*, especially when the product of calcium and phosphate concentrations exceeds 5.65 mmol/L. The administration of aluminium hydroxide or other phosphate binders to reduce serum phosphate levels is, however usually unnecessary. Skeletal resistance to parathyroid hormone and calcium sequestration in injured tissues may also contribute to hypocalcaemia. Mild *hyperuricaemia* and *hypermagnesaemia* (1–2 mmol/L) are to be expected and rarely require treatment.

Many of the systemic manifestations of uraemia may be due to 'middle molecules'; blood urea and creatinine levels are only an approximate guide to blood levels of these and other toxic substances. *Gastrointestinal disturbances* are prominent and include stomatitis, gastritis, anorexia, nausea, vomiting, hiccups and diarrhoea or constipation. The introduction of routine antacid prophylaxis, improved nutritional support and more aggressive dialysis may all have contributed to the virtual disappearance of gastrointestinal haemorrhage as an immediate cause of death.

Central nervous system (CNS) effects may progress from mild confusion, with decreased responsiveness, to agitation, disorientation, hyperreflexia, twitching, irritability and, occasionally, frank convulsions. The electroencephalogram changes usually indicate a non-specific metabolic disturbance. These CNS manifestations tend to occur only in severe uraemia and may resolve slowly, even when uraemia has been controlled with dialysis.

Acute uraemic fibrinous pericarditis, which can cause cardiac tamponade, is now rarely encountered because of the ready availability of dialysis. *Arrhythmias* are seen in 10–30% of patients with ARF.

Haemopoietic disturbances are common. Erythropoiesis is depressed, presumably by uraemic toxins, and this, sometimes exacerbated by haemolysis and haemorrhage, is responsible for the inevitable normocytic, normochromic anaemia in which the haemoglobin concentration falls inexorably to around 7 g/100 mL. Decreased erythropoietin production may also contribute to the development of anaemia in ARF, as may DIC, thrombotic microangiopathy and frequent blood sampling. This anaemia is not, in itself, an indication for blood transfusion. *Coagulopathies*, manifested as a purpuric rash or frank haemorrhage, are also common and are usually caused by a defect in platelet function with a prolonged bleeding time, although they may occasionally be related to DIC (see Chapter 5). Uraemic bleeding can be treated with 1-deamine-8-D-arginine *vasopressin*, an analogue of ADH which transiently releases endogenous stores of factor VIII–von Willebrand factor complexes from endothelial cells, thereby increasing platelet adhesion to the vessel wall. The effect is maximal within 1 hour and lasts 4–8 hours. *Cryoprecipitate* is an alternative, although onset of action is delayed (8–24 hours). These haematological abnormalities resolve during the diuretic phase, when the patient may require supplements of iron, folic acid or, rarely, vitamin B_{12}.

Patients with ARF are very susceptible to *infection* as a result of immune suppression caused by uraemia and poor nutrition. The infection may have been present initially (e.g. following trauma or surgery) or may arise during the period of ARF (e.g. peritonitis or related to invasive procedures). Pulmonary infections are also common, particularly in those requiring mechanical ventilation (see Chapter 7).

A number of events may precipitate *respiratory failure* in patients with ARF, including:

■ pulmonary oedema;
■ pneumonia;
■ a variety of cerebral disorders (e.g. hypertensive encephalopathy and cerebral oedema, the effects of marked uraemia or the accumulation of sedative drugs).

The combination of acute respiratory failure and ARF is difficult to manage and is associated with a poor prognosis.

Blood purification
INDICATIONS
In general, one of the blood purification techniques discussed below should be started early and performed frequently or continuously since this not only controls hyperkalaemia and uraemia, but also facilitates adequate nutritional support and simplifies drug and fluid therapy. In this way the incidence of complications may be reduced and outcome improved (Schiffl *et al.*, 2002).

Active intervention is required when there are uraemic symptoms or signs, salt and water overload, dangerous hyperkalaemia or severe acidosis. Some biochemical criteria for initating blood purification include urea > 30–50 mmol/L, creatinine > 0.7–1.5 mmol/L and bicarbonate < 12 mmol/L. Elective removal of water and electrolytes may be required to accommodate the fluid load of parenteral nutrition or blood transfusion. In non-catabolic ARF, these limits may not be exceeded for up to 6 days after the onset of oliguria, whereas early intervention is usually required (within 24–48 hours) in hypercatabolic patients.

There is evidence to suggest that in those with chronic renal failure, periprocedural haemofiltration can prevent the deterioration in renal function caused by radiocontrast agents (Marenzi *et al.*, 2003).

TECHNIQUES USING DIFFUSION (DIALYSIS) (Fig. 13.2)
The choice between peritoneal and haemodialysis depends on a number of factors, including the available facilities, the expertise of the staff and the type of patient requiring treatment.

PERITONEAL DIALYSIS (PD)
Indications and contraindications. PD is relatively simple and requires the minimum of expertise and equipment. It can be used when haemodialysis is contraindicated or the facilities for its use are not available, when vascular access is difficult and when there is a risk of bleeding or circulatory instability. It is also indicated in the management of some cases of pancreatitis. It should generally be avoided in those with respiratory difficulty (since it impedes diaphragmatic movement) and in the presence of faecal fistulae, abdominal wall infection, colostomy or tense ascites, as well as following aortic surgery. In patients with intra-abdominal adhesions from previous surgery or distended bowel, there is a significant risk of perforating the bowel during insertion of the

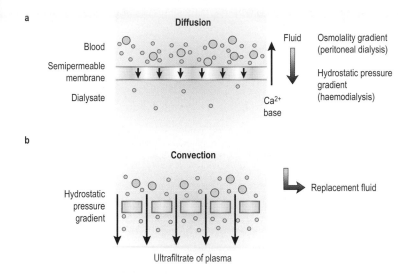

Fig. 13.2 Principles of blood purification. (a) Diffusion: solutes are removed by diffusion across a semipermeable membrane (synthetic in haemodialysis, peritoneum in peritoneal dialysis) according to their concentration gradient. Fluid is removed by hydrostatic pressure (haemodialysis) or osmosis (peritoneal dialysis). (b) Convection: the ultrafiltrate is replaced by a sterile electrolyte solution that has a similar composition to the dialysate used in haemodialysis.

catheter. PD can be relatively inefficient, may not control uraemia in the hypercatabolic patient and, when compared to pumped venovenous haemofiltration, has been associated with increased mortality (Phu *et al.*, 2002).

Technique

- Before inserting the PD catheter the bladder must be emptied.
- Using an aseptic technique and local anaesthesia, a trocar and semirigid Teflon catheter is usually inserted in the midline 2–10 cm below the umbilicus, although positions more laterally near the iliac fossae may also be used.
- Once the parietal peritoneum has been penetrated, the catheter is directed downwards into the pelvis. The catheter can be sited more easily, and the risk of bowel perforation reduced by filling the peritoneal cavity with 1–2 litres of dialysis fluid before manoeuvring the catheter.
- Movement of the catheter in relation to the anterior abdominal wall must be restricted by firmly enclosing the exposed portion of the catheter within a foam-rubber pad and an adhesive dressing.

For long-term PD, a soft Silastic Tenckhoff catheter is placed surgically.

In adults, a continuous-flow system, with minimal dwell time, should be used to reduce the risk of catheter blockage. The aim is to achieve a total exchange of approximately 40 L/day using cycles of 1–2L. For example, 1–2 litres of dialysate is run in as rapidly as possible, is left in the peritoneal cavity for about 30 minutes and then allowed to drain by gravity over about 20 minutes. Each cycle therefore lasts approximately 60 minutes. During early cycles the entire volume instilled may not be removed because a pelvic reservoir of 1–2 litres of fluid may be required.

Water is removed in proportion to the osmotic pressure gradient created by the glucose content of the dialysate. A glucose concentration of about 1.5% is approximately isotonic, while solutions containing up to about 4% glucose can be substituted in patients with fluid overload. Dialysate is usually supplied without potassium, but this may be added in the appropriate concentration should there be a tendency to hypokalaemia. During early cycles 500–1000 units heparin can be added to each dialysate exchange to prevent occlusion of the catheter by fibrin clots.

Monitoring. Cycle times as well as the volumes of fluid instilled and removed must be closely monitored. The circulating volume should be regularly assessed and plasma electrolytes, urea and creatinine should be determined at least daily. The most reliable means of assessing fluid balance is, however, body weight. The blood glucose level should be checked frequently, especially when hypertonic solutions, which may precipitate hyperglycaemia, are used. The returned dialysate should be inspected for turbidity and cultured daily.

Complications

- *Inadequate drainage of dialysate* is usually due to malposition of the catheter or obstruction by a fibrin clot. The catheter should be flushed with saline and repositioned or replaced.
- *Leakage of dialysate* around the catheter can usually be controlled with a purse string suture, but when pleural effusions develop, PD should be discontinued.
- *Pain* is usually felt deep in the pelvis and requires repositioning of the catheter, but may also occur at the end of inflow due to overdistension. Persistent pain and tenderness may be indicative of *peritonitis,* in which case a sample of the dialysate return should be sent for Gram stain, culture and sensitivities, while broad-spectrum antibiotics are instilled into the peritoneal cavity and dialysis is continued. In those with severe infection, antibiotics should also be administered systemically.

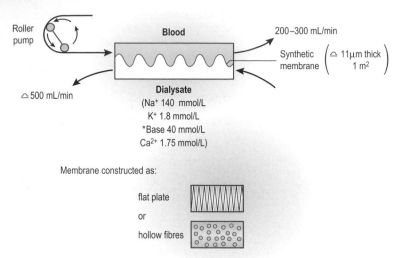

Fig. 13.3 Principles of haemodialysis.

Peritonitis can be due to *bowel perforation*, which may be associated with sudden watery diarrhoea and faeculent dialysate return. A conservative approach with antibiotic administration and continued PD via a different catheter is usually adequate, but surgical exploration is indicated in those who fail to respond.

- *Significant bleeding* is an unusual complication of PD.
- *Cardiorespiratory disturbances* may be precipitated by PD and include hypovolaemia, arrhythmias (due to hypokalaemia and increased vagal tone due to abdominal distension), basal atelectasis and chest infections.
- *Metabolic disturbances* associated with PD include hyperglycaemia, hypokalaemia and hypernatraemia.

HAEMODIALYSIS (Fig. 13.3)
Practical considerations. Haemodialysis removes solutes primarily by passive diffusion across a synthetic semipermeable membrane, the rate of removal depending on solute size and its concentration gradient between plasma and dialysate. Clearance of small molecules such as electrolytes, urea and creatinine is proportional to the permeability of the dialysing membrane, the duration of dialysis and blood and dialysate flow rates. Clearance of larger molecules such as the 'middle molecules' is primarily related to membrane porosity and dialysis duration, and is fairly independent of flow rates. Solute removal can therefore be controlled by adjusting the membrane surface area and the duration of dialysis. Membrane permeability depends on the type of artificial kidney used; dialysate flow is not normally a limiting factor for solute clearance, although blood flow may be limited by vascular access and cardiovascular status.

Removal of plasma water (ultrafiltration) is achieved by applying a hydrostatic pressure gradient across the dialysis membrane. The rate of water removal is determined primarily by the pressure gradient, but also depends on the permeability and surface area of the membrane. The pressure gradient is increased by raising the pressure on the blood side (by increasing the resistance to blood outflow) or by applying a negative pressure on the dialysate side of the membrane.

Vascular access is achieved using either a percutaneous double-lumen central venous catheter or an arteriovenous shunt created, for example, between the radial artery and the cephalic vein or the posterior tibial artery and the long saphenous vein. The rates of flow through arteriovenous shunts are usually less than can be achieved via large-bore venous catheters. The jugular vein is preferred to the subclavian for venous access not only because of the reduced risk of pneumothorax but also because of the lower frequency of vascular stenosis in the long term. The femoral vein is an alternative but a cannula at this site limits mobilization.

Anticoagulation is usually achieved by administering heparin as a low-dose infusion (500–1000 u/hour) or as a bolus injection of 70–100 u/kg followed by smaller doses every 1–3 hours.

Haemodialysis is performed intermittently for periods of 4–6 hours either on alternate days or daily.

Indications. Haemodialysis is a more efficient technique than PD, and corrects the metabolic disturbances more rapidly. It can also be used when there are contraindications to PD such as intra-abdominal pathology. Other advantages of haemodialysis include early mobilization of the patient between sessions and a lower risk of infection.

Complications. The incidence of bleeding due to heparinization is small, but invasive procedures should be avoided just before, during or immediately after haemodialysis. Significant bleeding usually only arises in those with pre-existing pathology such as peptic ulceration or a coagulopathy. In those particularly at risk (e.g. patients who have recently had a cerebrovascular accident or a severe head injury) in whom

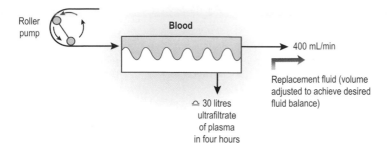

Fig. 13.4 Principles of intermittent haemofiltration. The anion most commonly used in replacement fluid is lactate which is normally converted to bicarbonate. In those with lactic acidosis, lactate-free replacement fluids can be used (e.g. Na$^+$ 140 mmol/L, Cl$^-$ 109.5 mmol/L, Ca^{2+} 1.75 mmol/L, Mg^{2+} 0.5 mmol/L, lactate 3 mmol/L, HCO$_{3+}^-$ 32 mmol/L). Increasingly lactate-free fluids are used as a routine in the critically ill.

haemodialysis is essential, anticoagulation with prostacyclin may be a safer alternative, although this is expensive and may cause hypotension. Regional heparinization, in which protamine is infused into the blood returning to the patient, has been recommended, but this is a difficult technique and a low-dose heparin infusion is probably equally effective.

The major disadvantage of haemodialysis is *hypotension*, which may perpetuate the renal injury and delay repair of tubular cells. Hypotension is most marked when attempts are made to remove large volumes of fluid by ultrafiltration, especially in those with cardiovascular instability or autonomic dysfunction. The cause has not yet been established, but it is thought that the combination of a non-sterile dialysate, a cuprophane membrane and acetate as the base in the dialysate solution in some way prevents the normal vasoconstrictor response to hypovolaemia (Bradley *et al.*, 1990). If simultaneous dialysis and ultrafiltration lead to cardiovascular instability, the ultrafiltration can be performed as a separate procedure (Bradley *et al.*, 1990), either on different days or sequentially on the same day.

There is some suggestion that in ARF outcome is worse in patients treated using a cuprophane membrane, which induces complement and activates leukocytes and the lipoxygenase pathway, than in those dialysed with a biocompatible polyacrylonitrile membrane (Schiffl *et al.*, 1994). These findings are controversial, however (Vanholder and Lameire, 1999), and in a more recent trial there was no difference in outcome between those treated with cuprophane membranes and those dialysed using polymethyl-methacrylate membranes (Jörres *et al.*, 1999). A subsequent meta-analysis has suggested that synthetic membranes may be associated with a lower mortality (Subramanian *et al.*, 2002). One study has demonstrated that daily, as opposed to alternate-day, haemodialysis is associated with fewer hypotensive episodes, better control of uraemia, more rapid resolution of ARF and a reduced mortality rate (Schiffl *et al.*, 2002). The authors concluded that alternate-day haemodialysis should no longer be considered adequate for critically ill patients. A recent prospective, randomized, multicentre study demonstrated that, provided strict guidelines to improve tolerance and metabolic control are used, almost all patients with ARF can be treated successfully with intermittent haemodialysis (Vinsonneau *et al.*, 2006).

Dialysis disequilibrium is related to the rapid onset of hypo-osmolality and causes headache, nausea, vomiting, cramps, restlessness, hypotension, and, when severe, seizures and coma. The syndrome is thought to be caused by cerebral oedema induced by a fall in plasma osmolality in the absence of changes in intracellular osmolality.

Hypoxaemia can be precipitated by microembolization of aggregated leukocytes and diffusion of carbon dioxide into the dialysate leading to hypoventilation.

Other problems associated with haemodialysis include the removal of water-soluble drugs and vitamins, and difficulties related to vascular access.

HAEMOFILTRATION

Haemofiltration relies on massive convection (see **Fig. 13.2**) of plasma water across a porous membrane and its replacement with an electrolyte solution. Solutes are removed only in proportion to their concentration in plasma, and large volumes of ultrafiltrate must therefore be produced to control uraemia and hyperkalaemia. Membranes may be made of polysulfone, polyamide or polyacrylonitrile, configured either as flat plates or, most often currently, as hollow fibres. The pores in the membrane only allow the passage of molecules with molecular weights of up to about 30 000; therefore, albumin and other proteins are not lost from the circulation.

When performed *intermittently* (**Fig. 13.4**), a pumped flow rate of 400 mL/min can produce approximately 30 litres of ultrafiltrate in about 4 hours. This technique is particularly effective in the treatment of diuretic-resistant fluid overload in patients with or without renal failure since large amounts of fluid can be removed without significantly altering osmolality, and acetate uptake is avoided. Hypotension is uncommon during isolated ultrafiltration, probably because the integrity of the peripheral vascular responses to hypovolaemia is not disrupted by dialysis (Bradley *et al.*, 1990). The length of each session is determined by the volume of ultrafiltrate required to control uraemia, while the volume of infusate used to replace the fluid loss is adjusted to achieve the appropriate fluid balance.

Continuous haemofiltration (Forni and Hilton, 1997) (Fig. 13.5). These techniques provide gradual continuous fluid removal and blood purification, thereby perhaps avoiding haemodynamic disturbances and disequilibrium. They are therefore well tolerated by critically ill patients with cardiovascular or respiratory instability, although in one crossover study there was no difference between intermittent

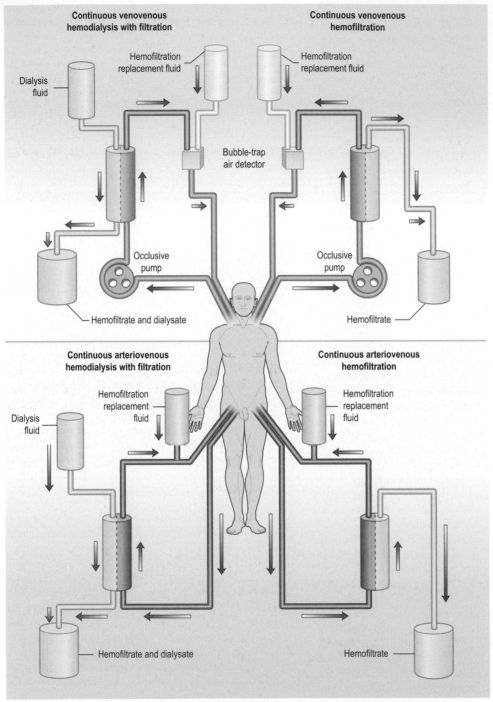

Fig. 13.5 Techniques for continuous haemofiltration and dialysis. Adapted from Forni LG, Hilton PJ 1997 Continuous Hemofiltration in the Treatment of Acute Renal Failure NEJM 336: 1303–1309 with permission.

haemodialysis and continuous renal replacement therapy in the incidence of hypotension or the need for vasopressors (Misset *et al.*, 1996). On the other hand, in critically ill patients with multiple-organ dysfunction intermittent haemodialysis was associated with increased inotropic requirements and intestinal intramucosal acidosis (Van der Schueren *et al.*, 1996). Additional fluid loads such as parenteral nutri-

tion are easily accommodated, there is considerable flexibility in achieving the desired fluid balance and blood chemistry is well controlled. Continuous techniques also avoid the need for dedicated dialysis staff and can be used in neonatal and paediatric patients, as well as in adults. Occasionally they are useful in patients without renal failure who are fluid-overloaded or receiving large volumes of fluid.

Continuous haemofiltration has been shown to remove inflammatory mediators such as cytokines (Bellomo et al., 1993), from the circulation of patients with sepsis, septic shock and acute respiratory distress syndrome, an observation that some believe should encourage the early use of these techniques in such patients. It has also been suggested that short-term, high-volume isovolaemic haemofiltration may be beneficial in patients with intractable cardiocirculatory failure complicating septic shock (Honore et al., 2000) and it seems that survival may be improved in patients undergoing continuous venovenous haemofiltration by increasing the rate of ultrafiltration to at least 35 mL/h per kg (Ronco et al., 2000). Such treatment doses would be difficult to achieve, and are likely to be poorly tolerated, with intermittent haemodialysis. Moreover there is some evidence to suggest that continuous renal replacement therapy may be associated with a lower mortality than intermittent techniques (Kellum et al., 2002), although a large multicentre trial is required to confirm or refute this finding. In one relatively small, randomized controlled trial, however, neither the use of high ultrafiltrate volumes nor early initiation of haemofiltration appeared to improve outcome (Bouman et al., 2002).

Continuous arteriovenous haemofiltration (CAVH) (see Fig. 13.5). This entails the creation of an arteriovenous shunt or percutaneous cannulation of the femoral artery and vein, the haemofilter being positioned between the arterial and venous limbs of a simple extracorporeal circuit without pumps. CAVH has been shown to be a safe and effective technique in critically ill septic patients with ARF (Ossenkoppele et al., 1985), although there is a significant risk of arterial haemorrhage.

The ultrafiltration rate and solute clearance are determined by the balance between the hydrostatic and oncotic transmembrane pressure gradients. Blood flow through the filter and the hydrostatic pressure generated are dependent primarily on the patient's systemic blood pressure, but are also influenced by blood viscosity and the quality of vascular access. Adequate filtration rates can usually be achieved with MAPs above 50–70 mmHg. Larger, shorter, more centrally positioned cannulae are associated with higher filtration rates. There is, however, an increased risk of vascular damage and infection with femoral cannulation; also patient movement can obstruct blood flow and this may restrict mobilization. Many therefore prefer a percutaneous shunt using the smaller distal vessels of the arm or leg.

The hydrostatic pressure gradient can be increased by adjusting the height of the ultrafiltration column. By raising the filter and placing the collecting system on the floor the negative gravitational pressure can be increased by 0.74 mmHg for every 1 cm of additional column height. This effect can be maximized by elevating the patient's bed. Venous back pressure (e.g. due to poor venous access or raised intrathoracic pressure) decreases flow through the filter and predisposes to clotting.

When conditions are optimal, flow rates through the filter may be sufficient to produce as much as 15–20 litres of ultrafiltrate per day. This volume can be reduced, if necessary, by applying a gate clamp to the collecting system tubing. The volume removed as ultrafiltrate is then replaced with blood, plasma, nutrients and crystalloid replacement fluid to achieve the desired fluid balance. Haemofiltration inevitably tends to produce viscous blood of high haematocrit and colloid osmotic pressure at the distal end of the filter. It is therefore generally unwise to produce a filtration rate of more than 30% of the blood flow rate. An alternative approach is upstream (predilutional) administration of replacement fluid, which has the advantage of reducing oncotic pressure and viscosity, thereby increasing clearance and reducing the risk of clotting. This technique has the disadvantage of reducing the efficiency and increasing the cost of haemofiltration because a proportion of the ultrafiltrate is in fact replacement fluid.

In patients without a bleeding diathesis, anticoagulation can be achieved with a bolus of 15–20 units/kg of heparin followed by a maintenance infusion into the arterial side of the filter to maintain the activated partial thromboplastin time at approximately 45 seconds. Alternatively, and certainly in those with a coagulopathy, thrombocytopenia or an increased risk of haemorrhagic complications, heparin can be administered as a low-dose continuous prefilter infusion at a rate of 5–10 units/kg per hour. It has been suggested that the use of *prostacyclin* (2–3 ng/kg per min) in combination with *low-dose heparin* (250 units/h) may limit platelet activation, prolong the life of the filter and reduce the risk of bleeding. In those who develop heparin-induced thrombocytopenia and in other high-risk cases, prostacyclin may be used alone in a dose of 2.5–5 ng/kg per min. Experience with low-molecular-weight heparin is at present limited. Patients at high risk of bleeding who require continuous CVVH(D) can often be safely managed without circuit anticoagulation (Tan et al., 2000).

Continuous arteriovenous haemofiltration with dialysis (CAVHD) (see Fig. 13.5) (Stevens et al., 1988). In catabolic critically ill patients biochemical control with CAVH may only be achieved by exchanging very large volumes of fluid, up to 20–40 L/day, or by using supplemental intermittent haemodialysis (Ossenkoppele et al., 1985). CAVHD, which combines diffusion with convection to produce more effective biochemical control, is therefore preferred in catabolic patients, when systemic blood pressure is low and when vascular access is suboptimal.

Dialysate, usually warmed to 37°C, is administered countercurrent to blood flow using an infusion pump at a rate of 1 L/h. Provided blood flow is greater than dialysate flow there should be complete equilibration of small solutes across the membrane. Creatinine clearances range between approximately 13 and 20 mL/min. Solute transfer from dialysate to blood also occurs and the composition of the dialysate can be altered by adding bicarbonate to correct acidosis or potassium to control hypokalaemia.

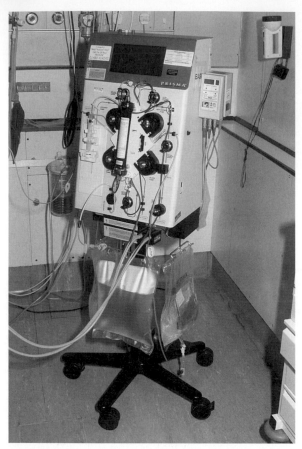

Fig. 13.6 Continuous venovenous haemodialfiltration using an automated device.

Continuous venovenous haemofiltration (CVVH) (Figs 13.5 and 13.6). Pump-driven haemofiltration allows better control of ultrafiltration, especially in those with poor vascular access and hypotension. CVVH may be associated with improved survival compared to CAVH, perhaps because the larger volumes of ultrafiltrate clear significant quantities of toxins and mediators from the circulation (Storck *et al.,* 1991). The increased complexity related to the inclusion of a pump in the circuit does not seem to result in increased complications or an increase in nursing staff requirements. Indeed the risks are reduced by the inclusion of safety devices and the use of a single venous cannula appears to reduce the incidence of access-related complications. A dialysis component can be added (CVVHD) to improve biochemical control with only a minimal further increase in complexity.

Arteriovenous haemofiltration is now rarely used and most consider CVVHD to be the technique of choice for managing ARF in the critically ill, although others contend that more than adequate clearance rates can be achieved with CVVH alone.

Complications of continuous haemofiltration. The relative ease with which CAVH(D) and CVVH(D) can be instituted belies the fact that they are potentially extremely dangerous, labour-intensive techniques that require considerable expertise. In particular there is an ever-present danger of serious errors in fluid and electrolyte balance. The risk of such errors is, however, markedly reduced by the use of modern automated machines (**Fig. 13.6**). Complications related to vascular access include infection, thrombosis, haemorrhage and aneurysm formation. The incidence of catheter-related sepsis is, however, low (in the region of 2%) and replacement of catheters only when clinically indicated seems to be as safe as routine replacement every 5 days (Wester *et al.,* 2002). It is important to consider the potential for continuous haemofiltration/dialysis to alter profoundly the pharmacokinetics of drugs administered to patients with renal failure. Lastly there is some concern that renal replacement therapy may delay renal recovery. Postulated mechanisms include treatment-associated haemodynamic instability, catheter-related sepsis and cytokine activation by bioincompatible membranes.

Nutritional support

Malnutrition is common and may be a consequence of anorexia, restricted access to food, the catabolic response, loss of nutrients in drainage fluids or dialysate, or, most often, a combination of these. The provision of adequate nutritional support is essential (see Chapter 11). In general, patients should receive appropriate quantities of protein and energy, either enterally or parenterally, regardless of the amount of fluid and nitrogen required. Dialysis or haemofiltration should then be used to prevent fluid overload and control uraemia. There is some evidence to suggest that the use of continuous haemofiltration to facilitate parenteral nutrition with a high-protein feed leads to improved survival in surgical ARF (Bartlett *et al.,* 1986).

Haemofiltration is associated with significant losses of non-urea nitrogen across the filter, while the use of a glucose-containing dialysate provides an important source of carbohydrate (Bellomo *et al.,* 1991). It may therefore be appropriate to increase the nitrogen content of feeds given to patients on continuous haemofiltration. Lipids are not removed during haemofiltration and do not appear to be trapped in the filter.

General management considerations

Patients with ARF are extremely susceptible to infection. Meticulous mouth care is required to prevent oral candidiasis and, in those who are essentially anuric, the urethral catheter should be removed to minimize the risk of urinary tract infection. Careful adjustment of drug doses, particularly H_2-receptor antagonists and antibiotics, has already been mentioned. If possible, the patient should be weighed daily to assess fluid balance, although in practice this can be difficult in intensive care patients. Finally, it is clearly essential to treat the underlying condition (e.g. by performing a laparotomy in those with intra-abdominal infection) since ARF rarely recovers in the presence of persistent sepsis.

DIURETIC PHASE

In patients with ATN, kidney function will normally recover spontaneously. This is heralded by the onset of a diuresis, usually 5–20 days after the initial insult, although in some cases this may occur within 48 hours or be delayed for up to 8–10 weeks.

Initially, the GFR remains relatively low; consequently blood urea and creatinine levels may continue to rise for a few days after the onset of a diuresis. Because tubular function is still impaired, the patient may lose large quantities of sodium, potassium and water, as well as phosphate and magnesium, although in some cases the diuresis may largely represent mobilization of accumulated solutes and water. Urinary losses of sodium and potassium must therefore be closely monitored; as an approximate guide, half the total fluid and electrolytes excreted should be replaced. Usually a combination of 0.9% saline and 5% dextrose in a 1:2 ratio is appropriate, since the urinary sodium concentration may be up to 70 mmol/L. Replacement of potassium, calcium and magnesium is also often required. Frequent careful assessment of each individual is, however, essential to avoid water and electrolyte (particularly potassium) depletion on the one hand, or persistent polyuria and oedema due to excessive fluid administration on the other.

Renal vascular autoregulation remains impaired for some weeks after the initial event. Consequently further haemodynamic, septic or nephrotoxic insults are poorly tolerated.

NON-OLIGURIC ARF

Non-oliguric ARF probably represents a less severe form of vasomotor nephropathy in which the GFR is maintained at approximately 2–5 mL/min, urine continues to be produced and the urinary sodium concentration is approximately 50 mmol/L. This form of ARF is becoming more common, possibly due to improved management of prerenal oliguria and incipient ARF (see above), as well as the increasing number of cases of tubular necrosis induced by toxic drugs. Approximately 20% of patients develop non-oliguric ARF, most commonly in the context of radiocontrast or aminoglycoside toxicity. Dialysis is required less frequently or not at all, complications (gastrointestinal bleeding, sepsis, acidosis, and neurological disturbances) are reduced, recovery is more rapid and the mortality may be lower.

INTERMEDIATE RENAL FAILURE

The increasing recognition of this less severe form of ARF in recent years may reflect improved management of prerenal and incipient ARF. Patients present with non-oliguric renal impairment, a low urinary sodium and FENa, urinary granular or epithelial cell casts, and a partial response to fluid challenge. The maintenance phase is abbreviated and the prognosis may be improved.

MANAGEMENT OF SOME SPECIFIC TYPES OF ARF

Rhabdomyolysis (Holt and Moore, 2001)

Restoration of intravascular volume is the single most important measure. The use of mannitol in order to promote a diuresis (> 200–300 mL/h) and reduce elevated compartment pressure is controversial. Loop diuretics should be avoided since they have the theoretical disadvantage of acidifying the urine. Although the efficacy of bicarbonate and mannitol administration remains unproven, laboratory studies support their use and such treatment is generally safe. Most therefore recommend that the urine should be maintained alkaline (e.g. pH > 7.0) by the systemic administration of sodium bicarbonate to inhibit precipitation of myoglobin in the renal tubules, lipid peroxidation and renal vasoconstriction. Necrotic muscle may require surgical excision, whilst fasciotomy may be required in those with compartment syndrome (see Chapter 10).

Acute interstitial nephritis

When nephritis is due to an acute hypersensitivity reaction to a drug, removal of the offending agent may prevent further deterioration in renal function. Recovery can, however, be slow and incomplete. The administration of corticosteroids may encourage recovery, although the rate of rise of urea will be increased and immune suppression is a potential danger. Some believe that the risks associated with steroid therapy outweigh the benefits in this situation.

Hyperuricaemic ARF

Treatment consists of rehydration and haemodialysis, followed by alkalinization and the administration of allopurinol.

ARF due to glomerular disease

Specialist nephrological advice should be obtained as a matter of urgency. Most cases of acute crescentic glomerulonephritis progress rapidly and inexorably to end-stage renal failure. This is also generally the case in Goodpasture's syndrome, although high-dose steroids, immunosuppressants and plasma exchange may be beneficial. Although the combination of these measures can usually rapidly control pulmonary haemorrhage, the outcome of the renal lesion is related to the severity of renal impairment at presentation. In Wegener's granulomatosis treatment with a combination of prednisone and cyclophosphamide leads to complete remission in more than 90% of cases.

Vascular ARF

Immediate intervention is required to avoid permanent loss of renal function. Acute renal artery occlusion requires urgent surgery or fibrinolytic therapy, followed by heparinization. In acute renal vein thrombosis, the patient should be heparinized and/or receive streptokinase.

ARF due to obstruction

The extent of renal parenchymal damage is related to the duration, degree and site of the obstruction, as well as the presence of infection. It is therefore imperative to confirm the diagnosis and relieve the obstruction as quickly as possible, although urinary tract instrumentation or surgery may be complicated by bacteraemia, endotoxaemia and septic shock. Urethral or bladder neck obstruction can usually be relieved temporarily by transurethral or suprapubic bladder catheterization. Ureteric obstruction may be treated initially by percutaneous catheterization of the dilated pelvis or ureter, and obstructing lesions are often removed percutaneously or bypassed by insertion of a ureteric stent. Surgery can be preceded by dialysis. Obstruction due to an inflammatory aortic aneurysm can be successfully treated with corticosteroids when surgery is not an option.

Following relief of the obstruction there may be a massive diuresis (often between 4 and 20 litres/day), primarily due to defective tubular function, but also as a result of the accumulation of urea and other osmotically active molecules. Approximately 5% develop a transient salt-wasting syndrome. Some will develop hyperkalaemic, hyperchloraemic tubular acidosis, the onset of which is usually indolent, and the abnormality tends to persist after relief of obstruction. Intravenous fluids are required to maintain blood pressure and glomerular filtration. Infection is common and should be treated with appropriate antibiotics, modified, if necessary, according to sensitivities obtained later (see Chapter 12).

PROGNOSIS OF ARF

The final outcome of ARF depends on the aetiology; mortality rates range from approximately 35 to 60% in medical, surgical or trauma patients, 0–30% in those cases related to obstetric disasters, and 75% or more in burns patients. When renal failure is the only problem, mortality rates may be as low as 8%, but in the remainder (i.e. those patients likely to require intensive care), the average mortality is higher than 60%. The presence of sepsis, particularly intra-abdominal sepsis, and multiorgan failure also adversely affects the prognosis (the combination of ARF and sepsis is associated with a mortality of around 70%), but age does not. Another factor affecting outcome is the site of surgery, mortality rates being particularly high following gastrointestinal surgery, especially when the bowel rather than the stomach is involved.

Although the overall mortality may have improved only slightly, if at all, over the last 25 years or so, this may be partly explained by changes in the type of patients being treated. Improvements in resuscitation, evacuation of casualties and surgical techniques have resulted in the survival of more seriously ill patients, while there has been a reduction in the number of obstetric patients with ARF (who have the best prognosis) and an increase in those associated with generalized sepsis, liver failure and cardiac arrest. An overall mortality of 53% was reported in one large series of intensive care patients with ARF treated by continuous haemofiltration, and there was evidence that survival rates increased during the course of the study (Barton et al., 1993). In a more recent series of patients who had received renal replacement therapy for ARF the 28-day mortality was 41%, but this had increased to 57% at 1 year and 70% after 5 years (Åhlström et al., 2005). It is worth noting that many patients die as a result of the precipitating cause, rather than as a direct result of the renal failure, although the development of ARF is independently associated within an increased risk of death (Levy et al., 1996).

In patients who do recover, tubular lesions usually heal completely and histological appearances may be normal 3–4 weeks after the insult. About 50% of survivors have subclinical abnormalities of renal function or structure but there is usually no obvious residual renal impairment and kidney function has normally recovered to about 80% of normal after 1 year. A few (< 5%) will require long-term renal replacement therapy, probably because of complete cortical necrosis. An additional 5% of patients experience a slow, progressive deterioration in renal function.

REFERENCES

Åhlström A, Tallgren M, Peltonen S, et al. (2005) Survival and quality of life of patients requiring acute renal replacement therapy. *Intensive Care Medicine* **31**: 1222–1228.

Allgren RL, Marbury TC, Rahman SN, et al. (1997) Anaritide in acute tubular necrosis. *New England Journal of Medicine* **336**: 828–834.

Baldwin L, Henderson A, Hickman P (1994) Effect of postoperative low-dose dopamine on renal function after elective major vascular surgery. *Annals of Internal Medicine* **120**: 744–747.

Barry KG, Cohen A, Knochel JP, et al. (1961) Mannitol infusion II: the prevention of acute functional renal failure during resection of an aneurysm of the abdominal aorta. *New England Journal of Medicine* **264**: 967–971.

Bartlett RH, Mault JR, Dechert RE, et al. (1986) Continuous arteriovenous hemofiltration: improved survival in surgical acute renal failure? *Surgery* **100**: 400–408.

Barton IK, Hilton PJ, Taub NA, et al. (1993) Acute renal failure treated by haemofiltration: factors affecting outcome. *Quarterly Journal of Medicine* **86**: 81–90.

Bellomo R, Martin H, Parkin G, et al. (1991) Continuous arteriovenous haemodiafiltration in the critically ill: influence on major nutrient balances. *Intensive Care Medicine* **17**: 399–402.

Bellomo R, Tipping P, Boyce N (1993) Continuous veno-venous hemofiltration with dialysis removes cytokines from the circulation of septic patients. *Critical Care Medicine* **21**: 522–526.

Bellomo R, Kellum JA, Wisniewski SR, et al. (1999) Effects of norepinephrine on the renal vasculature in normal and endotoxemic dogs. *American Journal of Respiratory and Critical Care Medicine* **159**: 1186–1192.

Bellomo R, Chapman M, Finfer S, et al. (2000) Low-dose dopamine in patients with early renal dysfunction: a placebo-controlled randomised trial. Australian and New Zealand Intensive Care Society (ANZICS) clinical trials group. *Lancet* **356**: 2139–2143.

Bellomo R, Kellum J, Ronco C (2001) Acute renal failure: time for consensus. *Intensive Care Medicine* **27**: 1685–1688.

Birck R, Krzossok S, Markowetz F, et al. (2003) Acetylcysteine for prevention of contrast nephropathy: meta-analysis. *Lancet* **362**: 598–603.

Bouman CSC, Oudermans-van Straaten HM, Tijssen TGP, et al. (2002) Effects of early high-volume continuous venovenous hemofiltration on survival and recovery of renal function in intensive care patients with acute renal failure: a prospective, randomized trial. *Critical Care Medicine* **30**: 2205–2211.

Bradley JR, Evans DB, Cowley AJ (1990) Comparison of vascular tone during combined haemodialysis with ultrafiltration and during ultrafiltration followed by haemodialysis: a possible mechanism for dialysis hypotension. *British Medical Journal* **300**: 1312.

Brezis M, Rosen S (1995) Hypoxia of the renal medulla – its implications for disease. *New England Journal of Medicine* **332**: 647–655.

Brezis M, Rosen S, Stoff JS, et al. (1986) Inhibition of prostaglandin synthesis in rat kidney perfused with and without erythrocytes: implication for analgesic nephropathy. *Mineral and Electrolyte Metabolism* **12**: 326–332.

Dawson JL (1964) Jaundice and anoxic renal damage: protective effect of mannitol. *British Medical Journal* **1**: 810–811.

Forni LG, Hilton PJ (1997) Continuous hemofiltration in the treatment of acute renal failure. *New England Journal of Medicine* **336**: 1303–1309.

Franklin SC, Moulton M, Sicard GA, et al. (1997) Insulin-like growth factor I preserves renal function postoperatively. *American Journal of Physiology* **272**: F257–F259.

Friedrich JO, Adhikari N, Herridge MS, et al. (2005) Meta-analysis: low-dose dopamine increases urine output but does not prevent renal dysfunction or death. *Annals of Internal Medicine* **142**: 510–524.

Herget-Rosenthal S, Marggraf G, Hüsing J, et al. (2004) Early detection of acute renal failure by serum cystatin C. *Kidney International* **66**: 1115–1122.

Hirschberg R, Kopple J, Lipsett P, et al. (1999) Multicenter clinical trial of recombinant human insulin-like growth factor I in patients with acute renal failure. *Kidney International* **55**: 2423–2432.

Ho KM, Sheridan DJ (2006) Meta-analysis of furosemide to prevent or treat acute renal failure. *British Medical Journal* **333**: 420.

Holt SG, Moore KP (2001) Pathogenesis and treatment of renal dysfunction in rhabdomyolysis. *Intensive Care Medicine* **27**: 803–811.

Honore PM, Jamez J, Wauthier M, et al. (2000) Prospective evaluation of short-term, high-volume isovolaemic hemofiltration on the hemodynamic course and outcome in patients with intractable circulatory failure resulting from septic shock. *Critical Care Medicine* **28**: 3581–3587.

Ichai C, Soubielle J, Carles M, et al. (2000) Comparison of the renal effects of low to high doses of dopamine and dobutamine in critically ill patients: a single-blind randomized study. *Critical Care Medicine* **28**: 921–928.

Jörres A, Gahl GM, Dobis C, et al. (1999) Haemodialysis-membrane biocompatibility and mortality of patients with dialysis-dependent acute renal failure: a prospective randomised multicentre trial. *Lancet* **354**: 1337–1341.

Juste RN, Panikkar K, Soni N (1998) The effects of low-dose dopamine infusions on haemodynamic and renal parameters in patients with septic shock requiring treatment with noradrenaline. *Intensive Care Medicine* **24**: 564–568.

Kellum JA, Angus DC, Johnson JP, et al. (2002) Continuous versus intermittent renal replacement therapy: a meta-analysis. *Intensive Care Medicine* **28**: 29–37.

Khan IH, Catto GR, Edward N, et al. (1997) Acute renal failure: factors influencing nephrology referral and outcome. *Quarterly Journal of Medicine* **90**: 781–785.

Kleinknecht D, Ganeval D, Gonzales-Duque LA, et al. (1976) Furosemide in acute oliguric renal failure. A controlled trial. *Nephron* **17**: 51–58.

Kopple JD, Hirschberg R, Guber HP, et al. (1996) Lack of effect of recombinant human insulin-like growth factor-1 (IGF-1) in patients with acute renal failure (ARF). *Journal of the American Society of Nephrologists* **7**: 1375.

Kron IL, Harman PK, Nolan SP (1984) The measurement of intra-abdominal pressure as a criterion for abdominal re-exploration. *Annals of Surgery* **199**: 28–30.

Lameire N, Van Biesen W, Vanholder R (2005) Acute renal failure. *Lancet* **365**: 417–430.

Levy EM, Viscoli CM, Horwitz RI (1996) The effect of acute renal failure on mortality. A cohort analysis. *Journal of the American Medical Association* **275**: 1489–1494.

Lindner A (1983) Synergism of dopamine and furosemide in diuretic-resistant, oliguric acute renal failure. *Nephron* **33**: 121–126.

MacAllister R, Vallance P (1994) Nitric oxide in essential and renal hypertension. *Journal of the American Society of Nephrology* **5**: 1057–1065.

McDonald RH, Goldberg LI, McNay JL, et al. (1964) Effect of dopamine in man: augmentation of sodium excretion, glomerular filtration rate and renal plasma flow. *Journal of Clinical Investigation* **43**: 1116–1124.

Marenzi G, Marana I, Lauri G, et al. (2003) The prevention of radiocontrast-agent-induced nephropathy by hemofiltration. *New England Journal of Medicine* **349**: 1333–1340.

Mehta RL, Pascual MT, Soroko S, et al. (2002) Diuretics, mortality, and nonrecovery of renal function in acute renal failure. *Journal of the American Medical Association* **288**: 2547–2553.

Merten GJ, Burgess WP, Gray LV, et al. (2004) Prevention of contrast-induced nephropathy with sodium bicarbonate: a randomized controlled trial. *Journal of the American Medical Association* **291**: 2328–2334.

Minuth AN, Terrell JB Jr, Suki WN (1976) Acute renal failure: a study of the course and prognosis of 104 patients and of the role of furosemide. *American Journal of the Medical Sciences* **271**: 317–324.

Mishra J, Dent C, Tarabishi R, et al. (2005) Neutrophil gelatinase associated lipocalin (NGAL) as a biomarker for acute renal injury after cardiac surgery. *Lancet* **365**: 1231–1238.

Misset B, Timsit JF, Chevret S, et al. (1996) A randomized cross-over comparison of the hemodynamic response to intermittent hemodialysis and continuous hemofiltration in ICU patients with acute renal failure. *Intensive Care Medicine* **22**: 742–746.

Olson D, Pohlman A, Hall JB (1996) Administration of low-dose dopamine to nonoliguric patients with sepsis syndrome does not raise intramucosal gastric pH nor improve creatinine clearance. *American Journal of Respiratory and Critical Care Medicine* **154**: 1664–1670.

Ossenkoppele GJ, Van der Meulen J, Bronsveld W, et al. (1985) Continuous arteriovenous hemofiltration as an adjunctive therapy for septic shock. *Critical Care Medicine* **13**: 102–104.

Parker S, Carlon GC, Isaacs M, et al. (1981) Dopamine administration in oliguria and oliguric renal failure. *Critical Care Medicine* **9**: 630–632.

Phu NH, Hien TT, Mai NTH, et al. (2002) Hemofiltration and peritoneal dialysis in infection-associated acute renal failure in Vietnam. *New England Journal of Medicine* **347**: 845–902.

Redl-Wenzl EM, Armbruster C, Edelmann G, et al. (1993) The effects of norepinephrine on hemodynamics and renal function in severe septic shock states. *Intensive Care Medicine* **19**: 151–154.

Ronco C, Bellomo R, Homel P, et al. (2000) Effects of different doses in continuous veno-venous haemofiltration on outcomes of acute renal failure: a prospective randomised trial. *Lancet* **356**: 26–30.

Schiffl H, Lang SM, König A, et al. (1994) Biocompatible membranes in acute renal failure: prospective case-controlled study. *Lancet* **344**: 570–572.

Schiffl H, Lang SM, Fischer R (2002) Daily hemodialysis and the outcome of acute renal failure. *New England Journal of Medicine* **346**: 305–310.

Schrier RW, Wang W (2004) Acute renal failure and sepsis. *New England Journal of Medicine* **351**: 159–169.

Segal JM, Phang PT, Walley KR (1992) Low-dose dopamine hastens onset of gut ischemia in a porcine model of hemorrhagic shock. *Journal of Applied Physiology* **73**: 1159–1164.

Shilliday IR, Quinn KJ, Allison ME (1997) Loop diuretics in the management of acute renal failure: a prospective, double-blind, placebo-controlled, randomized study. *Nephrology, Dialysis, Transplantation* **12**: 2592–2596.

Shusterman N, Strom BL, Murray TG, et al. (1987) Risk factors and outcome of hospital-acquired acute renal failure. Clinical epidemiologic study. *American Journal of Medicine* **83**: 65–71.

Solomon R, Werner C, Mann D, et al. (1994) Effects of saline, mannitol, and furosemide on acute decreases in renal function induced by radiocontrast agents. *New England Journal of Medicine* **331**: 1416–1420.

Stevens PE, Riley B, Davies SP, et al. (1988) Continuous arteriovenous haemodialysis in critically ill patients. *Lancet* **2**: 150–152.

Stevens MA, McCullough PA, Tobin KJ, et al. (1999) A prospective randomized trial of prevention measures in patients at high risk for contrast nephropathy: results of the PRINCE study. *Journal of the American College of Cardiology* **33**: 403–411.

Stevens PE, Tamimi NA, Al Hasani MK, et al. (2001) Non-specialist management of acute renal failure. *Quarterly Journal of Medicine* **94**: 533–540.

Storck M, Hartl WH, Zimmerer E, et al. (1991) Comparison of pump-driven and spontaneous continuous haemofiltration in postoperative acute renal failure. *Lancet* **337**: 452–455.

Subramanian S, Venkataraman R, Kellum JA (2002) Influence of dialysis membranes on outcomes in acute renal failure: a meta-analysis. *Kidney International* **62**: 1819–1823.

Tan HK, Baldwin I, Bellomo R (2000) Continuous veno-venous hemofiltration without anticoagulation in high-risk patients. *Intensive Care Medicine* **26**: 1652–1657.

Tepel M, van der Giet M, Schwarzfeld C, et al. (2000) Prevention of radiographic-contrast-agent-induced reductions in renal function by acetylcysteine. *New England Journal of Medicine* **343**: 180–184.

Thompson BT, Cockrill BA (1994) Renal-dose dopamine: a siren song? *Lancet* **344**: 7–8.

Uchino S, Doig GS, Bellomo R, *et al.* (2004) Diuretics and mortality in acute renal failure. *Critical Care Medicine* **32**: 1669–1677.

Van der Schueren G, Diltoer M, Laureys M, *et al.* (1996) Intermittent hemodialysis in critically ill patients with multiple organ dysfunction syndrome is associated with intestinal intramucosal acidosis. *Intensive Care Medicine* **22**: 747–751.

Vanholder R, Lameire N (1999) Does biocompatibility of dialysis membranes affect recovery of renal function and survival? *Lancet* **354**: 1316–1318.

Vinsonneau C, Camus C, Combes A, *et al.* (2006) Continuous venovenous haemodiafiltration versus intermittent haemodialysis for acute renal failure in patients with multiple-organ dysfunction syndrome: a multicentre randomised trial. *Lancet* **368**: 379–385.

Wester JP, de Koning EJ, Geers AB, *et al.* (2002) Catheter replacement in continuous arteriovenous hemodiafiltration: the balance between infections and mechanical complications. *Critical Care Medicine* **30**: 1261–1266.

14 Acute liver failure

TYPES OF ACUTE LIVER FAILURE

ACUTE LIVER FAILURE

Acute hepatitis with jaundice and coagulopathy without hepatic encephalopathy is referred to as *severe acute hepatitis*. The prognosis is generally good. The term *fulminant hepatic failure* (FHF) was originally defined as a clinical syndrome developing as a result of massive necrosis of liver cells or any other sudden and severe impairment of hepatic function (Trey and Davidson, 1970). This definition included the stipulation that there should be no history or evidence of pre-existing liver disease and that the signs of encephalopathy should appear within 8 weeks of the onset of the first symptoms. *Late-onset hepatic failure* was diagnosed when the onset of encephalopathy was delayed by 8–26 weeks from the onset of symptoms.

More recently, in an attempt to standardize the nomenclature a different terminology has been proposed. This is based on the interval between jaundice and encephalopathy, the terms *hyperacute, acute or subacute liver failure* being applied depending on whether this interval is 0–7 days, 8–28 days or 29 days to 12 weeks respectively (O'Grady et al., 1993). In this classification, in contrast to Trey and Davidson's original definition, cases with pre-existing chronic liver disease are included, although when the acute and chronic phases are due to the same process those with a previous history of symptomatic liver disease are normally excluded. This new terminology did not, however, receive universal approval (Bernuau and Benhamou, 1993). These authors suggest that patients with encephalopathy developing within 2 weeks of the onset of jaundice should be categorized as FHF, whereas the term *subfulminant hepatic failure* (SFHF) should be applied to those in whom the onset of encephalopathy is delayed for 2–12 weeks.

ACUTE-ON-CHRONIC LIVER FAILURE

Acute-on-chronic liver failure occurs when an acute illness causes decompensation of pre-existing symptomatic chronic liver disease. Usually the chronic liver impairment is related to hepatic cirrhosis (e.g. alcoholic, primary biliary, postnecrotic, sclerosing cholangitis), but is occasionally associated with infiltrative processes such as nodular regenerative hyperplasia, sarcoid or metabolic disorders.

ISCHAEMIC/HYPOXIC HEPATOCELLULAR DAMAGE

Ischaemic/hypoxic hepatocellular damage can occur in acute or chronic cardiac failure as well as following an episode of severe shock (haemorrhagic, septic or cardiogenic) or hepatic vascular occlusion. It is now a very rare complication of cardiac surgery. Characteristically there is hepatomegaly and a marked rise in transaminases (> 1000 u/L) with a prolonged prothrombin time, but bilirubin levels are usually only moderately elevated. Acute liver failure (ALF) is, however, rare following ischaemic liver damage and when it does occur the prognosis is poor, unless cardiovascular function can be improved.

CAUSES OF LIVER DYSFUNCTION IN CRITICAL ILLNESS

The causes of liver dysfunction in critical illness include:

- liver impairment associated with systemic inflammation and multiple-organ dysfunction (see Chapter 5);
- drug-induced liver damage;
- fatty infiltration of the liver precipitated by high-calorie total parenteral nutrition (TPN);
- biliary sepsis;
- liver trauma (including iatrogenic, e.g. following liver biopsy);
- jaundice of the critically ill.

The latter may be due to a reduced ability to transport conjugated bilirubin and is usually associated with an increased bilirubin load (e.g. massive blood transfusion, resolving haematomas). Jaundice usually develops 7–10 days after the initiating event. Mortality rates are closely related to bilirubin levels and may be as high as 50%.

ACUTE LIVER FAILURE

CAUSES (Table 14.1)

The most common cause of ALF in the UK was for many years *paracetamol* hepatotoxicity (see Chapter 19), which in one series accounted for 48% of cases. Viral hepatitis was responsible for 37%, with hepatitis A being diagnosed in

Table 14.1 Some causes of acute liver failure

Infections	Viral hepatitis (type A, type B, type C, type D, type E)
	Yellow fever
Poisons/chemicals	Ecstasy
	Paracetamol
	Monoamine oxidase inhibitors
	Tetracycline
	Sodium valproate
	Statins
	Non-steroidal anti-inflammatory agents
	Methyldopa
	Isoniazid
	Nucleoside analogues (e.g. zidovudine)
	Ethanol
	(Halothane)
	Phosphorus
	Carbon tetrachloride
	Amanita phalloides
	Aflatoxins
	Herbal medicines
Ischaemia	Shock
	Hepatic vascular occlusion
	Cardiac surgery
Miscellaneous	Fatty liver of pregnancy
	Reye's syndrome
	Wilson's disease
	Galactosaemia
	Autoimmune hepatitis
	Budd–Chiari syndrome
	Acute hepatic vein thrombosis
	Malignant infiltration

32% and hepatitis B in 24% (Gimson and Williams, 1983). Other infective causes of ALF include hepatitis D (always occurs as a coinfection in those with hepatitis B, most often in drug abusers or following transfusion), hepatitis C virus (implicated in sporadic ALF only rarely), hepatitis E (similar to hepatitis A, prevalent in travellers to the Indian subcontinent) and *yellow fever*. *Epstein–Barr virus, cytomegalovirus, herpes simplex viruses* 1 and 2, and *varicella-zoster* cause liver failure only rarely, but may contribute to the death of immunocompromised patients. In many cases of presumed viral ALF, no specific agent can be identified. The newly described hepatotrophic viruses, hepatitis G and transfusion-transmitted virus are unlikely to be important aetiological agents.

Outside the UK, viral hepatitis is the most frequent cause of ALF worldwide, accounting for about 70% of cases, while drug-induced liver failure is slightly less common. As well as paracetamol hepatotoxicity, idiosyncratic reactions to *antituberculosis drugs* (especially isoniazid), *monoamine oxidase inhibitors, tetracycline, sodium valproate, non-steroidal anti-inflammatory agents, statins* and *methyldopa* can cause ALF. Recently hepatotoxicity caused by *ecstasy* has become increasingly important, especially in young adults (see Chapter 19) and in some cases *nucleoside analogues*, such as zidovudine, can cause ALF with extreme lactic acidosis as a consequence of impaired hepatic mitochrondrial function (see Chapter 12).

In the past severe hepatic necrosis occasionally followed *halothane* anaesthesia (Editorial, 1986); the incidence was higher in females, the elderly and the obese, and was increased by multiple exposure. In addition, approximately 20% of patients undergoing repeated halothane anaesthesia were found to have less severe forms of liver injury (Wright *et al.*, 1975).

ALF occurring during *pregnancy* (Williams and Ede, 1981) may be related to viral hepatitis or acute fatty liver. Severe hepatic dysfunction may also occasionally be associated with toxaemia of pregnancy (haemolysis, elevated liver enzymes and low platelets (HELLP) syndrome; see Chapter 18) and can be caused by localized or systemic intravascular coagulation.

Poisoning with carbon tetrachloride, yellow phosphorus, mushrooms (*Amanita phalloides*), aflatoxins, some herbal medicines and alcohol can also be complicated by the development of ALF. In children and young adults it is worth remembering that *Wilson's disease* can present acutely, although usually there is evidence of haemolysis and underlying chronic liver disease (chronic active hepatitis, cirrhosis) and characteristically the alkaline phosphatase level is low. *Reye's syndrome* and *galactosaemia* may also cause ALF, as may replacement of normal hepatocytes with *tumour cells*.

MECHANISMS OF FHF
Viral hepatitis

It is unclear why only some of those with *viral hepatitis* develop ALF while in others the infection pursues a more benign course. Hepatitis B virus has no direct cytopathic effect and the onset of massive hepatocellular necrosis does not appear to be related to either the strain of virus or the size of the inoculum. There is, however, some evidence to suggest that those who develop liver failure produce an enhanced immune response to all three antigenic determinants of the virus and that the excess antibody leads to the formation of immune complexes. The latter may then obstruct hepatic sinusoids and cause ischaemic necrosis of liver cells. In contrast, cellular damage following hepatitis A or non-A non-B infection is probably due to a direct cytopathic effect of the virus and in these cases it is likely that an impaired immune response contributes to the fulminant course. It has also been suggested, however, that activation of the host's immune responses with liberation of proinflammatory cytokines may contribute to liver injury in viral hepatitis.

Hepatitis B virus may be reactivated when chronic asymptomatic carriers are given chemotherapy, in some cases precipitating ALF. This complication can be largely prevented by pretreatment with lamivudine.

Drug- and toxin-induced hepatotoxicity

Risk factors for drug-induced hepatotoxicity include the extremes of age, abnormal renal function, obesity, pre-existing liver disease and concurrent use of other hepato-toxic agents. Some drug toxicities occur in an intrinsic, dose-dependent, predictable manner (e.g. paracetamol) but most are idiosyncratic, immunologically mediated reactions, usually to a metabolite.

Hepatocellular damage following *paracetamol overdose* is related to the production of a toxic metabolite of paracetamol (*N*-acetyl-para benzoquine imide), which accumulates when hepatic glutathione has been overwhelmed (Black, 1980), although individuals vary considerably in their susceptibility to liver damage induced by this agent. Paracetamol toxicity is dose-dependent, but its effects are exaggerated by drugs that induce cytochrome P-2ε1 such as phenytoin, and especially by alcohol (which not only induces cytochrome P-2ε1 but also depletes hepatic glutathione both directly and as a consequence of malnutrition). Therefore, alcoholics taking therapeutic doses of paracetamol, for example, are at risk of developing ALF, particularly after an episode of binge drinking. Prolonged fasting is also a risk factor for paracetamol hepatoxicity. Management of paracetamol overdose is discussed further in Chapter 19.

PATHOLOGICAL CHANGES IN ALF

ALF is the result of cytotoxic and/or cytopathic injury. Hepatotoxic viruses, drugs or their toxic metabolites and other toxins can cause direct cytotoxic injury. Cytopathic injury, on the other hand, is caused by an immune-mediated injury to hepatocytes that express abnormal cell surface antigens (e.g. idiosyncratic drug reactions).

In ALF there is massive coagulative necrosis of liver cells throughout the hepatic lobule, often with preservation of the reticular framework, although ultimately the normal reticulin architecture of the lobule collapses. There may be infiltration with polymorphonuclear cells, lymphocytes, mononuclear cells or eosinophils, interspersed with islands of regenerating hepatocytes. In viral ALF the initial injury involves the periportal region, but then spreads to encompass all zones. In contrast, drug-induced injury and ischaemic damage begin around the central vein and spread rapidly to involve the periportal region. Severe fatty degeneration with accumulation of microventricular fat in intact cells is seen in ALF associated with pregnancy, Reye's syndrome and sodium valproate or tetracycline administration.

CLINICAL FEATURES, INVESTIGATIONS AND DIAGNOSIS (Tables 14.2 and 14.3)

The clinical features of ALF are largely attributable to failure of the normal functions of the liver (synthesis, storage and detoxification). Typically patients present with jaundice, coagulopathy, marked elevation of liver aminotransferases and, by definition, encephalopathy. Certain patterns of presentation, which may be indicative of the aetiology, have been described. For example, patients with paracetamol overdose typically present with severe coagulopathy and encephalopathy, but may not be jaundiced, whereas those with non-A, non-B hepatitis are usually deeply jaundiced at presentation and are less likely to develop cerebral oedema. Many patients subsequently develop sepsis, cardiovascular instability, metabolic acidosis, renal failure, cerebral oedema and multiple-organ failure.

Hepatic encephalopathy

The syndrome of ALF is differentiated from severe acute hepatitis by the development of encephalopathy. This presents as an acute mental disturbance which usually progresses over several days, but deep coma may develop in just a few hours. Occasionally the evolution of the disease is prolonged over several months. Often, the initial changes are subtle (e.g. a change in personality, lack of attention to personal detail, perhaps with euphoria or depression and some slowing of mentation). Later, the patient may become confused and begin to behave inappropriately. Drowsiness is a prominent feature and some patients will sleep continually, although at this stage they can be roused. Difficulty with writing and an inability to reproduce shapes (e.g. a star) accurately are characteristic (*constructional apraxia*); these skills can be tested repeatedly in order to follow the patient's progress. A 'flapping' tremor (*asterixis*) can often be demonstrated at this stage and is associated with a rigid facies, muscle stiffness and dysarthria. Some patients may become extremely agitated as their level of coma deepens; they may require sedation and mechanical ventilation to ensure their safety. Many patients will then lose consciousness and progress to deep coma with hypertonia, decerebrate and/or decorticate posturing and disturbances of vital reflexes.

Hepatic encephalopathy can be classified clinically into five grades, as shown in **Table 14.4**. In practice, however, such classifications are complicated by spontaneous fluctuations in coma grade and the necessity to administer sedatives to patients who are agitated or aggressive or to enable invasive procedures to be performed.

The *electroencephalographic (EEG) changes* (**Fig. 14.1**) correlate with the degree of cerebral dysfunction and, although not necessary to establish the diagnosis, serial EEGs can be performed, together with regular clinical assessment of the grade of encephalopathy, in order to follow the patient's progress.

Cerebral oedema may be present in over 80% of patients with grade IV encephalopathy, although more recent studies suggest that the incidence has fallen to around 40%. Cerebral oedema is uncommon in patients with SFHF and chronic liver disease.

Other clinical features

In the early stages, the liver may be palpable, although later in the illness it becomes small. Signs of chronic liver disease such as palmar erythema, spider naevi, splenomegaly and

Table 14.2 Clinical features of fulminant hepatic failure

Encephalopathy	
Cerebral oedema	
Jaundice	
Hepatic foetor, nausea, vomiting, right-upper-quadrant pain	
Coagulopathy and bleeding	Reduced synthesis of clotting factors Thrombocytopenia Upper gastrointestinal haemorrhage Haemorrhage from nasopharynx, respiratory tract and into retroperitoneal space
Metabolic disturbances	Hypoglycaemia Metabolic alkalosis Lactic acidosis
Electrolyte disturbances	Hypokalaemia Hyponatraemia Hypernatraemia (unusual) Hypomagnesaemia Hypocalcaemia Hypophosphataemia

Cardiovascular dysfunction	Hypotension
	Vasodilatation
	Increased cardiac output
	Microcirculatory dysfunction:
	    Maldistribution of flow
	        Increased capillary permeability
	        Tissue hypoxia

Respiratory dysfunction	Hyperventilation Intrapulmonary shunts Acute lung injury/acute respiratory distress syndrome Pulmonary aspiration Atelectasis Bronchopneumonia
Impaired host defences and sepsis	Bacteraemia Spontaneous bacterial peritonitis Pneumonia Urinary tract infections Translocation of gut-derived organisms and cell wall components
Renal dysfunction	Prerenal Acute tubular necrosis (Hepatorenal syndrome)
Pancreatitis	
Rare complications	Myocarditis Pneumonia caused by atypical organisms Aplastic anaemia Transverse myelitis Peripheral neuropathy

ascites are usually absent, but when ALF follows a more protracted course, both spider naevi and ascites may occur. In some cases, the patient may present with nausea, vomiting and abdominal pain (often in the right upper quadrant), suggestive of an 'acute abdomen'.

The signs of encephalopathy are usually accompanied by rapidly increasing *jaundice* and a characteristic *hepatic foetor*, an unpleasant sweetish smell due to exhalation of mercaptans. The rise in serum bilirubin concentration is associated with the appearance of bilirubin and its breakdown products in the urine. The diagnosis may, however, be difficult if the mental disturbance precedes the development of clinical jaundice. This occurs particularly in children with ALF and in adults who have taken a paracetamol overdose.

Table 14.3 Investigations in fulminant hepatic failure

Daily	Bilirubin, alkaline phosphatase, aminotransferases
	Haemoglobin, white blood count
	Prothrombin time, platelet count
	Urea, creatinine, sodium, potassium, magnesium
	Total protein, albumin, calcium, phosphate
	Chest radiograph, ECG
More frequently	Blood sugar
	Blood gases
	Acid–base
When indicated	Cultures of blood, urine, sputum, intravascular cannulae
	ECG, CT scan, ultrasonography
	Ammonia levels
	Liver biopsy
To establish aetiology	Serological investigations for viral hepatitis
	Drug screen (especially paracetamol)
	Plasma caeruloplasmin concentration and urinary copper excretion for Wilson's disease

CT, computed tomography; ECG, electrocardiogram.

Serum aminotransferase levels are initially nearly always markedly elevated, often to more than 2000 u/L, but the alkaline phosphatase level is usually only moderately raised. Serum albumin, because of its long half-life, generally remains normal until later in the illness. A fall in aminotransferase levels despite increasing hyperbilirubinaemia and a worsening coagulopathy indicate total destruction of liver cells and is associated with a very poor prognosis. Plasma levels of α-fetoprotein, prealbumin and factor V, as well as the prothrombin time, have been used as prognostic indicators (see below). Blood ammonia levels are usually increased, although routine determination of ammonia levels is not recommended (see below).

BLEEDING

Patients with ALF invariably develop a severe *coagulopathy*. The prothrombin time (or the international normalized ratio (INR) for prothrombin) is always markedly prolonged, reflecting reduced hepatic synthesis of clotting factors (V, VII, IX and X). Later this may be compounded by a fall in fibrinogen levels. The production of factors XI and XII may also be impaired. The prothrombin time and coagulation factor V levels (Izumi *et al.*, 1996) can be a useful guide to the progress and prognosis of ALF. Factor VIII, which is synthesized in vascular endothelium, is markedly elevated in ALF and a ratio of factor VIII to V of more than 30 has been associated with a poor prognosis (Pereira *et al.*, 1992). A number of anticoagulation factors, such as protein C and protein S, are also synthesized by the liver and the coagulation profile in ALF may become difficult to distinguish from DIC, especially since *thrombocytopenia* is also common. The latter may be due to hypersplenism, bone marrow

Table 14.4 A grading system for hepatic encephalopathy

Grade	Level of consciousness	Personality and intellect	Neurological signs	Electroencephalographic abnormalities
0	Normal	Normal	None	None
Subclinical	Normal	Normal	Abnormalities only on psychometric analysis	None
1	Inverted sleep pattern, restlessness	Forgetfulness, mild confusion, agitation, irritability	Tremor, apraxia, incoordination, impaired handwriting	Triphasic waves (5 cycles/second)
2	Lethargy, slow responses	Disorientation as regards time, amnesia, decreased inhibitions, inappropriate behaviour	Asterixis, dysarthria, ataxia, hypoactive reflexes	Triphasic waves (5 cycles/second)
3	Somnolence but rousable, confusion	Disorientation as regards place, aggressive behaviour	Asterixis, hyperactive reflexes, Babinski signs, muscle rigidity	Triphasic waves (5 cycles/second)
4	Coma	None	Decerebration	Delta activity

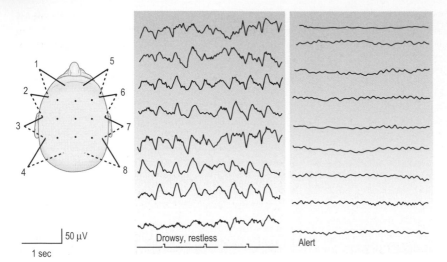

Drowsy, restless

Alert

Fig. 14.1 Electroencephalographic changes in hepatic coma. High-voltage slow waves with some triphasic components best seen at the front of the head.

suppression or DIC. Functional platelet abnormalities have also been described in association with morphological changes; platelet adhesion is increased, but aggregation decreased. The platelet count tends to decrease progressively during the course of ALF and is lower in those who die.

Upper gastrointestinal haemorrhage is a potentially lethal complication of ALF and may be related to oesophagitis, gastric erosions or duodenal ulceration. Acute portal hypertension commonly develops after about 3 weeks and may result in variceal haemorrhage. Bleeding may also occur from the nasopharynx, the respiratory tract or into the retroperitoneal space. Intracerebral haemorrhage is unusual.

METABOLIC DISTURBANCES

Hypoglycaemia is common and may be due to raised plasma insulin levels combined with depletion of glycogen stores and a failure of hepatic gluconeogenesis. The development of a *metabolic alkalosis* is probably related to hypokalaemia and defective urea synthesis. In the later stages of ALF a *lactic acidosis* is common, probably reflecting both anaerobic metabolism and reduced clearance of lactate. The development of a metabolic acidosis is associated with a poor prognosis.

ELECTROLYTE DISTURBANCES

In the absence of renal failure there is a marked tendency to *hypokalaemia* due to inadequate potassium intake, vomiting and secondary hyperaldosteronism. *Hypomagnesaemia* can be precipitated by the excessive use of diuretics. *Hyponatraemia* is also common, especially later in the course of ALF, and is due to redistribution of sodium into the cells combined with increased renal retention of water. *Hypernatraemia*, on the other hand, is unusual but can be precipitated by the sodium load in transfusions of fresh frozen plasma (FFP), human albumin solution (HAS) or colloidal solutions and is sometimes exacerbated by dehydration due to hyperglycaemia or diuretic administration. *Hypocalcaemia* may occur. *Hypophosphataemia* is common. Interestingly, in

patients with severe paracetamol-induced hepatotoxicity, hyperphosphataemia (perhaps caused by renal dysfunction in the absence of hepatic regeneration) has been associated with a poor outcome (Schmidt and Dalhoff, 2002).

CARDIOVASCULAR DYSFUNCTION (see Chapter 5)

Hypotension is common, even in the absence of haemorrhage or obvious sepsis, and is associated with a poor prognosis. The *peripheral resistance is low and cardiac output is usually increased*. Even when blood pressure is normal, severe tissue hypoxia may be present, as evidenced by a metabolic acidosis and raised blood lactate levels. Furthermore, there is an inverse correlation between the mixed venous lactate concentration and both the systemic vascular resistance and the oxygen extraction ratio, suggesting that vasodilation is associated with *maldistribution of microcirculatory flow* and tissue hypoxia (Bihari *et al.*, 1985). There is also a generalized *increase in capillary permeability* leading to hypovolaemia and interstitial oedema. It has been postulated that the hyperdynamic circulation that is characteristic of liver failure may be related to induction of nitric oxide (NO) synthase, possibly in response to endotoxaemia (Vallance and Moncada, 1991). Certainly impaired Kupffer cell function and the presence of portosystemic shunts may promote bacteraemia/endotoxaemia and exaggerate the inflammatory response.

Arrhythmias are also common and may be related to hypoxia, acid–base disturbances or electrolyte abnormalities.

RESPIRATORY DYSFUNCTION

A *respiratory alkalosis* due to hyperventilation is common in the early stages of ALF and may be a result of stimulation of the respiratory centre by toxins or an intracellular acidosis. Later, hypoxic depression of the respiratory centre may supervene and sudden unexpected *respiratory arrest* may occur, in some cases related to severe intracranial hypertension.

Many patients with ALF will be *hypoxaemic* and this may be due to intrapulmonary shunts (associated with diffuse dilatation of the pulmonary vasculature and, in some cases, pleural spider naevi) or pulmonary oedema. The commonest abnormality is *non-cardiogenic pulmonary oedema* (acute lung injury/acute respiratory distress syndrome (ALI/ARDS); see Chapter 8), which occurred in more than a third of patients in one series and is often associated with cerebral oedema (Baudouin *et al.*, 1995). It has been suggested that precapillary arteriolar dilatation disrupts pulmonary capillaries by exposing them to an increased hydrostatic pressure, but it seems more likely that the development of ALI/ARDS is simply a manifestation of the generalized increase in capillary permeability.

The presence of ascites may contribute to respiratory difficulty. Respiratory dysfunction may also be related to *pulmonary aspiration, atelectasis* or *bronchopneumonia*.

IMPAIRED HOST DEFENCES AND SEPSIS

A number of abnormalities have been identified as contributing to the increased susceptibility of patients with ALF to infection. These include a *deficiency of complement* factors involved in both the classical and alternative pathways (Wyke *et al.*, 1980), impaired opsonization, a *reduced chemoattractant activity* of patients' sera for normal polymorphonuclear leukocytes (Wyke *et al.*, 1982a) and a *reduction in plasma fibronectin levels* (Gonzalez Calvin *et al.*, 1982). It has also been suggested that decreased hepatic production of hepatocyte growth factor-like/macrophage-stimulating protein might cause impaired Kupffer cell phagocytosis in ALF (Harrison *et al.*, 1994). Consequently, bacteraemia/bacterial infections are relatively common and are most often due to Gram-positive organisms (mainly streptococci and *Staphylococcus aureus* in the early stages, with coagulase-negative staphylococci and enterococci being encountered later), whereas *Escherichia coli* is the commonest type of Gram-negative organism isolated (Wade *et al.*, 2003; Wyke *et al.*, 1982b). Common sites of infection include peritoneum, lung, intravascular devices and urinary tract. Line sepsis, cholangitis and endocarditis also occur. Fungal infections are sometimes seen, usually after the first week of intensive care. The usual signs of infection such as fever and leukocytosis are often absent.

RENAL DYSFUNCTION (Eckardt, 1999)

Renal impairment is common in patients with ALF and occurs in up to 75% of cases secondary to paracetamol overdose and in 30% of all other cases. The aetiology is usually multifactorial. Prerenal factors such as intravascular volume depletion due to gastrointestinal haemorrhage, diarrhoea or excessive diuretic administration are frequently implicated. Acute tubular necrosis (ATN) may be precipitated by hypotension, sepsis, DIC or the administration of nephrotoxic drugs. Patients with jaundice generally appear to be at increased risk of developing ATN. Occasionally combined liver and renal disease may be due to a common pathogenic mechanism which directly or indirectly affects both organs (e.g. glomerulonephritis associated with viral hepatitis). Paracetamol may cause direct renal toxicity and renal failure occurs in more than 75% of cases of paracetamol poisoning.

Hepatorenal syndrome (Epstein, 1992) (see also Chapter 13). This is a diagnosis of exclusion and can be defined as renal failure occurring in a patient with liver failure in the absence of clinical, laboratory or anatomical evidence of other possible causes. In clinical practice it can be difficult to distinguish hepatorenal syndrome from other causes of acute renal failure. Renal impairment is considered to be *functional* and *reversible* because:

- pathological lesions are minimal and inconsistent;
- normal function returns if the liver recovers;
- kidneys from patients with hepatorenal syndrome function normally after transplantation into recipients with normal liver function (Koppel *et al.*, 1969);
- renal function recovers when patients with hepatorenal syndrome undergo successful liver transplantation (Gonwa *et al.*, 1991).

The pathogenesis of hepatorenal syndrome remains obscure, but renal dysfunction appears to be related to intense intra-renal vasoconstriction with preferential cortical ischaemia and reduced glomerular filtration which is unresponsive to expansion of the circulating volume. The factors responsible for these changes have not yet been fully elucidated, but possibilities include:

- diminished perfusion pressure;
- endotoxaemia;
- hepatorenal and portorenal reflexes;
- activation of the renin–angiotensin system;
- increased sympathetic nervous system activity;
- alterations in the balance between vasodilator prostaglandins and vasoconstrictor thromboxanes;
- a relative impairment of renal kallikrein production.

There is also some evidence to suggest that *endothelins* are involved in the pathogenesis of the hepatorenal syndrome (Moore *et al.*, 1992; Soper *et al.*, 1996).

Since renal tubular function is preserved in the face of a reduced GFR, the capacity for sodium reabsorption and the concentration of urine are relatively normal. In contrast to ATN, therefore, urine sodium is low (< 10 mmol/L), urine osmolality is high (> 1000 mosmol/kg) and the urine-to-plasma creatinine ratio is higher than 10. Blood urea may be deceptively low because of the reduced capacity of the liver to metabolize ammonia to urea. Nevertheless, using electron microscopy some degree of tubular damage can be demonstrated (Mandal *et al.*, 1982) and most believe that hepatorenal syndrome can evolve into ATN. The prognosis of hepatorenal syndrome is poor.

PANCREATITIS

Biochemical and radiological evidence of pancreatitis may be found in more than 30% of patients with ALF and should be suspected in those with cardiovascular instability or hypocalaemia. Pancreatitis is associated with more severe multiple-organ dysfunction, more rapid deterioration and an increased mortality.

RARE COMPLICATIONS

Rare complications of ALF include:

- myocarditis;
- pneumonia due to atypical organisms;
- aplastic anaemia;
- transverse myelitis;
- peripheral neuropathy.

Establishing the cause of ALF

It is important to determine the cause of ALF because:

- in some cases specific therapy may be indicated;
- there may be implications for the spontaneous recovery of liver function;
- screening of family members (e.g. Wilson's disease) or close contacts (e.g. viral hepatitis) may be required.

Clinical examination is usually unhelpful but the likely cause of ALF can often be ascertained from a careful history.

Hepatitis B infection is associated with intravenous drug abuse, blood transfusion and inoculation injuries, while *hepatitis A and E* arise from ingestion of contaminated food or water and often occur in epidemics. The hepatitis B virus may also be spread via contaminated acupuncture needles, by tattooing and by close personal contact (e.g. sexual intercourse, particularly in homosexuals).

Serological investigations should include hepatitis A immunoglobulin M (IgM) antibody, hepatitis B core antigen antibody (HBcAb), hepatitis B surface antigen (HBsAg), hepatitis B e antigen (HBeAg) and hepatitis B DNA, as well as hepatitis C, D and E serology.

There may be a history of drug ingestion (intentional, with or without suicidal intent, or accidental) or exposure to poisons or chemicals. Appropriate *drug screening*, especially for paracetamol, should then be performed.

Halothane hepatitis should be suspected when the signs of hepatocellular necrosis, often accompanied by fever and chills, develop within 2 weeks of exposure.

Acute fatty liver of pregnancy usually presents as nausea, repeated vomiting and abdominal pain between the 30th and 38th week of gestation, and may continue to deteriorate even following delivery.

When *Wilson's disease* is suspected, plasma caeruloplasmin levels and urinary copper excretion should be determined pre- and post-penicillinamine challenge. The eyes should be examined for Kayser–Fleischer rings. If present they confirm the diagnosis, but their absence does not exclude the condition.

Liver biopsy may confirm the aetiology of ALF and can determine the degree of hepatocyte necrosis. This may provide some indication of prognosis, although sampling error may misrepresent the overall degree of necrosis. More-

over the presence of coaglopathy usually precludes the percutaneous approach and the transjugular route may therefore be preferred. In practice liver biopsy is indicated only very occasionally, usually to exclude underlying cirrhosis or malignancy (e.g. lymphoma).

Imaging the liver by ultrasound or computed tomography (CT) scanning may be useful to exclude hepatic vein thrombosis, chronic liver disease, space-occupying lesions or biliary obstruction, as well as to determine liver size and to assess liver vasculature if transplantation is contemplated.

PATHOGENESIS OF ENCEPHALOPATHY AND CEREBRAL OEDEMA

Altered cerebral metabolism, abnormal neurotransmitter function, direct effects on neuronal membranes, disturbed activity of Na^+/K^+ ATPase or, most likely, a combination of these factors, are thought to be responsible for the disturbance of neurotransmission that precipitates hepatic encephalopathy (Riordan and Williams, 1997). These abnormalities are in turn largely related to the accumulation of toxic substances normally metabolized by the liver. Although there are many similarities between the clinical and biochemical features of encephalopathy in ALF and chronic liver impairment, there are also a number of respects in which they differ; in particular, cerebral oedema is a common and important complication of ALF, but is extremely rare in chronic liver disease. In both cases, the disturbance of cerebral function is often exacerbated by:

- hypoglycaemia;
- alterations in acid–base homeostasis;
- fluid and electrolyte abnormalities;
- hypoxia and hypercarbia;
- systemic inflammation (usually sepsis).

In addition, patients with ALF are very sensitive to the effects of analgesics and sedatives, not only because of impaired drug metabolism, but also because of increased cerebral sensitivity and changes in plasma protein binding.

Examples of recognized toxins that accumulate in liver failure include:

- ammonia (colonic bacteria probably play a limited role in ammonia production, whereas enterocytes are a major source of ammonia);
- fatty acids;
- bile acids (unlikely to play a role in the pathogenesis of encephalopathy);
- mercaptans (derived from methionine);
- phenols;
- various aromatic amino acids.

The serum *amino acid* profile is abnormal in both chronic liver impairment and ALF. In patients with chronic liver disease and superimposed acute insults, there is an increase in blood levels of the aromatic amino acids and a reduction in the concentrations of the branched-chain amino acids.

This abnormality is probably the result of increased catabolism as well as impaired liver function. Circulating levels of aromatic amino acids are also markedly increased in ALF, but in this situation the concentration of branched-chain amino acids is normal. It is thought that this altered amino acid profile is caused by massive hepatocellular necrosis with release of amino acids into the circulation and that catabolism plays a less important role. The high circulating levels of aromatic amino acids combined with their enhanced uptake by active carrier systems and disruption of the blood–brain barrier could lead to increased intracerebral concentrations of phenylalanine, tyrosine and tryptophan. The excess tyrosine might then be converted to *octopamine*, while phenylalanine could be metabolized first to phenylethylamine and then *phenylethanolamine*. These substances are thought to act as weak (or *false*) *neurotransmitters*, displacing some of the normal transmitter compounds such as dopamine and noradrenaline (norepinephrine). Furthermore, tryptophan can be converted into the inhibitory neurotransmitter *serotonin*, and the intracerebral formation of normal excitatory transmitters may be reduced by competition for enzyme systems.

Although blood levels of *ammonia* are elevated in hepatic failure, there is a poor correlation between the blood ammonia concentration and the grade of encephalopathy. Moreover, it is difficult to reconcile the central nervous system depression that characterizes hepatic encephalopathy with the neuroexcitatory properties of ammonia. Nevertheless when urea synthesis is impaired by severe liver dysfunction, an alternative detoxification pathway involves the synthesis of *glutamine* from ammonia and glutamate. The consequent intracellular accumulation of glutamine causes brain swelling (Balata *et al.*, 2003) and may result in a rapid exchange of brain glutamine for neutral plasma amino acids; this provides a possible link between the neurotoxicity of ammonia and the false-neurotransmitter hypothesis (James *et al.*, 1979).

There is, however, some evidence against the false-transmitter theory, and a number of other mechanisms have been postulated. For example, it has been suggested that in ALF blood levels of γ-aminobutyric acid (GABA)-like compounds are markedly increased, probably because of reduced hepatic metabolism. In addition, the number of postsynaptic binding sites for GABA in the brain is increased (Schafer and Jones, 1982). Since the blood–brain barrier is disrupted in ALF, the concentration of GABA-like compounds within the brain could rise, thereby contributing to neural inhibition. The increase in GABA binding sites may also partly explain the enhanced sensitivity of these patients to sedatives. Postsynaptic GABA receptors are coupled to benzodiazepine receptors and there is now evidence that in a subpopulation of patients with ALF, GABAergic neurotransmission is enhanced by elevated levels of *benzodiazepine receptor agonist* ligands, perhaps derived from the patient's diet or enteric flora (Basile *et al.*, 1991; Editorial, 1991; Mullen, 1991). This hypothesis is supported by the observation that benzodiaz-

epine receptor antagonists can improve conscious level in hepatic encephalopathy (Grimm *et al.*, 1988).

The cause of *cerebral oedema* also remains uncertain but the permeability of the blood–brain barrier may be increased by circulating toxins (vasogenic oedema), and inhibition of $Na^+ K^+$ ATPase may lead to intracellular accumulation of sodium and water (cytotoxic oedema). As has been mentioned, the osmotic effects of glutamine, a product of cerebral ammonia detoxification, may also contribute. In support of this hypothesis, arterial ammonia levels have been shown to correlate with the development of brain herniation in ALF patients (Clemmesen *et al.*, 1999). Cerebral autoregulation is lost, cerebral blood flow becomes pressure-dependent (Larsen *et al.*, 2000), and in contrast to many other conditions associated with intracranial hypertension, cerebral blood flow is often reduced. In some studies, however, cerebral blood flow was found to be normal and others have suggested that cerebral hyperaemia may precede or coincide with the presence of cerebral oedema on CT scan. In patients with grade IV encephalopathy cerebral blood flow varies widely and, in those who developed clinical signs of cerebral oedema, correlates with the cerebral metabolic rate for oxygen ($CMRO_2$). Moreover in many of these patients the brain produces lactate, providing further evidence that cerebral oxygen delivery is frequently inadequate (Wendon *et al.*, 1994). Substantial increases in cerebral blood flow can be demonstrated following infusion of mannitol and N-acetylcysteine; this is associated with a rise in cerebral oxygen utilization and a reduction in anaerobic metabolism.

MANAGEMENT (Table 14.5) (Caraceni and Van Thiel, 1995)
General aspects
In the great majority of those who survive an episode of ALF, liver architecture returns essentially to normal and the development of cirrhosis is very unusual (Karvountzis *et al.*, 1974). Aggressive management of ALF is therefore based on the premise that if the patient is supported through the acute illness, regeneration of the liver will be associated with complete recovery. There is some support for the hypothesis that a number of hepatocytes usually survive the initial insult, but are functionally impaired by persisting ischaemia/hypoxia, perhaps related in part to vascular obstruction. Reversal of haemodynamic and respiratory abnormalities is therefore a fundamental aspect of supportive care for the patient with ALF. It is likely, however, that at least in some cases, hepatic necrosis will be so extensive that liver regeneration is not possible.

Patients with ALF should be admitted to an intensive care unit as soon as their conscious level deteriorates and should then, if possible, be transferred to a specialist centre once they have been resuscitated and stabilized. If transfer to a specialized unit is not indicated, or is logistically impossible, the case must at least be discussed with a specialist from a liver unit. It has been suggested that those with worsening encephalopathy, metabolic acidosis and hypoglycaemia in

Table 14.5 Management of fulminant hepatic failure

Monitoring	Temperature Electrocardiogram Intra-arterial pressure Central venous pressure
In selected cases	Pulmonary artery catheterization or other invasive haemodynamic monitoring Cardiac output Oxygen delivery (Do_2), oxygen consumption ($\dot{V}o_2$), lactate Intracranial pressure Cerebral function monitor
Cardiovascular system	Expand circulating volume (colloids: albumin, fresh frozen plasma; blood) Inotropes and vasopressors (dopamine, noradrenaline, adrenaline) Treat arrhythmias conventionally *N*-acetylcysteine
Respiratory support	Secure airway Protect lungs from aspiration Avoid hypoxia and hypercarbia Endotracheal intubation ± continuous positive airways pressure (CPAP) Mechanical ventilation ± positive end-expiratory pressure (PEEP)
Renal dysfunction	Prevent renal failure (volume replacement, optimize cardiac output and blood pressure) Continuous haemofiltration
Cerebral oedema	Mannitol ± furosemide Hyperventilation (beware excessive cerebral vasoconstriction) Thiopental or propofol Moderate hypothermia
Encephalopathy	Correct precipitating factors Avoid sedatives Treat convulsions If blood is suspected in gastrointestinal tract, give enema (e.g. 80 mL magnesium sulphate in 50% solution w/v) 2–3 times a day until no melaena Lactulose 60 mL followed by 30 mL 8-hourly, p.o. or nasogastric may also be given Elective ventilation for those with grade 3 or 4 encephalopathy
Hypoglycaemia	Continuous intravenous infusion 10–20% dextrose Intravenous boluses of 50% dextrose as required to maintain blood sugar > 4 mmol/L
Bleeding	Fresh frozen plasma for active bleeding Platelets if platelet count < 50 000 × 10^6 cells/L (depending on the circumstances) Fresh frozen plasma and platelets before invasive procedures Vitamin K 10 mg daily H_2-receptor blockade or proton pump inhibitor in all cases
Fluids and electrolytes	Large quantities intravenous potassium chloride Restrict sodium intake to < 50 mmol/day Hydration with dextrose solutions
Prevention of infection	Prophylactic antibiotics Oral antifungal agents
Extracorporeal liver assist	
Liver transplantation	
Precautions to minimize risk of cross-infection	

the presence of a coagulopathy and/or renal failure require urgent transfer to a specialist unit (Rahman and Hodgson, 2001).

Successful management depends largely on the quality of supportive care combined with an awareness of the potential complications, so that they can be either prevented or recognized early and treated appropriately. It is also important to be aware of the effects of ALF and the often associated acute renal failure, on the actions and elimination of drugs.

Precautions against cross-infection

All intensive care unit staff should be vaccinated against hepatitis B virus. In the event of an inoculation injury or permucosal exposure to blood or high-risk body fluids, those whose immune status is unknown should receive hepatitis B immune globulin as soon as possible. They should then be tested for HBsAb and, if negative, vaccination should be started immediately. Following exposure to hepatitis A virus a single intramuscular dose of immune globulin should be given as soon as possible.

Stringent measures to prevent cross-infection and minimize the dangers to staff should be instituted in all cases of viral hepatitis or when the aetiology of liver failure is uncertain. Initially all cases of ALF should be considered to be infectious. Particular care is required when handling blood, urine or faeces, and it is most important to avoid contamination of conjunctivae, cuts or abrasions, as well as self-inoculation. Safe practice for handling sharps includes:

- Discard immediately into approved containers.
- Never resheath a needle.
- Do not leave needles on syringes.
- Never overfill a sharps box.
- Do not leave loose sharps on trolleys or towels following procedures.

Saliva and tears are also potentially infective. Staff should wear an impermeable apron and gloves when performing medical or nursing procedures; masks and protective goggles should be used when the risk of conjunctival inoculation is considered to be high. Frequent handwashing is essential; cuts and abrasions should be covered with a waterproof dressing. Because staff are frequently unaware that a particular patient is carrying a blood-borne virus it is now recommended that these safe practices should be adopted universally (*universal precautions*).

Excreta should be disposed of immediately. Hypochlorite is the disinfectant of choice, and a hypochlorite detergent (1000 parts per million) should be used for cleaning the bed area and equipment. Contaminated items, excreta and laboratory specimens should be clearly labelled as high-risk. Automated analysers should be similarly labelled.

Hypoglycaemia

Blood sugar levels should be determined at least 2 hourly. Hypoglycaemia can be avoided by giving a continuous intra-venous infusion of 10% or 20% dextrose, supplemented as necessary by bolus doses of 50 mL 50% dextrose, to maintain the blood sugar level above 4 mmol/L. There is also, however, a danger of precipitating hyperglycaemia because of impaired glucose uptake by the liver, a complication that may be associated with lactic acidosis.

Nutrition

Feeding should be instituted as soon as possible. Enteral nutrition is nearly always well tolerated. There is no evidence to support protein restriction in ALF; calories and protein should be given as indicated by the clinical circumstances. Calorie requirements are increased in ALF. Branched-chain amino acid solutions have not been shown to improve encephalopathy or overall mortality rate.

Bleeding

Spontaneous haemorrhage is uncommon. Prophylactic correction of the clotting factor deficiency with infusions of FFP does not appear to influence the overall mortality and may precipitate sodium overload and possibly DIC. Also the fall in INR which may follow administration of FFP limits the value of this variable as a prognostic indicator. Administration of FFP is only indicated in those with active bleeding. Platelet transfusions are rarely indicated, but, depending on the circumstances, are often given if the platelet count is less than $50\,000 \times 10^6$ cells/L. FFP should also be administered prior to surgical procedures and vascular cannulation. Vitamin K 10 mg should be administered daily, although this generally has little demonstrable effect. Blood losses should be replaced as indicated.

Upper gastrointestinal haemorrhage can be virtually eliminated if gastric pH is maintained above 5 by the administration of an H_2-receptor antagonist (Macdougall *et al.*, 1977). Alternatively a proton pump inhibitor can be used (see Chapter 11).

Electrolyte disturbances

Large quantities of intravenous potassium chloride are usually required to correct hypokalaemia. Hydration should be maintained with 5%, 10% or 20% glucose as required to maintain blood sugar levels above 4 mmol/L. In hyperacute liver failure hyponatraemia may be precipitated by excessive volumes of glucose solutions. Hypernatraemia normally responds to careful rehydration. Excessive sodium administration must be avoided.

Cardiovascular support

Adequate expansion of the circulating volume with colloids and blood as indicated is essential, guided by the central venous pressure (CVP), the urine output and, in some cases, the pulmonary artery occlusion pressure (PAOP). If this fails to restore the blood pressure, there should be no hesitation before instituting treatment with a pressor agent, particularly since, in the presence of raised intracranial pressure (ICP), hypotension can precipitate cerebral ischaemia.

Dopamine is often chosen initially, although high doses may be necessary to produce some vasoconstriction and reverse hypotension. Many now recommend the use of noradrenaline to restore the systemic vascular resistance, while others suggest that adrenaline (epinephrine) is a suitable agent. Pulmonary artery catheterization or other forms of invasive haemodynamic monitoring may be indicated (see Chapter 4).

Administration of *N-acetylcysteine* to patients with ALF has been shown to increase cardiac output, oxygen delivery (DO_2), oxygen extraction and oxygen consumption ($\dot{V}O_2$). Despite a fall in systemic resistance, blood pressure also increased (Harrison *et al.*, 1991). The authors suggest that these effects might account for the improved survival associated with delayed administration of acetylcysteine to patients with paracetamol-induced ALF (Harrison *et al.*, 1990). There is also evidence to suggest that *N*-acetylcysteine can improve liver blood flow and function in patients with septic shock (Hein *et al.*, 2004; Rank *et al.*, 2000). The mechanism of these beneficial effects of *N*-acetylcysteine is unclear, although this agent is a potent antioxidant and repletes tissue sulphydryl groups, perhaps thereby promoting NO production in the microcirculation. In a controlled, prospective study, however, *N*-acetylcysteine had no significant haemodynamic effects in a small group of patients with advanced encephalopathy, neither was there any suggestion of clinically relevant improvements in global $\dot{V}O_2$, or in clinical markers of tissue hypoxia (Walsh *et al.*, 1998). The results of large prospective, randomized, controlled, clinical trials are awaited. In the meantime some specialist units recommend *N*-acetylcysteine, given for 5 days only, for paracetamol-induced ALF.

Respiratory support

Control of the airway and protection of the lungs from aspiration of blood or stomach contents is essential, and patients with ALF should be intubated early – certainly as soon as the airway-protective reflexes are depressed. Because the conscious level can deteriorate rapidly it has been recommended that patients should be sedated and intubated if encephalopathy progresses to grade III (Rahman and Hodgson, 2001). Continuous positive airways pressure (CPAP) can be used to maintain adequate oxygenation in spontaneously breathing patients. Hypercarbia and hypoxaemia should be avoided by early institution of mechanical ventilation, although it is important to remember that the institution of intermittent positive pressure ventilation (IPPV) may be associated with a marked reduction in hepatic perfusion if cardiac output is allowed to fall. Mechanical ventilation is also indicated when there is evidence of respiratory muscle fatigue (see Chapters 7 and 8). Positive end-expiratory pressure (PEEP) may be required and the underlying pulmonary abnormality should be treated as outlined in Chapter 8. Sedation is normally with propofol or, if haemodynamic function is compromised, a benzodiazepine such are lorazepam combined with an opiate such

as fentanyl. On the rare occasion that muscle relaxation is required, atracurium has been recommended (Riordan and Williams, 1997).

Renal support

Even though the development of renal failure is not necessarily related to the severity of liver impairment (ATN may occur without encephalopathy, for example), its onset is associated with an increased mortality. Prevention of renal failure is therefore of paramount importance. Maintenance of an adequate circulating volume, blood pressure and cardiac output is essential. Volume expansion may increase renal ammonia excretion, thereby ameliorating encephalopathy. Continuous haemodiafiltration is indicated for those with established renal failure or resistant fluid overload. High-volume haemofiltration may also be used (see Chapter 13). Care must be taken in the selection of replacement fluids since patients will not be able to metabolize many of the standard solutions in which lactate or acetate is the predominant buffer. Bicarbonate buffered solutions are well tolerated. Anticoagulation can be difficult, not least because of heparin resistance caused by concurrent antithrombin III deficiency. Supplemental antithrombin III can decrease heparin requirements and platelet consumption. Regional heparinization, in which blood returning to the patient from the machine is infused with protamine sulphate, or the use of prostacyclin is an alternative strategy.

There is evidence to suggest that terlipressin, especially when combined with albumin administration, can reverse hepatorenal syndrome in a high proportion of patients (Ortega *et al.*, 2002) and there is some indication that early administration of *N*-acetylcysteine can improve renal function in such cases (Holt *et al.*, 1999). It is important to appreciate that the hepatorenal syndrome is usually fatal if liver function does not improve and transplantation is not possible. In some patients with acute-on-chronic liver failure and no expectation of significant liver regeneration it may be appropriate, therefore, to withhold renal replacement therapy.

Prevention of infection

Prevention and early treatment of infectious episodes are crucial. Daily samples of urine, sputum and blood should be sent for microscopy and culture. Ascitic fluid and wound swabs should be examined at regular intervals and cultured when clinically indicated. Prophylactic antibiotics decrease the incidence of infectious episodes (Rolando *et al.*, 1996) but have not been shown to improve survival and the value of selective decontamination of the digestive tract remains uncertain (see Chapter 12). All patients should be given local oral antifungal treatment.

Cerebral oedema

Clinical features such as systemic hypertension, decerebrate posturing, hyperventilation and pupillary abnormalities are late signs of raised ICP. Some therefore recommend ICP measurement to detect significant cerebral oedema and rationalize management of intracranial hypertension in all patients with grade 3 or 4 encephalopathy, especially those who are candidates for transplantation. Others feel that the complications, in particular intracranial bleeding, outweigh the benefits. It has also been suggested that a cerebral perfusion pressure persistently less than 40 mmHg despite aggressive treatment should preclude transplantation, although it has been reported that 4 patients with ALF survived neurologically intact despite persistent intracranial hypertension (> 35 mmHg for 24–38 hours) refractory to standard therapy associated with a cerebral perfusion pressure of less than 50 mmHg for 2–72 hours (Davies et al., 1994). The aim should be to maintain the ICP below 20 mmHg and the cerebral perfusion pressure above 60 mmHg, although in many cases this may prove to be impossible because of loss of autoregulation (see Chapter 15).

Prior to insertion of an ICP monitoring device, sufficient FFP and platelets should be given to achieve an INR ≤ 2 and a platelet count > 50 > 10^9/L. Extradural devices are preferred since the complication rates are lower (see Chapter 15).

In the absence of ICP monitoring, intracranial hypertension should be suspected and treated if the pupils dilate or become unequal, react sluggishly or cease to react to light, and in the presence of decorticate/decerebrate posturing, hyperventilation, profuse sweating, opisthotonos or hypertension. Papilloedema is unusual.

CT scanning is neither reliable nor useful for the detection of cerebral oedema, although it may demonstrate the focal intracranial lesions that sometimes accompany ALF.

Jugular venous bulb blood sampling to determine oxygen saturation (S_vO_2) and arteriojugular lactate difference can provide an indirect indication of cerebral oxygen consumption and extraction. Cerebral blood flow and perfusion pressure can be assumed to be adequate when S_vO_2 is between 55 and 75% (see Chapter 15). Transcranial Doppler measurements have also been used for monitoring cerebral blood flow in this situation.

The administration of steroids is of no value in controlling the cerebral oedema associated with ALF, but mannitol is extremely effective in reducing ICP and may improve survival in those with intracranial hypertension (Canalese et al., 1982). Low doses of mannitol (0.5 g/kg over 10 minutes) are effective and can lead to an increase in $CMRO_2$ and a decrease in cerebral lactate production (Wendon et al., 1994). The serum osmolality should not be allowed to increase to above 320 mosmol/kg. Furosemide administration may be required to maintain the osmotic gradient and to allow transfusions of FFP, platelets and blood while avoiding hypervolaemia. In those with renal failure, continuous haemofiltration may create 'space' for the administration of mannitol. Although hyperventilation can restore cerebral autoregulation in patients with ALF (Strauss et al., 1998), the already subnormal cerebral blood flow may be further reduced. The use of hyperventilation therefore remains controversial, although it may have a role in the short-term

management of intracranial hypertension, closely guided by jugular venous oxygen saturation (Rahman and Hodgson, 2001).

Other measures to control intracranial hypertension, including positioning with a 10–20° head-up tilt, can be instituted as outlined in Chapter 15.

Thiopental, or, now more often propofol, may be useful in the treatment of intractable raised ICP associated with ALF (Forbes et al., 1989), although these agents may exacerbate hypotension and hypothermia. N-acetylcysteine increases cerebral blood flow and may reduce the incidence of cerebral oedema, whilst a bolus injection of indometacin has been shown to reduce ICP, and increase cerebral perfusion pressure, without compromising cerebral perfusion or oxidative metabolism (Tofteng and Larsen, 2004). Preliminary evidence suggests that induction of moderate hypothermia by active cooling may help to control refractory intracranial hypertension, whilst reducing circulating ammonia, cerebral ammonia uptake and cerebral metabolic rate (Jalan et al., 1999). Because hypothermia may inhibit hepatic regeneration, this technique should be reserved for patients scheduled for transplantation. It may, however, be sensible to maintain body temperature at or below 36°C in all patients with ALF who are at risk of cerebral oedema.

The value of cerebral function monitoring has been emphasized by the identification of subclinical seizure activity in patients with grade 3 and 4 encephalopathy (Ellis et al., 2000). Importantly, prophylaxis with phenytoin in patients with severe encephalopathy not only decreased the incidence of seizure activity but also reduced cerebral oedema. Lorazepam and propofol are now often used as alternatives to phenytoin.

Encephalopathy (Shawcross and Jalan, 2005)

Identifiable precipitating factors, such as infection/systemic inflammation, dehydration, haemorrhage, drug toxicity, electrolyte disturbances, constipation, hypoxaemia, hypercarbia, hypoglycaemia and acid–base disturbances must be corrected. Sedatives and analgesics may also precipitate or exacerbate coma, as well as hypotension, and should in general be avoided. If sedation is essential, small doses of a benzodiazepine such as lorazepam are recommended. Fentanyl, and if necessary atracurium, can be used in those receiving mechanical ventilation. Convulsions are relatively common and should be treated aggressively (see above and Chapter 15). There is no evidence to support the use of protein restriction in patients with encephalopathy.

Although it is traditional to institute measures designed to minimize the nitrogenous load absorbed from the bowel, this practice is based on the apparent improvement produced in chronic hepatic encephalopathy and there are no controlled data to suggest that such treatment is beneficial in ALF. Nevertheless, if blood is suspected in the gastrointestinal tract, the bowel should be emptied with an enema (e.g. 80 mL magnesium sulphate in 50% solution w/v) repeated 2–3 times a day until there is no melaena. Lactulose may also be given in a starting dose of 60 mL, followed by 30 mL 8-hourly or more frequently, in order to produce two soft bowel motions a day. It is not necessary to induce diarrhoea. Lactulose is a non-absorbable synthetic disaccharide that is not metabolized in the small bowel. It is hydrolysed in the colon to lactic and acetic acid, thereby causing a fermentative diarrhoea, and may act by trapping ammonia in the bowel by virtue of the fall in pH of the colonic contents. A second-generation disaccharide (*lactitol*) is available in more convenient powder form and is more palatable, and less liable to produce flatulence, than lactulose, while being equally effective in chronic stable encephalopathy. In a systematic review, however, it was concluded that there is insufficient evidence to recommend or refute the value of lactulose/lactitol in encephalopathic patients (Als-Nielsen *et al.*, 2004). Further trials are required to establish the effect of these agents not only on the severity of encephalopathy but also on outcome. Oral *neomycin*, 1 g 6-hourly, can be used to sterilize the bowel, but because significant amounts of this drug are absorbed, there is a risk of ototoxicity in those with renal impairment and most centres have now discontinued its routine prescription in ALF. Metronidazole is an alternative.

It has been suggested that manipulation of the abnormal plasma amino acid profile by intravenous infusion of branched-chain amino acids might be beneficial in hepatic encephalopathy, although controlled studies have produced conflicting results. Treatment with benzodiazepine receptor antagonists is not recommended. *L-ornithine L-aspartate* provides intermediates that increase the availability of glutamate, thereby enhancing the ability of muscle to detoxify ammonia and perhaps improving encephalopathy. *Probiotic therapy* may also prove to be useful.

Extracorporeal liver-assist techniques

These are based on the principle that removal of the toxins that accumulate in ALF, together with control of the inflammatory response, may prevent the development of cerebral oedema and provide a more favourable environment for hepatic regeneration (Zieve *et al.*, 1985). Extracorporeal techniques may also support the patient until the native liver regenerates or until transplantation can be performed, perhaps especially if the synthetic and metabolic functions of the liver can be replicated.

Early techniques included exchange transfusions, plasma exchange, cross-circulation with healthy volunteers or patients in irreversible coma, and extracorporeal perfusion of isolated animal (or human) livers. Cross-circulation with healthy humans was, of course, only applicable to those with ALF of non-infectious origin and even then exposed the volunteer to significant risk; its use was soon abandoned.

More recently developed systems rely on the perfusion of hepatocytes within a bioreactor to provide metabolic and synthetic function, in series with a charcoal or resin column. Recently such a device was found to be safe and seemed to improve survival in a subgroup of patients with FHF/SFHF (Demetriou *et al.*, 2004). Non-biological liver support systems are simpler to use but do not provide metabolic or synthetic function. *Charcoal haemoperfusion* was used with considerable enthusiasm in the past. Activated charcoal adsorbs a wide range of water-soluble substances, including those of middle molecular weight. In an early study remarkable results were obtained by instituting charcoal haemoperfusion early (i.e. in grade III encephalopathy) (Gimson *et al.*, 1982), but subsequently a large study indicated that this technique did not significantly influence the overall survival of patients in either grade III or IV hepatic encephalopathy (O'Grady *et al.*, 1988). *Plasmapharesis* is advocated by some groups but controlled clinical trials are required to establish whether this technique has a role in the management of liver failure (Hayes and Lee, 2001). *Haemodialysis* is no longer used for liver support.

The *molecular adsorbent recirculating system (MARS)* uses a double-sided albumin-impregnated, hollow-fibre dialysis membrane as a molecular adsorbent in a closed-loop dialysis circuit (**Fig. 14.2**) (Stange *et al.*, 2000). In patients with liver failure due to a variety of causes (mainly chronic hepatic failure and hepatorenal syndrome but also ALF), treatment with MARS was found to be well tolerated, with no serious adverse events, and was associated with a significant reduction in plasma levels of bilirubin, bile acids, tryptophan, short- and middle-chain fatty acids, aromatic amino acids and ammonia. At the same time the degree of hepatic encephalopathy decreased, mean arterial pressure increased and indices of renal and liver function improved (Mitzner *et al.*, 2001). In patients with hepatorenal syndrome survival was prolonged (Mitzner *et al.*, 2000). In a small study of patients with acute exacerbations of chronic liver disease MARS treatment was associated with a reduction in ICP and jugular bulb oxygen saturation, and an increase in cerebral perfusion pressure (Sorkine *et al.*, 2001).

A meta-analysis concluded that, although artificial liver support systems seem to reduce mortality in acute-on-chronic liver failure, neither artificial nor bioartificial systems appear to influence outcome in ALF (Kjaergard *et al.*, 2003). Nevertheless, larger randomized, controlled trials are required to clarify the role of these techniques in the management of both acute and chronic liver failure (Hayes and Lee, 2001; Kjaergard *et al.*, 2003).

Hepatocyte and stem cell transplantation

Transplantation of isolated fresh and cryopreserved human hepatocytes has been used successfully as a bridge to transplantation (Strom *et al.*, 1997) in patients with decompensated cirrhosis and metabolic disorders. Pluripotent hepatocyte stem cells derived from bone marrow may also prove useful and have been used successfully as temporary support for children with ALF.

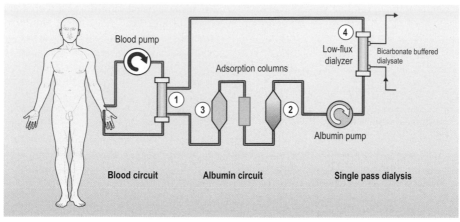

Fig. 14.2 Schematic depiction of a molecular adsorbent recirculating system (MARS). Blood from the patient is pumped through an albumin impermeable hollow fibre dialyser (1). The dialysate contains human albumin (15 g/dL) which binds molecules that diffuse through the pores of the membrane. Molecules that are bound to the albumin in the dialysate are removed by passing through a charcoal column (2) and an anion exchange column (3). The albumin solution is also subjected to a conventional single pass dialysis procedure (4) to remove dialysable ions of low molecular weight.

Liver transplantation

Liver transplantation is an effective treatment for ALF, with 1-year and 5-year survival rates of 80–90% and more than 70% respectively. Orthotopic liver transplantation (OLT) is now considered to be the treatment of choice for a subgroup of patients with ALF for whom the prognosis is poor, although unfortunately there is an ever-increasing shortage of donor organs. Contraindications to OLT include ischaemic cerebral injury, refractory hypotension, overwhelming sepsis, acquired immunodeficiency syndrome (AIDS) and advanced cardiopulmonary disease. Relative contraindications include untreatable psychiatric illness, current alcohol or substance abuse, severe pulmonary hypertension (usually only seen in chronic liver disease), cholangiocarcinoma and age over 70 years.

To improve patient selection and increase the time available for obtaining a donor organ, criteria have been devised (Table 14.6) that can be used to assist early identification of those patients with a poor prognosis who are most likely to benefit from transplantation, preferably before the development of advanced encephalopathy or other complications that could adversely affect the outcome (O'Grady *et al.*, 1989). Liver transplantation has been shown to have a limited but definite role in the management of patients with paracetamol-induced ALF, selected according to these criteria (O'Grady *et al.*, 1991). An alternative is to use the criteria developed by Bernuau and Benhameau (1993) (the 'Clichy criteria') (Table 14.7). Neither of these sets of criteria is applicable to children or to specific conditions such as Budd–Chiari syndrome, Wilson's disease or fatty liver of pregnancy. More recently it has been suggested that the

Table 14.6 Suggested criteria for liver transplantation in fulminant hepatic failure
Paracetamol
pH < 7.30 (irrespective of grade of encephalopathy)
or
Prothrombin time > 100 s and creatinine > 300 µmol/L in patients with grade III or IV encephalopathy
Non-paracetamol
Prothrombin time > 100 s (irrespective of grade of encephalopathy)
or any three of the following (irrespective of grade of encephalopathy): Age < 10 or > 40 years Aetiology: non-A non-B hepatitis, halothane hepatitis, idiosyncratic drug reaction Duration of jaundice before onset of encephalopathy > 7 days
Prothrombin time > 50 s
Serum bilirubin > 300 µmol/L

Reproduced from O'Grady *et al.* (1989).

admission Acute Physiology and Chronic Health Evaluation (APACHE) II score may be a useful means of identifying candidates for transplantation, since a score of more than 15 was associated with a transplant-free survival of only 10% (Mitchell *et al.*, 1998). Although further prospective studies are required, such scoring systems certainly provide a useful and objective means of identifying those patients who should be urgently transferred to a transplant centre. It is important to emphasize that decisions regarding transplantation must be individualized.

OLT does, however, suffer from a number of disadvantages: in particular, it is a major surgical procedure associated with considerable blood loss and if the graft does not function the patient either dies or must be retransplanted immediately. In addition, in those with ALF in whom there is a possibility of spontaneous recovery of liver function, removal of the native liver obviates any chance of such an outcome. These considerations have led to the concept of *auxiliary liver transplantation*, in which healthy liver tissue is placed somewhere in the body while the native liver is left *in situ* (Terpstra, 1993). This has the advantage that, once the native liver has regenerated sufficiently, immunosuppression may be withdrawn and the graft either resected or allowed to atrophy. This technique appears to increase the likelihood of a life free of immunosuppression without jeopardizing the patient's overall chances of survival (van Hoek *et al.*, 1999), although there is an increased risk of vascular and technical complications.

Recently there has been some interest in the use of *living donor liver transplantation (LDLT)*, in which a graft is obtained from a living donor (usually a parent) by partial hepatectomy. This technique has the potential to minimize the delay between listing and transplantation and may reduce mortality on the transplantation waiting list. There are, however, some concerns about the validity of the informed consent obtained from donors under such difficult circumstances. The risks of partial hepatectomy include prolonged recovery, long-term morbidity and a mortality rate of 0.1–0.5%. Because outcomes may be worse the advisability of using LDLT for adult patients with ALF in centres where cadaveric livers are readily available has been questioned.

PROGNOSIS

The mortality of ALF remains high. This condition therefore represents an important challenge because, although rare, it is a disease that affects young people and from which those who survive will make a complete recovery.

Overall survival rates in patients with ALF who progress to stage 3 or 4 encephalopathy are approximately 10–40%

with medical therapy and 60–80% with liver transplantation (Caraceni and Van Thiel, 1995), although the individual prognosis is very dependent on the aetiology of the hepatocellular damage. In a large series of patients treated between 1973 and 1985, for example, mortality rates varied from 55% for hepatitis A, 65% for paracetemol-induced hepatic necrosis and 76% for hepatitis B, to as high as 85% for reactions to drugs (including halothane) and more than 90% for non-A non-B hepatitis (O'Grady *et al.*, 1989).

Prognosis is also poor for those with fulminant Wilson's disease, whilst acute fatty liver of pregnancy has a relatively good prognosis. Survival is also influenced by the delay between the onset of jaundice and the development of encephalopathy. Paradoxically spontaneous recovery is more likely when the onset of encephalopathy is rapid. Using their proposed classification the group from King's College Hospital found that survival was 36% in those with hyperacute liver failure, despite the fact that all progressed to grade IV coma and 69% had evidence of cerebral oedema. Those with ALF also had a high incidence of cerebral oedema (56%), but only 7% survived and only 14% of those with subacute hepatic failure, in whom the frequency of cerebral oedema was low, survived (O'Grady *et al.*, 1993). It is worth noting that, although the King's College criteria have a high specificity and positive predictive value for non-survival, their negative predictive value is poor (Riordan and Williams, 2000).

Prognosis is also related to the age of the patient, the grade of encephalopathy, the bilirubin level and the creatinine concentration. Serum aminotransferases are of no value in assessing the prognosis, but the prothrombin time at presentation and the direction and rapidity of its change, as well as the peak level, provide a reasonable guide to the likely outcome. Coagulation factor V levels and the ratio of factor VIII to factor V may also provide a useful guide to prognosis (see above). The presence of a metabolic acidosis is associated with an extremely poor prognosis, and the longer the duration of jaundice before the onset of encephalopathy, the higher the mortality. The relative importance of these variables seems to depend on whether or not FHF was precipitated by paracetamol (see **Table 14.6**). In one recent study persistently elevated arterial blood lactate levels, despite adequate fluid resuscitation, were indicative of a poor outcome, whereas serum phosphate levels were of limited value as prognostic markers (MacQuillan *et al.*, 2005). Not surprisingly, the prognosis is better when the coma has an identifiable precipitating cause such as the administration of sedatives. Clearly the development of serious complications such as respiratory failure (Baudouin *et al.*, 1995), renal failure, hypotension, convulsions or haemorrhage will adversely affect the outcome.

CAUSES OF DEATH

In one series of 132 consecutive patients in grade IV encephalopathy, autopsy was performed in 96 of the 105 who died. In only 25 of these was death thought to be solely attributable to massive hepatic necrosis. In 36% of cases, cerebral oedema was considered to be the main contributory factor, while in 28 patients, death was due to major gastrointestinal haemorrhage and, in 12, sepsis was a contributory factor. Most importantly, in 10 of these patients, liver function appeared to be improving at the time of death, suggesting that if these major complications could have been prevented or successfully treated, a number of patients might have survived (Gazzard et al., 1975).

ACUTE DECOMPENSATION OF CHRONIC LIVER DISEASE

Acute decompensation of chronic liver disease requiring admission to the intensive care unit is most often the result of shock, usually related to gastrointestinal haemorrhage. Other precipitating factors include infection (particularly with *Escherichia coli* and spontaneous bacterial peritonitis), portal vein thrombosis, alcohol, sedative or hepatotoxic drugs, increased dietary protein, metabolic disturbances (especially hypokalaemic alkalosis caused by the excessive use of diuretics), constipation, anaesthesia and surgery. Hepatocellular carcinoma is often not initially recognized as a cause of decompensation. Most patients have portal hypertension with portosystemic collaterals (shunts), which allow circulating toxins to bypass the liver and contribute to the development of portosystemic encephalopathy. The creation of a portosystemic shunt via the transjugular route to relieve portal hypertension is associated with a 25% overall incidence of chronic hepatic encephalopathy (Riordan and Williams, 1997).

CLINICAL FEATURES

Acute decompensation of chronic liver disease is characterized by *jaundice* and *encephalopathy*. *Ascites* is common and is almost invariable in those with bleeding varices or advanced encephalopathy. Other signs of chronicity such as *palmar erythema* and *spider naevi* are usual. The encephalopathy tends to develop more gradually than in ALF and cerebral oedema is rare. Characteristically the circulation is hyperdynamic, at least in part because of increased production of NO (La Villa et al., 2001).

MANAGEMENT

Patients in whom there is thought to be a reversible component and those being considered for transplantation should be admitted for intensive care.

Measures to reduce the absorption of nitrogenous compounds from the bowel should be instituted and combined with general supportive care, as outlined above for ALF. Although restriction of dietary protein is effective, patients with cirrhosis often require a minimal daily protein intake of 0.8–1.0 g/kg to maintain nitrogen balance. Long-term restriction to below these levels should therefore be avoided (Riordan and Williams, 1997). There is some suggestion that

lactulose and neomycin may have an additive effect in cirrhotics with encephalopathy. Zinc deficiency is common in patients with cirrhosis and may precipitate overt hepatic encephalopathy by compromising the activity of enzymes responsible for metabolism of ammonia to urea. Under these circumstances oral zinc supplements may reverse the encephalopathy. It has also been suggested that deposition of manganese in the basal ganglia may contribute to the development of chronic hepatic encephalopathy and that chelation of manganese might therefore be beneficial. The results of clinical trials of this approach are awaited.

The management of gastrointestinal haemorrhage is discussed in Chapter 16. Infection must be identified and treated appropriately.

Diagnostic paracentesis should be performed to exclude spontaneous bacterial peritonitis, which occurs in 4–15% of cirrhotic patients with ascites. Broad-spectrum antibiotics should be given if there are more than 250×10^6 neutrophils/L of fluid, and if organisms are identified on a Gram stain or are cultured. The antibiotic regimen can be altered appropriately when sensitivities are available.

Control of ascites involves salt and water restriction (e.g. sodium intake < 50 mmol/day or even < 20 mmol/day), combined with administration of diuretics (e.g. furosemide 40 mg combined with amiloride 5 mg daily). There is, however, a danger of sodium depletion with excessive diuretic administration and rapid mobilization of ascitic fluid should normally be avoided. Nevertheless, when severe ascites is causing respiratory embarrassment, paracentesis of up to 3–5 L/day can be performed and appears to be safe. Paracentesis must be accompanied by intravascular volume replacement and some recommend intravenous administration of albumin solutions. There is evidence that in those with spontaneous bacterial peritonitis treatment with intravenous albumin reduces the incidence of renal failure and mortality (Sort et al., 1999). Ultrafiltration or insertion of a Levine shunt may be of value in resistant cases.

In patients with hepatorenal syndrome associated with cirrhosis the use of splanchnic vasoconstrictors, especially terlipressin, has been shown to reverse deteriorating renal function (Hadengue et al., 1998) (see above and Chapter 13). Current evidence suggests that artificial liver support systems such as MARS may reduce mortality in acute-on-chronic liver failure (Kjaergard et al., 2003), although the results of larger randomized, controlled trials are awaited.

PROGNOSIS

Resource utilization and mortality rates for cirrhotic patients admitted to the intensive care unit are high; in a recent series the in-unit and hospital mortality rates were 36.6% and 49% respectively (Aggarwal et al., 2001). In this study the APACHE III score, mechanical ventilation and use of pressors were independent predictors of unit mortality, whilst APACHE III score, use of pressors and acute renal failure were independent predictors of in-hospital mortality. Notably the Child Pugh score, which indicates the severity of the underlying liver disease, did not independently predict mortality. In another series of critically ill patients with cirrhosis, in which mortality rates were very similar, the Sequential Organ Failure Assessment (SOFA) was found to have greater discriminative power than APACHE II and the Child–Pugh system. The SOFA score was also closely related to resource utilization (Wehler *et al.*, 2001). In a recent study in the UK, hospital mortality was 94% in patients with decompensated alcoholic liver disease requiring acute renal replacement therapy (Mackle *et al.*, 2006).

REFERENCES

Aggarwal A, Ong JP, Younossi ZM, *et al.* (2001) Predictors of mortality and resource utilization in cirrhotic patients admitted to the medical ICU. *Chest* **119**: 1489–1497.

Als-Nielsen B, Gluud LL, Gluud C (2004) Non-absorbable disaccharides for hepatic encephalopathy: systematic review of randomised trials. *British Medical Journal* **328**: 1046.

Balata S, Damink SW, Ferguson K, *et al.* (2003) Induced hyperammonemia alters neuropsychology, brain MR spectroscopy and magnetization transfer in cirrhosis. *Hepatology* **37**: 931–939.

Basile AS, Hughes RD, Harrison PM, *et al.* (1991) Elevated brain concentrations of 1,4 benzodiazepines in fulminant hepatic failure. *New England Journal of Medicine* **325**: 473–478.

Baudouin SV, Howdle P, O'Grady JG, *et al.* (1995) Acute lung injury in fulminant hepatic failure following paracetamol poisoning. *Thorax* **50**: 399–402.

Bernuau J, Benhamou JP (1993) Classifying acute liver failure. *Lancet* **342**: 252–253.

Bihari D, Gimson AE, Lindridge J, *et al.* (1985) Lactic acidosis in fulminant hepatic failure. Some aspects of pathogenesis and prognosis. *Journal of Hepatology* **1**: 405–416.

Black M (1980) Acetaminophen hepatotoxicity. *Gastroenterology* **78**: 382–392.

Canalese J, Gimson AES, Davis C, *et al.* (1982) Controlled trial of dexamethasone and mannitol for the cerebral oedema of fulminant hepatic failure. *Gut* **23**: 625–629.

Caraceni P, Van Thiel DH (1995) Acute liver failure. *Lancet* **345**: 163–169.

Clemmesen JO, Larsen FS, Kondrup J, *et al.* (1999) Cerebral herniation in patients with acute liver failure is correlated with arterial ammonia concentration. *Hepatology* **29**: 648–653.

Davies MH, Mutimer D, Lowes J, *et al.* (1994) Recovery despite impaired cerebral perfusion in fulminant hepatic failure. *Lancet* **343**: 1329–1330.

Demetriou AA, Brown RS, Basuttil RW, *et al.* (2004) Prospective, randomized, multicenter, controlled trial of a bioartificial liver in treating acute liver failure. *Annals of Surgery* **239**: 660–670.

Eckardt K-U (1999) Renal failure in liver disease. *Intensive Care Medicine* **25**: 5–14.

Editorial (1986) Halothane associated liver damage. *Lancet* **1**: 1251–1252.

Editorial (1991) The brain in fulminant hepatic failure. *Lancet* **338**: 156–157.

Ellis AJ, Wendon JA, Williams R (2000) Subclinical seizure activity and prophylactic phenytoin infusion in acute liver failure: a controlled clinical trial. *Hepatology* **32**: 536–541.

Epstein M (1992) The hepatorenal syndrome – newer perspectives. *New England Journal of Medicine* **327**: 1810–1811.

Forbes A, Alexander GJ, O'Grady JG, *et al.* (1989) Thiopental infusion in the treatment of

intracranial hypertension complicating fulminant hepatic failure. *Hepatology* **10**: 306–310.

Gazzard BG, Portmann B, Murray-Lyon IM, *et al.* (1975) Causes of death in fulminant hepatic failure and relationship to quantitative histological assessment of parenchymal damage. *Quarterly Journal of Medicine* **44**: 615–626.

Gimson AES, Williams R (1983) Acute hepatic failure: aetiological factors, pathogenic mechanisms and treatment. In: Thomas HC, MacSween RNM (eds) *Recent Advances in Hepatology*, vol. 1, pp 57–69. Churchill Livingstone: Edinburgh.

Gimson AES, Braude S, Mellon PJ, *et al.* (1982) Earlier charcoal haemoperfusion in fulminant hepatic failure. *Lancet* **2**: 681–683.

Gonzalez Calvin J, Scully MF, Sanger Y, *et al.* (1982) Fibronectin in fulminant hepatic failure. *British Medical Journal* **285**: 1231–1232.

Gonwa TA, Morris CA, Goldstein RM, *et al.* (1991) Long-term survival and renal function following liver transplantation in patients with and without hepatorenal syndrome – experience in 300 patients. *Transplantation* **51**: 428–430.

Grimm G, Ferenci P, Katzenschlager R, *et al.* (1988) Improvement of hepatic encephalopathy treated with flumazenil. *Lancet* **ii**: 1392–1394.

Hadengue A, Gadano A, Moreau R, *et al.* (1998) Beneficial effects of the 2-day administration of terlipressin in patients with cirrhosis and hepatorenal syndrome. *Journal of Hepatology* **29**: 565–570.

Harrison PM, Wendon JA, Gimson AES, *et al.* (1990) Improved outcome of paracetamol-induced fulminant hepatic failure by late administration of acetylcysteine. *Lancet* **335**: 1572–1573.

Harrison PM, Wendon JA, Gimson AE, *et al.* (1991) Improvement by acetylcysteine of hemodynamics and oxygen transport in fulminant hepatic failure. *New England Journal of Medicine* **324**: 1852–1857.

Harrison P, Degen SJ, Williams R, *et al.* (1994) Hepatic expression of hepatocyte-growth-factor-like/macrophage-stimulating protein mRNA in fulminant hepatic failure. *Lancet* **344**: 27–29.

Hayes PC, Lee A (2001) What progress with artificial livers? *Lancet* **358**: 1286–1287.

Hein OV, Ohring R, Schilling A, *et al.* (2004) N-acetylcysteine decreases lactate signal intensities in liver tissue and improves liver function in septic shock patients, as shown by magnetic resonance spectroscopy: extended case report. *Critical Care* **8**: R66–R71.

Holt S, Goodier D, Marley R, *et al.* (1999) Improvement in renal function in hepatorenal syndrome with N-acetylcysteine. *Lancet* **353**: 294–295.

Izumi S, Langley PG, Wendon J, *et al.* (1996) Coagulation factor V as a prognostic indicator

in fulminant hepatic failure. *Hepatology* **23**: 1507–1511.

Jalan R, Damink SW, Deutz NE, *et al.* (1999) Moderate hypothermia for uncontrolled intracranial hypertension in acute liver failure. *Lancet* **354**: 1164–1168.

James JH, Ziparo V, Jeppsson B, *et al.* (1979) Hyperammonaemia, plasma aminoacid imbalance, and blood–brain aminoacid transport: a unified theory of portal-systemic encephalopathy. *Lancet* **ii**: 772–775.

Karvountzis GG, Redeker AG, *et al.* (1974) Long term follow-up studies of patients surviving fulminant viral hepatitis. *Gastroenterology* **67**: 870–877.

Kjaergard LL, Liu J, Als-Nielsen B, *et al.* (2003) Artificial and bioartificial support systems for acute and acute-on-chronic liver failure. A systematic review. *Journal of the American Medical Association* **289**: 217–222.

Koppel MH, Coburn JW, Mims MM, *et al.* (1969) Transplantation of cadaveric kidneys from patients with hepatorenal syndrome. Evidence for the functional nature of renal failure in advanced liver disease. *New England Journal of Medicine* **280**: 1367–1371.

Larsen FS, Strauss G, Knudsen GM, *et al.* (2000) Cerebral perfusion, cardiac output, and arterial pressure in patients with fulminant hepatic failure. *Critical Care Medicine* **28**: 996–1000.

La Villa G, Barletta G, Pantaleo P, *et al.* (2001) Hemodynamic, renal, and endocrine effects of acute inhibition of nitric oxide synthase in compensated cirrhosis. *Hepatology* **34**: 19–27.

Macdougall BR, Bailey RJ, Williams R (1977) H$_2$-receptor antagonists and antacids in the prevention of acute gastrointestinal haemorrhage in fulminant hepatic failure. Two controlled trials. *Lancet* **1**: 617–619.

Mackle IJ, Swann DG, Cook B (2006) One year outcome of intensive care patients with decompensated alcoholic liver disease. *British Journal of Anaesthesia* **97**: 496–498.

MacQuillan GC, Seifern MS, Nightingale P, *et al.* (2005) Blood lactate but not serum phosphate levels can predict outcome in fulminant hepatic failure. *Liver Transplantation* **11**: 1073–1079.

Mandal AK, Lansing M, Fahmy A (1982) Acute tubular necrosis in hepatorenal syndrome: an electron microscopy study. *American Journal of Kidney Diseases* **2**: 363–374.

Mitchell I, Bihari D, Chang R, *et al.* (1998) Earlier identification of patients at risk from acetaminophen induced acute liver failure. *Critical Care Medicine* **26**: 279–284.

Mitzner SR, Stange J, Klammt S, *et al.* (2000) Improvement of hepatorenal syndrome with extracorporeal albumin dialysis MARS: results of a prospective, randomised, controlled clinical trial. *Liver Transplantation* **6**: 277–286.

Mitzner SR, Stange J, Klammt S, *et al.* (2001) Extracorporeal detoxification using the molecular adsorbent recirculating system for critically ill patients with liver failure. *Journal* of the American Society of Nephrology 12: S75–S82.

Moore K, Wendon J, Frazer M, et al. (1992) Plasma endothelin immunoreactivity in liver disease and the hepatorenal syndrome. New England Journal of Medicine 327: 1774–1778.

Mullen KD (1991) Benzodiazepine compounds and hepatic encephalopathy. New England Journal of Medicine 325: 509–511.

O'Grady JG, Gimson AE, O'Brien CJ, et al. (1988) Controlled trials of charcoal hemoperfusion and prognostic factors in fulminant hepatic failure. Gastroenterology 94: 1186–1192.

O'Grady JG, Alexander GJ, Hayllar KM, et al. (1989) Early indicators of prognosis in fulminant hepatic failure. Gastroenterology 97: 439–445.

O'Grady JG, Wendon J, Tan KC, et al. (1991) Liver transplantation after paracetamol overdose. British Medical Journal 303: 221–223.

O'Grady JG, Schalm SW, Williams R (1993) Acute liver failure: redefining the syndromes. Lancet 342: 273–275.

Ortega R, Ginès P, Uriz J, et al. (2002) Terlipressin therapy with and without albumin for patients with hepatorenal syndrome: results of a prospective, nonrandomized study. Hepatology 36: 941–948.

Pereria LM, Langley PG, Hayllar KM, et al. (1992) Coagulation factor V and VIII/V ratio as predictors of outcome in paracetamol induced fulminant hepatic failure: relation to other prognostic indictors. Gut 33: 98–102.

Rahman T, Hodgson H (2001) Clinical management of acute hepatic failure. Intensive Care Medicine 27: 467–476.

Rank N, Michel C, Haertel C, et al. (2000) N-acetylcysteine increases liver blood flow and improves liver function in septic shock patients: results of a prospective, randomized, double-blind study. Critical Care Medicine 28: 3799–3807.

Riordan SM, Williams R (1997) Treatment of hepatic encephalopathy. New England Journal of Medicine 337: 473–479.

Riordan SM, Williams R (2000) Use and validation of selection criteria for liver transplantation in acute liver failure. Liver Transplantation 6: 170–173.

Rolando N, Wade JJ, Stangou A, et al. (1996) Prospective study comparing the efficacy of prophylactic parenteral antimicrobials, with or without enteral decontamination, in patients with acute liver failure. Liver Transplantation and Surgery 2: 8–13.

Schafer DF, Jones EA (1982) Hepatic encephalopathy and the γ-aminobutyric acid neurotransmitter system. Lancet 1: 18–20.

Schmidt LE, Dalhoff K (2002) Serum phosphate is an early predictor of outcome in severe acetaminophen-induced hepatotoxicity. Hepatology 36: 659–665.

Shawcross D, Jalan R (2005) Dispelling myths in the treatment of hepatic encephalopathy. Lancet 365: 431–433.

Soper CP, Latif AB, Bending MR (1996) Amelioration of hepatorenal syndrome with selective endothelin-A antagonist. Lancet 347: 1842–1843.

Sorkine P, Ben Abraham R, Szold O, et al. (2001) Role of the molecular adsorbent recycling system (MARS) in the treatment of patients with acute exacerbation of chronic liver failure. Critical Care Medicine 29: 1332–1336.

Sort P, Mavasa M, Arroyo V (1999) Effect of intravenous albumin on renal impairment and mortality in patients with cirrhosis and spontaneous bacterial peritonitis. New England Journal of Medicine 341: 403–409.

Stange J, Mitzner SR, Klammt S, et al. (2000) Liver support by extracorporeal blood purification: a clinical observation. Liver Transplantation 6: 603–613.

Strauss G, Hansen BA, Knudsen GM, et al. (1998) Hyperventilation restores cerebral blood flow autoregulation in patients with acute liver failure. Journal of Hepatology 28: 199–203.

Strom SC, Fisher RA, Thompson MT, et al. (1997) Hepatocyte transplantation as a bridge to orthotopic liver transplantation in terminal liver failure. Transplantation 63: 559–569.

Terpstra OT (1993) Auxiliary liver grafting: a new concept in liver transplantation. Lancet 342: 758.

Tofteng F, Larsen FS (2004) The effect of indomethacin on intracranial pressure, cerebral perfusion and extracellular lactate and glutamate concentrations in patients with fulminant hepatic failure. Journal of Cerebral Blood Flow and Metabolism 24: 798–804.

Trey C, Davidson CS (1970) The management of fulminant hepatic failure. In: Popper H, Schaffner F (eds) Progress in Liver Diseases, vol. 3, pp 282–298. Grune and Stratton: New York.

Vallance P, Moncada S (1991) Hyperdynamic circulation in cirrhosis: a role for nitric oxide? Lancet 337: 776–778.

Van Hoek B, de Boer J, Boudjema K, et al. (1999) Auxiliary versus orthotopic liver transplantation for acute liver failure. Journal of Hepatology 30: 699–705.

Wade J, Rolando N, Philpott-Howard J, et al. (2003) Timing and aetiology of bacterial infections in a liver intensive care unit. Journal of Hospital Infection 53: 144–146.

Walsh TS, Hopton P, Philips BJ, et al. (1998) The effect of N-acetylcysteine on oxygen transport and uptake in patients with fulminant hepatic failure. Hepatology 27: 1332–1340.

Wehler M, Kokoska J, Reulbach U, et al. (2001) Short-term prognosis in critically ill patients with cirrhosis assessed by prognostic scoring systems. Hepatology 34: 255–261.

Wendon JA, Harrison PM, Keays R, et al. (1994) Cerebral blood flow and metabolism in fulminant liver failure. Hepatology 19: 1407–1413.

Williams R, Ede RJ (1981) Hepatitis in pregnancy. British Medical Journal 283: 1074–1075.

Wright R, Eade OE, Chisholm M, et al. (1975) Controlled prospective study of the effect on liver function of multiple exposures to halothane. Lancet 1: 817–820.

Wyke RJ, Rajkovic IA, Eddleston AL, et al. (1980) Defective opsonisation and complement deficiency in serum from patients with fulminant hepatic failure. Gut 21: 643–649.

Wyke RJ, Yousif-Kadaru AG, Rajkovic IA, et al. (1982a) Serum stimulatory activity and polymorphonuclear leucocyte movement in patients with fulminant hepatic failure. Clinical and Experimental Immunology 50: 442–449.

Wyke RJ, Canalese JC, Gimson AE, et al. (1982b) Bacteraemia in patients with fulminant hepatic failure. Liver 2: 45–52.

Zieve L, Shekleton M, Lyftogt C, et al. (1985) Ammonia, octanoate and a mercaptan depress regeneration of normal rat liver after partial hepatectomy. Hepatology 5: 28–31.

15 Neurological disorders

HEAD INJURIES AND RAISED INTRACRANIAL PRESSURE

INTRODUCTION

Traumatic brain injury (TBI) is the commonest cause of raised intracranial pressure (ICP) requiring intensive therapy. Often the same principles can be applied to those with elevated ICP due to other causes. This includes not only patients with meningoencephalitis and spontaneous intracranial haemorrhage (see later in this chapter), but also a number of other causes of intracranial hypertension such as acute liver failure (see Chapter 14), near-drowning (see Chapter 10), eclampsia (see Chapter 18) and Reye's syndrome.

In the UK as many as one million people a year attend an emergency department because of a head injury. Of those 90% are classified as minor or mild, 5% as moderate and 5% as severe. In most western countries head injury accounts for about 250 hospital admissions per 100 000 of the population annually, of whom approximately 15 will require intensive hospital treatment. In the USA it is estimated that more than 250 000 patients are admitted to hospital with TBI every year (Marik et al., 2002). The annual death rate is about 9/100 000 of the population, of whom about a third die before reaching hospital. The prevalence of major disability after TBI is estimated at 100/100 000 of the population and in the USA it is thought that 70 000–90 000 head-injured patients survive with permanent neurological disabilities every year (Marik et al., 2002).

Despite the introduction of a variety of road safety measures, such as seatbelt legislation, penalties against those who drink and drive, and more recently strict enforcement of speed limits, motor vehicle accidents remain the commonest cause of TBI and most often involve teenagers and young adults. Falls are the next most frequent cause of head injury and are more common at the extremes of age. The incidence of TBI is two to three times higher in males than in females. Alcohol consumption is a contributing factor in approximately 40% of cases.

PATHOPHYSIOLOGY (Table 15.1)

At the time of injury, a variable amount of *primary cerebral damage* is sustained, which is largely irreversible. This may be *focal* (e.g. lacerations, contusions, intracranial haemorrhage) or *diffuse* (diffuse axonal injury). These two types of injury frequently coexist.

Diffuse axonal injury is due to shearing or rotational forces in high-kinetic-energy, acceleration/deceleration injuries and can cause dysfunction of the reticular activating system leading to immediate and prolonged unconsciousness. It seems that axonal injury is a result of damage to the axolemma that allows calcium influx with local cytoskeletal and mitochondrial damage within the axon. Apoptosis may also play a role in the pathogenesis of diffuse brain injury. Subsequently downstream disconnected fibres degenerate. Lesser degrees of stretch injury with reversible loss of function are responsible for the transient cerebral disturbance known as concussion.

Intracranial haemorrhage can be classified on the basis of location as being intracerebral, extradural, subdural or, not infrequently, a combination of these. Epidural haematomas are relatively uncommon, being present in fewer than 1% of all head-injured patients and fewer than 10% of those who are comatose. They are most often located in the temporal or temperoparietal region. Subdural haematomas are more common, occuring in around 30% of severe head injuries, and are more frequently associated with significant underlying brain injury. Intracerebral haemorrhage is common in those with moderate or severe TBI and usually produces a mass effect. The majority occur in the frontal and temporal lobes and their appearance is often delayed for more than 24 hours following the initial injury. Contusions most commonly involve the frontal and temporal lobes.

It is most important to appreciate that *secondary brain damage*, caused by neuronal ischaemia and/or hypoxia, is a common and potentially preventable cause of mortality and residual disability (Adams et al., 1980; Chesnut et al., 1993); evidence of such ischaemic injury has been found at necropsy in 88% of a series of patients who had died following

Table 15.1 Mechanisms of cerebral damage following head injury

Primary cerebral damage
Lacerations
Contusions
Intracranial haemorrhage
Diffuse axonal injury
Secondary cerebral damage
Inadequate cerebral perfusion
Traumatic arterial disruption
Cerebral vasospasm
Vascular distortion
Intracranial hypertension
Hypotension
Arterial hypoxaemia
Anaemia
Release of proinflammatory mediators, excitatory amino acids, free radicals, nitric oxide
Hyperthermia
Seizures
Hyperglycaemia
Infection
Iatrogenic

severe head injury (Graham *et al.,* 1989). Secondary brain injury is associated with episodes of inadequate cerebral perfusion (focal or diffuse), which may be caused by traumatic arterial disruption, cerebral vasospasm or vascular distortion, but most importantly by episodes of hypotension and raised ICP. Arterial hypoxaemia and anaemia can exacerbate the brain injury, as may hyperthermia, seizures, hyperglycaemia, iatrogenic insults and infections.

Various cellular and molecular events have been identified as being involved in the pathogenesis of TBI. The release of excitatory amino acids, such as glutamate and aspartate, from injured brain tissue activates the *N*-methyl-D-aspartate (NMDA) receptor complex, allowing calcium to enter the cells. Calcium-dependent enzymes are stimulated with activation of proteases, kinases and phospholipases. Inflammation with release of cytokines, free radical formation and increased production of nitric oxide also contributes to the development of vasogenic and cytotoxic oedema, vascular dysfunction and, eventually, cell death. Many other mediators have been implicated in secondary brain injury, including catecholamines, adenosine, opioid peptides and thyrotrophin-releasing hormone. Lastly a number of factors, including DNA and mitochondrial damage, as well as free radical production, can initiate apoptosis following TBI. In general, however, the metabolic derangement following TBI is complex and poorly understood.

Changes in cerebral blood flow
CEREBRAL PERFUSION PRESSURE
Cerebral blood flow (CBF) is dependent on the difference between the mean arterial blood pressure (MAP) and the mean ICP – the *cerebral perfusion pressure* (CPP). The normal value of CPP is between 70 and 100 mmHg. When CPP falls below a critical level, conventionally 60 mmHg (the lower limit for autoregulation in normal brain), CBF falls; there is then a danger of ischaemic cerebral damage. Electrical abnormalities indicative of cerebral ischaemia are detectable when CPP falls below approximately 25–30 mmHg, or regional cortical blood flow values are less than 20 mL/min per 100 g of brain tissue. Nevertheless, perfusion pressures of this order can be tolerated for several minutes, provided effective measures to restore CBF are instituted immediately (Prior, 1985). In practice, the calculated value for CPP is derived from a measurement which usually reflects global ICP and therefore only provides a guide to the adequacy of overall cerebral perfusion. In reality, pressures may be much higher locally in areas of contusion or intracerebral haemorrhage and deep to haematomas. These are only reflected as a measurable rise in ICP when the increased pressure has been dissipated by brain shifts. Moreover, MAP recorded from a systemic artery is not necessarily an accurate reflection of the pressure within intracranial vessels. Therefore, critical reductions in perfusion may occur locally in the most seriously damaged areas of brain even when overall CPP is apparently adequate. Importantly, ischaemic lesions are frequently identified in the arterial boundary zones where perfusion is always most precarious.

AUTOREGULATION
In health the cerebral circulation autoregulates, maintaining CBF constant over a wide range of perfusion pressure (**Fig. 15.1**). This is an intrinsic property of the smooth muscle in the walls of the cerebral arterioles and is independent of their nerve supply. Diseased, for example atheromatous, vessels lose the ability to autoregulate, while in patients with long-standing hypertension both the lower and upper limits for autoregulation are elevated. In drug-induced hypotension, CBF remains constant at lower pressures than usual. Loss of autoregulation is common in comatose head-injured patients so that CBF is directly related to perfusion pressure. Even when autoregulation is intact, the response of the cerebral vessels is delayed by 1.5–2 min so that sudden increases in blood pressure may nevertheless produce surges of intracranial hypertension. The upper and lower limits of autoregulation are also influenced by changes in $Pa\text{CO}_2$.

FLOW–METABOLISM COUPLING
CBF is normally closely matched to cerebral oxygen requirements (see **Fig 15.1**). In head-injured patients, however, this relationship is frequently disrupted (Lee *et al.,* 2001) and wide variations in CBF may occur, despite a consistent reduction in the cerebral metabolic rate for oxygen ($CMR\text{O}_2$). In one study, for example, 55% of patients exhibited

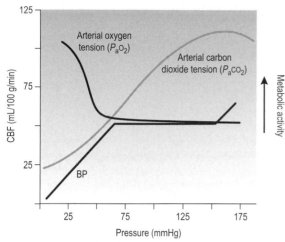

Fig. 15.1 Factors influencing cerebral blood flow (CBF). BP, blood pressure. From McDowall (1976), with permission.

transient relative *cerebral hyperaemia* or *'luxury perfusion'* (defined as a normal or increased CBF in the presence of a reduced $CMRO_2$), while in 45% flows were subnormal (Obrist *et al.*, 1984). In addition, there was little or no evidence of ischaemia in the latter group; rather, they exhibited the normal coupling of CBF and $CMRO_2$. This hyperaemia is probably caused by a loss of vasomotor tone with impaired autoregulation and seems to be at least partly related to the cerebrospinal fluid (CSF) lactic acidosis that can occur in head-injured patients.

INFLUENCE OF BLOOD GAS TENSIONS

Hypercarbia increases the concentration of hydrogen ions in the interstitial spaces, causing cerebral vasodilatation, loss of autoregulation and a rise in CBF (see **Fig. 15.1**). In *severe hypoxaemia*, with an arterial oxygen tension (P_aO_2) of less than 8 kPa (60 mmHg), CBF increases in response to the fall in oxygen content (see **Fig. 15.1**), possibly by a direct effect or via chemoreceptor stimulation and neurogenic influences. Finally, it is important to remember that most inhalational anaesthetic agents cause cerebral vasodilatation.

STEAL AND REVERSE STEAL

The phenomena of steal and reverse steal, which cause local alterations in the distribution of CBF, are also relevant to the management of head-injured patients. Vessels in damaged areas of brain are often relatively unresponsive to the factors that normally influence vascular tone and simply respond passively to alterations in perfusion pressure. In contrast, vessels in intact brain react normally to such stimuli. Hypercarbia will therefore cause dilatation of responsive vessels, diverting blood flow away from areas of cerebral damage and possibly precipitating ischaemia (steal). Conversely, hypocarbia will increase flow and hydrostatic pressure in damaged vessels, and this may potentiate oedema formation as well as increase pressure in injured areas of brain (reverse steal).

INTRACRANIAL PRESSURE

The rise in ICP that can occur following severe head injury may be caused by:

- intracranial haemorrhage;
- an increase in intracranial blood volume;
- cerebral oedema;
- a combination of these.

Alterations in *intracranial blood volume*, associated with the loss of cerebrovascular tone and hyperaemia mentioned previously, are probably largely responsible for intracranial hypertension occurring in the early stages of head injury and for phasic changes in ICP (see below). In one study, there was a highly significant association between hyperaemia and the presence of intracranial hypertension (ICP > 20 mmHg) (Obrist *et al.*, 1984).

Cerebral oedema develops later and may be vasogenic or cytotoxic.

- *Vasogenic oedema* is related to loss of capillary integrity exacerbated by vasodilatation, either locally in areas of contusion or globally; it is associated with a massive increase in capillary hydrostatic pressure and extravasation of protein-rich fluid into the interstitial spaces. This generates pressure gradients and the oedema then spreads, mostly through the white matter, to produce more generalized swelling.
- *Cytoxic/cellular oedema* is intracellular and is related to a failure of cellular ion homeostasis and membrane function due to ischaemic/hypoxic injury and mitochondrial dysfunction.

Not only do haematomas and oedema cause intracranial hypertension, which may be associated with global reductions in cerebral perfusion, as well as local impairment of microcirculatory flow, but they also produce *brain shifts* and *herniation* (**Fig. 15.2**). Unilateral mass lesions above the tentorium cause lateral distortion of the brain with local increases in pressure and impaired perfusion. Initially, the relatively rigid falx cerebri acts as a barrier to mass movements, but eventually brain may herniate beneath this structure, damaging the corpus callosum. If the supratentorial pressures exceed approximately 40 mmHg, uncal transtentorial herniation, or coning, may occur, jeopardizing brainstem perfusion and compressing the third cranial nerve. Initial pupillary constriction is followed by dilatation and absent responses to light. Herniation of the cerebellar tonsil(s) may occur through the foramen magnum and the brainstem itself may be forced downwards. These brain shifts cause vascular distortion and ischaemic cerebral injury.

INTRACRANIAL COMPLIANCE

It is important to appreciate the relationship between the volume of the contents of the skull and the ICP – the *intracranial compliance curve* (**Fig. 15.3**). The cranial cavity is a fixed space containing brain tissue, CSF, extracellular fluid and blood, all of which are essentially incompressible. As

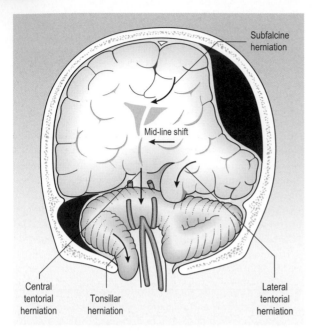

Fig. 15.2 Brain shifts and herniation caused by intracranial haematomas.

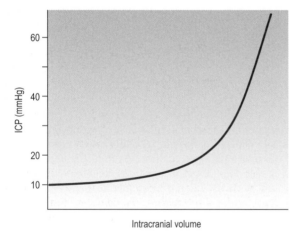

Fig. 15.3 Intracranial compliance curve. ICP, intracranial pressure.

intracranial volume increases, as a consequence, for example, of cerebral oedema or intracranial haemorrhage, there is at first only a gradual rise in ICP because of a compensatory reduction in the volume of blood and CSF within the skull. The CSF is displaced largely into the spinal compartment, where a reduction in the volume of blood within the extradural venous plexuses prevents local increases in pressure. If intracranial volume continues to increase, however, intracranial compliance falls progressively until further compensation is impossible and ICP rises rapidly. In addition, when intracranial compliance is reduced, stimuli such as coughing, physiotherapy and tracheal intubation, which normally cause only small transient increases in ICP, produce more pronounced and sustained intracranial hypertension.

IMMEDIATE CARE (Bartlett *et al.*, 1998) (see Chapter 10 and Advanced Trauma Life Support (ATLS) guidelines) (Table 15.2)

A significant proportion of deaths attributable to TBI occur before admission to hospital, a few from avoidable airway obstruction, and others arrive at emergency departments with partially obstructed airways or having inhaled gastric contents. Furthermore resuscitation at referring hospitals is sometimes inadequate and recognition and treatment of complications, particularly intracranial haematomas, may be delayed, although management may be improved by the introduction of referral policies and guidelines. The quality of the immediate care received by patients with TBI, not only following admission to hospital but also at the scene of the accident and during transfer, can therefore profoundly influence the final outcome. Ideally patients should be transferred directly from the scene of the accident to a specialized trauma centre with a neurosurgical unit.

Initial assessment and management should be in accordance with the ATLS system. Cervical spine immobolization is required for all patients whose Glasgow Coma Scale (GCS) is less than 15 at any time following the injury (see Chapter 10). In patients who are fully conscious the cervical spine should be immobolized if there is:

■ neck pain or tenderness;
■ focal neurological deficit;
■ paraesthesiae in the extremities;
■ any other clinical reason to suspect cervical spine injury.

The *airway* must be secured and protected immediately, if necessary by tracheal intubation and, because patients in traumatic coma are frequently hypoxic (Miller *et al.*, 1981), supplemental *oxygen* should always be given. There is some evidence to suggest that tracheal intubation in the field decreases the risk of death for patients with isolated severe head injury (Winchell and Hoyt, 1997), although some have reported an increase in mortality amongst patients undergoing rapid-sequence intubation by paramedics. This increased mortality seemed to be associated with hyperventilation and episodes of severe hypoxia (Davis *et al.*, 2004). In some cases, immediate institution of *positive-pressure ventilation* will be necessary to control the arterial carbon dioxide tension (P_aCO_2) and reduce acute severe intracranial hypertension. Tracheal intubation and mechanical ventilation are indicated for patients with:

■ GCS ≤ 8;
■ loss of protective laryngeal reflexes;
■ ventilatory insufficiency;
■ spontaneous hyperventilation;
■ respiratory arrhythmia.

It must be assumed that the stomach is full and the cervical spine unstable (the incidence of concomitant spinal injury in head-injured patients ranges from 6 to 8%: see Chapter

Table 15.2 Management of severe head injuries

Immediate care

Stabilize cervical spine

Secure and protect airway

Administer oxygen

Consider positive-pressure ventilation

Secure vascular access

Restore blood pressure

Consider intravenous mannitol

Pass orogastric tube

Insert urinary catheter

Investigations
  Skull radiograph
  Computed tomography scan

Intensive care management

Monitoring

Intracranial pressure

Jugular bulb venous oxygenation

Cerebral function monitor

Evoked potentials

Electroencephalogram

(Implantable sensors)

Prevention of ischaemic/hypoxic injury and brain shifts

Control/restore blood pressure

Control intracranial pressure
  Reduce intracranial blood volume
  Mechanical ventilation
  Sedation
  Ensure unobstructed cerebral venous drainage
  Control cerebral oedema
  Osmotic diuretic (e.g. mannitol)
  Loop diuretic (e.g. furosemide)
  Other measures
  Remove cerebrospinal fluid via intraventricular catheter
  Decompressive craniectomy
  Excise injured brain tissue

Control seizure activity

General measures

Peptic ulcer prophylaxis

Prophylaxis for thromboembolic complications

Antibiotics

Physiotherapy

Nutritional support

Management of pulmonary dysfunction

Management of diabetes insipidus, inappropriate antidiuretic hormone (ADH) secretion

Management of coagulopathy

---

10). During laryngoscopy, the head and neck should therefore be stabilized by an assistant or using sandbags and a rapid-sequence induction performed. Increases in ICP should be prevented or minimized by ensuring adequate oxygenation and prior hyperventilation and by administering sufficient intravenous anaesthetic agent and muscle relaxant. Etomidate, a rapidly acting anaesthetic agent with a short duration of action and minimal haemodynamic effects, is often preferred (although many are increasingly concerned about the possible consequences of the associated adrenal suppression), whilst rocuronium is considered by many to be the muscle relaxant of choice. Because etomidate has no analgesic properties and may not suppress the sympathetic response to tracheal intubation, fentanyl is often used in addition. The patient should be ventilated to achieve normoxia and mild hypocapnia, while maintaining sedation, analgesia and muscle relaxation as necessary.

Hypotension is associated with a 50% increase in mortality (Chesnut *et al.*, 1993) and must be prevented or corrected as rapidly as possible with intravenous volume replacement using normal saline, colloid (fluid resuscitation with albumin has been associated with higher mortality rates than resuscitation with saline in TBI, The SAFE Study Investigators, 2007) or blood and if necessary inotropes. The observation that early restoration of blood pressure may worsen outcome in penetrating thoracic injuries (see Chapter 10) is not relevant to the management of head-injured patients who are most often victims of blunt trauma. There is evidence to suggest that patients with TBI complicated by hypotension who received *hypertonic saline/dextran* are about twice as likely to survive as those who receive standard care (Wade *et al.*, 1997), but in a more recent randomized, controlled trial the use of *hypertonic saline* for the resuscitation of such patients did not appear to improve long-term neurological outcome (Cooper *et al.*, 2004).

At this stage, intravenous *mannitol* can be administered to control intracranial hypertension. A *urinary catheter* is then required and the stomach should be emptied using an *orogastric tube* (the nasal route can only be used when a basal skull fracture has been excluded).

Most patients with a severe head injury not admitted directly to a specialist centre will require urgent transfer to a neurosurgical unit. Since the time from injury to evacuation of an intracranial haematoma is critical for a good outcome (4 hours is considered to be the maximum permissible delay), rapid transfer is essential. Nevertheless, the patient should not be transferred or undergo investigations until adequate resuscitation has been completed. The patient must always be accompanied by a suitably qualified doctor whose priority should be to avoid further episodes of hypotension or hypoxia. As well as the indications listed above tracheal intubation and ventilation will be required prior to transfer when:

■ conscious level is deteriorating;
■ there are bilateral mandibular fractures;

- there is copious bleeding into the mouth;
- the patient has had a seizure.

Comprehensive guidelines for the resuscitation and transfer of head-injured patients are available (Gentleman *et al.*, 1993) (see Chapter 21).

HISTORY, EXAMINATION AND INVESTIGATIONS

Enquiries should be made about the circumstances of the injury and retrieval, the occurrence of seizures and the possibility of intoxication, as well as pre-existing medical problems and medications. Patients with a normal conscious level, no signs of external injury and a history of a trivial blow to the head can be discharged.

Other injuries must be excluded, which in the unconscious patient will often require abdominal ultrasound or computed axial tomography (CT) scan (see Chapter 10). Scalp lacerations, bruising and abrasions suggest an underlying fracture, while ecchymoses behind the ears (Battle's sign) or around the eyes are suggestive of a basal skull fracture.

Skull radiographs should be obtained in those with:

- an inadequate history;
- a history of loss of consciousness;
- a history of a fall more than 60 cm in height;
- loss of memory;
- neurological signs or symptoms;
- leakage of CSF or blood from the nose or ear;
- suspected penetrating injury;
- pronounced bruising/swelling or a full-thickness laceration of the scalp.

(Occasionally midline shift of a calcified pineal gland is seen on the anteroposterior film.)

Skull fractures may be linear or stellate, depressed or non-depressed. Linear fractures can cause haemorrhage from torn extradural vessels, and the presence of a linear vault fracture is associated with an increased risk of intracranial haematoma (Mendelow *et al.*, 1983), while those with depressed fractures may develop intracranial infection if untreated. Sometimes there is leakage of CSF through base-of-skull fractures, which may be seen as clear fluid trickling from the nose or ear. A positive test for sugar using a Dextrostix will confirm that the fluid is indeed CSF. *Cervical spine radiographs* should also be obtained at this time.

Immediate CT scan is indicated in resuscitated head-injured patients with:

- GCS < 13 at any time since the injury;
- GCS equal to 13 or 14 at 2 hours after the injury;
- a focal neurological deficit or other neurological signs (e.g. seizures);
- coma;
- a skull fracture;
- multiple injuries;
- more than one episode of vomiting;
- amnesia of greater than 30 minutes for events before injury.

It is debatable whether a CT scan is indicated for patients with a GCS of 15 but who have a history of loss of consciousness or amnesia. Certainly a CT scan should be performed in such cases when additional risk factors (e.g. age > 65 years, coagulopathy, dangerous mechanism of injury) are also present. A decision rule has been developed for patients with minor head injury (witnessed loss of consciousness, definite amnesia or witnessed disorientation in a patient with a GCS of 13–15) which might standardize and improve patient care, and could reduce the number of such patients who undergo CT scanning. Stiell and colleagues identified five high-risk factors ((1) failure to reach GCS 15 within 2 hours; (2) suspected open skull fracture; (3) any sign of basal skull fracture; (4) ≥ 2 episodes of vomiting; (5) age ≥ 65 years) and suggested that a CT scan is mandatory in patients with one or more of these features. Patients with either of two additional medium-risk factors (amnesia before impact > 30 minutes, dangerous mechanism of injury) can, they suggest, be managed with CT scanning or close observation, depending on local resources (Stiell *et al.*, 2001). When a CT scan is to be performed it is reasonable to forgo the skull radiograph. The opportunity may be taken to scan the cervical spine.

The CT scan may demonstrate cerebral swelling and reveal and localize intracranial haematomas, lacerations and contusions (**Fig. 15.4**). Compression of the ventricles may also be visible on CT scan and suggests significantly raised ICP (**Fig. 15.5**), while midline shift is seen in the presence of significant unilateral mass lesions (see **Fig. 15.4**). Areas of ischaemic infarction, contusions and intracranial air may also be revealed. The absence of an intracranial haematoma on the initial scan does not exclude the possibility that this complication will develop subsequently, particularly if the scan is performed soon after injury. Consequently, frequent neurological assessment, monitoring of ICP and repeat scans may be required to ensure that delayed intracranial haemorrhage is not missed. Some advocate routine repeat scanning of patients with moderate or severe head injury 4–8 hours afer presentation. A classification of head injuries based on the CT scan appearances has been described (Marshall *et al.*, 1992).

The place of *magnetic resonance imaging* (MRI) in the management of TBI is limited, not least because of the logistical difficulties in supporting and monitoring patients during the procedure. MRI may be more sensitive than CT scanning for the detection of small extracerebral haematomas not requiring surgery, non-haemorrhagic contusions, ischaemic areas and diffuse axonal injury. CT scanning is superior for detecting intracranial air, intraventricular and subarachnoid blood and foreign bodies, as well as for measuring bone depression. CT scanning remains the procedure of choice for the investigation of TBI whilst MRI scanning is only indicated if there is a focal neurological deficit or a prolonged period of unconsciousness not explained by CT scan. *Cerebral angiography* (or carotid Doppler ultrasound) is sometimes indicated if vascular injury is suspected.

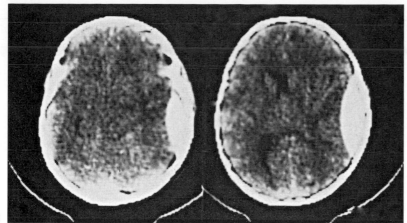

(a)

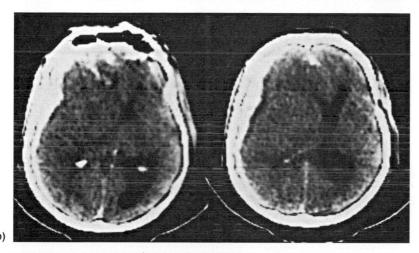

(b)

Fig. 15.4 Intracranial haematomas demonstrated by computed axial tomography. (a) Acute extradural haematoma: biconvex or lenticular high-attenuation collection with associated ipsilateral ventricular compression from oedema. (b) Acute subdural haematoma: high-attenuation collection concave outer and convex inner margin (i.e. crescent-shaped), and marked midline shift. (Courtesy of Dr K. Hall.) (c) Acute subdural haematoma with 'burst' temporal lobe. (Courtesy of Dr P.J.D. Andrews.) (d) Intracerebral contusions and haemorrhage. (Courtesy of Dr P.J.D. Andrews.)

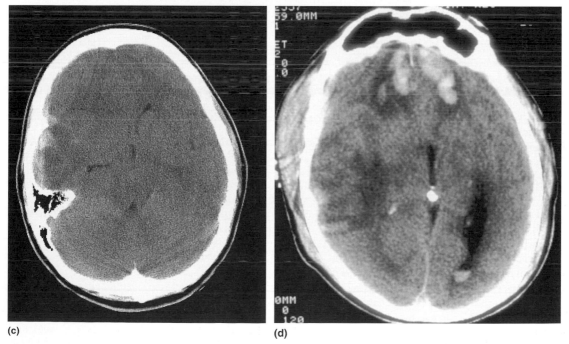

(c)

(d)

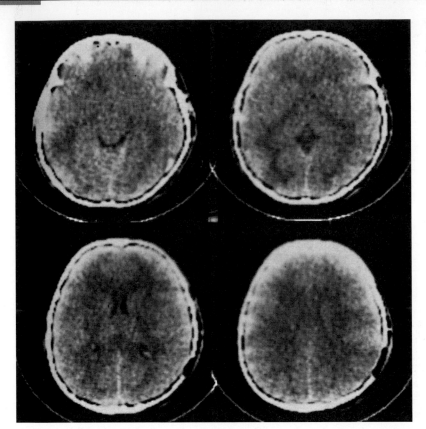

Fig. 15.5 Diffuse cerebral swelling in a patient with severe head injury. Note the ventricular compression. (Courtesy of Dr K. Hall.)

The *electrocardiogram (ECG)* may reveal bizarre ST-segment, T-wave changes such as those shown in **Figure 15.6**.

Laboratory investigations should normally include:

- full blood count;
- coagulation screen;
- urea and electrolytes;
- blood sugar;
- toxicology screen;
- blood gas analysis.

MONITORING
Clinical

In the unsedated patient, a clinical assessment of neurological status is possible. The *level of consciousness* can be graded according to whether the patient is alert and oriented, drowsy but rousable, and obeys simple commands or reacts to painful stimuli. A more sophisticated assessment is possible using the *GCS* (**Table 15.3**), which correlates closely with outcome. Patients with a score of 15 or 14 are classified as having a mild head injury, 13 to 9 as moderate and 8 to 3 (with no eye opening) as severe. This scoring system was, however, designed primarily to allow meaningful comparisons between the results obtained in different centres and with alternative treatment regimens; therefore, although it is

undoubtedly valuable for research, when used in isolation it can be insufficiently sensitive for clinical use. It is also important to beware of dismissing a patient's obtunded state as being solely due to intoxication; in such cases significant intracranial pathology is easily overlooked. *Localizing signs*, such as weakness and hypertonicity of the limbs on one side of the body, should also be sought, and the size and reactivity of the *pupils* assessed. When there is no history of ocular or local trauma, a single fixed and dilated pupil indicates temporal lobe herniation. Bilateral fixed, dilated pupils are a poor prognostic sign since they are often indicative of transtentorial brain herniation affecting the brainstem. These signs warrant the urgent intravenous administration of mannitol (see below). Pupillary signs are late indicators of intracranial compression and the aim should always be to detect deterioration before such changes occur. Papilloedema is uncommon in the acute phase of a head injury. Brainstem reflexes (oculocephalic and oculovestibular responses) should also be assessed. The importance of repeating the neurological examination at intervals cannot be overemphasized.

Patients who develop an extradural haematoma, usually due to laceration of a middle meningeal artery or vein, may present with a deteriorating conscious level following a *lucid interval*. Prompt evacuation of an extradural haematoma is not only life-saving but is often associated with a good recov-

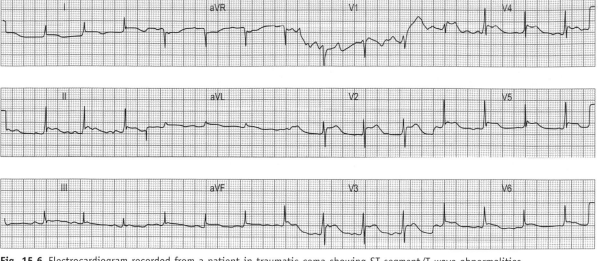

Fig. 15.6 Electrocardiogram recorded from a patient in traumatic coma showing ST-segment/T-wave abnormalities.

Table 15.3 Glasgow Coma Scale	
Function	**Score (maximum 15, minimum 3)**
Eye opening	
Spontaneous	4
To voice	3
To pain	2
None	1
Verbal response	
Oriented	5
Confused	4
Inappropriate words	3
Incomprehensible sounds	2
None	1
Best motor response	
Follows commands	6
Localizes pain	5
Withdraws from pain	4
Abnormal flexion	3
Abnormal extension	2
None	1

Intracranial pressure monitoring (Andrews and Citerio, 2004; Citerio and Andrews, 2004)

Because head injured patients admitted to the intensive care unit for controlled ventilation are usually sedated and may be paralysed, the clinical signs of rising ICP and neurological deterioration, except the haemodynamic and late pupillary changes, are masked. Most authorities (Brain Trauma Task Force, 2000; Ghajar, 2000; Marik et al., 2002) therefore believe that it is important to measure ICP, both as a guide to therapy aimed at its control and to detect increasing intracranial compression. If there is a sustained rise in ICP resistant to treatment, a repeat CT scan may reveal an intracranial haematoma requiring evacuation. ICP monitoring also enables nurses, physiotherapists and medical staff to assess the effects of procedures on intracranial dynamics. Suggested indications for ICP monitoring include:

- the need for mechanical ventilation;
- GCS ≤ 8;
- the presence of a small haematoma seen on CT scan;
- following decompressive surgery.

Despite convincing evidence to suggest that monitoring and treatment of ICP increase the likelihood of a favourable outcome (Murray et al., 1999), a survey by the European Brain Injury Consortium (Murray et al., 1999b) found that the frequency of ICP monitoring in comatose patients averaged only 43% and varied from 5% to 53% in different countries.

TECHNIQUES FOR MONITORING ICP

ICP should be monitored contralateral to any focal pathology in order to reflect pressures in undamaged brain. ICP may be monitored most sensitively, accurately and cost-effectively by introducing a fluid-filled catheter into a lateral ventricle, although this may be difficult in those in whom the ventricles are compressed by cerebral swelling. There is

ery because the underlying brain is usually relatively uninjured. Subdural haematomas, on the other hand, are usually seen in those with a severe head injury and laceration of the brain, whereas intracerebral haemorrhage is a feature of penetrating or very severe closed injuries.

also a risk of introducing infection and of obstruction of the catheter. An *intraventricular catheter* can, however, be periodically re-zeroed and does enable the clinician to remove CSF in order to control intracranial hypertension; many believe this to be the technique of choice and the 'gold standard' for monitoring ICP (Ghajar, 2000; Marik *et al.*, 2002). In the past *hollow bolts*, which could be threaded into the skull to measure subdural pressure, and *catheter tip transducers inserted subdurally* were used as alternatives. These devices are no longer used, however, because subdural pressures often differ significantly from intraventricular measurements, tending to underestimate, especially when ICP is high. *Extradural measurements* have also been abandoned because of their extremely poor correlation with intraventricular pressures. More recently, miniaturized fibreoptic catheter-tip devices have been introduced that can be inserted to a depth of 1 cm into the brain to measure *intraparenchymal pressure*. These read slightly higher than ventricular pressure, but are perhaps the best alternative to catheterization of the ventricles. Intraparenchymal solid-state systems, based on silicon chips with pressure-sensitive resistors forming a Wheatstone bridge, are also available. Progressive zero drift, which cannot be detected or corrected, is a problem during longer-term monitoring with these devices (> 4–5 days).

Complications of ICP monitoring include:

■ malfunction;
■ catheter obstruction;
■ malposition;
■ infection (the risk of bacterial colonization increases over time);
■ haemorrhage.

INTERPRETATION

Correct interpretation of ICP recordings depends on an appreciation of the *intracranial compliance curve* (see **Fig. 15.3**). Even during the initial phase of intracranial volume expansion, compensation is not perfect and ICP in fact rises from a normal value of less than 10 mmHg to about 20–25 mmHg. Above this level there is a danger of decompensation, and an ICP of less than 20–25 mmHg is therefore often used as a target for treatment aimed at controlling intracranial hypertension. There is, however, some evidence that outcome may be improved by controlling ICP to lower values (e.g. 15 mmHg). It must also be recognized that the absolute value of the ICP provides only an approximate guide to the degree of cerebral compression.

Intracranial compliance can be assessed by injecting a small volume of fluid into the ventricles (no longer recommended) or can be inferred from the response of the ICP to stimuli such as endotracheal suction (an increase in ICP of more than 15 mmHg during the latter manoeuvre indicates that intracranial compliance is markedly reduced). Recently a modified intraventricular catheter has been described which can continuously monitor cerebral compliance by automatically injecting and withdrawing small pulses (0.2 mL) of air through a pouch located at the tip of the catheter (Spiegelberg device) (Portella *et al.*, 2005). Also as intracranial compliance falls, there is an increase in the amplitude of the fluctuations in ICP, which occur in phase with the pulse and with ventilation. This is a valuable sign of intracranial compression. Finally, large (50–100 mmHg) spontaneous increases in ICP lasting between 5 and 20 minutes (*A waves* or *plateau waves*) as well as rhythmic oscillations at 0.5–2 cycles/min (*B waves*) and fluctuations related to blood pressure at about 6/min (*C waves*) all suggest that intracranial compliance is significantly reduced. An analogue monitoring device is required to appreciate these alterations in the character of the ICP waveform. When calculating CPP it is important that the arterial pressure transducer is at the same level as the ICP monitor.

Jugular bulb venous oxygen saturation, oxygen content and lactate levels *(Macmillan and Andrews, 2000)*

A thin radiopaque catheter can be inserted percutaneously into the internal jugular vein and passed retrogradely until it lies high in the jugular bulb. Simultaneous sampling of jugular venous and systemic arterial blood allows determination of the cerebral arteriovenous oxygen content difference ($C_{a-J}O_2$). The jugular bulb oxygen saturation (S_JO_2), and the jugular venous lactate level can also be determined (the normal $C_{a-J}O_2$ in adults is around 7 mL O_2/100 mL and the normal S_JO_2 is 54–75%). Fibreoptic catheters allow continuous S_JO_2 monitoring *in vivo*. If CBF is also determined (e.g. using the intravenous or inhaled [133]xenon method) cerebral oxygen consumption ($CMRO_2$) can be calculated. Although S_JO_2 monitoring is simple in principle, the successful use of this technique requires attention to detail. Complications are rare and usually minor, but include internal jugular vein thrombosis.

INTERPRETATION

A low $C_{a-J}O_2$ and/or a high S_JO_2 indicate that cerebral oxygen supply exceeds demand (e.g. when CBF is increased due to loss of autoregulation or when cerebral metabolism is reduced by administering hypnotics). Conversely a fall in S_JO_2 and/or a high $C_{a-J}O_2$ indicate that cerebral oxygen supply is inadequate, perhaps because CPP and therefore CBF are low or $CMRO_2$ is increased (e.g. by seizure activity).

Determination of $C_{a-J}O_2$ and S_JO_2 can be used clinically to detect episodes of global ischaemia and to assist in the selection of the most appropriate therapy for ICP reduction (see later in this chapter). It has also been suggested that these measurements can provide prognostic information. In one study, for example, a high S_JO_2 was found in about 19% of patients and was associated with a worse outcome (Cormio *et al.*, 1999), whilst poor outcomes have also been associated with low S_JO_2. It is important to appreciate that jugular venous oxygenation is only a reflection of the global balance between cerebral oxygen supply and demand; episodes of regional cerebral ischaemia will not necessarily be detected.

Importantly, in one study intermittent S_jO_2 monitoring did not influence the management of head-injured patients (Latronico et al., 2000) and it remains to be seen whether the identification and treatment of changes in S_jO_2 will alter outcomes.

Implantable sensors

Recent technical advances have allowed the development of implantable sensors that can measure the local partial pressure of oxygen in the cerebral extracellular space (P_bO_2) as an indication of the regional balance between oxygen supply and demand. Local carbon dioxide tension (P_bCO_2), pH and temperature can also be measured with these devices. Microdialysis techniques can be used to sample extracellular fluid for determination of lactate, pyruvate, glycerol and glucose concentrations. The lactate/pyruvate ratio provides an indication of the balance between aerobic and anaerobic metabolism, whilst glycerol is thought to be a marker of cell membrane breakdown. Interpretation is complicated, however, by the suggestion that astrocytes may provide lactate for neuronal metabolism. These techniques are being used increasingly to monitor patients with TBI, both to aid recognition of secondary ischaemic/hypoxic injury and to guide therapeutic interventions (Haitsma and Maas, 2002; Johnston and Gupta, 2002).

Transcranial near-infrared spectroscopy

Near-infrared light penetrates the skull and during transmission through or reflection from brain tissue undergoes wavelength changes, which are dependent on the relative concentrations of oxygenated and deoxygenated haemoglobin. This technique has limited clinical value and results correlate poorly with S_jO_2.

Monitoring cerebral blood flow

Methods include laser Doppler flowmetry, xenon-enhanced CT scanning, single-photon emission CT, thermal diffusion and position emission tomography. None allows reliable continuous bedside assessment of CBF.

Transcranial Doppler ultrasonography measures blood velocity, rather than flow, usually in the middle cerebral artery, and has been used to detect vasospasm.

Neurophysiological monitoring (Prior, 1985)

A number of neurophysiological techniques can be used to assess the functional state of the nervous system in patients with severe head injury.

Conventional bedside electroencephalograms (EEGs) can be recorded at intervals to obtain diagnostic and prognostic information. They may reveal the presence of seizure activity, can suggest hypoxic/ischaemic damage and will localize any dysfunction as well as indicate its severity and progress. The use of conventional EEGs for continuous monitoring of intensive care patients is, however, impractical. Some form of data reduction is required to monitor the EEG for prolonged periods automatically and to produce information that can be readily interpreted by clinicians.

In critically ill patients, the fundamental requirement is to monitor the serial EEG changes that accompany depression and recovery of neuronal function; these are similar whatever their aetiology (drugs, anaesthesia, hypothermia or hypoxia/ischaemia). Depression of neuronal function is accompanied by a reduction in the overall level of cortical electrical activity until electrical silence occurs. The most significant early warning of deterioration is the appearance of burst suppression activity (i.e. the breaking up of previously continuous EEG waves by increasingly long periods of electrical silence). The associated EEG frequency changes are more complex and less consistent, although there is a general tendency for frequencies to decrease. Both frequency and time domain analyses have been used to extract and display the most clinically relevant features of the EEG. Time domain analyses involve processing the EEG as a continuous signal (e.g. voltage plotted against time), whereas a frequency domain analysis averages the potentials present during a time period (epoch) and then plots frequency against another variable such as power.

FREQUENCY DOMAIN ANALYSIS

Because the frequency plots provide no time information, serial plots are conventionally displayed sequentially in the compressed spectral array (**Fig. 15.7**). A number of instruments are available that will perform this type of analysis. Although such techniques provide detailed information regarding frequency alterations, the output is relatively complex and difficult to interpret (see **Fig. 15.7**). In addition, it is possible to miss isolated events of short duration such as a brief seizure discharge, or the periods of electrical silence that are characteristic of burst suppression. Frequency-based EEG data are therefore most useful for the detection of subtle changes that may occur, for example, during sleep or with light levels of anaesthesia.

TIME DOMAIN ANALYSIS

For a more generally applicable monitoring system, a recording of the voltage range and the amount of activity is a better indication of the brain's energy output.

Continuous monitoring of the EEG can be performed using the cerebral function monitor (CFM). This is a relatively simple, robust, portable apparatus. It produces a continuous filtered and compressed paper trace of cortical electrical activity at 6–30 cm/h. This is recorded from two electrodes, which are generally positioned over the parietal region on either side, while a third electrode is placed in the midline to help rejection of interference. The recording electrodes are positioned close to the arterial boundary zones, which are particularly vulnerable to reductions in cerebral perfusion, to maximize their sensitivity to ischaemic events.

The CFM will detect subclinical seizure discharges and non-convulsive status epilepticus (**Fig. 15.8**). Episodes of cerebral ischaemia are associated with reductions in CFM voltage (**Fig. 15.9**) and, if not rapidly corrected, cortical activity is permanently extinguished (**Fig. 15.10**). It has been suggested, therefore, that the CFM may provide an early warning of ischaemia induced by hypocapnic vasospasm. The extent of depression of the CFM can be used as a guide to the level of sedation achieved with intravenous anaesthetic agents (**Fig. 15.11**). Thus, depression of the baseline of the CFM trace to below 5 μV is generally equivalent to a burst suppression pattern seen on the conventional EEG and indicates that $CMRO_2$ is maximally reduced. Under these circumstances, increasing the level of sedation is unlikely to produce further significant decreases in CBF and ICP (Bingham *et al.*, 1985). Many authorities believe that continuous monitoring of the CFM is mandatory when intravenous anaesthetic agents (especially barbiturates) are being used to control intracranial hypertension (see below). Finally the absence of reactivity to external stimuli during continuous EEG monitoring is a poor prognostic sign.

COMBINED TIME AND FREQUENCY DOMAIN ANALYSIS

An example of this type of analysis is the *cerebral function-analysing monitor* (CFAM). This records the amplitude of electrical activity as a mean, together with the 90th and 10th percentile values, as well as peaks and troughs that exceed these. In addition, frequency analysis is provided as the percentage of power falling into the traditional frequency bands (beta, alpha, theta and delta).

EVOKED POTENTIALS (Fig. 15.12)

Averaged evoked potentials to external sensory stimuli (visual, auditory and somatosensory) are easy to perform and can provide useful prognostic information. They are particularly valuable in traumatic coma because the short-latency brainstem components of the auditory and somatosensory responses are unaffected by heavy sedation or anaesthesia, even when the EEG has been rendered isoelectric, and they can assess the functional integrity of lower pathways. They are, however, affected by hypothermia. The most useful are the somatosensory evoked potentials (SEPs), which are obtained by electrical stimulation at a peripheral site (e.g. the median nerve). Auditory brainstem (click) stimuli may also give valuable information. Provided a peripheral response is obtained, which may not always be possible (e.g. if the eyes or ears have sustained direct traumatic damage), the conduction time through the brainstem to the appropriate cortical site can be measured. Delayed central somatosensory conduction times may indicate a transient functional disturbance (e.g. due to white-matter oedema). Major asymmetries or absence of potentials are associated with serious neurological deficits, vegetative survival or death. In one study (Sleigh *et al.*, 1999) outcome was good in 57% of patients in whom the control conduction time (CCT) was normal bilaterally, whereas any delay in CCT was associated with a decrease in those with a good outcome to only 30% of cases. Unilateral absence of the cortical component of the SEP was usually associated with severe disability or death, whilst bilateral absence was always associated with a poor outcome. A systematic review confirmed that bilaterally absent SEPs are a powerful predictor of a poor outcome, with a low rate of false positives (Carter and Butt, 2001). SEPs can, however, change over time and these authors cautioned against acting on the basis of bilaterally absent SEPs obtained in the first 24 hours after injury. They also recommended repeating the test in any patient with bilaterally absent SEPs.

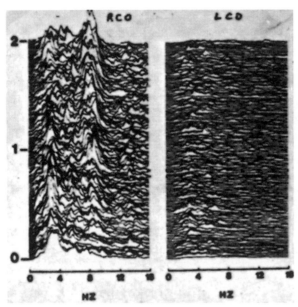

Fig. 15.7 Compressed spectral array recording from right and left centro-occipital regions showing interhemisphere asymmetry. Note the relative lack of activity from the left hemisphere recording compared with the large waves over a relatively wide frequency range on the right. The persistent reduction of left-sided activity in this patient, 4 days after a head injury, suggests that contusion has led to some permanent left hemisphere damage. (Unpublished data of A. Bricolo and S. Turazzi, reproduced with permission.)

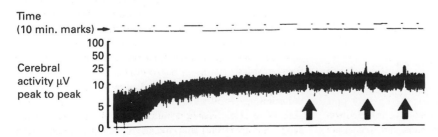

Fig. 15.8 Recording of cortical electrical activity obtained using the cerebral function monitor. Activity increases as the patient emerges from a period of heavy sedation. Seizure discharges are then seen and are indicated by the arrows.

Time
(10 min. marks) ➔

Cerebral
activity µV
peak to peak

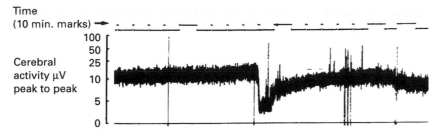

Fig. 15.9 A brief episode of profound cerebral ischaemia occurring in a patient with severe head injury. Rapid institution of measures to improve cerebral oxygenation is associated with partial recovery of cortical electrical activity.

Time
(10 min. marks) ➔

Cerebral
activity µV
peak to peak

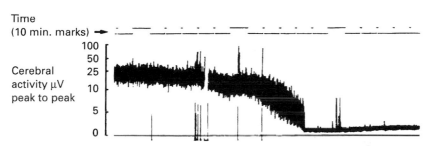

Fig. 15.10 In this cardiac surgery patient, postoperative failure of cerebral perfusion culminates in permanent extinction of cortical electrical activity.

ICP
mm Hg

BP
mm Hg

hours

Cerebral
activity µV
peak to peak

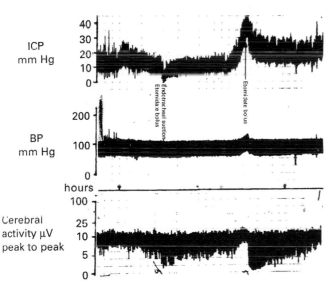

Fig. 15.11 The effects of administering bolus doses of the intravenous anaesthetic agent etomidate (0.2 mg/kg) on intracranial pressure (ICP), systemic blood pressure (BP) and cortical electrical activity as recorded by the cerebral function monitor (CFM). Etomidate administration reduces ICP on both occasions and this is associated with a fall in the baseline of the CFM trace to below 5 µV. There is also a small reduction in systemic blood pressure. There is no increase in ICP following endotracheal suction subsequent to the first bolus dose of etomidate.

MANAGEMENT (Brain Trauma Task Force, 2000; Ghajar, 2000; Marik *et al.*, 2002)

Indications for admission of brain-injured patients to intensive care include:

- comatose patients with diffuse brain injury;
- postoperative patients who have undergone neurosurgery;
- patients requiring tracheal intubation with or without mechanical ventilation;
- patients with multiple injuries and/or cardiovascular or respiratory complications;
- patients thought to be brainstem-dead (see below).

Intensive care management of severe head injuries is primarily concerned with the prevention of secondary ischaemic/hypoxic cerebral insults and minimizing brain shifts. This is based on maintaining adequate cerebral perfusion by controlling ICP, reducing brain swelling and optimizing systemic blood pressure. Outcomes are significantly worse in patients with a CPP < 60 mmHg and are better when CPP is above 80 mmHg in the first 48 hours after head injury. Available evidence suggests that CPP should be maintained at 60–70 mmHg (Brain Trauma Task Force, 2000; Ghajar, 2000). In one recent study, however, augmentation of CPP from around 70 mmHg to approximately 90 mmHg was associated with a significant increase in brain tissue oxygen, although there were no signficant changes in cerebral glucose, lactate, pyruvate or glycerol levels (Johnston *et al.*, 2005). It is important to appreciate that when autoregulation

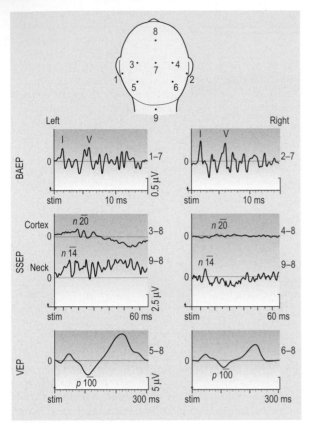

Fig. 15.12 Averaged sensory evoked potentials in traumatic coma. Brainstem auditory evoked potentials (BAEP), somatosensory evoked potentials (SSEP) over second cervical vertebra and contralateral somatosensory cortex following median nerve stimulation at the wrist and visual evoked potentials (VEP) to binocular flash stimulation. Note slight delay of BAEP wave I on the right, but otherwise normal BAEP, depressed cortical SSEP and reduced-amplitude VEP over the right hemisphere. Six weeks later the patient was conscious and active, but with a left hemiparesis. Stim, stimulation. From Prior (1985), with permission.

is even partly intact, perfusion pressures below a critical threshold can provoke cerebral vasodilatation and a rise in ICP. Cerebral metabolic demands should also be minimized and in this respect it is particularly important to detect and control seizure activity and fever.

An alternative approach aims to promote reabsorption of intracerebral water by maintaining colloid osmotic pressure (with blood and albumin infusions) and reducing intracapillary hydrostatic pressure. The latter is achieved by administering a β_1-antagonist (metoprolol) in combination with an α_2-agonist (clonidine). Intracapillary pressure may also be reduced by precapillary vasoconstriction (low-dose thiopental, dihydroergotamine), whilst intracranial blood volume may be reduced by arterial and large-vein vasoconstriction. Enthusiasts have reported positive clinical experiences with this approach (Eker *et al.*, 1998), which has nevertheless failed to gain general acceptance.

There is evidence to suggest that outcome from TBI can be improved by protocol-driven, targeted treatment in specialist centres, involving in particular manipulation of CPP (Bulger *et al.*, 2002; Patel *et al.*, 2005; Rosner *et al.*, 1995). Unfortunately, despite the availability of evidence-based guidelines, there remains considerable institutional variation in the management of patients with severe head injury (Bulger *et al.*, 2002).

Blood pressure control

Hypotension will usually respond to expansion of the circulating volume with blood, normal saline or colloid guided by central venous pressure (CVP) measurements. In a few complicated cases (e.g. those with multiple injuries, acute respiratory distress syndrome (ARDS) or pre-existing cardiac disease), pulmonary artery catheterization, or other invasive monitoring techniques, may be indicated. There is some concern that when the blood–brain barrier is compromised, colloidal solutions may leak into the extravascular space, thereby increasing ICP.

In those who fail to respond to volume expansion, inotropic support should be instituted. Dopamine can be used initially since this agent has been shown experimentally to increase CBF within and around injured brain without significantly increasing hemispheric swelling or water content (Kroppenstedt *et al.*, 2000). Administration of noradrenaline (norepinephrine) may produce more predictable and consistent increases in CPP than dopamine (Steiner *et al.*, 2004). The aim should be to maintain an MAP ≥ 90 mmHg (or a systolic pressure greater than 120 mmHg) while avoiding excessively high blood pressures, which, when autoregulation is impaired, may directly injure the capillary bed and increase ICP. Moreover vasopressors may cause cerebral vasoconstriction and could precipitate local reductions in CBF, despite apparently adequate CPP.

In some patients the hyperadrenergic state that can follow severe head injury causes extreme hypertension, but specific treatment (e.g. with an intravenous β-blocker) should only be used when all other measures (sedation, control of intracranial hypertension) have failed. Vasodilators may cause catastrophic falls in CPP and should be avoided. Cerebral vasodilators such as L-arginine can increase CBF (Cherian *et al.*, 1999) but their role in the management of head-injured patients remains uncertain.

Reduction of intracranial pressure

ICP can be reduced by decreasing intracranial blood volume, reducing cerebral oedema or both.

REDUCING INTRACRANIAL BLOOD VOLUME

Intracranial blood volume can be reduced by manipulating CBF. Because this produces relatively small alterations in intracranial volume, the change in ICP is greatest when cerebral compliance is significantly reduced.

Mechanical ventilation. There is no conclusive evidence that the routine use of mechanical ventilation, with or without induced hypocarbia, affects outcome in those with severe head injury. Nevertheless, because of the effects of alterations in blood gas tensions on cerebral vascular tone, including the steal phenomenon, which may be induced by a rising P_aCO_2 (see earlier in this chapter) and because hypoxaemia can precipitate neuronal damage in marginally ischaemic areas, it is clearly essential to avoid both hypercarbia and hypoxaemia. It is therefore universally accepted that maintenance of a patent airway with adequate ventilation and oxygenation is vital. This may require tracheal intubation and, in most cases, controlled ventilation. It is also generally agreed that mechanical ventilation should be instituted in head-injured patients who are hypoventilating or have respiratory arrhythmia, and in those with pulmonary dysfunction (see later). Patients who remain hypoxaemic despite administration of supplemental oxygen should also be ventilated, and may benefit from a positive end-expiratory pressure (PEEP) (see Chapter 7). The application of PEEP is unlikely to increase ICP (McGuire et al., 1997) unless P_aCO_2 is allowed to rise, although the lowest level that maintains adequate oxygenation and prevents end-expiratory alveolar collapse should be used. Some head-injured patients will hyperventilate in response to an increased CSF hydrogen ion concentration caused by cerebral ischaemia; controlled ventilation should also be instituted in these cases. Other suggested indications for controlled ventilation include spontaneous flexor or extensor posturing, convulsions and significant intracranial hypertension (e.g. ICP ≥ 15 mmHg) (**Table 15.4**).

Table 15.4 Some suggested indications for mechanical ventilation in head-injured patients

Coma with inadequate airway protection, but unable to tolerate endotracheal tube without sedation/paralysis

Spontaneous extensor posturing

Spontaneous flexor posturing

Glasgow Coma Scale ≤ 8

Repeated convulsions

Spontaneous hyperventilation with arterial carbon dioxide tension (P_aCO_2) < 3.5 kPa (25 mmHg)

Arterial oxygen tension (P_aO_2) < 10.0 kPa (75 mmHg) on air or P_aO_2 < 13 kPa (100 mmHg) on supplemental oxygen

P_aCO_2 > 6.0 kPa (45 mmHg)

Underventilating or showing respiratory arrhythmia in the acute phase

Associated pathology (e.g. chest injury, respiratory pathology) for which mechanical ventilation is indicated

Persistent hyperpyrexia unresponsive to conventional therapy

An intracranial pressure (ICP) of more than 25 mmHg for greater than 25% of a 30-minute period (others suggest a mean ICP persistently > 15 mmHg)

Potential advantages of controlled ventilation for patients in traumatic coma include:

- avoidance of fluctuations in blood gas tensions;
- abolition of the work of breathing;
- greater cardiovascular stability;
- sedatives and analgesic drugs can be administered without the risk of precipitating hypercarbia.

Elective hyperventilation can be used to induce hypocarbia, thereby achieving a reduction in CBF and ICP. The fall in ICP is, however, often relatively short-lived, at least in normal volunteers, because interstitial pH, and therefore cerebrovascular tone, approaches control levels after about 4 hours and is at its previous value within 12–24 hours. Although it is not certain that these time relations apply in those with head injury, it would seem that hyperventilation is of most benefit as a means of rapidly reducing acutely raised ICP. Other possible benefits of induced hypocarbia include the 'inverse steal' phenomenon, which might increase blood flow to damaged areas of brain, and correction of cerebral tissue acidosis, which may increase neuronal survival and improve autoregulation. On the other hand, excessive hypocarbia may produce a massive increase in blood flow through damaged areas of brain and this could enhance oedema formation, precipitate intracerebral haemorrhage and produce local pressure effects. Furthermore, vasoconstriction could precipitate cerebral ischaemia. Indeed, in one prospective, randomized, clinical study, prolonged hyperventilation was associated with a significantly worse outcome when compared to patients in whom normocarbia was maintained (Muizelaar et al., 1991).

Currently it is difficult to make firm recommendations, but it would seem reasonable to aim routinely to achieve only moderate hypocarbia (P_aCO_2 4–4.5 kPa), thereby avoiding the dangers of extreme cerebral vasoconstriction, and to reserve aggressive hyperventilation (P_aCO_2 not less than 3.3 kPa) for those in whom other methods of controlling ICP have failed. In such cases the adequacy of CBF must be monitored (see above). Prolonged hyperventilation is not recommended, although short-term hyperventilation may have a role in reducing elevated ICP in patients who are deteriorating before other measures can be instituted. To avoid a rebound increase in ICP P_aCO_2 must be allowed to rise gradually after a period of hyperventilation. Although some have suggested that a high P_aO_2 may improve brain tissue oxygenation, there is a danger that excessively high oxygen tensions may promote the formation of reactive oxygen species and increase lipid peroxidation. Continuous pulse oximetry and capnography are valuable guides to the ventilatory management of these patients.

Another approach is to use hyperventilation selectively in the management of traumatic coma since in those in whom CBF is already reduced, such treatment is more likely to precipitate brain ischaemia. Conversely, patients with hyperaemia, who remain particularly responsive to alterations in arterial carbon dioxide tension, are more likely to benefit from hyperventilation and are at least risk of developing cerebral ischaemia (Obrist *et al.*, 1984). Determination of the $C_{a-j}O_2$ (see earlier in this chapter) may enable patients with hyperaemia to be identified, whilst cerebral ischaemia precipitated by excessive hyperventilation may be detected as a reduction in S_jO_2.

Sedation. Sedation is commonly achieved by administering a continuous intravenous infusion of a benzodiazepine such as midazolam, accompanied by an opiate infusion to provide analgesia and suppress airway reflexes. Muscle relaxants are sometimes given, usually as a continuous infusion, to minimize the increases in intrathoracic pressure that may otherwise occur in response to positive-pressure ventilation and physiotherapy, as well as to prevent coughing and resisting the ventilator. It should be noted that continuous infusions of benzodiazepines, including midazolam, may be associated with prolonged recovery times and that such treatment has little intrinsic effect on ICP. There is also evidence to suggest that early routine paralysis does not improve outcome from severe head injury and may be detrimental because intensive care stay is prolonged and the incidence of extracranial complications, especially pneumonia, is increased (Hsiang *et al.*, 1994). It would seem sensible to reserve prolonged neuromuscular blockade for those with resistant intracranial hypertension or hypoxaemia. Adequate sedation can usually obviate the need for muscle relaxants.

Anaesthetic induction agents can be administered as continuous intravenous infusions to provide a constant controllable level of sedation. In addition, most have been shown to decrease CBF, probably secondary to a reduction in $CMRO_2$. (An important exception is ketamine, which causes hypertension and a rise in ICP.) It is also possible that the reduction in $CMRO_2$ will protect relatively ischaemic areas of brain from further damage, and seizure activity may be controlled. A disadvantage of all intravenous anesthetics is that they produce a variable degree of cardiovascular depression and can thereby adversely affect CPP (Prior *et al.*, 1983). A beneficial response to the administration of an intravenous anaesthetic agent (a significant reduction in ICP associated with a rise in CPP) is most likely when the baseline voltage of the CFM is greater than 5 μV, the cardiovascular system is stable, the circulating volume is adequate and in the presence of significant intracranial hypertension (ICP ≥ 25 mmHg) (Bingham *et al.*, 1985).

Of all the intravenous anaesthetic agents, *barbiturates* have received most attention, but their use in traumatic coma remains controversial. Although they can undoubtedly control intracranial hypertension and may redistribute blood flow to ischaemic areas as well as abolish seizure activity, the reduction in ICP is often transient and their effects on functional neurological outcome are unclear. Furthermore, barbiturates are particularly potent cardiovascular depressants and continuous infusions may have to be accompanied by the administration of pressor agents to maintain haemodynamic stability. Invasive haemodynamic monitoring may

then be indicated. A further disadvantage of the barbiturates is that they are redistributed to fat stores and as a consequence their sedative effect may persist for some time (at least 48 hours) after the infusion has been discontinued. Neurological assessment, and in particular examination of brainstem function, must therefore be considerably delayed. Prophylactic barbiturate therapy does not influence the incidence or duration of raised ICP, neither does it seem to affect outcome (Ward *et al.*, 1985); most would suggest that barbiturates should only be used, if at all, when other methods have failed to control severe intracranial hypertension. In this small subset of head-injured patients, high-dose barbiturates seem to be effective adjunctive therapy for the control of ICP and there is some suggestion that outcome may be improved (Eisenberg *et al.*, 1988). Barbiturate therapy is likely to be most effective in those with hyperaemia, in the presence of electrical activity and retained carbon dioxide reactivity.

In the past, the short-acting intravenous anaesthetic agents *althesin* and *etomidate* were used in a number of centres for sedation and control of ICP in traumatic coma (Bingham *et al.*, 1985; Prior *et al.*, 1983). These agents caused less cardiovascular depression than barbiturates and recovery was relatively rapid once the infusion had been discontinued. These drugs are no longer available for prolonged intravenous infusion. *Propofol*, which also has a rapid metabolic clearance, is now the hypnotic agent of choice in this situation (Farling *et al.*, 1989; Kelly *et al.*, 1999). This agent has a number of additional properties which may be beneficial in head-injured patients, including a decrease in cerebral metabolic rate (Alkire *et al.*, 1995), potentiation of GABAergic activity, inhibition of NMDA/glutamate receptors and voltage-dependent calcium channels and potent antioxidant activity (Bao *et al.*, 1998). It is believed that propofol maintains, or even improves, cerebral autoregulation but the effect of this agent on flow–metabolism coupling is more controversial. In one study, however, flow–metabolism coupling remained intact during a step increase in propofol, suggesting that achieving burst suppression with this agent may not ameliorate regional ischaemia, at least in the short term and in the absence of refractory intracranial hypertension (Johnston *et al.*, 2003). There has also been some concern that long-term, high-dose infusions (> 5 mg/kg per hour) of propofol may be associated with severe metabolic acidosis, hyperkalaemia, rhabdomyolysis and myocardial failure (Cremer *et al.*, 2001), comparable to that reported in children receiving high doses of this agent (see Chapter 11). Finally, the continuous infusion of anaesthetic induction agents is associated with immune suppression and an increased risk of infection.

Tracheostomy. Some centres perform a tracheostomy early in order to facilitate weaning and reduce sedation requirements, especially in those who remain comatose and in the presence of cervical cord injury.

Cerebral venous drainage. Clearly, intracranial blood volume will rise if cerebral venous drainage is impeded.

The tapes securing the endotracheal or tracheostomy tube must not constrict the neck veins and the patient's head should be centrally positioned. It has been demonstrated that elevation of the head to 30° lowers ICP without decreasing CPP or CBF (Feldman *et al.*, 1992) and that increased intra-abdominal pressure can exacerbate intracranial hypertension (Citerio *et al.*, 2001).

CONTROLLING CEREBRAL OEDEMA

Increases in capillary hydrostatic pressure will exacerbate oedema formation. Control of CBF and systemic blood pressure therefore has the additional theoretical advantage of minimizing cerebral oedema. Most clinicians also restrict intravenous administration of crystalloid solutions (e.g. to 20 mL/kg per day). Hypotonic solutions predispose to cerebral oedema and should not be used.

Diuretics. The fall in ICP that can follow the administration of an osmotic diuretic is probably largely due to a reduction in brain water secondary to the creation of an osmotic gradient between the intravascular and interstitial spaces. In brain-injured patients, administration of mannitol has been shown to reduce cerebral white-matter water content (Nath and Galbraith, 1986) and this is associated with a reduction in ICP, an increased CPP and improved CBF. The maximum effect is seen 10–30 minutes after the infusion and may last for up to 8 hours, but is often transient; its duration depends on the rate at which the gradient is dissipated as osmotically active molecules diffuse into brain tissue, and this in turn is influenced by the integrity of the blood–brain barrier. Fluid might therefore be removed predominantly from normal areas of brain, and this could accentuate brain shift. In addition, repeated doses are usually progressively less effective and eventually the increasing concentration of osmotically active molecules in the interstitial space may actually enhance oedema formation – *the rebound phenomenon*. It has also been suggested that the reduction in ICP produced by mannitol is due primarily to cerebral vasoconstriction, possibly as a compensatory response to an increase in CBF produced by the fall in blood viscosity (Muizelaar *et al.*, 1983). The latter mechanism would explain the early (within a few minutes) reduction in ICP that can follow the administration of mannitol. Mannitol is also a free radical scavenger and may reduce the production of CSF.

Overzealous use of mannitol can precipitate dehydration, electrolyte disturbances and overexpansion of the intravascular compartment. The latter is particularly liable to occur in patients with impaired renal function and will be especially dangerous in the presence of heart disease. Hypovolaemia as well as fluid and electrolyte disturbances can compromise renal function and may be associated with a metabolic acidosis.

To reduce the risk of rebound and fluid overload, the volume of osmotic agent administered should be carefully controlled. Continuous infusions are not recommended. If a patient is deteriorating rapidly in the early stages following a head injury, an intravenous bolus of 20% mannitol can be given in a dose of 0.6–0.7 g/kg. Subsequently 20% mannitol should be administered not more often than every 6 hours, and then only if the ICP is unacceptably high. If on any occasion intracranial hypertension fails to respond, there is no diuresis or the plasma osmolality rises to more than 320 mosm/L, further mannitol should be withheld. If the serum osmolality is allowed to rise to more than 350 mosm/L there is a risk of serious cellular damage.

Mannitol is not recommended as a means of reducing ICP in patients with posttraumatic hyperaemia since the expansion of the circulating volume and fall in viscosity may further increase CBF. Mannitol is most effective when pressure autoregulation is preserved and is superior to barbiturates when $C_{a-j}O_2$ is normal. It is particularly useful in the first few hours after intracranial haemorrhage when the risk of secondary ischaemic damage is greatest (Schrot and Muizelaar, 2002). Diuretics should be used cautiously in those with vascular lesions and in the elderly because decompression may encourage further intracranial bleeding.

If osmotic diuretics and heavy sedation fail to control ICP, it may be worth trying the effect of a *loop diuretic* such as furosemide. This may enhance and prolong the reduction in ICP produced by mannitol (Pollay *et al.*, 1983) by reducing brain water and ion content (irrespective of blood–brain barrier integrity), slowing the formation of CSF and reducing the CVP. Diuretics and mannitol can be used in combination and the losses replaced by colloids, thus maintaining normovolaemia whilst promoting intracellular dehydration. Some have used hypertonic 7.5% saline, sometimes combined with dextran as an alternative to mannitol (Wade *et al.*, 1997). These solutions expand the intravascular volume, reduce intracellular water content, decrease ICP and improve cardiac contractility (see earlier in this chapter). Nevertheless the precise indications for the administration of hypertonic saline have yet to be determined, as have the optimal timing, concentration and volume to be administered.

Steroids. Although steroids are thought to reduce the swelling surrounding a space-occupying lesion such as a cerebral metastasis, they seem to be less effective in controlling intracranial hypertension, and in two relatively small trials failed to improve outcome following severe head injury (Braakman *et al.*, 1983; Cooper *et al.*, 1979). Complications of steroid therapy include salt and water retention and an increase in both the incidence and severity of infectious complications (DeMaria *et al.*, 1985). Twenty-one amino steroids are much more potent antioxidants, without hormonal effects, but clinical trials of these have also proved disappointing. Nevertheless, uncertainty and controversy about the role of steroids in the management of TBI have continued for many years (Alderson and Roberts, 1997). In particular there was concern that the randomized trials of corticosteroids were too small to demonstrate or refute the possibility of only moderate, albeit clinically important, benefit, or indeed of moderate harmful effects (Yates and Roberts, 2000). This uncertainty has been largely resolved by the recent publication of a large (> 10 000 patients), international, multicentre trial which clearly demonstrated that the early administration of a continuous intravenous infusion of methylprednisolone for 48 hours is associated with an increased risk of death or severe disability in adults with clinically significant head injury (Edwards *et al.*, 2005; Roberts *et al.*, 2004). The administration of steroids to patients with severe TBI should therefore be abandoned.

HYPOTHERMIA

ICP is reliably reduced by hypothermia. Moreover, experimental and initial clinical studies suggested that moderate hypothermia (33°C) for 24 hours after the insult might improve the outcome from severe head injury (Marion *et al.*, 1997). On the other hand a more recent randomized, controlled, multicentre study found that hypothermia (33°C) reached within 8 hours of the injury and maintained for 48 hours did not improve outcome from acute brain injury, and perhaps even worsened outcome in those more than 45 years of age (Clifton *et al.*, 2001). In a systematic review, however, it was reported that the relative risk of death and a poor neurological outcome are reduced by hypothermia, and that outcomes are influenced by the depth and duration of hypothermia, as well as the rate of rewarming (McIntyre *et al.*, 2003). The evidence is by no means conclusive, however, and others have concluded that iatrogenic hypothermia confers only marginal benefit in terms of neurological outcome, although prolonged hypothermia may be more effective, particularly in those with raised ICP refractory to other measures (Henderson *et al.*, 2003). It has been suggested therefore that further randomized trials are required in which patients with severe TBI are cooled to 32–34°C within 4 hours of injury, maintained at this temperature for 48–72 hours, and then warmed only if ICP is < 20 mmHg and does not rise with gradual rewarming (Shann, 2003). Avoidance of side effects particularly hypotension, will also be important. In the meantime routine use of therapeutic hypothermia outside a clinical trial cannot be recommended. Nevertheless active warming of patients who are hypothermic on admission, as performed in the control group of the trial by Marion *et al.* (1997) is thought to be potentially harmful and is not recommended.

OTHER MEASURES

In resistant cases, intracranial hypertension may only be controlled by removal of a bone flap or by excising damaged areas of brain. Not only does this allow further expansion of brain substance, but the latter manoeuvre may remove a potential source of oedema fluid. In one series of patients with intractable intracranial hypertension who were treated with decompressive craniectomy, 25% attained social rehabilitation at 1 year (Albanèse *et al.*, 2003).

Finally, if an intraventricular catheter is *in situ*, CSF can be removed intermittently or continuously into a drainage system, although this is unlikely to reduce oedema within brain tissue. Potential problems include ventricular collapse,

with midline shift and obstructive hypdrocephalus in the contralateral ventricle, as well as increased CBF. Nevertheless some recommend drainage of CSF as the first-line manoeuvre in those with a ventricular catheter *in situ*.

Neuroprotective agents (*Royo* et al., 2003)

A wide variety of agents (more than 150) have been investigated for their potential to ameliorate secondary or delayed damage to the injured brain. These have included:

- glutamate antagonists;
- calcium channel blockers;
- magnesium;
- anti-inflammatory compounds (e.g. prostacyclin, cyclo-oxygenase inhibitors, bradykinin receptor antagonists);
- cannabinoids (which inhibit release of glutamate, reactive oxygen species and cytokines, as well as the activity of vasoconstrictors such as endothelin);
- free radical scavengers;
- inhibitors of nitric oxide synthase;
- immunosuppressants;
- caspase inhibitors;
- neurotrophic factors.

So far, however, the results of clinical trials of these agents have been disappointing (Dickinson *et al.*, 2000), perhaps in part because some have been of poor quality and most have been underpowered. In a phase III clinical trial the synthetic cannabinoid dexarabinol was shown to be safe and well tolerated. A single administration of this drug resulted in a significant improvement in ICP and CPP and a trend toward a better neurological outcome (Knoller *et al.*, 2002).

Control of seizure activity

Periods of unprovoked cardiovascular instability may be indicative of seizure activity. Seizures increase cerebral oxygen demands, CBF and, if intracranial compliance is reduced, ICP; prevention, early detection and rapid treatment of seizures are therefore vital.

Most recommend prophylactic administration of phenytoin (100 mg 8-hourly intravenously or orally, preceded by a loading dose of 18 mg/kg infused at a rate not exceeding 50 mg/min). The aim should be to achieve serum drug levels of 10–20 mg/L. If fitting occurs despite phenytoin administration, intravenous diazepam or clonazepam should be given. Occasionally a thiopental infusion may be required. Alternative anticonvulsants such as sodium valproate are sometimes prescribed (see later in this chapter).

Pulmonary dysfunction

Specific causes of pulmonary dysfunction include:

- neurogenic pulmonary oedema;
- prolonged respiratory depression or apnoea leading to atelectasis;
- airway obstruction;
- lung contusion;
- aspiration pneumonitis;

- fat embolism;
- nosocomial pneumonia.

In many patients, however, the cause is not obvious and it has been suggested that in such cases ventilation/perfusion (V/Q) mismatch (possibly related to hypothalamic injury), microemboli and depletion of surfactant may contribute to impaired gas exchange. This may represent a spectrum of lung injury associated with cerebral damage, of which neurogenic pulmonary oedema is the extreme example.

NEUROGENIC PULMONARY OEDEMA (Editorial, 1985; Macmillan et al., 2002)

In 1918, Moutier published a series of cases of rapidly fatal pulmonary oedema occurring in soldiers who had suffered severe head injury. Later, pulmonary oedema was reported in battle casualties in Vietnam who died almost immediately following a major head injury (Simmons *et al.*, 1969). Neurogenic pulmonary oedema is less common in civilian head injuries except in young patients who have sustained massive and usually rapidly fatal brain damage, and is seen most frequently in association with intracranial, especially subarachnoid, haemorrhage. Pulmonary oedema associated with intracranial pathology has also been described in patients with cerebral emboli, cerebral tumours and cysts, and chronically raised ICP. Neurogenic pulmonary oedema may also occur in association with spinal cord injury (see Chapter 10).

Mechanisms. Neurogenic pulmonary oedema develops extremely rapidly, is particularly associated with hypothalamic lesions and does not occur in the presence of cervical cord transection. It is thought to be related to acute hypothalamic dysfunction with medullary ischaemia and brainstem distortion causing a massive sympathetic discharge. It seems that initially this produces marked vasoconstriction and a dramatic rise in pulmonary and systemic arterial pressures, with a fall in cardiac output. As a consequence, there is a shift of circulating volume, pulmonary venous constriction and a rise in pulmonary capillary pressure. The transient, but massive, increase in pulmonary capillary pressure disrupts the endothelium, producing a 'permeability' oedema, which persists even though intravascular pressures rapidly return to normal. Other causes of increased capillary permeability such as microemboli may also be implicated.

Haemodynamic changes. Pulmonary artery occlusion pressure (PAOP), mean pulmonary artery pressure, systemic vascular resistance and pulmonary vascular resistance are characteristically substantially elevated. Reversible myocardial dysfunction, with impaired global and segmental left ventricular systolic function and reductions in cardiac output and left ventricular stroke work, is common (Deehan and Grant, 1996).

Management. Management is supportive and consists of mechanical ventilation, with or without PEEP, together with aggressive therapy to reduce ICP. (Mannitol should probably be avoided. It is preferable to use loop diuretics, ventricular drainage, an intravenous anaesthetic agent or surgical decompression.) Vasodilatation (e.g. using α-blockers, sodium nitroprusside (SNP) or chlorpromazine) may be beneficial, although associated hypotension might jeopardize cerebral perfusion in this vulnerable population of patients. Dobutamine is probably the inotrope of choice because it produces both systemic and pulmonary vasodilatation, reduces PAOP and increases cardiac output (Deehan and Grant, 1996). Despite these measures, mortality amongst those with neurogenic pulmonary oedema remains high, mainly because of the severity of the associated brain injury.

PULMONARY EMBOLISM

There is a considerable risk of deep-vein thrombosis in head-injured patients as a result of hypercoagulability and reduced muscular activity. The incidence has been estimated at 30–40%, with fatal pulmonary embolism occurring in 2–3%.

General measures

PEPTIC ULCER PROPHYLAXIS

Peptic ulcer prophylaxis should be instituted in all head-injured patients (see Chapter 11).

THROMBO-EMBOLIC PROPHYLAXIS

Deep-vein thrombosis and pulmonary embolism are common in head-injured patients. Because of the dangers of anticoagulation, initial preventive measures should include graduated compression stockings and intermittent compression devices. Prophylaxis with heparin can be started after 10–14 days (see Chapter 11).

ANTIBIOTICS

Prophylactic antibiotics are usually prescribed for patients with a CSF leak or an ICP monitoring device *in situ*, as well as postcraniotomy. Some centres do not now give prophylactic antibiotics to those with a CSF leak. It is worth noting that severe head injury precipitates significant immunological deficiencies within 72 hours of the event (Wolach *et al.*, 2001).

PHYSIOTHERAPY

Head-injured patients require expert physiotherapy, not only to prevent and treat pulmonary complications, but also to prevent contractions and to assist rehabilitation.

FLUID AND ELECTROLYTE BALANCE

Hyponatraemia is relatively common after head injury and may be due to cerebral salt wasting or the syndrome of inappropriate antidiuretic hormone (ADH). It is important to distinguish between these two possibilities because the former is treated by administering saline, whereas the latter requires fluid restriction (see Chapter 11). Hypomagnesaemia lowers the seizure threshold and must be corrected, especially since magnesium is neuroprotective.

NUTRITIONAL SUPPORT

Severe head injury is associated with a hypermetabolic state and in some cases the metabolic rate may increase by as much as 40–100%. This leads to a marked negative nitrogen balance and dramatic weight loss. Patients are hyperdynamic with increased $\dot{V}o_2$ and $\dot{V}co_2$. The greatest increase in $\dot{V}o_2$ is seen in those with brainstem involvement, possibly related to increases in catecholamine levels. Fever, agitation and the release of mediators, such as cortisol and interleukin-1, may also be involved in the production of the hypermetabolic state.

Nutritional support is therefore vital and should be started early, preferably within 48 hours. As always the enteral route is preferred. A systematic review has demonstrated a 55% reduction in the risk of infection when head-injured patients receive enteral nutrition within 36 hours, compared to those in whom initiation of enteral feeding was delayed (Marik and Zaloga, 2001) (see Chapter 11).

Other complications

Diabetes insipidus (see later in this chapter and Chapters 11 and 17) is a relatively common complication of severe head injury, but the syndrome of *inappropriate ADH* secretion is unusual.

Coagulopathies, particularly disseminated intravascular coagulation (DIC), can complicate head injury and must be managed aggressively to reduce the risk of intracranial haemorrhage.

PROGNOSIS OF SEVERE HEAD INJURY

The Glasgow Outcome Scale (Jennett and Bond, 1975) can be used to assess recovery from severe head injury in terms of five broad categories (**Table 15.5**). This scale has been criticized as being too insensitive to accommodate the complexities and variability of individual outcomes following TBI. The Extended Glasgow Outcome Scale (Wilson *et al.*, 1998) has therefore been developed that subdivides each of the last three categories into two in order to improve sensitivity for those patients with ratings in the upper end of the scale.

Although some patients may continue to improve for up to a year or even longer after their injury, the majority reach their ultimate outcome category within 3 months, and 90% fail to improve further beyond 6 months. Outcome is related to the GCS, the age of the patient and the nature of the intracranial lesion (Gennarelli *et al.*, 1982). Prognosis is

worst in those with acute subdural haematomas, whereas epidural haematomas and diffuse injury with coma lasting less than 24 hours are associated with a much better outcome (Gennarelli *et al.*, 1982). When the pupils are fixed and dilated mortality is around 90% and hypotension on admission is associated with a doubling of the mortality risk. Subarachnoid haemorrhage (SAH) around the base of the brain can provoke cerebral vasospasm, with poor perfusion leading to death or significant disability. Patients with diffuse axonal injury have a high mortality and, if they survive, are often severely disabled, many remaining in a persistent vegetative state. There is also some evidence to suggest that outcome may be influenced by the patient's genotype (Teasdale and Graham, 1998).

Mortality from severe TBI has fallen dramatically over the last three decades from more than 50% in the 1970s, to about 30% following the advent of intensive care, routine CT scanning, ICP monitoring and reorganization of trauma services. Most recently mortality rates as low as 20% have been reported from some centres. This improvement is probably largely a result of early recognition and treatment of cerebral hypoperfusion. In the early 1980s the overall mortality from severe head injury was in the region of 40–50%, with about 25% making a good recovery, around 17% being moderately disabled and 12–17% being severely disabled or vegetative (Gennarelli *et al.*, 1982; Jennett *et al.*, 1980). Fears that improved survival rates would be associated with an increase in the numbers of vegetative or severely disabled patients have proved to be unfounded. In fact there has been an increase in the numbers of patients with a good outcome, whilst the proportion of vegetative and severely disabled patients has remained essentially unchanged.

It is important to appreciate, however, that even those who are categorized as having made a 'good recovery' may experience considerable difficulties as a result of behavioural and cognitive changes. In some cases, mental disturbances such as anxiety, depression, fatigue, slowness of thinking and personality disorders are disabling and can be quite devastating for patients and their families (Fleminger and Ponsford, 2005). Active rehabilitation of survivors is considered to be essential to achieve the best possible outcomes following head injury.

 ## ACUTE BACTERIAL MENINGITIS
(see Chapter 12)

EPIDEMIOLOGY

The annual incidence of bacterial meningitis in the developed world is about 3–5 cases per 100 000 of the population, with around 75% of all cases occurring in children under 15 years of age. The causative organisms vary according to the age of the population studied but currently *Neisseria meningitidis* and *Streptococcus pneumoniae* are most common outside the neonatal age group (van de Beek *et al.*, 2004). In older children and adults nosocomial meningitis, caused by

Table 15.5 Outcome after brain injury (Glasgow Outcome Scale)
Dead
Persistent vegetative state – awake, but non-sentient
Severe disability – conscious, but dependent on daily support
Moderate disability – independent, but disabled (e.g. able to use transport independently and to work in a sheltered environment)
Good recovery – non-disabling sequelae

organisms such as *Pseudomonas aeruginosa*, enterococci, *Staphylococcus aureus* and coagulase-negative staphylococci, is increasingly common, often as a complication of neurosurgical interventions or trauma.

PATHOPHYSIOLOGY

In order to cause meningitis, bacteria must colonize and penetrate through the nasopharyngeal or oropharyngeal mucosa, survive and multiply in the bloodstream and then invade across the blood–brain barrier. There follows an inflammatory response in the CSF, with disruption of the integrity of the blood–brain barrier and the development of vasogenic, cytotoxic and interstitial oedema. In the early phase CBF autoregulation is impaired (Moller *et al.*, 2000) and cerebral blood volume and ICP are increased. Following this hyperaemic phase CBF may fall as a consequence of intracranial hypertension, the loss of autoregulation and systemic hypotension caused by bacterial sepsis. Vasculitis, vascular spasm and thrombosis also occur in bacterial meningitis and may cause cerebral infarction. As is the case in patients with head injury (see above) increased levels of excitatory amino acids such as glutamate may contribute to neuronal injury.

CLINICAL FEATURES

Patients with bacterial meningitis classically present with:

- fever;
- headache;
- photophobia;
- neck stiffness;
- vomiting;
- altered mental status.

Cranial nerve palsies, focal neurological signs and seizures may also occur. In severe cases there may be signs of raised ICP such as bradycardia, hypertension, altered respiratory pattern and coma. The presentation may be insidious or acute and fulminating. Approximately 50% of patients with meningococcal meningitis, and the majority of those with systemic meningococcal sepsis, will have a *maculopapular*, *petechial* or *purpuric rash*.

DIAGNOSIS

The diagnosis can be confirmed by examining CSF obtained by *lumbar puncture*. Contraindications to lumbar puncture include:

- signs of raised ICP;
- coagulopathy;
- cardiovascular compromise;
- infection of the skin at the proposed site of puncture.

A cranial *CT scan* should be performed before lumbar puncture in order to exclude brain shift in patients with coma, papilloedema or hemiparesis. In many cases, therefore, it may be prudent to defer lumbar puncture, especially in severe meningococcal disease with septic shock and coagu-

loapathy. In most cases of bacterial meningitis examination of the CSF will reveal:

- a white cell count > 1000/μL with a predominance of neutrophils;
- a glucose concentration < 2 mmol/L;
- a ratio of CSF to serum glucose below 0.23;
- a CSF protein > 2.2 g/L.

Any one of these findings alone should raise the possibility of meningitis. The CSF Gram stain is positive in 60–90% of cases and culture is positive in up to 85% of patients, depending on whether they have received prior antibiotic therapy. The use of latex agglutination tests and polymerase chain reaction (PCR) can assist in identification of the causal organism.

The differential diagnosis includes:

- chemical meningitis (e.g. due to intrathecal administration of chemotherapeutic agents);
- carcinomatous meningitis;
- parameningeal focus of infection;
- adverse drug reactions;
- cerebral abscess or tumour;
- intracranial haemorrhage;
- chronic meningitis (e.g. tuberculosis, cryptococcus).

MANAGEMENT

Delayed treatment of bacterial meningitis is associated with a worse outcome.

Antimicrobial therapy (see Chapter 12)
(Moller and Skinhoj, 2000)

Appropriate antimicrobial therapy must be given as soon as possible (ideally within 30 minutes of presentation) and should not be delayed whilst awaiting a CT scan or until lumbar puncture can be performed. A third-generation cephalosporin, such as ceftriaxone, is currently recommended as first line empirical treatment for bacterial meningitis. Ampicillin should be added if listerial meningitis cannot be excluded. In patients with obvious meningococcal disease penicillin is the agent of choice. Vancomycin can be included when pneumococcal meningitis is suspected since this agent acts synergistically with cephalosporins against penicillin-resistant pneumococci. Rifampicin may also have a role in such cases.

Anti-inflammatory treatment

A prospective, randomized, double-blind trial in adults demonstrated that intravenous dexamethasone (10 mg given 15–20 minutes before the first dose of an antimicrobial agent and then every 6 hours for 4 days) reduced the risk of an unfavourable outcome and death (de Gans and van de Beek, 2002). These benefits were most striking in patients with pneumococcal meningitis and in those with moderate to severe disease. In addition impairment of consciousness, seizures and cardiorespiratory failure developed less frequently in those treated with dexamethasone. Importantly, the risk of other adverse events, such as gastrointestinal bleeding, was not increased. The routine use of early adjunctive dexamethasone therapy therefore seems to be warranted in most adults with suspected pneumococcal meningitis (Tunkel and Scheld, 2002). The dexamethasone should be given with, or just before, the first dose of an antimicrobial agent. Delayed treatment is not recommended and, if meningitis is found not to be caused by *Streptococcus pneumoniae*, dexamethasone should be discontinued. In adults with tuberculous meningitis treatment with dexamethasone seems to improve survival but probably does not prevent severe disability (Thwaites *et al.*, 2004).

Supportive care

Many patients with acute bacterial meningitis warrant intensive care admission to monitor and treat cerebral and extracerebral complications. MAP should be restored and ICP controlled as outlined above for TBI. In particular adequate fluid replacement maintains cardiac output and CPP. Patients who require tracheal intubation and mechanical ventilation should be sedated as described above for those with TBI. Seizures must be controlled. Some patients develop the syndrome of inappropriate ADH or diabetes insipidus.

PROGNOSIS

In a recent study the overall mortality rate in adults with community-acquired acute bacterial meningitis was 21%. The mortality rate was higher in patients with pneumococcal meningitis than in those with meningococcal meningitis (30% versus 7%). An unfavourable outcome was more likely in those with evidence of systemic compromise, a low level of consciousness and infection with *S. pneumoniae* (van de Beek *et al.*, 2004).

◾ ENCEPHALITIS

PATHOPHYSIOLOGY

The term encephalitis is applied to conditions in which there is inflammation of neural parenchyma; when the covering of the brain or its myelinated neural tracts are involved the terms meningoencephalitis or encephalomyelitis, respectively, may be used. Neurological damage in encephalitis may be caused not only by the direct cytotoxic effects of the specific pathogen but also, as in acute bacterial meningitis (see above), by inflammation, cerebral oedema and vascular obstruction, with associated hypoxic/ischaemic injury.

CAUSES

Paraneoplastic and parainfectious (or postvaccinial) encephalitis are rare conditions, whilst aseptic meningitis (which may occur in association with a variety of viral upper respiratory or gastrointestinal infections) rarely requires intensive care. The majority of cases of encephalitis seen in the intensive care unit will be viral in origin, the most common

lethal, non-epidemic form being due to *herpes simplex* virus. Acute encephalitis may also be caused by small RNA viruses which move between blood-sucking insect vectors and a vertebrate host, usually small mammals or birds (arthropod-borne or arboviruses). Horses and humans are incidental hosts. *Cytomegalovirus* encephalitis is largely confined to immunosuppressed individuals. It is important to be aware that toxoplasmosis, caused by the protozoan *Toxoplasma gondii*, is one of the most frequent opportunistic central nervous system infections in patients with acquired immunodeficiency syndrome (AIDS). Otherwise acute encephalitis caused by parasitic infection (and by rabies) is now rare in North America and western Europe.

TREATMENT

In patients with herpes simplex encephalitis early treatment with aciclovir can dramatically reduce morbidity and mortality. Since aciclovir is generally a safe drug, empirical administration is justified when the diagnosis of herpes simplex encephalitis is suspected on clinical grounds. It may be possible to confirm the diagnosis later by EEG, MRI scan or PCR for viral DNA in CSF. The role of brain biopsy is controversial.

Supportive treatment should include:

- airway protection and mechanical respiratory support in selected cases;
- measures to control ICP (including mannitol) and maintain CPP;
- clinical and electrophysiological monitoring and control of seizures;
- ventriculostomy for obstructive hydrocephalus or surgical decompression in refractory cases;
- steroids (e.g. dexamethasone 10 mg i.v. followed by 4–6 mg every 6 hours i.v.) are sometimes used for life-threatening raised ICP caused by cerebral swelling.

PROGNOSIS

Despite treatment with aciclovir, the morbidity and mortality of herpes simplex encephalitis remain high and approximately 25% of those who present with stupor or coma will not survive. The prognosis for good functional recovery is also poor. Mortality rates of between 2 and 12% have been reported in epidemics of arboviral encephalitis, whilst rabies encephalitis is almost always fatal.

◾ NON-TRAUMATIC INTRACRANIAL HAEMORRHAGE

CAUSES

Intracranial haemorrhage may originate in the supratentorial region or in the posterior fossa and may occur:

- within the subarachnoid space (SAH);
- within the brain parenchyma (intracerebral or cerebellar haemorrhage);

- into the ventricular system (intraventricular haemorrhage);
- into the subdural or epidural space (rarely).

Often SAH is associated with an intracerebral haematoma and primary intracerebral haematomas may rupture into the subarachnoid space. Intraventricular haemorrhage is often associated with either a haematoma or subarachnoid bleeding.

Most frequently SAH is due to rupture of a saccular or berry cerebral aneurysm, although in some cases no cause is found. In younger patients an arteriovenous malformation may be the source. Intracerebral haemorrhage is more common in older patients, and is usually a consequence of hypertension, when it is usually located in the basal ganglia, pons, cerebellum or subcortical white matter. Lobar haemorrhages may occur in normotensive individuals and are often related to amyloid angiopathy. More unusual causes of intracranial haemorrhage include tumours, drug abuse, mycotic aneurysms and coagulopathy.

PATHOPHYSIOLOGY

Primary cerebral damage is caused by haemorrhagic destruction of brain tissue, whilst secondary brain injury is a consequence of cerebral ischaemia/hypoxia and is therefore potentially preventable. Intracranial hypertension is common and may be due to the space-occupying effect of an intracerebral haematoma, cerebral oedema or hydrocephalus. Hydrocephalus may be caused by intraventricular haemorrhage into the third or fourth ventricle with obstruction of CSF outflow, but extrinsic compression of the fourth ventricle by haematoma in the posterior fossa may also be responsible. Global CPP and CBF may be further compromised by systemic hypotension. Focal ischaemia may develop in the penumbra surrounding an intracerebral haematoma. In those with SAH the potential for ischaemic injury is exacerbated by cerebral vasospasm. *Delayed ischaemic neurological deficit* (DIND) occurs in up to 40% of patients with aneurysmal SAH and is an important cause of morbidity and mortality, with approximately half of these cases developing cerebral infarction.

INVESTIGATIONS

The diagnosis can usually be confirmed by *CT scan*, which also provides accurate information about the location, extent and sequelae of the haemorrhage. When the diagnosis is in doubt *lumbar puncture* may be indicated. *Cerebral angiography* provides detailed images of the cerebral vasculature and can be used to confirm the presence of cerebral vasospasm. *Magnetic resonance angiography* and *CT angiography* are increasingly being used to identify an underlying vascular cause. *Transcranial Doppler* monitoring can be used to detect vasospasm.

MANAGEMENT

Supportive care should include securing the airway, maintenance of oxygenation, blood pressure control, correction of coagulopathy, prevention of seizures and control of ICP. In general active measures to reduce blood pressure are hazardous and should be avoided, although extreme hypertension may exacerbate vasogenic oedema, precipitate left ventricular failure and increase the risk of rebleeding. Urgent surgical evacuation of the haematoma is sometimes indicated.

In those with aneurysmal SAH, hypertensive, hypervolaemic, haemodilution (*triple-H*) and/or endovascular therapy (coiling and balloon angioplasty) is frequently employed, together with prophylactic nimodipine (Barker and Ogilvy, 1996), in an attempt to decrease the incidence of DIND and improve functional outcomes. The mechanism by which nimodipine improves clinical outcomes in aneurysmal SAH is unclear but may be related to a neuroprotective effect since the rate of vasospasm is not altered; it is therefore particularly important to avoid hypotension during treatment with this agent. Complications of triple-H therapy include cardiac failure, pulmonary oedema, respiratory failure and cerebral oedema. Other complications which may be encountered in those with SAH include neurogenic pulmonary oedema, pneumonia, ARDS, arrhythmias and cardiogenic shock. Cardiogenic shock has been successfully treated with intravenous inotropes and intra-aortic balloon counterpulsation (Parr *et al.*, 1996). In some centres dexamethasone is used to control cerebral oedema.

PROGNOSIS

The best predictor of outcome in intracerebral haemorrhage is the size of the haematoma. Massive haemorrhage is rapidly fatal, whereas the prognosis for those with small haematomas is good, provided risk factors are controlled and anticoagulants are avoided. In patients with intermediate-size haemorrhage aggressive treatment may improve outcome, although the prognosis is poor in the elderly and in those with multiple bleeds. Younger patients can make surprisingly good recoveries and recurrence is unusual, provided hypertension is controlled.

Nearly half of the cases of SAH are either dead or moribund before they reach hospital. Of the remainder a further 10–20% die in the early weeks in hospital from rebleeding. Global hyperaemia has been associated with a favourable outcome following aneurysmal SAH (Rothoerl *et al.*, 2004). Prognosis is generally poor in those who remain comatose or have persistent severe neurological defects.

BRAIN DEATH AND IRREVERSIBLE CEREBRAL DAMAGE
(Park, 2004; Wijdicks, 2001)

Death is best viewed not as a single event, but rather as a process during which the function of various organs deteriorates progressively, the precise sequence and time course depending on the nature of the underlying disease, in some cases modified by treatment interventions. A confident diagnosis of death therefore depends on defining with certainty the point beyond which this process becomes irreversible, a decision which, particularly in the context of modern intensive care, is not always straightforward. The traditional signs of death (unconscious, not breathing, no pulse) are easily detectable, major events following which the process of dying normally rapidly accelerates and passes the point of no return. The institution of cardiopulmonary resuscitation can, of course, interrupt, and sometimes reverse, this process so that cessation of heart beat and breathing are no longer necessarily terminal, whilst in patients whose respiratory centre has ceased to function as a result of irreversible brain injury mechanical ventilation can prolong the process of dying. Clearly, therefore, not only do cessation of breathing and the absence of a detectable heart beat not necessarily indicate that the process of dying has become irreversible but there are other 'points of no return' that can precede cardiac arrest.

HISTORY OF BRAIN DEATH

Brain death was first described in 1959 by two French physicians, Mollaret and Goulon (1959), in 23 patients who were comatose, with absent brainstem reflexes, apnoea and an isoelectric EEG. These authors also mentioned various other consequences of brain death such as poikilothermia, diabetes insipidus, hypotension and acidosis. They used the term 'coma dépassé' (a state beyond coma) to describe such cases, which they differentiated from 'coma prolongé', the latter being the condition which is now termed 'persistent vegetative state'. In 1968 the Ad Hoc Committee of the Harvard Medical School defined brain death as irreversible coma (the cause of which had been identified), the patient being totally unreceptive and unresponsive, with absent reflexes and no spontaneous respiratory effort during a 3-minute period of disconnection from the ventilator. The report clearly indicated that this clinical state should be accepted as death. A few years later Mohandas and Chou (1971) suggested that in patients with known but irreparable intracranial lesions irreversible damage to the brainstem was 'the point of no return' and that the diagnosis 'could be based on clinical judgement', thereby introducing the important concepts of aetiological preconditions and a purely clinical diagnosis. Another key contribution was the memorandum issued in the UK by the Conference of Medical Royal Colleges and their Faculties in 1976 which has underpinned clinical practice in the UK, and in many other countries ever since. This emphasized that 'permanent functional death of the brainstem constitutes brain death' and that this should only be diagnosed in the context of irremediable structural brain damage, after exclusion of certain specified conditions which might contribute to or cause the coma (Conference of Medical Royal Colleges and their Faculties, 1976). This report also described the use of simple clinical tests to establish the permanent loss of brainstem function. A second memorandum in 1979 equated brainstem death with death itself and a code of practice was produced by the Academy of Medical Royal Colleges in 1998. In the USA guidelines

---

Table 15.6 Criteria for the diagnosis of death in the USA

Either:

A. An individual with irreversible cessation of circulatory and respiratory functions is dead
1. Cessation is recognized by an appropriate clinical examination
2. Irreversibility is recognized by persistent cessation of functions during an appropriate period of observation and/or trial of therapy

Or:

B. An individual with irreversible cessation of all functions of the entire brain, including the brainstem is dead
1. Cessation is recognized when evaluation discloses findings of a and b:
   a. Cerebral functions are absent and
   b. Brainstem functions are absent
2. Irreversibility is recognized when evaluation discloses findings of a and b and c:
   a. The cause of coma is established and is sufficient to account for the loss of brain functions and
   b. The possibility of recovery of any brain functions is excluded and
   c. The cessation of all brain functions persists for an appropriate period of observation and/or trial of therapy

---

issued by a government commission state that an individual who has sustained either irreversible cessation of circulatory and respiratory functions or irreversible cessation of all function of the *entire* brain, including the brainstem, is dead (**Table 15.6**).

Thus the means by which the diagnosis of death can be established with certainty has evolved from recognition of the traditional signs of death (coma, absent heart sounds, pulse and breathing) to the diagnosis of total brain death and, in the UK and many European countries, to establishing death of only the brainstem. Death, it has been suggested, should now be conceived as a state in which there is irreversible loss of the capacity for consciousness combined with irreversible loss of the capacity to breathe (and hence maintain a heartbeat) (Pallis, 1983). Alone neither would be sufficient. Both are essentially brainstem functions and death of the brainstem is therefore considered by many to be equivalent to death of the individual.

ETHICAL CONSIDERATIONS

If the brainstem is destroyed consciousness is lost and respiration ceases; independent existence is then impossible and in the absence of therapeutic intervention cardiac arrest rapidly supervenes. It is now widely accepted, therefore that 'brainstem death' is a definition of death itself. The recommendations of the Conference of Royal Colleges and their Faculties in the UK, or similar guidelines elsewhere in the world, are believed by most practising clinicians to be a correct and ethical means of diagnosing brain death. Death can therefore be declared once death of the brainstem has been confirmed (not some time later when the heart stops or the ventilator is switched off) and most would argue that mechanical ventilation should then be discontinued as soon as possible. This should not be viewed as withdrawing support to allow a patient to die but rather as ceasing a futile intervention in a patient who is already dead. To continue to ventilate a brain-dead patient until asystole supervenes can be undignified for the patient, is often unnecessarily distressing for the relatives, and can adversely affect staff morale. It is also an inefficient and uneconomical use of resources. Most clinicians therefore find the decision to discontinue ventilating a brain-dead patient relatively straightforward when compared to the more difficult ethical dilemmas involved in withdrawing or limiting treatment for patients in a persistent vegetative state or critically ill patients whose prognosis is considered to be hopeless (see Chapter 2). The only situation in which it might be considered inappropriate to discontinue ventilating a brainstem-dead patient is when she is pregnant. In some such cases it has proved possible to support the mother, for up to 3 months, to permit growth of the fetus until delivery by caesarean section can be performed safely.

It is a common misconception that the concept of brainstem death was developed in order to facilitate organ donation. Not only is this not the case but it should be clear that, even if transplantation therapy did not exist, the ability to diagnose brain death with confidence plays an important role in the humane practice of intensive care.

DIAGNOSIS

Before considering the diagnosis of brainstem death it is essential that certain preconditions and exclusions are fulfilled. (*These recommendations should not replace clinical judgement and may be modified in the light of clinical circumstances.*)

Preconditions

The diagnosis of brainstem death should only be considered when:

- The patient is in *apnoeic coma* (i.e. unresponsive and on a ventilator, with no spontaneous respiratory efforts).
- *Irremediable structural brain damage* due to a disorder that can cause brainstem death has been diagnosed with certainty (e.g. head injury, intracranial haemorrhage).

In most cases a CT scan will have clearly identified the cause of the coma and the extent of cerebral injury.

Exclusions

Exclusions for diagnosing brainstem death are as follows.

- The possibility that unresponsive apnoea is the result of *poisons, sedative drugs* or *neuromuscular-blocking agents*

must be excluded. Narcotics, hypnotics and tranquillizers may have a prolonged duration of action, especially in those with hypothermia, or renal or hepatic failure. The benzodiazepines in particular are cumulative and their actions may be persistent, as may those of thiopental. It is therefore essential that the drug history is carefully reviewed and adequate time is allowed for the persistence of drug effects to be excluded. A nerve stimulator may be used to ensure that the patient is not paralysed. Some have suggested that testing of the neuromuscular junction should be compulsory. Blood and urine should be tested for the presence of drugs if there is any doubt, although it should be recognized that plasma concentrations can be misleading when sedatives have been infused for prolonged periods and that they may not correlate with effect. Antagonist drugs such as naloxone or flumazenil may cause sudden changes in CPP and should only be used after the first set of tests has demonstrated brainstem death.

- *Hypothermia* must be excluded as a cause of coma. It is recommended that the central body temperature should be more than 35°C.
- There must be no significant *metabolic or endocrine disturbance* that could produce or contribute to coma or cause it to persist. There should be no profound abnormality of the plasma electrolytes, acid–base balance or blood glucose levels.

It is recognized that some metabolic and endocrine disturbances are common accompaniments of brainstem death (e.g. hypernatraemia, diabetes inspidius) but that these are the effect rather than the cause of the patient's condition and do not necessarily preclude the diagnosis of brainstem death.

A variety of acquired neuropathies and myopathies may complicate critical illness (see below). These conditions can cause profound weakness affecting all muscle groups, including the respiratory muscles, but should not be confused with true apnoea. They do not affect papillary, corneal, oculocephalic or vestibulo-ocular reflexes and are therefore easily distinguished from brainstem death. On the other hand variant forms of Guillain–Barré syndrome (GBS: see below) have been reported as mimicking brainstem death. In such cases, however, brainstem death criteria are not satisfied because the diagnosis of a disorder that can lead to brain death has not been established, neither is there evidence of irremediable structural brain damage.

Assessment of brainstem function

Next it is necessary to establish that all brainstem reflexes are absent. (The tests should not be performed in the presence of seizures or abnormal decorticate or decerebrate postures.)

- The *pupils* should be fixed and unresponsive to bright light. Both direct and consensual light reflexes should be examined. (Difficulty in interpretation may be experienced when there has been direct trauma to the eye and/or optic nerve, and if topical mydriatics have been used.) Pupil size is irrelevant, although most often they will be dilated.

- *Corneal reflexes* should be absent. (Again, there may be difficulty when the eyelids are bruised and oedematous due to trauma.)
- *Oculocephalic reflexes* should be absent (i.e. when the head is rotated from side to side, the eyes move with the head and therefore remain stationary relative to the orbit). In a comatose patient whose brainstem is intact, the eyes will rotate relative to the orbit (i.e. doll's-eye movements are present).
- *Vestibulo-ocular reflexes* should be absent ('caloric testing'). If 20 mL of ice-cold water is slowly instilled into the external auditory meatus it will stimulate the tympanic membrane. If the patient's brainstem is intact, reflex eye movements will occur within 20–30 seconds, provided that access to the tympanic membrane is not prevented (e.g. by blood or wax in the meatus). This possibility should be excluded by direct inspection. It should be remembered that gentamicin can cause end-organ poisoning, and central pathways may be impaired by drugs. Severe trauma may prevent caloric testing on one side or the other, but this does not invalidate the tests.
- There should be *no motor responses within the cranial nerve territory* to painful stimuli applied centrally or peripherally. Spinal reflex movements of the limb and trunk may be present. The doctor must be able to explain the significance of such movements to the patient's family, including the fact that they are reflex rather than voluntary.
- There must be no *gag or cough reflexes* in response to pharyngeal, laryngeal or tracheal stimulation.
- *Spontaneous respiration* should be absent. This test is crucial to the diagnosis of brainstem death. The patient should be ventilated with 5% carbon dioxide in 95% oxygen for 10 minutes and then disconnected from the ventilator for a further 10 minutes. Oxygenation is maintained by insufflation with 100% oxygen at high flows via a catheter placed in the endotracheal tube. The patient is observed for any signs of spontaneous respiratory efforts. A blood gas sample should be obtained during this period to ensure that the P_aCO_2 is sufficiently high to stimulate spontaneous respiration (≥ 6.7 kPa, 50 mmHg). It must be remembered that a few patients with severe chronic obstructive pulmonary disease (COPD) are dependent on a hypoxic drive to respiration. (In the USA a higher threshold P_aCO_2 of 60 mmHg or 20 mmHg above the baseline value is recommended.) It is essential to disconnect the patient from the mechanical ventilator to prevent 'auto-triggered' breaths which can simulate spontaneous respiration (Willatts and Drummond, 2000).

In the UK it is recommended that the examination should be performed by two doctors a minimum of 6 hours after the onset of coma, or if due to cardiac arrest, hypoxia or severe circulatory insufficiency at least 24 hours after restoration of an adequate circulation. Similarly it may take longer to establish the diagnosis in those suspected of having cerebral air or fat embolism. The logic of delaying tests under these circumstances has, however, been questioned.

UK guidelines also suggest that the tests should be performed on two separate occasions, the interval between the two being agreed by all the staff involved. The doctors should be either the consultant in charge of the case and one other (clinically independent of the first and registered for more than 5 years), or the consultant's deputy, provided he or she has been registered at least 5 years and has adequate appropriate experience, and one other. Neither should be a member of the transplant team. In some cases the primary pathology may be unclear and a confident diagnosis may only be reached by continued clinical observation and further investigations. A neurologist should be consulted if the underlying diagnosis is in doubt.

CONFIRMATORY TESTS

In the UK, and a number of other European countries and some states in the USA, confirmatory tests are optional and are normally reserved for those cases in which there is uncertainty regarding the cause and the reversibility of the coma. In several other European, Central and South American and Asian countries, confirmatory testing is required by law. Certain countries, such as Sweden, require only cerebral angiography.

Electroencephalography

Some still consider it to be important to confirm absence of cerebral electrical activity on serial EEG before concluding that a patient is brain-dead, and indeed this is mandatory in some jurisdictions. Others recommend the use of evoked potentials to assist in the diagnosis since these will be preserved when EEG silence is attributable to drugs (see above). This technique is, however, prone to errors of interpretation in inexperienced hands. In the UK most argue that an EEG would only be relevant if the objective was to establish death of the whole brain, not just the brainstem, and that, in any case, an isoelectric EEG cannot exclude activity in deeper areas of the brain and may have other causes, such as barbiturate coma. Patients have been reported in whom the EEG was isoelectric but brainstem reflexes were preserved, although this is extremely unusual. Moreover intensive care units are a hostile environment in which to record an EEG and considerable expertise is required to avoid multiple artefacts which might be falsely interpreted as residual electrical activity. In a patient who meets all the clinical criteria for brain death such residual activity might unnecessarily delay confirmation of the diagnosis in some patients. Finally the equipment and expertise to obtain and correctly interpret an EEG are not available in all hospitals.

Demonstrating absence of cerebral blood flow

Absence of CBF may also be used to confirm death of the whole brain. Four-vessel cerebral angiography can be used but more recently nuclear imaging with technetium (Tc99m) has been introduced. Transcranial Doppler ultrasonography may prove to be a useful bedside method for confirming the absence of CBF. Although total absence of CBF provides compelling evidence of brain death, findings can be equivocal in the presence of unequivocal clinical signs of brain death.

Recently, it has been suggested that some aspects of the UK code of practice (and some other national guidelines) would benefit from further refinement and greater clarity (Bell et al., 2004). In particular there is considerable variation in clinicians' interpretation of the guidance relating to elimination of confounding variables (such as biochemical disturbances and the residual effects of sedative drugs), the timing, repetition of and interval between the tests and the conduct of the apnoea test. It has also been suggested (Bell et al., 2004) that confirmatory tests could play a more prominent role, especially when clinical testing is delayed by the presence of long-acting sedative drugs.

ORGAN DONATION

As a result of advances in immunosuppression, surgical techniques and intensive care, transplantation of cadaveric organs is now a life-saving and life-enhancing treatment for patients with end-stage organ failure. Unfortunately the increase in the numbers undergoing transplant surgery has failed to keep pace with the accumulation of patients with end-stage organ failure who might benefit from transplantation, largely because of a persistent shortfall in the availability of donor organs. This long standing shortage of organs may have been exacerbated by a fall in donor numbers, possibly as a consequence of a reduction in deaths from motor vehicle accidents, improved trauma care and exclusion of some potential donors by human immunodeficiency virus (HIV) screening (although an HIV-positive donor could donate to an HIV-positive recipient). The shortfall has also been compounded by patients confirmed as brainstem-dead failing to donate organs because of general medical contraindications to organ donation, relatives' refusal to consent to organ retrieval and, rarely, failure to ask about organ donation. Non-performance of brainstem tests when brainstem death is a possibility may also account for a significant number of missed donors. Finally, in some cases lack of facilities or organizational difficulties prevent the procurement of offered, suitable organs and it has been noted that in many cases where consent is obtained for multiple organ donation, only the kidneys are retrieved. Clearly, therefore, there is considerable scope for improving organ retrieval rates from suitable brainstem-dead patients, although it seems that even if the proportion of such patients who become donors were to increase substantially, the yield would still be insufficient to satisfy the demand for cadaveric

organs (Gore et al., 1989, 1992). Suggested measures have included:

- further publicity and education to increase the proportion of cases where consent is obtained;
- increased discussion to allow multiple rather than limited organ retrieval;
- required discussion with the transplant coordinator;
- the avoidance of non-procurement of suitable organs by improved organization of retrieval teams;
- the provision of adequate facilities in transplant units.

Certainly early referral of potential donors is strongly recommended to allow time for discussions about donor care, as well as agreement on medical contraindications to donation and the suitability of specific organs for tranplantation. Prompt completion of brainstem testing should reduce the number of organs which become unsuitable due to deterioration of the donor. The likely impact of introducing required request or 'opting-out' legislation is less certain (Gore et al., 1989) and many believe that the best course of action would be to improve the efficiency of the 'opting-in' system, for example by establishing a comprehensive computer database and expanding the local registers. Coroner's refusal should rarely prevent donation. Finally consent rates are higher when the request is made by experienced personnel, in conjunction with the transplant coordinator, in a private setting and when the interview is separated from the pronouncement of brain death.

Recently attempts have been made to increase the number of cadaveric kidneys available for transplantation by using non-heart-beating donors. Certainly transplantation of kidneys from donors whose hearts have stopped beating, especially trauma victims, is often successful (Cho et al., 1998).

Securing permission for organ retrieval. Should it not be possible to determine the previously stated wishes of the deceased then permission for, or lack of objection to, organ retrieval is sought from the next of kin. On occasions there may be difficulty in deciding who this is, in which case the most senior, the closest, or at least the most concerned, relative should be identified and asked to canvass views within the family and to act as spokesperson. In the event of disagreement amongst the relatives it is normally acceptable to accede to the wishes of the nearest or most interested, or, in a situation where there are several close relatives, the majority view. If there is serious, unresolvable disagreement it may be wiser not to proceed to organ donation.

Difficulties may also be encountered when the next of kin attempt to override the clearly stated wish of the deceased to donate organs in the event of death. This may arise for example when the patient was carrying a donor card or had registered such wishes on a computer database. Currently the generally accepted legal view in the UK is that the person lawfully in possession of the body is the hospital management and that the relatives cannot therefore veto the patient's wishes. In practice, however, once the issues have been fully discussed it is almost always advisable to concur with the relatives' wishes.

All potential donors must be tested for HIV; it is recommended that permission to perform this test, and any other invasive procedure performed for the purpose of organ donation, should be obtained from the relatives. A positive HIV test must be revealed to those at risk of contracting the disease from the deceased. This requires sensitivity and tact, combined with the provision of appropriate counselling and follow-up services.

It is important that discussion with the relatives should specifically address the issue of multiple rather than limited organ retrieval.

Multiple organ donation

Because of the shortage of donors, retrieval of multiple organs, which can be performed without jeopardizing the function of individual organs, should now be the objective in all suitable brainstem-dead patients. In such cases, assiduous supportive treatment is essential to prevent deterioration of initially suitable donors as this will both increase donation rates and improve graft survival and function (Timmins and Hinds, 1991).

SUPPORTING THE ORGAN DONOR
(Wood *et al.*, 2004)

Complications related to the profound physiological consequences of brainstem death are common and include:

- hypotension;
- arrhythmias;
- cardiac arrest requiring cardiopulmonary resuscitation;
- requirement for multiple transfusions;
- diabetes insipidus;
- DIC;
- pulmonary oedema;
- hypoxia;
- acidosis;
- seizures;
- bacteraemia.

Since these complications may jeopardize organ function, potential donors should be carefully monitored and corrective measures instituted early. The incidence of complications increases progressively after brainstem death and, although adequate time must be allowed to confirm the diagnosis, unnecessary delays must be avoided. In the meantime meticulous intensive care is required to sustain organ perfusion and to improve graft survival and function. In particular a high level of nursing care is required. The introduction of a comprehensive standardized donor management regimen, which included pulmonary artery catheterization and hormone replacement (triiodothyronine (T_3), ADH, insulin and steroids), has been shown to increase the proportion of hearts which are suitable for transplantation (Wheeldon *et al.*, 1995). Similarly a policy of aggressive donor management which included pulmonary artery catheterization, fluid resuscitation, early use of vasopressors and the liberal use of thyroid hormone in haemodynamically

unstable donors was associated with a significant increase in the number of organs available for transplantation (Salim *et al.*, 2005). Such strategies may allow the recovery of organs that were initially assessed as unsuitable, minimize the loss of donors during maintenance and increase the number of organs that can be procured and transplanted with a favourable outcome.

Cardiovascular system
PATHOPHYSIOLOGY

When brainstem death is precipitated by intracranial hypertension, the sudden onset of brainstem ischaemia is associated with an agonal period of intense autonomic activity and considerable increases in circulating catecholamine levels. This can precipitate vasoconstriction, hypertension, myocardial ischaemia, tachycardia and various arrhythmias, including ventricular ectopics, supraventricular tachycardia and heart block. Left atrial pressure may increase sufficiently to cause pulmonary oedema. There may also be significant myocardial damage which can be severe and irreversible, especially when the rise in ICP is sudden. Moreover the myocardial cells are depleted of high-energy phosphates and glycogen, and lactate levels are increased. It has been suggested that this defect in oxidative metabolism might be caused by mitochondrial inhibition mediated by endocrine disturbances, in particular reductions in T_3 (see below). These changes, combined with desensitization of β-receptors and alterations in β-adrenergic signal transduction, are accompanied by impaired right and left ventricular function, which could contribute to early posttransplantation cardiac failure. Administration of high-dose catecholamines could exacerbate myocardial dysfunction by decreasing β-adrenergic receptor numbers. The period of intense autonomic activity is followed by a fall in catecholamine levels, loss of sympathetic tone and vasodilatation, sometimes with bradycardaia and a nodal rhythm unresponsive to atropine. ECG abnormalities, including ST-segment and T-wave changes, are common.

MONITORING

Assessment of cardiovascular function in brainstem-dead patients can be difficult. Central venous and intra-arterial pressure monitoring, as well as hourly measurements of urine volume, are essential and the core–peripheral temperature gradient should be monitored routinely, but these variables may be misleading as indicators of tissue perfusion. Pulmonary artery catheterization or oesophageal Doppler monitoring may therefore be helpful when blood pressure and urine output fail to improve despite an apparently adequate circulating volume, as well as for patients with pre-existing cardiac disease, pulmonary oedema or left ventricular dysfunction caused, for example, by direct cardiac trauma or cardiac tamponade. Echocardiography can also be useful. Because of the order in which the great vessels are ligated during harvesting of organs the arterial line is best located in the left radial or brachial artery and the pulmonary artery catheter in the right internal jugular vein.

MANAGEMENT

The initial sympathetic overactivity can be attenuated by the short-acting β-blocker esmolol. Hypotension may precipitate acute tubular necrosis and decrease graft survival. Initially hypotension should be treated with fluid resuscitation using normal saline or lactated Ringer's, although many prefer to use colloidal solutions. Starch solutions, however, should be avoided (see Chapter 5). Care should be exercised because organs that have been damaged during the sympathetic storm and by subsequent systemic inflammation (particularly the lungs) are susceptible to volume overload. Inotropes and/or vasopressors are indicated in those who fail to respond to volume expansion, although the use of high-dose inotropes may depress myocardial β-adrenergic receptors and adversely affect tissue blood flow. Most recommend dopamine in the first instance because at low infusion rates it causes vasodilation of renal and mesenteric vessels and might, therefore, help to preserve intra-abdominal organs. The direct tubular effect of dopamine could, however, exacerbate polyuria and, at higher doses, vasoconstriction might impair graft survival. Because the release of endogenous catecholamines is thought to be an important factor in the development of myocardial damage after brain death the use of dopamine, which can release noradrenaline from adrenergic nerve endings, might theoretically exacerbate myocardial injury. Dobutamine can be used in those who fail to respond to a moderate dose of dopamine and when specifically indicated (e.g. in patients with myocardial contusion), although β-mediated peripheral vasodilation may precipitate hypotension. Noradrenaline and more recently vasopressin have been recommended as a short-term measure in potential organ donors with profound vasodilation in order to maintain systemic blood pressure during fluid resuscitation. Adrenaline (epinephrine) may be useful in those with refractory hypotension. In the unlikely event of donor surgery involving only the heart, it has been suggested that a pure α-agonist which would maintain coronary perfusion pressure and limit tachycardia might be the ideal choice. In the event of cardiac arrest resuscitation should be attempted because recovery of cardiac function in the potential donor can result in successful transplantation.

Endocrine changes (Bittner *et al.*, 1995)
DIABETES INSIPIDUS (see Chapter 17)

Deficiency of ADH leads to loss of free water, dehydration, hypovolaemia, hyperosmolality, and other electrolyte disturbances. Treatment initially involves replacing measured urine volume and electrolyte losses with appropriate fluids. Hypernatraemia must be avoided by using hypotonic solutions such as 0.45% saline or 5% dextrose with added electrolytes, guided by plasma levels and urinary losses. It should be remembered that most colloidal solutions contain considerable quantities of sodium.

In view of the complications associated with the infusion of large volumes of crystalloid some have recommended that diabetes insipidus complicating brain death should be corrected by administering *vasopressin*. This approach has been controversial, however. Vasopressin causes a dose-dependent vasoconstriction that can decrease cardiac output, coronary, pulmonary and mesenteric blood flow and might be associated with a higher incidence of acute tubular necrosis and a lower rate of graft survival. On the other hand a continuous infusion of arginine vasopressin, in the lowest dose (0.5–6 units/hour) required to reduce urine output to 1.5–3 mL/kg per hour, can decrease plasma hyperosmolality, reduce electrolyte imbalance, improve haemodynamic stability and reduce inotrope requirements. There is, however, considerable disagreement about the volume of urine output above which vasopressin should be administered. Compared with vasopressin, *desmopressin* has a longer duration of action, coupled with a greater antidiuretic effect relative to its pressor activity and has therefore been recommended as an alternative to vasopressin. In a randomized controlled study desmopressin (1 μg bolus every 2 hours when diuresis was more than 300 mL/hour) had no adverse effects on the function of the grafted kidney (Guesde *et al.*, 1998).

THYROID HORMONES, ACTH, CORTISOL, INSULIN

Circulating levels of thyroxine (T_4) and T_3 fall in brain-dead experimental animals, while thyroid-stimulating hormone (TSH) levels remain unchanged. Similar reductions in T_3 have been reported in human donors. This reduction in circulating levels of thyroid hormones could be responsible for the inhibition of mitochondrial function, reduced aerobic metabolism and deterioration in myocardial function seen after brainstem death. In support of this hypothesis, administration of T_3 can reverse donor myocardial dysfunction. The fall in T_3 levels in brainstem-dead patients is, however, similar to that found in most severe illnesses (sick euthyroid syndrome: see Chapter 17) and, in such patients, replacement is of no proven benefit. T_3 supplementation may therefore be unnecessary and it is possible that the fall in T_3 is a protective mechanism.

Circulating levels of adrenocorticotrophic hormone (ACTH) and cortisol also fall after brain death in experimental animals and lesser falls have been recorded in organ donors. Reductions in serum cortisol levels following brainstem death do not, however, seem to be related to the incidence of hypotension. Glucagon and insulin levels also fall.

The administration of supplementary T_3, cortisol and insulin to organ donors may improve haemodynamics, reduce lactate levels and reverse acidosis, thereby increasing retrieval rates of transplantable organs and improving graft function. Nevertheless it has been recommended that, until the results of prospective clinical trials are available, hormone replacement therapy should be reserved for donors who remain unstable despite moderate doses of inotropes/vasopressors.

HYPERGLYCAEMIA

Hyperglycaemia is a frequent complication of brain death because of the administration of hypotonic glucose-containing fluids to replace large urinary losses, combined with reduced insulin secretion, and increased levels of catecholamines. The consequent increase in extracellular osmolality may lead to intracellular dehydration, an osmotic diuresis and electrolyte disturbances; hyperglycaemia may be associated with decreased pancreatic allograft survival. It is therefore important to control blood glucose levels with an intravenous insulin infusion.

Renal support

Episodes of hypotension can precipitate acute tubular necrosis and reduce graft survival. A donor urine output of less than 100 mL/h in the hour preceding nephrectomy has been shown to be associated with an increased incidence of acute tubular necrosis in the transplanted kidney. If urine output is low, despite an adequate circulating volume and perfusion pressure, some suggest that a low-dose dopamine infusion should be administered. If this fails to produce a diuresis, small intravenous doses of furosemide (10 mg) or a furosemide infusion may be given. Administration of mannitol (0.5 g/kg) 1 hour before harvest has been recommended.

Respiratory support

Respiratory function may be compromised by lung contusion, neurogenic pulmonary oedema, aspiration pneumonitis or pneumonia. The aim of respiratory support is to optimize oxygen delivery to vital organs by ensuring adequate oxygenation with minimal cardiovascular depression. The risk of pulmonary infection should be minimized by aseptic tracheal suction and postural drainage, there being no constraints on these procedures once brainstem death has been established. If low the P_aCO_2 should be allowed to return to normal levels in order to avoid the vasconstriction associated with hypocarbia. Since carbon dioxide production falls after brainstem death, this may require a considerable reduction in minute volume or the addition of dead space. The inspired oxygen concentration should be adjusted to achieve adequate saturation of haemoglobin with oxygen, but, especially if the lungs are to be transplanted, the fractional inspired oxygen concentration should, if possible, be maintained below 0.5–0.6 to avoid oxygen toxicity. High tidal volumes and airway pressures, which can reduce cardiac output and may exacerbate ventilator-associated lung injury (see Chapters 7 and 8), should be avoided, although if the lungs are to be transplanted, a low level of PEEP (5 cm H_2O) is recommended to prevent alveolar collapse. Despite these measures there is a high incidence of pulmonary dysfunction in brain-dead patients, which frequently excludes donation of the lungs for transplantation. There is evidence that lung injury in this situation is in part related to enhanced pulmonary inflammation caused by a systemic inflammatory response to severe brain injury (Fisher et al., 1999); it has been suggested that this inflammatory reaction is likely to involve other vital organs.

Coagulation

Tissue fibrinolytic agents and plasminogen activators are released from areas of ischaemic or necrotic brain. Fibrin deposits and free haemoglobin may jeopardize the function of transplanted organs. DIC occurs in as many as 28% of brain-dead organ donors. To minimize these problems, support with blood products and early procurement of organs is advised. Epsilon aminocaproic acid should not be given because of the risk of microvascular thrombosis in donor organs.

Hypothermia

Temperature regulation is markedly impaired after brain death by loss of hypothalamic control, with a reduction in heat production secondary to the fall in metabolic rate and loss of muscular activity, as well as peripheral vasodilation. Although mild hypothermia may protect vital organs, temperatures below 32°C can result in decreased cardiac performance and coagulopathy. Moreover, brainstem death cannot be diagnosed in a hypothermic (core temperature < 35°C) patient. The core temperature should be maintained above 35°C by increased insulation and active warming of the patient.

Intraoperative management

The principles of donor management described above should be continued into the intraoperative period. To avoid reflex neuromuscular activity a muscle relaxant that does not depress the cardiovascular system should be used. Nitroglycerine, nitroprusside and isoflurane have all been recommended to control reflex hypertension. Hypotension may be precipitated by manipulation of the heart and great vessels or flushing donor organs with cold preservation solution. Blood loss may be considerable. Administration of pressor agents, especially in high doses, may jeopardize organ perfusion and some recommend pulmonary artery catheterization or oesophageal Doppler monitoring during retrieval surgery to minimize the use of inotropes and vasopressor drugs. If cardiac arrest occurs, cardiopulmonary resuscitation should be instituted while procurement of liver and kidneys proceeds rapidly with cross-clamping of the aorta at diaphragm level and infusion of cold preservation solution into the distal aorta and portal vein.

Criteria for organ donation

In all cases brain death must have been established and the consent of the next of kin and the coroner must have been obtained. Blood samples should be taken for screening for hepatitis and HIV, as well as blood group determination and tissue typing. Although overwhelming infection generally precludes donation, bacteraemia and fungaemia are not absolute contraindications to donation. Organs from donors infected with hepatitis B and C may be transplanted into recipients infected with the same virus and may be considered for those who are not infected but are in urgent need of a life-saving transplantation. The organs must be removed by a surgeon who has examined the donor and is satisfied with the diagnosis of brainstem death. The procedure must be performed under full operating conditions in theatre.

Kidney

Guidelines for selecting a suitable kidney donor are shown in **Table 15.7**.

Heart and heart/lung

Guidelines for selecting a suitable heart or heart/lung donor are shown in **Table 15.7**.

A chest radiograph and 12-lead ECG should be obtained. Echocardiography should be performed to exclude structural abnormaliites that would preclude cardiac transplantation and to provide an estimate of the ejection fraction. Occasionally coronary angiography will be requested. Myocardial dysfunction associated with brain death may be reversible and is not necessarily a contraindication to donation.

Liver

Most suitable kidney donors are also suitable liver donors. There should be no history of drug or alcohol abuse.

Cornea

All adults are suitable donors provided there is no history of eye disease, intraocular surgery, syphilis, hepatitis, HIV infection or postinfectious polyneuritis. The eyes can be removed up to 24 hours after cardiorespiratory arrest, but preferably within 1 hour.

THE PERMANENT VEGETATIVE STATE

Once the diagnosis of brain death has been firmly established, the vast majority of clinicians accept that there is no ethical dilemma involved in discontinuing mechanical ventilation. A much more difficult problem arises when the brainstem remains intact, but the cerebral cortex ceases to function, either because of direct ischaemic/hypoxic damage (e.g. following cardiac arrest) or because of severe disruption of the white matter, such as may occur following head injury. These patients may breathe adequately unaided and can survive for long periods in a cognitively unresponsive state.

A working group convened by the Royal College of Physicians (1996) has defined this *vegetative state* as 'a clinical condition of unawareness of self and environment in which the patient breathes spontaneously, has a stable circulation and shows cycles of eye closure and eye opening which may simulate sleep and waking. This may be a transient stage in the recovery from coma or it may persist until death' (Review by a Working Group convened by the Royal College of Physicians, 1996). The *continuing vegetative state* can be diagnosed when the vegetative stage continues for more than 4 weeks, whilst *the permanent vegetative state* is diagnosed when irreversibility can be established with a high degree of certainty, for example after 6–12 months have elapsed. This working group also specified criteria for establishing the diagnosis. They recommend that the diagnosis of persistent vegetative state should be made by two medical practitioners experienced in assessing disturbances of consciousness and that the assessment be repeated when there is uncertainty. The

Table 15.7 Guidelines for the selection of suitable donors

Kidney

Brainstem dead

2–70 years old

Adequately perfused and hydrated

Artificially ventilated

Free from:
  Hepatitis antigen and HIV
  Malignant disease (except primary brain tumour and non-melanoma skin cancers)
  Overwhelming bacterial or fungal infection
  Systemic viral infection
  Prion-related disease
  Herpetic meningoencephalitis
  Chronic urinary tract infection (acute urinary tract infection related to catheterization is not a contraindication)
  Renal disease

The following are not necessarily contraindications:
  Diabetes
  Pneumonia
  Hypertension
  Hypotension

Heart or heart/lung

Brainstem dead

Preferably under 50 years old

Adequately perfused and hydrated

Artificially ventilated

Free from:
  Hepatitis antigen and HIV
  Malignant disease (except primary brain tumour and non-melanoma skin cancers)
  Overwhelming bacterial or fungal infection
  Systemic viral infection
  Prion-related disease
  Herpetic meningoencephalitis
  Diabetes mellitus
  Ischaemic heart disease
  Cardiac murmers

No family history of heart disease

No history of heavy smoking

HIV, human immunodeficiency virus.
In male donors over 35 years old and female donors over 40 years old, coronary angiograms may rarely be requested by the cardiac transplant team.
If there is any doubt, the local transplant coordinator should be contacted early for advice on donor/individual organ suitability.

Table 15.8 Differentiation of vegetative state from other conditions

Condition	Vegetative state	Coma	Brainstem dead	Locked-in syndrome
Self-awareness	Absent	Absent	Absent	Present
Cyclical eye opening	Present	Absent	Absent	Present
Glasgow Coma Scale	E4, M1–4, V1	E1–2, M1–4, V1–2	E1, M1–2, V1	E4, M1, V1
Motor function	No purposeful movement	No purposeful movement	None or only reflex spinal movement	Eye movement preserved in the vertical plane and able to blink volitionally
Pain perception	No/little	No/little	No	Yes
Respiratory function	Normal	Depressed or varied	Absent	Normal
Electroencephalogram activity	Polymorphic delta or theta – sometimes slow alpha	Polymorphic delta or theta, sometimes silent	Electrocerebral silence or theta	Normal or minimally abnormal
Cerebral metabolism	Reduced by 50% or more	Reduced by 50% or more	Absent or greatly reduced	Minimally or moderately reduced
Prognosis	Depends on cause and length	Recovery, vegetative state or death within 2–4 weeks	No recovery	Depends on cause, though recovery unlikely

differential diagnosis includes coma, brainstem death and locked-in syndrome (**Table 15.8**).

Once the diagnosis of persistent vegetative state has been established and after appropriate discussions with the family (see Chapter 2), the decision may be made to withhold or withdraw life-sustaining treatment. For some this decision may be complicated by case reports of emergence from persistent vegetative state (Childs and Mercer, 1996), although even in these cases the patient is likely to remain severely disabled and totally dependent. Currently the law requires, as a matter of practice, that the decision to withdraw nutrition and hydration under these circumstances should be referred to the court before any action is taken.

STATUS EPILEPTICUS
(Chapman *et al.*, 2001)

Status epilepticus is a common medical emergency which affects approximately 14 000 people each year in the UK. In the USA the frequency has been estimated as 50 patients per 100 000 residents per annum.

Status epilepticus can be defined as *persistent or recurrent seizure activity without intervening periods of consciousness*, lasting 30 minutes or more. Some have suggested that specifying the duration as 10–20 minutes would result in a safer definition. The interval between fits is usually in the order of 5–15 minutes. The term can also be applied to continuous seizures lasting at least 30 minutes, even when consciousness is not impaired.

CLINICAL PRESENTATION (Table 15.9)

Major (or grand mal) status epilepticus presents with loss of consciousness and typical tonic and clonic convulsions involving the whole body (*generalized* seizures). Tongue biting and urinary incontinence are common. Sometimes, however, exhaustion when seizures are prolonged or structural lesions within the central nervous system partially terminate the convulsions, which may then become purely clonic or asymmetrical. In some cases, the location of the seizures varies, whereas in others the only manifestations are loss of consciousness with spasmodic twitching or flickering of the eyelids. These *modified forms* of status epilepticus are commonly encountered in critically ill patients. In *partial status epilepticus*, there is repetitive focal twitching, but this may sometimes become secondarily generalized with loss of consciousness. Some patients suffer a particularly prolonged grand mal seizure in which the protracted clonic and tonic phases can cause extreme hypoventilation and hypoxaemia. In others, there are frequent convulsive episodes, but consciousness is regained between seizures. Treatment is nevertheless equally urgent. Status epilepticus may also be *non-convulsive* and either generalized (absence attacks or petit mal) or partial (complex partial seizures).

The differential diagnosis of convulsive status epilepticus includes myoclonic jerks, generalized dystonia, rigors and pseudo status epilepticus. The seizures in the latter are psychogenic in origin and may be flamboyant; consciousness is often retained. Non-convulsive status epilepticus is more difficult to diagnose. Clinical features may include agitation,

Table 15.9 Classification of status epilepticus

	Convulsive	Non-convulsive
Generalized	Tonic-clonic (grand mal) seizures Tonic seizures Myoclonic seizures	Absence attacks (petit mal)
Partial	Partial motor seizures	Complex partial seizures

abnormal eye movements, aphasia, abnormal limb posturing and fluctuating conscious level.

Unremitting myoclonic jerks may occur in isolation and are almost exclusively related to degenerative, hypoxic, toxic or metabolic encephalopathies. The twitching may be generalized or localized, rhythmic or disorganized, infrequent or occurring in bursts. They may arise spontaneously or be triggered by external stimuli.

CAUSES AND PRECIPITATING FACTORS

Status epilepticus is relatively unusual in patients with *pre-existing epilepsy*, but may be precipitated by:

- trauma;
- lack of sleep;
- fasting;
- excessive alcohol;
- intercurrent infection;
- failure to take antiepileptic medication;
- interference with the absorption or metabolism of antiepileptic medication (liver failure, renal failure, pregnancy, interaction with other drugs);
- electrolyte imbalance.

When patients with *no previous history of epilepsy* present in status epilepticus, an underlying cause should be suspected. There are many possibilities, including:

- head injury;
- postcraniotomy;
- cerebral tumour (primary or secondary);
- brain abscess;
- cerebrovascular thrombosis or haemorrhage;
- encephalitis/meningitis;
- fat embolism;
- drug toxicity/toxins;
- withdrawal syndromes;
- hypoxic/ischaemic cerebral damage;
- hypoglycaemia;
- water intoxication;
- extreme dehydration.

PATHOPHYSIOLOGY

In the early stages of status epilepticus the metabolic requirements of discharging neurones are satisfied by an increase in CBF. During prolonged seizures lasting for more than about 30 minutes, however, cerebral autoregulation fails. ICP rises and in the most severe cases cerebral oedema may develop as a consequence of impaired autoregulation, venous congestion, neuronal hypoxia and an increase in the permeability of the blood–brain barrier. Hypoxaemia may be caused by airway obstruction, apnoeic episodes, an aspiration pneumonitis or the development of pulmonary oedema, while CBF can be decreased by hypotension and cardiac arrhythmias. Hypercarbia and the accumulation of lactic acid produce an intracerebral acidosis. A variety of mechanisms have been implicated in the neuronal damage which may follow status epilepticus, including the release of the excitatory amino acid glutamate and $GABA_A$ receptor inhibition (see above).

Initially, patients are usually *hyperglycaemic*, but later blood sugar levels may be low. A *lactic acidosis* develops in severe cases and is probably largely a consequence of widespread anaerobic muscle metabolism. In some patients, life threatening *autonomic dysfunction* supervenes with hyperthermia, excessive sweating, salivation, dehydration, hypertension and, later, hypotension. The violent muscular contractions may produce myolysis, myoglobinuria and, in some cases, renal failure.

MANAGEMENT (Lowenstein, 2003)
(Table 15.10)

Status epilepticus is a medical emergency. Seizure activity must be controlled immediately and vital functions preserved. Decompensation occurs after about 30 minutes of uncontrolled convulsions. Also there is evidence to suggest that the longer the episode continues, the more refractory to treatment the seizures become and the greater is the possibility of chronic epilepsy. Importantly in this context, out-of-hospital administration of benzodiazepines to patients with status epilepticus by paramedics appears to be safe and effective (Alldredge *et al.*, 2001), although for most patients the time from onset of seizures to arrival in the emergency department is short. Remediable underlying disorders, and complications, must be identified and treated.

General aspects

The patient must be *protected from injury*, without using excessive restraint, and should be placed in the *lateral position*. The *airway* must be cleared and *oxygen* should be administered if available. *Tracheal intubation* may be required to secure the airway and protect the lungs from aspiration; in these cases, the nasal route may be preferred since this avoids the danger of the patient biting on the tube. A short-acting muscle relaxant should be used to facilitate tracheal intubation since prolonged neuromuscular blockade will obscure

Table 15.10 Management of status epilepticus

Immediate measures

Protect patient from injury

Place patient in lateral position

Secure and protect airway

Administer oxygen

Establish venous access

Restore blood pressure

General measures

Identify and treat remediable causes

Correct:
  Fluid and electrolyte abnormalities
  Hyper-/hypoglycaemia
  Hypocalcaemia
  Hypomagnesaemia
  Persistent acidosis

Control hyperpyrexia

Treat cerebral oedema

Prevent acute renal failure

When indicated:
  Mechanical ventilation
  Muscle relaxation

Administer anticonvulsants

Benzodiazepines
  Lorazepam (now drug of choice)
  Diazepam
  Midazolam

Phenytoin in selected cases

Phenobarbital in those who fail to respond to a
  benzodiazepine and phenytoin

Thiopental or

Propofol (now preferred to thiopental)

Sodium valproate

Management of complications

Pulmonary aspiration

Neurogenic pulmonary oedema

Arrhythmias

Hyperthermia

Rhabdomyolysis

clinical evidence of seizure activity. An intravenous infusion should be established and at this time blood can be obtained for determination of anticonvulsant levels, blood glucose, urea and electrolytes, creatine kinase levels and a full blood count. Liver function tests and a toxicology screen should also be performed. If necessary, the circulating volume is

then expanded to *restore the systemic blood pressure*. In some cases inotropes/vasopressors may be required in order to ensure that CPP is adequate (see earlier in this chapter).

Abnormalities of *fluid and electrolyte balance*, including *hyperglycaemia, hypoglycaemia, hypocalcaemia* and *hypomagnesaemia*, must be corrected. The *acidosis* usually resolves spontaneously, but may require correction if it persists. It is important to avoid fluid overload in those receiving a continuous infusion of anticonvulsant. *Hyperpyrexia* can exacerbate cerebral damage and should be vigorously treated with fanning, tepid sponging, axillary ice packs and nasogastric or rectal antipyretics.

Mechanical ventilation is indicated if there is:

- respiratory depression (often induced by large doses of anticonvulsant);
- refractory hypoxaemia;
- increasing acidosis;
- cerebral oedema;
- hyperpyrexia;
- the seizures are not controlled within 50–60 minutes.

Muscle relaxation may be required in those with prolonged uncontrolled seizures, but it is then essential to monitor the EEG (e.g. by using a CFM – see above) to detect continued seizure activity. Because in some cases subclinical seizure activity may not be detected by the CFM, a formal EEG should be performed at intervals.

It may be reasonable to administer mannitol to those with prolonged status in whom *cerebral oedema* is suspected. Attempts to prevent *acute renal failure* in those with DIC and/or myoglobinuria may involve fluid loading, alkalinization of the urine and the administration of mannitol or furosemide (see Chapter 13).

Anticonvulsants

Convulsive status should not be allowed to continue; if it persists for more than 30 minutes, severe permanent brain damage may occur. Specific treatment is therefore urgent and should be instituted as soon as the airway has been secured and intravenous access has been established. The aim is the rapid and safe termination of seizure activity and prevention of recurrence without, if possible, causing significant cardiovascular or respiratory depression, or further decreasing the level of consciousness. Treatment should be tailored to the individual patient.

BENZODIAZEPINES

These GABA$_A$ receptor agonists potentiate inhibition of neuronal firing. They are potent and rapidly acting, but cause sedation and respiratory depression; repeated doses have a cumulative effect. Intravenous lorazepam, which has a substantially longer duration of antiseizure activity than diazepam, is now widely considered to be the drug of choice for generalized convulsive status epilepticus. As initial treatment lorazepam (0.1 mg/kg) alone is at least as effective as diazepam followed by phenytoin in controlling seizures during the first 12 hours, is easy and quick to administer and recurrence rates are probably similar to those seen with pheno-barbital and phenytoin (Treiman *et al.*, 1998). In an early study lorazepam successfully terminated clinical seizure activity in 85% of cases, with a mean time to cessation of seizures of 3 minutes (Leppik *et al.*, 1983). For treatment out of hospital both lorazepam and diazepam were found to be safe and effective but there was some evidence that loraze-pam was superior (Alldredge *et al.*, 2001). Furthermore diaz-epam has a very short effective duration of action and must therefore be followed within 20 minutes by administration of a long-acting drug such as phenytoin. Diazepam can, however, be administered rectally by family members, thereby potentially decreasing the time to treatment for patients with recurrent seizures. Importantly, there is evi-dence to suggest that GABA receptors become less respon-sive to benzodiazepines during prolonged seizures.

Intravenous midazolam 0.2 mg/kg has also been used as initial therapy but is rapidly metabolized. Continuous infu-sions may be useful for the treatment of refractory status epilepticus (Kumar and Bleck, 1992).

PHENYTOIN (DIPHENYLHYDANTOIN)

Phenytoin (or the prodrug fosphenytoin) remains the agent of choice for status epilepticus which fails to respond to lorazepam (e.g. if seizure activity fails to stop within 10 minutes of administering lorazepam or if intermittent sei-zures continue for more than 20 minutes). A single loading dose of phenytoin (18 mg/kg) should be administered slowly into a large vein. Phenytoin is highly lipid-soluble and peak brain levels are achieved within 15 minutes; serum levels are generally maintained in the therapeutic range for 24 hours. The loading dose should be followed by a daily dose of 200–500 mg. The serum phenytoin level should be moni-tored, although it must be appreciated that patients often require levels above the therapeutic range to achieve control of status epilepticus, without apparent side-effects. The main dangers of intravenous phenytoin are hypotension, prolongation of the QT interval and arrhythmias. The 'purple-glove' syndrome (a soft-tissue reaction characterized by profound swelling of the hand, sometimes complicated by arterial occlusion and tissue necrosis) has been reported in more than 5% of patients who have received an intrave-nous infusion of phenytoin distal to the antecubital fossa (O'Brien *et al.*, 1998). Fosphenytoin may be a safer means of achieving an effective serum concentration of phenytoin. Because fosphenytoin is water-soluble there are no adverse consequences of extravasation. The incidence of hypoten-sion and arrhythmias may also be reduced. Although fosphe-nytoin can be infused more rapidly than phenytoin, the time required for conversion of the prodrug to the active com-pound means that therapeutic concentrations are not achieved significantly earlier. Because of the additional cost fosphenytoin is not yet widely used in clinical practice. It has been suggested that the use of this agent should be restricted to children, the elderly and those in whom secure venous access cannot be obtained.

PHENOBARBITAL

High doses of phenobarbital are usually required to control seizures. This drug has a long half-life and side-effects such as hypotension, respiratory depression and prolonged seda-tion are common. Its use is now generally limited to the treatment of refractory status epilepticus when it is given in a dose of 10 mg/kg by intravenous injection at a rate of not more than 100 mg/min to a maximum dose of 1 g.

SODIUM VALPROATE

Sodium valproate can be given nasogastrically, rectally or intravenously. It causes little respiratory depression and is more effective in focal and complex partial epilepsy. High doses (12–15 mg/kg) of the intravenous preparation can be effective in refractory status epilepticus.

NMDA RECEPTOR ANTAGONISTS

There is increasing interest in the potential of NMDA recep-tor antagonists such as ketamine for the treatment of refrac-tory status epilepticus.

GENERAL ANAESTHESIA

General anaesthesia is indicated for patients with refractory status epilepticus and should be titrated using continuous EEG monitoring. Although conventionally the aim is to achieve a burst suppression pattern, in many cases this is not necessary to control seizure activity, whereas in others status epilepticus is only controlled by rendering the EEG isoelec-tric. The level of anaesthesia can be reduced once the patient has been free of seizure activity for 24–96 hours (depending on local policy). If seizures recur the depth of anaesthesia should be increased and the regime of long-acting epileptic agents adjusted appropriately.

Long acting anticpileptic agents such as phenytoin should be continued during this phase of treatment and blood levels should be maintained at the upper limit of the therapeutic range.

Thiopental is an effective anticonvulsant at doses lower than those normally required to induce anaesthesia. Never-theless, there is a risk of cardiovascular and respiratory depression, and tracheal intubation is necessary. Many patients will require mechanical ventilation and some vaso-pressors. Thiopental should be given as an initial bolus of 1–3 mg/kg intravenously. This should be followed by a con-tinuous infusion titrated to control seizure activity; this may require more than 3 mg/min in some cases. Blood thiopental levels should be monitored. Elimination is delayed (see earlier in this chapter).

Propofol is a potent anticonvulsant which, because of its rapid clearance, is now often preferred to thiopental for the control of refractory status epilepticus (see earlier in this chapter). An initial bolus of 1 mg/kg is given over 5 minutes and is repeated as necessary until seizure activity is abol-ished. A maintenance infusion (usually 2–10 mg/kg per hour) is then titrated to eliminate seizure activity on the EEG. Rapid discontinuation of the propofol infusion can precipitate recurrence of seizures; gradual withdrawal is therefore recommended. Some still prefer thiopental, however, because barbiturates have intrinsic anticonvulsant properties whereas propofol does not.

Isoflurane has been used successfully to treat refractory status epilepticus but practical difficulties have limited the use of volatile agents in the intensive care unit (see Chapter 11).

Identify and treat the underlying cause

Once the seizures have been controlled and the patient has been stabilized it is important to attempt to identify the underlying cause. A careful history from relatives, friends or ambulance personnel may suggest precipitating factors such as alcohol withdrawal, drug overdose, cerebrovascular accident, infection or a recent change in anticonvulsant medication.

Further investigations may include a CT scan to identify intracranial space-occupying lesions, and a lumbar puncture when meningoencephalitis, SAH or an intracranial abscess is suspected. An EEG can identify and localize seizure activity and may assist in the diagnosis of the underlying disorder.

Manage complications

Complications of status epilepticus include:

- pulmonary aspiration;
- neurogenic pulmonary oedema;
- arrhythmias;
- hyperthermia;
- rhabdomyolysis.

Management of these complications is discussed elsewhere.

PROGNOSIS

Most deaths are a consequence of the underlying disorder, only about 2% being directly attributable to the epilepsy. When seizures are precipitated by drug withdrawal or alcohol the majority of patients will make a good recovery, whereas when cerebrovascular accidents or cerebral hypoxia are the cause the prognosis is poor. Outcome is also influenced by age and the speed with which seizures are terminated. Survivors of status epilepticus may suffer significant neuropsychological sequelae, impaired cognitive function and memory loss.

TETANUS (Cook *et al.*, 2001)

The advent of effective prophylactic immunization has virtually eliminated tetanus in the developed world. In these countries, this condition now occurs mainly in those who have failed to maintain an adequate level of immunity. In the UK, for example, 12–15 cases are notified each year and 50–70 are reported annually in the USA. Recently, however, there has been an increase in the number of cases of tetanus seen in injecting drug users in the UK (Beeching and Crow-

croft, 2005). On the other hand, tetanus is common in most developing countries, where hundreds of thousands die of this disease every year. Overall as many as 1 million individuals may succumb to tetanus each year, many of the victims being neonates and young children. In Europe, the disease occurs most frequently in women and in the elderly.

PATHOGENESIS

Tetanus is caused by *Clostridium tetani*, an anaerobic Gram-positive, motile, spore-bearing bacillus found mainly in cultivated soil and as an inhabitant of the lower gastrointestinal tract in domestic animals and humans. This organism produces two potent exotoxins. *Tetanolysin* is capable of locally damaging tissue surrounding the wound and optimizing the conditions for bacterial multiplication. *Tetanospasmin* is responsible for the clinical manifestations of the disease. This toxin travels from the site of infection to the spinal cord, mainly via the perineurium of motor nerves, but also sometimes within autonomic and sensory nerve fibres, at a rate of approximately 75 mm/day. It then accumulates preferentially in the ipsilateral ventral root of the spinal cord where it passes into the presynaptic terminals of the inhibitory spinal interneurones and blocks release of the transmitter substances GABA and glycine. Further retrograde intraneural transport of toxin may lead to involvement of the brainstem and midbrain. Gamma motor neurones, interneurones and gamma segments of the medulla are therefore disinhibited and discharge spontaneously. Simultaneous contraction of both agonist and antagonist muscle groups produces the characteristic muscle rigidity and spasms. Later preganglionic sympathetic neurones in the lateral horns and the parasympathetic centres are also affected. The release of acetylcholine from motor neurones is also inhibited, which may lead to considerable weakness between spasms. Tetanospasmin may also have cortical convulsant activity.

CLINICAL FEATURES AND INVESTIGATIONS

Contamination of a wound with soil, manure or rusty metal can cause tetanus. Often, the site of entry is a trivial wound, which in some cases may even be invisible. In others, the organism gains access via ulcers, areas of ischaemic gangrene (particularly in diabetics), burns, middle-ear infections, necrotic snake bites, intramuscular injections or following intra-abdominal, pelvic or obstetric surgery. In developing countries, uterine and neonatal tetanus are relatively frequent, as is tetanus associated with injuries to the feet.

The incubation period for tetanus averages 7–10 days, with a range of 1–60 days, and tends to be shorter in more severe cases. Nevertheless, severe attacks can also occur following a long incubation period. Investigations are generally unhelpful in identifying cases of tetanus and the diagnosis is made clinically, based on the triad of rigidity, muscle spasms and, in severe cases, autonomic dysfunction. The majority of patients present with classical trismus (*lockjaw*). Initially, there is only some slight difficulty in opening the mouth, but this may progress until the patient is unable to eat and develops a characteristic *risus sardonicus*. Dysphagia, sore throat and neck stiffness with retraction of the head may also be present at this stage. More unusual presentations include *cephalic tetanus*, in which a wound in the head and neck region is associated with local cranial nerve involvement, or *local tetanus*, where spasms are confined to the injured area. The differential diagnosis includes local causes of trismus (e.g. an abscess), hysteria, dystonic drug reactions, hypocalcaemia and strychnine poisoning.

All these forms of tetanus may then progress at a variable rate through the various grades of severity. Usually, the paroxysms gradually become more generalized to involve the muscles of the neck, the trunk and, to a lesser extent, the limbs. During contractions, the neck may become rigid and hyperextended, while spasm of the paravertebral muscles can produce a marked lumbar lordosis (*opisthotonos*). Ventilation may be seriously impaired and respiratory arrest can occur, either due to involvement of the thoracic and abdominal musculature or because of glottic spasm. In addition, swallowing becomes impossible and this contributes to the risk of asphyxia and aspiration. Ventilation/perfusion mismatching causes hypoxia, even when the lungs are radiologically clear. Some patients develop ARDS. Hyperventilation and hypocarbia may occur as a consequence of fear, autonomic disturbance or altered brainstem function. Limb involvement usually consists of tonic spasms, occurring particularly on the same side as the offending wound. In some cases spasms may be severe enough to cause fractures and tendon avulsions. Spasms may be spontaneous or triggered by touch, visual, auditory or emotional stimuli.

In severe, uncomplicated tetanus tachycardia is universal with hypertension, increased stroke volume and a high cardiac output. Right and left ventricular filling pressures are usually normal and systemic vascular resistance is normal or low. In more serious cases, there may be continuous, but fluctuating, *overactivity of the sympathetic nervous system* (Kerr *et al.*, 1968). This autonomic instability is associated with profuse sweating, salivation, increased bronchial secretions, paroxysmal hypertension, tachycardia, arrhythmias, vasoconstriction, pyrexia and gastrointestinal stasis. Basal catecholamine levels are elevated. Occasionally, dangerous episodes of bradycardia and hypotension occur, either spontaneously or in response to stimuli such as endotracheal suction, and these may culminate in cardiac arrest. Neuronal, rather than adrenal, medullary activity seems to predominate, with levels of noradrenaline being higher than those of adrenaline. The role of the parasympathetic nervous system is less clear, although hypotension, bradycardia and asystole may be precipitated by increased vagal tone. The signs of autonomic dysfunction usually develop 2–4 days after the spasms and resolve within 1–2 weeks. Spasms begin to resolve after 2–3 weeks, but stiffness may persist considerably longer.

Material from wounds should be Gram-stained and cultured anaerobically for *C. tetani*, which can be identified in about one-third of cases.

Table 15.11 Management of tetanus

Eradication of infection

Incise, clean, lay open and debride wound

Antibiotics: metronidazole (alternatives include erythromycin, chloramphenicol, clindamycin, tetracycline or benzylpenicillin)

Neutralize toxin

Booster dose of tetanus toxoid in those previously immunized

Passive immunization with tetanus immunoglobulin of human origin and first dose of tetanus toxoid in those who have not previously been immunized

Passive immunization with tetanus immunoglobulin of human origin in all patients with established tetanus

Intensive care

Isolated trismus

Avoid disturbance (no oral fluids, no gastric tube)

Sedate (benzodiazepine)

Close observation

Generalized tetanus

Tracheal intubation

Sedation

Muscle relaxation

Treat autonomic disturbances

Ensure adequate hydration

Nutritional support

Thromboembolism prophylaxis

MANAGEMENT (Table 15.11)
Eradication of infection

The source of infection is identified in only about two-thirds of tetanus cases and many appear very trivial (e.g. an ingrowing toenail). Nevertheless, potentially infected wounds must be incised, cleaned and laid open, and all the dead tissue excised. Frequently, if even apparently minor puncture sites are explored, a deep-seated necrotic area will be found, often surrounding a foreign body. When tetanus develops following an abortion, dilatation and curettage or a hysterectomy should be performed, while in cases associated with limb ischaemia, amputation may be required.

For many years *benzylpenicillin* (penicillin G) has been used (in a dose of 3.6–7.2 g/day or more for at least 1 week), but this antibiotic is a GABA antagonist and has been associated with convulsions. Erythromycin, chloramphenicol, clindamycin or tetracycline can be used as alternatives. There is some evidence that metronidazole is equally or even more effective than penicillin and this agent is now probably the antibiotic of choice. Hyperbaric oxygen is of little value.

Neutralization of toxin

Patients at risk of developing tetanus who have previously been immunized should receive a *booster dose of tetanus toxoid*. Such active immunization must be combined with thorough wound debridement and antibiotic prophylaxis, as outlined above. The rare at-risk patient who has never been vaccinated will require *passive immunization* with *tetanus immunoglobulin of human origin (HTIG)*, as well as the first dose of tetanus toxoid.

Most authorities recommend that patients with established tetanus should be passively immunized with HTIG (3000–6000 iu) administered intramuscularly. This may reduce the mortality, possibly by neutralizing circulating toxin, thereby preventing relapse or further deterioration. Others consider that systemic passive immunization is unhelpful in the established case since toxin is already fixed within the spinal cord. In a prospective randomized trial the addition of intrathecal administration (1000 iu of a lyophilized human immunoglobulin, free of preservative) to standard intramuscular treatment with HTIG (3000 iu) seemed to be associated with an improvement in clinical progression of the disease (Miranda-Filho *et al.*, 2004).

Intensive care

All patients with tetanus should be admitted to an intensive care unit for observation, assessment and treatment. The priorities are to control the spasms, prevent aspiration and/or asphyxia by tracheal intubation or tracheostomy and avoid complications. Those with *isolated trismus* should be disturbed as little as possible to avoid precipitating a paroxysm. In particular, oral fluids should not be permitted, nor should a nasogastric tube be passed since both can precipitate laryngeal spasm. The patient should be sedated with a benzodiazepine to control muscle spasms, and should be closely observed. Facilities for emergency intubation and respiratory support must be immediately available at the bedside.

Patients with *generalized tetanus* will require tracheal intubation, followed by early tracheostomy combined with sedation to control spasms. *Diazepam* has excellent muscle-relaxant properties with minimal cardiovascular effects, and has been used extensively to sedate patients with tetanus. It can be administered as a continuous intravenous infusion, although it is important to remember that active metabolites of diazepam are cumulative. *Midazolam* and *propofol* have also been used successfully in patients with tetanus. Intravenous *opiates* can be added to the regimen. *Barbiturates* (e.g. an intravenous dose of thiopental followed by regular phenobarbital) may also be effective. Because all these agents can cause respiratory depression controlled ventilation is often required. *Chlorpromazine* may also be valuable, whilst *dantrolene* has been used successfully to control refractory spasms.

If this regimen is unsuccessful (spasms lasting more than 15–20 seconds persist), the patient should be paralysed, preferably using a continuous infusion of a *non-depolarizing muscle relaxant*. Pancuronium has been used most frequently, but this agent could worsen autonomic instability and atracurium or rocuronium may be more suitable alternatives. Because neuromuscular blockade and mechanical ventilation may have to be maintained for 15–20 days, this is a potentially hazardous approach and should only be used in those unresponsive to alternative measures. Finally intrathecal *baclofen* has been used with varying success, although a significant number of patients develop coma and respiratory depression. In the future *sodium valproate* may prove to be useful.

Autonomic disturbances can be minimized by fluid loading and heavy sedation with benzodiazepines, opiates and chlorpromazine (which has anticholinergic and α-adrenergic antagonist properties).

β-adrenergic blockers have been used extensively to control episodes of hypertension and tachycardia, but these agents have been associated with profound hypotension, pulmonary oedema and sudden death. Labetalol is an alternative, but has not been shown to be superior to propranolol. More recently the short-acting agent esmolol has been used successfully. Because sudden cardiac death is a feature of severe tetanus, and may be related to sudden loss of sympathetic drive and/or increased parasympathetic activity, the use of long-acting β-blockers in isolation is no longer recommended. Moreover β-blockade could exacerbate cardiac failure caused by catecholamine-induced myocardial injury.

Postganglionic and α-adrenergic blocking agents (e.g. bethanidine, guanethidine, phentolamine, phenoxybenzamine) have been used successfully in combination with propranolol but induced hypotension may be difficult to reverse, tachyphylaxis occurs and withdrawal can lead to rebound hypertension. The use of high-dose *atropine* to produce both muscarinic and nicotinic blockade, with central sedation and neuromuscular relaxation, has been reported, as has the administration of the α₂-adrenergic agonist *clonidine*. *Epidural* and *spinal blockade* have also been reported to reduce cardiovascular instability, although catecholamine infusions may be required to maintain an adequate arterial blood pressure. In one study, for example, epidural bupivacaine and sufentanil was reported to be effective in controlling sympathetic overactivity and the associated complications (Bhagwanjee *et al.*, 1999). A number of other agents have a potential role in the control of autonomic disturbances, including *angiotensin-converting enzyme inhibitors, dexmedetomidine* (a potent α₂-adrenergic agonist) and *adenosine*.

A number of centres have used *magnesium sulphate* to limit autonomic disturbance and to control spasms in patients with tetanus. Potentially beneficial actions of magnesium in this situation include neuromuscular relaxation, inhibition of catecholamine release, reduced receptor responsiveness to catecholamines and vasodilatation. Magnesium antagonizes calcium in the myocardium and at the neuromuscular junction, lowers serum calcium by inhibiting parathyroid hormone release and has anticonvulsant properties. In high doses magnesium may produce severe weakness, central sedation, hypotension and bradyarrhythmia. In a prospective observational study intravenous magnesium controlled spasms in 38 of 40 patients within a serum magnesium range of 2–4 mmol/L and sympathetic overactivity was controlled without supplementary sedation. Two patients required additional neuromuscular blockade and 17 were mechanically ventilated, whilst 36 patients remained cooperative and conscious throughout. No deaths were attributable to autonomic dysfunction (Attygalle and Rodrigo, 2002). A recent prospective randomized controlled trial indicated that an infusion of magnesium sulphate can reduce the requirement for other drugs to control muscle spasms and maintain cardiovascular stability, although the need for mechanical ventilation was not reduced (Thwaites et al., 2006).

GENERAL MEASURES
The general principles of managing the immobile ventilated intensive care patient are outlined in Chapter 11. Patients with tetanus lose relatively large quantities of salt and water as a result of excessive sweating and salivation. These losses are difficult to quantify and careful daily assessment of *fluid and electrolyte balance* is particularly important. Tetanus patients are often hypovolaemic when first seen, and this may be unmasked by sedation and/or mechanical ventilation; rapid *volume expansion* is then required. Renal function may be impaired not only by hypovolaemia but also as a consequence of sepsis, rhabdomyolysis and alterations in renal blood flow caused by sympathetic overactivity. *Nutritional support* can usually be provided via the enteral route (a percutaneous gastrostomy may be useful), but constipation can be a problem and paralytic ileus may occur in those receiving muscle relaxants. Occasionally, therefore, parenteral feeding is necessary. Weight loss is invariable. Prophylaxis against thromboembolism, gastrointestinal haemorrhage and pressure sores should be provided as usual. Psychological support is also important.

PROGNOSIS
The acute phase of tetanus persists for 3–4 weeks, and complete recovery may take up to a further 4 weeks. The disease is most severe during the first week, plateaus during the second and wanes in the third. Provided patients receive extensive rehabilitation, a full recovery without neurological sequelae can be anticipated. Some patients, however, will have sustained crush fractures of one or more vertebral bodies, or tendon avulsion as a result of their spasms. Psychological problems are frequent.

In developing countries without facilities for prolonged intensive care and ventilatory support mortality rates may exceed 50%, most deaths being attributable to airway obstruction, respiratory failure or renal failure. Trujillo and colleagues (1987) have reported a reduction in mortality from 44 to 15% following the introduction of intensive care management and it has been suggested that in developed

countries it should be possible to achieve mortality rates of 10% or less. Mortality rates do vary with age, however, and may exceed 50% in those over 60 years old. The majority of deaths in those receiving intensive care are a result of unexpected cardiac arrest. Other important causes of morbidity and mortality include nosocomial infections, especially ventilator-associated pneumonia, generalized sepsis, thromboembolism and gastrointestinal haemorrhage.

Occasionally, severe generalized tetanus develops extremely rapidly with continuous spasms, high fever, hypertension and tachycardia. In such cases, death usually follows within 24–48 hours due to major circulatory disturbances.

MYASTHENIA GRAVIS
(Vincent et al., 2001)

Myasthenia gravis is relatively rare, with an annual incidence of between 0.25 and 2 per 100 000 and a prevalence of up to 400 per million. The majority of cases in the younger age groups are female but there has been a substantial increase in the number of patients presenting beyond 60 years of age, the majority of whom are men.

PATHOGENESIS
Myasthenia gravis is an *autoimmune disorder* which in most cases is due to a reduction in the effective number of acetylcholine receptors (AChR) at skeletal muscle motor endplates caused by *autoantibodies* specific for the human nicotinic AChR. These antibodies bind to the extracellular domains of the native molecule, increasing the rate of breakdown and internalization of the receptor, as well as perhaps blocking the action of acetylcholine. In addition the antibody initiates complement-mediated lysis of the postjunctional folds. Seronegative myasthenia gravis also seems to be antibody-mediated and in a high proportion of such cases antibodies to muscle-specific receptor tyrosine kinase (MuSK) can be detected. MuSK is an essential component of the developing neuromuscular junction and may be involved in the maintenance of the high density of AChRs at the neuromuscular junction. MuSK antibodies may induce complement-mediated damage to the neuromuscular junction. Antibodies to striated muscle are detected in approximately one-third of patients with myasthenia, usually in those with a thymic tumour, but are also found in association with thymic tumours in the absence of muscle weakness. It is therefore unlikely that their presence is of pathogenic significance.

Genetic predisposition appears to be important in the development of myasthenia gravis, which in susceptible individuals may be precipitated by several largely unidentified environmental factors. In this context it is of interest that patients with early-onset and late-onset disease have different human leukocyte antigen (HLA) associations, that there is an increased frequency of other autoimmune diseases in those with early-onset disease, and that monozygotic twins are at increased risk of concordancy. Lastly it is not unknown for more than one family member to be affected and frequently other family members suffer from autoimmune diseases.

The thymus gland is thought to be necessary for the deletion of autoreactive T cells and seems to play an important role in the pathogenesis of myasthenia gravis. In early-onset disease there is often histological evidence of a thymic abnormality, usually germinal centre hyperplasia, but in about 10% there is a thymoma, the majority of which are benign. About 30–60% of thymomas are associated with myasthenia gravis.

CLINICAL FEATURES

The *muscle weakness* in myasthenia gravis is typically painless, exacerbated by exertion and improved by rest. Some patients complain of fatigue rather than weakness. The onset may be acute or subacute and there may be relapses and remissions. Weakness has a characteristic distribution affecting, in descending order of frequency, the extraocular, bulbar, neck, limb girdle, distal limb and trunk muscles. Involvement of the extraocular and levator palpebrae muscles presents as diplopia and ptosis, whilst bulbar and facial muscle weakness causes limited facial expression (e.g. a snarling appearance when attempting to smile) and difficulty with speech, chewing and swallowing. Neck muscle weakness leads to head droop. Limb weakness is most pronounced proximally, although often with specific weakness of the hand muscles. Weakness of the respiratory muscles can be life-threatening (see below). Weakness sometimes remains localized to one group of muscles for many years (this is common with ocular myasthenia) or may become generalized. There is no sensory involvement and tendon reflexes are normal. *Other autoimmune disorders* such as thyroid disease and pernicious anaemia are significantly associated with myasthenia gravis.

Myasthenia gravis can present first during pregnancy, postnatally, or after general anaesthesia and on occasions seems to be precipitated by infection. *Neonatal myasthenia gravis* occurs in about 10% of babies born to women with the disease, and occasionally occurs when the mother is free of symptoms. *Childhood myasthenia gravis* is rare in Caucasians, but relatively common in oriental populations. *Early-onset myasthenia gravis* (onset before 40 years of age) is more common in women and usually presents in adolescence or early adult life. In most cases the thymus gland is enlarged and AChR antibodies can be detected. About 60% of these patients are HLA-B8 DR3. *Late-onset myasthenia* gravis (onset after 40 years of age) is slightly more common in men; the thymus gland is usually not enlarged and may be atrophic. There is an association with HLA-B7 DR2. In *ocular myasthenia gravis* AChR antibody titres tend to be low and are undetectable in 40–60% of cases. The peak onset of *thymoma-associated myasthenia gravis* is during the fourth to sixth decades, there are no clear HLA associations and antibodies to other muscle antigens are usually detectable.

A number of myasthenic syndromes have been described and may be encountered on the intensive care unit when such a patient fails to breathe following an anaesthetic during which muscle relaxants were used. For example, the *Lambert–Eaton syndrome* (Lambert *et al.*, 1956) is caused by antibodies to voltage-gated calcium channels on the presynaptic motor nerve terminal. In about 50% of patients there is an associated small-cell lung cancer. The syndrome is characterized by muscle weakness with aching and stiffness which, in contrast to true myasthenia, improve on exertion and spare the ocular and bulbar muscles. Nevertheless, these patients are also exquisitely sensitive to non-depolarizing muscle relaxants, and anticholinesterases have little beneficial effect. 3,4-Diaminopyridine, which prolongs the motor nerve action potential, thereby increasing neurotransmitter release, is often effective in Lambert–Eaton syndrome. This agent can be used in combination with an anticholinesterase. In those who fail to respond, immunosuppressants can be effective.

INVESTIGATIONS
Acetylcholine receptor antibodies
When detected these are diagnostic for myasthenia gravis.

Edrophonium test
The diagnosis of myasthenia gravis can be established and the adequacy of treatment assessed using an intravenous test dose of the short-acting anticholinesterase *edrophonium*. To perform this test an intravenous cannula should be inserted, the ECG should be monitored continuously and atropine should be available to counteract bradycardia. Facilities for resuscitation should also be available. An indicator of muscle function, appropriate for the particular patient, should be chosen for assessment before and after edrophonium. Usually, the most severely affected muscle group is selected. Therefore, if extraocular muscle weakness is most prominent, eye movement and/or diplopia can be evaluated, while straight-arm-raising time can be used for those with predominantly limb involvement. Many of the patients admitted to the intensive care unit will have respiratory muscle weakness and in these cases *forced vital capacity (FVC)* provides an excellent objective indicator of the response to an anticholinesterase. Edrophonium should be administered slowly intravenously, initially in a dose of 2 mg, followed 1 minute later by a further 8 mg, provided no adverse effects are seen. Improvement is rapid (within 2 minutes), but short-lived (less than 5 minutes). False-positive and false-negative results may occur.

Electromyography
Electromyography shows characteristic changes (increased decrement of the evoked compound muscle action potential in response to repetitive supramaximal stimulation) in 90% of patients with generalized myasthenia gravis, as well as in many of those with only ocular symptoms. Single-fibre electromyography may be more sensitive.

Table 15.12 Management of myasthenia gravis
Treatment
Anticholinesterase
Pyridostigmine bromide
Neostigmine
Anticholinergics
Propantheline
Immunosuppressants
Steroids
Azathioprine
Plasma exchange
Immunoglobulins
Thymectomy
Intensive care
Myasthenic or cholinergic crisis
Secure airway
May require ventilatory support
Anticholinergics may be required
Treat precipitating factors
Physiotherapy
Management post thymectomy

Imaging
Once the diagnosis has been established CT or MRI is indicated to exclude an associated thymoma.

TREATMENT (Table 15.12)
Anticholinesterases
These agents are used to produce symptomatic improvement. Oral *pyridostigmine bromide* (60 mg tablets) is the treatment of choice; initially, 60 mg four times daily, and then gradually increased to achieve the optimal response. If required, pyridostigmine can be taken during the night. In difficult cases, pyridostigmine can be combined with *neostigmine* (15 mg tablets), which has a more rapid onset of action and can therefore be particularly useful first thing in the morning. It may not be possible to abolish muscle weakness completely, and if the dose of anticholinesterase is progressively increased in an attempt to achieve complete relief of symptoms, a 'cholinergic crisis' may be precipitated. The daily dose of pyridostigmine should not normally exceed 450 mg. In the long term these drugs may damage the neuromuscular junction.

Anticholinergics
Muscarinic anticholinergics (e.g. propantheline) may be required to control side-effects such as salivation, lacrimation, colic and diarrhoea. In general, however, these drugs are best avoided in the routine management of myasthenia since they may mask the onset of a cholinergic crisis.

Immunosuppressants
Corticosteroids (usually alternate-day prednisolone) may be useful in those who fail to improve following thymectomy and preoperatively in the most seriously ill patients. They are also valuable in ocular myasthenia and in those who are unsuitable for surgery. Because the administration of corticosteroids in high doses may be associated with an initial, sometimes severe deterioration, treatment should be started at a low dose, which is then gradually increased. Improvement may not be apparent for several weeks. Subsequently the dose can be reduced to that required to maintain remission. Corticosteroids can precipitate hypokalaemia by increasing urinary potassium excretion, and thereby may exacerbate muscle weakness. Plasma potassium levels should be maintained in the upper normal range.

Azathioprine can be used as a steroid-sparing agent in those with severe myasthenia unresponsive to other measures, but can also produce an initial deterioration. Improvement may be delayed for up to 6–12 weeks, and is maximal at 6–15 months. Azathioprine can cause bone marrow depression and liver dysfunction. The combination of prednisolone and azathioprine seems to be more effective and better tolerated than prednisolone alone. Ciclosporin, methotrexate and cyclophosphamide are alternatives in those who cannot tolerate, or do not respond to, azathioprine.

Plasma exchange
In some patients, plasma exchange produces a dramatic, albeit temporary improvement. Exchange is usually performed on 5 successive days, the maximum response is normally seen at 7–10 days and improvement persists for about 1 month. Plasma exchange can be a useful technique for managing acute problems (e.g. severe acute myasthenia during the perioperative period), to improve muscle weakness prior to thymectomy and to facilitate weaning from ventilatory support. Azathioprine can be used to prevent a rebound increase in antibody levels.

Immunoglobulins
Intravenous immunoglobulins can also produce a striking but temporary improvement. They are easier to administer than plasma exchange and are therefore the treatment of first choice in many units. The precise mechanisms underlying their beneficial effect are unclear.

Thymectomy
Early thymectomy seems to produce a more rapid onset of remission and a lower mortality than medical therapy and is now the recommended treatment for early-onset, AChR antibody-positive patients with generalized myasthenia. The explanation for this improvement is unclear, although when the thymus appears histologically active antibody levels fall following thymectomy. Thymectomy is not normally performed in patients with isolated ocular disease and is not

usually beneficial in late-onset disease. Some centres will not perform thymectomy in antibody-negative patients. Thymectomy alone, or with chemotherapy and radiotherapy, can also be used to treat thymoma, but weakness usually does not improve and may even worsen.

Intensive care

As a result of improvements in the medical management of myasthenia, respiratory support is required less frequently, although patients continue to be admitted for postoperative care following thymectomy.

MANAGEMENT OF MYASTHENIC AND CHOLINERGIC CRISES

A crisis may arise when bulbar and respiratory muscle weakness (with an inability to breathe deeply, cough effectively and protect the airway) causes respiratory failure requiring control of the airway and ventilatory support. Such deterioration may be precipitated by:

- treatment with corticosteroids, azathioprine or radiotherapy;
- inability to swallow or absorb anticholinesterase tablets (e.g. vomiting, coma, perioperative starvation);
- mental or physical stress;
- hormonal changes (such as occur during menstruation or pregnancy and in thyrotoxicosis);
- intercurrent infection;
- surgery;
- various drugs – respiratory depressants, diuretics (probably as a result of hypokalaemia), aminoglycosides (which can inhibit acetylcholine release), laxatives (which can decrease the absorption of anticholinesterases), antiarrhythmics such as procainamide, lidocaine, propranolol and quinidine, as well as the quinine present in tonic water (which reduce the excitability of muscle membrane and probably also inhibit neuromuscular transmission), ciprofloxacin and penicillamine.

It may be difficult to distinguish between an *exacerbation of myasthenia* and a *cholinergic crisis*; both can result in respiratory failure, bulbar palsy and virtually complete paralysis. Cholinergic crisis is characterized by sweating, hypersalivation, lacrimation, vomiting and miosis; respiratory difficulty may be exacerbated by excessive secretions. The most common cause is anticholinesterase overdose in a self-medicating patient who misjudges the cause of the weakness. Medical misjudgements may also occur.

In severe cases, immediate tracheal intubation and mechanical ventilation will be required, whereas in others an edrophonium test (see above) can be performed to establish the aetiology of the crisis. Particular care is required when a cholinergic crisis is suspected since in this situation edrophonium may cause sudden severe deterioration.

The indications for instituting mechanical ventilation and for weaning patients with myasthenia and other neuromuscular causes of ventilatory failure are discussed in Chapters 7 and 8. Ventilatory function assessed by FVC may be the best guide to the ability to wean from controlled ventilation, while the adequacy of bulbar muscle function largely determines the timing of extubation and the need for a tracheostomy.

When mechanical ventilation has been initiated, anticholinesterases should be withdrawn and reintroduced 24–48 hours later, if necessary guided by the response to edrophonium. Pyridostigmine can be administered as an elixir via the nasogastric tube. Some believe that a period without anticholinesterase therapy allows the motor endplate to regain its sensitivity, but there is little evidence to support this theory. If the response to anticholinesterases is unsatisfactory, the use of plasma exchange or immunoglobulins, with or without azathioprine or corticosteroids, should be considered.

Secretions must be controlled with frequent physiotherapy and, if necessary, anticholinergics; some patients will require a tracheostomy, particularly if bulbar muscles are involved. Plasma potassium and magnesium levels should be maintained in the high-normal range and adverse drug effects (see earlier in this section) must be avoided. Precipitating factors should be corrected.

Antithromboembolic prophylaxis should be instituted.

MANAGEMENT POSTTHYMECTOMY

The appropriate management for patients admitted to intensive care following thymectomy depends on the severity and distribution of their preoperative muscle weakness. Therefore, mild myasthenics without respiratory or bulbar muscle involvement may be extubated immediately. Those with more severe disease will require elective postoperative ventilation until respiratory function is adequate (FVC > 10–15 mL/kg). The endotracheal tube should remain in place until both respiratory and bulbar muscle function are considered to be satisfactory and the risk of unexpected deterioration is minimal (i.e. approximately 48 hours postoperatively). Nasal endotracheal tubes are sometimes preferred in these cases because they are more easily tolerated by the alert patient. Some centres have rigid protocols for postoperative care following thymectomy; others adjust their treatment regimen to suit the individual patient.

ACUTE INFLAMMATORY POLYRADICULONEUROPATHY
(Hahn, 1998)

In 1916, Guillain, Barré and Strohl described two cases of paralysis with muscle tenderness and areflexia associated with a high protein content, but normal white cell count, in the CSF. Both patients eventually recovered. Landry had previously described a similar case in 1859, although he had not obtained CSF, and the condition should therefore properly be called the Landry–Guillain–Barré–Strohl syndrome. Common practice, however, is to omit the names of both

Landry and Strohl from this eponym. The term *acute inflammatory polyneuropathy* (AIP) encompasses this well-known syndrome as well as other causes of acute polyneuritis not associated with an identifiable preceding infection or CSF changes. Acute neuropathies due to toxic, metabolic or nutritional causes, as well as those associated with collagen diseases and vasculitis, are excluded from this definition.

PATHOLOGY

Guillain-Barré syndrome (GBS) is generally viewed as a reactive, self-limited, autoimmune disorder triggered by an antecedent event which is most often infective. In the early stages there is deposition of activated complement components along the outer Schwann-cell surface membrane of myelinated nerve fibres and local infiltration with lymphocytes. The affected myelin sheaths then undergo vesicular disruption progressing from outside inwards. Later macrophages are recruited to the sites of inflammation and complete the process of segmental demyelination. Various antibodies to neural tissues (e.g. ganglioside surface components) have been detected in serum from GBS patients and it is postulated that binding of such antibodies to epitopes on the Schwann-cell surface membrane might lead to complement activation and initiation of inflammatory demyelination, although a direct causal link has yet to be shown. In many patients, particularly those with severe disease, inflammatory demyelination is accompanied by variable disruption and loss of nerve axons, probably as a consequence of intense inflammation, oedema and nerve swelling. The extent of this axonal injury is an important determinant of the speed of resolution and the prospects for long-term recovery. Because the inflammatory process involves the spinal roots as well as peripheral nerves this form of GBS has been termed *acute inflammatory demyelinating polyradiculoneuropathy* (AIDP). In western countries AIDP accounts for 85–90% of cases of GBS.

It is now recognized that the clinical spectrum encompassed by the term GBS also includes acute neuropathies in which the autoimmune response is directed primarily against the nerve axons. In *acute motor-sensory axonal neuropathy* (AMSAN) there is severe axonal degeneration of motor and sensory fibres with minimal lymphocytic infiltration and little demyelination. The condition is characterized by rapid onset of severe paralysis and sensory loss, severe generalized muscle atrophy and delayed, often very poor recovery. Sporadic cases of an *acute motor axonal neuropathy* (AMAN) without sensory involvement also occur and a predominantly sensory form of GBS has been recognized (Hughes, 2001). Interestingly patients with the more severe, axonal form of GBS (whether primary or secondary to demyelination) are more likely to have been infected with *Campylobacter jejuni* (Rees *et al.*, 1995).

CLINICAL FEATURES

The annual incidence of GBS is 1–2 cases per 100 000 population, with a slight peak in late adolescence and young adults (perhaps coinciding with an increased risk of infection with cytomegalovirus or *C. jejuni*), and a second peak in the elderly (perhaps related to dysregulation of the immune response in old age). Although all age groups can be affected, GBS is rare in infancy. The sex incidence is equal. A *precipitating event* can be identified in approximately two-thirds of cases, often a minor respiratory tract infection or gastrointestinal upset. GBS is particularly associated with *Campylobacter* infection (the most frequent antecedent pathogen), cytomegalovirus, Epstein–Barr and varicella-zoster virus, but probably can also follow *Mycoplasma* or bacterial infections, as well as surgery. An association between HIV infection and AIP is now well recognized but the link with immunization is less clear.

Weakness can develop acutely (within days) or subacutely (up to 4 weeks) and then reaches a plateau, following which there is spontaneous resolution. Weakness is normally distal initially and is generally relatively symmetrical (although some asymmetry is not inconsistent with the diagnosis). *Ascending paralysis* often progresses rapidly to involve proximal muscle groups, including the respiratory and bulbar muscles. Tendon reflexes are absent or markedly reduced. Although motor involvement predominates, sensory symptoms such as paraesthesiae and numbness are common, and marked sensory loss is occasionally seen. In some cases, *muscle pain and tenderness* are severe, while sphincter function is usually preserved. Sometimes a patient will present with *cranial nerve involvement*; for example, the combination of ophthalmoplegia, ataxia and areflexia is a well-recognized variant of AIP (Miller Fisher syndrome) which is most frequently triggered by *C. jejuni* infection. The presence of muscle fibrillation indicates complete denervation and suggests that recovery will be delayed or incomplete. Occasionally fulminant GBS may mimic brain death (Vargas *et al.*, 2000) (see earlier in this chapter).

The autonomic nervous system may also be involved (Lichtenfeld, 1971), most commonly in those with extensive disease or cranial nerve involvement. The manifestations of *autonomic neuropathy* are complex and can be lethal. Sinus tachycardia is a common feature and may be punctuated by periods of profound bradycardia or even asystole occurring either spontaneously or in response to stimulating procedures such as tracheal suction. These episodes are often accompanied by sweating and flushing. Blood pressure is labile and prolonged periods of hypertension may occur. These are associated with vasoconstriction and may be interspersed with episodes of hypotension, with or without tachycardia. Associated ECG abnormalities include flattening of T waves, ST-segment depression, an increased QRS voltage, left-axis deviation and prolongation of the Q-T interval. Gastrointestinal disturbances and genitourinary dysfunction may also occur, as may profuse sweating and salivation. Both the syndrome of inappropriate ADH secretion and diabetes insipidus may be encountered. Hallucinations are sometimes associated with these autonomic disturbances.

The differential diagnosis includes:

- porphyria;
- diphtheria;
- heavy-metal poisoning;
- volatile solvent abuse;
- other toxic neuropathies;
- poliomyelitis;
- botulism;
- hysteria.

AIDP must also be distinguished from the chronic form (CIDP), which follows a more insidious course with progressive deterioration or stepwise relapses and is not usually preceded by an infection.

INVESTIGATIONS

An *elevated CSF total protein* concentration (> 0.4 g/L), with a normal white cell content (< 10/mL) is characteristic of GBS, but is not invariable. The CSF protein content is elevated in more than 90% of those with GBS within 1 week of the onset of symptoms. *Electrophysiological studies* may demonstrate reduced nerve conduction velocities, prolongation of distal latencies and conduction block. In some cases features consistent with axonal loss may be seen.

MANAGEMENT (Table 15.13)
Specific treatment
PLASMA EXCHANGE
Plasma exchange is effective in GBS, provided treatment is instituted within 1–2 weeks of the onset of the disease (Winer, 1992). Although overall mortality is not affected, plasma exchange reduces the likelihood of patients requiring mechanical ventilation, decreases the time to onset of motor recovery, to weaning from ventilatory support and to walking, and also shortens hospital stay (French Co-

Table 15.13 Management of Guillain–Barré syndrome

Specific treatment
Plasma exchange
Immunoglobulin

Intensive care
Serial assessment of respiratory reserve and airway-protective reflexes
Secure airway
Mechanical ventilation
Monitoring and control of autonomic neuropathy
Pain control
Bowel care
Nutritional support
Prevent complications (thromboembolism, pressure area care)
Psychological support

operative Group on Plasma Exchange in Guillain–Barré Syndrome, 1987; Guillain–Barré Syndrome Study Group, 1985). The incidence of complications also seems to be reduced, possibly due to a reduction in the duration and severity of the acute phase. Moreover in the long term more treated patients recover full muscle strength at 1 year (French Cooperative Group on Plasma Exchange in Guillain–Barré Syndrome, 1992). Plasma exchange also seems to be beneficial in milder cases of GBS (French Cooperative Group on Plasma Exchange in Guillain–Barré Syndrome 1987, 1992).

Current recommendations are to use two plasma exchange treatments for mild GBS and four or five for severe GBS, starting as soon as possible after the onset of disease on an alternate-date schedule. Relapses may be seen in about 10% of patients, usually 1–2 weeks after the initial improvement. They should be treated with additional exchanges or with intravenous immunoglobulin (see below). Plasma exchange is not recommended for those with infectious complications. It is not an entirely innocuous procedure, especially in haemodynamically unstable patients, and should only be performed when experienced staff and appropriate facilities are available. Plasma exchange is also costly.

Although the mechanism for the beneficial effect of plasma exchange in Guillain–Barré syndrome remains uncertain, it is assumed to be related to removal of immune mediators. Its efficacy does not seem to depend on the administration of immunoglobulins or complement fractions as replacement fluid since either fresh frozen plasma (FFP) or diluted albumin is equally effective (French Cooperative Group on Plasma Exchange in Guillain–Barré Syndrome, 1987). In this study several of the patients given FFP developed viral hepatitis, and the incidence of fever and skin rashes was higher in this group. The use of FFP as replacement fluid during plasma exchange is not therefore recommended.

HIGH-DOSE INTRAVENOUS IMMUNOGLOBULIN
Intravenous immunoglobulin is an effective, safe and easy-to-use treatment for GBS, with obvious practical advantages when compared to plasma exchange (Van der Meché et al., 1992). The efficacy of intravenous immunoglobulin appears to be equivalent to that of plasma exchange, but combining the two treatments does not seem to confer any significant additional advantage (Plasma Exchange/Sandoglobulin Guillain Barré Syndrome Trial Group, 1997). Limited relapses may be seen in about 10% of patients and may respond to repeat doses of immunoglobulin. Intravenous immunoglobulin is currently the preferred tretment for GBS.

CORTICOSTEROIDS
Contrary to expectations corticosteroids, either alone (Hughes, 1991), or when added to standard treatment with intravenous immunoglobulin (van Koningsveld et al., 2004), seem to be ineffective in GBS (Hughes, 2004) and are not currently recommended.

FUTURE TREATMENTS

The use of immunological treatments targeted specifically at the underlying pathological processes may lead to further improvements in outcome. It will be particularly important to develop treatments capable of minimizing the number of patients with severe residual disability, perhaps by promoting axonal regeneration with, for example, nerve growth factors. Preventive measures, in particular to control or eliminate certain *C. jejuni* infections, could contribute to a reduction in the incidence of GBS.

Intensive care
MECHANICAL VENTILATION

About 30% of patients with GBS will require mechanical ventilation. Respiratory and bulbar muscle function must be closely monitored so that the airway can be secured and controlled ventilation instituted before lung function deteriorates or respiratory arrest supervenes. Aspiration pneumonia is common. The FVC should be measured at least twice a day in all cases, and more frequently in those who develop respiratory muscle weakness. As well as the absolute value of FVC, the speed with which ventilatory impairment progresses influences the decision to intervene. If lung function is also impaired (e.g. due to recurrent aspiration or secondary pneumonia) the patient may require respiratory support before the FVC has fallen below the conventional 10–15 mL/kg. Mechanical ventilation should also be considered if the patient complains of breathlessness and must be instituted immediately if the P_aCO_2 is elevated or rising (hypoxia and hypercarbia are late signs of respiratory failure in these patients). The presence of abdominal paradox (indrawing of the abdominal wall during inspiration) and respiratory difficulty when supine is indicative of significant diaphragm weakness. Nasotracheal intubation is more easily tolerated by awake patients and may be preferred in those with GBS. Tracheostomy should be performed early

MANAGEMENT OF AUTONOMIC NEUROPATHY

Autonomic disturbances can be minimized by achieving and maintaining an adequate circulating volume, by ensuring satisfactory oxygenation, especially during tracheal suction, and by adequate sedation. Suxamethonium should be avoided when intubating patients with GBS. β-blockade can be used to control episodes of hypertension and tachycardia, although high doses may be required. Insertion of a pacemaker should be considered in those with significant bradycardia and is essential if the patient has an episode of asystole. Atropine may alleviate the situation until the pacemaker is in place. Because severe autonomic disturbances can occur suddenly and unexpectedly, some routinely administer regular atropine and a β-blocking agent to all patients with GBS who require intensive care. Others simply treat the haemodynamic abnormalities appropriately as they arise.

PAIN CONTROL

Limb pains are common and may be severe during the recovery phase, particularly during passive movements.

Administration of quinine, non-steroidal anti-inflammatory drugs (NSAIDs) and tricyclics may help to control the pain, but opiates are often required. Nasogastric methadone has been recommended and even epidural opiates have been suggested if the pain is very severe. Carbamezepine has been shown to be an effective adjuvant for pain control in patients with GBS (Tripathi and Kaushik, 2000).

PREVENTION OF COMPLICATIONS
Potentially lethal complications of GBS include:

- thromboembolism;
- pulmonary infection;
- gastrointestinal haemorrhage.

Prophylactic anticoagulants and frequent passive limb movement minimize the risk of deep-vein thrombosis and pulmonary embolism. Antacid prophylaxis (see Chapter 11) and measures to reduce the risk of aspiration, atelectasis and pulmonary infection are also important aspects of the care of patients with severe GBS. Patients with paralytic ileus may require parenteral nutrition. Psychological disturbances should be prevented or managed as outlined in Chapter 11. The visiting and counselling services offered by past patients through the *Guillain–Barré Syndrome Support Group* can be enormously helpful in this regard. Excellent nursing care and physiotherapy are essential for a successful outcome.

PROGNOSIS

Evolution of the disease is usually complete within 3 weeks (75% of patients reach their nadir within 2 weeks, 92% within 3 weeks and 94% within 4 weeks), but the speed of recovery is variable. Some improvement is generally seen within a few days of the period of maximum disability, but sometimes several weeks elapse before recovery begins. About half the survivors will have improved substantially within 3–6 months, and 70% will have completely recovered within 1 year. Approximately 16% will have a significant permanent residual handicap, while about 3% develop a chronic or relapsing course. A few, usually elderly, patients may remain bedridden or ventilator-dependent. These latter patients are distinguished by having a higher prevalence of certain HLA antigens and responding to immunosuppression (Winer, 1992). It is possible to achieve an overall mortality rate of around 3–8% or less. A poor outcome is associated with more rapidly progressive disease, the need for mechanical ventilation, the presence of small distal evoked muscle action potentials and older age (Winer, 1992). Infection with *C. jejuni* is associated with axonal degeneration, slow recovery and severe residual disability (Rees *et al.*, 1995).

CRITICAL ILLNESS POLYNEUROMYOPATHY
(Deem *et al.*, 2003; Kennedy *et al.*, 2000)

Neuromuscular weakness is a common, but underrecognized, complication of critical illness. More than 50% of patients mechanically ventilated for more than 7 days and around 70% of those with sepsis or systemic inflammatory response syndrome (SIRS) will develop electrophysiological abnormalities, whilst myopathic changes are seen in 48–96% of such cases and weakness is clinically obvious in about a third. Acquired neuromuscular weakness prolongs weaning from mechanical ventilation, delays mobilization and discharge from the intensive care unit and hospital and adds considerably to the cost of care, not least because of the need in many cases for prolonged rehabilitation. These disorders have also been associated with increased mortality.

CAUSES

In the 1980s it became clear that neuromuscular weakness complicating critical illness was a result not only of severe catabolic muscle wasting, but was in some cases also attributable to acquired polyneuropathies (*critical illness polyneuropathy*) (Bolton *et al.*, 1984), myopathies or a combination of both. Because it is often difficult to distinguish between a motor neuropathy and a myopathy, and because the two frequently coexist, many now use the term *critical illness polyneuromyopathy* (CIPNM) to describe neuromuscular weakness syndromes complicating critical illness. Indeed, more recent studies have indicated that in the majority of patients with CIPNM there is evidence of non-neuropathic myopathy (Trojaborg *et al.*, 2001), although a follow-up study of unselected long-term survivors of prolonged critical illness revealed persisting neurophysiological evidence of widespread chronic partial denervation/reinnervation in 20 of the 22 cases, suggesting that myopathic changes rarely occur in the absence of neuropathy (Fletcher *et al.*, 2003).

The profound myopathic weakness which can complicate acute severe asthma treated with corticosteroids and neuromuscular-blocking agents has been described as a distinct entity and is often called *acute quadriplegic myopathy* (AQM), although there is probably a degree of overlap between AQM and CIPNM. Muscle histology in AQM reveals either selective thick (myosin) filament loss or widespread myonecrosis, which may represent two ends of the spectrum of the same injury, since occasionally the two seem to coexist. In a few cases muscle necrosis may be sufficiently severe to cause rhabdomyolysis. Occasionally *prolonged neuromuscular blockade* may be responsible for profound, persistent weakness, especially when vecuronium or pancuronium is given to patients with renal impairment.

AETIOLOGY AND PATHOGENESIS

The precise site and nature of the lesion(s) which cause weakness in the critically ill remain uncertain. The motor abnormalities found in CIPNM have been associated with SIRS, sepsis and multiple-organ failure and it has been suggested that neuromuscular failure may represent just another organ damaged by uncontrolled inflammation. On the other hand neuromyopathy can also occur in patients who do not fulfil conventional criteria for sepsis and in those with only single-organ failure (Coakley *et al.*, 1992). It may be that, as well as impaired perfusion of peripheral nerves, the increased vascular permeability associated with systemic inflammation allows neurotoxic substances, including steroids and neuromuscular-blocking agents easy passage across the blood–nerve barrier. Other factors that have been implicated include osmolal shifts, decreased albumin levels resulting in endoneural oedema, hyperalimentation, hyperpyrexia and a circulating low-molecular-weight toxin. Disturbances of glycolysis and consequent impairment of axonal transport, if prolonged, could also cause axonal degeneration. The recent observation that tight glycaemic control (see Chapter 17) dramatically reduces the incidence of CIPNM supports previous suggestions that hyperglycaemia is an important cause of motor weakness in the critically ill. As with other organ failures, many of these insults might be reversible in the early stages and this could explain the sometimes rapid recovery of motor function when sepsis resolves.

Treatment with corticosteroids and neuromuscular-blocking agents has been implicated in the development of CIPNM, and in particular the acute myopathic changes. Possible additional risk factors include aminoglycoside antibiotics, catecholamines/vasopressors, parenteral nutrition and renal replacement therapy, although because these potential risk factors are all related to sepsis and the severity of illness, it is difficult to establish a direct causal link to CIPNM. The risk of CIPNM seems to be increased in females and in the elderly. It has also been suggested that a number of hitherto unexplored molecular mechanisms, such as axonal channelopathies and disorders of myofibrillar excitation–contraction coupling and cross-bridge formation, could contribute to neuromuscular dysfunction. Abnormalities of neurotransmitter synthesis, packaging, release and reuptake, or loss of synaptic cleft integrity could also account for motor weakness.

The pathogenesis of AQM is unclear. Initial reports of acute myopathy in severe asthma concentrated on the potential role of corticosteroids but it later became clear that the prolonged use of neuromuscular-blocking agents was also associated with this syndrome. Indeed, the degree of clinical weakness seemed to be related to the total dose and duration of administration of neuromuscular-blocking agents, particularly when administered by infusion. Because vecuronium and pancuronium contain an aminosteroid nucleus, it was suggested that these agents might have an additive toxic effect with corticosteroids. More recently, however, there have been a number of reports of myopathy developing after the use of structurally unrelated neuromuscular-blocking agents such as atracurium and cisatracurium. Morever the development of AQM is not confined to patients with asthma and there have been reports of patients with acute respiratory failure developing acute myopathy in the absence of corticosteroids and neuromuscular-blocking agents. It may be that pharmacological denervation produced by neuromuscular-blocking agents potentiates the toxic effects of other agents such as corticosteroids or inflammatory mediators. Experimentally denervation results in proliferation of glucocorticoid receptors in skeletal muscle cytosol, with preferential atrophy of type II B-muscle fibres, and subsequent steroid administration results in muscle thick filament loss with a reduction in membrane excitability. Denervation also appears to potentiate the acute catabolic effects of corticosteroids on skeletal muscle. It also seems possible that the functional denervation seen in CIPNM may provide a link between this condition and AQM.

CLINICAL FEATURES

During the acute phase of critical illness the clinical manifestations of neuromuscular dysfunction may be masked by the administration of sedatives and muscle relaxants, as well as by cerebral dysfunction caused, for example, by septic encephalopathy or head injury. In unconscious patients reduced limb movements are often ascribed to central neurological dysfunction, even though neuromyopathy has been shown to be extremely common in such cases (Latronico et al., 1996), emphasizing the importance of recognizing these disorders in order to avoid unnecessary investigations and overly pessimistic prognoses. Neuromuscular weakness may only become readily apparent during the recovery phase of critical illness, usually some weeks after admission to the intensive care unit, when the earliest indications are often diminished limb movements and/or difficulty weaning from mechanical ventilation. Deep painful stimulation of a distal extremity may then reveal symmetrical weakness, especially in the lower limbs, despite strong facial grimacing. Loss or reduction of deep tendon reflexes is common, but not invariable, and muscle wasting, although difficult to quantify, is mentioned by many authors. In the most severe cases (e.g. acute necrotizing myopathy) there may be severe areflexic paralysis and ophthalmoplegia. Prolonged neuromuscular blockade is more often accompanied by weakness of cranial as well as limb muscles. When CIPNM is the cause of difficulty with weaning from mechanical ventilation, spontaneous breathing is typically rapid and shallow and is associated with carbon dioxide retention.

The diagnosis of AQM should be suspected when unexplained quadriplegia develops in a patient with respiratory failure who has received corticosteroids and/or neuromuscular-blocking agents. Both proximal and distal muscles, including the diaphragm, are affected and weakness can be profound. Reflexes may be present or absent, but sensation remains intact.

INVESTIGATION OF NEUROMUSCULAR WEAKNESS
Electrophysiological testing

Nerve conduction velocities and *distal latencies* are almost always normal, thus excluding demyelination, whilst *compound muscle action potentials* (CMAPs) are usually markedly reduced. These findings are compatible with denervation due to an axonal neuropathy, but similar features may be seen in acute myopathies and in combined neuromyopathy. *Sensory action potentials* (SAPs) may also be reduced, suggesting that these changes could be due to a generalized sensorimotor axonal polyneuropathy. Indeed, the detection

of reduced SAPs (albeit usually of much less magnitude than the reduction in CMAPs) in the presence of weakness and clearly reduced CMAPs has generally been regarded as diagnostic of critical illness polyneuropathy (CIP). In order to establish a precise diagnosis, and in particular to distinguish between neuropathic and myopathic disorders, *electromyography* should be performed. This may reveal abnormal spontaneous activity (fibrillation and positive sharp waves) which is indicative of significant neuromuscular dysfunction but can occur in both polyneuropathy and myopathy. These two conditions can be differentiated by analysing motor unit potentials (MUPs) and fibre recruitment generated by voluntary effort, an investigation which is only possible when the patient is able to cooperate with the neurophysiologist. Following denervation, as occurs in axonal polyneuropathy, MUPs are of increased amplitude and duration, with a high firing pattern as recruitment increases. These features can persist for several years (Fletcher et al., 2003). In myopathy, on the other hand, MUPs are decreased in amplitude and are of short duration, with early recruitment. These changes may be rapidly reversible (< 6 weeks) in toxic myopathies. *Single-fibre electromyography* is difficult and time consuming but in one follow-up study findings supported other evidence of widespread denervation/reinnervation in a significant proportion of unselected long term survivors of prolonged intensive care (Fletcher et al., 2003).

Nerve biopsy

This investigation is rarely indicated because a degree of permanent neurological deficit is inevitable. Acute axonal degeneration has been seen in patients with sepsis and those requiring prolonged mechanical ventilation, as well as at postmortem in patients who died with sepsis and multiple-organ failure.

Muscle biopsy

A variety of histological abnormalities of muscle have been described in critically ill patients. In one study (Coakley et al., 1993) neurophysiological abnormalities were always associated with abnormal muscle histology. The incidence of muscle necrosis varies considerably between studies (9–55%) as does the proportion of patients with significant fibre atrophy (39–96%). The incidence of generalized fibre atrophy increases with the duration of critical illness, whilst type II fibre atrophy is known to occur with disuse and is associated with corticosteroid administration. AQM is associated with thick filament (myosin) loss. Raised serum creatine kinase levels do not always correlate with the presence of myopathy.

PATTERNS OF NEUROPHYSIOLOGICAL ABNORMALITY

Although the most common neurophysiological abnormality is a combination of reduced CMAPs and a less marked reduction in SAPs (findings typical of CIP), a few patients have sensory abnormalities alone and in some cases CMAPs are profoundly reduced in the presence of normal SAPs (Coakley *et al.*, 1998). This 'critical illness motor syndrome' has been described by others (Hund *et al.*, 1997) and termed 'respiratory failure neuropathy' (Gorson and Ropper, 1993). Such isolated motor dysfunction could be explained by an abnormality in the distal portion of the motor axon, at the neuromuscular junction or motor endplate and in some cases by a severe myopathy (such as AQM) with inexcitable muscle membranes or extreme loss of muscle bulk. It seems possible that the classical neurophysiological features of CIP could be explained, at least in some cases, by a combination of an acquired motor abnormality and a mild, non-specific or pre-existing sensory neuropathy.

PREVENTION AND TREATMENT

Currently prevention of CIPNM depends on prompt and effective treatment of the underlying disease, in particular the control of sepsis, and avoidance, when possible, of corticosteroids and neuromuscular-blocking agents, especially in combination. Recent evidence suggests that tight control of blood sugar levels can dramatically reduce the incidence of CIPNM (see Chapter 17). Intensive physiotherapy and rehabilitation remain the mainstay of treatment of the established condition.

PROGNOSIS

Although the outlook for recovery of muscle strength is generally good and complete recovery can occur within weeks, many patients take several months to achieve an acceptable level of mobility and independence after hospital discharge. Clinical weakness, with neurophysiological evidence of partial denervation, may persist for more than a year (Fletcher *et al.*, 2003). Disturbingly, in a few cases tetraplegia may persist for years and some of these patients die without recovering muscle strength (De Sèze *et al.*, 2000).

REFERENCES

Adams JH, Graham DI, Scott G, *et al.* (1980) Brain damage in fatal non-missile head injury. *Journal of Clinical Pathology* **33**: 1132–1145.

Albanèse J, Leone M, Alliez J-R, *et al.* (2003) Decompressive craniectomy for severe traumatic brain injury: evaluation of the effects at one year. *Critical Care Medicine* **31**: 2535–2538.

Alderson P, Roberts I (1997) Corticosteroids in acute traumatic brain injury: systematic review of randomised controlled trials. *British Medical Journal* **314**: 1855–1859.

Alkire MT, Haier RJ, Barker SJ, *et al.* (1995) Cerebral metabolism during propofol anesthesia in humans studied with positron emission tomography. *Anesthesiology* **82**: 393–403.

Alldredge BK, Gelb AM, Isaacs SM, *et al.* (2001) A comparison of lorazepam, diazepam, and placebo for the treatment of out-of-hospital status epilepticus. *New England Journal of Medicine* **345**: 631–637.

Andrews PJ, Citerio G (2004) Intracranial pressure. Part one: Historical overview and basic concepts. *Intensive Care Medicine* **30**: 1730–1733.

Attygalle D, Rodrigo N (2002) Magnesium as first line therapy in the management of tetanus: a prospective study of 40 patients. *Anaesthesia* **57**: 811–817.

Bao YP, Williamson G, Tew D, *et al.* (1998) Antioxidant effects of propofol in human hepatic microsomes: concentration effects and clinical relevance. *British Journal of Anaesthesia* **81**: 584–589.

Barker FG, Ogilvy CS (1996) Efficacy of prophylactic nimodipine for delayed ischemic deficit after subarachnoid hemorrhage: a metaanalysis. *Journal of Neurosurgery* **84**: 405–414.

Bartlett J, Kett-White R, Mendelow AD, *et al.* (1998) Guidelines for the initial management of head injuries: recommendations from the Society of British Neurological Surgeons. *British Journal of Neurosurgery* **12**: 349–352.

Beeching NJ, Crowcroft NS (2005) Tetanus in injecting drug users. *British Medical Journal* **330**: 208–209.

Bell MD, Moss E, Murphy PG (2004) Brainstem death testing in the UK – time for reappraisal? *British Journal of Anaesthesia* **92**: 633–640.

Bhagwanjee S, Bösenberg AT, Muckart DJ (1999) Management of sympathetic overactivity in tetanus with epidural bupivacaine and sufentanil: Experience with 11 patients. *Critical Care Medicine* **27**: 1721–1725.

Bingham RM, Procaccio F, Prior PF, *et al.* (1985) Cerebral electrical activity influences the effects of etomidate on cerebral perfusion pressure in traumatic coma. *British Journal of Anaesthesia* **57**: 843–848.

Bittner HB, Kendall SW, Chen EP, *et al.* (1995) Endocrine changes and metabolic responses in a validated canine brain death model. *Journal of Critical Care* **10**: 56–63.

Bolton CF, Gilbert JJ, Hahn AF, *et al.* (1984) Polyneuropathy in critically ill patients. *Journal of Neurology, Neurosurgery, and Psychiatry* **47**: 1223–1231.

Braakman R, Schouten HJ, Blaauw-Van-Dishoeck M, *et al.* (1983) Megadose steroids in severe head injury. Results of a prospective double-blind clinical trial. *Journal of Neurosurgery* **58**: 326–330.

Brain Trauma Task Force (2000) Management and prognosis of severe traumatic brain injury. *Journal of Neurotrauma* **17**: 451–553.

Bulger EM, Nathens AB, Rivara FP, *et al.* (2002) Management of severe head injury: institutional variations in care and effect on outcome. *Critical Care Medicine* **30**: 1870–1876.

Carter BG, Butt W (2001) Review of the use of somatosensory evoked potentials in the prediction of outcome after severe brain injury. *Critical Care Medicine* **29**: 178–186.

Chapman MG, Smith M, Hirsch NP (2001) Status epilepticus. *Anaesthesia* **56**: 648–659.

Cherian L, Chacko G, Goodman CJ, *et al.* (1999) Cerebral hemodynamic effects of phenylephrine and L-arginine after cortical impact injury. *Critical Care Medicine* **27**: 2512–2517.

Chesnut RM, Marshall LF, Klauber MR, *et al.* (1993) The role of secondary brain injury in determining outcome from severe head injury. *Journal of Trauma* **34**: 216–222.

Childs NL, Mercer WN (1996) Late improvement in consciousness after post-traumatic vegetative state. *New England Journal of Medicine* **334**: 24–25.

Cho YW, Terasaki PI, Cecka JM, *et al.* (1998) Transplantation of kidneys from donors whose hearts have stopped beating. *New England Journal of Medicine* **338**: 221–225.

Citerio G, Andrews PJ (2004) Intracranial pressure Part two: clinical applications and technology. *Intensive Care Medicine* **30**: 1882–1885.

Citerio G, Vascotto E, Villa F, *et al.* (2001) Induced abdominal compartment syndrome increases intracranial pressure in neurotrauma patients: a prospective study. *Critical Care Medicine* **29**: 1466–1471.

Clifton GL, Miller ER, Choi SC, *et al.* (2001) Lack of effect of induction of hypothermia after acute brain injury. *New England Journal of Medicine* **344**: 556–563.

Coakley JH, Nagendran K, Ormerod IE, *et al.* (1992) Prolonged neurogenic weakness in patients requiring mechanical ventilation for acute airflow limitation. *Chest* **101**: 1413–1416.

Coakley JH, Nagendran K, Honavar M, *et al.* (1993) Preliminary observations on the neuromuscular abnormalities in patients with organ failure and sepsis. *Intensive Care Medicine* **19**: 323–328.

Coakley JH, Nagendran K, Yarwood GD, *et al.* (1998) Patterns of neurophysiological abnormality in prolonged critical illness. *Intensive Care Medicine* **24**: 801–807.

Conference of Medical Royal Colleges and their Faculties in the United Kingdom (1976) Diagnosis of brain death. *British Medical Journal* **2**: 1187–1188.

Cook TM, Protheroe RT, Handel JM (2001) Tetanus: a review of the literature. *British Journal of Anaesthesia* **87**: 477–487.

Cooper PR, Moody S, Clark WK, *et al.* (1979) Dexamethasone and severe head injury. A prospective double-blind study. *Journal of Neurosurgery* **51**: 307–316.

Cooper DJ, Myles PS, McDermott FT, *et al.* (2004) Prehospital hypertonic saline resuscitation of patients with hypotension and severe traumatic brain injury: a randomized controlled trial. *Journal of the American Medical Association* 291: 1350–1357.

Cormio M, Valadka AB, Robertson CS (1999) Elevated jugular venous oxygen saturation after severe head injury. *Journal of Neurosurgery* 90: 9–15.

Cremer OL, Moons KG, Bouman EA, *et al.* (2001) Long-term propofol infusion and cardiac failure in adult head-injured patients. *Lancet* 357: 117–118.

Davis DP, Dunford JV, Poste JC, *et al.* (2004) The impact of hypoxia and hyperventilation on outcome after paramedic rapid sequence intubation of severely head-injured patients. *The Journal of Trauma* 57: 1–10.

Deehan SC, Grant IS (1996) Haemodynamic changes in neurogenic pulmonary oedema: effect of dobutamine. *Intensive Care Medicine* 22: 672–676.

Deem S, Lee CM, Curtis JR (2003) Acquired neuromuscular disorders in the intensive care unit. *American Journal of Respiratory and Critical Care Medicine* 168: 735–739.

de Gans J, van de Beek D for the European Dexamethasone in Adulthood Bacterial Meningitis Study Investigators (2002) Dexamethasone in adults with bacterial meningitis. *New England Journal of Medicine* 347: 1549–1556.

DeMaria EJ, Reichman W, Kenney PR, *et al.* (1985) Septic complications of corticosteroid administration after central nervous system trauma. *Annals of Surgery* 202: 248–252.

De Sèze M, Petit H, Wiart L, *et al.* (2000) Critical illness polyneuropathy: a 2-year follow-up study in 19 severe cases. *European Neurology* 43: 61–69.

Dickinson K, Bunn F, Wentz R, *et al.* (2000) Size and quality of randomised controlled trials in head injury: review of published studies. *British Medical Journal* 320: 1308–1311.

Editorial (1985) Neurogenic pulmonary oedema. *Lancet* 1: 1430–1431.

Edwards P, Arango M, Balica L, *et al.* (2005) Final results of MRC CRASH, a randomised placebo-controlled trial of intravenous corticosteroid in adults with head injury – outcomes at 6 months. *Lancet* 365: 1957–1959.

Eisenberg HM, Frankowski RF, Contant CF, *et al.* (1988) High-dose barbiturate control of elevated intracranial pressure in patients with severe head injury. *Journal of Neurosurgery* 69: 15–23.

Eker C, Asgeirsson B, Grände PO, *et al.* (1998) Improved outcome after severe head injury with a new therapy based on principles for brain volume regulation and preserved microcirculation. *Critical Care Medicine* 26: 1881–1886.

Farling PA, Johnston JR, Coppel DL (1989) Propofol infusion for sedation of patients with head injury in intensive care. A preliminary report. *Anaesthesia* 44: 222–226.

Feldman Z, Kanter MJ, Robertson CS, *et al.* (1992) Effect of head elevation on intracranial pressure, cerebral perfusion pressure, and cerebral blood flow in head-injured patients. *Journal of Neurosurgery* 76: 207–211.

Fisher AJ, Donnelly SC, Hirani N, *et al.* (1999) Enhanced pulmonary inflammation in organ donors following fatal non-traumatic brain injury. *Lancet* 353: 1412–1413.

Fleminger S, Ponsford J (2005) Long term outcome after traumatic brain injury. *British Medical Journal* 331: 1419–1420.

Fletcher SN, Kennedy DD, Ghosh IR, *et al.* (2003) Persistent neuromuscular and neurophysiologic abnormalities in long-term survivors of prolonged critical illness. *Critical Care Medicine* 31: 1012–1016.

French Cooperative Group on Plasma Exchange in Guillain–Barré Syndrome (1987) Efficiency of plasma exchange in Guillain–Barré syndrome: role of replacement fluids. *Annals of Neurology* 22: 753–761.

French Cooperative Group on Plasma Exchange in Guillain–Barré Syndrome (1992) Plasma exchange in Guillain–Barré syndrome: one-year follow-up. *Annals of Neurology* 32: 94–97.

Gennarelli TA, Spielman GM, Langfitt TW, *et al.* (1982) Influence of the type of intracranial lesion on outcome from severe head injury. *Journal of Neurosurgery* 56: 26–32.

Gentleman D, Dearden M, Midgley S, *et al.* (1993) Guidelines for resuscitation and transfer of patients with serious head injury. *British Medical Journal* 307: 547–552.

Ghajar J (2000) Traumatic brain injury. *Lancet* 356: 923–929.

Gore SM, Hinds CJ, Rutherford AJ (1989) Organ donation from intensive care units in England. *British Medical Journal* 299: 1193 1197.

Gore SM, Cable DJ, Holland AJ (1992) Organ donation from intensive care units in England and Wales: two year confidential audit of deaths in intensive care. *British Medical Journal* 304: 349 355.

Gorson KC, Ropper AH (1993) Acute respiratory failure neuropathy: a variant of critical illness polyneuropathy. *Critical Care Medicine* 21: 267–271.

Graham DI, Ford I, Adams JH, *et al.* (1989) Ischaemic brain damage is still common in fatal non-missile head-injury. *Journal of Neurology, Neurosurgery, and Psychiatry* 52: 346–350.

Guesde R, Barrou B, Leblanc I, *et al.* (1998) Administration of desmopressin in brain-dead donors and renal function in kidney recipients. *Lancet* 352: 1178–1181.

Guillain–Barré Syndrome Study Group (1985) Plasmapheresis and acute Guillain–Barré syndrome. *Neurology* 35: 1096–1104.

Guillain G, Barré JA, Strohl A (1916) Sur un syndrome de radiculo-nivrite avec hyperalbuminose du liquide encephalora-chidien sans réaction cellulaire. *Bulletins et memoires de la Société Médicale des Hopitaux de Paris* 40: 1462–1470 (translated *Archives of Neurology* (1968) 18: 450–452).

Hahn AF (1998) Guillain–Barré syndrome. *Lancet* 352: 635–641.

Haitsma IK, Maas AI (2002) Advanced monitoring in the intensive care unit: brain tissue oxygen tension. *Current Opinion in Critical Care* 8: 115–120.

Henderson WR, Dhingra VK, Chittock DR, *et al.* (2003) Hypothermia in the management of traumatic brain injury. A systematic review and meta-analysis. *Intensive Care Medicine* 29: 1637–1644.

Hsiang JK, Chesnut RM, Crisp CB, *et al.* (1994) Early, routine paralysis for intracranial pressure control in severe head injury: is it necessary? *Critical Care Medicine* 22: 1471–1476.

Hughes RA (1991) Ineffectiveness of high dose intravenous methylprednisolone in Guillain–Barré syndrome. *Lancet* 338: 1142.

Hughes RA (2001) Sensory form of Guillain–Barré syndrome. *Lancet* 357: 1465.

Hughes RA (2004) Treatment of Guillain–Barré syndrome with corticosteroids: lack of benefit? *Lancet* 363: 181–182.

Hund E, Genzwurkar H, Bohrer H, *et al.* (1997) Predominant involvement of motor fibres in patients with critical illness polyneuropathy. *British Journal of Anaesthesia* 78: 274–278.

Jennett B, Bond M (1975) Assessment of outcome after severe brain damage. *Lancet* i: 480–484.

Jennett B, Teasdale G, Fry J, *et al.* (1980) Treatment for severe head injury. *Journal of Neurology, Neurosurgery, and Psychiatry* 43: 289–295.

Johnston AJ, Gupta AK (2002) Advanced monitoring in the neurology intensive care unit: microdialysis. *Current Opinion in Critical Care* 8: 121–127.

Johnston AJ, Steiner LA, Chatfield DA, *et al.* (2003) Effects of propofol on cerebral oxygenation and metabolism after head injury. *British Journal of Anaesthesia* 91: 781–786.

Johnston AJ, Steiner LA, Coles JP, *et al.* (2005) Effect of cerebral perfusion pressure augmentation on regional oxygenation and metabolism after head injury. *Critical Care Medicine* 33: 189–195.

Kelly DF, Goodale DB, Williams J, *et al.* (1999) Propofol in the treatment of moderate and severe head injury: a randomized, prospective, double-blinded pilot trial. *Journal of Neurosurgery* 90: 1042–1052.

Kennedy DD, Fletcher N, Hinds CJ (2000) Neuromuscular dysfunction in critical illness: what are we dealing with? *Current Opinion in Anaesthesiology* 13: 93–98.

Kerr JH, Corbett JL, Prys-Roberts C, *et al.* (1968) Involvement of the sympathetic nervous system in tetanus. Studies on 82 cases. *Lancet* 2: 236–241.

Knoller N, Levi L, Shoshan I, *et al.* (2002) Dexanabinol (HU-211) in the treatment of severe closed head injury: a randomized placebo-controlled phase II clinical trial. *Critical Care Medicine* 30: 548–554.

Kroppenstedt S-N, Stover JF, Unterberg AW (2000) Effects of dopamine on posttraumatic cerebral blood flow, brain edema and cerebrospinal fluid glutamate and hypoxanthine concentrations. *Critical Care Medicine* 28: 3792–3798.

Kumar A, Bleck TP (1992) Intravenous midazolam for the treatment of refractory status epilepticus. *Critical Care Medicine* 20: 483–488.

Lambert EH, Eaton LM, Rooke ED (1956) Defect of neuromuscular conduction associated with malignant neoplasms. *American Journal of Physiology* 187: 612–613.

Latronico N, Fenzi F, Recupero D, *et al.* (1996) Critical illness myopathy and neuropathy. *Lancet* 347: 1579–1582.

Latronico N, Beindorf AE, Rasulo FA, *et al.* (2000) Limits of intermittent jugular bulb oxygen saturation monitoring in the management of severe head trauma patients. *Neurosurgery* 46: 1131–1139.

Lee JH, Kelly DF, Oertel M, *et al.* (2001) Carbon dioxide reactivity, pressure autoregulation, and metabolic suppression reactivity after head injury: a transcranial Doppler study. *Journal of Neurosurgery* 95: 222–232.

Leppik IE, Derivan AT, Homan RW, *et al.* (1983) Double-blind study of lorazepam and diazepam in status epilepticus. *Journal of the American Medical Association* **249**: 1452–1454.

Lichtenfeld P (1971) Autonomic dysfunction in the Guillain–Barré syndrome. *American Journal of Medicine* **50**: 772–780.

Lowenstein DH (2003) Treatment options for status epilepticus. *Current Opinion in Pharmacology* **3**: 6–11.

Macmillan CS, Andrews PJ (2000) Cerebrovenous oxygen saturation monitoring: practical considerations and clinical relevance. *Intensive Care Medicine* **26**: 1028–1036.

Macmillan CS, Grant IS, Andrews PJ (2002) Pulmonary and cardiac sequelae of subarachnoid haemorrhage: time for active management? *Intensive Care Medicine* **28**: 1012–1023.

McDowall DG (1976) Neurosurgical anaesthesia and intensive care. In: Hewer CL and Atkinson RS (eds) *Recent Advances in Anaesthesia and Analgesia* 12. Edinburgh: Churchill Livingstone, pp. 16–43.

McGuire G, Crossley D, Richards J, et al. (1997) Effects of varying levels of positive end-expiratory pressure on intracranial pressure and cerebral perfusion pressure. *Critical Care Medicine* **25**: 1059–1062.

McIntyre LA, Fergusson DA, Hébert PC, et al. (2003) Prolonged therapeutic hypothermia after traumatic brain injury in adults: a systematic review. *Journal of the American Medical Association* **289**: 2992–2999.

Marik PE, Zaloga GP (2001) Early enteral nutrition in acutely ill patients: a systematic review. *Critical Care Medicine* **29**: 2264–2270.

Marik PE, Varon J, Trask T (2002) Management of head trauma. *Chest* **122**: 699–711.

Marion DW, Penrod LE, Kelsey SF, et al. (1997) Treatment of traumatic brain injury with moderate hypothermia. *New England Journal of Medicine* **336**: 540–546.

Marshall LF, Marshall SB, Klauber MR, et al. (1992) The diagnosis of head injury requires a classification based on computed axial tomography. *Journal of Neurotrauma* **9**: S287–S292.

Mendelow AD, Teasdale G, Jennett B, et al. (1983) Risks of intracranial haematoma in head-injured adults. *British Medical Journal* **287**: 1173–1176.

Miller JD, Butterworth JF, Gudeman SK, et al. (1981) Further experience in the management of severe head injury. *Journal of Neurosurgery* **54**: 289–299.

Miranda-Filho DB, Ximenes RA, Barone AA, et al. (2004) Randomised controlled trial of tetanus treatment with antitetanus immunoglobulin by the intrathecal or intramuscular route. *British Medical Journal* **328**: 615.

Mohandas A, Chou SN (1971) Brain death – a clinical and pathological study. *Journal of Neurosurgery* **35**: 211–218.

Mollaret P, Goulon M (1959) Le coma dépasse (memoire preliminaire). *Rev Neurol* **101**: 3–15.

Moller K, Skinhoj P (2000) Guidelines for managing acute bacterial meningitis. *British Medical Journal* **320**: 1290.

Moller K, Larsen FS, Qvist J, et al. (2000) Dependency of cerebral blood flow on mean arterial pressure in patients with acute bacterial meningitis. *Critical Care Medicine* **28**: 1027–1032.

Moutier F (1918) Hypertension et mort par oedème pulmonaire aigu chez les blessés cranio-encéphaliques. *Presse Medicale* **26**: 108–109.

Muizelaar JP, Wei EP, Kontos HA, et al. (1983) Mannitol causes compensatory cerebral vasoconstriction and vasodilation in response to blood viscosity changes. *Journal of Neurosurgery* **59**: 822–828.

Muizelaar JP, Marmarou A, Ward JD, et al. (1991) Adverse effects of prolonged hyperventilation in patients with severe head injury: a randomized clinical trial. *Journal of Neurosurgery* **75**: 731–739.

Murray GD, Teasdale GM, Braakman R, et al. (1999a) European Brain Injury Consortium Survey of Head Injuries. *Acta Neurochirurgica* **141**: 223–236.

Murray LS, Teasdale GM, Murray GD, et al. (1999b) Head injuries in four British neurosurgical centres. *British Journal of Neurosurgery* **13**: 546–549.

Nath F, Galbraith S (1986) The effect of mannitol on cerebral white matter water content. *Journal of Neurosurgery* **65**: 41–43.

O'Brien TJ, Cascino GD, So EL, et al. (1998) Incidence and clinical consequence of the purple glove syndrome in patients receiving intravenous phenytoin. *Neurology* **51**: 1034–1039.

Obrist WD, Langfitt TW, Jaggi JL, et al. (1984) Cerebral blood flow and metabolism in comatose patients with acute head injury. Relationship to intracranial hypertension. *Journal of Neurosurgery* **61**: 241–253.

Pallis C (1983) ABC of brainstem death. *British Medical Journal* ••.

Park GR (2004) Death and its diagnosis by doctors. *British Journal of Anaesthesia* **92**: 625–628.

Parr MJ, Finfer SR, Morgan MK (1996) Reversible cardiogenic shock complicating subarachnoid haemorrhage. *British Medical Journal* **313**: 681–683.

Patel HC, Bouamra O, Woodford M, et al. (2005) Trends in head injury outcome from 1989 to 2003 and the effect of neurosurgical care: an observational study. *Lancet* **366**: 1538–1544.

Plasma Exchange/Sandoglobulin Guillain–Barré Syndrome Trial Group (1997) Randomised trial of plasma exchange, intravenous immunoglobulin, and combined treatments in Guillain Barré syndrome. *Lancet* **349**: 225–230.

Pollay M, Fullenwider C, Roberts PA, et al. (1983) Effect of mannitol and furosemide on blood–brain osmotic gradient and intracranial pressure. *Journal of Neurosurgery* **59**: 945–950.

Portella G, Cormio M, Citerio G, et al. (2005) Continuous cerebral compliance monitoring in severe head injury: its relationship with intracranial pressure and cerebral perfusion pressure. *Acta Neurochirurgica* **147**: 707–713.

Prior PF (1985) EEG monitoring and evoked potentials in brain ischaemia. *British Journal of Anaesthesia* **57**: 63–81.

Prior JGL, Hinds CJ, Williams J, et al. (1983) The use of etomidate in the management of severe head injury. *Intensive Care Medicine* **9**: 313–320.

Rees JH, Soudain SE, Gregson NA, et al. (1995) *Campylobacter jejuni* infection and Guillain–Barré syndrome. *New England Journal of Medicine* **333**: 1374–1379.

Review by a Working Group convened by the Royal College of Physicians and endorsed by the Conference of Medical Royal Colleges and their Faculties of the United Kingdom (1996) The permanent vegetative state. *Journal of the Royal College of Physicians of London* **30**: 119–121.

Roberts I, Yates D, Sandercock P, et al. (2004) Effect of intravenous corticosteroids on death within 14 days in 10008 adults with clinically significant head injury (MRC CRASH trial): randomised placebo-controlled trial. *Lancet* **364**: 1321–1328.

Rosner MJ, Rosner SD, Johnson AH (1995) Cerebral perfusion pressure: management and clinical results. *Journal of Neurosurgery* **83**: 949–962.

Rothoerl RD, Woertgen C, Brawanski A (2004) Hyperemia following aneurysmal subarachnoid hemorrhage: incidence, diagnosis, clinical features and outcome. *Intensive Care Medicine* **30**: 1298–1302.

Royo NC, Shimizu S, Schouten JW, et al. (2003) Pharmacology of traumatic brain injury. *Current Opinion in Pharmacology* **3**: 27–32.

Salim A, Velmahos GC, Brown C, et al. (2005) Aggressive organ donor management significantly increases the number of organs available for transplantation. *Journal of Trauma* **58**: 991–994.

Schrot RJ, Muizelaar JP (2002) Mannitol in acute traumatic brain injury. *Lancet* **359**: 1633–1634.

Shann F (2003) Hypothermia for traumatic brain injury: how soon, how cold, and how long? *Lancet* **362**: 1950–1951.

Simmons RL, Martin AM Jr, Heisterkamp CA 3rd, et al. (1969) Respiratory insufficiency in combat casualties. II. Pulmonary edema following head injury. *Annals of Surgery* **170**: 39–44.

Sleigh JW, Havill JH, Frith R, et al. (1999) Somatosensory evoked potential in severe traumatic brain injury: a blinded study. *Journal of Neurosurgery* **91**: 577–580.

Steiner LA, Johnston AJ, Czosnyka M, et al. (2004) Direct comparison of cerebrovascular effects of norepinephrine and dopamine in head-injured patients. *Critical Care Medicine* **32**: 1049–1054.

Stiell IG, Wells GA, Vandemheen K, et al. (2001) The Canadian CT head rule for patients with minor head injury. *Lancet* **357**: 1391–1396.

Teasdale GM, Graham DI (1998) Craniocerebral trauma: protection and retrieval of the neuronal population after injury. *Neurosurgery* **43**: 723–738.

The SAFE Study Investigators (2007) Saline or albumin for fluid resuscitation in patients with traumatic brain injury? *New England Journal of Medicine* **357**: 874–884.

Thwaites GE, Nguyen DB, Nguyen HD, et al. (2004) Dexamethasone for the treatment of tuberculous meningitis in adolescents and adults. *New England Journal of Medicine* **351**: 1741–1751.

Thwaites CL, Yen LM, Loan HT, et al. (2006) Magnesium sulphate for treatment of severe tetanus: a randomised controlled trial. *Lancet* **368**: 1436–1443.

Timmins AC, Hinds CJ (1991) Management of the multiple organ donor. *Current Opinion in Anaesthesiology* **4**: 287–292.

Treiman DM, Meyers PD, Walton NY, et al. (1998) A comparison of four treatments for generalised convulsive status epilepticus. *New England Journal of Medicine* **339**: 792–798.

Tripathi M, Kaushik S (2000) Carbamazepine for pain management in Guillain–Barré syndrome patients in the intensive care unit. *Critical Care Medicine* **28**: 655–658.

Trojaborg W, Weimer LH, Hays AP (2001) Electrophysiologic studies in critical illness associated weakness: myopathy or neuropathy – a reappraisal. *Clinical Neurophysiology* **112**: 1586–1593.

Trujillo MH, Castillo A, Espana J, *et al.* (1987) Impact of intensive care management on the prognosis of tetanus: Analysis of 641 cases. *Chest* **92**: 63–65.

Tunkel AR, Scheld WM (2002) Corticosteroids for everyone with meningitis? *New England Journal of Medicine* **347**: 1613–1615.

van de Beek D, de Gans J, Spanjaard L, *et al.* (2004) Clinical features and prognostic factors in adults with bacterial meningitis. *New England Journal of Medicine* **351**: 1849–1859.

Van der Meché FG, Schmitz PI and the Dutch Guillain–Barré Study Group (1992) A randomized trial comparing intravenous immune globulin and plasma exchange in Guillain–Barré syndrome. *New England Journal of Medicine* **326**: 1123–1129.

van Koningsveld R, Schmitz PIM, van der Meché FGA, *et al.* (2004) Effect of methylprednisolone when added to standard treatment with intravenous immunoglobulin for Guillain–Barré syndrome: randomised trial. *Lancet* **365**: 192–196.

Vargas F, Hilbert G, Gruson D, *et al.* (2000) Fulminant Guillain–Barré syndrome mimicking cerebral death: case report and literature review. *Intensive Care Medicine* **26**: 623–627.

Vincent A, Palace J, Hilton-Jones D (2001) Myasthenia gravis. *Lancet* **357**: 2122–2128.

Wade CE, Grady JJ, Kramer GC, *et al.* (1997) Individual patient cohort analysis of the efficacy of hypertonic saline/dextran in patients with traumatic brain injury and hypotension. *Journal of Trauma* **42**: S61–S65.

Ward JD, Becker DP, Miller JD, *et al.* (1985) Failure of prophylactic barbiturate coma in the treatment of severe head injury. *Journal of Neurosurgery* **62**: 383–388.

Wheeldon DR, Potter CD, Oduro A, *et al.* (1995) Transforming the 'unacceptable' donor: outcomes from the adoption of a standardized donor management technique. *Journal of Heart and Lung Transplantation* **14**: 734–742.

Wijdicks EF (2001) The diagnosis of brain death. *New England Journal of Medicine* **344**: 1215–1221.

Willatts SM, Drummond G (2000) Brainstem death and ventilator trigger settings. *Anaesthesia* **55**: 676–677.

Wilson JT, Pettigrew LE, Teasdale GM (1998) Structured interviews for the Glasgow Outcome Scale and Extended Glasgow Outcome Scale: guidelines for their use. *Journal of Neurotrauma* **15**: 573–585.

Winchell RJ, Hoyt DB (1997) Endotracheal intubation in the field improves survival in patients with severe head injury. *Archives of Surgery* **132**: 592–597.

Winer J (1992) Guillain–Barré syndrome revisited. Pathogenesis still unknown. *British Medical Journal* **304**: 65–66.

Wolach B, Sazbon L, Gavrieli R, *et al.* (2001) Early immunological defects in comatose patients after acute brain injury. *Journal of Neurosurgery* **94**: 706–711.

Wood KE, Becker BN, McCartney JG, *et al.* (2004) Care of the potential organ donor. *New England Journal of Medicine* **351**: 2730–2739.

Yates D, Roberts I (2000) Corticosteroids in head injury. *British Medical Journal* **321**: 128–129.

16 Gastrointestinal disorders

Not only may dysfunction of organs perfused by splanchnic vessels contribute significantly to the development and lethality of multiple-organ failure (see Chapter 5), but primary pathology involving the gastrointestinal tract is a frequent cause of critical illness.

GASTROINTESTINAL HAEMORRHAGE

Acute gastrointestinal bleeding is an important cause of in-hospital morbidity and mortality. In the intensive care unit, gastrointestinal haemorrhage may be encountered under two circumstances:

1. patients who initially present with massive upper or lower gastrointestinal haemorrhage;
2. critically ill patients, often with multisystem involvement, in whom gastrointestinal haemorrhage develops as a secondary complication.

UPPER GASTROINTESTINAL HAEMORRHAGE

The reported incidence of upper gastrointestinal bleeding in the UK varies from 47 per 100 000 to 116 per 100 000, and rises to around 485 per 100 000 in the elderly (Rockall *et al.*, 1995).

Causes *(Lewis* et al., *2000)*

The commonest causes of upper gastrointestinal haemorrhage are:

- gastric or duodenal ulceration;
- reflux oesophagitis;
- gastritis and gastric erosions;
- stress ulceration;
- oesophageal and gastric varices;
- Mallory–Weiss tear (gastric or gastro-oesophageal tear).

Certain lesions are more common in particular categories of patients. For example, *angiodysplasia* of the stomach and duodenum is the most common cause of acute or recurrent bleeding in patients with chronic renal failure, while patients with aortic grafts may bleed from *aortoenteric fistulae*, and in cirrhotics a high percentage of bleeding originates from *varices*, although in many cases bleeding is from a non-variceal site, such as *Mallory–Weiss* tears or *peptic ulceration*. *Gastric carcinoma* is an unusual cause of gastrointestinal bleeding.

Clinical presentation

Most commonly patients present with *haematemesis* and/or *melaena*, combined, when bleeding is severe, with signs and symptoms of *shock*, including anxiety, sweating, dizziness, pallor and confusion (see Chapter 5). Haematemesis occurs in about one-half to two-thirds of patients with upper gastrointestinal haemorrhage, and melaena is seen in around two-thirds of cases. Although bright-red rectal bleeding is almost always a sign of colonic haemorrhage, upper gastrointestinal bleeding may result in the passage of maroon-coloured, rather than black, stools when large quantities of blood in the gastrointestinal tract increase intestinal motility.

The presence of *pain* is suggestive of peptic ulceration, pancreatitis or biliary disease, while a history of protracted retching and vomiting raises the possibility of Mallory–Weiss syndrome. *Dysphagia, anorexia* and *weight loss* may suggest the diagnosis of carcinoma, and in those who have previously undergone aortoiliac reconstructive surgery, bleeding may be due to an aortoenteric fistula. Finally, a meticulous drug history should always be taken, including the use of aspirin or other non-steroidal anti-inflammatory drugs (NSAIDs) and alcohol. The combined use of steroids and NSAIDs appears to increase the risk of upper gastrointestinal haemorrhage considerably, while treatment with anticoagulants can exacerbate bleeding from any source. It is unclear whether steroids alone are associated with an increased risk of upper gastrointestinal bleeding.

Bleeding from ulcers ceases spontaneously in at least 80% of patients, most of whom make an uneventful recovery without specific interventions.

Physical examination

Physical examination should include an assessment of the severity of blood loss and the patient's physiological response to haemorrhage and resuscitation. The patient should also be examined for clues as to the source of bleeding, such as hepatosplenomegaly, epigastric tenderness, abdominal masses and wasting. The stigmata of chronic alcoholic liver disease should be sought, as should the mucocutaneous changes of diseases known to be associated with gastrointestinal haemorrhage (*hereditary haemorrhagic telangiectasia, Ehlers–Danlos syndrome* and *Peutz–Jeghers syndrome*).

Investigations

Initial evaluation of patients with suspected gastrointestinal haemorrhage, including those with rectal bleeding not clearly due to lower gastrointestinal haemorrhage, should include *placement of a nasogastric tube*. Gastric aspirates and stool may be tested for blood if not obviously bloody. Only rarely (< 1% of cases) does upper gastrointestinal haemorrhage occur without a positive bloody nasogastric aspirate, usually when there is active bleeding from the duodenum without reflux into the stomach. Gastric lavage can help to determine the severity and rapidity of bleeding.

Initial laboratory investigations should include haemoglobin and haematocrit determinations together with a request for cross-matching. A full blood count and electrolyte determinations together with liver function tests and coagulation studies are essential in all patients. Routine chest and abdominal radiographs should be obtained. Because silent myocardial infarction may complicate significant gastrointestinal bleeding, an electrocardiogram is indicated in older patients.

ENDOSCOPY

In the majority of patients the site of bleeding is most likely to be identified by endoscopy, which may provide clues as to the source of haemorrhage even when the stomach cannot be entirely cleared of blood. Measures must be taken to avoid aspiration in those with a full stomach, including the avoidance of excessive sedation, as well as ensuring the availability of adequate suctioning apparatus and skilled assistance. In some instances endotracheal intubation may be required before endoscopy can proceed.

The timing of endoscopy is important. All resuscitative measures should have been instituted and the patient should be stable before the procedure is begun. An exception may be made in those with massive haemorrhage who require an immediate life-saving procedure. In stable patients who continue to bleed, endoscopy should be performed as soon as possible, and certainly within 24 hours to determine the most appropriate intervention.

When bleeding has stopped or has been easily controlled by conservative measures (see below) endoscopy can be performed as a semielective procedure, although its value in such patients has been questioned. Specific endoscopic signs may, however, be helpful in predicting the likelihood that an ulcer will rebleed. For example, when an actively bleeding ulcer is seen at endoscopy the risk of rebleeding is high, even though in a proportion of cases haemorrhage can be controlled by electrocoagulation of the ulcer base and multiple injections of adrenaline (epinephrine) in normal saline.

Similarly, the finding of a non-bleeding 'visible vessel' (*sentinel clot* or *pigmented protuberance*) in an ulcer base is associated with an increased risk of recurrent haemorrhage whether treated with perendoscopic injection of sclerosants or with intravenous omeprazole. Endoscopic findings suggesting that the risk of rebleeding is low (< 10%) include ulcers with a clean base or containing flat pigmented spots (Kovacs and Jensen, 1987). The size and location of the ulcer may also influence the risk of rebleeding; ulcers located on the posterior wall of the duodenal bulb and those larger than 1 cm in diameter have an increased chance of rebleeding (Branicki *et al.*, 1990).

ANGIOGRAPHY

When endoscopy fails to locate the source of haemorrhage in a patient who continues to bleed, angiography may be indicated. Emergency angiography allows localization of the bleeding site and subsequent administration of vasopressin or embolization (see later in this chapter). When angiography is not immediately available or the patient is in danger of exsanguination, emergency surgery is indicated to control bleeding.

Management *(Table 16.1)*

Management is influenced by:

- the patient's age;
- the amount of blood lost/severity of bleeding;
- continuing visible blood loss;
- signs of chronic liver disease;
- evidence of comorbidity (e.g. cardiac failure, ischaemic heart disease, renal disease, malignant disease);
- presence of shock.

When a patient presents with gastrointestinal bleeding, the primary initial consideration is resuscitation and haemodynamic stabilization: rapid restoration of the patient's vascular volume is of paramount importance. Large-bore intravenous access should be established and consideration given to central venous and urinary catheterization in patients who are shocked, in the elderly and in those with significant cardiopulmonary disease. More invasive monitoring is occasionally indicated, although oesophageal Doppler monitoring is often impractical or contraindicated. Pending cross-matching of blood, volume losses should be replaced with crystalloid or colloidal solutions. Supplemental oxygen should be given in all cases (see Chapter 5). Patients with severe haemorrhage and those who are shocked are best managed in a high-dependency or intensive care unit.

Some authorities recommend that ice-water lavage be commenced through the nasogastric tube after an initial aspiration of bloody or coffee-ground contents. Cooling of the stomach may reduce the rate of blood loss (although there is no convincing evidence to support this contention), as well as facilitating any subsequent endoscopy.

No absolute rules exist to guide blood transfusion. In general, a haemoglobin concentration greater than 8 g/dL is

Table 16.1 Management of upper gastrointestinal haemorrhage

Resuscitation	
Rapidly restore circulating volume	Large-bore intravenous access In selected cases monitor central venous pressure More invasive monitoring may be indicated in the most complex cases
Supplemental oxygen	
Investigations	
	Pass nasogastric tube (not universally recommended) Test stool and gastric aspirate for blood if not obviously bloody Haemoglobin concentration/haematocrit Urea and electrolytes Coagulation studies Liver biochemistry Chest and abdominal radiographs Electrocardiogram Endoscopy Angiography
Continued management	
Blood transfusion to maintain haemoglobin above 8 g/dL	Consider surgery in those patients with ongoing or haemodynamically important bleeding
Fresh frozen plasma, platelets and clotting factor concentrates as indicated	

a reasonable goal. Packed red blood cells are sufficient to meet transfusion requirements in most cases. Fresh frozen plasma, platelets and clotting factor concentrates may be required. Patients with ongoing or haemodynamically important bleeding require a surgical opinion.

Specific management decisions are best made jointly between gastroenterologists and surgeons. Immediate endoscopic or surgical assessment is recommended for:

- patients with persisting shock;
- those over 60 years of age who have received more than 4 units of blood;
- any patient transfused with more than 8 units of blood.

Patients with significant, unresponsive hypotension (e.g. systolic blood pressure < 80 mmHg) should be referred immediately for surgical consideration.

Prognosis

The 5–10% mortality from gastrointestinal haemorrhage has not improved over the years despite changes in management such as early therapeutic endoscopy, mainly because an increasing proportion of patients are elderly with concurrent illness (Rockall et al., 1996). A number of readily identifiable presenting features are associated with an increased mortality. For example, patients who report red haematemesis, with or without melaena, or coffee-grounds emesis with melaena have a higher mortality rate than those presenting with melaena alone, as do those in whom red blood is aspirated from the nasogastric tube. Haemorrhage occurring as a complication of hospitalization and associated with hypo-

tension is also associated with a greatly increased mortality rate compared with bleeding in the absence of hypotension or tachycardia. A haematocrit less than 30% or a haemoglobin less than 8 g/dL on presentation is associated with a worse outcome, although the increase in risk is less than that associated with hypotension. Perhaps the best predictor of mortality is continued bleeding after admission (Lewis et al., 2000). In one study age, the presence of shock, comorbidity, the underlying diagnosis, major stigmata of recent haemorrhage and rebleeding were all independent predictors of mortality (Rockall et al., 1996). From these variables a numerical score for calculating risk standardized mortality was developed (**Table 16.2**).

Specific causes of upper gastrointestinal haemorrhage
BLEEDING PEPTIC ULCER (Saltzman and Zawacki, 1997; Jenkins, 1999) (Table 16.3)
Approximately half of all upper gastrointestinal bleeds are due to peptic ulceration. Patients with bleeding peptic ulcer should initially be managed and resuscitated as outlined above.

Pharmacological therapy. Haemorrhage may be controlled by decreasing gastric blood flow, increasing gastric pH, stabilizing the blood clot or a combination of these. A variety of agents have been studied.

H_2-receptor antagonists and proton pump inhibitors have been extensively investigated. Although pooled data indicated that rates of rebleeding and emergency surgery may be

Table 16.2 Contributors to the Rockall score

Contributor	Score			
	0	1	2	3
Age (years)	< 60	60–79	> 80	
Shock	None	Pulse > 100 beats/min BP > 100 mmHg	BP < 100 mmHg	
Comorbidity	None		CCF/IHD or other	Renal/liver failure, disseminated malignancy
Diagnosis	None or Mallory–Weiss	All others	Upper GI tract malignancy	
Endoscopic stigmata	None		Blood in upper GI tract/ adherent clot/visible vessel	

BP, blood pressure; CCF, congestive cardiac failure; GI, gastrointestinal; IHD, ischaemic heart disease.

Table 16.3 Management of bleeding peptic ulcer

Pharmacological treatment

Proton pump inhibitors

H₂-receptor antagonists

(Somatostatin/octreotide)

(Vasopressin analogues)

(Tranexamic acid)

Endoscopic techniques

Thermal coagulation

Injection therapy

Mechanical (e.g. clips)

Laser

Arteriography

Surgery

reduced and survival improved by H₂-receptor blockade (Collins and Langman, 1985), a randomized placebo-controlled trial failed to show any influence of the H₂-receptor antagonist famotidine on the morbidity and mortality associated with bleeding from peptic ulcer (Walt et al., 1992). Proton pump inhibitors (e.g. omeprazole) are usually given to patients with bleeding ulcers in view of their longer-term benefits in ulcer healing when combined with *Helicobacter pylori* eradication therapy. High-dose (40 mg 12-hourly for 5 days) oral treatment or continuous intravenous infusion (8 mg/h for up to 72 hours following an 80-mg bolus dose) of omeprazole reduces the rate of further bleeding and the need for surgery, both when used alone (Khuroo et al., 1997) and in combination with therapeutic

endoscopy (Lau et al., 2000). A recent meta-analysis confirmed that treatment with a proton pump inhibitor reduces the risk of rebleeding and the requirement for surgery but does not influence overall mortality (Leontiadis et al., 2005). Neither antacids nor sucralfate have a place in the initial management of acute upper gastrointestinal haemorrhage.

Somatostatin is a potent inhibitor of gastric acid secretion and reduces splanchnic blood flow. Several randomized trials (Christiansen et al., 1989; Magnusson et al., 1985) and a meta-analysis (Imperiale and Bergisson, 1997) have evaluated the use of somatostatin in ulcer haemorrhage as either the natural hormone or the commercially available long-acting analogue *octreotide*. Overall there are few published data to support a clear role for somatostatin in the treatment of ulcer haemorrhage. Similarly, no trials have documented the efficacy of *vasopressin* or its analogues in ulcer haemorrhage.

The antifibrinolytic agent *tranexamic acid* decreased mortality in a randomized controlled trial, despite having no effect on the rates of rebleeding or surgery (Barer et al., 1983). A later study (von Holstein et al., 1987) and meta-analysis (Henry and O'Connell, 1989) concluded that this agent reduced the proportion of patients who required emergency surgery. There was a high rate of thrombophlebitic complications in those given tranexamic acid and, since the rate of recurrent bleeding was not significantly reduced, this agent is not currently widely used. Tranexamic acid is not approved for the treatment of bleeding ulcers in the UK.

Endoscopic techniques are preferred in the first instance to control bleeding and can be repeated in those with recurrent bleeding. The two most extensively studied endoscopic means of achieving haemostasis of bleeding ulcers are thermal coagulation and injection therapy (Chung et al., 1997). The former may be accomplished by monopolar, bipolar or multipolar electrocautery and by heater probe. Injection therapy is the simplest and least expensive means of achieving haemostasis. A variety of solutions, both scle-rosants and vasoactive agents, have been used to control haemorrhage by a combination of thrombosis, inflamma-tion and sclerosis (British Society of Gastroenterology Endoscopy Committee, 2002). There is little evidence that the addition of agents other than adrenaline reduces the rate of rebleeding. The injection of these agents may be compli-cated by necrosis of the injected tissue. Although laser therapy is effective, this technique can be complicated by transmural injury and therefore requires considerable tech-nical expertise. Mechanical methods such as suturing, clip-ping or stapling are generally less effective than thermal coagulation. Heater probe treatment after endoscopic adren-aline injection may be more effective in those with spurting haemorrhage.

As mentioned above, the single most important determi-nant of outcome in those with gastrointestinal haemorrhage originating from ulcer disease is whether bleeding persists or recurs (Branicki et al., 1990). Various randomized trials of endoscopic therapy for ulcer bleeding have concluded that outcome is indeed improved, largely through a reduction in the rate of recurrent bleeding but also because fewer patients need emergency surgery (Sacks et al., 1990). Fortunately the two major complications of endoscopic therapy (perforation and uncontrollable bleeding) are rare.

Surgery (Lau et al., *1999).* Surgical intervention has long been a mainstay of therapy for bleeding ulcers, although the precise indications for surgery, its timing and the relative merits of the various procedures remain controversial. Surgery is usually performed for continued or recurrent bleeding when endoscopic therapy has failed or is unavail-able. There is also no question that immediate operative intervention, with or without previous endoscopy, is the procedure of choice for exsanguinating haemorrhage. Con-versely, emergency surgery has little to offer in the manage-ment of ulcers that have been found endoscopically to have a low risk of rebleeding. Some suggested indications for surgical management of bleeding ulcers include:

- immediate surgery for exsanguinating haemorrhage;
- immediate surgery for those with active bleeding despite attempts at endoscopic haemostasis;
- early elective operation after initial endoscopic haemostasis for elderly patients with comorbidities and/or haemodynamic instability due to arterial ulcer haemorrhage;
- surgery is usually advised for elderly patients with comor-bidities and/or haemodynamic instability who have a visible vessel in an ulcer crater treated endoscopically, particularly for those with a positive arterial Doppler signal in the ulcer crater, a large posterior duodenal ulcer or a large high lesser curvature gastric ulcer;
- surgery is advised for elderly patients with comorbidities and/or haemodynamic instability who develop recurrent ulcer bleeding while hospitalized or who require a blood transfusion of 5 units or more.

For bleeding gastric ulcer most authors recommend gastric resection with or without vagotomy (Welch et al., 1986), although others have suggested that simple oversewing may be equally effective (McGuire and Horsley, 1986). Ligation of the artery, with undersewing of the ulcer, is currently the recommended operative treatment for bleeding duodenal ulcer.

Arteriography. This procedure has a limited though well-defined role in the management of massive bleeding in patients who are poor surgical risks and in whom endo-scopic therapy has failed or is unavailable. In such cases over 50% of bleeding ulcers can be controlled by embolization of the bleeding artery or by intra-arterial infusion of vasopres-sin. Procedural complications such as gastric necrosis, perforation, ischaemic stenosis or abscess formation can, however, be life-threatening (Lieberman et al., 1984).

Most deaths from peptic ulcer bleeding are now due to respiratory, cardiac or renal decompensation rather than exsanguinating haemorrhage. The goal of reducing the number of deaths from peptic ulcer bleeding may ultimately be achieved by improvements in supportive care and strate-gies to prevent initial bleeding, as well as by improving tech-niques for stopping the bleeding once it has started.

ACUTE GASTRIC EROSIONS (Durham and Shapiro, 1991)

Gastritis or multiple acute gastric erosions may cause bleeding:

- in patients who ingest substances that irritate the gastric mucosa, such as aspirin and other NSAIDs or alcohol;
- as a complication of critical illness – *stress ulceration* (see Chapter 11).

The incidence of stress-related gastric mucosal injury increased from the 1950s and through the 1970s, as did the recognition of this clinical entity. Initially it was considered to be a surgical disease occurring in patients with trauma, shock, abdominal sepsis, severe burns or central nervous system injury. It is now appreciated, however, that stress-induced injury to the gastric mucosa may also be seen in medical patients in the intensive care unit. The ageing popu-lation as well as the increasing number of critically ill patients with multiple-organ failure has led to an increase in the number of patients susceptible to stress-related gastric mucosal injury.

Pathogenesis. The presence of acid and pepsin in the stomach lumen are prerequisites for the development of stress ulceration. The major inciting events impair the mech-anisms that normally preserve the integrity of the gastric mucosa and may include:

- a reduction in mucosal blood flow;
- impaired production of gastric mucus;
- a decrease in the pH gradient from the gastric lumen to the intracellular space;
- a disturbed acid–base balance;

- a reduction in mucosal prostaglandins;
- impaired epithelial cell renewal.

Mucosal injury may be enhanced by:

- reflux of bile acids from the duodenum;
- uraemia.

Pathology. Initially there is submucosal haemorrhage, which results in gastric petechiae or areas of haemorrhagic gastritis. Microscopic erosions then develop followed by ulceration superficial to the submucosa. Multiple asymptomatic superficial lesions occur in the areas of functioning oxyntic gland mucosa (i.e. the fundus and midbody of the stomach). The lesions do not extend through the mucosa and bleeding arises from the superficial capillaries. There is no fibrous base or intense inflammatory reaction. This contrasts with peptic ulcer disease, in which the lesions are few in number, are more commonly located in non-acid-producing areas, penetrate deeply beneath the mucosa, are associated with chronic inflammatory changes and can cause massive bleeding from a large single vessel.

Clinical course. Intensive care patients have endoscopic evidence of gastric injury within 24–48 hours of admission. Approximately 20% of these patients will develop bleeding, which may be overt or occult, but in only 2–5% will this be clinically significant (Cook *et al.,* 1991). The ultimate prognosis depends upon correcting the underlying disease.

Prevention. Prevention is discussed in Chapter 11.

Management of acute haemorrhage from stress ulcers. Occasionally stress ulcers may give rise to life-threatening gastric bleeding. Following effective resuscitation, patients should undergo emergency endoscopy to define the source. Therapeutic endoscopy with coagulation probes is less helpful when there are multiple bleeding points. H$_2$-receptor blockers should be administered if not already prescribed; otherwise the addition of omeprazole may prove to be effective.

In cases of massive bleeding, *emergency arteriography* can be performed. *Selective embolization* of the left gastric artery may then control the bleeding. Alternatively an *intra-arterial infusion of vasopressin* for 48–72 hours at a dosage of 0.2–0.4 units/min has been used.

Surgery plays a limited role because of the diffuse nature of the bleeding. Furthermore, there is no consensus as to which operation should be performed. Vagotomy and pyloroplasty and subtotal and total gastrectomy are all associated with a high mortality and rebleeding is common except when a total gastrectomy is performed.

GASTROINTESTINAL HAEMORRHAGE FROM OESOPHAGEAL VARICES (Garcia-Tsao, 2001; Sharara and Rockey, 2001)

Approximately 90% of patients with cirrhosis will develop oesophageal varices over a 10-year period, but only about one-third will be complicated by variceal haemorrhage.

The presentation of patients with bleeding varices is often not substantially different from that of patients with upper gastrointestinal haemorrhage of other aetiologies. Sometimes, however, variceal haemorrhage is characterized by its *sudden onset* and *massive quantity* in the *absence of upper abdominal pain.* Occasionally, *painless melaena* for several days may be the only sign.

On physical examination, signs of chronic liver disease and/or portal hypertension may be present, but do not of course confirm the diagnosis of variceal bleeding. Endoscopic studies have demonstrated that, even in those with documented varices, bleeding may be from other sources in a significant proportion of cases (e.g. gastric ulceration). *Portal hypertensive (or congestive) gastropathy* (a term used for the chronic gastric congestion, punctate erythema and gastric erosions sometimes seen at endoscopy) may in some cases prove to be the source of bleeding.

The general approach to managing a patient with variceal bleeding differs little from that described above, although it is important to note that these patients may have disorders of acid–base balance, coagulation, blood glucose levels, fluid status and conscious level as a result of associated liver disease (see Chapter 14). The management of variceal haemorrhage involves primary prophylaxis (by non-selective beta-blockade with the aim of decreasing the hepatic venous pressure gradient), management of acute variceal haemorrhage and secondary prophylaxis (banding and beta-blockers). Urgent endoscopy should be performed to confirm the diagnosis of varices and exclude bleeding from other sites.

According to the current UK guidelines, specific medical therapy (**Table 16.4**) for variceal haemorrhage may include (Jalan and Hayes, 2000):

- vasopressin analogues, e.g. terlipressin;
- somatostatin analogues, e.g. octreotide;
- endoscopic therapy;
- balloon tamponade;
- invasive radiological procedures, including transjugular intrahepatic portosystemic shunting (TIPS);
- surgery.

Pharmacotherapy is aimed at lowering intravariceal pressure by reducing portal venous pressure and blood flow. *Vasopressin* lowers portal venous pressure by causing splanchnic arteriolar constriction. Significant complications of vasopressin can occur at any dose and this agent is now rarely used, even in combination with a nitrate. Common side-effects include abdominal colic, defecation, facial pallor, bradycardia and hypertension. Vasopressin in high doses also reduces coronary blood flow and cardiac output and should not be used in patients with ischaemic heart disease. *Terlipressin,* a derivative of vasopressin, appears to be more effective and has a lower complication rate. Terlipressin is administered by intravenous injection of 2 mg followed by 1 or 2 mg every 4–6 hours for the first 24 hours, then 1 mg every 4 hours. A recent study comparing terlipressin and

Table 16.4 Management of variceal bleeding

Active variceal bleeding

Resuscitation

Pharmacological therapy (vasopressin or somatostatin analogues)

Endoscopic band ligation or sclerotherapy

If bleeding continues

Repeat banding or sclerotherapy

Consider balloon tamponade

Consider transjugular intrahepatic portosystemic shunting (TIPS)

Consider oesophageal transection

Long-term obliteration of oesophageal varices

Endoscopic band ligation or sclerotherapy

β-blockade

Recurrent variceal bleeding

TIPS

Consider portosystemic shunt

Consider transplantation

Gastric varices

Attempt endoscopic therapy

TIPS

Portosystemic shunt

---

endoscopic therapy in patients with oesophageal varices showed the two methods to be equally effective, both in controlling bleeding and in terms of outcome (Escorsell et al., 2000).

Somatostatin. Somatostatin and its synthetic analogues octreotide and vapreotide decrease both splanchnic blood flow and gastric acid secretion, but have few side-effects. These agents have been used for bleeding from variceal (Kravetz et al., 1984) and non-variceal sources (Magnusson et al., 1985) and are as effective as vasopressin (Feu et al., 1996) or sclerotherapy (Jenkins et al., 1997) for controlling the initial variceal bleed. They can also be used in conjunction with sclerotherapy or band ligation therapy (Cales et al., 2001). Octreotide is usually administered as an infusion of 25–50 µg/h (unlicensed indication).

Endoscopic sclerosis. This involves injecting the varices with a sclerosing agent (e.g. ethanolamine) through a flexible endoscope. Complications include:

- oesophageal motility disturbances;
- oesophageal ulceration;
- oesophageal stenosis;
- oesophageal perforation;
- decreased lower oesophageal sphincter pressures.

Bleeding gastric varices are more difficult to treat than oesophageal varices and depending on their position sclerotherapy, cyanoacrylate (tissue glue) and thrombin injections have been used.

Endoscopic oesophageal variceal banding, a technique first reported in 1990 (Goff, 1990), has largely superseded sclerotherapy. A prospective randomized controlled comparision of oesophageal variceal banding and emergency injection sclerotherapy showed that the two treatments were equally effective in controlling variceal bleeding but that ligation was associated with fewer treatment-related complications and a lower mortality (Stiegmann et al., 1992). It is recommended that patients who continue to bleed despite repeat attempts at endoscopic therapy should have their variceal haemorrhage temporarily controlled by balloon tamponade and then be considered for a shunt procedure or operative oesophageal transection. Endoscopic therapy is less successful when bleeding arises from gastric varices.

Balloon tamponade. This is indicated when drug or endoscopic therapy has failed or is contraindicated or if there is exsanguinating haemorrhage. A variety of balloons are available, including the Sengstaken–Blakemore tube, which incorporates a 300-mL gastric balloon, a 45–60 mL oesophageal balloon and gastric aspiration ports. The Patten–Johnson (Minnesota) quadruple tube is a modification of the Sengstaken–Blakemore tube and has an additional port for suctioning the secretions that usually accumulate above the oesophageal balloon.

Balloon tamponade should only be used in an intensive care unit; the majority of patients require tracheal intubation to prevent aspiration of secretions and many also require mechanical ventilation. Complications of balloon tamponade include *oesophageal ulceration* or *rupture* and *pulmonary aspiration* (Pitcher, 1971). The danger of rupture and/or ulceration can be minimized by carefully monitoring the balloon position and pressure, endeavouring to control bleeding with the gastric balloon only and limiting the duration of its use to 12 hours.

Although balloon tamponade has been reported to be effective in controlling haemorrhage in the majority of patients, rebleeding is unfortunately common. Balloon tamponade, like pharmacotherapy, is usually only a temporary measure until definitive treatment can be undertaken.

Invasive radiological procedures. In the past portosystemic shunting could only be achieved by major surgery. TIPS is a non-operative interventional radiological technique that has proved to be useful in those with persistent bleeding. A catheter is passed into the hepatic vein via the jugular vein and a tract is opened into a major portal branch with a rigid needle followed by a guidewire. The tract is dilated and patency is maintained by an expandable metal stent (Ring *et al.*, 1992). TIPS has been useful in the short-term control of refractory variceal haemorrhage, especially in poor-risk patients. In the longer term, portal hypertension may recur owing to shunt stenosis or thrombosis. TIPS has not yet been conclusively shown to alter mortality rates.

Surgical procedures. Surgical procedures such as variceal ligation (e.g. transoesophageal stapling) or emergency decompressive procedures (e.g. portocaval shunting) can also effectively control variceal bleeding.

Regardless of the specific treatment used to control haemorrhage, hepatic encephalopathy secondary to the increased intestinal protein load is common in patients with compromised liver function (see Chapter 14).

In addition *prophylactic antibiotic therapy* (e.g. ciprofloxacin 500 mg b.d. for 7 days) should be given to patients with cirrhosis and active variceal bleeding (Jalan and Hayes, 2000). Sucralfate 1 g q.d.s. can be given to reduce oesophageal ulceration following endoscopic therapy. Prevention of later recurrent variceal bleeding may be achieved by non-selective beta-blockade (Lo *et al.*, 2000). This appears to be as effective as sclerotherapy (Villanueva *et al.*, 1996) and ligation (Villanueva *et al.*, 2001) as it also prevents bleeding from portal hypertensive gastropathy. Preventive strategies which employ a combination of methods are likely to gain in popularity.

The *prognosis* depends largely on the severity of the underlying liver disease, with an overall mortality of around 25%.

LOWER GASTROINTESTINAL HAEMORRHAGE

Lower gastrointestinal bleeding accounts for only 20% of all episodes of acute gastrointestinal bleeding. Massive bleeding from the lower gastrointestinal tract is rare.

Causes

Lower gastrointestinal haemorrhage is most common in the elderly (Boley *et al.*, 1981). Causes include:

- colorectal carcinoma;
- colonic polyps;
- colonic ischaemia;
- inflammatory bowel disease;
- diverticular disease;
- colonic vascular ectasias (angiodysplasia).

Diverticular bleeding is arterial and thought to be due to erosion of an arteriole at the base of a single diverticulum by a faecolith. *Vascular ectasias* are degenerative lesions associated with ageing. It is believed that they result from repeated partial low-grade obstruction of the colonic sub-mucosal veins, especially where they pierce the muscular layer of the colon. The obstruction causes dilatation and tortuosity of the vein and subsequently of the arteriocapillary–venular unit, with the development of a small arteriovenous communication. Bleeding from vascular ectasias is characteristically recurrent and may stop spontaneously.

Clinical presentation

Both the rate and the pattern of bleeding depend on the underlying cause. Bleeding from diverticulosis, for example, is usually acute and severe and in most patients occurs without preceding symptoms. On the other hand, approximately one-quarter of patients with ectatic bleeding have had previous melaena or anaemia due to blood loss.

Investigations

Every patient should undergo immediate *nasogastric aspiration* to exclude upper gastrointestinal haemorrhage. The most suitable investigation for a patient with suspected lower gastrointestinal haemorrhage is usually dictated by the rate of bleeding. *Massive* bleeding may preclude any direct examination other than rectal examination, proctoscopy and *rigid sigmoidoscopy*. If large quantities of blood are originating from a source above the sigmoidoscope, *angiography* should be considered to localize the site of bleeding. The value of angiography is not, however, confined to those with massive haemorrhage since it is capable of detecting active bleeding at rates as low as 0.5–1.0 mL/min. Selective angiography can be performed not only for diagnostic purposes, but also therapeutically. Vasoconstrictors such as vasopressin may be administered intra-arterially at the time of angiography, and bleeding vessels can be selectively embolized with autologous clot, gelfoam emboli or metal spring coils. *Barium examinations* should not be performed before angiography as this may mask the angiographic findings.

When acute bleeding is less severe, *colonoscopy* after bowel preparation by lavage (Gostout, 2000) can be performed after sigmoidoscopy. The advantage of colonoscopy under these circumstances is that individual lesions such as angiodysplasia or a bleeding diverticulum can often be identified and treated. Even if a specific lesion cannot be seen, the general area of bleeding can frequently be ascertained. Furthermore, it may be possible to control the bleeding with injection (adrenaline, sclerosant), cautery, laser coagulation or polypectomy. Endoscopes to visualize the small bowel (enteroscopy) are now available at specialist centres and may be useful in the assessment of patients who have unexplained recurrent bleeding (Gostout, 2000).

In patients with intermittent or small-volume bleeding, angiography may be negative and in such cases *administration of an intravascular tracer* such as [99m]technetium (Tc)-labelled red blood cells has been recommended. With the gastrointestinal scintiscan the patient can then be monitored for gastrointestinal bleeding after a single injection (Markisz *et al.*, 1982). In some institutions this examination is used in preference to arteriography in those with lower gastrointestinal bleeding.

Management *(Table 16.5)*

Patients with lower gastrointestinal haemorrhage should initially be managed and resuscitated as outlined earlier.

Table 16.5 Management of lower gastrointestinal haemorrhage

Investigations

Nasogastric aspiration (to exclude upper gastrointestinal haemorrhage)

Rectal examination and proctoscopy

Rigid sigmoidoscopy

Colonoscopy

Barium enema

Angiography

Administration of an intravascular tracer

Treatment

Selective angiography
  Vasopressin
  Embolization

Colonoscopy
  Injection (sclerosant, adrenaline)
  Cautery
  Laser coagulation
  Polypectomy

Surgery

DIVERTICULAR HAEMORRHAGE

Despite the large number of diverticula often found in the left or sigmoid colon, the source of bleeding is most frequently a single diverticulum in the right colon. Although diverticular haemorrhage is often severe, bleeding either stops spontaneously or is controlled with medical therapy in over three-quarters of patients. Conventional endoscopic therapy by means of injection, coagulation or both for the control of bleeding from a visible vessel may prevent recurrent bleeding and decrease the need for surgery (Jensen et al., 2000). As a consequence a low proportion of patients with diverticular bleeding require operative treatment and only rarely is emergency intervention indicated.

BLEEDING FROM VASCULAR ECTASIAS

Similarly, bleeding from vascular ectasias is characteristically recurrent and may stop spontaneously. Otherwise patients may require colonoscopy and coagulation biopsy (Howard et al., 1982). Bleeding that fails to stop with general measures may respond to an intra-arterial infusion of vasopressin following angiographic diagnosis. Patients whose bleeding continues or recurs are candidates for either segmental colectomy or hemicolectomy.

ABDOMINAL EMERGENCIES

ABDOMINAL EMERGENCIES ARISING IN HOSPITAL

The clinical features, management and prognosis of abdominal crises developing *de novo* in an inpatient are distinctly different from those of the acute abdomen typically seen in the emergency department. It is also important to appreciate that, despite their differing aetiologies and anatomy, all major gastrointestinal emergencies may be complicated by the development of endotoxaemia/bacteraemia and peritonitis. Subsequent deterioration may then be related to dissemination of the inflammatory response and, in the most severe cases, progression to multiple-organ dysfunction (see Chapter 5). Since many of these conditions are amenable to surgery, the prompt advice of an experienced surgeon is essential. Surgical delay has long been recognized as an important predictor of mortality and the crucial role of timely surgical evaluation and intervention in treating the acute abdomen in intensive care patients has recently been re-emphasized (Gajic et al., 2002).

Causes

Patients recovering from major abdominal, orthopaedic, cardiovascular or thoracic procedures may develop intra-abdominal catastrophes either primarily or secondary to specific surgical complications. *Perforated peptic ulcer, diverticulitis, appendicitis and acalculous cholecystitis* can all complicate extensive surgery, while *pancreatitis* can be precipitated by any intra-abdominal procedure, but most often complicates renal transplantation, cardiopulmonary bypass or endoscopic retrograde cholangiopancreatography (ERCP). Patients may also develop a perforated viscus as a complication of a procedure (e.g. colonoscopy, gastroscopy). *Intestinal or colonic ileus* can occur after spinal fractures, trauma, burns or myocardial infarction, and may also be caused by sepsis, metabolic disturbances or medications (especially opiates). Mural thrombosis complicating cardiac arrhythmias or recent myocardial infarction may embolize to the mesenteric vessels, causing *acute ischaemia and bowel infarction*. Low cardiac output states such as congestive heart failure, myocardial infarction, hypovolaemia and arrhythmias can also produce *bowel ischaemia* (see Chapter 5).

Clinical presentation and diagnosis

It is important to enquire about all medications, as well as to obtain a history of all previous medical conditions and surgical procedures. Absence of typical clinical findings because of altered mental state, medications, immunosuppression or underlying disease is now recognized as a reason for delays in surgical intervention (Gajic et al., 2002). Often a change in vital signs such as an increased pulse rate or the development of metabolic acidosis may be the only indication of an intra-abdominal problem. Vague abdominal discomfort, distension, loss of appetite and oliguria are important indications that all is not well. Bowel obstruction, ileus and gastric dilatation may not be accompanied by vomiting in an unconscious, sedated and ventilated patient in whom the only signs may be frequent small episodes of regurgitation or failure to absorb enteral feed.

On physical examination such a patient may not grimace on palpation and peritonitis may be masked by a flaccid distended abdominal wall. Radiological and laboratory investigations are essential to avoid missing a treatable abdominal catastrophe. The computed tomography (CT) scan has higher sensitivity for the detection of free air compared with plain radiographs but may lack specificity with regard to other findings (bowel wall thickening, ileus, ascites) (Jacobs and Birnbaum, 1997). Abdominal ultrasound may be more sensitive than CT scanning in the diagnosis of gallbladder disease.

INTRA-ABDOMINAL SEPSIS

The commonest causes of intra-abdominal sepsis are:

- leaking enteric suture lines;
- bowel perforation, e.g. benign and malignant ulcers;
- infected haematoma;
- incomplete eradication of septic foci, e.g. pelvic inflammatory disease, Crohn's disease and ulcerative colitis, diverticulitis, pancreatitis.

Clinical presentation

Most commonly patients present with abdominal distension, pain and tenderness with pyrexia. The clinical diagnosis can, however, be difficult, especially in postoperative patients. The clinical assessment of critically ill patients by surgeons and intensivists requires a high index of suspicion based on the history and clinical findings, supplemented by appropriate investigations.

Investigations

Routine investigations should include white cell count, C-reactive protein, microbiology and assessment of acid–base status (see Chapter 5). Imaging techniques can be classified into those that detect anatomical abnormalities, such as CT or ultrasound scanning, and radionuclide methods such as isotopic uptake scans which detect areas of inflammation.

ULTRASOUND

Ultrasound is the technique of choice for investigating the perihepatic region, whereas CT scanning is preferred for imaging the retroperitoneum. Ultrasound has the advantage of being rapid and portable. Real-time imaging allows monitoring of diaphragmatic movement and, provided the patient has a full bladder, it is also possible to detect collections in the pouch of Douglas and rectovesical pouch. The major disadvantages of ultrasound in postoperative patients relate to the restricted access due to abdominal wounds and drains, together with interference from air-filled bowel loops accompanying postoperative ileus.

CT SCANNING

If there is a high index of suspicion and ultrasound is equivocal, a CT scan should be performed. CT scanning is also regarded as the technique of choice for imaging the pancreas, particularly when combined with oral and intravenous contrast media (see below). The main disadvantage of CT scanning is the need to transport the patient to the radiology department.

RADIONUCLIDE SCANNING

Among the nuclear medicine techniques radiolabelled leukocyte scanning is the most commonly used method for detecting sepsis and inflammation. Technetium-99m-labelled white cell imaging can be sensitive and specific for abdominal sepsis (and inflammatory bowel disease) within a few hours following injection, although a disadvantage is that the patient must be transferred to the nuclear medicine department.

MAGNETIC RESONANCE IMAGING (MRI)

MRI provides high-quality images of soft-tissue inflammation (e.g. retroperitoneal space) but again an important limitation is that the patient has to be transported to the radiology department. Moreover, monitoring devices and medical equipment within the field of the scan have to be of a non-magnetic material.

Management

Treatment of the septic abdomen involves antibiotic therapy together with eradication of the source of infection and debridement of necrotic tissue in an attempt to prevent recurrent sepsis. Patients usually also require multiple-organ support, including enteral or parenteral nutrition.

ERADICATION OF SEPSIS

Source control and drainage can be accomplished surgically, percutaneously or endoscopically. Although percutaneous drainage is appropriate for subphrenic or pelvic unilocular collections, multilocular, inaccessible retroperitoneal collections and those associated with fistulae require more definitive measures to prevent recurrence of sepsis. Relaparotomy with laparostomy, where the whole abdomen is left open and treated as an abscess cavity, is now frequently undertaken when sepsis has recurred following conventional surgical drainage and when the abscesses are too extensive or their contents too thick, for drainage by interventional radiology or conventional surgical procedures. This approach also prevents the development of the abdominal compartment syndrome (ACS).

Prognosis

Multiple-organ failure accompanying intra-abdominal sepsis has a poor prognosis.

ABDOMINAL COMPARTMENT SYNDROME
(Moore et al., 2004)

ACS can be defined as an abnormally high intra-abdominal pressure (IAP) with associated organ dysfunction (Meldrum et al., 1997) and occurs when there is a discrepancy between the volume of the abdominal cavity and its contents. Although the abdominal wall is not a rigid structure, compliance decreases with increasing distension so that eventually small changes in volume will cause large increases in

Table 16.6 Common causes of increased intra-abdominal pressure

Abdominal trauma
    Use of abdominal packs
    Postresuscitation visceral oedema
    Pelvic or retroperitoneal bleeding
    Intraperitoneal bleeding

Tense ascites
Liver transplantation
Postoperative intra-abdominal haemorrhage
Acute pancreatitis
Ileus
Intestinal obstruction
Laparoscopy with pneumoperitoneum
Ruptured abdominal aortic aneurysm

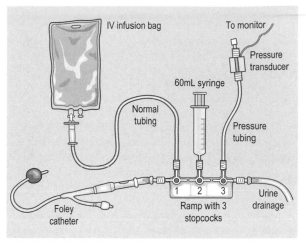

Fig. 16.1 A system for determining intravesical pressure.

pressure. Perfusion of abdominal organs is impaired as occurs in other well-recognized compartment syndromes such as increased intracranial pressure, pericardial tamponade, tension pneumothorax and those involving the extremities. Blood flow to the abdominal wall may also be compromised.

Causes and consequences (Table 16.6)

Primary ACS is a recognized complication of laparotomy. Retained abdominal packs, ongoing bleeding, progressive oedema of reperfused bowel, ileus and gaseous distension all contribute to increased abdominal content.

Secondary ACS occurs in the setting of severe haemorrhage. The abdominal content may be increased in volume by bowel oedema and ascites. Alternatively the volume of the abdominal cavity may be decreased by space-occupying haematomas, e.g. retroperitoneal blood originating from pelvic fractures.

The consequences of increased IAP include:

- decreased venous return due to compression of the inferior vena cava and portal vein, combined with increased intrathoracic pressure, an increased afterload and cardiac compression, lead to a reduction in cardiac output;
- increased cardiac filling pressures;
- decreased thoracic volume and compliance and increased work of breathing;
- compression atelectasis;
- pulmonary hypertension;
- oliguria despite aggressive fluid resuscitation. Mechanisms responsible for the impairment of renal function include direct compression of the renal parenchyma, as well as decreased renal perfusion as a consequence of reduced cardiac output and compression of renal veins, perhaps exacerbated by raised circulating levels of renin, antidiuretic hormones and aldosterone. Ureteric com-

pression is not considered to be an important mechanism;
- impaired splanchnic function is a consequence of the reduction in cardiac output and increased splanchnic vascular resistance;
- increased intracranial pressure and consequently decreased cerebral blood flow;
- predisposition to thromboembolic disease.

ACS may be preventable if primary fascial closure after damage control laparotomy is avoided by using a prosthetic mesh closure, laparostomy or vacuum-assisted technique (see below).

Epidemiology

Since the definition of ACS has not been standardized the incidence is not easily determined. The development of ACS is, however, a predictor of both multiple organ dysfunction and mortality.

Measurement of IAP

Clinical examination is an insensitive means of detecting raised IAP, especially in the early stages (Malbrain, 2004). IAP can be measured by filling the urinary bladder with 50 mL normal saline through a previously drained and clamped standard urinary catheter (Kron *et al.*, 1984). A transducer is connected to the urethral catheter and measurements are taken relative to the level of the symphysis pubis. Alternatively a new disposable modified urinary collection system connected to the urinary catheter can act as a precalibrated manometer, thereby enabling the determination of intravesical pressure (**Fig. 16.1**). Other less popular techniques for determining IAP include transgastric pressure measurement via a nasogastric tube, measurement of venous pressure via the femoral vein and rectal pressure measurement (Malbrain, 2004). It has been suggested that IAP should be measured every 8 hours in patients at risk.

Management

Early recognition and treatment are essential since prolonged ACS may not be completely reversible by decompression and untreated ACS is fatal. There is some debate as to the level of IAP that should be considered abnormal in humans but a value above 20 mmHg is nearly always significant. The normal value for IAP ranges from around 0 to 16 mmHg with a mean value of about 6 mmHg. An IAP above 18 mmHg is important in most cases, a level above 15 mmHg is often significant and organ dysfunction may even occur when IAP is in the region of 12 mmHg (Moore *et al.*, 2004).

The timing of surgical intervention can also be difficult. Some suggest intervening when IAP exceeds 25 or 26 mmHg, whereas others suggest a threshold of 20 mmHg when there is associated oliguria, high inflation pressures and a reduced oxygen delivery.

ACS can be prevented by leaving the abdomen open at laparotomy and can be treated by abdominal decompression by laparotomy and laparostomy. Both approaches clearly require management with an open abdomen, which may in itself be associated with significant morbidity and mortality. Following intestinal cover with a Bogota bag (a transparent, impervious sheet) healing by secondary intention or delayed fascial closure may still leave large fascial defects necessitating repeated plastic surgical interventions. In this regard a vacuum-assisted wound closure system has been developed to assist with fascial closure (Garner *et al.*, 2001). Abdominal coverage may also be achieved with a mesh, cut to size and sutured to the wound edges, enabling slow plication as abdominal distension resolves. Various forms of mesh are available; some are absorbable whilst others incorporate a 'zipper' for repeat laparotomy.

Decompression may precipitate haemodynamic instability, sudden respiratory alkalosis, hyperkalaemia, bleeding, cardiac arrhythmias or asystolic cardiac arrest. It is important to appreciate that laparostomy may be followed by extremely large fluid losses.

Prognosis

Although more than 80% of patients respond to abdominal decompression with a dramatic improvement in organ function, only around 50% survive.

GASTRODUODENAL EMERGENCIES
Perforated ulcer
CLINICAL FEATURES

Perforation of a duodenal ulcer is a common cause of *sudden, severe abdominal pain*. In the majority of patients there will be no history of previous symptoms compatible with peptic ulcer disease. Perforation may occur at any age, but the peak incidence is between the ages of 20 and 40 years. Patients in whom perforation complicates treatment with steroids or NSAIDs are usually older and may present with minimal symptoms and signs.

A patient with a perforated ulcer will *lie still* and take *shallow breaths* to avoid exacerbating abdominal pain.

The abdomen is *board-like* on palpation, although older patients and those on steroids may not exhibit peritonism. *Liver dullness may be lost* because of free air between the liver and the chest wall. *Bowel sounds will be absent* after a few hours.

DIAGNOSIS

The most important investigation is an *erect plain chest radiograph* and an upright or left lateral *decubitus view of the abdomen*; in the majority of cases this will demonstrate free air within the abdominal cavity. In about one-third of cases, however, no free air is seen on plain X-ray and a *CT scan* will be required to confirm the diagnosis.

MANAGEMENT

A perforated peptic ulcer is a surgical emergency and demands immediate attention. A *nasogastric tube* should be inserted; *antibiotics, fluid resuscitation* and *surgery* are indicated. In the presence of concurrent medical illness, sepsis or perforation existing for more than 48 hours, a simple closure is the most prudent course. In stable patients with pre-existing ulcer disease proximal to the duodenum, resection of ulcers and vagotomy are generally preferred.

INTESTINAL EMERGENCIES
Small-bowel obstruction
CLINICAL FEATURES

The diagnosis of small-bowel obstruction is suggested by:

- cramping abdominal pain;
- vomiting;
- constipation;
- varying degrees of abdominal distension.

Physical examination may also yield clues to the aetiology of bowel obstruction. In adults, the most common causes are:

- adhesions from previous surgery;
- herniation;
- volvulus;
- intussusception;
- Crohn's disease;
- malignancy.

INVESTIGATIONS

The confirmatory diagnostic investigations are plain and decubitus *abdominal radiographs. Contrast studies with barium* are only performed to distinguish mechanical obstruction from paralytic ileus and partial from complete bowel obstruction and in those patients in whom therapy will be changed if the cause is known (e.g. Crohn's disease, irradiation enteritis or extrinsic pressure from abscesses). Abdominal *CT scanning* can provide information about the presence, site, severity and cause of the obstruction.

MANAGEMENT

Initial management should consist of *intravenous fluids, correction of electrolyte disturbances* and *gastric decompression*. Controversy exists as to whether decompression is best performed by a long intestinal tube or nasogastric tube. Most surgeons prefer a nasogastric tube.

Indications for *surgery* in a patient with small-bowel obstruction are dependent on the cause and degree of obstruction (partial or complete) but include:

- persistent abdominal tenderness;
- pain after decompression;
- failure to improve clinically 12–24 hours after successful decompression;
- the presence of tachycardia and fever.

A longer period of decompression and observation may be indicated in patients recovering from surgery since under these circumstances it is frequently difficult to differentiate bowel obstruction from prolonged ileus.

Acute mesenteric ischaemia and infarction
(Brands and Boley, 2000)
CAUSES

Transmural ischaemia following acute occlusion of the superior mesenteric artery is usually due to an *embolus* originating from the heart. The superior mesenteric artery is more susceptible to embolism than the inferior because of its larger lumen and more direct origin from the aorta. Partial intestinal ischaemia may also be related to *low cardiac output, spontaneous thrombosis* or *systemic embolism. Mesenteric venous thrombosis* may be idiopathic or may evolve as a result of an intra-abdominal catastrophe such as appendicitis, diverticulitis, abscess or pancreatitis. It may also complicate hypercoagulable states such as polycythaemia rubra vera and the use of oral contraceptives.

CLINICAL FEATURES

Small- and large-bowel embolism cause *severe pain* that is unrelieved by narcotics and is out of proportion to the physical findings. More peripheral emboli cause less severe pain and their presence may not be detected until there are peritoneal signs of infarction intolerance to enteral feeding or vital signs deteriorate. Ischaemia due to low cardiac output may be precipitated by congestive heart failure, cardiac arrhythmias, acute myocardial infarction and severe hypovolaemia, while sepsis/septic shock may be associated with mucosal hypoxia despite a high cardiac output (see Chapter 5).

INVESTIGATIONS

There may be a profound metabolic acidosis associated with leukocytosis and raised lactate dehydrogenase (LDH) and lactate concentrations. *Plain X-ray films of the abdomen* should be obtained to exclude other identifiable causes of abdominal pain such as perforated ulcer. *Abdominal CT scanning* with or without contrast enhancement may be undertaken, although sometimes an abdominal tap in a patient who is suspected of having necrotic bowel produces foul-smelling blood-stained fluid and therefore hastens surgery. In a few cases angiography performed as soon as possible after the onset of abdominal pain may allow various therapeutic approaches, including the infusion of vasodilators or thrombolytics, or surgery. *Echocardiography* should also be performed in selected cases to exclude mural thrombi.

MANAGEMENT

Following effective resuscitation and administration of *antibiotics*, gangrenous bowel must be *resected*. In some cases when large segments of intestine are involved and its viability is questionable the patient may be re-explored 24 hours later, by which time demarcation may be more obvious. Treatment in the meantime is directed towards correcting the primary cause, except if there is extensive infarction or the prognosis of the underlying disease is hopeless, when continued aggressive therapy may be inappropriate.

PROGNOSIS

Mortality may approach 90%, but can be decreased by early diagnosis.

Acute colonic ischaemia (Brands and Boley, 2000)

Colonic ischaemia is the most common form of intestinal ischaemia.

CAUSES

Ischaemic colitis may follow surgical procedures, e.g. cardiac surgery, but can also present *de novo*. Primary colonic ischaemia due to vascular disease usually affects the splenic flexure where the collateral circulation is most precarious. Embolic ischaemic colitis is unusual (see earlier). Interruption of the inferior mesenteric artery and its collateral vessels may follow abdominal aortic aneurysmectomy or resection of the left hemicolon. An increasing number of young people are being identified in whom colonic ischaemia is associated with long distance running, cocaine use or infections (e.g. *Escherichia coli*) and coagulopathies.

CLINICAL FEATURES AND DIAGNOSIS

Clinical features include *abdominal distension, burgundy-coloured stools* and *tenesmus*. Although in some cases the condition is self-limiting, in others ischaemia may progress to necrosis with *peritonitis, fever, leukocytosis, sepsis, shock, raised blood lactate* with *metabolic acidosis* or *lower intestinal bleeding*. In the early stages a plain radiograph of the abdomen may show 'thumbprinting' of the oedematous mucosa. *Proctoscopy* or *colonoscopy* may confirm oedematous, dusky, necrotic mucosa. *Abdominal CT scanning* or *mesenteric angiography* may also be undertaken in selected cases to exclude acute mesenteric ischaemia.

MANAGEMENT

Although in some instances management can be expectant with *bowel rest* and *antibiotics, resection* of the affected area and proximal colostomy/ileostomy are essential if the patient demonstrates peritonism. The most seriously ill patients may present with septic shock as a consequence of faecal peritonitis; they will require fluid resuscitation and, usually, administration of inotropes/vasopressors perioperatively.

Colonic pseudo-obstruction *(Laine, 1999)*
CLINICAL FEATURES
In colonic pseudo-obstruction there is dilatation of the colon in the absence of a mechanical cause. Pseudo-obstruction may be seen following operations in the retroperitoneal area, as well as in debilitated medical patients and those with electrolyte imbalance. The diagnosis is suggested by extreme abdominal distension, which can be seen to involve the whole colon, including the rectum, on abdominal radiography. The greatest danger is perforation of the caecum, which is associated with significant mortality (Strodel and Brothers, 1989). A caecal diameter of 9 cm may be used as a threshold for diagnosis and perforation becomes a serious concern when the diameter exceeds 12 cm.

MANAGEMENT
If the colon is not greatly distended treatment should include:

- intestinal decompression by nasogastric tube, rectal tube or colonoscopy;
- discontinuation of narcotics and sedatives if possible;
- correction of metabolic imbalance and electrolyte disturbances.

If symptoms persist or worsen and if the colonic diameter increases or remains above around 12 cm, colonoscopy is generally performed. Although colonoscopic decompression reduces the diameter of the caecum in the majority of patients repeated colonoscopy may be required. Colonoscopy of unprepared bowel can be technically difficult and is not without risk of iatrogenic perforation. It has been suggested that following 24 hours of conservative measures neostigmine should be given, provided there are no contraindications, such as bradycardia. Neostigmine (2 mg intravenously over a period of 3–5 minutes) may speed the resolution of pseudo-obstruction and reduce the need for colonoscopy and surgery (Ponec *et al.*, 1999). Continuous intravenous administration of neostigmine (0.4–0.8 mg/h over 24 hours) may also be useful in critical illness-related colonic ileus (Van der Spoel *et al.*, 2001). Surgical decompression is generally recommended for patients with persistent or worsening colonic pseudo-obstruction despite colonoscopic decompression. If perforation has occurred, a *limited right hemicolectomy* with construction of an ileostomy and a mucous fistula is advised.

BILIARY TRACT EMERGENCIES
Acute acalculous cholecystitis *(Williamson, 1988)*
Detection of sepsis originating from the gallbladder (calculous or acalculous cholecystitis) is particularly difficult in critically ill patients who are sedated and unresponsive and often have multiple-organ dysfunction.

AETIOLOGY
A variety of factors have been implicated (Howard, 1981), including:

- burns;
- trauma;
- previous surgery;
- sepsis;
- shock;
- multiple transfusions;
- prolonged ventilation;
- opiate sedation;
- long-term parenteral nutrition.

Biliary sludge is commonly found in these patients and is composed of calcium bilirubinate with an increased proportion of unconjugated bilirubin. The precise role of sludge in the development of acalculous cholecystitis is, however, unclear.

PATHOGENESIS
A combination of the above factors may lead to *ischaemia* and *necrosis of the gallbladder mucosa*, which may then become secondarily infected.

CLINICAL PRESENTATION
Clinical and laboratory features are similar to those of calculous cholecystitis and include:

- fever and rigors;
- pain;
- vomiting;
- tender right upper quadrant mass on abdominal examination;
- a raised white cell count;
- elevated bilirubin;
- raised alkaline phosphatase.

INVESTIGATIONS
Ultrasound scanning and *cholescintigraphy* are widely used in the diagnosis of cholecystitis. Ultrasound findings of diagnostic significance in acalculous cholecystitis include:

- thickening of the gallbladder wall to 5 mm or more (in the absence of hypoalbuminaemia);
- transverse gallbladder diameter of 5 cm or more;
- a sonolucent layer within the gallbladder wall;
- sediment or sludge within the gallbladder lumen;
- pericholecystic fluid collections.

TREATMENT
In addition to antibiotic therapy *open cholecystectomy* or *cholecystostomy* may be performed, although *percutaneous cholecystostomy* is less invasive, and may be useful in critically ill patients (Lee *et al.*, 1991).

ACUTE PANCREATITIS
The incidence of acute pancreatitis appears to be increasing, perhaps in part as a consequence of more accurate diagnosis and greater awareness, but probably also due to an increase

in the prevalence of risk factors such as excessive alcohol consumption. The quoted incidence varies widely from 5.4 to 79.8 per 100 000 of the population per annum. (Glazer and Mann, 1998; Kingsnorth and O'Reilly, 2006; Nathens *et al.*, 2004; Swaroop *et al.*, 2004; Whitcomb, 2006).

Causes

The most common associated aetiological factor is *gallstones*, although most patients with cholelithiasis never develop evidence of pancreatitis. *Alcohol*, the other major associated factor, causes predominantly chronic damage to the pancreas but has also been implicated in the increasing number of hospital admissions for acute pancreatitis (Goldacre and Roberts, 2004). At least 30 other causes of pancreatitis have been identified, encompassing an array of anatomical and metabolic abnormalities, drugs, toxins and infections. These include hypercalcaemia, hypertriglyceraemia, hypothermia, pancreatic tumour, trauma, viral infection (including human immunodeficiency virus (HIV)), drugs (e.g. thiazides), ERCP and pancreas divisum. The substantial number of cases labelled as '*idiopathic*' (around 20%) serves to emphasize the lack of understanding of the causes of this disease.

Pathogenesis *(Barry, 1988)*

Pancreatitis is believed to be due to *autodigestion* by activated enzymes within the gland. In particular there is inappropriate activation of trypsinogen to trypsin and a failure to eliminate active trypsin from within pancreatic tissue. *Duodenopancreatic reflux* may be a common factor underlying many of the aetiological associations since duodenal contents contain enzymes capable of activating proenzymes in the pancreas. They would normally also contain bacteria, raising the possibility that pancreatic infection is a triggering event.

The factors that determine whether a given attack will be mild or severe are also incompletely understood. Clinical and experimental evidence suggests that the degree of protease activation early in the course of the disease is a key factor in determining the outcome. In severe cases dissemination of the inflammatory response is associated with the development of systemic inflammation, sepsis (when complicated by infection) and multiple-organ failure (see Chapter 5).

Clinical features

Patients with pancreatitis frequently describe *abdominal pain* that is central, radiates to the back and is eased by sitting forward. Typically the pain increases in severity over a few hours before reaching a plateau that may last for several days. In gallstone pancreatitis, the pain may be sudden, epigastric and 'knife-like'. *Nausea and vomiting* are invariable accompaniments to the pain. There may be a history of heavy alcohol intake. It is important to take a detailed drug history.

On examination the patient is usually agitated with *epigastric tenderness*. In some cases there may be signs of generalized peritonitis. Pleural effusions may be suspected from examination of the chest. Retroperitoneal haemorrhage is evidenced by a blue-grey discoloration in the flanks (*Grey Turner's sign*) or in the umbilicus (*Cullen's sign*). The abdomen is usually distended due to an associated *ileus*. The differential diagnosis includes:

- perforated peptic ulcer;
- perforated bowel;
- mesenteric ischaemia;
- acute cholecystitis;
- bowel obstruction;
- renal colic;
- myocardial infarction;
- pneumonia;
- ketoacidosis.

Overall about 20% of patients have severe acute pancreatitis (SAP), which is defined by the presence of organ failure, local complications (e.g. peripancreatic fluid collection, necrosis, abscess, pseudocyst) or both. The clinical course of SAP consists of two distinct phases.

1. *An early toxaemic phase* characterized by a disseminated inflammatory response with marked fluid shifts related to the systemic release of activated enzymes and toxic substances from the pancreas. This phase may be complicated by multiple-organ failure (see Chapter 5 – systemic inflammatory response syndrome and multiple-organ dysfunction syndrome).
2. *A late necrotic phase*. Pancreatic necrosis is the presence of a diffuse or focal area of non-viable pancreatic parenchyma, often associated with peripancreatic necrosis. SAP with such areas of necrosis is also referred to as *necrotizing pancreatitis*. Intra-abdominal necrosis creates a culture medium for bacterial invasion from the digestive tract and in 40–70% of cases necrotizing pancreatitis becomes infected. In some cases a *pancreatic abscess* is formed which may contain gas. *Pancreatic pseudocysts* (collections of pancreatic juice enclosed by a wall of fibrous or granulation tissue) may also develop.

Eleven clinical features identified by Ranson *et al.* (1976) correlate with morbidity, length of stay in intensive care and eventual mortality. The following five can be assessed on admission:

1. age greater than 55 years;
2. blood glucose greater than 11 mmol/L;
3. white blood cell count greater than 16 000/mm^3;
4. serum LDH greater than 350 iu/L;
5. serum aspartate aminotransferase greater than 250 u/L.

The other six features are evaluated within 48 hours of admission:

1. serum calcium level less than 2 mmol/L;
2. arterial oxygen tension (P_aO_2) less than 8 kPa (60 mmHg);
3. base deficit greater than 4 mmol/L;

4. blood urea increase greater than 2 mmol/L;
5. haematocrit fall greater than 10%;
6. fluid sequestration greater than 6 litres.

Fewer than three of the criteria correlate with the benign form of pancreatitis. SAP is diagnosed if three or more of Ranson's criteria are present, if the Acute Physiology and Chronic Health Evaluation (APACHE) II score is 8 or more and in the presence of organ failure with one or more of shock, renal insufficiency, pulmonary insufficiency or gastrointestinal bleeding. Those who develop local complications such as necrosis, pseudocyst or abscess may also be classified as having SAP (Swaroop *et al.*, 2004). The Glasgow score (Imrie's signs) is assessed on the basis of nine clinical and laboratory values also obtained during the initial 48 hours. This system has been shown to provide similar accuracy to the Ranson score for the assessment of disease severity. In particular, as with Ranson scoring, the presence of fewer than three signs is a reliable indicator of mild disease.

Patients who need monitoring during large-volume fluid administration, patients who require ventilatory support and those with metabolic imbalance, renal insufficiency, cardiovascular instability and impending multiple organ failure should be admitted for higher-dependency care. Thirst, oliguria, progressive tachycardia, tachypnoea, hypoxaemia, agitation, confusion, a rising haematocrit and a lack of improvement in symptoms have been identified as warning signs of impending severe disease and should prompt admission to a critical care area (Whitcomb, 2006). Patients who have undergone pancreatic surgery may also be admitted for postoperative care.

Investigations (Table 16.7)

A raised serum amylase (e.g. more than three to four times the upper limit of normal), in conjunction with a compatible history and clinical signs, strongly suggests a diagnosis of acute pancreatitis. It is important to appreciate, however, that serum amylase concentrations decline quickly over 3–4 days and that levels may be raised in other acute abdominal conditions. Measurement of serum lipase levels is more sensitive and specific for acute pancreatitis. Elevated liver enzymes, especially alanine aminotransferase, to more than three times the upper limit of normal suggests a biliary cause.

Plain radiographs may provide clues as to the cause of acute pancreatitis (e.g. calcified gallstones or pancreatic calcification on the plain abdominal film) or reveal complications (e.g. acute respiratory distress syndrome or pleural effusions on the chest radiograph).

Abdominal ultrasound will readily identify gallstones, sludge and bile duct dilatation but is less sensitive for detecting stones in the distal bile duct. Visualization of the pancreas by ultrasonography in acute disease is often limited by overlying bowel gas caused by associated ileus. Endoscopic ultrasonography may be a more accurate means of visualizing biliary tract abnormalities.

Table 16.7 Management of severe acute pancreatitis
Investigations
Serum amylase, C-reactive protein
Computed tomography (CT) scan
Abdominal ultrasound
General principles of management
Nasogastric intubation
Nutritional support: enteral if possible
Control symptoms (e.g. pain, nausea and vomiting)
Prevent and treat vital organ dysfunction
Endoscopy
Endoscopic retrograde cholangiopancreatography (ERCP)
Interventional radiology
CT-guided fine-needle aspiration or catheter drainage
Surgery

CT of the abdomen is the best means of visualizing the pancreas and can be used to confirm the diagnosis of pancreatitis. It may also suggest the cause of the attack (e.g. gallstones, fatty infiltration of the liver if related to alcohol, pancreatic tumour, pancreas divisum (London *et al.*, 1989)). The severity of pancreatitis can also be inferred from the extent of pancreatic enlargement and the presence of peripancreatic inflammatory changes, as well as from the number and location of fluid collections (**Table 16.8; Fig. 16.2**). Not all patients with acute pancreatitis require an immediate CT scan unless the initial diagnosis is in doubt since documentation of pancreatic or peripancreatic necrosis (non-perfused areas) or pseudocysts does not by itself influence treatment. Nevertheless dynamic contrast-enhanced CT remains the most valuable investigation for evaluating patients between 3 and 10 days after admission (Glazer and Mann, 1998). Pancreatic necrosis (Table 16.9), defined as diffuse or focal areas of non-viable parenchyma with accompanying fever and leukocytosis, is an indication for CT-guided fine-needle aspiration and microbiological examination of the aspirate. The finding of intrapancreatic gas pockets increases the likelihood of identifying infected pancreatic necrosis.

MRI is better than CT for distinguishing between an uncomplicated pseudocyst and one that contains necrotic debris and may identify early duct disruption not seen on CT.

Management (see Table 16.7)

General supportive measures should include:

■ control of symptoms (e.g. pain, nausea and vomiting);
■ prevention and treatment of vital organ dysfunction (adequate fluid resuscitation is essential; some patients

Table 16.8 Revised computed tomography (CT) grading system for acute pancreatitis (Balthazar *et al.*, 1994; Balthazar, 2002)

Grade	Contrast-enhanced CT scan findings	CT severity index points	Morbidity (%)	Mortality (%)
A	Normal	0	} 4	} 0
B	Focal or diffuse pancreatic enlargement	1		
C	Peripancreatic changes (without fluid collection)	2		
D	Single extra pancreatic fluid collection	3	} 54	} 14
E	Two or more fluid collections or gas in and around the pancreas	4		

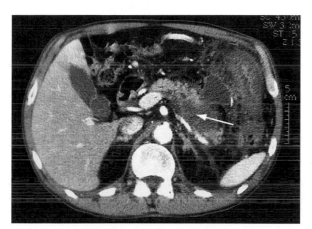

Fig. 16.2 Computed tomography scan appearances in a patient with severe acute pancreatitis showing necrosis of the pancreatic parenchyma (arrow) and a fluid collection extending outside the gland with inflammatory thickening of the colon. Reproduced from Kumar P, Clark M 2005 Clinical Medicine 6E Elsevier with permission.

may require mechanical ventilation, inotropic support and blood purification);

■ a nasogastric tube is not recommended routinely but may be helpful if protracted vomiting occurs in the presence of a radiologically demonstrated ileus.

NUTRITIONAL SUPPORT (Marik and Zaloga, 2004)

Although in the past standard practice was to administer nutritional support parenterally in order to avoid stimulating the pancreas, most now recommend early institution of enteral nutrition. When compared to parenteral nutrition the enteral route seems to be associated with fewer infectious complications, a reduction in the need for surgical intervention, a shorter length of hospital stay and reduced costs. The nasojejunal route is usually preferred in the belief that pancreatic stimulation can be avoided (Nathens *et al.*, 2004), although there is some evidence to suggest that nasogastric feeding is equally safe and effective. Parenteral nutrition is reserved for those who do not tolerate enteral feeding or in whom an adequate nutritional intake cannot be achieved within 2–4 days (see Chapter 11).

ENDOSCOPY AND PERCUTANEOUS DRAINAGE

Initial clinical trials provided no convincing evidence that early endoscopy for detecting common bile duct stones, sphincterotomy and stone extraction moderated disease severity (Fan *et al.*, 1993; Neoptolemos *et al.*, 1988). Similarly, another trial failed to demonstrate any benefit from early ERCP in patients who had acute gallstone pancreatitis without evidence of either biliary obstruction or acute cholangitis (Folsch *et al.*, 1997). Indeed, this multicentre study was closed early because of a non significant increase in the severity of complications and mortality rates following ERCP. Nevertheless most centres still proceed to ERCP in patients with severe acute gallstone pancreatitis with evidence of cholangitis, a dilated common bile duct, progressive jaundice or liver function tests suggestive of biliary tract obstruction. This approach is supported by a meta-analysis which indicated that ERCP and sphincterotomy reduced complications and mortality in patients with SAP in the presence of biliary obstruction or cholangitis (Sharma and Howden, 1999). The role of early ERCP in patients without biliary obstruction or cholangitis remains unclear.

Increasingly local complications, such as pseudocysts, are successfully treated using endoscopic or percutaneous techniques. Contraindications to endoscopic drainage of pancreatic pseudocysts include abscess formation, the presence of necrotic tissue within the cyst, gastric or duodenal varices, coagulopthy and a thick (> 1 cm) cyst wall. Echoendoscopes are now available that allow direct drainage without the need for a separate endoscopic procedure. Percutaneous drainage, performed using ultrasound or CT guidance, can be used to drain peripancreatic fluid collections, non-communicating pseudocysts and abscesses.

ADJUNCTIVE THERAPY

Although as mentioned above, many of the systemic effects of pancreatitis are mediated through kinins found in the peritoneal exudate, there is no evidence to support the administration of antiproteases or inhibition of pancreatic exocrine secretions (e.g. with somatostatin and its long-acting analogues).

ANTIMICROBIAL THERAPY (Bassic et al., 2003)

Pancreatic infection is the leading cause of morbidity and mortality in patients with SAP. Infection usually develops at least 10 days after the onset of pancreatitis.

Prophylactic antibiotics may promote selection of resistant organisms and encourage opportunistic fungal infection, particularly when given for more than 5–7 days. Although an Italian cooperative trial suggested that prophylactic imipenem reduced the rate of infection in pancreatic necrosis, this was not associated with a reduction in mortality (Pederzoli *et al.*, 1993) and in a more recent double-blind trial antibiotic prophylaxis with ciprofloxacin and metronidazole failed to influence the development of infected pancreatic necrosis (Isenmann *et al.*, 2004). The most appropriate approach remains unclear (Nathens *et al.*, 2004). Many now recommend that antibiotic treatment should be reserved for those who develop sepsis, failure of two or more organs, proven infection or an increase in C-reactive protein levels in combination with other evidence of infection. Others suggest that those with proven pancreatic necrosis on CT scan should receive agents active against enteric organisms (e.g. imipenem or ofloxacin with metronidazole) for 1–2 weeks. Some centres use antifungal agents in combination with antibacterial therapy.

Selective decontamination of the digestive tract (see Chapter 12) warrants further investigation as a means of preventing infection in SAP (Nathens *et al.*, 2004).

PERITONEAL LAVAGE

Early and prolonged peritoneal lavage has been claimed to reduce both the frequency and mortality from pancreatic sepsis (Ranson and Berman, 1990), although this finding contradicts those of previous studies (Mayer *et al.*, 1985). It seems that, although peritoneal lavage may reduce inflammation, outcome is not improved. Moreover lavage is incompatible with the 'open-abdomen' approach.

SURGERY

Since many cases of acute pancreatitis are due to gallstones, and because passage of stones through the ampulla is thought to be an important initiating event, there has been a long-standing interest in the potential role of *early biliary tract surgery* in arresting progression of acute pancreatitis secondary to gallstones. Despite initial enthusiasm, a controlled study (Kelly and Wagner, 1988) concluded that cholecystectomy and common bile duct exploration within 48 hours of diagnosis was associated with a prohibitive morbidity and mortality.

Major pancreatic resection has also become obsolete except in a very few cases of total pancreatic necrosis because

of the technical difficulty, as well as the high morbidity and mortality. Instead a surgical approach similar to that for advanced peritonitis (*planned re-laparotomies, prolonged drainage and open packing of wounds*) may be required. Infection of pancreatic necrosis can be confirmed or excluded by percutaneous aspiration guided by ultrasound or CT, followed by culture and Gram stain. Standard treatment of infected pancreatic necrosis is by *surgical debridement*, although good outcomes have been reported using radiologically positioned percutaneous drains or endoscopy. This approach is particularly useful for postsurgical candidates or those who have well-contained infection. Once necrosis develops the ultimate outcome is determined by the amount of pancreatic and extrapancreatic injury (**Table 16.9**), the presence of bacterial contamination, and, perhaps most importantly, the general condition of the patient. Surgical, percutaneous or endoscopic decompression may also be indicated when fluid collections continue to enlarge, cause pain, become infected or compress adjacent organs.

The optimum treatment of *sterile necrosis* (Rattner *et al.*, 1992) is still debated but management is usually conservative. It is unclear whether surgical debridement improves the outcome for those with sterile necrosis who are unstable, demonstrate signs of raised IAP or exhibit a significant systemic inflammatory response.

The main surgical approaches to debridement of pancreatic necrosis include:

- necrosectomy and continuous lavage of the lesser sac (Beger *et al.*, 1988);
- blunt debridement with open packing of the resulting cavity and wound (D'Egidio and Schein, 1991) or the use of an abdominal 'zipper' (see above);
- blunt debridement with closed packing and closed-system suction catheters.
- planned, staged laparotomies with repeated lavage.

With all these techniques operative procedures vary according to the expertise of individual surgeons. The thoroughness of the initial debridement is the most important determinant of the need for subsequent re-explorations and survival. Since infection is clearly associated with mortality in necrotizing pancreatitis, control of bacterial and fungal colonization of devitalized tissue is essential.

Table 16.9 Relationship between a computed tomography (CT) grading system for pancreatic necrosis, morbidity and mortality in severe pancreatitis

Necrosis	% Pancreas failing to enhance with intravenous contrast	CT severity index points	Morbidity (%)	Mortality (%)
None	None	0	6	0
Mild	0–30%	2	48	0
Moderate	30–50%	4	} 94	} 29
Extensive	> 50%	6		

(Balthazar *et al.* 1994, Balthazar 2002).

It is generally accepted that early surgical management of acute pancreatitis should be limited to patients with unrelenting diffuse peritonitis and multiple-organ failure after 2–3 days of intensive non-operative management. Ideally surgery should be postponed to the second or third week in order to allow sequestrectomy of necrotic pancreas and facilitate debridement. In some patients earlier surgical intervention will be necessary to ameliorate the cardiovascular, pulmonary and renal effects of raised IAP.

Prognosis

Mortality rates for patients hospitalized with acute pancreatitis have changed little since the 1980s (Goldacre and Roberts, 2004); around 10–30% of those with SAP will die. During the acute phase pancreatitis is associated with major local or systemic complications in about 10% of patients, half of whom will die despite conventional supportive treatment. Pancreatic infection is the commonest cause of death, sterile necrosis being much less often associated with a fatal outcome: a significant proportion of patients with infected necrosis die (Bassic et al., 2003).

REFERENCES

Balthazar EJ (2002) Acute pancreatitis: assessment of severity with clinical and CT evaluation. Radiology 223: 603–613.

Balthazar EJ, Freeney PC, van Sonnenberg E (1994) Imaging and intervention in acute pancreatitis. Radiology 193: 297–306.

Barer D, Ogilivie A, Henry D, et al. (1983) Cimetidine and tranexamic acid in treatment of acute upper gastrointestinal-tract bleeding. New England Journal of Medicine 308: 1571–1575.

Barry RE (1988) The pathogenesis of acute pancreatitis. British Medical Journal 296: 589.

Bassic C, Larvin M, Villatoro E (2003) Antibiotic therapy for prophylaxis against infection of pancreatic necrosis in acute pancreatitis. Cochrane Database of Systematic Reviews 4: CD002941.

Beger HG, Buchler M, Bittner R, et al. (1988) Necrosectomy and postoperative local lavage in necrotizing pancreatitis. British Journal of Surgery 75: 207–212.

Boley SJ, Brandt LJ, Frank MS (1981) Severe lower intestinal bleeding: diagnosis and treatment. Clinics in Gastroenterology 10: 65–91.

Brands LJ, Boley SJ (2000) AGA technical review on intestinal ischemia. Gastroenterology 118: 954–968.

Branicki FJ, Boey J, Fok PJ, et al. (1990) Bleeding duodenal ulcer: a prospective evaluation of risk factors for rebleeding and death. Annals of Surgery 211: 411–418.

British Society of Gastroenterology Endoscopy Committee (2002) Non-variceal upper gastrointestinal haemorrhage: guidelines. Gut 51: 1–6.

Cales P, Masliah C, Bernard B, et al. (2001) Early administration of vapreotide for variceal bleeding in patients with cirrhosis. New England Journal of Medicine 344: 23–28.

Christiansen J, Ottenjann R, Von-Arx F (1989) Placebo-controlled trial with the somatostatin analogue SMS 201–995 in peptic ulcer bleeding. Gastroenterology 97: 568–574.

Chung SS, Lau JY, Sung JJ, et al. (1997) Randomised comparison between adrenaline injection alone and adrenaline injection plus heat probe treatment for actively bleeding ulcers. British Medical Journal 314: 1307–1311.

Collins R, Langman M (1985) Treatment with histamine H₂ antagonists in acute upper gastrointestinal hemorrhage. Implications of randomized trials. New England Journal of Medicine 313: 660–666.

Cook D, Pearl RG, Cook RJ (1991) Incidence of clinically important bleeding in mechanically ventilated patients. Intensive Care Medicine 6: 167–174.

D'Egidio A, Schein M (1991) Surgical strategies in the treatment of pancreatic necrosis and infection. British Journal of Surgery 78: 133–137.

Durham RM, Shapiro MJ (1991) Stress gastritis revisited. Surgical Clinics of North America 71: 791–810.

Escorsell A, Ruiz del Arbol L, Planas R, et al. (2000) Multicenter randomized controlled trial of terlipressin versus sclerotherapy in the treatment of acute variceal bleeding: the TEST study. Hepatology 32: 471–476.

Fan S-T, Lai EC, Mok FP, et al. (1993) Early treatment of acute biliary pancreatitis by endoscopic papillotomy. New England Journal of Medicine 328: 228–232.

Feu F, Ruiz del Arbol L, Banares R, et al. (1996) Double-blind randomized controlled trial comparing terlipressin and somatostatin for acute variceal hemorrhage. Gastroenterology 111: 1291–1299.

Folsch UR, Nitsche R, Ludtke R, et al. (1997) Early ERCP and papillotomy compared with conservative treatment for acute biliary pancreatitis. New England Journal of Medicine 336: 237–242.

Gajic O, Urratia LE, Sewani H, et al. (2002) Acute abdomen in the medical intensive care unit. Critical Care Medicine 30: 1187–1190.

Garcia-Tsao G (2001) Current management of the complications of cirrhosis and portal hypertension. Gastroenterology 120: 726–748.

Garner GB, Ware DN, Cocanour CS, et al. (2001) Vacuum-assisted wound closure provides early fascial reapproximation in trauma patients with open abdomens. American Journal of Surgery 182: 630–638.

Glazer G, Mann DV (1998) United Kingdom guidelines for the management of acute pancreatitis. British Society of Gastroenterology Gut 42 (Suppl. 2): S1–S13.

Goff JS (1990) Esophageal variceal ligation. Canadian Journal of Gastroenterology 4: 639–642.

Goldacre MJ, Roberts SE (2004) Hospital admission for acute pancreatitis in a English population, 1963–98: database study of incidence and mortality. British Medical Journal 328: 1466–1469.

Gostout CJ (2000) The role of endoscopy in managing acute lower gastrointestinal bleeding. New England Journal of Medicine 342: 125–127.

Henry DA, O'Connell DL (1989) Effects of fibrinolytic inhibitors on mortality from upper gastrointestinal haemorrhage. British Medical Journal 298: 1142–1146.

Howard RJ (1981) Acute acalculous cholecystitis. American Journal of Surgery 141: 194–198.

Howard OM, Buchanan JD, Hunt RH (1982) Angiodysplasia of the colon. Experience of 26 cases. Lancet 2: 16–19.

Imperiale TF, Birgisson S (1997) Somatostatin or octreotide compared with H₂ receptor antagonists and placebo in the management of acute nonvariceal upper gastrointestinal hemorrhage: a meta-analysis. Annals of Internal Medicine 127: 1062–1071.

Isenmann R, Runzi M, Kron M, et al. (2004) Prophylactic antibiotic treatment in patients with predicted severe acute pancreatitis: a placebo-controlled, double-blind trial. Gastroenterology 126: 997–1004.

Jacobs JE, Birnbaum BA (1997) Abdominal computed tomography of intensive care unit patients. Seminars in Roentgenology 32: 128–141.

Jalan R, Hayes PC (2000) UK guidelines on the management of variceal haemorrhage in cirrhotic patients. Gut 46 (Suppl. III): iii 1–iii 15.

Jenkins DM (1999) Management of severe ulcer rebleeding. New England Journal of Medicine 340: 799–801.

Jenkins SA, Shields R, Davies M, et al. (1997) A multicentre randomised trial comparing octreotide and injection sclerotherapy in the management and outcome of acute variceal haemorrhage. Gut 41: 526–533.

Jensen DM, Machicado GA, Jutabha R, et al. (2000) Urgent colonoscopy for the diagnosis and treatment of severe diverticular hemorrhage. New England Journal of Medicine 342: 78–82.

Kelly TR, Wagner DS (1988) Gallstone pancreatitis: a prospective randomized trial of the timing of surgery. Surgery 104: 600–605.

Khuroo MS, Yattoo GN, Javid G, et al. (1997) A comparison of omeprazole and placebo for bleeding peptic ulcer. New England Journal of Medicine 336: 1054–1058.

Kingsnorth A, O'Reilly D (2006) Acute pancreatitis. British Medical Journal 332: 1072–1076.

Kovacs TO, Jensen DM (1987) Endoscopic control of gastroduodenal hemorrhage. Annual Review of Medicine 38: 267–277.

Kravetz D, Bosch J, Teres J, et al. (1984) Comparison of intravenous somatostatin and vasopressin infusions in treatment of acute variceal hemorrhage. *Hepatology* 4: 442–446.

Kron IL, Harman PK, Nolan SP (1984) The measurement of intra-abdominal pressure as a criterion for abdominal re-exploration. *Annals of Surgery* 199: 28–30.

Laine L (1999) Management of acute colonic pseudo-obstruction. *New England Journal of Medicine* 341: 192–193.

Lau JY, Sung JJ, Lam Y-H, et al. (1999) Endoscopic retreatment compared with surgery in patients with recurrent bleeding after initial endoscopic control of bleeding ulcers. *New England Journal of Medicine* 340: 751–756.

Lau JY, Sung JJ, Lee KK, et al. (2000) Effect of intravenous omeprazole on recurrent bleeding after endoscopic treatment of bleeding peptic ulcers. *New England Journal of Medicine* 343: 310–316.

Lee MJ, Saini S, Brink JA, et al. (1991) Treatment of critically ill patients with sepsis of unknown cause: value of percutaneous cholecystostomy. *American Journal of Roentgenology* 156: 1163–1166.

Leontiadis GI, Sharma VK, Howden CW (2005) Systematic review and meta-analysis of proton pump inhibitor therapy in peptic ulcer bleeding. *British Medical Journal* 330: 568.

Lewis JD, Shin EJ, Metz DC (2000) Characterization of gastrointestinal bleeding in severely ill hospitalized patients. *Critical Care Medicine* 28: 46–50.

Lieberman DA, Keller FS, Katon RM, et al. (1984) Arterial embolization for massive upper gastrointestinal tract bleeding in poor surgical candidates. *Gastroenterology* 86: 876–885.

Lo G, Lai KH, Cheng JS, et al. (2000) Endoscopic variceal ligation plus nadolol and sucralfate compared with ligation alone for the prevention of variceal rebleeding: a prospective, randomized trial. *Hepatology* 32: 461–465.

London NJM, Neopotolemos JP, Lavelle J, et al. (1989) Serial computed tomography scanning in acute pancreatitis: a prospective study. *Gut* 30: 397–403.

McGuire HH Jr, Horsley JS 3rd (1986) Emergency operations for gastric and duodenal ulcers in high risk patients. *Annals of Surgery* 203: 551–557.

Magnusson I, Ihre T, Johansson C, et al. (1985) Randomised double blind trial of somatostatin in the treatment of massive upper gastrointestinal haemorrhage. *Gut* 26: 221–226.

Malbrain ML (2004) Different techniques to measure intra-abdominal pressure (IAP): time for a critical re-appraisal. *Intensive Care Medicine* 30: 357–371.

Marik PE, Zaloga GP (2004) Meta-analysis of parenteral nutrition versus enteral nutrition in patients with acute pancreatitis. *British Medical Journal* 328: 1407.

Markisz JA, Front D, Royal HD, et al. (1982) An evaluation of ^{99m}Tc-labeled red cell scintigraphy for the detection and localization of gastrointestinal bleeding sites. *Gastroenterology* 83: 394–398.

Mayer AD, McMahon MJ, Corfield AP, et al. (1985) Controlled clinical trial of peritoneal lavage for the treatment of severe acute pancreatitis. *New England Journal of Medicine* 312: 399–404.

Meldrum DR, Moore FA, Moore EE, et al. (1997) Prospective characterization and selective management of the abdominal compartment syndrome. *American Journal of Surgery* 174: 667–672.

Moore AFK, Hargest R, Martin M, et al. (2004) Intra-abdominal hypertension and the abdominal compartment syndrome. *British Journal of Surgery* 91: 1102–1110.

Nathens AB, Curtis JR, Beale RJ, et al. (2004) Management of the critically ill patient with severe acute pancreatitis. *Critical Care Medicine* 32: 2524–2536.

Neoptolemos JP, Carr-Locke DL, London NJ, et al. (1988) Controlled trial of urgent endoscopic retrograde cholangiopancreatography and endoscopic sphincterotomy versus conservative treatment for acute pancreatitis due to gallstones. *Lancet* 2: 979–983.

Pederzoli P, Bassi C, Vesentini S, et al. (1993) A randomized multicenter clinical trial of antibiotic prophylaxis of septic complications in acute necrotizing pancreatitis with imipenem. *Surgery, Gynecology and Obstetrics* 176: 480–483.

Pitcher JL (1971) Safety and effectiveness of the modified Sengstaken–Blakemore tube: a prospective study. *Gastroenterology* 61: 291–298.

Ponec RJ, Saunders MD, Kimmey MB (1999) Neostigmine for the treatment of colonic pseudo-obstruction. *New England Journal of Medicine* 341: 137–141.

Ranson JH, Berman RS (1990) Long peritoneal lavage decreases pancreatic sepsis in acute pancreatitis. *Annals of Surgery* 211: 708–718.

Ranson JH, Rifkind JM, Turner JW (1976) Prognostic signs and nonoperative peritoneal lavage in acute pancreatitis. *Surgery, Gynecology and Obstetrics* 143: 209–219.

Rattner DW, Legermate DA, Lee MJ, et al. (1992) Early surgical debridement of symptomatic pancreatic necrosis is beneficial irrespective of infection. *American Journal of Surgery* 163: 105–110.

Ring EJ, Lake JR, Roberts JP, et al. (1992) Using transjugular intrahepatic portosystemic shunts to control variceal bleeding before liver transplantation. *Annals of Internal Medicine* 116: 304–309.

Rockall TA, Logan RF, Devlin HB, et al. (1995) Incidence and mortality from acute upper gastrointestinal haemorrhage in the United Kingdom. *British Medical Journal* 311: 222–226.

Rockall TA, Logan RF, Devlin HB, et al. (1996) Risk assessment after acute upper gastrointestinal haemorrhage. *Gut* 38: 316–321.

Sacks HS, Chalmers TC, Blum AL, et al. (1990) Endoscopic hemostasis. An effective therapy for bleeding peptic ulcers. *Journal of the American Medical Association* 264: 494–499.

Saltzman JR, Zawacki JK (1997) Therapy for bleeding peptic ulcers. *New England Journal of Medicine* 336: 1091–1093.

Sharara AI, Rockey DC (2001) Gastroesophageal variceal hemorrhage. *New England Journal of Medicine* 345: 669–681.

Sharma VK, Howden CW (1999) Metaanalysis of randomized controlled trials of endoscopic retrograde cholangiography and endoscopic sphincterotomy for the treatment of acute biliary pancreatitis. *American Journal of Gastroenterology* 94: 3211–3214.

Stiegmann GV, Goff JS, Michaeltz-Onody PA, et al. (1992) Endoscopic sclerotherapy as compared with endoscopic ligation for bleeding esophageal varices. *New England Journal of Medicine* 326: 1527–1532.

Strodel WE, Brothers T (1989) Colonoscopic decompression of pseudo-obstruction and volvulus. *Surgical Clinics of North America* 69: 1327–1335.

Swaroop VS, Chari ST, Clain JE (2004) Severe acute pancreatitis. *Journal of the American Medical Association* 291: 2865–2868.

Van der Spoel J, Oudemans-van Straaten H, Stoutenbeek C, et al. (2001) Neostigmine resolves critical illness-related colonic ileus in intensive care patients with multiple organ failure – a prospective, double-blind placebo-controlled trial. *Intensive Care Medicine* 27: 822–827.

Villanueva C, Balanzo J, Novella MT, et al. (1996) Nadolol plus isosorbide mononitrate compared with sclerotherapy for the prevention of variceal rebleeding. *New England Journal of Medicine* 334: 1624–1629.

Villanueva C, Minana J, Ortiz J, et al., (2001) Endoscopic ligation compared with combined treatment with nadolol and isosorbide mononitrate to prevent recurrent variceal bleeding. *New England Journal of Medicine* 345: 647–655.

von Holstein CC, Eriksson SB, Kallen R (1987) Tranexamic acid as an aid to reducing blood transfusion requirements in gastric and duodenal bleeding. *British Medical Journal* 294: 7–10.

Walt RP, Cottrell J, Mann SG, et al. (1992) Continuous intravenous famotidine for haemorrhage from peptic ulcer. *Lancet* 340: 1058–1062.

Welch CE, Rodkey GV, Von Ryall Gryska P (1986) A thousand operations for ulcer disease. *Annals of Surgery* 204: 454–467.

Whitcomb DC (2006) Acute pancreatitis. *New England Journal of Medicine* 354: 2142–2150.

Williamson RCN (1988) Acalculous disease of the gall bladder. *Gut* 29: 860–872.

17 Endocrine emergencies

The involvement of intensive care specialists in the management of endocrine emergencies has led to the application of new techniques and clinical practice to conditions that in the past were managed almost exclusively by physicians on general wards. This has inevitably led to some controversy, particularly in the care of diabetic emergencies, which are the most frequently encountered acute endocrine disorders. Some are still reluctant to admit such patients routinely to an intensive care unit (ICU), despite the potential advantages of a high nurse-to-patient ratio, the availability of constant monitoring and ready access to repeated biochemical and blood gas analysis, together with the immediate availability of skilled medical staff.

DIABETES MELLITUS

DEFINITION
Diabetes mellitus is a group of metabolic disorders characterized by hyperglycaemia due to an absolute or relative deficiency of insulin.

NORMAL PHYSIOLOGY
In normal healthy individuals the blood glucose concentration is controlled within narrow limits, even after a meal when glucose may be stored in muscle or liver cells as glycogen, taken up into fat cells and converted into lipid, or metabolized via glycolysis to produce energy. This regulation is achieved by alterations in insulin secretion, which promote anabolic processes involving the storage of glucose, amino acids and fat, and corresponding changes in the counterregulatory hormones, including glucagon, thyroid hormones, adrenaline (epinephrine), noradrenaline (norepinephrine), cortisol and growth hormone. Glucose may subsequently be released from the liver by glycogenolysis or gluconeogenesis, but during prolonged fasting the body's energy needs may have to be met by lipolysis and oxidation of fatty acids.

TYPES OF DIABETES MELLITUS
Diabetes may be *primary* or *secondary*. Although secondary diabetes accounts for only 1–2% of new cases it must not be missed because the cause can often be treated (see below).

Type 1 diabetes mellitus
Patients with type 1 diabetes mellitus have pancreatic beta-cell destruction. Insulin deficiency and subsequent hyperglycaemia necessitate exogenous insulin administration. The risk of developing insulin-dependent diabetes mellitus (IDDM) is human leukocyte antigen (HLA)-linked and genetic susceptibility is polygenic, although environmental factors are also important. Autoimmune processes with antibodies directed against antigens present in the islet cells play an important role in the pathogenesis of type 1 diabetes (Gale, 2001) and this condition is associated with other autoimmune diseases, including thyroid disorders, Addison's disease and pernicious anaemia. About two-thirds of patients with IDDM present before 30 years of age. A variant form, sometimes called latent autoimmune diabetes of adults (LADA), occurs in later life and can be difficult to distinguish from type 2 diabetes. The incidence of type 1 diabetes appears to be increasing.

Type 2 diabetes mellitus
Type 2 diabetes is characterized by both insulin hyposecretion and insulin resistance. Patients with non-insulin-dependent diabetes mellitus (NIDDM) usually present over the age of 40 years. Although the tendency to develop type 2 diabetes is also inherited (Lo *et al.*, 1991), the age at which the disease is manifest is influenced by body weight, diet, level of physical activity and intercurrent illness. Such patients do not normally require maintenance insulin treatment, at least initially. Their risk of myocardial infarction, intracerebral haemorrhage and peripheral vascular disease is much higher than in similarly aged non-diabetics. A rare variant of type 2 diabetes, which has an early onset and is dominantly inherited, is called maturity-onset diabetes of the young (MODY).

DIABETIC KETOACIDOSIS
Diabetic ketoacidosis (DKA) is the most common endocrine emergency and is the hallmark of uncontrolled type 1 diabetes. In almost three-quarters of all cases DKA can be traced to one of three causes:

1. previously undiagnosed diabetes;
2. infection or intercurrent illness (e.g. gastroenteritis, myocardial infarction) in a known diabetic patient;
3. a decrease in insulin dosage made by the physician or the patient (often because the patient feels unable to eat because of nausea and vomiting).

Less frequently DKA may be precipitated by:

- trauma;
- acute pancreatitis.

Pathophysiology

The combination of insulin deficiency, oversecretion of glucagon and excess production of stress hormones (e.g. adrenaline, cortisol) promotes accelerated hepatic glucose production via glycogen breakdown and unrestrained gluconeogenesis. Combined with a reduction in cellular uptake and use of glucose, this leads to a rise in blood sugar levels, which precipitates glycosuria and an osmotic diuresis, with loss of water, sodium, potassium, phosphate and other electrolytes. Typically more water than sodium is lost. Initially the loss of glucose in the urine limits the rise in blood sugar levels, while the fluid losses are replaced by drinking. Eventually, however, nausea and vomiting exacerbate dehydration and prevent adequate fluid intake. Fever and diarrhoea may further increase fluid losses. The same hormonal changes promote lipolysis with release of triglycerides and non-esterified fatty acids from fat cells. The fatty acids are metabolized to ketones in hepatic mitochondria and this contributes to the development of a metabolic acidosis.

Clinical features

When IDDM develops *de novo*, ketoacidosis is usually heralded by several days of *polyphagia, polydipsia* and *polyuria* followed by *weakness, prostration, anorexia* and finally *nausea and vomiting*. In those with established diabetes mellitus, however, ketoacidosis can develop in a matter of hours. *Confusion* and *stupor* are common, while up to 5% present in *coma*.

Examination reveals the *musty, fruity odour* of ketones on the breath. The patient may hyperventilate (*Kussmaul breathing or 'air hunger'*) in an attempt to compensate for progressive metabolic acidosis. There may be signs of extreme *dehydration* and *hypovolaemia*. In severe cases shock with impaired tissue perfusion may be associated with *lactic acidosis. Abdominal pain, a rigid abdomen* and *rebound tenderness* may simulate intra-abdominal pathology. Examination of the lower limbs may reveal signs of *peripheral vascular insufficiency* and superimposed *infection*. Diabetic patients with infection are not necessarily febrile and may be mildly *hypothermic*.

Whenever diabetes mellitus is newly diagnosed the possibility that it might be secondary to another endocrine disorder (e.g. *Cushing's syndrome, acromegaly, phaeochromocytoma, thyrotoxicosis, glucagonoma*) should be considered. *Pancreatic carcinoma* is a possibility in any patient with recent-onset diabetes mellitus associated with abdominal pain, jaundice and weight loss. *Pancreatitis* and *cirrhosis* are other possibilities. *Drug therapy* (e.g. thiazide diuretics and steroids) and *parenteral or enteral feeding* may also reveal glucose intolerance.

Particular care should be taken to detect problems associated with the underlying diabetes (e.g. neuropathy, retinopathy and vascular insufficiency), as well as likely causative factors such as abscess, cellulitis, ulceration, urinary tract infection, pneumonia or myocardial infarction.

Some patients present with ketoacidosis but only slightly elevated blood sugar levels – *euglycaemic ketoacidosis*. Such patients are typically young insulin-dependent diabetics who have developed a concurrent illness, but whose glycogen stores are depleted so that mild hypoglycaemia is maintained solely by gluconeogenesis.

Diagnosis and investigations

The diagnosis of hyperglycaemia can be rapidly established by bedside testing, but must always be confirmed by laboratory analysis. Ketosis is diagnosed when urinalysis reveals ketones (++ or greater) or when undiluted plasma produces a positive result on near-patient dipstick testing that measures ketones. A venous plasma concentration of bicarbonate less than 15 mmol/L or an anion gap ($[Na^+ + K^+]$ − $[HCO_3^- + Cl^-]$) (see Chapter 6) greater than 16 mmol/L provides confirmatory evidence. In this context an acidosis is defined as an arterial pH of less than 7.30. Patients who are well hydrated may present with an anion gap and a hyperchloraemic acidosis (see Chapter 6). Plasma osmolality is increased, but is generally less than 320 mosmol/L.

A full blood count should be obtained, together with blood glucose, urea and electrolytes (specify chloride if out of hours) and plasma osmolality. The serum sodium may be high, normal or low, hyperkalaemia is common initially, whilst magnesium and phosphate levels are often low. Hypokalaemia at presentation is associated with a worse prognosis. Arterial blood should be analysed for acid–base status. Urinalysis should be undertaken and specimens of urine and blood sent for culture. A chest radiograph should be organized and an electrocardiogram (ECG) recorded. Since repeated investigations are likely to be required, all results should be carefully recorded in the notes or on a flow chart. It is important to remember that a neutrophil leukocytosis is common in diabetic patients with DKA and does not necessarily indicate infection, while a low or normal temperature does not rule out infection. Furthermore, the serum amylase may be spuriously elevated. The differential diagnosis in an unconscious patient should include alcohol or drug intoxication, intracerebral or subarachnoid haemorrhage, and meningitis.

Management

PHASE 1 (RESUSCITATION PHASE) (Table 17.1)

DKA is a medical emergency associated with significant morbidity and mortality (2–5%) (Lebovitz, 1995). In devel-

Table 17.1 Guidelines for the management of diabetic ketoacidosis in phase 1

Confirm the diagnosis	**Underlying disorders** 　Cardiac disease 　Renal impairment
Blood glucose level	**Insulin**
Measure ketones in urine/blood	6–10 units/hour intravenously
Take blood	**Further investigations**
Glucose, sodium, potassium, plasma osmolality	Chest radiograph
Urea, bicarbonate, chloride	Electrocardiogram
Amylase	Urinalysis
Full blood count	Midstream urine specimen
Blood cultures	**Other measures**
Cardiac enzymes, troponin estimation	Supplemental oxygen to unobstructed airway in all cases
Arterial blood gas analysis	Nasogastric tube
Intravenous fluids	Coma position if stuporose
Colloidal solutions to restore intravascular volume and an adequate circulation	Urinary catheter
	Blood/plasma expander for persistent hypotension
Large volumes of 0.9% saline are often required.* For example: 　1 litre in 30 minutes then 　1 litre in 1 hour then 　1 litre in 2 hours then 　1 litre every 4 hours	Prophylactic heparin in the obese, the elderly, in comatose or severely dehydrated patients and in those with a coincidental haemoglobinopathy
Potassium replacement (e.g. potassium chloride 20–30 mmol/hour, not more than 80 mmol/hour)	Consider central venous pressure measurement, oesophageal Doppler monitoring or pulmonary artery catheterization in those who are hypotensive or at risk of developing pulmonary oedema
History and examination	Consider bicarbonate if pH less than 7.0 (e.g. 500 mL 1.26% $NaHCO_3$ plus 10 mmol KCl)
Precipitating cause 　? Stopping insulin 　? Infection 　? Myocardial infarction 　? Drug therapy	Consider antibiotics
	Reassess
Assessment of dehydration 　Blood pressure 　Capillary refill 　Peripheral cyanosis 　Peripheral temperature 　Reduced tissue turgor	Hourly blood glucose
	Hourly assessment of circulating volume
	2-hourly sodium and potassium levels
	2-hourly arterial blood gas analysis
	Record results on flow chart

*Fluid replacement must be carefully tailored to the individual patient.

oped countries the majority of deaths are related to sepsis or pulmonary and cardiovascular complications. Corrective measures must not be delayed and should start in the emergency department (Foster and McGarry, 1983). Normal resuscitative priorities apply to diabetic emergencies as for all critically ill patients. Oxygen should be administered to an unobstructed airway, respiratory function should be assessed and adequate intravenous fluids must be administered immediately to restore vital signs. Patients with a Glasgow Coma Scale < 9 will require tracheal intubation. Because cardiovascular function may be impaired in diabetic patients (autonomic neuropathy, coronary artery disease,

cardiomyopathy), measurement of central venous pressure (CVP), oesophageal Doppler monitoring and in some cases pulmonary artery catheterization may be indicated in hypotensive diabetic patients with DKA, particularly those over 60 years of age. Urine output may be a misleading guide to haemodynamic function because of the osmotic diuresis induced by the high sugar load; oliguria is a late sign of hypovolaemia. Specific management of the patient with DKA involves:

■ controlled rehydration;
■ provision of insulin and potassium;

- the avoidance of complications (e.g. hypoglycaemia, hypokalaemia, hypothermia).

Fluid replacement. The admission of patients with unstable diabetes into intensive therapy units has led to considerable debate regarding the management of volume replacement and rehydration. Particular controversy has surrounded the relative merits of crystalloids or colloids (Hillman, 1987), the use of 0.9% saline or 0.18% saline in dextrose 4% for rehydration, as well as the rate of fluid administration and the most sensitive means of detecting unwanted effects (e.g. the use of pulse oximetry on the wards to identify pulmonary flooding).

The average fluid deficit in patients with DKA is of the order of 6–10 litres. Although restoration of these losses is essential for reversing hyperglycaemia, acidosis and hypotension, injudicious administration of large volumes of crystalloid solutions may precipitate tissue oedema and worsen pulmonary gas exchange (Fein *et al.*, 1982; Sprung *et al.*, 1980). Most would accept that immediate, rapid expansion of the circulating volume with colloidal solutions, with or without whole blood to maintain the haemoglobin concentration, is indicated if the patient is hypotensive. Although large volumes of 0.9% saline are also usually required, a more cautious approach should be adopted in the elderly and in those with pre-existing cardiovascular or respiratory disease. Later 0.18% saline in dextrose 4% can be substituted for 0.9% saline if the plasma sodium exceeds 160 mmol/l. Persistent or recurrent hypotension and oliguria should be corrected with additional intravenous colloid. In less severe cases and when there is no hypotension, 0.18% saline in dextrose 4% can be used as the initial fluid therapy. It is, however, always important to *tailor fluid resuscitation to the individual patient.*

Potassium. Patients with DKA are almost always potassium-depleted due to a combination of osmotic diuresis, polydipsia and vomiting. Potassium levels are, however, usually elevated initially because of an acidosis-induced potassium shift from the intracellular to the extracellular space, but quickly fall when insulin is given and the acidosis is corrected. In most patients, therefore, intravenous potassium replacement (5–30 mmol of potassium chloride/hour) should be given to prevent hypokalaemia when insulin treatment is started. If the initial plasma potassium concentration is low, replacement can be given more rapidly, but generally not faster than 80 mmol/hour. Regular monitoring of electrolyte concentrations (e.g. every 2 hours) is essential during the initial phases of treatment.

Insulin. Bolus doses of insulin, which may cause rapid falls in blood sugar levels, should not be given. Instead various fixed low-dose intravenous insulin regimens are used by most clinicians treating DKA. An initial infusion rate of 6–10 units insulin/hour may be given through a separate vein or by 'piggyback' into the intravenous line carrying the replacement fluid. Again, insulin dosage should be adjusted to the individual's requirements. Adsorption of insulin to the plastic tubing of the giving set is not a problem in clinical practice.

Rapid alterations in blood glucose levels and pH can cause cerebral oedema (Hammond and Wallis, 1992), particularly in children and adolescents, perhaps because changes in the cerebrospinal fluid lag behind those in the blood. Accordingly a reduction in blood glucose of not more than 5 mmol/l per hour is an appropriate target. Cerebral oedema has also been associated with either a reduction in serum sodium levels or a failure of sodium concentrations to increase. The diagnosis of cerebral oedema can be established by computed tomography (CT) scan and treatment is with intravenous mannitol.

It is important to appreciate that the movement of glucose into the cells in response to insulin administration is accompanied by a shift of potassium from the extracellular to the intracellular space, with potentially disastrous consequences if significant hypokalaemia supervenes. There is also a danger of precipitating hypoglycaemia, the clinical signs of which include *sweating, tachycardia, hypotension* and an *obtunded level of consciousness* (see later in this chapter). Current treatment with lower doses of insulin which reduce blood glucose by suppressing hepatic glucose output rather than stimulating peripheral uptake are much less likely to produce hyoglycaemia.

Bicarbonate. Although severe metabolic acidosis has a number of adverse consequences, rapid correction with bicarbonate is also associated with some risks, including a reduction in peripheral oxygen unloading, exacerbation of hypokalaemia, intracellular acidosis and hypernatraemia (see Chapter 5). In those with mild or moderate acidosis, the blood pH will usually normalize within a few hours without the need for bicarbonate administration. Severe acidosis, however, may impair myocardial contractility, diminish vascular responsiveness to pressor amines and predispose to cardiac arrhythmias. Therefore, bicarbonate should be reserved for patients with an initial pH of less than 7.0; in such cases 8.4% sodium bicarbonate can be added to the dextrose saline used as replacement fluid or administered as 1.26% sodium bicarbonate solution, which is iso-osmolar with normal plasma.

Other measures. Because DKA may be associated with gastric atony, comatose or lethargic patients should have a nasogastric tube inserted to minimize the risk of aspiration of gastric contents. Clinically significant hypophosphataemia and hypomagnesaemia may require correction.

Antibiotics should not be routinely prescribed, although in the most seriously ill patients broad-spectrum antibiotics may be considered according to local policy (see Chapter 12) following a careful search for infection, and after urine and blood cultures have been sent to the microbiology laboratory. Infections that are easily overlooked include:

- otitis media;
- mastoiditis;

Table 17.2 Guidelines for the management of diabetic ketoacidosis in phase 2 (blood glucose < 12 mmol/l)

Change fluids (e.g. to 1 litre 0.18% saline in dextrose 4%, 5% dextrose or 10% dextrose as required to maintain blood glucose concentrations, with 20 mmol potassium chloride per litre 6-hourly)

Continue intravenous insulin infusion for 24 hours after clearance of ketonuria. Change fixed-dose to a variable-dose intravenous regimen, for example:

Blood glucose (mmol/L)	Insulin infusion (units/h)
0–3.5	0.5 (give glucose rather than discontinue insulin)
3.6–6.0	1
6.1–9.0	2
9.1–12.0	3
12.1–16.0	4
16.1–20.0	5
20.1 or above	6 (call doctor)

Table 17.3 Guidelines for the management of diabetic ketoacidosis in phase 3 (ketoacidosis resolved for more than 24 hours and there is no doubt that the patient is able to eat and drink normally)

Stop all intravenous fluid therapy. The insulin infusion should not be stopped before subcutaneous (s.c.) insulin has been started

Start regular pre-meal subcutaneous insulin 3 or 4 times daily (24-hour total dose of insulin should be equal to the previous 24 hours' insulin consumption) or resume previous insulin regimen

Arrange patient education and follow-up

- sinusitis;
- perirectal abscess.

Prophylactic subcutaneous heparin should be prescribed in comatose or severely dehydrated patients, the elderly, the obese and in those with coincidental haemoglobinopathy.

PHASE 2 (MONITORING PHASE) (Table 17.2)

The postresuscitation phases of DKA are generally not well managed unless a diabetic specialist is involved, and errors commonly occur about 24–48 hours after admission. Once the blood glucose level has fallen to less than 12 mmol/L, the 0.9% saline infusion can be changed for 0.18% saline in dextrose 4%, 5% dextrose or 10% dextrose 1 litre 6-hourly, with continued intravenous potassium and an insulin infusion adjusted to maintain the blood glucose in the range 6–10 mmol/litre. This regimen should be continued for 24 hours after clearance of ketonuria, even if the patient is well recovered clinically.

PHASE 3 (RECOVERY PHASE) (Table 17.3)

When the ketoacidosis has resolved for more than 24 hours and there is no doubt that the patient is able to eat and drink normally, established diabetic patients can usually resume their previous insulin therapy, while new patients can be managed using Actrapid insulin subcutaneously at least 8-hourly. Intravenous insulin has a very short half-life of only 4 minutes and an *insulin infusion should never be discontinued without giving a depot subcutaneous dose*. This is one of the most common serious mistakes made during the management of this phase. Arrangements should be made to provide patient education and follow-up, e.g. through the local diabetic nurse specialist.

HYPERSOMOLAR NON-KETOTIC DIABETIC EMERGENCIES

Hyperosomolar non-ketotic (HONK) decompensation usually complicates uncontrolled, often undiagnosed type 2 diabetes and is characterized by:

- extreme hyperglycaemia;
- hyperosmolality;
- severe dehydration, but minimal acidosis.

Pathophysiology

It should be appreciated that non-ketotic coma and ketoacidosis represent two ends of a spectrum rather than being two distinct disorders.

Residual insulin secretion probably determines whether a patient presents with DKA or with HONK. Those who develop HONK usually have sufficient insulin to inhibit unrestrained ketogenesis, but not to prevent hyperglycaemia. Initially, compensation for polyuria may be achieved by increased oral intake of water and this may in turn lead to hyponatraemia. In undiagnosed diabetes mellitus the consumption of sweet drinks in response to thirst often contributes to the rapid development of hyperglycaemia. Later, however, increased oral intake fails to keep pace with the continued urinary losses, particularly during the night. The elderly experience thirst less acutely and more readily become dehydrated. Hypernatraemia, hyperglycaemia and hyperosmolality combine to diminish conscious level and eventually the patient becomes comatose.

Causes

As in DKA, decompensation is often precipitated by stressful stimuli such as *infection* (e.g. pneumonia, pyelonephritis) or *surgery*. *Drug administration* can also precipitate hyperosmolar crisis; potassium-losing diuretics (hypokalaemia decreases insulin secretion), phenytoin (directly inhibits insulin secretion) and glucocorticoids (increased gluconeogenesis and peripheral insulin antagonism) have all been implicated in this regard. In some cases consumption of glucose rich fluids (e.g. Lucozade) may be implicated. *Myocardial infarction, cerebrovascular accidents* and *subdural haematomas* must also be considered when searching for precipitating factors. In hospitalized patients, *hyperalimentation* or *infusion of concentrated glucose solutions* can cause hyperosmolar crisis.

Clinical presentation and diagnosis

Most patients are middle-aged or elderly individuals with mild to moderate NIDDM or no previous history of diabetes mellitus.

Polyuria and *polydipsia* may be present, but may not be obvious in older, less alert patients. Extreme *dehydration* and *disturbances in consciousness* (e.g. stupor or coma) are characteristic. Some patients present with seizures or focal neurological deficits, including hemiparesis. The hyperventilation and abdominal pain seen in patients with DKA are unusual in HONK. *Mild renal insufficiency* is common.

The diagnosis of a HONK crisis is usually not difficult once the plasma glucose is measured and the plasma osmolality (which is usually extremely high) is determined. Serum sodium levels of 155–160 mmol/L are common.

Management (Table 17.4)
INITIAL MEASURES

Oxygen should be administered to an unobstructed *airway*. *Ventilatory support* is occasionally required, particularly if

Table 17.4 Guidelines for the management of hyperosmolar non-ketotic decompensation of diabetes mellitus

Initial measures

Secure airway, administer oxygen

Mechanical ventilation may be required

Invasive cardiovascular monitoring

Pass nasogastric tube

Catheterize the bladder

Specific treatment

Rehydration
  Synthetic gelatin combined with hypotonic saline or 5% dextrose *or* 0.9% saline (3/4 to 1/2 estimated fluid deficit in first 12 hours, approximately 2/3 over next 12 hours and correct any remaining deficit over next 12 hours)

Potassium replacement
  Deficits are generally less than in diabetic ketoacidosis (DKA)

Insulin
  As in DKA, except start with lower dose (e.g. 3 units/ hour) and monitor blood glucose very closely

General measures

Must include subcutaneous heparin

Treat precipitating cause (e.g. infection)

pneumonia is implicated as a precipitating factor. Vital signs should be monitored and invasive cardiovascular monitoring instituted. A *nasogastric tube* and *urinary catheter* should be inserted. Many of those who succumb have Gram-negative infection and this must be considered when searching for a precipitating factor or selecting antibiotic therapy in patients thought to be infected.

SPECIFIC MANAGEMENT

Therapy is directed at producing predictable gradual reductions in circulating and tissue glucose concentrations, which, together with a fall in plasma sodium, will lower plasma osmolality.

Fluid and electrolyte therapy. Overzealous intravascular resuscitation with large volumes of hypotonic crystalloid solutions such as 0.18% saline in dextrose 4% may promote generalized extracellular oedema. Pulmonary oedema will be associated with hypoxia, while cerebral oedema may produce life-threatening rises in intracranial pressure, and rapid falls in plasma sodium may precipitate acute myelinolysis (see Chapter 11). It has been suggested that careful expansion of the intravascular volume with synthetic gelatin solutions can produce slow and controlled falls in plasma and extracellular sodium concentrations when combined with hypotonic saline or 5% dextrose administration (Hillman, 1987) without significant risk of pulmonary oedema, acute myelinolysis or cerebral complications. Others give approximately one-third to one-half of the estimated fluid deficit in the first 12 hours as 0.9% saline, approximately two-thirds of the deficit over the next 12 hours as 0.9% saline, with repletion of any remaining deficit in the following 12 hours also with 0.9% saline. Rehydration of these patients with 0.9% saline, combined with the effects of secondary hyperaldosteronism, is usually associated with further rises in serum sodium concentrations as water leaves the vascular compartment to correct intracellular dehydration. This increase in serum sodium should be accepted as an inevitable consequence of correcting the intracellular environment and should not inhibit continued administration of 0.9% saline or synthetic gelatin solutions, provided plasma sodium levels do not exceed 165 mmol/L and there are no signs of peripheral or pulmonary oedema. In difficult cases more invasive cardiovascular monitoring may be indicated.

Potassium replacement is also necessary but, because acidosis is usually only mild, deficits are generally less than with DKA. Underlying renal disease when present also reduces urinary potassium losses.

Insulin. Insulin is administered as in DKA, although some patients with HONK are particularly sensitive to insulin and it may be safer to commence the infusion at 3 units/hour with very careful blood sugar monitoring for the first 2–3 hours. If the plasma glucose concentration fails to fall satisfactorily, the insulin infusion rate can be increased to 6 units/ hour. The aim should be to avoid rapid changes and return the plasma glucose concentration to normal within 6–10 hours.

Immobile patients with hyperosmolar states are at significant risk of thromboembolism and arterial thrombotic episodes (e.g. mesenteric ischaemia) and should receive regular prophylactic *heparin*.

Continued management. Diabetic patients should never be discharged from the ICU or hospital without establishing the cause of the decompensation and initiating measures to prevent recurrence. Survivors of HONK coma typically require long-term management of type 2 diabetes.

Prognosis

In some series the mortality rate for HONK coma has been as high as 30–50%. This reflects in part the coexistence of severe disease in elderly patients.

Unlike ketoacidosis, non-ketotic hyperglycaemia is not an absolute indication for subsequent insulin therapy.

PERIOPERATIVE MANAGEMENT OF THE PATIENT WITH DIABETES MELLITUS (Husband *et al.*, 1986; McAnulty and Hall, 2003)

Diabetic patients may be admitted to ICUs not only for management of an acute diabetic emergency but also as a consequence of an unrelated disorder (e.g. surgery, major trauma).

For the purposes of this discussion, surgery may be broadly divided into minor procedures, following which the patient is able to resume oral intake on the same day, or major interventions, which preclude oral intake in the early postoperative period. The latter inevitably includes thoracic, cardiac and neurosurgical operations, as well as major intra-abdominal procedures. Certain types of surgical procedure may precipitate particularly rapid and large fluctuations in blood sugar levels (e.g. when there are associated metabolic changes, as may occur during hypothermic cardiopulmonary bypass and when surgery is performed as an emergency). Diabetic patients can also be categorized into three broad groups:

1. diet-controlled type 2 NIDDM;
2. oral hypoglycaemic-controlled type 2 NIDDM;
3. type 1 or insulin-treated type 2 IDDM.

Using these definitions, a straightforward scheme of perioperative management can be prepared, such as that outlined in Table 17.5.

INSULIN THERAPY IN CRITICALLY ILL PATIENTS

Critically ill patients commonly require exogenous insulin to combat hyperglycaemia and insulin resistance. Recent evidence has indicated that more intensive insulin therapy, with tighter control of blood sugar levels, is associated with improved outcomes among surgical patients (the majority postcardiac surgery with low Acute Physiology and Chronic Health Evaluation (APACHE) scores) admitted to intensive

care (Van den Berghe *et al.*, 2001). In this prospective, randomized trial the treatment group received sufficient insulin to maintain their blood glucose level between 4.4 and 6.1 mmol/L, whereas in the conventional group the target value for blood glucose was 10.0–11.1 mmol/L. Importantly, all patients also received continuous intravenous glucose infusions on admission to intensive care and parenteral or enteral nutrition thereafter.

There was a significant mortality reduction in the intensive treatment group (mortality 4.6%) compared with the conventional group (mortality 8.0%), although this survival advantage was only apparent in patients who stayed in the ICU for more than 5 days. The greatest reduction in mortality was in deaths due to multiple-organ failure associated with a septic focus. Intensive insulin therapy also reduced episodes of sepsis by over 40% and lowered mortality rates in those surgical patients with bacteraemia. There were fewer patients with a length of ICU stay greater than 5 days in the intensive treatment group compared to those patients managed conventionally and in-hospital deaths were also significantly reduced. Interestingly, the incidence of critical illness polyneuropathy was also dramatically reduced by intensive insulin therapy (see Chapter 15).

In a more recent study of patients admitted to a medical ICU 'tight glycaemic control', but with less aggressive nutritional support, failed to influence mortality on an intention-to-treat basis, but did significantly reduce morbidity by preventing newly acquired kidney injury and accelerating weaning from mechanical ventilation, discharge from the ICU and discharge from hospital. Moreover, among those who remained in the ICU for more than 3 days, mortality was significantly reduced, from 52.5 to 43% (Van den Berghe *et al.*, 2006). In those who received less than 3 days of intensive care, however, mortality was increased in the protocol group, making it difficult to decide which patients should receive intensive insulin therapy as they are admitted to the ICU. There is also concern that this approach is associated with an unacceptably high incidence of hypoglycaemia (5.1% of patients in the surgical study, 18.7% in the medical patients). Indeed, one multicentre trial in medical and surgical patients with severe sepsis was suspended because tight glycaemic control was associated with a considerably higher incidence of hypoglycaemia and no reduction in mortality (Brunkhorst *et al.*, 2005) (see also Chapter 5). It is hoped that the results of further multicentre trials already in progress will clarify the most appropriate approach to adopt in the various categories of critically ill patients. In the meantime many recommend adopting a less aggressive approach in which blood glucose values of < 8.3–8.5 mmol/L are targeted, although it might be reasonable to adopt a policy of tight control in critically ill patients after elective surgery in ICUs with aggressive feeding policies and a high staffing ratio.

The mechanism of benefit with intensive insulin therapy requires further elucidation, for example with regard to the interrelationship between hyperglycaemia and oxidative stress and lung injury (Leverve, 2003; Philips and Baker,

Table 17.5 Suggested guidelines for the management of diabetic patients undergoing surgery

Classification of diabetes mellitus	Minor surgery protocol	Major surgery protocol
Type 2 diabetes – diet-controlled NIDDM (often middle-aged and overweight. Pathological process is one of peripheral insulin resistance)	Monitor blood sugar level (BSL). Normal stress response causes elevation of fasting BSL, but acidosis unlikely and therefore no intervention required	Monitor BSL. Normal stress response causes elevation of BSL, thereby avoiding any possibility of hidden hypoglycaemia. Insulin may be required, especially in those receiving parenteral nutrition
Type 2 diabetes – oral hypoglycaemic controlled NIDDM (may initially have been controlled by diet alone, but now requires oral agents daily)	Omit oral hypoglycaemic agent the night before surgery and the morning of operation. Schedule for morning theatre list Monitor BSL pre-, per- and postoperatively Recommence therapy after first meal	Omit oral hypoglycaemic agent the night before surgery and the morning of operation Schedule for morning theatre list Monitor BSL perioperatively May need preoperative insulin infusion Glucose-insulin-potassium (GIK) regimen likely to be required postoperatively
Type 1 or 2 diabetes – insulin-dependent (usually juvenile or middle-aged. Pathological process is absolute insulin insufficiency. Associated autonomic neuropathy and widespread vascular disorders possible)	Consider converting the patient from long-acting insulins to three-times-daily short-acting insulin Monitor BSL On the morning of surgery establish secure intravenous access and commence a GIK infusion e.g. 1 mL/kg per hour. K = 10 mmol potassium chloride (provided that the patient is not hyperkalaemic), I = 10 units insulin, G = 500 mL 10% glucose Monitor BSL and potassium and adjust the GIK prescription accordingly Continue GIK until after first meal	Consider converting the patient from long-acting insulins to three-times-daily short-acting insulin. Monitor BSL On the morning of surgery establish secure intravenous access and commence a GIK infusion e.g. 1 mL/kg per hour (provided that the patient is not hyperkalaemic) Monitor BSL and potassium and adjust the GIK prescription accordingly Continue GIK until after first meal

NIDDM, non-insulin-dependent diabetes mellitus.

2003). Current evidence suggests that the beneficial effects of this regimen are related to achieving normoglycaemia, rather than the increased dose of insulin (Van den Berghe *et al.*, 2003) and that prevention of the direct toxic effects of intracellular glucose overload on hepatic mitochondria may be important (Vanhorebeek *et al.*, 2005). Other suggested mechanisms of benefit have included prevention of immune dysfunction, reduction of systemic inflammation and endothelial protection.

HYPOGLYCAEMIA

Hypoglycaemia is defined as a circulating venous plasma glucose level less than 2 mmol/L. It is a potentially life-threatening emergency. Hypoglycaemia occurs due to a mismatch between insulin, glucose or food intake and physical activity and may complicate *insulin therapy, oral hypoglycaemic treatment* or *systemic disease.*

Causes

While *intentional overdosage* with intravenous insulin or oral hypoglycaemic tablets may occur in those with suicidal intent, the more usual circumstances surrounding insulin-induced hypoglycaemia are *accidental* (e.g. complicating routine self-treatment in brittle diabetic subjects) or *iatrogenic* during management of DKA, hyperalimentation or diabetic patients undergoing surgery. Islet-cell neoplasms of the pancreas (*insulinomas*) also present as recurrent hypoglycaemic episodes. Hypoglycaemia can also occur as a complication of:

- hepatic failure (see Chapter 14);
- hypothermia (see Chapter 20);
- hypopituitarism (see later in this chapter);
- Addisonian crisis (see later in this chapter);
- salicylate poisoning in children (see Chapter 19);
- Reye's syndrome.

Repeated hypoglycaemic episodes in a diabetic patient whose insulin dosage has been decreasing may indicate the development of renal insufficiency, adrenal failure, hypothyroidism or hypopituitarism.

Clinical features

Patients may complain of *weakness, lethargy, incoordination* and *confusion*. This may ultimately progress to *seizures* and *coma*. Rapid falls in blood sugar levels produce *adrenergic symptoms* such as tremulousness, sweating, palpitations and anxiety, which are attributable to the increased sympathetic drive. *Faintness* and *sweating* with *tachycardia, variable blood pressure* and *pupillary dilatation* are easily overlooked or mistaken for alternative pathologies. Measurement of blood glucose is therefore essential in any patient presenting with 'funny turns', hypothermia or altered consciousness.

It has been suggested that the warning signs of hypoglycaemia are less well appreciated by patients receiving human insulin than by those using animal insulins. This phenomenon, which is probably related to more rapid absorption of human insulin, was extensively investigated, but no clear differences between the hypoglycaemic effects of human and animal insulin emerged (Gale, 1989). It is also important to appreciate that loss of awareness of hypoglycaemia occurs over time in many diabetics, regardless of the type of insulin prescribed.

Hypoglycaemia from the long-acting sulphonylureas is especially dangerous because glucose levels can be suppressed for many hours. Chlorpropamide is excreted mainly unmetabolized by the kidney and coexisting renal insufficiency greatly prolongs its half-life, thereby increasing the risk of hypoglycaemia. It is no longer recommended.

Management

Simultaneously with the usual resuscitative measures, any insulin infusion should be discontinued and *25 mL 50% dextrose (or 50 mL 20% dextrose) injected intravenously*. This usually produces an immediate improvement in conscious level and vital signs. The circulating blood glucose level can then be maintained by the continuous administration of 10% or 20% dextrose. To avoid superficial thrombophlebitis concentrated dextrose solutions should be administered via a central vein.

Accidental or deliberate overdose with sulphonylureas can be refractory to an infusion of concentrated dextrose alone and may require the additional administration of *hydrocortisone, glucagon* or *diazoxide*. Glucocorticoids increase glucose levels by stimulating gluconeogenesis and antagonizing the effects of insulin. Glucagon is a polypeptide hormone produced by the alpha cells of the islets of Langerhans, which increases plasma glucose concentration by mobilizing glucose from hepatic glycogen stores. Diazoxide acts directly on the pancreas to decrease insulin secretion. Haemodialysis is not helpful since sulphonylureas are protein-bound.

Intentional overdosage with intravenous insulin injections may prove impossible to reverse, especially when there is significant delay in discovering the collapsed hypoglycaemic patient. Parenteral administration of insulin has, nevertheless, been successfully treated by surgical resection of the subcutaneous tissue into which the insulin had been injected.

Malnourished alcoholic patients are susceptible to hypoglycaemia as a consequence of alcohol-induced suppression of gluconeogenesis. Furthermore, glucagon administration is usually not effective in reversing hypoglycaemia in such patients since liver glycogen stores are often depleted.

Prolonged coma despite treatment of hypoglycaemia should prompt consideration of other potential causes of unconsciousness such as hypoxic cerebral injury, intracerebral haemorrhage, drug or alcohol intoxication, meningitis or hypothermia.

Clearly, whatever the aetiology of hypoglycaemia, subsequent treatment and investigations should be aimed at the primary disorder.

Prognosis

The prognosis after severe prolonged hypoglycaemia depends on the duration of coma and corresponding cerebral injury.

THYROID EMERGENCIES

THYROID CRISIS (Ringel, 2001)
Causes

Thyroid crisis (or 'storm') is a life-threatening hypermetabolic condition which can involve every organ/system (Jiang et al., 2000). A precipitating event such as *infection, surgery, trauma* or other *intercurrent illness* (e.g. stroke, DKA) can usually be identified in a patient with partially treated or untreated hyperthyroidism. Thyroid crisis may also follow *massive overdose of thyroid hormone preparations, radioiodine therapy* and the *administration of iodinated contrast dyes*.

The mechanism underlying thyroid crisis remains unclear, but may involve an increase in β-adrenergic receptor numbers.

Clinical presentation

In thyroid crisis, the characteristic features of hyperthyroidism are accentuated (Burch and Wartofsky, 1993). Cardiovascular manifestations include *tachycardia, arrhythmias* (e.g. *atrial fibrillation), heart block* and *cardiac failure*. There is *profuse sweating, extreme irritability, tremor, nausea, vomiting, diarrhoea* and *abdominal pain*. *Delirium*, sometimes with a psychotic component, progresses to *coma or convulsions* in the most severe cases. Abnormalities of liver function and *jaundice* may also be seen. *Fever* is invariable and sets thyroid crisis apart from hyperthyroidism, but makes the distinction from sepsis extremely difficult. *Leukocytosis* is also well recognized in thyrotoxicosis, even in the absence of infection. *Myopathy* is common in both hyper- and hypo-thyroidism and *rhabdomyolysis* has been reported.

Amphetamine overdose also resembles severe thyrotoxicosis and a toxicology screen should be undertaken when drug abuse is suspected, especially if the thyroid gland is not palpable. Phaeochromocytoma can also present in a similar fashion, but severe hypertension and paroxysmal attacks usually dominate the clinical presentation of this condition.

Investigations

Blood should be collected for thyroid function tests and a cortisol level before commencing therapy. A toxicology screen should be performed and specimens should be sent for microscopy, culture and sensitivity. Liver function tests may be abnormal.

Management (Table 17.6)

In these extremely ill patients therapy for thyrotoxicosis must precede laboratory confirmation of the diagnosis. Treatment is aimed at decreasing the synthesis and secretion of thyroid hormone and countering the effects of thyroid hormone already in the circulation, as well as identifying and treating any precipitating illness and providing supportive

Table 17.6 Guidelines for the management of thyroid crisis

General measures

Oxygen administration

Intravenous fluids

Cooling blanket and/or tepid sponging

Chlorpromazine (25–50 mg intramuscularly)

Treat arrhythmias and cardiac failure

Specific treatment

Carbimazole (15–40 mg daily)

Propylthiouracil (500 mg loading dose followed by 250 mg every 6 hours PO, NG or PR)

Iodine preparations should be delayed for approximately 1 hour following the first dose of propylthiouracil. e.g.:
Potassium iodide (60 mg orally 8-hourly)
Lugol's iodine (10 drops of a solution containing 130 mg of iodine/mL 12-hourly)
Sodium iodide (250 mg intravenously 6-hourly if available)
Radiographic contrast dyes

Lithium carbonate (initially 300 mg 6-hourly) can be used in those with iodine sensitivity

Propranolol (80 mg orally 8-hourly or 2 mg intravenously as required) or atenolol

Dexamethasone (2 mg intravenously 6-hourly) or hydrocortisone 100 mg i.m. 6-hourly

Plasmapharesis in severe, unresponsive cases

NG, nasogastric; PO, orally; PR, per rectum.

therapy. A combination of antithyroid drugs and iodine may decrease serum triiodothyronine (T_3) levels in days but the metabolic response lags behind.

GENERAL MEASURES

Supplemental oxygen should be given to an unobstructed airway. Many patients are dehydrated and will require intravenous *fluid and electrolyte replacement*. A *cooling blanket* or *tepid sponging* can be used to decrease body temperature. **Salicylates should not be used since they displace thyroid hormone from binding proteins and may worsen hypermetabolism.**

Chlorpromazine (25–50 mg intramuscularly) can be given to reduce agitation and anxiety and may also facilitate cooling. Standard antiarrhythmic drugs can be used, including digoxin for atrial fibrillation, after correction of hypokalaemia (see Chapter 9). If sepsis is a possibility antibiotics should be given.

SPECIFIC MANAGEMENT

Carbimazole and *propylthiouracil* (PTU) impede formation of thyroid hormone and block peripheral conversion of thyroxine (T_4) to the metabolically active hormone T_3. A 500-mg loading dose followed by 250 mg of PTU every 6 hours is recommended and can be given by nasogastric tube or rectally if the patient is unable to take oral medication.

The administration of *iodine*, which blocks the synthesis and release of thyroid hormone, should be delayed for approximately 1 hour following the first dose of PTU to minimize the possibility of massive hormone release following iodination. Traditional preparations include *potassium iodide* (60 mg orally three times daily), Lugol's iodine (use 10 drops of a solution containing 130 mg of iodine/ml diluted in milk or water twice daily), or *sodium iodide* (250 mg intravenously every 6 hours). *Radiographic contrast dyes* containing iodine have also been used in place of traditional preparations (Burger and Philippe, 1992).

Lithium carbonate may be used to block thyroid hormone release in those with iodine sensitivity. There is a considerable risk of serious cardiovascular and central nervous system side-effects because of the narrow therapeutic ratio. The initial dose of 300 mg 6-hourly should be adjusted to maintain plasma lithium levels of approximately 1 mmol/L. Lithium should be avoided in those with cardiac failure or renal insufficiency.

Propranolol (80 mg orally 8-hourly or 2 mg intravenously as required) blocks the sympathetic effects of thyroid hormone and is especially useful to reduce sinus tachycardia (Hellman *et al.*, 1977). It inhibits release of thyroid hormone, impairs conversion of T_4 to T_3 and blocks sympathetic hyperactivity, which is responsible for many of the psychomotor and cardiovascular features of thyrotoxicosis. β-blockers are relatively contraindicated in patients with moderate or severe cardiac failure, as well as in peripheral vascular disease, and should not be used in those with reversible airflow limitation. More specific β-blockers such as atenolol can be used in such cases. *Dexamethasone* 2 mg intravenously every 6 hours, or hydrocortisone (100 mg intramuscularly 6-hourly), can also be used to reduce the conversion of T_4 to T_3 and may be useful because severe hyperthyroidism can cause relative hypoadrenalism due to accelerated cortisol metabolism.

In known or suspected causes of thyroid hormone overdose gastric lavage with charcoal, perhaps combined with the administration of cholestyramine to increase faecal elimination, may be indicated.

The response to treatment can be monitored by observation of clinical signs (e.g. pulse, temperature and agitation) and by regular serum T_3 estimations.

In extreme cases that are unresponsive to conventional therapy *plasmapharesis* has been undertaken.

Prognosis

When treated, thyroid crisis is associated with a mortality of 20–40%, mainly due to cardiac failure, arrhythmias or hyperthermia.

MYXOEDEMA COMA (Fliers and Wiersinga, 2003)

Myxoedema coma is an extreme decompensated form of hypothyroidism associated with a high mortality.

Causes

Frequent precipitating causes include:

- exposure to cold;
- surgery;
- trauma;
- infection (e.g. respiratory);
- cerebrovascular accident;
- drug administration (e.g. chlorpromazine, narcotics, β-blockers).

Coma may be secondary to the metabolic deficit induced by profound hypothyroidism, carbon dioxide narcosis, accentuated effects of sedative drugs or hypoglycaemia.

Clinical presentation and diagnosis

Myxoedema coma usually occurs in older patients with long-standing unrecognized hypothyroidism, most commonly caused by autoimmune thyroiditis, radioiodine therapy or thyroidectomy. A failure of thyrotrophin (thyroid-stimulating hormone: TSH) secretion due to pituitary disease is termed secondary hypothyroidism, while hypothalamic dysfunction is a tertiary disorder also associated with a low TSH level. There may be a history of previous thyroid disease or antithyroid, lithium or amiodarone therapy. A family history of thyroid or organ-specific autoimmune disease may be elicited.

Recognition of myxoedema coma may be difficult because of its low prevalence and non-specific symptoms. The classical manifestations of hypothyroidism are usually present and may include:

- characteristic facies;
- extreme bradycardia;

- hypotension;
- jeopardized respiratory function, including hypoventilation and upper-airway obstruction by tongue enlargement;
- delayed or absent relaxation of the tendon reflexes;
- paralytic ileus, megacolon and urinary retention;
- seizures and cerebellar signs.

Altered mental status, defective thermoregulation and a *precipitating event or illness* are the three essential elements in making a diagnosis of myxoedema coma. In fact most patients are not comatose, but altered mental status may manifest as disorientation, extreme lethargy, confusion or, occasionally, psychosis.

Hypothermia, due to an inability to produce heat and defective hypothalamic function, and *hyponatraemia* secondary to diminished free water clearance are common. Body temperature may be normal in those harbouring an infection. Occasionally the patient is *hypoglycaemic*. Routine investigations may also reveal a normocytic, normochromic or megaloblastic *anaemia* and *hypercholesterolaemia*. Raised *enzymes* (creatine phosphokinase; lactate dehydrogenase; aspartate aminotransferase) may cause confusion with an acute myocardial infarction or reflect a cardiac event in a susceptible patient. In myxoedema coma, however, these enzymes may remain high for several days, unlike the acute transient changes seen after a myocardial infarction, and troponin levels will not be elevated. An *ECG* is helpful in the differential diagnosis; typical changes in hypothyroidism include small voltages and a prolonged QT interval. Blood gas analysis often reveals *hypercapnia* and *hypoxia*. A *chest X-ray* should be obtained and specimens sent for culture and sensitivity.

Thyroid function tests should be requested urgently together with a serum cortisol. Most commonly the tests reveal a primary thyroid disorder (low T_3 and T_4, high TSH), but occasionally show secondary (pituitary) or tertiary (hypothalamic) hypothyroidism (low T_4, low TSH). Some patients may also have adrenal insufficiency. In some cases interpretation may be complicated by the presence of non-thyroidal illness syndrome (NTIS) (see below), in which case TSH may be inappropriately normal or low.

Management (Table 17.7)
GENERAL MEASURES

Myxoedema coma is an endocrine emergency. Once suspected, treatment can be life-saving and should start promptly, without waiting for laboratory confirmation of the diagnosis. Impaired myocardial performance and hypotension should be managed in accordance with the usual principles and patients with carbon dioxide retention or type II respiratory failure may require ventilatory support. The circulating volume should be expanded cautiously because these patients are at risk of congestive cardiac failure. It must be remembered that patients in myxoedema

Table 17.7 Management of myxoedema coma

General measures

Airway management: administer supplemental oxygen

Mechanical ventilation may be indicated

Haemodynamic support

Fluid restriction for hyponatraemia

Hypertonic saline rarely required

Intravenous glucose for hypoglycaemia

Gradual rewarming

Specific treatment

Triiodothyronine (T_3) 2.5 µg twice daily intravenously or
   nasogastrically/orally

Hydrocortisone 100 mg intramuscularly 8-hourly

Subsequently maintenance therapy with thyroxine
   (50–100 µg daily)

coma are particularly sensitive to central nervous system depressants. The mild hyponatraemia that is frequently present usually responds to fluid restriction (total input of less than 1 litre in 24 hours). Generally hypertonic saline (50–100 mL of 5% sodium chloride) should be avoided unless the plasma sodium concentration is less than 110 mmol/L or the hyponatraemia precipitates convulsions (see Chapter 11). Intravenous glucose 10 or 20% may be infused to reverse hypoglycaemia. In those with mild to moderate hypothermia, gradual rewarming with a covering blanket is all that is required. The rapid increase in body temperature that can be achieved with more active rewarming (see Chapter 20) may increase oxygen consumption, exacerbate hypoglycaemia and precipitate vasodilatation with cardiovascular collapse. Broad-spectrum antibiotics should be given while awaiting the results of cultures.

SPECIFIC THERAPY

The most appropriate thyroid hormone replacement regime continues to be debated. There are concerns that overzealous thyroid hormone replacement in myxoedema coma might increase oxygen consumption and cardiac workload and could precipitate myocardial ischaemia (Chernow et al., 1983). These authors recommend that T_3 is preferable to T_4 and that T_3 therapy should commence with a very low dose (2.5–5 µg twice daily) given intravenously. Some prefer a loading dose of T_4 (300–500 µg i.v.), followed by 50–100 µg T_4 i.v. daily.

Others are more cautious and recommend oral or nasogastric therapy. The dose of T_3 is increased in a stepwise fashion every 2–3 days (5, 10, 20 µg daily). Because thyroid replacement therapy can precipitate cardiac ischaemia and ventricular arrhythmias, continuous ECG monitoring is essential. In the most severe cases more invasive haemodynamic monitoring may be warranted. There is also a danger

that coexisting adrenal insufficiency could decompensate into adrenal crisis as the metabolic rate increases with thyroid replacement. Corticosteroids should therefore be given as hydrocortisone 100 mg intramuscularly 6-hourly. Blood should be obtained for determination of plasma cortisol concentration before treatment since this will guide further administration of hydrocortisone.

Maintenance with T_4 is commenced by some immediately, although the various regimens lack secure scientific justification and others switch to T_4 (50–100 µg/day) only when the dose of T_3 has been increased to at least 20 µg twice daily. The efficacy of therapy is gauged by repeated TSH estimations.

Prognosis

Estimated mortality rates vary between 20 and 60%. Persistent hypothermia and bradycardia, as well as greater age, cardiac complications and high-dose thyroid hormone replacement, have been associated with a worse prognosis (Yamamoto et al., 1999).

THE 'SICK EUTHYROID SYNDROME' ('LOW T_3 SYNDOME' OR 'NON-THYROIDAL ILLNESS SYNDROME') (McIver and Gorman, 1997; Van den Berghe, 2000)

More than 40 years ago Oppenheimer et al. (1963) first reported that thyroid function tests may be abnormal in seriously ill patients who do not have thyroid disease. During starvation and in early, or mild, acute illness or injury there is a reduction in T_3 and an increase in reverse T_3 (rT_3) levels, whilst T_4 and TSH levels rise initially but subsequently return to normal. In the more severely ill patients, circulating concentrations of T_4 and TSH may fall and rT_3 levels may normalize, whilst T_3 levels remain low (hence 'low T_3 syndrome') (**Fig. 17.1**). Tissue levels of T_3 are also dramatically reduced, although in some patients there may be unexplained, sporadically high tissue levels, especially in the heart and skeletal muscle (Arem et al., 1993). Possible mechanisms for these changes include:

- reduced uptake of T_4 and rT_3 into iodothyronine deiodinase 1 (D1)-containing tissues such as the liver;
- decreased availability of T_4 for peripheral conversion to T_3;
- reduced number and occupancy of nuclear receptors;
- reduced concentration of binding proteins;
- inhibition of hormone binding, transport and metabolism (e.g. by bilirubin, free fatty acids and heparin);
- differential regulation of the iodothyronine deiodinases (D1, D2 and D3) (Peeters et al., 2003):
  - Liver D1 is downregulated and skeletal muscle D1 and D2 activity is negligible or undetectable. This leads to decreased conversion of T_4 to T_3 and reduced clearance of rT_3;
  - D3 (not normally present in liver and skeletal muscle of healthy individuals) is induced, leading to enhanced clearance of T_3 and increased production of rT_3.

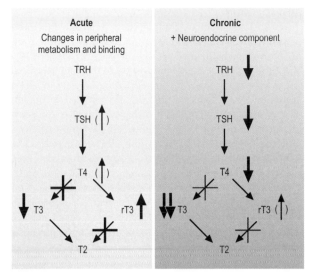

Fig. 17.1 The major changes occurring within the thyroid axis during the acute and chronic phases of critical illness. TRH, thyroid-releasing hormone; TSH, thyroid-stimulating hormone; T3, triiodothyronine; T4, thyroxine.

Whereas in acute critical illness these changes in peripheral metabolism and binding predominate, it seems that in prolonged critical illness a neuroendocrine component also contributes to the Non-Thyroidal Illness Syndrome (NTIS) (see **Fig. 17.1**), with a loss of the normal nighttime surge in TSH secretion, a blunted response to thyroid-releasing hormone (TRH) and a marked reduction in the pulsatility of the TSH secretory pattern. Moreover the extent of this reduction in pulsatility (Van den Berghe *et al.*, 1997) and the associated decrease in hypothalamic TRH and mRNA expression (Fliers *et al.*, 1997) correlate with the reduction in serum T_3 and TSH levels. In keeping with the concept of a central component to the NTIS, exogenous administration of TRH and growth hormone secretagogues to patients with prolonged critical illness restores TSH pulsatility and this is associated with an increase in circulating thyroid hormone levels, confirming peripheral responsiveness (Van den Berghe *et al.*, 1998).

Possible causes of NTIS include:

- nutritional factors;
- somatostatin – partial inhibition of TSH;
- glucocorticoids – reduce pituitary responsiveness to TRH, inhibit deiodinases;
- cytokines (interleukin-6, tumour necrosis factor, interleukin-1) – decrease activity of D1 via NF-κB activation, inhibit iodide uptake by the thyroid, inhibit thyroid hormone release;
- dopamine – exogenous administration suppresses TSH release (Van den Berghe *et al.*, 1994); possible role for endogenous dopamine.

Conventional wisdom has been that these abnormalities of thyroid function do not indicate hypothyroidism since TSH levels are normal or low and the patients do not appear to be clinically hypothyroid (hence the term 'sick euthyroid syndrome'). It has also been argued that NTIS may be an appropriate adaptive response designed to reduce energy expenditure during acute illness. On the other hand, mortality is closely related to the severity of the changes in thyroid hormones (Rothwell and Lawler, 1995), tissue availability of T_4 and T_3 is reduced, tissue levels of T_3 are low and the number and occupancy of nuclear receptors are reduced. Moreover the usual clinical features of hypothyroidism take several weeks to develop. Finally it is now clear that the low levels of TSH are due to a reduction in hypothalamic stimulation, at least in prolonged critical illness, rather than being a reflection of a euthyroid state (hence most now prefer the term 'non-thyroidal illness syndrome'). Some have therefore speculated that central hypothyroidism could contribute to the feeding-resistant catabolic state of prolonged critical illness and consequently might warrant intervention. Intravenous administration of thyroid hormones is, however, crude and may not be effective (Brent and Hershman, 1986).

More recently it has been suggested that treatment with hypothalamic-releasing factors may be intrinsically safer and more effective because feedback inhibition is preserved and the body is able to adjust peripheral hormone activity and metabolism. Moreover the need to define optimal circulating levels, and hence the dose, of peripherally active hormones is circumvented. Certainly there is evidence to suggest that such an approach can be effective and may eventually prove to be clinically useful (Van den Berghe *et al.*, 1999, 2002). Nevertheless further studies are required to resolve the continued controversy surrounding the clinical significance of NTIS and the possible role of therapeutic interventions.

CALCIUM METABOLISM

HYPERCALCAEMIA

Hypercalcaemia results from an imbalance between calcium influx (from gastrointestinal absorption and bone resorption) and efflux (by renal excretion).

Causes

The most frequent causes of hypercalcaemia are *primary hyperparathyroidism* and *malignancy,* e.g. squamous cell tumours of lung and breast, multiple myeloma. The former results most commonly from a parathyroid adenoma or hyperplasia, or rarely a carcinoma. In addition to osteolytic bony metastases a parathyroid hormone-related protein (PTHrP), that shares the parathyroid hormone (PTH) receptor and has similar physiological actions to PTH, has been identified in cases of paraneoplastic hypercalcaemia (Broadus *et al.*, 1988; Strewler, 2000). A number of less common causes have also been identified. Granulomatous diseases such as *sarcoidosis* and *tuberculosis* can be associated with unregulated production of 1,25-dihydroxycholecalciferol.

Table 17.8 Causes of hypercalcaemia

Malignancy

Hyperparathyroidism

Calcium therapy (e.g. milk-alkali syndrome)

Renal (renal failure or transplant)

Granulomatous disease

Immobilization

AIDS-related

Drug-induced (thiazides, lithium, oestrogens, tamoxifen, theophylline)

Endocrine (hyperthyroidism, multiple endocrine neoplasia syndrome, acromegaly, Addison's disease, phaeochromocytoma)

Other (hyperalimintation, chronic liver disease, overdose of vitamin A or D, idiopathic)

AIDS, acquired immunodeficiency syndrome.

Table 17.9 Symptoms and signs of hypercalcaemia

Central nervous system	Depression, memory loss, lethargy, psychosis, ataxia, stupor, confusion, coma, neuromuscular weakness, proximal myopathy, hypotonia, reduced deep tendon reflexes
Renal	Polyuria, renal stones, hyperchloraemic acidosis, nephrocalcinosis
Gastrointestinal	Anorexia, nausea, vomiting, constipation, peptic ulceration, pancreatitis
Cardiovascular	Hypertension, bradycardia (even asystole), short QT interval on electrocardiogram
Other	Tissue calcification (e.g. heart valves), bone disease, band keratopathy

Drugs such as *thiazide diuretics* may also worsen coincidental hyperparathyroidism (**Table 17.8**).

Clinical features

Symptoms and signs are non-specific and may vary from *gastrointestinal complaints* to *acute mental changes* with drowsiness, confusion, mania, psychosis and coma. *Pruritus* is a frequent accompaniment, together with *polyuria* and *polydipsia* (**Table 17.9**).

Investigations

Investigations should include a chest X-ray, an ECG and serum electrolytes. The total serum calcium concentration is normally maintained within a narrow range (2.2–2.7 mmol/L). Since a large proportion of the total measured calcium is bound to serum proteins, it is necessary to adjust for alterations in plasma albumin. An accepted correction factor is to add 0.02 mmol/L to the calcium level per gram of albumin below 40 g/L. Ionized serum calcium concentration can be measured using an ion-selective electrode. The normal range is 1.1–1.3 mmol/L.

Hyperparathyroidism produces typical radiographic appearances in the hand with subperiosteal erosions and bone cysts. Long-standing hypercalcaemia can result in nephrocalcinosis and renal calculi, both of which may be visible on plain abdominal radiographs. Once the diagnosis has been made, a search for the cause of hypercalcaemia must be undertaken. The hallmark of primary hyperparathyroidism is hypercalcaemia and hypophosphataemia, usually with elevated serum parathormone concentrations. When this combination is present then further investigations are usually unnecessary. Where serum parathormone levels are equivocal a number of other investigations are indicated, including protein electrophoresis (to exclude myeloma), thyroid function tests, morning cortisol and a bone scan. It is important to exclude familial benign hypocalciuric hypercalcaemia by measuring urine calcium concentration and serum parathormone level, which is usually modestly elevated.

Management

Patients with potentially life-threatening manifestations (bradycardia, prolonged QT, altered conscious level) require urgent intervention. Emergency management involves rehydration and the administration of agents that inhibit mobilization of calcium from the skeleton.

- Drugs such as thiazides and vitamin D compounds should be discontinued and dietary calcium should be restricted.
- Plasma osmolality should be restored to within the normal range of 280–290 mosmol/L with intravenous administration of high volumes of fluid (e.g. sodium chloride 0.9%). Osmolality can be measured directly or can be calculated approximately from the formula $2(Na^+ + K^+) +$ glucose + urea, all in mmol/L. The sodium load reduces calcium reabsorption in the proximal renal tubule.
- Once the patient is rehydrated forced saline diuresis, with furosemide as required, is initiated (furosemide inhibits calcium reabsorption in the distal tubules). In some cases invasive monitoring will be required.
- In renal failure haemodialysis or haemofiltration using a low-calcium dialysate is an effective alternative to forced diuresis.

- Serum calcium, electrolytes, magnesium and phosphate concentrations must be closely monitored.
- Biphosphonates inhibit bone resorption by binding to hydroxyapatite and inhibiting the dissolution of bone crystals (Davis and Heath, 1989). These slow effects take 2–3 days to decrease the serum calcium level and approximately 1 week to achieve the nadir (Bilezikian, 1992). The currently available agents include disodium pamidronate as a single 90-mg intravenous infusion over 24 hours or sodium clodronate 300 mg as an intravenous infusion over 4 hours, repeated daily for a maximum of 7–10 days or as a single-dose infusion of 1.5 g.
- Calcitonin is a potent inhibitor of osteoclastic bone resorption and can rapidly lower serum calcium levels. It is given in a dose of 3–4 units/kg intravenously over at least 6 hours initially, followed by 4 units/kg at 12–24-hour intervals by subcutaneous or intramuscular injection.
- Glucocorticoids such as hydrocortisone 100 mg 6-hourly by intramuscular injection or 60 mg prednisolone daily by mouth have beneficial effects in hypercalcaemia due to vitamin D intoxication, granulomatous disorders and haematological malignancy, but are not effective in those with primary hyperparathyroidism or solid cancers (Percival et al, 1984).
- Intravenous phosphates may be given in life-threatening hypercalcaemia, but should not be used in those with hyperphosphataemia.

- Parathyroidectomy may be indicated for hyperparathyroidism.

HYPOCALCAEMIA

Total serum calcium concentrations are low in 70–90% of intensive care patients, although ionized hypocalcaemia occurs in only about 15–20% of such cases.

Causes (Table 17.10)

Abnormal vitamin D metabolism. Disorders of vitamin D metabolism (e.g. impaired production of the active metabolite of vitamin D in renal disease and vitamin D-dependent rickets) cause hypocalcaemia, principally by reducing the absorption of calcium from the intestine and enhancing renal excretion. Vitamin D deficiency is increasingly being recognized as an important cause of hypocalcaemia in the critically ill, who are often malnourished, chronically ill and deprived of natural sunlight.

Hypoparathyroidism. Primary hypoparathyroidism is rare but secondary hypoparathyroidism is relatively common. Removal of all the parathyroid glands during thyroidectomy or of a single functional parathyroid adenoma during parathyroidectomy, for example, is likely to precipitate hypocalcaemia in the immediate postoperative period. In either event it is advisable to monitor the magnesium concentration as well as the calcium level since both the secretion of PTH and its activity are compromised by hypomagnesaemia.

Table 17.10 Causes of hypocalcaemia

Vitamin D deficiency (nutritional, malabsorption)	Osteomalacia/rickets
Vitamin D resistance	
Increased phosphate levels	Chronic renal failure Phosphate therapy
Drugs	Calcitonin Biphosphonates
Hypoparathyroidism	Surgical (transient, prolonged, permanent) Congenital (DiGeorge syndrome) Idiopathic (autoimmune) Severe hypomagnesaemia Infiltration (e.g. sarcoidosis, metastatic carcinoma, Wilson's disease, haemochromatosis)
Resistance to parathyroid hormone	Pseudohypoparathyroidism
Other	Acute pancreatitis Massive transfusion citrated blood Low plasma albumin Malabsorption (e.g. coeliac disease) Rhabdomyolysis Malignant hyperthermia Severe burns Tumour lysis syndrome

Sequestration of calcium. Hyperphosphataemia may precipitate hypocalcaemia as a result of calcium precipitation and suppression of renal I-hydroxylation of 25 hydroxyvitamin D. Muscle trauma, with sudden and massive release of phosphate from injured cells, caused by, for example, rhabdomyolysis, tumour lysis or malignant hyperthermia, as well as rapid transfusion with citrated blood and severe burns, may also precipitate hypocalcaemia. Sudden sequestration of circulating calcium can also occur in severe pancreatitis as a result of intra-abdominal saponification of fat and in fat embolism syndrome.

Occasionally hypocalcaemia may be due to an activating mutation of the parathyroid calcium receptor. It is important not to confuse this condition with primary hypoparathyroidism since treatment of the former can lead to renal tract calcification.

Clinical presentation
Hypocalcaemia presents with neuromuscular irritability and neuropsychiatric manifestations. General symptoms include *fatigue, irritability* and *anxiety*. Patients may give a history of *circumoral numbness*, peripheral *paraesthesiae* and *cramps*. When the serum calcium falls below 2.0 mmol/l, spontaneous indications of neuromuscular irritability such as *carpopedal spasm* may be observed. In addition, tapping the facial nerve may elicit the typical facial twitch that represents a *positive Chvostek's sign. Trousseau's sign* may be demonstrated by observing paraesthesiae and carpal spasm following inflation of a blood pressure cuff above the systolic pressure for 3 minutes. Characteristically adduction of the thumb precedes flexion of the metacarpophalangeal joints and extension of the interphalangeal joints, which is then followed by flexion of the wrist. Occasionally hypocalcaemia can precipitate *laryngeal spasm*. Some patients develop a *psychosis*. Hypocalcaemia is also a recognized cause of *seizures* and may contribute to the development of *cardiac failure* as well as tachyarrhythmias, bradycardia, *conduction defects* involving delays in ventricular repolarization and lengthening of the QT interval. Severe hypocalcaemia may cause *papilloedema*. Signs and symptoms of hypocalcaemia are notoriously difficult to elicit in critically ill patients, who are frequently intubated, sedated and sometimes paralysed. Calcium levels must therefore be monitored routinely in all patients.

Investigations
The clinical diagnosis can be confirmed by a low serum calcium. Parathormone levels are inappropriately low or absent in hypoparathyroidism but high in other causes of hypocalcaemia. 25-hydroxyvitamin D serum levels are low in vitamin D deficiency. Parathyroid antibodies may be detected in idiopathic hypoparathyroidism.

Management
Continuous ECG monitoring is recommended during intravenous replacement therapy to detect the development of cardiac arrhythmias. In hypocalcaemic tetany 10 mL of 10% (2.25 mmol) calcium gluconate is administered intravenously over 10 minutes. This can be followed by a continuous infusion of 40 mL of 10% (9 mmol) calcium gluconate in 1 litre of 0.9% saline solution daily. The rate of administration should be guided by frequent serum calcium determinations. Hypomagnesaemia should also be corrected by infusing 1–5 mmol of magnesium sulphate over 10 minutes intravenously. Drugs that might exacerbate hypocalcaemia (e.g. furosemide) should be discontinued. Potassium deficiency protects against hypocalcaemic tetany and hypokalaemia should not be corrected without treating the hypocalcaemia.

Once the patient has been stabilized, longer-term maintenance therapy can be achieved with oral or nasogastric calcium supplements (1–2 g of elemental calcium/day) and 1 α-hydroxylated derivatives of vitamin D (e.g. alfalcidol 1–3 μg/day), provided deficiency of vitamin D is confirmed.

PHAEOCHROMOCYTOMA

Phaeochromocytoma is a rare cause of hypertension (< 1 in 1000 cases), although it is recognized that a significant number remain unsuspected clinically and are only diagnosed at postmortem (Sutton *et al.*, 1981).

PATHOLOGY
Phaeochromocytomas arise from chromaffin cells, which are derivatives of neural crest tissue. Approximately 95% of these tumours are found in the abdomen, the vast majority (90%) in the adrenal gland. The most common extra-adrenal sites for phaeochromocytomas lie along the chain of sympathetic ganglia. Around 25% are multiple. A little less than 10% of phaeochromocytomas are malignant, although the presence of a phaeochromocytoma in an unusual location should suggest this possibility. Most tumours release both noradrenaline and adrenaline but large tumours and extra-adrenal tumours produce almost entirely noradrenaline.

CLINICAL FEATURES (Ross and Griffith, 1989)
The clinical features are those of catecholamine excess and are usually, but not invariably, intermittent. The *hypertension* associated with phaeochromocytoma is often sustained but even in these cases there may be marked *paroxysmal* increases in blood pressure. Some patients only develop hypertension during an attack. Other features include *headache, sweating* and *anxiety* with *palpitations* and *diarrhoea*.

Although crises often occur spontaneously, they may be precipitated by certain drugs such as metoclopramide and foods containing tyramine, such as beer. Some wines and cheeses may also precipitate an attack by directly stimulating the release of catecholamines from the tumour. Surgery, labour and delivery, deep palpation of the abdomen or micturition (in those with a bladder tumour) may also initiate an attack. *Hypotension* during a crisis should arouse suspicion of a *reduced cardiac output*, as a result of either catecholamine-induced myocardial damage or ventricular arrhythmias. Other life-threatening complications include *dissecting aneurysm, acute renal failure* and *stroke*.

There are several familial diseases associated with phaeochromocytoma. Multiple endocrine neoplasia (MEN) type 2a, for example, is characterized by medullary carcinoma of the thyroid, hyperparathyroidism and phaeochromocytoma. In patients with these disorders it is important to exclude a phaeochromocytoma before proceeding to parathyroidectomy or thyroid surgery. Other familial associations include neurofibromatosis (5% of patients), von Hippel–Lindau disease and the Sturge–Weber syndrome and familial paraganglioma syndromes.

INVESTIGATIONS (Bouloux and Fakeeh, 1995)

A full blood count may show an increased haematocrit, reflecting the plasma volume contraction caused by constant α-adrenergic stimulation. Glucose tolerance may be impaired. Hypercalcaemia is also a recognized association and may be related to secretion of a PTH-like peptide. The diagnosis is confirmed by directly measuring plasma or urine catecholamine levels or collecting 24 hour urine samples in acid for estimation of free catecholamines and catecholamine metabolites such as metanephrines or vanillylmandelic acid (Sheps *et al.*, 1990). Tumours can be located using CT scanning or magnetic resonance imaging (MRI) in conjunction with venous sampling for catecholamine measurements. Scanning with $[I^{131}]$-metaiodobenzylguanidine (mIBG) produces specific uptake in sites of sympathetic activity. Clonidine suppression and glucagon stimulation tests should only be performed in specialist centres.

MANAGEMENT

During a paroxysmal crisis continuous ECG and invasive blood pressure monitoring is recommended. Administration of *sodium nitroprusside* by infusion or *phentolamine* (1–5 mg boluses intravenously) will usually control the hypertensive surges. Tachycardia may be ameliorated by the simultaneous administration of β-*blocking agents* (e.g. intravenous infusion of esmolol or oral propranolol 80 mg 12-hourly).

There is a significant risk of cardiac arrhythmias, especially numerous premature ventricular contractions, ventricular tachycardia or ventricular fibrillation, particularly in those with pre-existing heart disease. Initial treatment should be with intravenous *lidocaine* as a 100-mg bolus followed by an infusion at 2–4 mg/min. In patients who fail to respond to lidocaine administration, propranolol should be given in a dosage of 2–10 mg intravenously as 1 mg increments every 4–5 min. If α stimulation remains unopposed, β-blockers can paradoxically worsen hypertension during acute episodes and most authorities therefore believe that these agents should not be administered unless the patient has already received an α-blocking drug.

Severe hypotension can complicate acute therapy for a hypertensive crisis. Reducing or discontinuing the hypotensive agent and expansion of the circulating volume is usually all that is required to restore the blood pressure. Treatment with vasoactive drugs such as adrenaline or noradrenaline should be avoided and may be ineffective because of adrenergic receptor downregulation.

Once the acute attack has been controlled, a long-acting α-adrenergic blocking agent such as phenoxybenzamine may be commenced at a dosage of 10 mg daily orally or infused intravenously over 2 hours. The dosage is then increased by 10 mg/day until the usual dose of 1–2 mg/kg daily in four divided doses is reached.

Once the patient has been stabilized on maintenance therapy with phenoxybenzamine and the circulating volume has been restored, further investigations can be undertaken. During the acute hypertensive crisis little consideration is usually given to biochemical confirmation of the diagnosis, although it is of course at this time that catecholamine secretion is at its highest.

Tumours should if possible be removed surgically. Preoperative preparation includes complete α- and β-blockade using phenoxybenzamine (20–80 mg daily initially in divided doses) and then propranolol (120–140 mg daily). The contracted circulating volume should be expanded with blood and colloidal solutions as indicated. Preoperatively phenoxybenzamine is often given as an intravenous infusion in an attempt to reduce the incidence and severity of intraoperative hypotension following exclusion of the tumour. Control of hypertension in the perioperative period is best achieved with sodium nitroprusside.

ADRENAL CRISIS

CAUSES (Table 17.11)

Adrenal crisis is most commonly seen in patients with chronic untreated primary adrenal disease (Oelkers, 1996), although adrenal insufficiency may also be secondary to hypothalamic–pituitary disease. Whatever the cause, adrenal failure may present acutely or when an acute stressful episode, which may be major, such as surgery, or relatively minor, such as gastroenteritis, precipitates rapid decompensation following a period of insidious deterioration. Adrenal failure may also occur when long-term corticosteroid therapy is discontinued (Schlaghecke *et al.*, 1992) and when treated patients fail to increase their glucocorticoid cover during an episode of major stress or illness. Adrenal haemorrhagic infarction due to bacteraemia is now rare except in children with meningococcaemia, although it may occasionally be seen in adults with staphylococcal or Gram-negative infections. Pituitary infarction may be associated with a sudden loss of adrenocorticotrophic hormone (ACTH) secretion and this may also precipitate an adrenal crisis.

Table 17.11 Causes of adrenal crisis

Primary hypoadrenalism	Autoimmune disease (approximately 90% of cases in UK)
	Tuberculosis (less than 10% of cases in UK)
	AIDS-related necrotizing adrenalitis
	Disseminated fungal infections
	Surgical removal
Bilateral haemorrhage/infarction	Meningococcal sepsis
	Venography
	Embolus
	Thrombosis
	Adrenal vein thrombosis
Infiltration	Malignant destruction
	Amyloid
Drugs	Ketoconazole
	Etomidate
	Phenytoin
Schilder's disease (adrenal leukodystrophy)	
Secondary hypoadrenalism	Hypothalamic–pituitary disease
	Pituitary infarction
	Long-term steroid therapy

AIDS, acquired immunodeficiency syndrome.

CLINICAL PRESENTATION

The onset of primary hypoadrenalism is usually insidious with non-specific symptoms such as weakness, fatigue, lassitude, myalgia, anorexia, constipation and weight loss.

Nausea, vomiting, weight loss and *abdominal pain* are prominent in both the primary and secondary forms of acute adrenal insufficiency. *Hypotension, postural changes in blood pressure* and *dehydration* are often most prominent in those with primary adrenal crisis, whereas in secondary hypocortisolism due to hypothalamic–pituitary disease, mineralocorticoid secretion is maintained and signs of volume depletion are minimal. *Hyperpigmentation* due to high circulating levels of ACTH also helps to distinguish primary adrenal disease from hypothalamic–pituitary failure. In the final stages of adrenal apoplexy, *apathy, confusion*, *depression, psychosis, delirium* and even *coma* develop, progressing to *shock* (which is often unresponsive to volume loading and vasopressor agents), *extreme weakness* and, if unrecognized, death. The possibility of adrenocortical insufficiency should be considered in all shocked patients. Fever, abdominal pain and tenderness can mimic an acute abdomen.

LABORATORY INVESTIGATIONS

Typical initial laboratory findings include *hyponatraemia* with a high urinary sodium concentration, *hyperkalaemia* and a mild *metabolic acidosis*. Hyponatraemia is due primarily to a diminished ability to excrete free water rather than mineralocorticoid deficiency. When adrenal failure occurs acutely, however, electrolyte levels may be normal. Fasting *hypoglycaemia* may occur since glucocorticoids are necessary

for gluconeogenesis. Although *hypercalcaemia* may be seen, this is secondary to dehydration and requires no treatment. The blood count may show a mild to moderate normocytic normochromic anaemia with leukocytosis and an eosinophilia. Blood should be taken for basal cortisol and aldosterone estimations. Plasma ACTH is raised in Addison's disease and low in pituitary disease. In a severely ill patient a plasma cortisol less than 275 mmol/L strongly suggests the diagnosis of adrenal insufficiency, whereas when the level is above 550 mmol/L the diagnosis is unlikely. An ACTH stimulation test can be performed later once the patient has recovered. A stimulated rise in serum cortisol to above 600 nmol/L by 30–60 minutes virtually excludes the diagnosis of primary adrenal insufficiency. Depot Synacthen testing has a slightly greater sensitivity for detecting milder degrees of adrenal insufficiency.

Diagnostic imaging (CT scan, MRI) can be used to identify anatomical lesions in the hypothalamic–pituitary–adrenal axis.

MANAGEMENT

Treatment for this life-threatening emergency must be instituted immediately following collection of blood samples for subsequent cortisol determination.

Intravenous hydrocortisone should be given as a 200-mg bolus followed by either an infusion of 200 mg over the next 16 hours or 100 mg intramuscularly every 6 hours. Once the precipitating event has resolved and the diagnosis has been confirmed, corticosteroid doses can be tapered over the following 4–5 days to replacement levels (e.g. oral hydrocortisone 10 mg in the morning, 5 mg at midday and 5 mg in the evening). Specific mineralocorticoid replacement will not be required until later because high-dose hydrocortisone possesses sufficient mineralocorticoid activity. Subsequently *fludrocortisone* replacement can be adjusted depending on postural symptoms, plasma electrolytes and renin activity. A typical dose range is 50–300 μg orally daily. Dexamethasone (4 mg i.v.), which does not significantly interfere with the plasma cortisol assay, is preferred when an ACTH stimulation test is to be performed later.

Fluid replacement should initially be with sodium chloride 0.9%. Usually 2–4 litres will be required over the first 24 hours in patients with primary adrenal insufficiency, especially if vomiting complicates the presentation. In those with hypopituitarism the fluid deficit is less severe and rarely requires replacement with more than 1–2 litres. If the patient is hypoglycaemic, an intravenous bolus of 50 mL of 50% dextrose should be given. Subsequently an infusion of a concentrated dextrose solution may be indicated. Invasive monitoring may be required to guide fluid management. After correction of hypovolaemia the circulation may become hyperdynamic, mimicking septic shock.

RELATIVE OR OCCULT ADRENAL INSUFFICIENCY
(see Chapter 5)

Systemic inflammation initiates reciprocal signalling between the neuroendocrine and peripheral immune system. For example, proinflammatory mediators stimulate the hypothalamic–pituitary–adrenal axis to counterregulate inflammation by synthesis and release of cortisol. It is well established that glucocorticoids modulate the stress response to sepsis by enhancing cardiovascular responsiveness to vasopressors and inhibiting cytokine synthesis in a dose-dependent manner (Sapolsky *et al.*, 2000). The immunological effects of continuously infused low doses of hydrocortisone (240 mg/day) in septic shock have been shown to include inhibition of proinflammatory mediators (reduced circulating levels of interleukin-6, interleukin-8 and plasma nitrate) (Keh *et al.*, 2003), although the anti-inflammatory immune response is also inhibited, with reductions in circulating levels of interleukin-10 and soluble tumour necrosis factor receptors.

Several randomized controlled trials have demonstrated that short-term (1–2 days) administration of high-dose glucocorticoids (up to 40 g of hydrocortisone equivalent per day) in early septic shock is without effect and may even be harmful (Lefering and Neugebauer, 1995), most probably because of immunosuppression and an increased incidence of secondary infection. In contrast, recent randomized controlled trials have indicated that prolonged (5 days or more) administration of 'low'-dose hydrocortisone (240–300 mg/day) in early or late septic shock improves shock reversal (Bollaert *et al.*, 1998; Briegel *et al.*, 1996) and perhaps outcome (Annane *et al.*, 2002). These results are in keeping with the concept that adrenocortical reserve is impaired in septic shock (Briegel *et al.*, 1996; Rothwell *et al.*, 1991; Soni *et al.*, 1995), although it has been reported that shock reversal

and clinical outcome following replacement doses of hydrocortisone are independent of adrenal function (Bollaert *et al.*, 1998). Other studies, however, suggest that the degree of adrenal dysfunction correlates with outcome (Annane *et al.*, 2000) and that hydrocortisone therapy reduces mortality in patients with relative adrenal insufficiency (Annane *et al.*, 2002). More recent evidence has fuelled the controversy surrounding the diagnosis and treatment of relative adrenal insufficiency in shock (see also Chapter 5).

PITUITARY EMERGENCIES

CAUSES

Long-standing pituitary insufficiency with multiple deficiencies may be associated with *pituitary tumours* and their treatment (*surgery or radiotherapy*), *infiltrative diseases* (e.g. granulomas) and *vascular lesions*. *Infective causes* include basal meningitis (e.g. tuberculosis), encephalitis and syphilis. Pituitary failure can also occur following an acute insult such as *postpartum infarction* (Sheehan's syndrome), *haemorrhage* or *infarction* of a *pituitary tumour* or *trauma*. Impairment of the control of vasopressin release from the posterior pituitary, as seen with severe intracranial hypertension following closed head injury, is by far the commonest cause of diabetes insipidus encountered on the ICU (see Chapter 15).

CLINICAL PRESENTATION

In general the symptoms and signs of deficiencies of pituitary-stimulating hormones are the same as those of a primary deficiency of the peripheral endocrine gland (see above).

Patients with hitherto undetected ACTH and TSH deficiency may *decompensate* in response to the stress of infection, trauma, surgery or sedation, particularly when they are currently being given or have recently received steroids. Some patients with pituitary failure present in *coma* preceded by a sudden onset of headache with visual impairment. In these cases the first indication that collapse may be related to an endocrine emergency is often the presence of clinical signs such as hypogonadism, galactorrhoea or characteristic appearances of the skin or hair such as those seen in myxoedema. *Hypothermia* is almost invariable and life-threatening *hypoglycaemia* can occur. Patients with posterior pituitary or hypothalamic diseases sometimes present with *diabetes insipidus*, with thirst, polyuria and nocturia being the main complaints.

INVESTIGATIONS

Once the patient has been resuscitated, a careful history and examination should be followed by baseline measurements of haemoglobin concentration, plasma electrolytes, urine and plasma osmolalities and glucose concentration. Circulating levels of cortisol, prolactin, testosterone, oestradiol, gonadotrophin and growth hormone should be determined for definitive diagnosis. Thyroid function tests will also be required.

MANAGEMENT

Hydrocortisone (100 mg i.v.) should then be given followed by 100 mg intramuscularly 6-hourly (or an i.v. infusion of hydrocortisone at 1–3 mg/h) pending detailed evaluation of the hypothalamopituitary–adrenal axis, including urgent CT scanning, and institution of appropriate replacement therapy with oral corticosteroids, T_4 and desmopressin as indicated.

REFERENCES

Annane D, Sebille V, Troche G, et al. (2000) A 3-level prognostic classification in septic shock based on cortisol levels and cortisol response to corticotrophin. *Journal of the American Medical Association* 283: 1038–1045.

Annane D, Sebille V, Charpentier C, et al. (2002) Effect of treatment with low doses of hydrocortisone and fludrocortisone on mortality in patients with septic shock. *Journal of the American Medical Association* 288: 862–871.

Arem R, Wiener GJ, Kaplan SG, et al. (1993) Reduced tissue thyroid hormone levels in fatal illness. *Metabolism* 42: 1102–1108.

Bilezikian JP (1992) Management of acute hypercalcemia. *New England Journal of Medicine* 326: 1196–1203.

Bollaert PE, Charpentier C, Levy B, et al. (1998) Reversal of late septic shock with supraphysiologic doses of hydrocortisone. *Critical Care Medicine* 26: 645–650.

Bouloux PG, Fakeeh M (1995) Investigation of phaeochromocytoma. *Clinical Endocrinology* 43: 657–664.

Brent GA, Hershman JM (1986) Thyroxine therapy in patients with severe nonthyroidal illnesses and low serum thyroxine concentration. *Journal of Clinical Endocrinology and Metabolism* 63: 1–8.

Briegel J, Schelling G, Haller M, et al. (1996) A comparison of the adrenocortical response during septic shock and after complete recovery. *Intensive Care Medicine* 22: 894–899.

Broadus AE, Mangin M, Ikeda K, et al. (1988) Humoral hypercalcemia of cancer. Identification of a novel parathyroid hormone-like peptide. *New England Journal of Medicine* 319: 556–563.

Brunkhorst FM, Kuhnt E, Engel C, et al. (2005) Intensive insulin therapy in patient with severe sepsis and septic shock is associated with an increased rate of hypoglycaemia-results from a randomised multicenter study (VSEP). *Infection* 33 (Suppl. 1): 19–20.

Burch HB, Wartofsky L (1993) Life-threatening thyrotoxicosis. *Endocrinology and Metabolism Clinics of North America* 22: 263–277.

Burger AG, Philippe J (1992) Thyroid emergencies. *Baillière's Clinical Endocrinology and Metabolism* 6: 77–93.

Chernow B, Burman KD, Johnson DL, et al. (1983) T_3 may be a better agent than T_4 in the critically ill hypothyroid patient: evaluation of transport across the blood–brain barrier in a primate model. *Critical Care Medicine* 11: 99–104.

Davis JR, Heath DA (1989) Comparison of different dose regimes of aminohydroxypropylidene-1,1-bisphosphanate (APD) in hypercalcaemia of malignancy. *British Journal of Clinical Pharmacology* 28: 269–274.

Fein IA, Rackow EC, Sprung CL, et al. (1982) Relation of colloid osmotic pressure to arterial hypoxemia and cerebral edema during crystalloid volume loading of patients with diabetic ketoacidosis. *Annals of Internal Medicine* 96: 570–575.

Fliers E, Wiersinga WM (2003) Myxedema coma. *Reviews in Endocrine and Metabolic Disorders* 4: 137–141.

Fliers E, Guldenaar SE, Wiersinga WM, et al. (1997) Decreased hypothalamic thyrotropin-releasing hormone gene expression in patients with nonthyroidal illness. *Journal of Clinical Endocrinology and Metabolism* 82: 4032–4036.

Foster DW, McGarry JD (1983) The metabolic derangements and treatment of diabetic ketoacidosis. *New England Journal of Medicine* 309: 159–169.

Gale EA (1989) Hypoglycaemia and human insulin. *Lancet* 2: 1264–1266.

Gale EA (2001) The discovery of type 1 diabetes. *Diabetes* 50: 217–226.

Hammond P, Wallis S (1992) Cerebral oedema in diabetic ketoacidosis. *British Medical Journal* 305: 203–204.

Hellman R, Kelly KL, Mason WD (1977) Propranolol for thyroid storm. *New England Journal of Medicine* 297: 671–672.

Hillman K (1987) Fluid resuscitation in diabetic emergencies – a reappraisal. *Intensive Care Medicine* 13: 4–8.

Husband DJ, Thai AC, Alberti KG (1986) Management of diabetes during surgery with glucose-insulin-potassium infusion. *Diabetic Medicine* 3: 69–74.

Jiang Y-Z, Hutchinson KA, Bartelloni P, et al. (2000) Thyroid storm presenting as multiple organ dysfunction syndrome. *Chest* 118: 877–879.

Keh D, Boehnke T, Weber-Cartens S, et al. (2003) Immunologic and hemodynamic effects of 'low dose' hydrocortisone in septic shock. *American Journal of Respiratory and Critical Care Medicine* 167: 512–520.

Lebovitz HE (1995) Diabetic ketoacidosis. *Lancet* 345: 767–772.

Lefering R, Neugebauer EA (1995) Steroid controversy in sepsis and septic shock: a meta-analysis. *Critical Care Medicine* 23: 1294–1303.

Leverve X (2003) Hyperglycemia and oxidative stress: complex relationships with attractive prospects. *Intensive Care Medicine* 29: 511–514.

Lo SS, Tun RY, Hawa M, et al. (1991) Studies of diabetic twins. *Diabetes/Metabolism Reviews* 7: 223–238.

McAnulty GR, Hall GM (2003) Anaesthesia for the diabetic patient. *British Journal of Anaesthesia* 90: 428–429.

McIver B, Gorman CA (1997) Sick euthyroid syndrome: an overview. *Thyroid* 7: 125–132.

Oelkers W (1996) Adrenal insufficiency. *New England Journal of Medicine* 335: 1206–1212.

Oppenheimer JH, Squef R, Surks MI, et al. (1963) Binding of thyroxine by serum proteins evaluated by equilibrium dialysis and electrophoretic techniques. Alterations in nonthyroidal illness. *Journal of Clinical Investigation* 42: 1769–1782.

Peeters RP, Wouters PJ, Kaptein E, et al. (2003) Reduced activation and increased inactivation of thyroid hormone in tissues of critically ill patients. *Journal of Clinical Endocrinology and Metabolism* 88: 3202–3211.

Percival RC, Yates AJ, Gray RE, et al. (1984) Role of glucocorticoids in management of malignant hypercalcaemia. *British Medical Journal* 289: 287.

Philips B, Baker E (2003) Hyperglycaemia and the lung. *British Journal of Anaesthesia* 90: 430–433.

Ringel MD (2001) Management of hypothyroidism and hyperthyroidism in the intensive care unit. *Critical Care Clinics* 17: 59–74.

Ross EJ, Griffith DN (1989) The clinical presentation of phaeochromocytoma. *Quarterly Journal of Medicine* 71: 485–496.

Rothwell PM, Lawler PG (1995) Prediction of outcome in intensive care patients using endocrine parameters. *Critical Care Medicine* 23: 78–83.

Rothwell PM, Udwadia ZF, Lawler PG (1991) Cortisol response to corticotropin and survival in septic shock. *Lancet* 337: 582–583.

Sapolsky RM, Romero LM, Munck AU (2000) How do glucocorticoids influence stress responses? Integrating permissive, suppressive, stimulatory and preparative actions. *Endocrine Reviews* 21: 55–89.

Schlaghecke R, Kornely E, Santen RT, et al. (1992) The effect of long-term glucocorticoid therapy on pituitary–adrenal responses to exogenous corticotrophin-releasing hormone. *New England Journal of Medicine* 326: 226–230.

Sheps SG, Jiang NS, Klee GG, et al. (1990) Recent developments in the diagnosis and treatment of pheochromocytoma. *Mayo Clinic Proceedings* 65: 88–95.

Soni A, Pepper GM, Wyrwinski PM, et al. (1995) Adrenal insufficiency occurring during septic shock: incidence, outcome and relationship to peripheral cytokine levels. *American Journal of Medicine* 98: 266–271.

Sprung CL, Rackow EC, Fein IA (1980) Pulmonary edema: a complication of diabetic ketoacidosis. *Chest* 77: 687–688.

Strewler GJ (2000) The physiology of parathyroid hormone-related protein. *New England Journal of Medicine* 342: 177–185.

Sutton MG, Sheps SG, Lie JT (1981) Prevalence of clinically unsuspected pheochromocytoma. Review of 50 year autopsy series. *Mayo Clinic Proceedings* 56: 354–360.

Van den Berghe G (2000) Euthyroid sick syndrome. *Current Opinion in Anaesthesiology* 13: 89–91.

Van den Berghe G, de Zegher F, Lauwers P (1994) Dopamine and the sick euthyroid syndrome in critical illness. *Clinical Endocrinology* 41: 731–737.

Van den Berghe G, De Zegher F, Veldhuis JD, et al. (1997) Thyrotropin and prolactin release in prolonged critical illness: dynamics of spontaneous secretion and effects of growth hormone-secretagogues. *Clinical Endocrinology* 47: 599–612.

Van den Berghe G, De Zegher F, Baxter RC, et al. (1998) Neuroendocrinology of prolonged critical illness; effects of exogenous thyrotropin-releasing hormone and its combination with growth hormone secretagogues. *Journal of Clinical Endocrinology and Metabolism* **83**: 309–319.

Van den Berghe G, Wouters P, Weekers F, *et al.* (1999) Reactivation of pituitary hormone release and metabolic improvement by infusion of growth hormone-releasing peptide and thyrotropin-releasing hormone in patients with protracted critical illness. *Journal of Clinical Endocrinology and Metabolism* **84**: 1311–1323.

Van den Berghe G, Wouters P, Weekers F, *et al.* (2001) Intensive insulin therapy in the critically ill patients. *New England Journal of Medicine* **345**: 1359–1367.

Van den Berghe G, Baxter RC, Weekers F, *et al.* (2002) The combined administration of GH-releasing peptide-2 (GHRP-2), TRH and GnRH to men with prolonged critical illness evokes superior endocrine and metabolic effects compared to treatment with GHRP-2 alone. *Clinical Endocrinology* **56**: 655–669.

Van den Berghe G, Wouters PJ, Bouillon R, *et al.* (2003) Outcome benefit of intensive insulin therapy in the critically ill: insulin dose versus glycemic control. *Critical Care Medicine* **31**: 359–366.

Van den Berghe G, Wilmer A, Hermans G, *et al.* (2006) Intensive insulin therapy in the medical ICU. *New England Journal of Medicine* **354**: 449–461.

Vanhorebeek I, De Vos R, Mesotten D, *et al.* (2005) Protection of hepatocyte mitochondrial ultrastructure and function by strict blood glucose control with insulin in critically ill patients. *Lancet* **365**: 53–59.

Yamamoto T, Fukuyama J, Fujiyoshi A (1999) Factors associated with mortality of myxedema coma: report of eight cases and literature survey. *Thyroid* **9**: 1167–1174.

18 Obstetric intensive care

Critical illness in the obstetric population may occur coincidentally or as a direct consequence of pregnancy. There are also a variety of emergencies that may involve the pregnant woman, such as trauma (including self harm and domestic violence), haemorrhage, sepsis, cardiopulmonary collapse and pulmonary embolism, as well as numerous medical conditions that carry an increased risk for the pregnant woman and her fetus (e.g. cardiopulmonary disease, diabetes mellitus and sickle-cell disease) (Campbell and Klocke, 2001). Women with life-threatening complications of pregnancy should be managed according to the same principles as any other patient with a similar condition, although some adjustments may be required to accommodate altered maternal physiology and fetal safety: for the majority the outcome is good (Bouvier-Colle, 1996; Hazelgrove *et al.*, 2001; Lewinsohn *et al.*, 1994; Wheatley *et al.*, 1996).

In the UK, reports from Confidential Enquiries into Maternal Deaths in England and Wales (2004; 2007) have recorded the changing pattern of ultimately fatal illnesses complicating pregnancy since a triennial system of reporting began in 1952 (now published by the Royal College of Obstetricians and Gynaecologists and available online from www.cemach.org.uk) (**Fig. 18.1**). Importantly, only a proportion of pregnant women who die in the UK are treated in an intensive care facility. Admission policies and case mix clearly differ from unit to unit (depending on the presence of high-dependency facilities), city to city and country to country (Collop and Sahn, 1993; Hazelgrove *et al.*, 2001; Platteau *et al.*, 1997; Tang *et al.*, 1997) but most admissions to high-dependency or intensive care units (ICUs) are unpredictable and follow postpartum complications such as hypertensive disease of pregnancy and surgery for postpartum major haemorrhage. By way of contrast, many women dying outside critical care facilities suffer cardiopulmonary collapse as a consequence of pulmonary embolism, amniotic fluid embolism (AFE), anaesthetic airway disasters or catastrophic peripartum haemorrhage. Although intensive care is indicated for many of these life-threatening disorders, estimates of the incidence of intensive care admissions vary between 1 and 9 for every 1000 obstetric deliveries (Bouvier-Colle *et al.*, 1996; Confidential Enquiry into Maternal and Child Health, 2004; 2007; Kilpatrick and Matthay, 1992;

Lapinsky *et al.*, 1995; Mabie and Sibai, 1990; Umo-Etuk *et al.*, 1996; Waterstone *et al.*, 2001; Wheatley *et al.*, 1996).

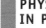 PHYSIOLOGICAL ALTERATIONS IN PREGNANCY

Cardiac output begins to rise in the first trimester and increases progressively to peak at 30–50% above pre-existing levels at 32 weeks' gestation (de Swiet, 1980). This rise in cardiac output is due to increases in both heart rate and stroke volume. *Plasma volume* expands by 40–50%, while red cell mass increases by only 20–30%, producing a dilutional 'physiological anaemia of pregnancy'. The placental bed serves as a large arteriovenous shunt, which reduces total *systemic vascular resistance.* There is also arteriolar vasodilation, which may be related to endothelial release of prostacyclin and nitric oxide (NO), together with increased circulating levels of progesterone.

These changes in cardiac output and systemic vascular resistance are associated with increases in blood flow to the kidneys, the uterus, the breasts and the skin. Mean arterial blood pressure (MAP) falls by 5–15 mmHg during the second trimester, returning to near-normal levels at term.

Similar alterations occur in the *pulmonary circulation*. There is vasodilation with an increased pulmonary blood volume while mean pulmonary artery pressure and pulmonary artery occlusion pressure (PAOP) remain within the normal range. Nevertheless the capacity of the pulmonary circulation to compensate for a further increase in circulating volume is reduced and the pregnant patient therefore has an increased risk of developing pulmonary oedema.

Minute ventilation is increased by 50% during pregnancy and *tidal volume* (V_T) increases to a greater extent than *respiratory rate* (**Table 18.1**). Functional residual capacity (FRC) is decreased by about 20% with a fall in both expiratory reserve volume (ERV) and residual volume (RV). Total lung capacity (TLC) is, however, only marginally reduced. Oxygen consumption ($\dot{V}O_2$) is increased by about 20%, with a further 60% increase during active labour. During late pregnancy mild hypoxaemia may occur, especially when the patient is

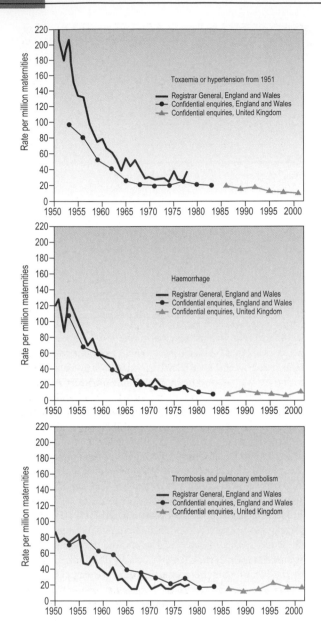

Fig. 18.1 Trends in rates of maternal deaths by leading cause reported to Confidential Enquiries: England and Wales, 1952–1984, UK 1985–2002 and rates of maternal death registered in England and Wales, 1950–1978.

supine, because of the reduction in FRC combined with the increased $\dot{V}o_2$.

SEVERITY-SCORING SYSTEMS IN THE OBSTETRIC POPULATION

Importantly, the physiological range of the variables used when calculating severity scores, and the weighting for deviation from normal, is usually derived from a healthy non-preg-

nant population. Young, previously fit pregnant women have significant physiological reserves which can mask the severity of important life-threatening illnesses, e.g. haemorrhage or infection. The changes in some of these physiological variables in pregnant women (e.g. tachycardia, alterations in pH and changes in haematocrit) could also confound outcome prediction and some have suggested that early warning and severity scoring systems should be developed specifically for pregnant patients (Lapinsky *et al.*, 1997; Scarpinato and Gerber, 1995; Confidential Enquiry into Maternal and Child Health 2007). Others have found, however, that a variety of existing severity of illness scoring systems (e.g. Acute Physiology and Chronic Health Evaluation (APACHE) II, APACHE III and Simplified Acute Physiology Score (SAPS)), accurately reflect the outcome of critically ill obstetric patients (El Solh and Grant, 1996; Hazelgrove *et al.*, 2001).

PRE-ECLAMPSIA

Pre-eclampsia is a condition unique to pregnancy that complicates approximately 2–8% of pregnancies. Eclampsia, which is a complication of severe pre-eclampsia, occurs in approximately 0.04% of deliveries in developed countries, whereas in developing countries estimates of the incidence vary from 1 in 100 to 1 in 1700. Pre-eclampsia and eclampsia are one of the commonest causes of maternal death in developed countries.

DEFINITIONS

Pre-eclampsia is defined as the onset of *hypertension* with *proteinuria* at more than 20 weeks' gestation. Hypertension is defined as a rise in systolic blood pressure of more than 15 mmHg or a blood pressure higher than 140/90 mmHg on more than two occasions 6 hours apart. *Eclampsia* is the occurrence of a *tonic-clonic seizure* in a patient with pre-eclampsia. *Severe pre-eclampsia* is diagnosed in the presence of:

- blood pressure higher than 170 mmHg systolic or 110 mmHg diastolic on two occasions;
- proteinuria greater than 0.5 g/24 hours or 3–4+ on a dipstick;
- cerebral or visual disturbances suggestive of imminent eclampsia.

PATHOPHYSIOLOGY

The pathophysiological changes of pre-eclampsia suggest that organ dysfunction is largely related to reductions in blood flow. Impaired perfusion of the kidney, liver, brain and intervillous spaces of the placenta can be demonstrated, and examination of retinal vessels, nailbeds and conjunctivae provides direct evidence of *vasoconstriction*. This vasoconstriction is accompanied by a *reduced plasma volume* and *activation of the coagulation cascade* (Mushambi *et al.*, 1996). In some cases these changes antedate clinically evident disease by several weeks.

Table 18.1 Respiratory changes in pregnancy

	Non-pregnant	Pregnant (at term)
Total lung capacity (TLC) (mL)	4200	↓ 4000
Tidal volume (V_t) (mL)	450	↑↑ 600
Inspiratory capacity (IC) (mL)	2500	↑ 2650
Expiratory reserve volume (ERV) (mL)	700	↓↓ 550
Residual volume (RV) (mL)	1000	↓↓ 800
Functional residual capacity (FRC) (mL)	1700	↓↓ 1350
Vital capacity (VC) (mL)	3200	→ 3200

Although there is some controversy about the changes in cardiac output in pre-eclampsia, a study of untreated cases found that *cardiac output was low to normal* (Wallenburg, 1988). This finding, in conjunction with documented hypertension, supports the suggestion that *increased systemic vascular resistance* is an important component of the clinical condition. Pre-eclampsia is also accompanied by a *low plasma volume*, with *reduced plasma renin* and *high atrial natriuretic peptide* concentrations (Malee et al., 1992), suggesting that profound vasoconstriction reduces the intravascular capacity. The vasoconstriction and consequent reduction in organ perfusion are possibly secondary to the increased sensitivity to circulating pressor substances observed in women with pre-eclampsia. Severe pre-eclampsia is also associated with abnormal tissue oxygen extraction (Belfort et al., 1993).

At postmortem, histological changes include *cerebral oedema, placental thrombotic lesions, pulmonary oedema* and a wide range of *hepatic abnormalities*. The electron microscopic changes observed in renal and placental vessels of women with pre-eclampsia and eclampsia sometimes reveal enlarged glomerular capillary endothelial cells with electron-dense cytoplasmic inclusions that may occlude the capillary lumen (Spargo et al., 1976). This *glomeruloendotheliosis* supports the concept that pre-eclampsia is a disorder in which generalized vascular endothelial injury plays a central role.

Eclampsia can complicate the severe clinical disorder, but not necessarily very high blood pressure, and is a reflection of neurovascular hyperreactivity. It is usually accompanied by *cerebral oedema* and *intracranial haemorrhages*. One report (Belfort et al., 2002) suggests that elevated cerebral perfusion pressure rather than decreased cerebral blood flow is the primary cause of injury. Increased cerebral perfusion pressure is believed to result in cerebral barotrauma and vasogenic oedema as a consequence of overperfusion.

AETIOLOGY

The aetiology of pre-eclamptic toxaemia (PET) and eclampsia is still poorly understood. Epidemiological data and animal experiments indicate that *impaired placental perfu-*sion, frequently secondary to *abnormal implantation*, is the initiating factor. It is proposed that blood-borne products originating from the poorly perfused fetoplacental unit affect the maternal circulation, primarily by causing vascular endothelial cell dysfunction. In particular *prostacyclin* formation appears to be reduced and there is a relative rise in the circulating concentrations of the vasoconstrictor *thromboxane A_2*. Furthermore there is some evidence to suggest that a systemic disorder of *NO* production may be involved in the aetiology of hypertension and thrombocytopenia in pre-eclampsia (De Belder et al., 1995). Indeed endothelial dysfunction, raised plasma concentrations of asymmetric dimethylarginine (an endogenous inhibitor of endothelial NO synthase) and increased circulating levels of antiangiogenic proteins have been shown to predate the development of pre-eclampsia (Levine et al., 2006; Savvidou et al., 2003). These changes are associated with *endothelial damage, loss of plasma volume, platelet activation, intravascular coagulation* and *diminished organ perfusion*. Vasospasm and microthrombi may then exacerbate the deficient placental perfusion and further disturb endothelial cell function. This autoacceleration of the disorder is compatible with the clinical presentation of pre-eclampsia. It is also suggested that there is an autosomal-recessive *genetic predisposition* to develop such an immune response within the placenta.

CLINICAL PRESENTATION

Although combinations of *headache, hypertension, proteinuria, hyperreflexia* and *oedema* are well recognized, there are other clinical presentations. A significant proportion of all *eclamptic seizures* still occur in hospital and may occur for the first time in the postpartum period. Furthermore a group of patients has been recognized with the constellation of *haemolysis, elevated liver enzymes* and *low platelets* (HELLP syndrome) (Weinstein, 1982). Patients manifesting this syndrome usually present before term (< 36 weeks' gestation) complaining of malaise, epigastric or right upper quadrant pain and nausea or vomiting. Some will have non-specific viral syndrome-like symptoms, while hypertension and proteinuria may be absent or slight (Sibai et al., 1993b). Any pregnant woman presenting with some or all of these

Table 18.2 Guidelines for the postdelivery management of pre-eclampsia and eclampsia

General measures

Prophylaxis against acid aspiration syndrome and venous thromboembolism

Routine analgesia and antiemesis

Mechanical ventilation in selected cases

Control of hypertension

Sympathetic antagonists

Vasodilators
  Hydralazine
  Sodium nitroprusside
  Glyceryl trinitrate

Calcium channel blockers

Prevention of seizures

Magnesium sulphate

Fluid balance

Restrict crystalloids

Careful expansion of circulating volume

Monitor central venous pressure (CVP) and, in selected cases, cardiac output and pulmonary artery occlusion pressure (PAOP)

Diurectics may be indicated (e.g. for pulmonary oedema)

symptoms should have a full blood count with platelet and liver enzyme determinations, irrespective of her blood pressure.

MANAGEMENT
Obstetric management
Peripartum treatment should include:

- control of severe hypertension;
- control of, and prophylaxis against, seizures;   } before delivery
- careful fluid balance.

Once hypertension and seizures are under control, the optimum timing and mode of delivery must be decided.

Management after delivery (Table 18.2)
Pre-eclampsia/eclampsia appears to be one of the most common conditions requiring postpartum admission to an ICU, especially in South Africa. Generally moderate haemodynamic instability is managed antenatally in the delivery unit by the anaesthetic and obstetric staff. Once the patient has delivered, however, the specialized services associated with fetal assessment and delivery are no longer the priority (Kilpatrick and Matthay, 1992).

Any patient with severe pre-eclampsia/eclampsia who has undergone caesarean section should be returned to a high-dependency unit or ICU. The need for mechanical ventilation is determined by the patient's mental state, and level of irritability, as well as the dosage of antihypertensives required. Sedation and analgesia are generally maintained with continuous infusions of an opiate and a benzodiazepine. Lateralizing signs or continued irritability post caesarean section are an indication for computed tomography (CT) scanning or magnetic resonance imaging (MRI).

CONTROL OF HYPERTENSION
It is recommended that postnatal patients are routinely admitted for high-dependency care if they require intravenous antihypertensive medication by infusion. It is increasingly accepted that such therapy should be monitored by indwelling intra-arterial and central venous cannulae as in the non-pregnant population. Modest systolic hypertension and oliguria with documented high urinary osmolality may be tolerated in the early postpartum period. It is, however, advisable to treat systolic blood pressure greater than 160 mmHg and diastolic blood pressures higher than 110 mmHg to minimize the risk of intracranial haemorrhage. Crystalloid solutions should be restricted to, for example, 1.2 L/day and colloids should be administered if there is oliguria (< 0.5 mL/kg per hour) associated with low cardiac filling pressures. A spontaneous diuresis heralds resolution of the condition. Indications for a pulmonary artery flotation catheter have included pulmonary oedema, persistent profound oliguria (< 0.5 mL/kg per hour) despite fluid challenge and life-threatening uncontrollable hypertension. In some cases alternative means of monitoring cardiac output may be indicated.

Sympathetic antagonists. Labetalol has been suggested as a suitable agent for the control of hypertension associated with pre-eclampsia. Chronic use of oral labetalol and intravenous administration of labetalol to women with pre-eclampsia have been shown not to decrease interplacental blood flow, despite producing significant falls in blood pressure (Jouppila *et al.*, 1986). One difficulty with the use of labetalol in severe pre-eclampsia, however, is its variable efficacy. Whereas in some reports a diastolic blood pressure of less than 100 mmHg was easily achieved (Mabie *et al.*, 1987), in others pressure control proved difficult (Ashe *et al.*, 1987). In the former study labetalol was administered as increasing boluses from 20 to 80 mg, while in the latter it was administered as a continuous infusion to a maximum of 160 mg/h. A more recent study has demonstrated the safety and efficacy of labetalol in the initial treatment of severe hypertension of pregnancy (Elatrous *et al.*, 2002).

Vasodilators (see Chapter 5). Hydralazine is widely used in the acute treatment of pre-eclampsia, despite the observation that in many antenatal patients it causes significant fetal distress (Mabie *et al.*, 1987). This can apparently be prevented by prior infusion of colloid (Paterson-Brown *et al.*,

Table 18.3 Guidelines for intravenous magnesium sulphate dosage in the management of pre-eclampsia and eclampsia

1 Give a loading dose of 4 g magnesium sulphate (equivalent to 16.3 mmol Mg^{2+}) intravenously over 5–10 minutes during eclamptic seizures or over 10–15 minutes for seizure prophylaxis

2 Start a continuous intravenous infusion of magnesium sulphate at the rate of 1 g/h (4 mmol/h) and continue the infusion for 24 h after delivery or after the last seizure

3 If convulsions persist, give 2 g magnesium sulphate intravenously over 5–10 minutes

4 Examine carefully every 30 minutes for the presence of limb reflexes, respiration rate of at least 16 breaths/min and urinary output of at least 25 mL/h. If reflexes are slow, urinary output diminished (100 mL in 4 hours) and respiratory rate diminished with the mother well oxygenated, halve the magnesium sulphate infusion. Measure serum magnesium concentrations if possible

Normal range	0.75–1.25 mmol/L
Effective anticonvulsant	2–3.5 mmol/L
Reflexes disappear	5.00 mmol/L
Respiratory depression	7.50 mmol/L
Cardiac arrest	15.00 mmol/L

If reflexes are absent, respiration depressed, urinary output inadequate or if serum magnesium is within an elevated or dangerous range, discontinue the magnesium sulphate infusion. In the event of cardiorespiratory arrest give 10 mL of 10% calcium gluconate intravenously slowly over 10 minutes in addition to advanced life support

5 Magnesium sulphate may enhance the action of non-depolarizing muscle relaxants. Anaesthetists and paediatricians must be told that the drug is being used. The magnesium ion crosses the placenta and may affect the newborn

1994). Although its use is therefore not without hazard, the risks can be minimized by ensuring an adequate circulatory volume and careful dosing to achieve a MAP less than 125 mmHg.

Sodium nitroprusside (SNP) is an extremely potent dilator of both the resistance and capacitance blood vessels and is administered by continuous infusion. Because of its rapid onset of action and short half-life, continuous intra-arterial blood pressure monitoring is essential. Experience with the use of SNP in the antenatal period is limited and there is concern that the capacity of the fetus to metabolize cyanide may be limited by relative immaturity of the hepatic enzyme systems. Nevertheless there have been a few case reports describing the use of SNP in severe pre-eclampsia complicated by pulmonary oedema. In four early cases reported by Stempel *et al.* (1982), SNP produced a marked decline in PAOP that paralleled the decrease in MAP. Three of these patients had

previously failed to respond to hydralazine. Cyanide was undetectable in blood samples obtained from one neonate and two mothers. When used carefully SNP appears to be a safe and effective hypotensive agent in resistant or complicated cases of severe pre-eclampisa. Because of the precarious state of hydration in these patients the infusion should be started at a very low dose (e.g. 0.25 μg/kg per min).

Glyceryl trinitrate (GTN) is also a suitable agent for controlling blood pressure in pre-eclampsia complicated by pulmonary oedema, although its efficacy may be limited in the well-hydrated patient. Like SNP, its rapid onset and short duration of action allow titration of a continuous infusion to achieve the desired blood pressure. Intra-arterial pressure monitoring is required. Early clinical reports of the use of GTN in severe pre-eclampsia were limited to small studies (Cotton *et al.*, 1986a).

As well as the fetal distress that can complicate excessive iatrogenic reductions in blood pressure, there are specific concerns about the potential of vasodilators to exacerbate intracranial hypertension. Nevertheless in view of the possible role of NO deficiency in the aetiology of pre-eclampsia, both GTN and SNP, being NO donors, may have a limited but important role in the more severe cases, especially those with pulmonary oedema.

Calcium channel blockers. These agents have a number of advantages as antihypertensive agents. They are easily administered in oral form but can also be administered intravenously (Elatrous *et al.*, 2002), and have a rapid onset of action with a duration of 3–5 hours. The ensuing reduction in MAP is proportional to the baseline blood pressure and serious hypotension is therefore rare. These agents also dilate the coronary vasculature and may improve subendocardial myocardial perfusion.

Diuretics. In the past diuretics were widely prescribed to control the physiological oedema of pregnancy; it was thought that these agents might also reduce the incidence of pre-eclampsia. It is now appreciated, however, that since the circulating volume is contracted in pre-eclampsia, diuretic therapy is contraindicated. Occasionally diuretic therapy is required for the treatment of specific complications such as pulmonary oedema, in which case the agent of choice is parenteral furosemide.

Steroids. There is some evidence to suggest that steroids (two doses of dexamethasone 10 mg 12 hours apart followed by 5 mg at 24 and 36 hours) may be beneficial when given to women with HELLP syndrome both before and after delivery (Clenney and Viera, 2004).

PREVENTION OF SEIZURES

In 1990 a report from South Africa suggested that *magnesium sulphate* is more effective than phenytoin for preventing seizures in eclampsia (Dommisse, 1990), a finding confirmed by a later landmark clinical study (Eclampsia Trial Collaborative Group, 1995). Magnesium sulphate had for some time been popular in North America (Pritchard *et al.*, 1984) and South Africa (Richards *et al.*, 1986), despite the risk of neuromuscular toxicity leading to respiratory arrest. It was suggested that the likelihood of this complication could be minimized by titrating the dose according to physical signs and that administration should be discontinued if there was oliguria or an absent patellar reflex.

Despite the fact that the mode of action of magnesium sulphate remains obscure, the results of the Eclampsia Trial Collaborative Group (1995) prompted speculation about whether the drug might also prevent the development of eclampsia in women with pre-eclampsia. The Magpie Trial (Altman *et al.*, 2002), which involved 10 141 women with pre-eclampsia in 175 hospitals in 33 countries over $3^1/_2$ years, has demonstrated beyond reasonable doubt that magnesium sulphate reduces the risk of eclampsia among women with pre-eclampsia, as well as controlling eclamptic convulsions should they occur. In this respect it has also been demonstrated that parenterally administered magnesium sulphate is significantly better than oral nimodipine at preventing eclamptic seizures in women with severe pre-eclampsia, especially in the postpartum period (Belfort *et al.*, 2003). Guidelines for the intravenous use of magnesium sulphate based on the study regimen are provided in **Table 18.3**.

FLUID BALANCE

Currently treatment usually involves a combination of volume expansion and vasodilators. Judicious volume replacement has been shown to increase cardiac output and oxygen delivery, as well as to reduce systemic vascular resistance (Cotton *et al.*, 1986b). Vasodilation in the face of hypovolaemia may precipitate hypotension and fetal distress. On the other hand, severe pre-eclampsia may be complicated by cerebral oedema, and cardiogenic or non-cardiogenic pulmonary oedema. In the more severe cases, central venous pressure (CVP) monitoring can be misleading as there may be significant disparity in the function of the left and right ventricles (Cotton *et al.*, 1985; Mabie *et al.*, 1989). Pulmonary artery catheterization may occasionally be warranted in such cases. Standardization of measured or estimated cardiac output to body surface area (i.e. calculating cardiac index), however, appears to be hampered by the poor correlation between cardiac output and body surface area in pregnancy (van Oppen *et al.*, 1995).

Complications

HAEMORRHAGE

A ruptured liver, intra-adrenal haemorrhage, life-threatening coagulopathy or rupture of a congenital intracerebral aneurysm are all possible life-threatening sequelae to pre-eclampsia.

ECLAMPSIA (Douglas and Redman, 1994)

Should a patient have a seizure, the airway must be protected, oxygenation maintained and the seizure terminated with the intravenous administration of magnesium sulphate. In complicated cases elective tracheal intubation and mechanical ventilation may be indicated so that anticonvulsants can be administered freely without the risk of respiratory depression or pulmonary aspiration and to control intracranial hypertension (Richards *et al.*, 1986) (see Chapter 15). As well as the immediate control of convulsions it is important that raised blood pressure is treated promptly. Management protocols should reflect the need to avoid very high systolic blood pressures and the associated risk of intracerebral haemorrhage. Many consider that the optimal MAP in obstetric patients with suspected cerebral oedema complicating severe pre-eclampsia/eclampsia is 80–100 mmHg. In those who develop eclampsia, optimal timing of the delivery of the baby is a priority following control of hypertension and seizures.

CEREBRAL ISCHAEMIA

The successful administration of nimodipine, a calcium channel blocker with specific cerebral vasodilator activity, to a moribund patient with eclampsia suggested that cerebral ischaemia in eclampsia is secondary to vasospasm (Duncan *et al.*, 1989; Lewis *et al.*, 1988). An alternative view is that elevated intracranial pressure, which is exacerbated by nimodipine but decreased by magnesium sulphate, is the primary cause of cerebral injury (Belfort *et al.*, 2002). In this regard it has been shown that oral nimodipine is no more effective than parenteral magnesium sulphate in preventing eclampsia (Belfort *et al.*, 2003).

ACUTE LUNG INJURY/ACUTE RESPIRATORY DISTRESS SYNDROME (see Chapter 8)

Acute respiratory distress syndrome (ARDS) remains a frequent mode of death in patients with hypertensive disorders of pregnancy, although severe acute lung injury (ALI) rarely complicates pre-eclampsia unless there are other complications such as coagulopathy, issues of fluid overload or pulmonary aspiration of gastric content.

ACUTE RENAL FAILURE (see Chapter 13)

Acute renal failure is now rare, but may complicate the HELLP syndrome (Drakeley *et al.*, 2002).

Prevention

The observation that pre-eclampsia is associated with endothelial damage (Roberts and Redman, 1993) accompanied by increased thromboxane concentrations and low prostacyclin levels provided a rationale for aspirin prophylaxis. Anecdotal reports were followed by two large trials (Italian Study of Aspirin in Pregnancy, 1993; Sibai *et al.*, 1993a) that failed to confirm efficacy, although both differed from earlier studies in that lower-risk women were recruited. Subsequently the large Collaborative Low-dose Aspirin Study in Pregnancy (CLASP) study also indicated that routine prophylactic low-dose aspirin (60 mg/day) is not effective in women at risk for pre-eclampsia or intrauterine growth retardation (CLASP Collaborative Group, 1994). A recent meta-analysis, however, suggested that the use of antiplatelet agents during pregnancy is associated with moderate but consistent reductions in the relative risk of pre-eclampsia, of birth before 34 weeks' gestation and of having a pregnancy with a serious adverse outcome (Askie *et al.*, 2007). Currently only the Magpie trial has shown efficacy in reducing the risk of eclampsia in women with pre-eclampsia and it now seems likely that magnesium sulphate also reduces the risk of maternal death.

DIFFERENTIAL DIAGNOSIS

Should the blood pressure prove refractory to antihypertensive therapy, including intravenous treatment, other causes of hypertension such as phaeochromocytoma should be considered.

OUTCOME

Pre-eclampsia contributes to 10% of maternal deaths in the UK and the HELLP syndrome carries a 1–4% mortality. Women should be counselled about the risk of recurrent pre-eclampsia and the HELLP syndrome affecting future pregnancies.

ACUTE LUNG INJURY/ACUTE RESPIRATORY DISTRESS SYNDROME IN OBSTETRIC PATIENTS (see Chapters 7 and 8)

In critically ill obstetric patients, ALI/ARDS may follow:

- amniotic fluid embolism;
- hypertensive disorders of pregnancy;
- haemorrhage, including placental abruption;
- dead-fetus syndrome;
- sepsis, including pneumonia;
- inhalation of gastric contents;
- β-adrenergic agonist therapy with or without corticosteroids for premature labour.

The incidence of ALI/ARDS complicating pregnancy appears to have increased. This may be due partly to its more frequent recognition by pathologists and partly to patients surviving longer, thereby allowing time for the disease to become established.

ASPIRATION OF GASTRIC CONTENTS DURING ANAESTHESIA

Although in the early Confidential Enquiries the proportion of deaths directly attributable to anaesthesia was small, their incidence remained disappointingly constant, and complications related to anaesthesia were a common cause of maternal death in the UK. These anaesthetic-related deaths were frequently a consequence of pneumonitis due to pulmonary aspiration of acidic gastric contents (Mendelson's syndrome) (Mendelson, 1946), and continued despite the widespread administration of antacids before delivery.

Pathogenesis

The severity of aspiration pneumonitis depends on the acidity of the gastric contents as well as the volume aspirated (see Chapter 8). In Mendelson's original series, women died from asphyxia, not from the aspiration pneumonitis that now carries his name. The increased lethality of this condition compared to Mendelson's original observations (Mendelson, 1946) may be due to the widespread practice of instituting intermittent positive-pressure ventilation in such cases. This may only serve to disseminate inhaled gastric contents throughout the lung, thereby enlarging the acid burn to the alveolar–capillary membrane. Moreover, the free and liberal administration of crystalloid solutions, either as an adjunct to epidural analgesia or as a nutritional supplement during labour, combined with the routine administration of ergometrine or Syntometrine, both of which are pulmonary vasoconstrictors, may exacerbate oedema formation.

Aspiration pneumonitis is associated with hypoxia and hypovolaemia, which may precipitate splanchnic vasoconstriction, exacerbate generalized tissue hypoxia and trigger the release of inflammatory mediators. Patients are therefore at risk of developing primary multiple-organ dysfunction syndrome (MODS), the systemic inflammatory response syndrome (SIRS) and eventually secondary MODS (see Chapter 5). The combination of a chemical burn to the alveolar–capillary membrane and a disseminated inflammatory response frequently leads to the development of ALI/ARDS.

Management

The management of pulmonary aspiration in obstetric patients should be the same as for the non-pregnant population. The airway must be secured and cleared of debris; this may require *bronchoscopy*, but bronchoalveolar lavage is not recommended. Appropriate *respiratory support* should be instituted (see Chapter 7), and in the most severe cases the use of *extracorporeal gas exchange* should be considered. *Steroid* administration is not thought to be of any benefit in aspiration pneumonitis. Insertion of an *oesophageal Doppler* probe, or less frequently *pulmonary artery catheterization* may be indicated to guide volume administration and haemodynamic support.

Prevention

Various studies discredited the particulate antacid magnesium trisilicate as effective prophylaxis against the consequences of aspirating gastric contents. A regimen involving the regular prescription of oral ranitidine (150 mg 6-hourly) together with the administration of 30 mL 0.3 M sodium citrate was shown to be an effective means of controlling the acidity and volume of the gastric contents (Gillett *et al.*, 1984). Results from national surveys revealed that routine prophylaxis in the UK generally consists of such a combination of H_2-receptor blockade (e.g. ranitidine) and a nonparticulate antacid (e.g. 0.3 M sodium citrate) (Greiff *et al.*, 1994; Tordoff and Sweeney, 1990). Organizational changes prompted by the recommendations of the Confidential Enquiries mean that unsupervised junior staff should no longer undertake anaesthesia for caesarean section without adequate training and skilled assistance. The importance of correctly applied cricoid pressure and a rehearsed failed intubation drill have been emphasized repeatedly in successive reports. There has also been a trend for the increased use of regional techniques for operative delivery.

AMNIOTIC FLUID EMBOLISM (AFE)

AFE is a rare but catastrophic complication of pregnancy. Although the number of maternal deaths due to AFE has fallen significantly over the last decade in the UK, the condition remains unpredictable, unpreventable and is rapidly progressive but not now universally fatal. The incidence of AFE has been estimated at between 1/8000 and 1/80000 deliveries.

Risk factors

Risk factors for AFE include:

- increasing maternal age;
- obstetric interventions, e.g. amniocentesis and medical induction of labour (Kramer *et al.*, 2006);
- women of high parity;
- strong uterine contractions.

Pathogenesis

Conventionally, the cardiorespiratory complications of AFE were thought to be a consequence of acute right-sided heart failure secondary to severe pulmonary hypertension following occlusion of, or vasospastic changes in, the pulmonary vasculature. This explanation has been questioned, however (Clark, 1990). In contrast to observations in experimental models, a review of published cases of AFE in humans has revealed only mild to moderate elevations in pulmonary artery pressure, variable increases in CVP, elevated PAOP and evidence of left ventricular dysfunction or failure (Clark *et al.*, 1985). Although the cause of the left ventricular failure remains obscure, it is the only significant haemodynamic abnormality that has been consistently documented in patients with AFE.

To reconcile these experimental and clinical findings, Clark (1990) postulates a biphasic pattern of cardiorespiratory disturbance. The initial response of the pulmonary vasculature to the presence of amniotic fluid is perhaps vasospasm, which produces transient pulmonary hypertension and profound hypoxia. This initial period of hypoxia might account for the approximately 50% of patients who succumb to AFE within the first hour after the onset of symptoms. The transient nature of this initial haemodynamic response could also account for the failure of subsequent invasive monitoring to document significant pulmonary hypertension. Those patients who survive this initial phase may experience a secondary phase of haemodynamic compromise, which involves left heart failure with right heart function returning to normal. While such a biphasic course is an attractive explanation, it must be recognized that the existence of the initial phase of transient pulmonary vasospasm in humans is speculative.

Some no longer consider the identification of fetal squames in the pulmonary vasculature (Plauche, 1983) to be pathognomonic for AFE. Some fetal squames probably normally enter the venous circulation of pregnant women, raising the possibility that it is only *abnormal* amniotic fluid or other fetal elements such as lanugo hair, mucin from meconium and fat from vernix caseosa that causes the clinical syndrome of AFE. Intriguingly, metabolites of arachidonic acid can produce many of the haemodynamic and haematological effects found in patients with clinical AFE. Such metabolites, including the prostaglandins and leukotrienes, are present in amniotic fluid in increasing concentrations during labour (Karim and Devlin, 1967).

Clinical features

AFE presents as a sudden life-threatening collapse with *respiratory distress, cyanosis, restlessness and altered behaviour, hypotension* and *hypoxia* (Steiner and Lushbaugh, 1941). This may progress rapidly to *refractory cardiorespiratory arrest*. Of those who survive the initial cardiovascular and respiratory insults, 45% will develop *life-threatening coagulopathy* within the next 4 hours, which may be compounded by *uterine atony*. Almost three-quarters of those who survive the initial haemodynamic collapse will develop a secondary *non-cardiogenic pulmonary oedema* (Koegler *et al.*, 1994) due to increased alveolar–capillary permeability. Patients surviving to receive invasive haemodynamic monitoring generally demonstrate *left ventricular dysfunction* or failure accompanied by moderate or severe elevations in PAOP and depressed left ventricular contractility (Vanmaele *et al.*, 1990). Superimposed *renal failure* worsens the prognosis.

Diagnosis

The diagnosis of AFE must be made on the basis of clinical presentation and supportive laboratory studies. There is no single clinical or laboratory finding that by itself can confirm or exclude AFE, even though fetal squamous cells may be detected in samples of pulmonary capillary blood (Masson and Ruggieri, 1985). At autopsy cells or debris may also be found in the pulmonary artery vasculature. Modern immunocytochemical techniques are now more sensitive than standard histochemical methods and it is recommended that maternal lung sections should be probed with cytokeratin markers when the clinical diagnosis of AFE has been suspected.

Laboratory abnormalities include coagulopathy (decreased fibrinogen and elevated levels of fibrin split products, prolonged partial thromboplastin and prothrombin times) and thrombocytopenia. It must be emphasized that not all these coagulation abnormalities will be present in every case (Quinn and Barrett, 1993).

The differential diagnosis of AFE includes:

- septic shock;
- aspiration pneumonia;
- acute myocardial infarction;
- pulmonary thromboembolism;
- placental abruption;
- air embolism;

- disseminated intravascular coagulation;
- thrombotic thrombocytopenic purpura.

History and examination should be supplemented with a 12-lead electrocardiogram (ECG) and chest radiograph. A right ventricular strain pattern on the ECG and perihilar infiltrates on the chest radiograph are suggestive, but not diagnostic. The onset of a haemorrhagic phase manifest by bleeding from venepuncture sites or surgical incisions is, however, strongly suggestive of AFE in these circumstances.

Management

In addition to normal resuscitative measures, mechanical ventilation and the administration of pressor agents are central to the acute management of AFE. Management of the coagulopathy associated with AFE should include replacement of the circulating blood volume as well as administration of platelets and clotting factors as indicated (Quinn and Barrett, 1993). Some have speculated that *cryoprecipitate* may be particularly beneficial in AFE. This plasma fraction contains not only significant levels of fibrinogen and other clotting factors, but also high concentrations of fibronectin. The latter facilitates clearance of cellular and particulate matter from the circulation by the reticuloendothelial system and might therefore improve outcome from AFE.

A report of successful management of AFE syndrome with *continuous haemofiltration* (see Chapter 13) raises the possibility that this technique can effectively remove substances that might play an important role in the genesis of left ventricular and respiratory dysfunction (Weksler *et al.*, 1994).

Prognosis

The overall mortality may be greater than 80%, and even in those patients who survive the initial cardiorespiratory events and subsequent multisystem organ dysfunction, the initial hypoxaemia may have caused irreversible damage to the maternal central nervous system.

THE AMNIOTIC FLUID EMBOLISM REGISTER

A confidential register of all cases of AFE is being established for the UK. The aim is to identify features commonly associated with survival or death, in the hope that these will suggest interventions which might help to improve survival.

Criteria for inclusion in the register are:

- acute hypotension or cardiac arrest;
- acute hypoxia (dyspnoea, cyanosis or respiratory arrest);
- coagulopathy (laboratory evidence of intravascular coagulation or severe haemorrhage);
- no other clinical condition or potential explanation for the symptoms and signs;
- a pathological diagnosis (presence of fetal squames or hair in the lungs).

All cases of suspected or proven AFE in the UK should be reported to the UK Obstetric Surveillance System (www.npeu.ox.ac.uk/ukoss).

PERIPARTUM CARDIOMYOPATHY
(de Beus *et al.*, 2003)

This is a rare cause of cardiac failure occurring late in pregnancy or in the postpartum period. Overall mortality rates vary between 25 and 50%, with nearly half of the deaths occurring in the first 3 months after delivery. In about 50% of patients cardiomegaly and left ventricular dysfunction have resolved at 6 months postpartum and the prognosis is favourable. Conversely, mortality may be as high as 85% amongst those in whom abnormalities persist at 6 months.

ACUTE COAGULOPATHY IN PREGNANCY

COAGULATION IN PREGNANCY

Although blood loss after placental separation is controlled primarily by arterial constriction, the deposition of a fibrin mesh over the placental site is also important. In anticipation of this requirement, levels of factor VII, IX and X increase throughout pregnancy and the fibrinogen level at term is almost twice that in the non-pregnant state. Fibrin deposition occurs in the placental matrix and the walls of the spiral arteries. Systemic fibrinolytic activity is not, however, increased, tissue plasminogen activator is not found in the placenta (Letsky, 1989) and plasma fibrinolytic activity is reduced in mid and late pregnancy. Pregnancy is therefore associated with a *procoagulant* state. The risk of thrombosis is increased in pregnancy and prophylaxis against deep venous thrombosis must be commenced at the earliest safe opportunity (www.cemach.org.uk).

COAGULATION FAILURE IN PREGNANCY

Endothelial damage unites the intravascular coagulation factors with their extravascular activators: the resultant fibrin formation is normally localized to the site of damage. If coagulation activators enter the circulation, however, uncontrolled fibrin deposition may lead to *disseminated intravascular coagulation* (DIC) (see Chapter 5). Placental tissue is rich in thromboplastin, and amniotic fluid is a devastatingly effective activator of coagulation that can produce DIC of sudden onset and life-threatening severity. By comparison, slow release of thromboplastic substances into the circulation occurs in conditions such as missed abortion or mild pre-eclampsia. Some other causes of coagulopathy such as hypovolaemia and incompatible transfusion are not exclusive to pregnancy. Complications of pregnancy such as placenta praevia, placental abruption, uterine rupture, and vaginal or perineal tears may be complicated by massive blood loss (defined as replacement of the whole blood volume within 24 hours or more than half the blood volume within 1 hour). Large-volume blood transfusion (> 4–5 litres) may exacerbate coagulopathy by haemodilution.

It is thought that thrombocytopenia in pre-eclampsia is a form of microangiopathic haemolytic anaemia, as diagnosed by the presence of fragmented red blood cells in the blood film, anaemia and increased serum haptoglobins or lactic dehydrogenase. This differs from DIC in that the primary defect is endothelial damage with resulting adhesion and aggregation of platelets, thrombin formation and secondary activation of the clotting cascade. Haemolysis (as in the HELLP syndrome) is caused by distortion of red cells as they pass through thrombosed blood vessels.

DIAGNOSIS OF COAGULATION FAILURE

Haemorrhage in the case of DIC may be localized to sites of tissue injury (venepunctures, intravenous and epidural cannulation sites, uterus and perineum) or may be generalized with bruising, epistaxis, haematemesis and intracranial haemorrhage.

When coagulopathy is suspected, blood should be obtained for coagulation tests, including prothrombin time, activated partial thromboplastin time, fibrinogen and fibrin split products, together with samples for a full blood count and cross-matching. A fresh venepuncture should always be used for tests of coagulation. The diagnosis of DIC is based on laboratory findings including thrombocytopenia (platelet count below 100×10^9/L), marked hypofibrinogenaemia and the presence of fibrin split products. Consultant haematologists should be involved in the care of women with coagulopathy.

Treatment of coagulation failure
GENERAL MEASURES
Treatment priorities for the bleeding pregnant woman are the same as for the non-pregnant patient, always keeping in mind the normal physiological changes of pregnancy, including the increased tissue oxygen demands of the fetoplacental unit. *The best therapy for the fetus is rapid and effective resuscitation of the mother.*

ANTEPARTUM COAGULOPATHY
DIC is always secondary to an underlying cause. If DIC is directly attributable to the gravid uterus as in pre-eclampsia, placental abruption or intrauterine death, then evacuation of the uterus and delivery of the fetus are indicated.

POSTPARTUM HAEMORRHAGE (Drife, 1997)
Resuscitation from life-threatening postpartum bleeding must be accompanied by definitive measures to control haemorrhage. Such treatment may include infusing oxytocics and intramyometrial prostaglandins together with attempts at surgical control of the haemorrhage. Early hysterectomy or internal iliac artery ligation or embolization can be life-saving in extreme cases.

SPECIFIC MANAGEMENT OF DIC
If DIC is severe enough to cause bleeding or if there is coagulation failure due to massive haemorrhage, replacement of the depleted coagulation components will be necessary following discussion with the haematology department.

Fresh frozen plasma (FFP). This plasma fraction is a source of coagulation factors but does not contain platelets. FFP does not require cross-match, but ABO compatibility is desirable to avoid transfusion of ABO antibodies. FFP is never indicated solely for volume replacement.

Platelet concentrates. Platelet concentrates do not require cross-match. They should be transfused as soon as they are received; their viability is greatly reduced by sedimentation and cooling. Platelets do not carry the rhesus (D) (Rh(D)) antigen but, because of the possibility of red cell contamination of the concentrate, the administration of Rh(D)-positive platelets to a Rh(D)-negative obstetric patient should be followed by prophylactic injection of anti-D. In the presence of bleeding platelet concentrates should be given to maintain a platelet count of greater than 50×10^9/L. Platelet transfusion may also be required prior to operative intervention.

Cryoprecipitate. This blood product contains almost all the factor VIII of one donor unit of blood in plasma and may be useful in the treatment of coagulation failure complicated by severe hypofibrinogenaemia (< 1.5 g/L). As with FFP, crycoprecipitate may contain red cells and when necessary should be followed by prophylactic anti-D therapy.

Blood product therapy should be given immediately and rapidly. The coagulation profile and platelet count are then repeated to ascertain the response and the need for further therapy.

REFERENCES

Altman D, Carroli G, Duley L, *et al.* (2002) Do women with pre-eclampsia and their babies benefit from magnesium sulphate? The Magpie trial: a randomised placebo-controlled trial. *Lancet* **359**: 1877–1890.

Ashe RG, Moodley J, Richards AM, *et al.* (1987) Comparison of labetalol and dihydralazine in hypertensive emergencies of pregnancy. *South African Medical Journal* **71**: 354–356.

Askie LM, Daley L, Henderson-Smart DJ, *et al.* (2007) Antiplatelet agents for prevention of

pre-eclampsia: a meta-analysis of individual patient data. *Lancet* **369**: 1791–1798.

Belfort MA, Anthony J, Saade GR, *et al.* (1993) The oxygen consumption/oxygen delivery curve in severe preeclampsia: evidence for a fixed oxygen extraction state. *American Journal of Obstetrics and Gynecology* **169**: 1448–1455.

Belfort MA, Varner MW, Dizon-Townson DS, *et al.* (2002) Cerebral perfusion pressure and not cerebral blood flow may be the critical determinant of intracranial injury in pre-

eclampsia: a new hypothesis. *American Journal of Obstetrics and Gynecology* **187**: 626–634.

Belfort MA, Anthony J, Saade GR, *et al.* (2003) A comparison of magnesium sulfate and nimodipine for the prevention of eclampsia. *New England Journal of Medicine* **348**: 304–311.

Bouvier-Colle MH, Salanave B, Ancel PY, *et al.* (1996) Obstetric patients treated in intensive care units and mortality. *European Journal of*

Obstetrics, Gynecology and Reproductive Biology **65**: 121–125.

Campbell LA, Klocke RA (2001) Update in nonpulmonary critical care: implications for the pregnant patient. *American Journal of Respiratory and Critical Care Medicine* **163**: 1051–1054.

Clark SL (1990) New concepts of amniotic fluid embolism: a review. *Obstetrical and Gynecological Survey* **45**: 360–368.

Clark SL, Montz FJ, Phelan JP (1985) Hemodynamic alterations associated with amniotic fluid embolism: a reappraisal. *American Journal of Obstetrics and Gynecology* **151**: 617–621.

CLASP (Collaborative Low-dose Aspirin Study in Pregnancy) Collaborative Group (1994) CLASP: a randomised trial of low-dose aspirin for the prevention and treatment of pre-eclampsia among 9364 pregnant women. *Lancet* **343**: 619–629.

Clenney TL, Viera AJ (2004) Corticosteroids for HELLP (haemolysis, elevated liver enzymes, low platelets) syndrome. *British Medical Journal* **329**: 270–272.

Collop NA, Sahn SA (1993) Critical illness in pregnancy. An analysis of 20 patients admitted to a medical intensive care unit. *Chest* **103**: 1548–1552.

Confidential Enquiry into Maternal and Child Health (2004) Why mothers die 2000–2002. CEMACH 2004. Available online at: www.cemach.org.uk.

Confidential Enquiry into Maternal and Child Health (2007). Saving mothers' lives: reviewing maternal deaths to make motherhood safer, 2003–2005. CEMACH 2007. Available on-line at: www.cemach.org.uk.

Cotton DB, Gonik B, Dorman K, et al. (1985) Cardiovascular alterations in severe pregnancy-induced hypertension: relationship of central venous pressure to pulmonary capillary wedge pressure. *American Journal of Obstetrics and Gynecology* **151**: 762–764.

Cotton DB, Jones MM, Longmire S, et al. (1986a) Role of intravenous nitroglycerin in the treatment of severe pregnancy-induced hypertension complicated by pulmonary edema. *American Journal of Obstetrics and Gynecology* **154**: 91–93.

Cotton DB, Longmire S, Jones MM, et al. (1986b) Cardiovascular alterations in severe pregnancy-induced hypertension: effects of intravenous nitroglycerin coupled with blood volume expansion. *American Journal of Obstetrics and Gynecology* **154**: 1053–1059.

De Belder A, Lees C, Martin J, et al. (1995) Treatment of HELLP syndrome with nitric oxide donor. *Lancet* **345**: 124–125.

de Beus E, van Mook WN, Ramsay G, et al. (2003) Peripartum cardiomyopathy: a condition intensivists should be aware of. *Intensive Care Medicine* **29**: 167–174.

de Swiet M (1980) The cardiovascular system. In: Hytten F, Chamberlain G (eds) *Clinical Physiology in Obstetrics*, pp. 3–42. Blackwell Scientific: Oxford.

Dommisse J (1990) Phenytoin sodium and magnesium sulphate in the management of eclampsia. *British Journal of Obstetrics and Gynaecology* **97**: 104–109.

Douglas KA, Redman CW (1994) Eclampsia in the United Kingdom. *British Medical Journal* **309**: 1395–1400.

Drakeley AJ, Le Roux PA, Anthony J, et al. (2002) Acute renal failure complicating severe preeclampsia requiring admission to an obstetric intensive care unit. *American Journal of Obstetrics and Gynecology* **186**: 253–256.

Drife J (1997) Management of primary postpartum haemorrhage. *British Journal of Obstetrics and Gynaecology* **104**: 275–277.

Duncan R, Hadley D, Bone I, et al. (1989) Blindness in eclampsia: CT and MR imaging. *Journal of Neurology, Neurosurgery, and Psychiatry* **52**: 899–902.

Eclampsia Trial Collaborative Group (1995) Which anticonvulsant for women with eclampsia? Evidence from the Collaborative Eclampsia Trial. *Lancet* **345**: 1455–1463.

Elatrous S, Nouira S, Ouanes Besbes L, et al. (2002) Short-term treatment of severe hypertension of pregnancy: prospective comparison of nicardipine and labetalol. *Intensive Care Medicine* **28**: 1281–1286.

El-Solh AA, Grant BJ (1996) A comparison of severity of illness scoring systems for critically ill obstetric patients. *Chest* **110**: 1299–1304.

Gillett GB, Watson JD, Langford RM (1984) Ranitidine and single-dose antacid therapy as prophylaxis against acid aspiration syndrome in obstetric practice. *Anaesthesia* **39**: 638–644.

Greiff JM, Tordorff SG, Griffiths R, et al. (1994) Acid aspiration prophylaxis in 202 obstetric anaesthetic units in the UK. *International Journal of Obstetric Anesthesia* **3**: 137–142.

Hazelgrove JF, Price C, Pappachan VJ, et al. (2001) Multicenter study of obstetric admissions to 14 intensive care units in southern England. *Critical Care Medicine* **29**: 770–775.

Italian Study of Aspirin in Pregnancy (1993) Low dose aspirin in prevention and treatment of intrauterine growth retardation and pregnancy-induced hypertension. *Lancet* **341**: 396–400.

Jouppila P, Kirkinen P, Koivula A, et al. (1986) Labetolol does not alter the placental and fetal blood flow or maternal prostanoids in pre-eclampsia. *British Journal of Obstetrics and Gynaecology* **93**: 543–547.

Karim SM, Devlin J (1967) Prostaglandin content of amniotic fluid during pregnancy and labour. *Journal of Obstetrics and Gynaecology of the British Commonwealth* **74**: 230–234.

Kilpatrick SJ, Matthay MA (1992) Obstetric patients requiring critical care. A five-year review. *Chest* **101**: 1407–1412.

Koegler A, Sauder P, Marolf A, et al. (1994) Amniotic fluid embolism: a case with non-cardiogenic pulmonary edema. *Intensive Care Medicine* **20**: 45–46.

Kramer MS, Rouleou J, Baskett TF, et al. (2006) Amniotic-fluid embolism and medical induction of labour: a retrospective, population-based cohort study. *Lancet* **368**: 1444–1448.

Lapinsky SE, Kruczynski K, Slusky AS (1995) Critical care in the pregnant patient. *American Journal of Respiratory and Critical Care Medicine* **152**: 427–455.

Lapinsky SE, Kruczynski K, Seaward GR, et al. (1997) Critical care management of the obstetric patient. *Canadian Journal of Anaesthesia* **44**: 325–329.

Letsky EA (1989) Coagulation defects. In: de Swiet M (ed.) *Medical Disorders in Obstetric Practice*, 2nd edn, pp. 104–165. Blackwell Scientific Publications: Oxford.

Levine RJ, Lam C, Yu KF, et al. (2006) Soluble endoglin and other circulating antiangiogenic factors in preeclampsia. *New England Journal of Medicine* **355**: 992–1005.

Lewinsohn G, Herman A, Leonov Y, et al. (1994) Critically ill obstetrical patients: outcome and predictability. *Critical Care Medicine* **22**: 1412–1414.

Lewis LK, Hinshaw DB Jr, Will AD, et al. (1988) CT and angiographic correlation of severe neurological disease in toxemia of pregnancy. *Neuroradiology* **30**: 59–64.

Mabie WC, Sibai BM (1990) Treatment in an obstetric intensive care unit. *American Journal of Obstetrics and Gynecology* **162**: 1–4.

Mabie WC, Gonzalez AR, Sibai BM, et al. (1987) A comparative trial of labetalol and hydralazine in the acute management of severe hypertension complicating pregnancy. *Obstetrics and Gynecology* **70**: 328–333.

Mabie WC, Ratts TE, Sibai BM (1989) The central hemodynamics of severe preeclampsia. *American Journal of Obstetrics and Gynecology* **161**: 1443–1448.

Malee MP, Malee KM, Azuma SD, et al. (1992) Increases in plasma atrial natriuretic peptide concentration antedate clinical evidence of preeclampsia. *Journal of Clinical Endocrinology and Metabolism* **74**: 1095–1100.

Masson RG, Ruggieri J (1985) Pulmonary microvascular cytology: a new diagnostic application of the pulmonary artery catheter. *Chest* **88**: 908–914.

Mendelson CL (1946) The aspiration of stomach contents into lungs during obstetric anesthesia. *American Journal of Obstetrics and Gynecology* **52**: 191–205.

Mushambi MC, Halligan AW, Williamson K (1996) Recent developments in the pathophysiology and management of pre-eclampsia. *British Journal of Anaesthesia* **76**: 133–148.

Paterson-Brown S, Robson SC, Redfern N, et al. (1994) Hydralazine boluses for the treatment of severe hypertension in pre-eclampsia. *British Journal of Obstetrics and Gynaecology* **101**: 409–413.

Platteau P, Engelhardt T, Moodley J, et al. (1997) Obstetric and gynaecological patients in an intensive care unit: a year review. *Tropical Doctor* **27**: 202–206.

Plauche WC (1983) Amniotic fluid embolism. *American Journal of Obstetrics and Gynecology* **147**: 982–983.

Pritchard JA, Cunningham FG, Pritchard SA (1984) The Parkland Memorial Hospital protocol for the treatment of eclampsia: evaluation of 245 cases. *American Journal of Obstetrics and Gynecology* **148**: 951–963.

Quinn A, Barrett T (1993) Delayed onset of coagulopathy following amniotic fluid embolism: two case reports. *International Journal of Obstetric Anesthesia* **2**: 177–180.

Richards AM, Moodley J, Graham DI, et al. (1986) Active management of the unconscious eclamptic patient. *British Journal of Obstetrics and Gynaecology* **93**: 554–562.

Roberts JM, Redman CW (1993) Pre-eclampsia: more than pregnancy-induced hypertension. *Lancet* **341**: 1447–1451.

Savvidou MD, Hingorani AD, Tsikas D, et al. (2003) Endothelial dysfunction and raised plasma concentrations of asymmetric dimethylarginine in pregnant women who subsequently develop pre-eclampsia. *Lancet* **361**: 1511–1517.

Scarpinato L, Gerber D (1995) Critically ill obstetrical patients. Outcome and predictability. *Critical Care Medicine* **23**: 1449–1451.

Sibai B, Caritis S, Phillips E, *et al.* (1993a) Prevention of pre-eclampsia: low-dose aspirin in nulliparous women: a double blind, placebo-controlled trial. *American Journal of Obstetrics and Gynecology* **167**: 286.

Sibai BM, Ramadan MK, Usta I, *et al.* (1993b) Maternal morbidity and mortality in 442 pregnancies with hemolysis, elevated liver enzymes and low platelets (HELLP syndrome). *American Journal of Obstetrics and Gynaecology* **169**: 1000–1006.

Spargo BH, Lichtig C, Luger AM, *et al.* (1976) The renal lesion in preeclampsia. In: Lindheimer MD, Katz AI, Zuspam FP (eds) *Hypertension in Pregnancy*, pp. 129–137. Wiley: New York.

Steiner PE, Lushbaugh CC (1941) Maternal pulmonary embolism by amniotic fluid. *Journal of the American Medical Association* **117**: 1340–1345.

Stempel JE, O'Grady JP, Morton MJ, *et al.* (1982) Use of sodium nitroprusside in complications of gestational hypertension. *Obstetrics and Gynecology* **60**: 533–538.

Tang LC, Kwok AC, Wong AY, *et al.* (1997) Critical care in obstetrical patients: an eight-year review. *Chinese Medical Journal* **110**: 936–941.

Tordoff SG, Sweeney BP (1990) Acid aspiration prophylaxis in 288 obstetric anaesthetic departments in the United Kingdom. *Anaesthesia* **45**: 776–780.

Umo-Etuk J, Lumley J, Holdcroft A (1996) Critically ill parturient women and admission to intensive care: a 5 year review. *International Journal of Obstetric Anesthesia* **5**: 79–84.

Vanmaele L, Noppen M, Vincken W, *et al.* (1990) Transient left heart failure in amniotic fluid embolism. *Intensive Care Medicine* **16**: 269–271.

van Oppen AC, van der Tweel I, Duvekot JJ, *et al.* (1995) Use of cardiac index in pregnancy: is it justified? *American Journal of Obstetrics and Gynecology* **173**: 923–928.

Wallenburg HCS (1988) Hemodynamics in hypertensive pregnancy. In: Rubin PC (ed.) *Hypertension in Pregnancy. Hand-book of Hypertension*, vol. 10, pp. 66–101. Elsevier: Amsterdam.

Waterstone M, Bewley S, Wolfe C (2001) Incidence and predictors of severe obstetric morbidity: case-control study. *British Medical Journal* **322**: 1089–1094.

Weinstein L (1982) Syndrome of hemolysis, elevated liver enzymes and low platelet count: a severe consequence of hypertension in pregnancy. *American Journal of Obstetrics and Gynecology* **142**: 159–167.

Weksler N, Ovadia L, Stav A, *et al.* (1994) Continuous arteriovenous hemofiltration in the treatment of amniotic fluid embolism. *International Journal of Obstetric Anesthesia* **3**: 92–96.

Wheatley E, Farkas A, Watson D (1996) Obstetric admissions to an intensive therapy unit. *International Journal of Obstetric Anaesthesia* **5**: 221–224.

19 Poisoning

In the UK patients admitted to hospital suffering from the effects of acute poisoning account for up to 15–20% of all medical admissions. Although only a proportion of poisoning victims require intensive observation and supportive care (with or without active treatment), management of such patients may account for up to one-third of admissions to a multidisciplinary intensive care unit. The total number of deaths from poisoning in the UK remains unchanged at approximately 4000 per year. The commonest cause of death by poisoning in the UK is carbon monoxide (CO) (Jones and Volans, 1999).

TYPES OF POISONING

SELF-POISONING

The vast majority of adult cases of acute poisoning are self-administered. Most of these are manipulative or represent 'a cry for help' rather than a genuine attempt at suicide and there is often a history of previous similar episodes. The mean age of patients admitted to hospital with an overdose is approximately 25 years, with a female to male ratio of 1.3 : 1, whereas the mean age of successful suicide is about 50 years. In females the peak incidence is in those less than 25 years of age, whereas in males self-poisoning is commonest between the ages of 20 and 35 years.

ACCIDENTAL POISONING

Accidental poisoning is most common in children between 1 and 5 years of age who ingest medicinal, domestic or cosmetic agents. In only a minority of such cases presenting to a hospital does the child develop symptoms, and fatalities are unusual. Accidental poisoning may also be the result of industrial or agricultural mishaps.

NON-ACCIDENTAL POISONING

Non-accidental poisoning may be related to experimentation with drugs or solvents (usually in young adults) or may represent part of the syndrome of child abuse, in which case poisoning is more often fatal than in accidental cases. Homicidal poisoning is rarely encountered in clinical practice.

Because the hospital mortality of acute poisoning is generally low, active measures to hasten the elimination of the poison (which can be associated with a significant morbidity and, in some cases, mortality) is recommended only in a few exceptional instances; indeed, the 'Scandinavian method' of elective supportive care was originally introduced because of the dangers associated with the use of analeptics in patients in barbiturate coma.

Above all else, therefore, the management of acute poisoning involves the application of the principles of *supportive care* detailed elsewhere in this book, including:

- maintenance and protection of the airway;
- respiratory support;
- expansion of the circulating volume;
- maintenance of fluid and electrolyte balance;
- correction of acid–base disturbances;
- occasionally the use of inotropes and/or vasopressors;
- provision of nutritional support;
- thromboembolic and stress ulcer prophylaxis;
- control of body temperature;
- skilled nursing care.

DIAGNOSIS AND ASSESSMENT

HISTORY

The diagnosis can often be established from the history, which may need to be supported by circumstantial evidence. The quantity and nature of the substances taken must be determined. In most cases, a history can be obtained from the patient, although this is frequently misleading and about half will exaggerate or, less often, minimize the severity of poisoning. Currently self-poisoning episodes in the UK most commonly involve the ingestion of benzodiazepines, paracetamol, aspirin or tricyclic antidepressants or the inhalation of motor exhaust fumes. In many cases a mixture of drugs will have been ingested, often including alcohol and a benzodiazepine. Sometimes patients refuse to divulge any information, while others are incoherent or unconscious. In all cases, therefore, the history should be corroborated by interviewing witnesses such as patients, carers or relatives, friends and paramedics, as well as by contacting the general practitioner when appropriate. Bottles, pills or other substances found on or about the patient may provide important clues as to the nature of the poisoning, although they can also be misleading (e.g. drugs may have been stored in incorrectly labelled bottles). Tablets can often be identified using the *Chemist and Druggist Directory,* or a computer-aided tablet and capsule identification system such as TicTac. In the UK this is available to authorized users such as poisons information centres. In some cases it may be appropriate to send a sample of the substance ingested to the laboratory for analysis. Clear documentation of all relevant information is essential.

TOXBASE is the primary clinical toxicology database of the National Poisons Information Service in the UK. It is also available on the internet to registered users (www.spib.axl.co.uk) and provides information about routine diagnosis, treatment and management of patients exposed to drugs, household products and agricultural chemicals.

Other important aspects of the initial enquiry include a history of previous psychiatric disorders and self-poisoning episodes, as well as evidence of complicating illnesses such as liver or renal disease, which might impair the patient's ability to handle poisons.

EXAMINATION
A detailed physical examination should be performed and should include a search for associated injuries (e.g. pressure necrosis, compartment syndrome) as well as medical conditions that might have precipitated the overdose (e.g. depression or psychosis) or could be responsible for coma. When indicated, body temperature should be recorded with a low-reading rectal thermometer. An assessment of the patient's conscious level is particularly important; this should be repeated at regular intervals to follow progress and, in some cases, indicate the need for active intervention. A simple clinical grading of conscious level suitable for use in cases of acute poisoning is shown in **Table 19.1**.

Organic brain damage should be suspected when there is no improvement in the depth of coma within 24 hours, especially when the history of poisoning is dubious. Although the signs and symptoms may suggest intoxication with a specific poison there is in practice often little relationship between the drugs suspected on admission and those detected in the blood.

INVESTIGATIONS (Table 19.2)
When possible, samples of gastric contents (50 mL of vomit, aspirate or first portion of gastric lavage), blood (10 mL lithium-heparinized blood, 10 mL clotted sample, 2 mL of fluoride blood for ethanol assay) and urine (50 mL of the first sample voided after admission) should be obtained for laboratory identification of the poisons involved. Preferably these samples should be collected before the administration of medications, which might complicate toxicological analysis.

Table 19.1 Clinical grading of conscious level in acute poisoning

Grade 0	Fully conscious
Grade I	Drowsy, but responsive to verbal commands
Grade II	Unconscious, but responding to painful stimuli
Grade III	Unconscious, but responding only to maximal painful stimulus
Grade IV	Unconscious, not responding to pain

Table 19.2 Investigations in acute poisoning

Toxicological analysis Gastric contents Blood Urine
Haemoglobin, white cell count
Blood sugar
Urea, creatinine and electrolytes
Liver function tests
Blood gas analysis
Chest radiograph

Since about 50% of those presenting to the emergency department with coma of unknown cause are suffering from self-poisoning it is often advisable to perform a toxicological screen in all such cases. Automated devices for measuring blood levels of some of the common poisons are now available and can be positioned within, or close to, the intensive care unit. Meticulous maintenance and quality control are, however, essential, and purchase of such a device can only be recommended when the unit admits large numbers of poisoned patients. Assistance is always available from the poisons information centre or TOXBASE.

Baseline determinations of haemoglobin concentration, blood sugar, urea and electrolyte levels and liver function tests should be performed in all cases. Blood gas analysis is also routine and may reveal hypercarbia due to respiratory depression or hypoxaemia related to pulmonary pathology such as infection, atelectasis, aspiration or oedema. A chest radiograph should also be obtained.

PRINCIPLES OF MANAGEMENT
(Table 19.3)

IMMEDIATE MANAGEMENT
It is worth reiterating that the majority of patients require only supportive treatment. This should include immediate

Table 19.3 Principles of management of acute poisoning
Immediate management
Secure and protect airway
Respiratory support
Expand circulating volume
Occasionally inotropes and/or vasopressors
Treat arrhythmias
Pass nasogastric tube
Control seizures
Supportive care
Cardiovascular support
Respiratory support
Renal support
Prevent and treat neurological complications
Skilled nursing care
Physiotherapy
Stress ulcer prophylaxis
Enteral nutrition (rarely parenteral)
Antithrombotic/antiembolic prophylaxis
Control body temperature
Prevent further absorption of poison
Activated charcoal
Gastric aspiration and lavage
Whole-gut irrigation
Accelerated elimination of poison
Repeated dose activated charcoal
Enhanced urinary excretion
Haemodialysis and/or haemoperfusion
Treat liver failure
Specific antidotes

life-saving measures and prevention of complications such as hypotension, pulmonary aspiration, acid–base disturbances, fluid and electrolyte imbalance and hypothermia.

Airway

Patients with impaired cough and gag reflexes, as well as those with borderline airway protection needing gastric lavage, require immediate tracheal intubation to secure their airway and prevent aspiration. All patients should be given supplemental oxygen.

Breathing

Mechanical ventilation should be instituted without delay in those with respiratory depression. Because hypoxia and hypercarbia can exacerbate intracranial hypertension and may cause or potentiate cardiac arrhythmias, prompt treatment is essential. Some patients may have developed aspiration or hypostatic pneumonia before admission (see Chapter 8).

Circulation

Acutely poisoned patients are frequently hypotensive, usually as a result of peripheral vasodilatation. Fluid depletion is also common with prolonged stupor or coma and is often exacerbated by vomiting, sweating and hyperventilation. In most cases blood pressure can be restored by intravascular volume expansion, although occasionally vasopressors will be indicated, and in a few inotropic support may be required to counteract myocardial depression (see Chapter 5). Hypertension occurs less frequently than hypotension but may be associated with poisoning by sympathomimetic drugs such as amphetamines, phencyclidine and cocaine.

Cardiac arrhythmias are common and may be due to hypoxia, hypercarbia, acid–base disturbances or electrolyte imbalance, as well as the direct effects of the toxin or drug (e.g. tricyclic antidepressants, some antipsychotics, some antihistamines and co-proxamol). A 12-lead electrocardiogram (ECG) should be obtained and the ECG should then be continuously monitored. Ventricular arrhythmias associated with significant hypotension may require treatment. If the QT interval is prolonged specialist advice should be sought because the use of some antiarrhythmic drugs may be contraindicated (see Chapter 9). Should cardiac arrest occur it is often resistant to attempts to restore sinus rhythm. It is therefore important to persist with cardiopulmonary resuscitation (if necessary using a mechanical support device), especially since fixed dilated pupils may be attributable to the direct effects of the toxin. When toxicity is likely to be prolonged (e.g. with tricyclic antidepressants or calcium antagonists), cardiovascular support in the form of intra-aortic balloon counterpulsation or cardiopulmonary bypass may be life-saving (Purkayastha *et al.*, 2006).

Gastrointestinal

Gastric stasis is common in comatose patients and may be exacerbated by the effects of opiates or drugs with anticholinergic properties. A nasogastric tube should therefore be passed to decompress the stomach and reduce the risk of regurgitation.

Neurological

Prolonged or recurrent convulsions should be treated with lorazepam up to 4 mg or diazepam (preferably as emulsion) up to 10 mg by slow intravenous injection in the first instance (see Chapter 15).

SUPPORTIVE CARE

As well as continued cardiovascular and respiratory support, subsequent management involves the institution of measures to prevent and treat complications. Intensive nursing care and physiotherapy are essential in prolonged coma. It is important to document the presence or absence of neuropraxias, corneal abrasions and injury to pressure areas on admission to the intensive care unit.

Gastrointestinal

Stress ulcer prophylaxis should be instituted in the most seriously ill patients (see Chapter 11). Enteral nutrition should be established early; if this is not possible parenteral nutrition should be considered (see Chapter 11).

Neurological

Neurological complications may include:

- coma;
- seizures (related to cerebral hypoxia, metabolic disturbances or the direct effects of the poison);
- cerebral oedema (due to severe hypoxia, cardiac arrest, profound hypotension, severe CO poisoning);
- peripheral nerve injuries (due to prolonged pressure).

The possibility that neurological abnormalities are unrelated to poisoning should be considered when:

- the reduction in conscious level is out of proportion to the severity of poisoning;
- the conscious level fails to improve;
- there are lateralizing signs.

In such cases further investigations, including a cerebral computed tomographic (CT) scan, are warranted to exclude, for example, an intracranial haemorrhage.

Renal

Renal failure may be related to the direct effects of the toxin (e.g. in those poisoned with non-steroidal anti-inflammatory drugs (NSAIDs) or heavy metals), to prolonged hypotension or to sepsis/septic shock (e.g. in patients with pneumonia). *Rhabdomyolysis* is a common cause of renal failure in patients with poisoning and should be suspected in those who have been immobile for a prolonged period before admission, especially when pressure areas are seen to be discoloured with poor capillary refill (see Chapter 10). Rhabdomyolysis may also be precipitated by the combination of prolonged seizures, hyperthermia, hypokalaemia and extreme tissue hypoxia.

A urinary catheter should be inserted in at-risk patients and measures instituted to reverse oliguria and prevent renal failure, as outlined in Chapter 13. Those who progress to established renal failure will require renal support (see Chapter 13).

Liver

Liver failure should be treated as outlined in Chapter 14.

Temperature regulation (see Chapter 20)

Hypothermia is a common complication of prolonged coma outside hospital in patients of any age and is particularly likely in those poisoned with drugs that prevent vasoconstriction and shivering (e.g. barbiturates and phenothiazines). Usually passive rewarming is sufficient, but occasionally active measures are warranted.

Hyperthermia may complicate intoxication with tricyclic antidepressants, monoamine oxidase inhibitors, cocaine, amphetamines or ecstasy, and is an important feature of the neuroleptic malignant syndrome. Children and the elderly are also at risk of raised body temperature when taking drugs with anticholinergic properties in therapeutic doses.

Initial management involves removing all unnecessary clothing and using a fan. Sponging with tepid water will also promote evaporation; iced water should not be used. In the severest cases active cooling measures with sedation, muscle relaxation and mechanical ventilation with unheated gases may be required (see Chapter 20). Advice should be sought from a poisons information centre on the management of severe hyperthermia.

Thromboembolic prophylaxis
(see Chapter 11)

PREVENTION OF ABSORPTION OF POISON
Activated charcoal

Activated charcoal is a powerful non-specific adsorbent that can bind many drugs and poisons within the gastrointestinal tract, thereby reducing absorption. It seems to provide a relatively safe and effective means of limiting drug absorption when given soon after ingestion of the poison.

Drugs that are well adsorbed to activated charcoal include:

- benzodiazepines;
- barbiturates;
- anticonvulsants, e.g. carbamazepine, phenytoin;
- theophylline;
- antidepressants;
- quinine;
- dapsone.

Salicylates and paracetamol are only moderately well adsorbed. Substances not well adsorbed to activated charcoal are listed in **Table 19.4**. Current recommendations are that 50 g of activated charcoal should be given to adults who have taken a substantial overdose of a toxic substance no more than 1 hour previously – longer in the case of modified-release preparations or drugs with anticholinergic properties (American Academy of Clinical Toxicology and European Association of Poisons Centres, 1997b). Charcoal should not be given if the airway cannot be protected. Repeated doses can be used for sustained-release preparations such as propranolol or theophylline, as well as for salicylates, phenobarbital and carbamazepine (see below).

Table 19.4 Substances not effectively adsorbed by activated charcoal
Ferrous salts
Lithium preparations
Potassium salts
Ethanol
Methanol
Ethylene glycol
Acids
Alkalis
Fluorides
Organic solvents
Mercury and its salts
Lead and its salts

Gastric aspiration and lavage

When performed in seriously poisoned patients, gastric aspiration and lavage are associated with a considerable risk of complications, including:

- pulmonary aspiration;
- seizures;
- arrhythmias;
- perforation of the stomach.

The procedure should therefore only be undertaken by experienced personnel with the facilities available to treat any complications, and then only if potentially life-threatening amounts of a toxic substance have been ingested within the preceding hour (American Academy of Clinical Toxicology and European Association of Poisons Centres, 1997c). This time limit can be extended in cases of poisoning with agents that delay gastric emptying such as salicylates and tricyclic antidepressants. It may also occasionally be considered in patients who have ingested drugs that are not adsorbed by charcoal such as iron or lithium. On the other hand, in those who have ingested agents that do not delay gastric emptying and are rapidly absorbed from the gastrointestinal tract (e.g. paracetamol), gastric aspiration and lavage may prove ineffective, even when performed early.

Gastric aspiration and lavage are contraindicated when corrosive substances or a petroleum distillate have been taken. Aspiration of kerosene or its derivatives can produce a particularly destructive form of *lipoid pneumonia*.

Procedure

Gastric aspiration and lavage should only be performed if the patient has adequate laryngeal and pharyngeal reflexes or has an endotracheal tube in place with the cuff inflated. The use of an intravenous anaesthetic agent and muscle relaxation to allow tracheal intubation of a semicomatose patient is only justified when gastric lavage is clearly indicated; in the majority of cases, it is not. The semiconscious patient should be positioned head-down, lying on the left side. Facilities for pharyngeal suction must be immediately available. Foreign matter should be removed from the mouth and pharynx before introducing a wide-bore tube into the mouth, which the patient is then persuaded to swallow (a large tube is less likely to enter the trachea and allows aspiration of particulate matter). The stomach contents are then aspirated and retained for analysis, following which lavage is performed with 250 mL warmed tap water. This procedure is repeated until the aspirate is clear of debris. Subsequently, the wide-bore tube is replaced by a Ryle's tube, which is aspirated hourly.

Whole-bowel irrigation

Whole-bowel irrigation has been used in poisoning with certain sustained-release medications, in severe poisoning with heavy metals, iron and lithium salts, and when button batteries or illicit drug packets have been ingested. The procedure involves isotonic polyethylene glycol administration (e.g. KleenPrep) (2 L/h) orally or via a nasogastric tube for 3–5 hours in adults to flush out gastrointestinal contents, but it is not yet clear whether outcome is improved. Advice should be sought from a poisons information centre. This technique is contraindicated in patients with bowel obstruction, perforation, ileus, haemodynamic instability or where the airway cannot be protected (American Academy of Clinical Toxicology and European Association of Poisons Centres, 1997a). Polyethylene glycol or laxatives are sometimes used in 'body packers' to remove packets that are beyond the pylorus, although one report described the death of a body packer when ingested condoms dissolved after paraffin was given (Visser *et al.*, 1998). Packets in the stomach are best removed endoscopically (Choudhary *et al.*, 1998) and packets in the small or large intestine that contain potentially lethal amounts of drugs may be removed surgically (Lancashire *et al.*, 1988).

Induction of vomiting

Induction of emesis (e.g. with ipecacuanha) is not now recommended because there is no evidence that it affects absorption or systemic toxicity (Vale *et al.*, 1986) and it may increase the risk of aspiration. It is also difficult to give activated charcoal after an emetic (American Academy of Toxicology and European Association of Poisons Centres, 1997d).

ACCELERATED ELIMINATION OF POISON

Active measures to increase the elimination of a poison are indicated if the patient is seriously ill and deteriorating, if significant amounts of the poison can be removed and if this is likely to produce worthwhile improvement. In fact only a small proportion of acutely poisoned patients merit such treatment and it is sensible to *first obtain the advice of a poisons information centre*.

Table 19.5 Indications for multiple dose activated charcoal

Modified-release preparations such as theophylline (but not lithium)
Carbamazepine
Dapsone
Digoxin
Paraquat
Phenobarbital
Quinine
The fungus *Amanita phalloides*

ACTIVATED CHARCOAL

Repeated administration of activated charcoal is a cheap, safe and effective means of reducing drug levels by creating a negative diffusion gradient between the gut lumen and blood – so-called gastrointestinal dialysis (Levy, 1982). Nevertheless pulmonary aspiration of activated charcoal can have serious consequences (Menzies *et al.*, 1988). There is also a risk of gastrointestinal obstruction and hypernatraemia from the sodium load.

Severely poisoned adults should be given 50 g orally or via a nasogastric tube then every 4 hours as repeated doses (Table 19.5).

In cases of intolerance the dose may be reduced and the frequency increased, e.g. 25 g every 2 hours or 12.5 g every hour. Vomiting and dose reductions may, however, compromise the efficacy of charcoal treatment. Other techniques intended to enhance the elimination of poisons after their absorption are only indicated for a small number of severely poisoned patients.

RENAL ELIMINATION

Urinary excretion can be enhanced by altering the pH of the urine to increase the degree of ionization of the substance and reduce its lipid solubility. In aspirin overdose alkalinization of the urine therefore increases salicylate elimination but forced alkaline diuresis is no longer recommended. In severe chlorpromazine poisoning maintaining acidic urine may be appropriate.

Haemodialysis and haemoperfusion
(Cutler et al.*, 1987)*

Haemodialysis and haemoperfusion are of dubious value, but are likely to be most effective when:

- the poison diffuses readily across the dialysis membrane or is avidly taken up by the adsorbent;
- the pharmacological effect of the toxin is closely related to blood levels;
- dialysis or haemoperfusion adds significantly to other routes of drug elimination.

On the other hand, drugs that are highly lipid-soluble and have a large volume of distribution are difficult to eliminate.

Haemodialysis may be of value in the management of severe salicylate overdose and poisoning with death cap mushrooms (*Amanita phalloides*). Clearance of barbiturates, anticonvulsants, benzodiazepines, lithium, cardiac glycosides and many other less commonly encountered poisons can certainly be enhanced with these techniques, but it is uncertain whether morbidity or mortality is reduced. In severe methyl alcohol (methanol) and ethylene glycol ingestion, it is logical to attempt removal of these water-soluble poisons before they are metabolized to potentially lethal formaldehyde and formic acid or glycolic and oxalic acids respectively. Large molecules and poisons that are highly protein-bound cannot be cleared efficiently by haemodialysis and in such cases haemoperfusion is preferred, e.g. chloral hydrate, theophylline. Such extracorporeal techniques are relatively complex and can be associated with a significant risk of complications. Clearance of paracetamol, paraquat and tricyclic antidepressants is not significantly enhanced.

Haemodialysis or haemofiltration may also be considered for renal failure or refractory acid–base disturbances. It is occasionally indicated when a patient is deteriorating despite adequate supportive care as a result of poisoning with a dialysable substance. Peritoneal dialysis has no established role in the management of poisoning.

SPECIFIC ANTIDOTES

An antidote can be defined as any substance that can favourably influence the onset, severity or duration of the toxic effects of a poison (Collee and Hanson, 1993). Only a few specific antidotes are available and some may themselves have toxic effects. They may act by:

- competing for drug receptor sites (e.g. flumazenil, naloxone);
- binding with the toxin to form less toxic chelates that are more easily excreted (e.g. digoxin-specific antibody fragments, snake antivenoms);
- influencing metabolism of a poison to prevent or reduce the formation of harmful metabolites (e.g. *N*-acetylcysteine in paracetamol overdose; ethanol or fomepizole in methanol or ethylene glycol poisoning).

The use of specific antagonists such as naloxone and flumazenil to reverse central nervous system depression is controversial and is discussed later in this chapter. Analeptics should never be used.

MANAGEMENT OF SPECIFIC POISONINGS

ALCOHOLS
Ethanol

Acute intoxication with alcohol (ethanol) is seen most commonly in adults but is also occasionally encountered in children. *Aspiration of vomitus, hypothermia and non-traumatic rhabdomyolysis* are special risks accompanying alcohol-induced coma, and *hypoglycaemia* may occur in children and some adults. Management is supportive. Glucose can be given if indicated.

Methanol

Acute methanol (methyl alcohol) poisoning occurs most frequently in vagrants, although cases of accidental ingestion are occasionally encountered. Methanol is a constituent of antifreeze (alone or with ethylene glycol), paint removers and varnish and is produced in some home-made beverages. Methylated spirit, however, is composed largely of ethanol with only 5% methanol. Methanol is metabolized to formic acid and formaldehyde, both of which are extremely toxic.

CLINICAL FEATURES

The central effects of acute methanol intoxication may be delayed for 12–36 hours after ingestion, at which time *nausea, vomiting, abdominal pain, headache* and *ataxia* can occur and may progress to *coma*. There is often a *profound metabolic acidosis* with Kussmaul respiration. If poisoning is severe (blood methanol > 500 mg/L, marked acidosis), the patient may develop an *acute optic nerve papillitis* with blurring of vision that can progress to blindness, dilatation of the pupils and papilloedema.

TREATMENT

Advice on the treatment of methanol or ethylene glycol poisoning should be obtained from a poisons information centre.

Gastric aspiration and lavage should be performed if the patient is seen within 1 hour of ingestion and any *metabolic acidosis should be corrected*. Because *ethanol* competes with methanol for the enzyme alcohol dehydrogenase, administration of the former (by mouth or intravenous infusion) can limit the production of formic acid. *Haemodialysis* has also been recommended if the patient fails to respond to these measures and has visual impairment, a severe metabolic acidosis or a blood methanol level greater than 1 g/L. There is no evidence, however, that dialysis is more effective than standard measures. *Fomepizole* (Antizol), available from poisons information centres, has also been used for the treatment of methanol or ethylene glycol poisoning (Brent et al., 1999). Like ethanol, fomepizole (4-methylpyrazole) is a competitive inhibitor of alcohol dehydrogenase. Compared with treatment with ethanol (by mouth or intravenous infusion) 4-methylpyrazole has the advantage of reduced central nervous system depression, although haemodialysis may still be required for the management of renal failure.

ANALGESICS
Salicylates

The increased use of paracetamol as a mild analgesic has resulted in a reduction in the incidence of salicylate poisoning. Nevertheless, it remains a relatively common cause of poisoning in children and adults. Many readily available salicylate preparations do not mention that they contain aspirin. Oil of wintergreen, for example, contains methyl salicylate and is potentially highly toxic.

MECHANISMS OF TOXICITY

Aspirin is normally deacetylated by plasma esterases and is eliminated by conjugation. Following overdose, however, the conjugation pathway is saturated, free salicylate has to be eliminated via the kidneys and excretion is prolonged.

Aspirin uncouples oxidative phosphorylation, leading to increased metabolism of glucose and fats with a rise in oxygen consumption ($\dot{V}O_2$) and carbon dioxide production. The respiratory centre is stimulated both directly and by the increased carbon dioxide production, thereby producing respiratory alkalosis. If salicylate levels are very high, however, respiratory depression may supervene. Blood levels of pyruvate, lactate and ketone bodies are increased and, combined with the fact that aspirin is itself an organic acid, this produces a metabolic acidosis.

CLINICAL FEATURES

The majority of patients present within 6 hours of ingestion and are conscious, alert and oriented, although some are *restless, irritable* and *confused. Hallucinations* may occur. Coma is rare and in adults drowsiness indicates severe poisoning. Confusion and drowsiness are more frequently seen in children.

Other clinical features include:

- sweating;
- tinnitus and deafness;
- blurred vision;
- tachycardia;
- hyperventilation.

Initially there is a respiratory alkalosis, although in severe cases respiratory acidosis may occur as a terminal event, whilst in children a *metabolic acidosis* can develop rapidly and usually becomes the dominant abnormality.

Less commonly, patients poisoned with aspirin have *epigastric pain* and *vomiting* with *severe dehydration* and *oliguria*. Rarely, they may develop acute renal failure. Gastrointestinal bleeding is uncommon, but may be related to *gastric erosions* and a *coagulopathy*. The latter is usually due to hypoprothrombinaemia, which can be corrected with fresh frozen plasma and vitamin K, but may also be due to thrombocytopenia, decreased production of factor VII or impaired platelet function.

In some cases, *pulmonary oedema* develops in association with an increase in capillary permeability, proteinuria and hypoproteinaemia. These patients may also be hypotensive and hypovolaemic. Administration of colloidal solutions is appropriate but care is required to avoid precipitating or worsening pulmonary oedema.

Salicylate poisoning may also be associated with hypokalaemia, hyperglycaemia or hypoglycaemia; the latter may be particularly severe in children. Some patients develop an *encephalopathy* and *hyperthermia*.

INVESTIGATIONS

Investigations should include:

- blood gas and acid–base analysis;
- urea and electrolytes;
- coagulation studies;
- blood glucose.

In severe poisoning, protein and calcium levels should be determined and liver function tests should be performed.

The diagnosis should be confirmed, and the severity of poisoning assessed, by measuring *plasma salicylate levels*. They should be related to the time of ingestion, bearing in mind that, after an overdose, absorption of aspirin continues for some time and peak levels may not be attained for 8 hours or more. Therefore, a level of 350 mg/L (2.5 mmol/L) may be significant 12 hours after ingestion, but is almost within the therapeutic range at 4–6 hours. Active treatment, including sodium bicarbonate (1.26%) given to enhance urinary salicylate excretion, should be considered if the level is more than 500 mg/L (3.6 mmol/L) within 12 hours of ingestion, and for levels greater than 350 mg/L (2.5 mmol/L) beyond this time. In children, measures to hasten elimination are indicated when the level is more than 350 mg/L (2.5 mmol/L) at 12 hours. Respiratory depression is a common mode of death when the plasma salicylate level exceeds 1000 mg/L (7.2 mmol/L).

TREATMENT

Gastric aspiration and lavage should be performed if the patient presents within 1 hour of ingestion. *Activated charcoal* should be administered in repeated doses via the nasogastric tube (although see comments earlier in this chapter).

When active treatment is indicated, it should be instituted immediately, since death can occur suddenly and unexpectedly. Intravascular volume must be replenished and any significant metabolic acidosis should be corrected. In selected cases, invasive monitoring may be indicated to guide volume replacement and avoid fluid overload. The clearance of salicylates is pH-dependent, increasing 10-fold when blood pH rises from 6.0 to 7.5. Salicylate levels and acid–base status should be measured repeatedly. If a moderate salicylate level has increased to greater than 700 mg/L (5.1 mmol/L), if a severe metabolic acidosis persists or the salicylate level has failed to decrease, *haemodialysis* is appropriate. If the salicylate level has fallen, however, activated charcoal with or without sodium bicaronate (1.26%) treatment should be continued.

Paracetamol

The incidence of poisoning with paracetamol has gradually increased over the last 20–30 years and is one of the commonest causes of fulminant hepatic failure (FHF) (see Chapter 14) (Routledge *et al.*, 1998).

CLINICAL FEATURES

Patients who have taken a paracetamol overdose normally *remain fully conscious*. Clinical features may include pallor, perspiration, epigastric pain, nausea and vomiting. Occasionally, a massive paracetamol overdose may directly damage the myocardium and cause peripheral vasodilatation with *shock*. In such cases metabolic acidosis may be severe.

The early symptoms are not a reliable indication of the severity of poisoning and there is a wide individual variability in tolerance to paracetamol, as well as in susceptibility to *hepatotoxicity*. When liver damage does occur, the signs of hepatic failure are not usually apparent until 48 hours after the overdose. At this time, the patient may become jaundiced with an enlarged and tender liver. Liver function tests are most abnormal 3–5 days after ingestion. In severe, but non-fatal hepatotoxicity a cholestatic picture is usually seen, and in the most serious cases FHF develops about 3–7 days after ingestion.

MECHANISMS OF HEPATOTOXICITY (see also Chapter 14)

Paracetamol hepatotoxicity is due to a toxic metabolite, which is formed via an oxidative pathway dependent on cytochrome P2E1 and is normally scavenged by intracellular glutathione. Following an overdose, this mechanism may be overwhelmed and the highly reactive metabolite combines with sulphydryl groups of liver cell proteins, producing a centrilobular necrosis. Increased intracellular concentrations of calcium appear to play an important role in causing cellular injury.

Paracetamol-induced liver damage is likely to be more severe in patients exposed to hepatic enzyme-inducing agents such as barbiturates, carbamazepine, isoniazid, phenytoin, rifampicin, ethanol and St John's wort. In patients who are malnourished (e.g. in anorexia, chronic alcoholism or those who are human immunodeficiency virus (HIV)-positive), however, increased susceptibility to paracetamol poisoning is probably related to decreased plasma and liver concentrations of glutathione.

INVESTIGATIONS

Plasma levels of paracetamol must be determined in any patient suspected of being poisoned with this agent. When related to the time since ingestion, they correlate closely with the subsequent risk of liver damage, provided this time interval is not less than 4 hours. Therefore, in the absence of treatment, a level of more than 200 mg/L (1.32 mmol/L) at 4 hours or more than 50 mg/L (0.33 mmol/L) at 12 hours is usually hepatotoxic (**Fig. 19.1**), while a level less than 100 mg/L (0.66 mmol/L) at 4 hours should be regarded as carrying a low risk of liver damage. It is worth noting that large overdoses of paracetamol can triple its plasma half-life from 2.4 to 7.3 hours.

Plasma paracetamol concentrations measured earlier than 4 hours from ingestion may be misleading. Furthermore, the prognostic accuracy of plasma paracetamol

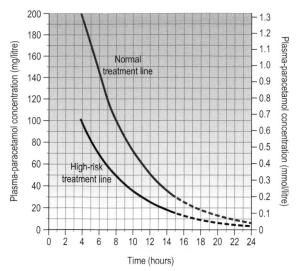

Fig. 19.1 Plasma paracetamol concentrations related to time since ingestion. Liver damage is likely to be severe above the upper line, severe to mild between the lines and clinically insignificant below the lower line (which joins points that are 50% of the plasma paracetamol concentrations of the normal treatment line). From University College of Wales College of Medicines, Therapeutics and Toxicology Centre (*British National Formulary*).

concentrations 15 hours or more after ingestion is uncertain, although values above the relevant treatment lines should be regarded as carrying a serious risk of significant liver damage. Plasma paracetamol concentrations may also be difficult to interpret when the history is unreliable or when paracetamol has been ingested over several hours. If there is any doubt the patient should be treated with an antidote (see below).

Laboratory investigations should include:

- urea and electrolytes;
- coagulation studies;
- blood sugar level;
- liver function tests.

Blood glucose levels should be determined hourly.

TREATMENT

Gastric lavage is recommended if the patient is seen within 1 hour of ingestion. Administration of activated charcoal should also be considered if paracetamol in excess of 150 mg/kg or 12 g (whichever is the smaller) is thought to have been ingested within the previous hour. Intravenous glucose should be administered if required. Early renal replacement therapy may also be necessary.

Preventive treatment is based on the principle that, by providing an alternative supply of sulphydryl groups, unstable precursors can be displaced from either glutathione or liver cell protein. Antidotes such as acetylcysteine and methionine protect the liver if given within 10–12 hours of ingestion; acetylcysteine is thought to be effective up to and possibly beyond 48 hours.

Oral methionine (2.5 g immediately followed by three further doses at 4-hourly intervals) may be used if acetylcysteine is not available in those who present within 10–12 hours of ingestion and are not vomiting.

Acetylcysteine, which repletes gluthathione stores, has fewer side-effects and is now the treatment of choice (Keays *et al.*, 1991). This agent should be given in a dose of 150 mg/kg intravenously over 15 minutes, followed by 50 mg/kg in 500 mL 5% dextrose over 4 hours and then 100 mg/kg in 1 litre of 5% dextrose over 16 hours.

Currently it is recommended that acetylcysteine is administered by intravenous infusion to all high-risk patients whose plasma paracetamol concentrations are above the lower line in **Figure 19.1**. Treatment is still indicated at least as late as 24 hours after ingestion (Smilkstein *et al.*, 1988) and there is evidence to suggest that acetylcysteine can improve outcome even when administered after the onset of paracetamol-induced FHF, possibly by improving oxygen delivery (DO_2) and $\dot{V}O_2$ and limiting the extent of vital organ dysfunction (Keays *et al.*, 1991) (see Chapter 14). Acetylcysteine is also a potent antioxidant, an action that partly underlies its protective effect in paracetamol overdose. Very occasionally acetylcysteine may precipitate a histamine-mediated reaction.

Referral to a centre specializing in the management of paracetamol intoxication should be considered when:

- pH is less than 7.3 more than 24 hours after ingestion;
- prothrombin time is longer than 45 seconds at 48 hours, or longer than 50 seconds at 72 hours;
- creatinine concentration is increasing;
- there is rapid development of grade II encephalopathy.

Liver transplantation may be considered when:

- pH is less than 7.3 (irrespective of grade of encephalopathy);
- prothrombin time is longer than 100 seconds;
- serum creatinine is higher than 300 μmol/L;
- there is grade III or IV encephalopathy (see Chapter 14).

Opiates

Opiate poisoning is usually encountered in drug abusers who have taken an overdose, either intentionally or accidentally. Overdose may also occur with inexperienced users, when there has been a change in the purity of the supplied drug or when loss of tolerance has occurred during a period of abstinence. Drug couriers who swallow opiates in containers (e.g. a condom or plastic bag) may develop severe toxicity if the package leaks ('body packers' – see earlier in this chapter). An abdominal radiograph often reveals the package, which may require surgical removal.

CLINICAL FEATURES

The triad of *coma, respiratory depression* (infrequent deep respirations) and *pinpoint pupils* (which are equal and reactive) is virtually diagnostic of opiate poisoning. *Cardiovascular depression* also occurs.

Physical examination may reveal *evidence of addiction* such as venepuncture scars, or the complications of intravenous drug abuse such as hepatitis and sepsis. Acute heroin intoxication can be complicated by *non-cardiogenic pulmonary oedema*, which may be related to hypoxia, hypersensitivity to the heroin or a contaminant, or to a direct toxic effect. Profound sedation may be associated with muscular compression which, especially when aggravated by hypoxia, acidosis and hypovolaemia, can precipitate *rhabdomyolysis*.

Death is usually due to respiratory depression, often combined with *pulmonary aspiration*.

TREATMENT

Coma and respiratory depression can be reversed by *naloxone* 0.4–1.2 mg intravenously or intramuscularly (in children 5–10 µg/kg). Because the half-life of naloxone is short (opiate reversal persists for only 15–30 minutes), repeated doses or an infusion may be required. Naloxone can precipitate an acute withdrawal syndrome in addicts and may cause laryngeal spasm. In addition, a number of adverse reactions to naloxone have been described, including ventricular fibrillation, hypertension and pulmonary oedema. These are presumably related to sympathetic nervous system responses to opiate withdrawal. Caution is therefore required in those with known cardiovascular disease and in some cases it may be safer to intubate the trachea and institute mechanical ventilation until the opiate effects have resolved spontaneously. Non-cardiogenic pulmonary oedema usually responds rapidly to mechanical ventilation with a positive end-expiratory pressure (PEEP).

It is important to recognize that some opioids such as methadone have a very long duration of action. Methadone also has cardiotoxic effects which may require treatment with sodium bicarbonate or magnesium sulphate or both: arrhythmias may occur for up to 12 hours.

ANTIDEPRESSANTS
Tricyclic and related antidepressants

Tricyclic and related antidepressants have been extensively prescribed for an 'at-risk' population of depressed patients. Furthermore, improvement in mood is often delayed for up to 2 weeks after the start of treatment. Consequently, acute poisoning with tricyclic antidepressants has been common.

CLINICAL FEATURES

The features of tricyclic antidepressant overdose are due to a mixture of *central excitation and depression* combined with *anticholinergic effects*. Although the conscious level may be decreased, coma is not common unless the overdose is large. Both pyramidal and extrapyramidal disturbances may occur

and convulsions are common. Some patients hallucinate, and rapid distorted speech is characteristic. Respiration is frequently depressed. *Anticholinergic effects* are manifested as:

- dilated pupils;
- dry mouth;
- tachycardia;
- absent sweating;
- urine retention;
- paralytic ileus.

The combination of central depression and an inability to sweat impairs temperature regulation and may lead to *hyperthermia*. Examination may reveal hyperreflexia and extensor plantar responses. The diagnosis can be confirmed by detecting the drug in the urine.

The *cardiovascular effects* of tricyclic antidepressants are complex. Sinus tachycardia is common and both hyper- and hypotension may occur. Terminally, hypotension may become refractory, culminating in pulseless electrical activity (PEA). The ECG changes include a dose-related prolongation of the QT interval, widening of the QRS complex, atrioventricular block, and intraventricular conduction disturbances; right bundle branch block is characteristic. When the QRS complex is longer than 0.1 seconds, convulsions are likely; when prolonged to more than 0.16 seconds there is a considerable risk of ventricular arrhythmias (Boehnert and Lovejoy, 1985). Although in one case death occurred 5 days after the overdose (Masters, 1967), a review of 72 consecutive cases of tricyclic antidepressant overdose suggested that late unexpected complications are very rare and in practice a 2-day period of intensive observation is probably sufficient (Stern *et al.*, 1985).

TREATMENT

Because stomach emptying may be delayed following an overdose of tricyclic antidepressants, *gastric aspiration/lavage* and administration of activated charcoal may be worthwhile in an attempt to prevent absorption even many hours after ingestion. Measures to hasten elimination of tricyclic antidepressants are however ineffective because these drugs are highly lipid-soluble, they are also strongly protein-bound and only small amounts are excreted in the urine. Management is therefore supportive.

The ECG should be monitored continuously following a serious overdose. It has been recommended that all patients with respiratory depression, twitching or cardiac arrhythmias should be intubated and mechanically ventilated (Collee and Hanson, 1993). In this way hypercarbia and hypoxia, which may precipitate cardiac arrhythmias, and acidosis (respiratory or metabolic), which enhances cardiotoxicity, can be avoided. Also tracheal intubation secures the airway, thereby allowing the safe use of anticonvulsants. Provided the patient is well oxygenated and the pH is maintained above 7.4 cardiac arrhythmias usually resolve. If hyperventilation alone fails to raise the pH above this level it has been suggested that small (50 mmol) doses of bicarbonate should be given.

If ventricular arrhythmias do occur, they may be resistant to conventional treatment, although some claim that they have experienced no difficulty in defibrillating such patients and that the subsequent infusion of amiodarone or lidocaine successfully prevents recurrence. Prophylactic antiarrhythmics have also been recommended for those with ventricular ectopics. Phenytoin may be useful since it can control both the ventricular arrhythmias and any accompanying convulsions, although it is a negative inotrope and as such could precipitate PEA.

Although it might seem logical to administer an anticholinesterase such as physostigmine, this is unwise in the acute phase since such treatment may precipitate seizures, bradycardia and cardiac failure. Similarly, administration of a β-blocker may cause extreme bradycardia and even asystole. Although a direct current shock should be used when clearly indicated, there is a risk of precipitating asystole or PEA.

A few patients may be hypotensive in the absence of arrhythmias, but expansion of the circulating volume will usually restore the blood pressure. Inotropes should in general be avoided because of the danger of precipitating arrhythmias. If inotropic support is required, dobutamine is a suitable agent. Pulmonary artery catheterization should be avoided because of the risk of precipitating arrhythmias.

Cardiac toxicity generally resolves quite rapidly, within about 6 hours, and mechanical ventilation for convulsions is rarely required for more than 24 hours.

Extrapyramidal symptoms can be controlled with benzatropine 1–2 mg intramuscularly or intravenously, while the agitation and convulsions that may occur during the recovery phase are best treated with diazepam or lorazepam either orally or by intravenous administration.

Selective serotonin reuptake inhibitors (SSRIs)

These antidepressants act by inhibiting serotonin reuptake but lack the antimuscarinic actions of tricyclics.

CLINICAL FEATURES

Even large overdoses of SSRIs appear to be relatively safe, unless combined with alcohol. In most patients there are no signs of toxicity. Drowsiness, nausea, diarrhoea, sinus tachycardia and influenza-like symptoms have been reported. Seizures, hypertension and functional bradycardia are rare. A *serotonin syndrome* (confusion, sweating, diarrhoea and cardiovascular instability – see Chapter 20) usually only occurs as a result of an interaction with another drug, rather than from an overdose of the SSRI alone.

TREATMENT

Management is supportive.

Monoamine oxidase inhibitors

An isolated overdose of these agents may produce a severe serotonin syndrome, and severe toxicity may occur when they are taken in combination with foods containing precursors of biogenic amines or with drugs such as amphetamines and sympathomimetic amines.

CLINICAL FEATURES

Signs and symptoms of toxicity include:

- tachycardia;
- fluctuating blood pressure;
- warm peripheries;
- sweating;
- pyrexia;
- dilated pupils.

Muscle twitching may progress to diffuse *muscle spasm, trismus* and *opisthotonos*. As with amphetamine analogues, severe cases may be complicated by *rhabdomyolysis, disseminated intravascular coagulation (DIC)* and *renal failure*.

The interaction between a monoamine oxidase inhibitor and another drug or food (the 'cheese' reaction) consists of a hypertensive crisis with headache, vomiting, abdominal pain and possibly heart failure.

TREATMENT

Management is *supportive* combined with *cooling, sedation* and administration of *muscle relaxants* when core temperature is 39°C or more. A hypertensive crisis can be managed with phentolamine.

Lithium intoxication

Toxicity may be precipitated by an overdose, dehydration, concomitant administration of NSAIDs or diuretics and, because lithium is cleared via the kidney, renal failure.

CLINICAL FEATURES

Features of intoxication include:

- confusion;
- agitation;
- hypertonia;
- hyperreflexia;
- ataxia and tremor;
- convulsions;
- vomiting.

Patients may also develop hyponatraemia, diabetes insipidus and renal failure.

INVESTIGATIONS

In acute lithium poisoning the plasma level is usually higher than 2 mmol/l (therapeutic range 0.4–1.0 mmol/L).

TREATMENT

Management should include *gastric lavage* up to 1 hour after ingestion and measures to increase urine output. *Haemodialysis* is indicated in those with neurological symptoms, renal failure or both. Whole-bowel irrigation should be considered for significant ingestion of a delayed-release formulation but advice should be sought from a poisons information centre.

CARDIOVASCULAR DRUGS

β-blocking drugs

β-blockers are extensively prescribed and readily available; poisoning with β-blockers is therefore relatively common.

CLINICAL FEATURES

Manifestations of profound β-blockade include *lassitude, drowsiness, bradycardia* and *hypotension. Peripheral vasospasm* and *Raynaud's phenomenon* may occur. *Bronchospasm* may be precipitated, particularly in those with asthma or chronic obstructive pulmonary disease.

TREATMENT

Gastric aspiration and lavage should be performed if the patient is seen within 1 hour of ingestion. *Intravenous atropine*, 1–3 mg, and an *isoprenaline* infusion can be given in an attempt to counteract the hypotension and bradycardia. Cardiogenic shock unresponsive to atropine is probably best treated with an intravenous injection of glucagon (2–10 mg) (unlicensed indication and dose) followed by an intravenous infusion of 50 μg/kg per hour in glucose 5% (with precautions to protect the airway in case of vomiting). The mechanism of action of glucagon is thought not to involve the β-adrenoreceptor. Some recommend dopamine or dobutamine as alternatives to isoprenaline. Ideally, *cardiac pacing* should be instituted in those with extreme bradycardia. Severe bronchospasm should be treated with *salbutamol*.

Calcium channel blockers

CLINICAL FEATURES

Calcium channel-blocking drugs (CCB) can cause fatal cardiovascular toxicity in overdose. They *slow sinoatrial and atrioventricular nodal conduction, decrease myocardial contractility* and cause *vasodilatation*. CCBs also *decrease insulin secretion* and cause *peripheral insulin resistance*, leading to *lactic acidosis* and *hyperglycaemia* and depriving the myocardium of carbohydrate substrate.

TREATMENT

Treatment of CCB poisoning is challenging as patients can deteriorate suddenly, with prolonged hypotension and bradyarrhythmias resistant to conventional treatments; inotropic and antiarrhythmic agents are largely ineffective. These drugs are well absorbed enterally, are highly protein-bound and have large volumes of distribution, so that extracorporeal removal is not effective. *Aggressive supportive* care has been the mainstay of treatment. The most effective specific treatment to date appears to be the use of high doses of insulin. Hyperinsulinaemic euglycaemia therapy involves the infusion of *high doses of insulin* (range 0.1–2.0 iu/kg per hour) together with appropriate amounts of dextrose to maintain normal blood glucose levels. Because insulin drives potassium into cells, potassium supplements may also be necessary (Lheureux *et al.*, 2006).

Digoxin

Digoxin has a narrow therapeutic index and is therefore particularly liable to produce life-threatening complications after accidental or deliberate overdose. Serious overdoses are frequently fatal: mortality is around 18% following ingestion of 15 mg digoxin and approximately 95% when more than 35 mg is taken. In general plasma levels do not correlate closely with the severity of poisoning but the likelihood of toxicity increases progressively through the range 1.5–3 μg/L.

CLINICAL FEATURES

Nausea and vomiting are constant features, while *diarrhoea* is less common. There may be *anorexia* and *abdominal pain*.

Digoxin overdose is associated with hyperkalaemia due to inhibition of Na^+/K^+ ATPase; the extent of the rise in plasma potassium is correlated with the clinical course. Any patient with a plasma potassium of over 5.3 mmol/L should be considered at high risk.

Cardiac toxicity may be associated with:

- bradycardia;
- varying degrees of atrioventricular block;
- supraventricular arrhythmias (with or without heart block);
- less commonly, ventricular arrhythmias, including ventricular tachycardia/ventricular fibrillation.

Other features of toxicity may include extreme *fatigue, weakness* and *visual disturbances*, often with abnormal red–green colour perception. Some patients complain of *headaches, dizziness* and *abnormal dreams*.

MANAGEMENT

Gastric lavage, when indicated, should only be performed with extreme care because of the risk that increased vagal tone will precipitate cardiac arrest. Tissue stores of cardiac glycosides are large; measures to enhance their elimination such as enhanced diuresis, haemodialysis or haemoperfusion are therefore generally ineffective and the risks outweigh the benefits.

Bradycardia should be treated with atropine or transvenous pacing. Infusion of catecholamines should be avoided.

Hypokalaemia, which is most likely in those receiving chronic diuretic therapy, should be corrected.

Hyperkalaemia may be treated with intravenous dextrose and insulin (see Chapter 13), but inhibition of Na^+/K^+ ATPase may limit its efficacy.

Lidocaine can be administered for the treatment of *ventricular arrhythmias*. In cases of paroxysmal supraventricular tachycardia with block, intravenous administration of a beta-blocker may be useful following specialist advice.

Severe digitalis intoxication should be treated with *digoxin-specific antibody fragments* (Martiny *et al.*, 1988). These have a greater affinity for digoxin than does digoxin for its receptors, they do not fix complement and they are not susceptible to immune degradation. The antibody fragments easily pass into the interstitial spaces where they bind to molecules of digitalis glycoside, leading to an improvement in signs and symptoms within about 30 minutes. At this time plasma digoxin levels rise, although, because the drug is now bound, it is pharmacologically inactive. Plasma potassium levels fall. The digoxin–antibody complex is then eliminated via the kidneys. The plasma half-life after intravenous administration of digoxin-specific antibody fragments is 16–34 hours in those with normal renal function. There is little experience of using digoxin-specific antibody fragments in renal failure and there is at least a theoretical danger that retained complex might be metabolized to release free digoxin, with recurrence of toxicity.

Suggested indications for digoxin-specific antibody treatment are:

- life-threatening cardiac arrhythmias;
- plasma digoxin concentration higher than 20 µg/L;
- rising or uncontrollable potassium levels.

HYPNOTICS AND SEDATIVES
Benzodiazepines
MECHANISMS
Many of the effects of benzodiazepines are mediated by occupation of specific receptor sites, thereby enhancing the effects of γ-aminobutyric acid (GABA), an inhibitory neurotransmitter.

CLINICAL FEATURES
When taken alone, benzodiazepines can produce *drowsiness, dizziness, ataxia* and *slurred speech*. More serious manifestations of overdose such as *coma* or *hypotension* are infrequently seen and death due to isolated benzodiazepine poisoning, which is usually related to *respiratory depression* and *pulmonary aspiration*, is unusual. Many cases of self-poisoning, however, involve ingestion of a number of drugs, and benzodiazepines are often one of these. Under these circumstances the clinical picture is often confusing and additive effects may aggravate or precipitate respiratory failure and hypotension.

Benzodiazepines are absorbed relatively slowly from the gastrointestinal tract and elimination of their active metabolites, as well as the parent compound, may take several days. In general, less than 5% of the ingested dose is recovered unchanged in the urine. However, acute tolerance occurs after an overdose and clinical recovery within hours is the rule. Nevertheless the performance of skilled tasks (e.g. driving a car or operating machinery) can be impaired for weeks after apparent recovery from benzodiazepine poisoning.

TREATMENT
In general, management of benzodiazepine poisoning involves *supportive care* only. Although the benzodiazepine antagonist *flumazenil* can reverse coma in such cases (Ashton, 1985), its value in clinical practice is uncertain. It has been suggested that, following isolated benzodiazepine overdose,

flumazenil might speed recovery, reduce after-effects and shorten hospital stay, while in multiple self-poisoning it could reverse respiratory depression and facilitate diagnosis.

Flumazenil can be given in aliquots of 100 µg to a dose of 1.0 mg and has a rapid onset of action in less than a minute, with a maximal effect at 5 minutes. Because it has a relatively short half-life (54 minutes), repeated administration or a continuous infusion at 100–400 µg/h may be required. Moreover, there is a danger of precipitating acute withdrawal symptoms. Convulsions may be produced, especially in epileptics and in the presence of proconvulsant agents such as tricyclic antidepressants, and rapid reversal may also precipitate ventricular fibrillation.

Many therefore now believe that flumazenil has little or no place in the management of benzodiazepine overdose. Others, however, have suggested that flumazenil is a safe aid to diagnosis in cases of multiple-drug overdose and that this agent reduces the requirement for interventions such as gastric lavage, tracheal intubation, mechanical ventilation and CT scan of the brain (Höjer *et al.*, 1990). Flumazenil should, therefore, be used on expert advice only.

Phenothiazines and related drugs
Although these major tranquillizers are often prescribed for the 'at-risk' population of patients with psychotic illnesses, they are a relatively uncommon cause of self-poisoning.

CLINICAL FEATURES
Following an overdose, the patient may become *drowsy* or *comatose* with *respiratory depression* and *hypotensive* with a *tachycardia*. Arrhythmias may occur (particularly with thioridazine) and the ECG may show prolongation of the QT interval and flattening of the T waves. Sudden death is a possibility, probably as a result of *torsades de pointes* (see Chapter 9). Impaired hypothalamic function combined with cardiovascular depression makes the patient susceptible to *hypothermia*. *Extrapyramidal disturbances* such as oculogyric crises, dystonia (particularly with prochlorperazine and trifluoperazine) and convulsions may also occur. Some may develop neuroleptic malignant syndrome (see Chapter 20).

TREATMENT
Methods to speed elimination are ineffective and treatment is therefore *supportive*. Plasma potassium should be maintained within the normal range and the pH should be kept above 7.4. Extrapyramidal disturbances can be treated with repeated intravenous administration of *benzatropine mesilate* 1–2 mg or diazepam (emulsion preferred). Acute dystonia is generally relieved by *procyclidine*, 5–10 mg intravenously. Arrhythmias may respond to correction of hypoxia, acidosis and other biochemical abnormalities; otherwise specialist advice should be sought. If hypotension requires specific treatment, an α *adrenoceptor stimulant* should be used.

Barbiturates

These drugs are now rarely prescribed as anticonvulsants. Consequently barbiturate overdose is uncommon.

CLINICAL FEATURES

Barbiturate overdose produces *generalized depression of the central nervous system*. The conscious level is reduced and this may progress to deep coma with flaccidity and hyporeflexia. The corneal reflex is often absent. The pupillary response to light is sluggish or absent and conjugate eye movement is lost. Unequal pupils suggest hypoxic cerebral damage, a diagnosis that is supported by the presence of other focal neurological signs, sometimes accompanied by seizures.

Profound cardiovascular depression may occur and is caused by a reduction in central vasomotor activity, a decrease in arteriolar tone and myocardial depression. Cardiac output and blood pressure are low, while central venous pressure (CVP) may be high (in those with myocardial failure) or low (in the presence of relative hypovolaemia). There may be a metabolic acidosis.

Respiratory depression causes hypoventilation with hypercarbia and hypoxaemia. Hypoxaemia may be exacerbated by increased capillary permeability leading to the development of acute respiratory distress syndrome (see Chapter 8) and/or ventilation/perfusion mismatch (Sutherland *et al.*, 1977).

The reduction in muscle tone combined with cardiovascular depression causes *vascular stasis and tissue hypoxia*. Ischaemic muscle damage may lead to *rhabdomyolysis*, which may in the long term be followed by muscle calcification. Local hypoxia may also be responsible for the development of *skin blisters*, which are seen in approximately 5% of patients with barbiturate poisoning. Although these blisters often develop over pressure areas, they are not necessarily related to trauma and may occasionally complicate even a relatively trivial overdose.

Gastrointestinal motility is often depressed. It is thought that the fluctuations in conscious level that sometimes occur in barbiturate poisoning are due to the intermittent recovery of intestinal function leading to further absorption of the drug.

Hypothermia is a common complication of barbiturate overdose and is a result of impaired hypothalamic function, a reduction in muscle tone and vasodilatation.

TREATMENT

The vast majority of those who reach hospital alive will survive with *aggressive supportive care*, provided they have not suffered irreversible cerebral damage. CVP and, in some cases, cardiac output monitoring are required in seriously poisoned patients to guide intravenous volume replacement. Hypothermia must be prevented or treated (see Chapter 20).

Repeated doses of activated charcoal may be used for barbiturate poisoning, combined in severe cases with haemodialysis. Charcoal haemoperfusion has been recommended for those who are deeply unconscious and failing to improve following a massive overdose of a long-acting barbiturate.

IRON SALTS

Iron tablets are most frequently prescribed to young women and they, or their children, therefore account for the majority of cases of poisoning.

Clinical features

Within the first 6 hours, symptoms are mainly due to gastrointestinal irritation with abdominal pain, nausea, vomiting, haematemesis, melaena and even *gastric perforation*. Some complain of a *metallic taste*. Those who are seriously poisoned become *hypovolaemic* and *shocked*. There is usually an asymptomatic interval from 8 to 24 hours after ingestion. *Convulsions, coma, hepatic necrosis, hypoglycaemia* and *metabolic acidosis* may supervene later due to the toxic effects of iron on the liver and other organs.

Treatment

Iron is slowly absorbed. *Gastric aspiration and lavage* should be performed within 1 hour of ingesting a significant quantity of iron or if radiography reveals tablets in the stomach. Whole-bowel irrigation may be considered in severe poisoning.

The severity of poisoning can be assessed by measuring the serum iron level, and if this is more than twice the upper limit of normal, 1–2 g of desferrioxamine which chelates iron should be administered intramuscularly and repeated 3–12 hours later. In severe toxicity or if the patient is shocked, this agent should be given intravenously (15 mg/kg per hour up to a total dose of 80 mg/kg in 24 hours – in severe cases higher doses may be used on advice from a poisons information centre).

STIMULANTS AND DRUGS OF MISUSE
Amphetamines

Amphetamines are now rarely prescribed; episodes of poisoning are therefore usually related to illicit use. Amphetamines can be injected, inhaled or taken orally.

CLINICAL FEATURES

In overdose, amphetamines produce:

- confusion and hallucinations;
- anxiety;
- restlessness and wakefulness;
- tremor;
- irritability.

The patient may be *hyperreflexic* with *dilated pupils*. An initial pallor is followed by *flushing, tachycardia* and *arrhythmias*. Hypertension may be associated with convulsions, hyperthermia and coma.

TREATMENT

Treatment is *supportive* and includes sedation with a *benzodiazepine* or, if this fails, a *phenothiazine*. Advice should be sought from a poisons information centre on the management of hypertension, convulsions and hyperpyrexia. Elimination of amphetamines can be enhanced by inducing an acid diuresis, although this is rarely necessary.

MDA and MDMA (ecstasy)

Methylenedioxyamphetamine (MDA) and methylenedioxymethamphetamine (MDMA) – known as *ecstasy* – are synthetic amphetamine derivatives with a mild amphetamine-like stimulant effect. They also induce a feeling of euphoria and increased sociability as well as enhanced perception. Their hallucinogenic potential is low (Henry, 1992), although many substances are added to ecstasy, including caffeine and ketamine (Winstock and King, 1996). Side effects include:

- loss of appetite, nausea;
- trismus and teeth grinding;
- muscle aches and stiffness;
- ataxia;
- sweating, dehydration;
- tachycardia, hypertension;
- hyponatraemia and catatonic stupor (Maxwell *et al.*, 1993).

The pharmacological effects of the drug can be compounded by relentless drug-stimulated physical exertion in a hot environment such as a nightclub. Afterwards there may be fatigue and insomnia. Under these circumstances acute severe complications may occur unpredictably and can include:

- hyperpyrexia;
- delirium, collapse, hyperreflexia, convulsions;
- rhabdomyolysis;
- DIC;
- acute renal failure;
- acute hepatitis;
- ventricular arrhythmias, hypotension;
- acute respiratory distress syndrome;
- cerebral haemorrhage or infarction due to uncontrolled hypertension or vasculitis;
- self-induced water intoxication.

The hyperthermic syndrome resembles malignant hyperpyrexia and heat stroke (see Chapter 20). Serotonin syndrome may occur.

MANAGEMENT

Management is urgent and should include:

- control of agitation and convulsions with diazepam (emulsion preferred);
- rapid rehydration;
- measurement of core temperature and active cooling measures if rectal temperature exceeds 40°C;
- paralysis and ventilation if muscle spasm is continuing to generate heat;
- cardiovascular and respiratory support;
- management of rhabdomyolysis, DIC and renal failure, as described elsewhere.

The extent to which dantrolene is of value (Denborough and Hopkinson, 1997) is in doubt (Watson *et al.*, 1993) and dose-dependent adverse effects such as hepatitis are a cause for concern. Hepatotoxicity has also occurred with ecstasy poisoning and has been successfully treated with liver transplantation (Henry *et al.*, 1992; Jones and Simpson, 1999). Advice should be sought from a poisons centre.

Cocaine

The recreational use of cocaine has increased dramatically. It can be taken intravenously or by intranasal insufflation and can be smoked. 'Crack' (so called because it crackles when burnt) is a more potent alkaloid of cocaine that is suitable for smoking and is very rapidly absorbed. Abuse of 'crack' has now reached epidemic proportions.

MECHANISMS

Unlike other local anaesthetics, cocaine also impairs the presynaptic uptake of catecholamines and upregulates postsynaptic receptors. It also has other poorly understood actions within the central nervous system. When mixed with alcohol, cocaine may be metabolized in the liver to a longer-lasting, more lethal metabolite, cocaethylene (Randall, 1992). Street cocaine is frequently contaminated with adulterants such as amphetamines, lysergic acid diethylamide (LSD), quinine and heroin.

CLINICAL FEATURES

The clinical features of cocaine intoxication are related to peripheral and central nervous system stimulation and include:

- euphoria (the effect desired by the user);
- dysphoria;
- chest pain;
- agitation, hyperactivity, confusion, headaches, aggression;
- delirium;
- paranoia;
- hallucinations;
- hyperreflexia, tremors, fasciculation, seizures;
- hyperthermia;
- dilated pupils.

Increased peripheral sympathetic activity may cause *tachycardia, cardiac arrhythmias* and *hypertension* associated with marked *vasoconstriction* (Cregler and Mark, 1986). Complications include myocardial infarction, dilated cardiomyopathy, cerebrovascular accidents and rhabdomyolysis with or without renal failure (Steingrub *et al.*, 1989).

When taken intravenously, impurities are filtered by the lungs, but all forms of cocaine abuse can be associated with *non-cardiogenic pulmonary oedema. Bronchiolitis obliterans* has also been reported. '*Crack lung*' is characterized by bronchospasm, fever and transient pulmonary infiltrates. Because it is associated with elevated serum immunoglobulin E levels and eosinophilia it has been attributed to a hypersensitivity reaction. Those who smoke cocaine may perform a deep, prolonged and forceful Valsalva manoeuvre, which can also be complicated by subcutaneous emphysema, pneumomediastinum and pneumothorax. Cocaine can also cause pulmonary haemorrhage.

Cocaine use in pregnancy has been associated with serious maternal and fetal complications, including abruptio placentae, spontaneous abortion and preterm labour. It may also cause placental ischaemia, as well as myocardial or cerebral infarction in the fetus.

DIAGNOSIS AND INVESTIGATIONS

The clinical features of cocaine toxicity are similar to those of neuroleptic malignant syndrome (see Chapter 20), acute withdrawal from alcohol, sedatives or hypnotics, and an overdose of anticholinergics, hallucinogens or amphetamine.

Investigations should include:

- ECG;
- blood glucose;
- creatine phosphokinase (CK) and troponin levels, urinary myoglobin;
- blood and urine cultures;
- in selected cases, cerebral CT scan and occasionally lumbar puncture;
- core temperature (should be measured frequently).

The metabolites of cocaine can be detected in the urine.

MANAGEMENT

The circulating volume should be expanded and adequate oxygenation ensured. Tracheal intubation and mechanical ventilation may be indicated in those with:

- extreme agitation;
- deep coma;
- seizures;
- hyperthermia.

Agitation should be controlled with an intravenous *benzodiazepine*. This will limit the severity of the cardiovascular disturbance as well as helping to prevent hyperthermia and acidosis. A benzodiazepine such as lorazepam is also indicated in those with *seizures*. More resistant cases will require a benzodiazepine infusion, usually combined with tracheal intubation and mechanical ventilation. In general phenytoin is not a particularly effective anticonvulsant in those with cocaine toxicity and *barbiturates* are preferred. *Dantrolene* may have a place in the management of severe *hyperthermia* (core temperature > 40°C). Neuroleptic agents should be avoided.

Supraventricular tachyarrhythmias may not require specific treatment. Importantly, lidocaine can aggravate cocaine

toxicity. Severe *hypertension* can be treated with an infusion of *sodium nitroprusside* or, possibly, *labetalol*. Pure β-blockers should be avoided because there is a danger that the unopposed α-activity will precipitate extreme vasoconstriction, hypertension and a fall in cardiac output.

Myocardial ischaemia should be treated with nitrates and morphine. Surprisingly, CCBs have not proved useful and thrombolytic therapy can be dangerous.

Non-cardiogenic pulmonary oedema should be managed as outlined in Chapter 8, while steroids may be indicated in patients with bronchiolitis obliterans and 'crack lung'.

OTHER POISONS
Carbon monoxide

The commonest sources of CO poisoning are motor vehicle exhaust fumes, incorrectly maintained and ventilated heating systems and smoke from fires (see Chapter 10). Approximately 300 people die from CO poisoning in England and Wales every year and CO is a common cause of death from poisoning in children. CO is a complex poison and the diagnosis is often difficult (Wright, 2002).

MECHANISMS

The affinity of CO for haemoglobin is some 200–250 times greater than that of oxygen, which it therefore displaces. It also shifts the oxyhaemoglobin dissociation curve to the left and may inhibit cellular respiration as a result of binding to other haem-containing proteins. Although CO only combines with cytochromes under hypoxic conditions, once binding occurs it is difficult to reverse with conventional oxygen therapy. These tissue effects may be the major cause of clinical toxicity and this may explain the discrepancy between clinical consequences and carboxyhaemoglobin (COHb) levels. The net effect is cellular hypoxia, which may be fatal.

CLINICAL FEATURES

The clinical course of CO toxicity is directly related to the degree and duration of exposure (Meredith and Vale, 1988). The diagnosis can be confirmed by estimating the percentage of COHb present in the blood, but this should be taken as only an approximate indication of severity as clinical findings are a better guide. In general COHb levels less than 10% produce no symptoms whereas levels above 50–60% are associated with coma and a risk of cardiovascular collapse or cardiac arrest. Arterial oxygen tension is usually normal.

Manifestations of *acute poisoning* include headaches, dizziness, hyperventilation, confusion, disorientation and, in severe cases, coma. Nausea, vomiting and faecal incontinence may also occur, as may hyperreflexia, convulsions and cardiac arrhythmias. Later, pulmonary oedema and respiratory depression may supervene, while extreme hypoxia may produce cerebral oedema and hyperpyrexia. Myocardial injury is common and is a predictor of long-term mortality (Henry *et al.*, 2006). Some patients develop rhabdomyolysis and renal failure. The *pink discoloration of the skin* caused by the presence of large amounts of COHb is generally only seen in postmortem cases. *Cyanosis* and *skin pallor* are more usual. *Skin blisters* may occur as a result of tissue hypoxia. Delayed sequelae may include neuropsychiatric disturbances such as memory loss, impaired intellect and cerebellar damage, which may appear several weeks after exposure. Repeated exposure may lead to headaches, poor concentration, dizziness, visual disturbances, paraesthesiae, chest pain, abdominal pain and diarrhoea. Repeated *chronic exposure* or a severe single exposure may be followed by fatigue, poor memory, impaired concentration and a change in personality.

TREATMENT

Administration of oxygen in high concentrations, and mechanical ventilation if indicated, should be instituted immediately. Cerebral oedema should be anticipated in severe poisoning and is treated with an intravenous infusion of mannitol.

Hyperbaric oxygen. The elimination half-life of CO is reduced from 250 minutes when breathing air to 59 minutes when 100% oxygen is administered and to 22 minutes when 100% oxygen is breathed at 2.2 atmospheric pressure. To date, however, the authors of several randomized trials have disagreed as to whether treatment with hyperbaric oxygen is effective in clinical practice (Ducasse *et al.*, 1995; Raphael *et al.*, 1989; Scheinkestel *et al.*, 1999; Thom *et al.*, 1995). Limitations of these trials have included too few patients, inclusion of patients exposed to other toxins in fires and differing protocols for delivering hyperbaric oxygen therapy.

Current recommendations for considering hyperbaric oxygen therapy include:

- recovery of consciousness after an initial high COHb concentration;
- neurological or psychiatric features other than headache;
- evidence of myocardial ischaemia;
- pregnancy (in view of the greater susceptibility of the fetus to CO).

Contraindications to hyperbaric oxygen are in the main related to the practical difficulties of managing patients in single-person (monoplace) chambers and include:

- mechanical ventilation;
- inability to maintain an airway;
- hypovolaemic or vasopressor-dependent patients;
- cardiac arrhythmias potentially requiring urgent intervention;
- asthma.

Larger (multiplace) chambers in which medical attendants can also be pressurized overcome most of these difficulties but are not widely available. The logistical difficulties of transporting patients to distant hyperbaric oxygen chambers should not be underestimated.

Cyanide

Cyanides are used industrially in electroplating and to clean or harden metals as well as in some chemical laboratories reagents. Most cases of poisoning encountered in clinical practice are caused by ingestion or inhalation of sodium or potassium cyanide; free hydrocyanic acid (prussic acid) is almost instantaneously fatal if taken orally. The effects of inhaled prussic acid depend on the concentration of the vapour. The direct-acting vasodilator sodium nitroprusside is a complex cyanide that releases free hydrogen cyanide (HCN) *in vivo* and may produce related toxic effects when a large amount has been administered (see Chapter 5).

MECHANISMS

Cyanide produces its toxic effects by reacting with cytochrome oxidase, thereby inhibiting the final steps in oxidative phosphorylation.

CLINICAL FEATURES

If large quantities (1–2 g) are ingested, there is a rapid *loss of consciousness*, followed by *convulsions* and *death*. Lesser amounts produce *drowsiness, dizziness, breathlessness, confusion, nausea, vomiting* and *shock*. Coma and death may follow. *Severe lactic acidosis* and a *reduced $C_{A-v}O_2$* are characteristic. Some individuals are able to detect an odour of bitter almonds on the breath of the victim. For obvious reasons expired-air resuscitation must *not* be given.

TREATMENT

When an unconscious patient is known to have ingested or inhaled cyanide, immediate treatment is imperative. A heparinized blood sample should be obtained for blood gas analysis and cyanide assay. General supportive measures including the administration of oxygen in high concentrations should be instituted and a specific antidote given. Immediately following massive exposure to cyanide (e.g. following an industrial accident) *intravenous dicobalt edetate* (300 mg over 1 minute) should be administered by intravenous injection, followed immediately by an infusion of 50 mL of 50% glucose (dicobalt edetate can cause hypoglycaemia). If the response is inadequate a second dose of both may be given. If there is still no response after a further 5 minutes a third dose of both may be administered. Dicobalt edetate is an effective antidote because it has a rapid action and, although it is itself toxic, in the presence of HCN a stable non-toxic complex is formed.

If the patient is conscious or has minimal symptoms after assumed exposure to cyanide, dicobalt edetate should not be given since in the absence of HCN it is likely to produce an anaphylactoid reaction, sometimes with severe laryngeal oedema. Dicobalt edetate may also precipitate atrial fibrillation, hypocalcaemia and hypomagnesaemia. Therefore, when some time has elapsed between ingestion and arrival in hospital or when there is doubt as to the nature of the poisoning, *sodium nitrite* followed by *sodium thiosulphate* are the antidotes of choice.

Sodium nitrite acts by converting haemoglobin to methaemoglobin, the ferric iron of which then combines with HCN. Sodium nitrite (300 mg) should be given intravenously in order to convert approximately 25% of the haemoglobin to methaemoglobin. However, this clearly reduces the amount of haemoglobin available for oxygen transport and is potentially hazardous, especially in children. In addition, nitrites can precipitate or exacerbate hypotension.

Sodium thiosulphate enables natural detoxification mechanisms to convert cyanide to thiocyanate. Sodium thiosulphate injection (500 mg/mL) should be administered in a dose of 12.5 g every 10 minutes. Both sodium nitrite and sodium thiosulphate are special-order (unlicensed) products used without restriction when administered to save life in an emergency. Advice should be sought from a poisons information centre, drug manufacturer or regional hospital manufacturing unit. Hydroxocobalamin is an alternative antidote for cyanide poisoning but its use should ideally be discussed with a poisons information centre. The usual dose is hydroxocobalamin 70 mg/kg by intravenous infusion (repeated once or twice according to severity).

Pesticides

PARAQUAT (Editorial, 1976)

Paraquat is a herbicide that is available commercially as a 10–20% concentrated liquid (e.g. *Gramoxone*) and to the general public in the form of solid granules containing 2.5% paraquat (e.g. *Weedol*).

Clinical features. Paraquat is a *strong cytotoxin* that will burn the skin, tongue, mouth and oesophagus. This may not be apparent until 24–48 hours after ingestion when large white necrotic areas develop; these are often painless. Inhalation of spray, mist or dust containing paraquat may cause nose bleeding and sore throat. Eye contamination will cause extreme irritation with ulceration of the conjunctivae and cornea. *Sweating, nausea, repeated vomiting* and *diarrhoea* are usual, and in some cases the vomitus will contain gastric and oesophageal epithelial cells. *Tremor* and *convulsions* may occur.

Ingestion of large amounts of paraquat may be associated with the development of multiorgan failure and death within 72 hours. When poisoning is less severe, evidence of myocardial, liver and renal dysfunction may be delayed for several days. Paraquat can, however, accumulate progressively in the lungs by an energy-dependent process (Rose *et al.*, 1974) even when plasma concentrations are relatively low. Subsequently, the alveolar epithelial lining is destroyed and this is followed by *progressive pulmonary fibrosis* culminating in hypoxaemic respiratory failure. Although this lung lesion may take 2–3 weeks to develop, it is irreversible and death is inevitable.

Investigations. The diagnosis of paraquat poisoning can be confirmed by a simple qualitative urine test. Moreover, there is a good correlation between early blood levels and the severity of poisoning.

Treatment. Treatment with activated charcoal should be started immediately, although severe vomiting may complicate its administration and an antiemetic may be required. Intravenous fluids and analgesics are given as necessary. Unduly high inspired oxygen levels should be avoided in the early stages of management since this may accentuate the lung damage, although high concentrations may be required later to palliate symptoms. Further measures to enhance elimination of absorbed paraquat should be discussed with a poisons information centre and guidance obtained on predicting the likely outcome based on plasma concentrations.

Prognosis. An oral dose of approximately 2–3 g is likely to be fatal if untreated. Although the ingestion of granular preparations for garden use have caused few deaths, the mortality from poisoning with the concentrated solution is approximately 90%.

ORGANOPHOSPHORUS PESTICIDES

Organophosphorus pesticides are usually supplied as powders or dissolved in organic solvents.

Mechanisms. Most of the organophosphorus compounds are highly lipid-soluble and are therefore well absorbed via all routes, including the bronchi and intact skin. They form very stable links with acetylcholinesterase, thereby prolonging and intensifying the effects of acetylcholine. Recovery of anticholinergic activity is therefore delayed until sufficient quantities of enzyme have been manufactured. This may take days or even months.

Clinical features. Poisoning with cholinesterase inhibitors causes:

- an increase in postganglionic parasympathetic nervous activity;
- muscle fasciculation followed by paralysis;
- central nervous stimulation followed by depression.

There is anorexia, salivation, rhinorrhoea, vomiting, abdominal colic and diarrhoea. The patient is restless with constricted pupils; coma and convulsions may occur. Later, respiratory depression supervenes with paralysis of respiratory and ocular muscles, laryngobronchospasm and increased tracheobronchial secretions. Cardiovascular manifestations include bradycardia and hypotension. Hyperglycaemia and glycosuria without ketonuria may also be present.

Treatment (Roberts and Aaron 2007). Immediate management must include measures to *prevent further exposure* to the poison, including the removal of contaminated clothing and thorough washing of contaminated skin with soap and water. Gastric lavage should be considered provided the airway is protected. *Atropine* should be administered in large doses (2 mg) repeated every 5–10 minutes until the skin becomes flushed and dry, the pupils dilate and tachycardia develops. Prolonged administration (2–3 days) may be required. *Pralidoxime mesilate*, a cholinesterase reactivator, is used as an adjunct to atropine in moderate or severe poisoning. It improves muscle tone within 30 minutes following intravenous injection in an initial dose of 30 mg/kg (repeated every 4–6 hours or as an intravenous infusion at 8 mg/kg per hour in severe case). A high-dose regimen, consisting of a continuous infusion of 1 g/h for 48 hours after a 2 g loading dose, may reduce morbidity and mortality in moderately severe cases (Pawar *et al*., 2006). Otherwise, treatment is *supportive* and may include mechanical ventilation.

Nerve agents. The course of nerve agent poisoning is shorter than that of organophosphorus insecticide poisoning, and although treatment is similar, patients reaching hospital alive have generally already recovered. In emergencies involving the release of nerve agents, kits which contain pralidoxime may be obtained from designated centres (see TOXBASE (www.spib.axl.co.uk) or contact the UK National Poisons Information Service on 0870 6006266). In very rare circumstances when exposure to tabun is suspected, obidoxime will also be supplied. In all instances involving nerve agents the risk of cross-contamination is significant and protective clothing and adequate decontamination are essential.

Corrosives
CLINICAL FEATURES
Acids and alkalis. Acids and alkalis are used for cleaning, both domestically and industrially, as well as being involved in chemical manufacturing processes. When swallowed, they can cause *extensive burns* of the mouth, tongue, pharynx, oesophagus and stomach. These are extremely painful and may lead to *perforation* of the oesophagus or stomach. Oedema of the epiglottis and larynx can produce severe *upper-airway obstruction* necessitating tracheal intubation. Systemic absorption produces profound *acid–base disturbances* and *shock*. Delayed deaths may be associated with necrosis and superimposed infection.

Long-term complications in survivors include *gastrointestinal scarring* and *stenosis*.

Phenolic compounds. Phenolic compounds are commonly found in antiseptics, disinfectants and preservatives. If swallowed, they cause blanching or erythema around the mouth and chin followed by *intense thirst, nausea, vomiting, diar-*

rhoea and *sweating*. Those who are severely poisoned may develop *abdominal pain, convulsions* and *coma*. *Acute renal failure* is common and *hepatic damage* may occur.

Treatment. Gastric lavage should probably be avoided because of the risk of aspiration, although some recommend this technique as a means of diluting the corrosive. Surgical intervention is required if there are signs of perforation. Otherwise, treatment is supportive and may include total parenteral nutrition. Prognosis is poor in severe cases.

Mushroom poisoning
Over 90% of those who die as a result of fungal poisoning have eaten *Amanita phalloides*. Earlier recognition of mushroom poisoning combined with aggressive treatment before liver failure has developed have been associated with mortality rates of 10–15% (Vesconi *et al*., 1985).

AMANITA PHALLOIDES (DEATH CAP)
Mechanisms. This fungus contains two toxins. The *phallotoxins* (heptapeptides) produce violent nausea, vomiting and diarrhoea, while the *amatoxins* (octapeptides) cause a fatal hepatorenal syndrome. The latter produce severe cellular damage by binding to the nuclear RNA polymerase B of eukaryotic cells, inhibiting enzyme activity and precipitating cell necrosis. In humans, amatoxins are specifically toxic to hepatocytes, intestinal epithelium and possibly the kidney.

Clinical features. Nearly all patients poisoned by *A. phalloides* first develop gastrointestinal symptoms some 6–18 hours after ingestion. There is *vomiting* and *abdominal pain*. *Diarrhoea* can be severe ('cholera-like') leading to hypovolaemia, dehydration and hypokalaemia.

The *signs of hepatocellular necrosis* become evident about 36 hours after ingestion with elevated transaminase levels and, a little later, prolongation of the prothrombin time.

Treatment. The patient should be rehydrated and the circulating volume should be expanded.

Removal of circulating toxins by inducing a *diuresis* is the most effective, safest and cheapest immediate intervention.

Although other techniques such as haemodialysis, haemofiltration and haemoperfusion are effective, they should probably only be used when it proves impossible to produce an enhanced diuresis. *Activated charcoal* can be given to bind toxins within the gastrointestinal tract.

No specific *antidotes* are available, although high-dose penicillin has been recommended. The mechanism of action of penicillin in this situation is unclear, but it may reduce hepatic uptake of amatoxins.

FHF should be managed as outlined in Chapter 14. Liver transplantation has been performed in patients with FHF associated with mushroom poisoning.

OTHER RARE MUSHROOMS

Other rare mushrooms include:

- *Gyromitra*, the effects of which are similar to those produced by amatoxins except that it also produces neurological symptoms such as restlessness, stupor, dizziness, tremor, seizures, diplopia and nystagmus;
- *Orellanus*, which rarely causes initial gastrointestinal symptoms; patients may develop renal failure 7–17 days after ingesting the mushrooms.

Snake bites and animal stings

Envenoming from snake bites is unusual in the UK but common worldwide. The only indigenous venomous snake in the British Isles is the adder (*Vipera berus*).

CLINICAL FEATURES

The bite may cause local and systemic effects, including early anaphylactoid symptoms and later persistent hypotension, ECG abnormalities, coagulopathy with spontaneous systemic bleeding, acute respiratory distress syndrome and acute renal failure.

TREATMENT

Early anaphylactoid symptoms should be treated with adrenaline (epinephrine) (for the management of anaphylaxis: see Chapter 5). Indications for antivenom treatment include systemic envenoming and marked local envenoming with increasing swelling and erythema within 4 hours of the bite. For both adults and children the contents of one vial (10 mL) of European viper venom antiserum is given by intravenous injection over 10–15 minutes or by intravenous infusion over 30 minutes after diluting in sodium chloride 0.9% (5 mL diluent/kg body weight). The dose can be repeated in 1–2 hours if symptoms of systemic envenoming persist. Adrenaline may be required for the management of anaphylactic reactions to the antivenom (see Chapter 5).

Antivenom is available for certain foreign snakes, spiders and scorpions. Specialist information will be required on identification, management and antivenom supply and administration (e.g. Arizona Poisons Centre (www.pharmacy.arizona.edu/centers/poison-center/); Rocky Mountain Poisons Center (www.rmpcdc.org/poisoncenter/index.cfm/)).

REFERENCES

American Academy of Clinical Toxicology and European Association of Poisons Centres (1997a) Whole bowel irrigation. *Journal of Clinical Toxicology* **35**: 699–709.

American Academy of Clinical Toxicology and European Association of Poisons Centres (1997b) Position statement: single-dose activated charcoal. *Journal of Clinical Toxicology* **35**: 721–741.

American Academy of Clinical Toxicology and European Association of Poisons Centres (1997c) Gastric lavage. *Journal of Clinical Toxicology* **35**: 711–719.

American Academy of Clinical Toxicology and European Association of Poisons Centres (1997d) Position statement: ipecac syrup. *Journal of Clinical Toxicology* **35**: 699–709.

Ashton CH (1985) Benzodiazepine overdose: are specific antagonists useful? *British Medical Journal* **290**: 805–806.

Boehnert MT, Lovejoy FH Jr (1985) Value of the QRS duration versus the serum drug level in predicting seizures and ventricular arrhythmias after an acute overdose of tricyclic antidepressants. *New England Journal of Medicine* **313**: 474–479.

Brent J, McMartin K, Phillips S, *et al.* (1999) Fomepizole for the treatment of ethylene glycol poisoning. *New England Journal of Medicine* **340**: 832–838.

Choudhary AM, Taubin H, Gupta T, *et al.* (1998) Endoscopic removal of a cocaine packet from the stomach. *Journal of Clinical Gastroenterology* **27**: 155–156.

Collee GG, Hanson GC (1993) The management of acute poisoning. *British Journal of Anaesthesia* **70**: 562–573.

Cregler LL, Mark H (1986) Medical complications of cocaine abuse. *New England Journal of Medicine* **315**: 1495–1500.

Cutler RE, Forland SC, Hammond PG, *et al.* (1987) Extracorporeal removal of drugs and poisons by hemodialysis and hemoperfusion. *Annual Review of Pharmacology and Toxicology* **27**: 169–191.

Denborough MA, Hopkinson KC (1997) Dantrolene and 'ecstasy'. *Medical Journal of Australia* **166**: 165–166.

Ducasse JL, Celsis P, Marc-Vergnes JP (1995) Non-comatose patients with acute carbon monoxide poisoning: hyperbaric or normobaric oxygenation? *Undersea Hyperbaric Medicine* **22**: 9–15.

Editorial (1976) Paraquat poisoning. *Lancet* **1**: 1057.

Henry JA (1992) Ecstasy and the dance of death. *British Medical Journal* **305**: 5–6.

Henry JA, Jeffreys KJ, Dawling S (1992) Toxicity and deaths from 3,4 methylenedioxymethamphetamine ('ecstasy'). *Lancet* **340**: 384–387.

Henry CR, Satran D, Lindgren B, *et al.* (2006) Myocardial injury and long-term mortality following moderate to severe carbon monoxide poisoning. *Journal of the American Medical Association* **295**: 398–402.

Höjer J, Baehrendtz S, Matell G, *et al.* (1990) Diagnostic utility of flumazenil in coma with suspected poisoning: a double-blind, randomised controlled study. *British Medical Journal* **301**: 1308–1311.

Jones AL, Simpson KJ (1999) Mechanisms and management of hepatotoxicity in ecstasy (MDMA) and amphetamine intoxications. *Alimentary Pharmacology and Therapeutics* **13**: 129–133.

Jones AL, Volans G (1999) Recent advances: management of self-poisoning. *British Medical Journal* **319**: 1414–1417.

Keays R, Harrison PM, Wendon JA, *et al.* (1991) Intravenous acetylcysteine in paracetamol-induced fulminant hepatic failure: a prospective controlled trial. *British Medical Journal* **303**: 1026–1029.

Lancashire MJ, Legg PK, Lowe M, *et al.* (1988) Surgical aspects of international drug smuggling. *British Medical Journal* **296**: 1035–1037.

Lheureux PE, Zahir S, Gris M, *et al.* (2006) Bench-to-bedside review: hyperinsulinaemia/euglycaemia therapy in the management of overdose of calcium-channel blockers. *Critical Care* **10**: 212.

Levy G (1982) Gastrointestinal clearance of drugs with activated charcoal. *New England Journal of Medicine* **307**: 676–678.

Martiny SS, Phelps SJ, Massey KL (1988) Treatment of severe digitalis intoxication with digoxin-specific antibody fragments: a clinical review. *Critical Care Medicine* **16**: 629–635.

Masters AB (1967) Delayed death in imipramine poisoning. *British Medical Journal* **3**: 866–867.

Maxwell DL, Polkey MI, Henry JA (1993) Hyponatraemia and catatonic stupor after taking 'ecstasy'. *British Medical Journal* **307**: 1399.

Menzies DG, Busuttil A, Prescott LF (1988) Fatal pulmonary aspiration of oral activated charcoal. *British Medical Journal* **297**: 459–460.

Meredith T, Vale A (1988) Carbon monoxide poisoning. *British Medical Journal* **296**: 77–79.

Pawar KS, Bhoite RR, Pillay CP, *et al.* (2006) Continuous pralidoxime infusion versus repeated bolus inection to treat organophosphorus pesticide poisoning: a randomised controlled trial. *Lancet* **368**: 2136–2141.

Purkayastha S, Bhangoo P, Athanasiou T, *et al.* (2006) Treatment of poisoning induced cardiac impairment using cardiopulmonary bypass: a review. *Emergency Medicine Journal* **23**: 246–250.

Randall T (1992) Cocaine, alcohol mix in body to form even longer lasting, more lethal drug. *Journal of the American Medical Association* **267**: 1043–1044.

Raphael J-C, Elkarrat D, Jars-Guincestre MC, *et al.* (1989) Trial of normobaric and hyperbaric oxygen for acute carbon monoxide intoxication. *Lancet* **2**: 414–419.

Roberts DM, Aaron CK (2007) Managing acute organophosphorus pesticide poisoning. *British Medical Journal* **334**: 629–634.

Rose MS, Smith LL, Wyatt I (1974) Evidence for energy-dependent accumulation of paraquat into rat lung. *Nature* **252**: 314–315.

Routledge P, Vale JA, Bateman DN, *et al.* (1998) Paracetamol (acetaminophen) poisoning. No need to change current guidelines to accident departments. *British Medical Journal* **317**: 1609–1610.

Scheinkestel CD, Bailey M, Myles PS, *et al.* (1999) Hyperbaric or normobaric oxygen for acute carbon monoxide poisoning: a randomised controlled clinical trial. *Medical Journal of Australia* **170**: 203–210.

Smilkstein MJ, Knapp GL, Kulig KW, *et al.* (1988) Efficacy of oral *N*-acetylcysteine in the treatment of acetaminophen overdose. Analysis of the national multicenter overdose (1976 to 1985). *New England Journal of Medicine* **319**: 1557–1562.

Steingrub JS, Sweet S, Teres D (1989) Crack-induced rhabdomyolysis. *Critical Care Medicine* **17**: 1073–1074.

Stern TA, O'Gara PT, Mulley AG, *et al.* (1985) Complications after overdose with tricyclic antidepressants. *Critical Care Medicine* **13**: 672–674.

Sutherland GR, Park J, Proudfoot AT (1977) Ventilation and acid–base changes in deep coma due to barbiturate or tricyclic antidepressant poisoning. *Clinical Toxicology* **11**: 403–412.

Thom SR, Taber RL, Mendiguren II, *et al.* (1995) Delayed neuropsychologic sequelae after carbon monoxide poisoning: prevention by treatment with hyperbaric oxygen. *Annals of Emergency Medicine* **25**: 474–480.

Vale JA, Meredith TJ, Proudfoot AT (1986) Syrup of ipecacuanha: is it really useful? *British Medical Journal* **293**: 1321–1322.

Vesconi S, Langer M, Iapichino G, *et al.* (1985) Therapy of cytotoxic mushroom intoxication. *Critical Care Medicine* **13**: 402–406.

Visser L, Stricker B, Hoogendoorn M, *et al.* (1998) Do not give paraffin to packers. *Lancet* **352**: 1352.

Watson JD, Ferguson C, Hinds CJ, *et al.* (1993) Exertional heat stroke induced by amphetamine analogues. Does dantrolene have a place? *Anaesthesia* **48**: 1057–1060.

Winstock AR, King IA (1996) Ecstasy and neurodegeneration. Tablets often contain substances in addition to, or instead of, ecstasy. *British Medical Journal* **313**: 423–424.

Wright J (2002) Chronic and occult carbon monoxide poisoning: we don't know what we're missing. *Emergency Medicine Journal* **19**: 386–390.

Disturbances of body temperature

ACCIDENTAL HYPOTHERMIA (Danzl and Pozos, 1994; Epstein and Anna, 2006)

DEFINITIONS

- Accidental hypothermia can be defined as an unintentional fall in core body temperature below 35°C (Danzl and Pozos, 1994). It can be classified as mild (body temperature, 32–35°C), moderate (body temperature 28 to < 32°C), or severe (temperature, < 28°C) and results in a clinical syndrome characterized by multiple systemic derangements that lead to decreased tissue oxygenation.
- *Frostbite* is due to local freezing of tissue with intracellular ice crystal formation and microvascular occlusion. It can be classified according to the depth of the injury.
- *Non-freezing cold injury* to the extremities is due to microvascular endothelial damage, stasis and vascular occlusion. With ambient temperature above freezing, prolonged exposure over several days leads to 'trench foot'. Although the entire foot may appear black, deep tissue destruction may not be present.

CAUSES

Accidental hypothermia may follow exposure to low environmental temperatures or immersion in cold water and is frequently associated with impaired temperature regulation. Factors predisposing to exposure hypothermia include inadequate or wet clothing, strong winds, contact with snow and strenuous exercise. Paradoxically, hypothermia is more common in relatively temperate regions where the dangers of, for example, hill walking in winter are often underestimated and preventive measures are consequently inadequate. The incidence of immersion hypothermia is rising, probably because of the widespread use of lifejackets, which support the head above water and prevent drowning, as well as the increasing popularity of water sports. The rate of heat loss in water is approximately 25 times greater than that in air at the same temperature and is accelerated by the increase in cutaneous blood flow that accompanies exertion (e.g. swimming) as well as a redistribution of the warmed water layer surrounding the body. Subcutaneous fat provides insulation so that obese subjects can generally survive longer periods of immersion; even non-waterproof conventional clothing is protective.

Diseases in which the metabolic rate is reduced (e.g. *myxoedema, hypopituitarism* and *malnutrition*) limit the ability to maintain body temperature by increasing heat production. Similarly, patients with *spinal cord lesions* are unable to produce thermal energy by increasing muscular activity, and this is exacerbated by an inability to adjust skin blood flow (see Chapter 10). *Hypothalamic lesions* can impair thermoregulation and patients in *coma* (e.g. due to a cerebrovascular accident, alcohol abuse or self-poisoning) are frequently hypothermic. Furthermore, *alcohol* and many *sedative drugs*, especially barbiturates, increase heat loss by causing cutaneous vasodilatation. The *elderly* are particularly vulnerable to cold because of inactivity, impaired shivering, low metabolic rate, malnutrition, reduced subcutaneous fat, decreased vasoconstriction in response to cold and poor social conditions (Editorial, 1977).

Debilitating conditions such as hepatic, renal or cardiac failure, as well as sepsis, may also contribute to hypothermia.

CLINICAL MANIFESTATIONS AND PATHOPHYSIOLOGY

The clinical manifestations of hypothermia at a particular body temperature are variable and probably depend on the rate of cooling and the duration of hypothermia. In cases of mild hypothermia, however, thermoregulatory mechanisms usually remain intact. At lower temperatures physiological dysfunction worsens progressively, while cooling to below 30°C produces severe cardiorespiratory and neurological abnormalities with failure of thermoregulation. Body temperatures of less than 27–28°C can mimic death, and extreme hypothermia (< 24–26°C) is usually incompatible with life, although some remarkable cases of survival under these circumstances have been reported (Gilbert *et al.*, 2000) (see Chapter 10).

Metabolic responses

Initially, metabolic rate increases as the victim shivers and increases voluntary muscle activity in an attempt to maintain body temperature. If this is unsuccessful, thermoregulation eventually fails and oxygen consumption ($\dot{V}O_2$) falls by around 7% for each degree Celsius reduction in body temperature (e.g. $\dot{V}O_2$ may be reduced to about 80 mL/min per m^2 at a core temperature of 32°C). Most enzymatic reactions slow by around 50% with a 10°C fall in core temperature. All enzymes are affected, including those involved in liver metabolism and Na$^+$/K$^+$ pumps. As would be expected, the reduction in metabolic rate is greater in those with myxoedema coma.

Neurological manifestations

The severity of the neurological disturbance depends on the rate of cooling. In general, cerebral metabolism is depressed and this minimizes cerebral damage during episodes of ischaemia or hypoxia (see Chapters 9 and 15 for a discussion of therapeutic hypothermia). At core temperatures below 35°C, the patient may be dysarthric, apathetic and ataxic with impaired judgement. Amnesia may occur at temperatures below 34°C and hallucinations may develop below 33°C. Conscious level falls progressively until at 30°C the victim is usually stuporose, with infrequent voluntary movements. Tendon reflexes are slowed, with prolonged contraction and relaxation phases. At core temperatures below 28°C, patients are usually comatose and hypotonic with absent tendon and plantar reflexes. The pupils are dilated and do not react to light; voluntary movements are absent. Muscle rigidity may supervene.

Cardiovascular changes

At first, cardiac output rises in response to sympathetic stimulation and to satisfy the increased metabolic demands, but subsequently the cardiovascular system is depressed in proportion to the fall in body temperature. Initial tachycardia and hypertension are followed by progressive bradycardia, probably due to a direct effect of cold on the sinus node (30–40 beats/min at 28–29°C, 10 beats/min at 25–26°C) so that cardiac output falls dramatically, despite a normal or increased stroke volume. Initially, blood pressure is maintained by vasoconstriction and an increase in viscosity, but hypotension usually supervenes at temperatures below 28°C. In addition, many hypothermic patients are hypovolaemic and vasodilatation induced by rewarming can precipitate serious hypotension. Blood pressure may also fall when the increase in viscosity is reversed by intravenous fluid administration.

Sinus rhythm is maintained during moderate hypothermia, although atrial flutter or fibrillation, sometimes with ventricular premature contractions, often supervenes in the more serious cases. With more profound falls in body temperature, an idioventricular rhythm is common and atrial activity may completely disappear. There is a risk of ventricular fibrillation (VF) when core temperature falls below 30°C; this arrhythmia may be precipitated by hypoxia or hypotension.

The electrocardiogram (ECG) in hypothermia shows evidence of a prolonged cardiac cycle and reduced conductivity with prolongation of the PR and QT intervals, as well as widening of the QRS complex. The ST segment is generally

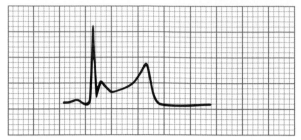

Fig. 20.1 The electocardiogram in accidental hypothermia. Lead V$_5$ showing J-wave and ST-segment changes.

depressed or concave, but is sometimes elevated. J waves may be seen at the junction of the QRS and ST segments (**Fig. 20.1**) when core temperature falls below 32–33°C but are neither sensitive nor specific, since they may also be seen in severe sepsis and subarachnoid haemorrhage. J waves are found consistently when core temperature falls below 25°C.

Respiratory changes

Hypothermia reduces the ventilatory response to hypoxaemia and hypercarbia so that tidal volume and respiratory rate fall progressively. The reduction in minute volume is, however, accompanied by a fall in both $\dot{V}O_2$ and carbon dioxide production. The arterial carbon dioxide tension (P_aCO_2) corrected to body temperature may therefore be low, normal or high depending on the balance between the reduction in alveolar ventilation and the fall in carbon dioxide production. On the other hand, hypothermic patients are consistently hypoxaemic (when arterial oxygen tension is corrected to body temperature), with an increased $P_{A-a}O_2$, largely due to ventilation–perfusion (V/Q) mismatch. Although the consequences of a reduction in arterial oxygen tension (P_aO_2) are minimized by the fall in $\dot{V}O_2$, and are generally well tolerated, a metabolic acidosis is common. Moreover, significant tissue hypoxia can develop when the metabolic rate rises during rapid rewarming or shivering, and restoration of blood flow to previously ischaemic areas washes accumulated acid into the general circulation. This metabolic acidosis is exacerbated by impaired hepatic clearance of lactic acid and a reduction in the capacity of the kidneys to excrete hydrogen ions.

Because airway reflexes are depressed and bronchial secretions are increased hypothermic patients are at risk of atelectasis, mucous plugging and aspiration. *Bronchopneumonia* is a relatively common complication of hypothermia; both its incidence and severity are related to the duration and the degree of hypothermia.

Renal dysfunction

Hypothermia is associated with a diuresis and haemoconcentration, despite a reduction in renal blood flow. Polyuria may be related to a central shift of the blood volume as well as impaired tubular function caused by inhibition of enzyme systems and a reduced responsiveness to antidiuretic hormone. Hypothermic patients therefore produce dilute, eventually almost iso-osmotic urine, with a reduced creatinine clearance, an elevated blood urea and increased sodium excretion owing to a shift of potassium into cells. Hypokalaemia is common unless hypothermia is associated with asphyxia or rhabdomyolysis.

A few patients develop established acute renal failure and require dialysis. This is unlikely to be the result of hypothermia alone and is probably related to associated abnormalities such as hypoxia, hypotension and hypovolaemia.

Other abnormalities

Initially, glucose is released from liver glycogen and its use is increased. Later, glucose uptake decreases, as a consequence of insulin resistance, reduced insulin secretion or inactivation of hexokinase. Hyperglycaemia is exacerbated by elevated cortisol levels. Synthesis of free fatty acids, ketones and glycerol is increased. Lactate levels rise.

Serum amylase levels are often raised in hypothermia, probably reflecting a mild acute pancreatitis. Occasionally a severe oedematous, haemorrhagic or necrotic pancreatitis may complicate hypothermia. Liver enzymes may be raised.

Gastrointestinal motility is decreased, leading to ileus and sometimes acute dilatation of the stomach and colon. Gastric ulcerations and haemorrhage are common (Wischnevsky lesions).

Thrombocytopenia, platelet dysfunction and various coagulation abnormalities (including reduced thromboxane A_2 levels, slowing of the coagulation cascade and fibrinolysis) have been described, but these are of doubtful clinical significance.

Immune function is compromised, increasing the patient's susceptibility to pneumonia and wound infections.

MANAGEMENT (Lazar, 1997)
Monitoring

The diagnosis can be established using a *low-reading rectal thermometer*. Subsequently, body temperature can be continuously monitored using a rectal probe. This must be inserted at least 10 cm beyond the anal sphincter and will record a temperature 0.25–0.5°C below that of blood. An oesophageal probe may more closely reflect the temperature of the blood and the myocardium but can be affected by warmed inhaled air. Tympanic measurements may more closely reflect central nervous system temperature. Thermistor-tipped urinary or central venous catheters are also reliable. It is recommended that body temperature should be recorded simultaneously at two different sites and continuously monitored to follow the response to treatment.

Blood pressure, central venous pressure (CVP), the ECG and urine output should also be monitored in all cases. Insertion of a pulmonary artery catheter is generally not recommended, not least because passage of the catheter may precipitate VF.

Glucose and electrolyte concentrations (particularly potassium) should be measured as soon as possible and fre-

quently thereafter. Other laboratory investigations should include a complete blood count, coagulation screen, liver and pancreatic enzymes, lactate and creatine phosphokinase. Drug and poisons screening and thyroid and/or adrenal function tests should be performed as indicated. Blood, urine and sputum should be sent for microscopy and culture when infection is suspected. Imaging, including computed tomography (CT) scanning, is performed as indicated.

Determination of blood gas tensions is complicated by the influence of alterations in body temperature on the position of the haemoglobin dissociation curve (see Chapter 3). Blood gas analyser measurements are made at 37°C and, if corrected, for example, to a body temperature of 25°C, a P_aO_2 of 13.3 kPa (100 mmHg) and a P_aCO_2 of 5.3 kPa (40 mmHg) become 6.7 and 3 kPa (50 and 22.5 mmHg) respectively. Changes in temperature also affect pH measurements; a fall of 1°C increases pH by 0.0147 units. In practice, however, most clinicians prefer to use uncorrected (alpha stat) blood gas measurements.

Supportive treatment

Patients who are profoundly hypothermic may survive despite appearing to be clinically dead on admission. Moreover, survival has been reported even following prolonged cardiac arrest or VF (Gilbert et al., 2000; Walpoth et al., 1997). Attempts at resuscitation should therefore continue until rewarming has been achieved or until it is clear that the situation is hopeless. Extreme hyperkalaemia has been described in hypothermia associated with asphyxia and cardiorespiratory arrest, as exemplified by snow avalanche victims, and in this situation seems to be an indicator of futility (Schaller et al., 1990).

Hypoxaemia must be corrected by securing the *airway* and administering warmed, humidified *oxygen*; this is particularly important during rewarming when oxygen requirements increase. In view of the depressed airway-protective reflexes *early tracheal intubation* is recommended to guard against aspiration. Some patients will require *mechanical ventilation*. To avoid extreme hypocarbia, which can exacerbate peripheral vasoconstriction and may precipitate VF, the minute volume must be adjusted to match the reduced carbon dioxide production.

Cannulation of a peripheral vein may be difficult because of cold-induced vasoconstriction. Central venous cannulation or, in cases of extreme difficulty, adult intraosseous infusion may therefore be required. Intravenous *fluid replacement* should be started with 5% or 10% dextrose, combined with sodium bicarbonate, if necessary, to correct severe metabolic acidosis. *Expansion of the circulating volume* is essential during rewarming. Intravenous fluids should be warmed. Subsequent fluid administration should be guided by frequent estimation of urea, electrolytes and blood sugar levels, and haematocrit.

Occasionally, hypothermic patients develop cardiac failure during rewarming, with an elevated CVP, persistent hypotension, oliguria and acidosis. This may require the administration of an *inotropic agent*, although there is a considerable risk of inducing arrhythmias. The heart rate normally increases progressively as body temperature rises and definitive treatment of the bradycardia is usually not indicated. Intracardiac pacing is generally ineffective and may increase the risk of VF. Patients in VF will require direct current *defibrillation*. Although successful defibrillation has been reported at temperatures as low as 24°C, in general restoration of an effective cardiac rhythm is unlikely until core temperature has reached 30°C. Vasoactive drugs such as adrenaline (epinephrine) and lidocaine are also not recommended until core temperature has reached 30°C (Soar et al., 2005).

Steroids are of no value in hypothermia, and antimicrobial therapy should be reserved for those with established infection. Thromboembolism prophylaxis should not be initiated in the early stages. In all cases, underlying diseases must also be treated.

Rewarming (Table 20.1)

The risk of complications such as myocardial failure, bronchopneumonia and neurological dysfunction increases the longer hypothermia persists. Furthermore, spontaneous rewarming takes place more slowly when hypothermia is prolonged. It is worth emphasizing, however, that there is no good evidence to suggest that the rate of rewarming influences outcome and that the objective of treatment must be a live patient rather than a given rate of heat transfer.

The first step is to prevent further heat loss. The patient should be removed from the cold environment, dressed in dry clothes and covered with insulating blankets or sleeping bags. Warm drinks can be given to conscious patients who are haemodynamically stable.

Table 20.1 Rewarming for accidental hypothermia

Further heat loss must be prevented

Record body temperature simultaneously from two different sites.

Repeatedly monitor to follow the response to treatment

Passive rewarming may be achieved in patients with mild hypothermia by covering the head and body with warm blankets, and administering warm humidified oxygen and hot drinks

External active warming techniques for patients with moderate or severe hypothermia include the forced-air rewarming (Bair Hugger) blanket

Internal active rewarming techniques include warmed intravenous fluids, warmed humidified oxygen via facemask or endotracheal tube, gastric or peritoneal lavage and extracorporeal rewarming

Cardiopulmonary bypass may be indicated for severely hypothermic patients in cardiac arrest

Spontaneous or passive rewarming is the rule in patients suffering mild hypothermia, and may be possible in a few with core temperatures as low as 26–27°C. Passive rewarming is also preferred by some for elderly patients with prolonged hypothermia and underlying disease (e.g. myxoedema). The patient should be moved to a warm room (25–30°C) with warm blankets and clothing. It is also important to insulate the patient's head since scalp vessels do not constrict in response to cold and considerable heat can be lost from this region. Reported rewarming rates range from 0.1 to 3.7°C/hour.

In other patients, particularly those with impaired thermoregulation and an inability to shiver, *active measures* are required to restore body temperature. This can be achieved with *surface heat* using hot water bottles, heat cradles, circulating water mattresses or electric blankets. These methods are usually suitable for young patients with moderate hypothermia of short duration and for elderly patients who fail to respond to passive rewarming. Warming rates vary from 1 to 4°C/hour. Surface rewarming can, however, produce abrupt vasodilatation and hypotension (*rewarming shock*), while reperfusion of cold ischaemic regions can cause a fall in central body temperature of as much as 3–4°C (*afterdrop*) as well as exacerbating metabolic acidosis. Surface warming techniques are also relatively inefficient and may cause skin burns. Complications can usually be avoided by adequate fluid resuscitation using warmed intravenous solutions. *Hot baths* (at 40–45°C), with the limbs out of the water to avoid afterdrop and minimize hypotension, are suitable for fit young adults, particularly following a short period of immersion in cold water, but should not be used in the elderly. Warming rates range from 5 to 7°C/hour. With this method, active rewarming should be discontinued when the core temperature reaches 33°C. Immersion in a hot bath does, however, place the patient in an uncomfortable and inaccessible position. Moreover cardiopulmonary resuscitation and defibrillation are impracticable in water. *Convective blankets* (e.g. Bair Huggers) are effective with less tendency to be associated with 'afterdrop' hypotension (Steele et al., 1996) or skin burns and can increase body temperature by more than 2–3°C per hour.

Theoretically, *central rewarming*, which warms the 'core' before the 'shell', should avoid some of the dangers of surface heating as well as ensuring that the myocardium warms early and is able to respond to the increasing metabolic demands. Moreover, it is the only practicable method in those with cardiac arrest. Central rewarming at a rate of up to 10°C/hour can be achieved using an *extracorporeal circulation*. Cardiopulmonary bypass via a femoral artery and vein is relatively complex and its use should be restricted to those with severe hypothermia (< 28°C) complicated by myocardial failure or cardiac arrest. Continuous haemodialysis can be effective in patients with moderate hypothermia complicated by haemodynamic instability, intoxication or renal failure and is technically feasible in most intensive care units. *Peritoneal lavage* with warm fluid is less efficient, but may also hasten drug elimination in cases of self-poisoning. Warmed solutions can also be administered via a nasogastric tube.

Intravenous administration of warm fluids and ventilation with warmed humidified gases are usually inadequate when used alone, but are useful adjuncts to other measures. Indeed, the optimal approach in an individual patient is often to use a carefully selected combination of the available techniques.

PROGNOSIS

In those whose temperature is above 32°C morbidity and mortality are determined not by the hypothermia but by the underlying disease. On the other hand hypothermia below 32°C may itself be fatal with mortality rates of up to 80%. Poor prognostic factors include old age, the presence of serious comorbidities, profound hypothermia, cardiorespiratory arrest and severe pancreatitis. Hypothermia associated with poisoning has a good prognosis.

■ HYPERTHERMIA

Although still uncommon, the incidence of severe hyperthermia has recently increased, due principally to the popularity of long-distance running events and the increased availability and use of amphetamine-like drugs such as ecstasy at nightclubs, raves and parties (see Chapter 19). Global warming has also been associated with an increase in the incidence of heat-related illness, including heat stroke.

DEFINITIONS

A variety of disorders can elevate body temperature; those resulting from thermoregulatory failure are termed hyperthermia whereas those resulting from intact homeostatic responses are categorized as fever. The latter is not considered in this chapter.

Hyperthermia is defined as a core body temperature above the hypothalamic set point when heat-dissipating mechanisms are impaired or overwhelmed by environmental or internal (metabolic) heat. *Severe hyperthermia* or *heat stroke* is defined as a core temperature of 40°C or higher accompanied by central nervous system abnormalities such as delirium, convulsions or coma. Hyperthermia occurs along a continuum of heat-related conditions starting with heat stress, progressing to heat exhaustion, then heat stroke and culminating in multiple-organ failure and cardiovascular collapse in some instances (Grogan and Hopkins, 2002).

CAUSES (Table 20.2)

Heat cramps occur in heavily exercised muscles, usually the calves, during unaccustomed exercise when the environmental temperature is high. They are caused by a combination of dehydration and sodium loss and are therefore more

Table 20.2 Causes of hyperthermia

Increased heat production
Increased muscular activity
Exercise
Seizures
Agitation
Rigidity
Uncoupling of oxidative phosphorylation
Salicylates
Stimulation of hepatic metabolism
Sympathomimetics
Alterations in brain chemistry
Reduced heat dissipation
Behavioural dysfunction
High ambient temperature and humidity
Pre-existing disease
Drug-related
Specific syndromes
Malignant hyperthermia
Neuroleptic malignant syndrome
Serotonin syndrome

common in those who sweat profusely and when lost fluids are replaced with water without added salts.

Most cases of *severe hyperthermia* are caused by a combination of exogenous and endogenous factors that result in an excessive heat load, impaired heat dissipation or a combination of both (Simon, 1993). A large number of predisposing factors have been identified (Table 20.3). Many cases follow extreme exertion such as long-distance running, training in the armed forces or prolonged dancing in association with drug abuse, and the incidence is higher when ambient temperature and humidity are high.

Drug toxicity is frequently implicated. Severe hyperthermia has, for example, been described following the use of many recreational drugs. It is not always certain, however, whether this is related to idiosyncratic reactions, overdose or a genetic predisposition to exertional heat stroke (Hopkins et al., 1991), and rhabdomyolysis (Wappler et al., 2001) or is simply a result of unremitting drug-stimulated exercise in hot and humid conditions with inappropriate clothing and inadequate hydration. Responsible drugs may include:

- amphetamines and amphetamine derivatives;
- cocaine;
- lysergic acid diethylamide (LSD);
- phencyclidine (PCP).

Drugs that reduce sweating such as the tricyclic antidepressants, atropine and antihistamines, as well as those that uncouple oxidative phosphorylation such as the salicylates

Table 20.3 Predisposing factors to hyperthermia

Pre-existing conditions

Cardiovascular disease

Endocrine disease

Autonomic dysfunction

Dehydration

Fever

Delirium tremens

Psychosis

Neonates/elderly

Malignant hyperthermia

Parkinsonism

Myopathy

Drugs

Anticholinergics

Phenothiazines

Tricyclic antidepressants

Monoamine oxidase inhibitors (MAOIs)

Selective serotonin reuptake inhibitors (SSRIs)

β-blockers

α-agonists

Sympathomimetics

Hallucinogens

Salicylates

Diuretics

Alcohol

Behaviour

Overexertion

Inappropriate clothing

Poor fluid intake

Poor acclimatization

have also been implicated in precipitating hyperthermia. Sympathomimetic agents increase heat production by stimulating hepatic metabolism of glucose and fat, while α-agonists such as phenylephrine and some appetite suppressants, as well as amphetamine and its derivatives (Logan et al., 1993), cocaine, PCP ('angel dust') and ketamine ('special K'), cause cutaneous vasoconstriction with reduced heat loss. Drugs that cause seizures or rigidity such as tricyclic antidepressants or monoamine oxidase inhibitors (MAOIs) may also increase heat production. *Malignant hyperthermia (MH), neuroleptic malignant syndrome (NMS)*

and the serotonin syndrome are related to the administration of specific drugs (see later in this chapter and Chapter 19).

Increased *centrally mediated thermogenesis* may also be due to dopamine hyperactivity (which causes extrapyramidal rigidity) and excess serotoninergic activity. These are additional mechanisms for temperature disturbances associated with amphetamine derivatives, MAOIs and selective serotonin reuptake inhibitors (SSRIs) such as citalopram and fluoxetine.

Failure to adapt to environmental conditions may also contribute to the development of hyperthermia (Stephan et al., 2005). For example, the mentally ill, small babies, the elderly or infirm and soldiers in training may fail to remove excess clothing or move to a cooler place. Ingestion of alcohol or drugs may also prevent appropriate responses to hot and humid environments.

The ability to increase cardiac output and therefore cutaneous blood flow is also crucial to the dissipation of heat and may be impaired in the elderly, those with pre-existing cardiac disease and by dehydration. Additionally exercise diverts blood to muscles, thereby further reducing cutaneous blood flow.

PATHOPHYSIOLOGY

When temperature regulation fails and core temperature exceeds 42°C, oxidative phosphorylation is uncoupled and enzymes cease to function. Simultaneously energy stores are depleted, membrane permeability increases and there is an influx of sodium into the cells. Adenosine triphosphate (ATP) depletion caused by increased membrane depolarization and neurotransmitter activity leads to further heat production. Therefore, as temperature control fails, hyperthermia is accelerated, proteins denature and there is widespread damage to vital organs. Tissues most at risk include vascular endothelium, nervous tissue and hepatocytes. In severe cases there may be coma, liver failure, renal failure, acute respiratory distress syndrome (ARDS), rhabdomyolysis and disseminated intravascular coagulation (DIC). Recent work suggests that heat stroke is associated with a systemic inflammatory response leading to multiorgan dysfunction in which encephalopathy predominates (Bouchama and Knochel, 2002).

HISTORY AND CLINICAL FEATURES

Usually it is not possible to obtain an adequate history from the patient, whilst family, friends or bystanders may be unable or reluctant to provide information, especially if drug abuse is involved. It is important to establish whether the patient has been exposed to excessive heat loads and whether drug abuse, medications or intercurrent illness are implicated.

Heat exhaustion is characterized by:

- intense thirst;
- headache;
- malaise;
- dizziness;
- nausea and vomiting;
- body temperature higher than 37°C, but less than 40°C.

Traditionally *severe hyperthermia* or *heat stroke* has been divided into *classical heat stroke*, which is seen in those with compromised homeostatic mechanisms when ambient temperature is high, and *exertional heat stroke*, which occurs in young previously healthy people, usually in association with extreme physical exertion. Classical heat stroke has a slower onset and is often associated with an absence of sweating, whereas exertional heat stroke has a rapid onset and sweating may be profuse.

The core temperature will be high (> 40°C), although the patient may already have begun to cool by the time of presentation and may feel deceptively cool as a result of cutaneous vasoconstriction.

The patient's mental state is invariably altered and *neurological changes* are the hallmark of severe hyperthermia. These may include:

- confusion/irritational behaviour;
- seizures;
- abnormal posturing;
- ataxia;
- syncope;
- focal neurological signs;
- coma.

The muscles are likely to be flaccid in those with exertional or environmental hyperthermia, but may be rigid or dystonic in patients with drug-induced hyperthermia. Most of these neurological symptoms and signs resolve, provided treatment is not delayed. Nevertheless, long-term sequelae do occur and may include cerebellar ataxia, paresis and personality changes.

Muscle damage and *rhabdomyolysis* are common, particularly when hyperthermia is secondary to drug abuse and/or unremitting exertion. Muscles are swollen and painful, creatine kinase levels are grossly elevated and there is myoglobinuria.

The *cardiovascular system* is usually hyperdynamic, with tachycardia, normotension with a wide pulse pressure or hypotension associated with hypovolaemia. Early cutaneous vasodilatation may be followed later by peripheral vasoconstriction. Eventually cardiac failure may supervene with a normal or high peripheral vascular resistance. It is worth noting that myocardial contractility is impaired when body temperature exceeds 40°C.

Hyperthermic patients are often *tachypnoeic* and their appearance has been likened to that of a panting dog. Later *pulmonary oedema* may develop. This may be the result of fluid overload, perhaps exacerbated by central redistribution of the circulating volume during cooling and myocardial dysfunction. Alternatively pulmonary endothelial injury may lead to the development of ARDS.

DIC is a common and sinister complication of hyperthermia. It is probably related to activation of the clotting cascade by endothelial damage and heat-induced denaturation of clotting factors.

Acute renal failure is also a common complication of severe hyperthermia and may be related to hypovolaemia, hypotension, direct thermal injury, rhabdomyolysis and haemolysis. Similarly *liver dysfunction* is almost universal and may be due to impaired perfusion, hypoxia or direct thermal injury. Liver failure will exacerbate the coagulopathy.

The combination of extreme exertion, muscle rigidity, seizures and circulatory insufficiency may precipitate *lactic acidosis*, while hypermetabolism and respiratory failure may be complicated by *respiratory acidosis*.

Electrolyte disturbances include hypernatraemia and hypokalaemia, which may be followed later by dangerous hyperkalaemia secondary to rhabdomyolysis and acute renal failure. Hypocalcaemia is common, but rarely requires intervention.

DIFFERENTIAL DIAGNOSIS

The most important differential diagnosis in a patient with the combination of fever and neurological signs is *meningoencephalitis*. If there are signs of meningeal irritation and the history is unclear, appropriate antibiotics should be administered until the diagnosis is clarified by CT scan and, when indicated, lumbar puncture. *Sepsis* may also cause fever and altered mental status. It is particularly important to enquire about foreign travel and the possibility of malaria or other tropical diseases. *Prolonged status epilepticus* or other disorders in which muscle tone is markedly increased such as *discontinuation of antiparkinsonian treatment*, as well as some *psychoses*, can also present as hyperthermia. The *serotonin syndrome* is characterized by hyperthermia, agitation, confusion, tremor, diarrhoea, tachycardia and hypertension (see Chapter 19).

Occasionally *cerebrovascular thrombosis or haemorrhage* involving the hypothalamus or *endocrine disorders* such as thyroid storm or phaeochromocytoma may present with severe hyperthermia and altered mental state (see Chapter 17).

INVESTIGATIONS

Investigations should include:

- full blood count (thrombocytopenia in DIC; elevated white cell count in hyperthermia, but may also indicate infection);
- coagulation screen (coagulopathy may develop rapidly);
- liver function tests;
- creatine kinase;
- urea and electrolytes, blood glucose;
- blood gas and acid–base analysis;
- ECG;
- chest radiograph;
- CT scan of head;
- lumbar puncture.

TREATMENT

The main therapeutic objectives in patients with heat stroke are to cool the patient rapidly (while maintaining oxygen

Table 20.4 Management of heat stroke

Out of hospital

If the core temperature is > 40°C, move the patient to a cooler place, remove clothing and begin external cooling with cold packs to neck, axillae and groin with fanning and spraying of the skin with tepid water

Coma position for stuporose patients

Administer oxygen

Give normal saline intravenously

Transfer to hospital

In hospital

Monitor rectal and skin temperatures

Continue cooling

Give benzodiazepines for seizures

Consider tracheal intubation for airway protection and deteriorating respiratory performance

Administer fluids. Consider invasive monitoring and vasopressors for hypotension

With myoglobin-induced renal injury, administer intravenous furosemide, mannitol and sodium bicarbonate. Monitor serum electrolytes and treat hyperkalaemia

After cooling continue supportive therapy for multiple-organ dysfunction

delivery) and to support vital organ function (**Table 20.4**). Depending on the cause of hyperthermia, specific therapy may be indicated.

Prehospital management

The victim should immediately be moved to a cooler environment and clothing removed. Cooling should be achieved by whatever means are available (e.g. the patient can be sprayed or splashed with water and evaporation encouraged by opening windows and doors, or by using a fan or even the down-draught from helicopter blades). Ice packs, when available, should be applied to the neck, axillae or groins. Vigorous massaging of the skin is also recommended since external cooling may result in cutaneous vasoconstriction. If possible oxygen should be given and an intravenous infusion of crystalloid established.

Management in hospital
COOLING
Aggressive measures to cool the patient should be started as soon as the diagnosis has been established. Immersion in ice-cold water is impractical and its efficacy is limited by cutaneous vasoconstriction, which diminishes the capacity for heat loss. The most effective methods combine evaporation and convection, most simply by splashing or sponging the patient with tepid (not cold) water and exposing him or

her to a continuous current of air (e.g. using a fan). The Mecca body-cooling technique is recommended as a means of reducing body temperature in heat stroke victims. It involves spraying the naked victim with lukewarm, atomized water (at 15°C) while warm air (at 40–50°C) is blown over the body and the skin temperature is maintained above 30°C to encourage cutaneous vasodilatation (Weiner and Khogali, 1980). As well as administering cold humidified oxygen and cold intravenous fluids, which contribute minimally to heat loss, iced gastric lavage is a relatively simple procedure that has been used in combination with evaporative techniques. Convective coolers and intravascular devices designed for induced hypothermia are effective.

If these measures fail to reduce core temperature to below 40°C within about 30 minutes then additional measures such as iced peritoneal lavage (instillation of 2 litres of iced 0.9% saline into the peritoneal cavity, which is drained after 30 minutes) or, rarely, extracorporeal cooling may be used.

Importantly, normalizing the body temperature may not prevent systemic inflammation, disseminated intravascular coagulation and progression to multiple-organ dysfunction.

DRUG THERAPY
Dantrolene is a direct-acting muscle relaxant that inhibits the release of calcium from the sarcoplasmic reticulum. It reduces heat production by preventing muscle contraction. Dantrolene reverses the clinical features of MH (Kolb *et al.*, 1982) and can prevent this condition when given prophylactically to susceptible patients undergoing general anaesthesia. Dantrolene seems to be of no benefit in heat stroke (Bouchama *et al.*, 1991) or NMS (Reulbach *et al.*, 2007) and there is little evidence to support its use in severe hyperthermia associated with the use of amphetamine analogues (see Chapter 19).

Serotonin antagonists such as ketanserin may be useful in the treatment of drug-induced hyperthermia due to agents such as fluoxitene, MAOIs and some amphetamine derivatives whose hyperthermic activity may be partially attributable to increased serotonin levels.

Calcium antagonists such as nimodipine may also be useful by virtue of inhibition of calcium-dependent serotonin release from storage vesicles (Azmitia *et al.*, 1990).

Drugs that *increase dopaminergic activity* such as bromocriptine, amantidine and levodopa and *anticholinergics* such as benzatropine may be useful in NMS, although there is no clear evidence for their efficacy.

In some cases the muscle-relaxant properties of a *benzodiazepine* may be useful.

SUPPORTIVE MEASURES
In severe cases supportive measures may include:

- tracheal intubation and mechanical ventilation, which can be combined with neuromuscular blockade to reduce muscular activity and heat production;

- expansion of the circulating volume (guided by CVP and, in selected cases, cardiac output monitoring);
- inotropic support, though this is rarely required (avoid α-agonists, which may cause cutaneous vasoconstriction and impair heat loss);
- management of pulmonary oedema and/or ARDS (see Chapter 8).
- management of rhabdomyolysis (see Chapters 10 and 13);
- prevention of agitation and seizures (which increase heat production) with prophylactic phenytoin and a benzodiazepine as indicated;
- early haemofiltration for severe rhabdomyolysis and/or renal failure (see Chapter 13);
- administration of blood and blood products as indicated to treat coagulopathy;
- supportive measures for liver impairment (see Chapter 14);
- if cardiac arrest occurs, follow standard procedures for basic and advanced life support. Cool the patient, attempt defibrillation, if appropriate, according to current guidelines while continuing to cool the patient.

PROGNOSIS

Morbidity and mortality are directly related to the peak temperature and the duration of hyperthermia. Recovery of central nervous system function during cooling is a favourable prognostic sign. This should be expected in the majority of patients who receive prompt and aggressive treatment. Prolonged coma and DIC, which is often associated with ARDS, are associated with a poor prognosis (Dematte et al., 1998).

MALIGNANT HYPERTHERMIA

MH is a rare inherited disorder of the calcium-release channel of the skeletal muscle sarcoplasmic reticulum (Loke and MacLennan, 1998). Genetic studies in MH families have found linkage to the locus of the ryanodine receptor gene which encodes the skeletal muscle sarcoplasmic reticulum Ca^{2+}-release channel (MacLennan et al., 1990). Mutations in the ryanodine receptor gene appear responsible for predisposition to MH in many susceptible individuals (Hopkins, 2000).

Pathogenesis

It appears that MH is precipitated when exposure of a susceptible individual to a triggering agent leads to a sudden increase in intracellular calcium concentrations, probably as a result of impaired uptake of calcium by the sarcoplasmic reticulum or inappropriate release of calcium from intracellular stores. The increase in intracellular calcium concentration accelerates hydrolysis of ATP, induces muscle rigidity and uncouples oxidative phosphorylation. These changes induce a hypermetabolic state (Hopkins, 2000) with increased heat production, impaired active transport mechanisms and eventual depletion of ATP.

Responsible agents include:

- succinylcholine;
- inhalational anaesthetic agents (except nitrous oxide);
- caffeine;
- halogenated radiographic contrast media (rarely);
- phenothiazines (increase intracellular calcium).

Ketamine is probably safe, but is best avoided because the hypertension and tachycardia that usually accompany its use might confuse management of a susceptible patient. The condition may also be triggered by strenuous exercise or massive muscle injury, especially in hot and humid conditions, as well as by emotional stress.

Clinical features

Susceptibility to MH is associated with subclinical and clinical myopathies such as Duchenne muscular dystrophy. There may be a history of previous episodes, unexplained perioperative fever or an aborted anaesthetic. MH often presents insidiously in a patient undergoing general anaesthesia. The earliest reliable indication is usually *increased carbon dioxide production*, which may be detected as a rise in the end-tidal carbon dioxide concentration in mechanically ventilated patients or as an increase in minute ventilation in those breathing spontaneously. Unusual and rapid exhaustion of the carbon dioxide absorbent may also be recognized. *Muscle rigidity* is often first noted in the jaw muscles, but later becomes generalized, although the specificity of masseter spasm as a sign of MH has been questioned. Tachycardia, arrhythmias and hypertension may be followed later by hypotension as cardiac function deteriorates. As the hypermetabolic state progresses *body temperature increases*, although this is usually a late sign, and the rate of temperature rise is variable (from 1°C/hour to 1°C every 5 minutes). The onset of fever is also influenced by the precipitating agent(s). Cyanotic mottling of the skin, especially over the head, neck and upper chest, may also be noted.

As the condition progresses patients may develop:

- pulmonary oedema and cardiac failure;
- DIC;
- rhabdomyolysis;
- haemolysis;
- acute renal failure;
- lactic acidosis;
- early and possibly prolonged hyperkalaemia;
- changes in serum calcium, phosphorus and magnesium levels;
- neurological damage.

Investigations and monitoring

Investigations may include:

- blood gas and acid–base analysis;
- plasma electrolytes, urea and glucose;
- creatine kinase;
- liver enzymes;

- coagulation screen and platelet count;
- tests for haemolysis;
- blood lactate.

Body temperature, end-tidal carbon dioxide, ECG, blood pressure, CVP and urine output should be continuously monitored.

Investigation of susceptibility to MH involves testing contractile responses to agents such as caffeine and halothane in a fresh viable muscle biopsy obtained from the patient (Ørding *et al.*, 1997). Testing is performed in a limited number of specialist centres and the results can be inconsistent.

Treatment *(http://www.anaesthesiauk.com/article.aspx?articleid=285)*

The treatment of MH is as follows:

- Terminate anaesthesia and surgery as soon as possible.
- Hyperventilate with oxygen, preferably through a vapour-free circuit.
- If surgery cannot be concluded immediately, use narcotics and non-depolarizing muscle relaxants.
- Administer dantrolene 1 mg/kg intravenously every 5 minutes to a total dose of 10 mg/kg followed by 4–8 mg/day in 3–4 divided doses orally, for 3–4 days as prophylaxis.
- Correct acidosis.
- Control potassium.
- Institute measures to cool the patient.
- Give mannitol and furosemide to promote a diuresis.
- Control arrhythmias.
- Minimize movement and handling of the patient since this may precipitate ventricular arrhythmias.

Drugs such as barbiturates, narcotics and antipyretics are probably of little value. Steroids have been recommended, but their role is unclear. *Chlorpromazine* may help to promote heat loss by reversing peripheral vasoconstriction and inhibiting shivering.

Drugs that should be avoided during an episode of MH include cardiac glycosides, belladonna alkaloids, vasopressors and calcium chloride.

Prognosis

In the 1960s the mortality from MH was around 80%, but improved treatment, earlier detection and increased recognition and understanding of the syndrome have reduced the mortality to less than 10%.

NEUROLEPTIC MALIGNANT SYNDROME

NMS is characterized by fever and muscle rigidity (Adnet *et al.*, 2000). NMS is a potentially fatal idiosyncratic response to neuroleptic drugs, including phenothiazines, butyrophenones, thioxanthenes and other major tranquillizers such as lithium. The condition has also occurred after metoclopramide and withdrawal of antiparkinsonian drugs. The estimated incidence is 0.2–2.0% of those taking neuroleptics and in susceptible patients the syndrome may be triggered by factors such as exhaustion, dehydration and organic brain disease. It affects people of all ages, but is commoner in males and in those less than 40 years of age.

Pathogenesis

NMS is thought to be precipitated by blockade of dopamine D_2 receptors in the basal ganglia and hypothalamus. Hyperthermia is probably related to impaired temperature regulation and sustained muscle contraction.

Clinical features *(Haddow et al., 2004)*

Frequently the syndrome occurs within 2 weeks of instituting treatment or when the dosage is increased; symptoms usually progress rapidly over 2–3 days. Characteristic features include:

- hyperthermia*;
- muscle rigidity and tremors*;
- akinesia;
- impaired consciousness and confusion†;
- autonomic dysfunction with tachycardia†, labile blood pressure† and sweating†;
- tachypnoea†;
- dysarthria and sialorrhoea;
- urinary retention/incontinence.

Investigations may reveal a leukocytosis†, abnormal liver function tests (increased transaminases), hypokalaemia, a raised creatinine kinase*, myoglobinuria and metabolic acidosis.

Three major (*) or two major and four minor (†) criteria plus supportive history have been suggested as a diagnostic threshold for the condition.

The differential diagnosis includes:

- MH;
- Parkinson's disease;
- catatonia;
- serotonin syndrome;
- heat stroke;
- central anticholinergic syndrome;
- drug interactions with MAOIs;
- sepsis;
- tetanus;
- meningoencephalitis.

Admission to intensive care may be precipitated by cardiac arrest (e.g. due to myocardial infarction), respiratory failure (pulmonary oedema, aspiration pneumonitis), seizures or acute renal failure (related to dehydration and/or myoglobinuria).

Treatment

The offending drug should be withdrawn and other dopamine antagonists such as metoclopramide should be avoided. Supportive therapy should include:

- cooling;
- rehydration;
- measures to prevent acute renal failure;
- cardiovascular support;
- mechanical ventilation if indicated.

Specific treatment is intended to alter the balance between dopaminergic and cholinergic activity in the basal ganglia as well as to provide muscle relaxation. Suggested pharmacological interventions have included:

- bromocriptine;
- amantidine;
- levodopa orally;
- benzatropine;
- other muscle relaxants such as diazepam and non-depolarizing agents.

Dantrolene may no longer be the evidence-based treatment of choice in cases of NMS (Reulbach *et al.*, 2007).

REFERENCES

Adnet P, Lestavel P, Krivosic-Horber R (2000) Neuroleptic malignant syndrome. *British Journal of Anaesthesia* **85**: 129–135.

Azmitia EC, Murphy RB, Whitaker-Azmitia PM (1990) MDMA (ecstasy) effects on cultured serotonergic neurons: evidence of $Ca^{2(+)}$ dependent toxicity linked to release. *Brain Research* **510**: 97–103.

Bouchama A, Knochel JP (2002) Heat stroke. *New England Journal of Medicine* **346**: 1978–1988.

Bouchama A, Cafege A, Devol EB, *et al.* (1991) Ineffectiveness of dantrolene sodium in the treatment of heatstroke. *Critical Care Medicine* **19**: 176–180.

Danzl DF, Pozos RS (1994) Accidental hypothermia. *New England Journal of Medicine* **331**: 1756–1760.

Dematte JE, O'Mara K, Buescher J, *et al.* (1998) Near-fatal heat stroke during the 1995 heat wave in Chicago. *Annals of Internal Medicine* **129**; 173–181.

Editorial (1977) The old in the cold. *British Medical Journal* **i**: 336.

Epstein E, Anna K (2006) Accidental hypothermia. *British Medical Journal* **332**: 706–709.

Gilbert M, Busund R, Skagseth A, *et al.* (2000) Resuscitation from accidental hypothermia of 13.7°C with circulatory arrest. *Lancet* **355**: 375–376.

Grogan H, Hopkins PM (2002) Heat stroke: implications for critical care and anaesthesia. *British Journal of Anaesthesia* **88**: 700–707.

Haddow AM, Harris D, Wilson M, *et al.* (2004) Clomipramine induced neuroleptic malignant syndrome and pyrexia of unknown origin. *British Medical Journal* **329**: 1333–1335.

Hopkins PM (2000) Malignant hyperthermia: advances in clinical management and diagnosis. *British Journal of Anaesthesia* **85**: 118–128.

Hopkins PM, Ellis FR, Halsall PJ (1991) Evidence for related myopathies in exertional heat stroke and malignant hyperthermia. *Lancet* **338**: 1491–1492.

Kolb ME, Horne ML, Martz R (1982) Dantrolene in human malignant hyperthermia: *Anaesthesiology* **56**: 254–262.

Lazar HL (1997) The treatment of hypothermia. *New England Journal of Medicine* **337**: 1545–1547.

Logan AS, Stickle B, O'Keefe N, *et al.* (1993) Survival following 'ecstasy' ingestion with a peak temperature of 42°C. *Anaesthesia* **48**: 1017–1018.

Loke J, MacLennan DH (1998) Malignant hyperthermia and central core disease: disorders of Ca^{2+} release channels. *American Journal of Medicine* **109**: 470–486.

MacLennan DH, Duff C, Zorzato F, *et al.* (1990) Ryanodine receptor gene is a candidate for predisposition to malignant hyperthermia. *Nature* **343**: 559–561.

Ørding H, Brancadaro V, Cozzelino S, *et al.* (1997) In vitro contracture test for diagnosis of malignant hyperthermia following the protocol of the European MH group: results of testing patients surviving fulminant MH and unrelated low-risk subjects. The European Malignant Hyperthermia Group *Acta Anaesthesiologica Scandinavica* **41**: 955–966.

Reulbach UK, Duetsch C, Biermann T, *et al.* (2007) Managing an effective treatment for neuroleptic malignant syndrome. *Critical Care* **11**: R4.

Schaller MD, Fischer AP, Perret CH (1990) Hyperkalaemia. A prognostic factor during acute severe hypothermia. *Journal of the American Medical Association* **264**: 1842–1845.

Simon HB (1993) Hyperthermia. *New England Journal of Medicine* **329**: 483–487.

Soar J, Deakin CD, Nolan JP, *et al.* (2005) European resuscitation council guidelines for resuscitation 2005. Section 7: cardiac arrest in special circumstances. *Resuscitation* **67**: S135–S170.

Steele MT, Nelson MJ, Sessler DI, *et al.* (1996) Forced air speeds rewarming in accidental hypothermia. *Annals of Emergency Medicine* **27**: 479–484.

Stephan F, Ghiglione S, Decailliot F, *et al.* (2005) Effect of excessive environmental heat on core temperature in critically ill patients. An observational study during the 2003 European heat wave. *British Journal of Anaesthesia* **94**: 39–45.

Walpoth BH, Walpoth-Aslan BN, Mattle HP, *et al.* (1997) Outcome of survivors of accidental deep hypothermia and circulatory arrest treated with extracorporeal blood warming. *New England Journal of Medicine* **337**: 1500–1505.

Wappler F, Fiege M, Steinfath M, *et al.* (2001) Evidence for susceptibility to malignant hyperthermia in patients with exercise-induced rhabdomyolysis. *Anesthesiology* **94**: 95–100.

Weiner JS, Khogali M (1980) A physiological body-cooling unit for treatment of heat stroke. *Lancet* **ii**: 507–509.

Transporting the critically ill

Critically ill patients may have to be transported to hospital from the site of illness or injury (*primary transport*) or be transferred from one hospital to another for specialist investigations and treatment (*secondary transport*); sometimes transfer is necessary because of a shortage of staffed intensive care beds. Seriously ill patients may also have to be moved within the hospital (e.g. to admit the patient to the intensive care unit (ICU), to the operating theatre for surgical procedures or for investigations such as computed tomography (CT) scanning or angiography).

Moving critically ill patients is hazardous, especially when they are receiving intensive haemodynamic and respiratory support and when unqualified or inexperienced staff are involved (Bion *et al.*, 1988). Not only is there a significant risk of mishaps such as accidental extubation, loss of intravascular access and discontinuation of vasoactive or sedative agents, but seriously ill patients are intolerant of lifting, tipping, abrupt movements, vibration and acceleration/deceleration. Transfer can be associated with a significant deterioration in oxygenation, while accelerational forces and vertical movements can precipitate cardiovascular instability, especially in those who are volume-depleted or vasodilated due to sepsis, sedation or drugs. The mechanisms underlying the reduction in cardiac output that often occurs under these circumstances have not been fully explained, but both venous pooling and vagally mediated responses via the eighth cranial nerve are possibilities. Transfer may also cause significant changes in intracranial pressure. Accelerational forces in the longitudinal plane, for example, will alter the pressure in central veins, intracranial sinuses and cerebrospinal fluid. Placing patients in the head-down position (e.g. when they are being loaded into an ambulance) may also exacerbate intracranial hypertension. Physical difficulties such as narrow corridors, small lifts and cramped vehicles, as well as poor weather conditions, may also be encountered.

In all cases, therefore, the decision to transfer a critically ill patient, either within or between hospitals, must be based on a careful assessment of the potential benefits weighed against the risks. A risk score has been described which can help to identify those patients most at risk of developing complications during transfer (Markakis *et al.*, 2006). Meticulous planning, the use of suitably qualified personnel and

the availability of appropriate equipment can minimize risk and improve outcomes. All hospitals should designate a senior clinician, responsible for transfers, who ensures that written policies and procedures are prepared (addressing, for example issues relating to communication), that equipment and staff are available and that standards are audited.

PRIMARY TRANSPORT

Most often, primary transport of critically ill patients is required for the victims of cardiorespiratory collapse or major trauma, including severe head injuries, and may involve extrication of trapped individuals, handling of mass casualties and evacuation from isolated locations. It may also be necessary to attend to the needs of relatives and bystanders who may be seriously distressed by the events they have witnessed.

COMPOSITION OF THE PRE-HOSPITAL TEAM

In many countries primary transport is normally performed using an ambulance staffed by medical technicians trained in simple first aid or by paramedics; the latter may be trained to provide basic life support (BLS) only or advanced life support (ALS). Some have questioned whether the additional skills of medically qualified personnel can be used to advantage in the pre-hospital environment, although most are now convinced that the inclusion of a doctor in the emergency team is valuable (Koppenberg and Taeger, 2002), and it has been claimed that the survival of patients with blunt trauma is improved when they are attended by flight crews that include a physician (Baxt and Moody, 1987). Those who advocate including a physician in the team argue that, although paramedics with advanced training may be competent to perform the commonly required practical procedures, the particular skills of a doctor are invaluable for diagnosis, assessing the severity of the injury, deciding priorities and triage. There are also reservations about those without medical knowledge using advanced resuscitation techniques unsupervised.

It is claimed that a number of other benefits may arise from specialist medical involvement in pre-hospital care. For example it becomes unnecessary to dispatch relatively inexperienced doctors in training, unsupervised, to the scene of an incident, and hospitals are not deprived of doctors when patients require transfer. Also the training of doctors in emergency medicine at the roadside is improved and experienced doctors are immediately available to respond to major disasters. Certainly the French have insisted that doctors should play a central role in the control and provision of pre-hospital emergency care and to this end have created an emergency medical assistance service – Service d'Aide Médicale Urgente (SAMU) – which each *département* is now legally required to provide. Every SAMU has a control room, offices and a garage for the rescue vehicles. The control room acts as a centre for the reception of medical emergency calls and is under the control of a fulltime *chef de service*. The main functions of the SAMU are:

- centralization of emergency medical calls;
- organization of the appropriate response;
- ensuring that medical assistance arrives rapidly;
- continuous radio link with the hospital during initial medical care;
- preparation of hospital reception;
- organization of interhospital and intrahospital transports;
- promotion of research and teaching in emergency and disaster medicine for medical, nursing and paramedical personnel.

In other countries separate accident, coronary and obstetric flying squads have been used to provide expert medical assistance at the scene, but in general their value has been difficult to establish and, at least in the UK, they are few in number and fragmented. Most hospitals do, however, have major accident protocols, which include the provision of suitably experienced and qualified medical and nursing staff at the scene of the incident. To ensure the appropriate level of response, it is essential to establish good communications and to ensure that the response is supervised and coordinated by a senior physician in the receiving hospital's emergency department.

CONDUCT OF PRIMARY TRANSPORT

Occupational fatality rates in the emergency medical services exceed those of the general population and most frequently involve transportation incidents (vehicle/air crashes or pedestrian accidents). Other causes of death have included smoke inhalation, electrocution, drowning and needlesticks (Maguire *et al.*, 2002). Even moderate injury to a member of the pre-hospital team reduces the help available at the scene and produces an additional patient requiring assessment and treatment. It is therefore important to take measures to secure the safety of personnel involved in pre-hospital care, including the provision of safe transport, as well as issuing protective, clearly visible, clothing and headgear, with clear identification. Environmental safety measures such as controlling fires and protection from oncoming traffic are also important.

Conventionally two broad approaches to the primary transport of seriously ill patients have been described.

- *Scoop and run* is intended to avoid wasting valuable time while inadequately trained personnel attempt complex life-saving measures.
- The alternative approach of *field stabilization* or *stay and play* is based on the premise that prior resuscitation may reduce morbidity and mortality, mainly by decreasing the risks of deterioration during transport, especially when journey times are long.

It remains unclear which of these approaches is to be preferred (Koppenberg and Taeger, 2002) and in practice the most appropriate course of action in an individual patient is dictated by the anticipated journey time, the nature of the illness or injury and whether or not the victim is trapped. Thus when the patient is close to a hospital in an urban environment, immediate transfer is often preferable, whereas when longer distances are involved, the patient should be fully resuscitated before being moved. If extended transport times are anticipated, treatment of life-threatening injuries may begin at the scene and continue during transport. In most cases it is possible to relieve the most serious problem(s) by simple, quick interventions, followed by rapid transfer, without delay to the most appropriate hospital (*play and run*). Patients with penetrating thoracic injuries involving the myocardium are best taken immediately to the nearest major hospital with only the minimum of pre-hospital care, whereas tracheal intubation before transfer is clearly indicated for many head injuries.

All patients should receive *supplemental oxygen* to an *unobstructed airway* and most will benefit from establishing venous access and *expansion of their circulating volume* before transfer. *Stabilization of the cervical spine* is quick and of proven value, whereas application of military antishock trousers (MAST) takes time and is of uncertain benefit (see Chapter 5). *Pleural drainage*, when indicated, is most easily established via the second intercostal space in the midclavicular line where the drain can be easily observed with the patient on a stretcher. A *Heimlich valve* connected to a simple wound drainage bag can be useful under these circumstances. Appropriate intravenous, gaseous or regional *analgesia* should usually be given, and gross angulated *fractures* with vascular compression should be corrected and splinted. Objects impaling the trunk should not be removed. *Hypothermia* may compromise the immune and haematopoietic responses to injury, may be complicated by coagulopathy and can jeopardize vital organ function. Importantly, hypothermia on admission has been shown to be independently associated with increased mortality after major trauma (Wang *et al.*, 2005). Except in certain special circumstances, for example following cardiopulmonary resuscitation (see Chapter 9) or traumatic brain injury (see Chapter 15), it is therefore important to institute measures to restore or maintain body temperature.

BENEFITS OF PRE-HOSPITAL EMERGENCY TREATMENT

The provision of pre-hospital emergency medical services is of proven value for victims of a cardiac arrest provided that cardiopulmonary resuscitation is initiated by a bystander, the paramedics arrive at the scene within a few minutes and the patient is rapidly transferred to hospital for definitive care. The benefits for trauma victims are less clear, except when a coordinated approach from primary transport to specialized trauma centres is established (see below; Biewener et al., 2004).

SECONDARY TRANSPORT

Considerably fewer seriously ill patients require secondary transport, although in the UK it is thought that at least 10 000 critically ill patients require interhospital transfer each year (Mackenzie et al., 1997). The increasing tendency to concentrate specialist services such as trauma, neurosurgery, plastic surgery, cardiothoracic surgery, nephrology and intensive care in regional centres is likely to increase the demand for secondary transfer of the most seriously ill patients (Wallace and Lawler, 1997).

PRINCIPLES OF SAFE SECONDARY TRANSPORT
(Tables 21.1 and 21.2) (Australian and New Zealand College of Anaesthetists, Joint Faculty of Intensive Care Medicine, Australasian College for Emergency Medicine, 2003; Intensive Care Society, 2002; Wallace and Ridley, 1999; Warren et al., 2004)

Optimize patient's condition before transfer

Prior stabilization is fundamental to the safe transfer of critically ill patients – the 'scoop and run' approach described above for primary transport is not appropriate in this

---

Table 21.1 Transporting critically ill patients: a checklist

Administration	Equipment
Administration	**Equipment**
Establish effective communication between transferring and receiving hospitals and ambulance authority	Provision of respiratory support and monitoring 　Equipment for airway management 　Gas supply: oxygen ± air 　Cylinders 　Portable liquid oxygen containers 　Air compressor 　Portable ventilator 　Heat and moisture exchanger 　Suction apparatus 　(Extracorporeal membrane oxygenation) 　Airway pressure gauge 　Pulse oximeter 　Capnography
Notify and explain reasons for transfer to relatives	
For the conscious patient, explain the reasons for the transfer	
Collect together patient records to accompany patient	
Ensure appropriately experienced and qualified staff accompany patient	
Select most appropriate mode of transport: surface ambulance, air transport (fixed-wing, helicopter), sea	Provision of cardiovascular monitoring and support 　Fluid administration: infusion pumps 　Vasoactive agents and inotropes: syringe pumps 　Portable defibrillator 　Continuous electrocardiogram monitoring 　Continuous direct intra-arterial pressure monitoring 　(Pulmonary artery pressures) 　(Intracranial pressure) 　(Cardiac output) 　(Intra-aortic balloon pump) 　(Continuous haemofiltration)
Before transfer, receiving location confirms that they are ready to receive the patient	
Document reasons for transfer in medical record	
Preparation of patient	
Optimize patient's condition 　Circulating volume 　Haemodynamic support 　Respiratory support 　Appropriate monitoring 　Evaluate need for sedation, analgesia and muscle relaxants 　Rarely need surgery before transfer	Drugs 　Resuscitation drugs 　Antiarrhythmics 　Sedatives/analgesics 　Muscle relaxants 　Crystalloids/colloids
Underwater seal drains: do not clamp or lift above patient	
Nutritional support: if this is discontinued, beware of hypoglycaemia	Mobile phones
Maintain body temperature (warming blanket)	
Investigations 　Radiographs to confirm position of endotracheal tube, intravascular cannulae and chest drains	

Table 21.2 Principles of safe transfer

Experienced staff
Appropriate equipment and vehicle
Full assessment and investigation
Comprehensive monitoring
Stabilize patient before transfer
Reassessment before transport
Continuing care during transfer
Direct handover
Documentation and audit

situation (Gebremichael *et al.*, 2000; Uusaro *et al.*, 2002). A detailed systems-based assessment of the patient's condition should be performed before instituting measures to prepare the patient for transfer. Most will require optimization of their circulating volume (hypovolaemic patients are intolerant of transfer), as well as institution of mechanical ventilation and appropriate monitoring if these are not already in progress. Needless to say, reliable venous access must be established. Because endotracheal intubation in transit can be extremely difficult it is advisable to intubate those at risk of developing a compromised airway or respiratory failure before departure. Intubated patients should be mechanically ventilated.

It is important to ensure adequate sedation, analgesia and, when indicated, muscle relaxation before moving the patient. A few may need surgery before transfer (e.g. to evacuate an acute intracranial haematoma). Investigations may include radiographs to confirm the positions of the endotracheal tube, intravascular cannulae and chest drains. These must be securely tied or sutured in place before moving the patient. Underwater seal drains should not be clamped or lifted above the patient during transfer. It is important to appreciate that abrupt cessation of glucose administration (e.g. if parenteral nutrition is discontinued) may precipitate dangerous hypoglycaemia. A nasogastric tube should be inserted in those with an ileus or intestinal obstruction and in patients requiring mechanical ventilation. Measures should be taken to maintain body temperature. If the patient is conscious the proposed transfer and all that is entailed should be explained to him or her.

Maintain a high standard of care during transfer

In general there should be no reduction in the level of care during transport; it is strongly recommended that a minimum of two people accompany all critically ill patients. Medically qualified personnel are nearly always involved in secondary transport, although occasionally it may be acceptable for a stable patient to be transferred by an experienced critical care nurse with another non-physician member of the critical care team (e.g. technician, paramedic). All unsta-

ble patients must, however, be accompanied by an appropriately trained doctor. In some countries (e.g. North America, Australia and France) comprehensive transport systems have been developed, but in the UK the provision of specialist services for secondary transfer remains poor and around 90% of patients are accompanied by staff from the referring hospital. Not only does this deprive the base hospital of on-call staff but the accompanying clinical team will usually have only limited experience of transferring critically ill patients.

This may partly account for the observation that medical care during transfer is often deficient. In a series of 50 mainly postoperative patients, for example, 7 developed life-threatening complications, including obstruction of an endotracheal tube, respiratory arrest, unrecognized disconnection of arterial and central venous cannulae and severe hypotension (Bion *et al.*, 1988). This study also suggested that patients under the care of experienced anaesthetists deteriorated less during transport than those supervised by other medical specialties (Bion *et al.*, 1988). It is therefore recommended that the patient should be accompanied by an experienced doctor competent in resuscitation, airway care, ventilation and other organ support. This doctor, usually an anaesthetist, should preferably have received training in intensive care and should ideally be trained and have experience in transport medicine (Koppenberg and Taeger, 2002). The doctor should be assisted by another doctor or a nurse, paramedic or technician familiar with intensive care procedures and equipment, although in many countries staff shortages mean that this ideal is not always achieved (Wallace and Ridley, 1999). A service for transporting extremely ill patients has been described in which the team consists of an attending physician with critical care training, a critical care nurse and a respiratory therapist. Even the driver has expertise and training in respiratory therapy, critical care medicine and transport physiology (Gebremichael *et al.*, 2000).

Personnel involved in patient transfer should not be prone to motion sickness, should not have ear or sinus disorders and should have no difficulty with working in a confined space. Although in general the patient's condition improves after initial resuscitation and, with careful medical care, does not usually deteriorate further during transport (Bion *et al.*, 1985), invasive monitoring, including pulmonary artery catheterization, has clearly demonstrated that transport can sometimes adversely affect even patients who have been adequately resuscitated.

The use of a *specialist transfer team* has been associated with significantly improved acute physiology of critically ill patients on arrival in the receiving unit and may reduce early mortality (Bellingan *et al.*, 2000). Certainly critically ill patients can be safely transferred provided that those involved are appropriately trained and equipped, with fewer than 1% dying during transfer and only 3% dying within 12 hours of arrival in the receiving unit (Bellingan *et al.*, 2000; Markakis *et al.*, 2006). Even the most seriously ill patients with severe, unstable respiratory and circulatory failure can be safely transferred over long distances by a dedicated transfer team using a customized, fully equipped ground transport vehicle (Gebremichael *et al.*, 2000; Uusaro *et al.*, 2002). It is even possible to transfer patients safely with severe acute respiratory distress syndrome (ARDS) without major complications (Gebremichael *et al.*, 2000; Uusaro *et al.*, 2002) and extracorporeal membrane oxygenation has been used during the transfer of hypoxaemic patients with severe ARDS (Rossaint *et al.*, 1997).

Communication and cooperation

Communication and cooperation between the transferring and receiving hospitals, as well as close liaison with the ambulance authority, are fundamental to the success of secondary transport. A decision to transfer should be made by senior clinicians only after a full assessment and discussion between referring and receiving hospitals, taking into account the balance of risk and benefit. The receiving unit should be informed of the estimated time of arrival. Continuity of patient care must be ensured by effective communication between medical and nursing staff at the referring and receiving institutions. Changes in the patient's condition and response to treatment during transfer should be recorded and this, together with a written summary of the patient's history (including the results of relevant laboratory investigations and imaging), and initial treatment and the indication for transfer, must be handed over to the receiving staff. When transfer is urgent, however, the preparation of written records should not delay departure – necessary documentation can be delivered later.

MODES OF TRANSPORT

Selection of the most appropriate mode of transport should be individualized and requires consideration of the following:

- the patient's diagnosis and the possible effects of transport on his or her condition;
- the degree of any instability;
- the urgency of the transfer;
- the level of medical care the patient is receiving;
- the level of medical care the patient requires;
- the availability and experience of staff,
- the distance and duration of the journey;
- the methods of transport available;
- the weather and traffic conditions;
- cost.

As a general principle transport should be performed smoothly, rather than at high speed.

SURFACE AMBULANCES

Surface ambulances are probably the most practical and efficient means of transport within urban areas and for journeys not exceeding 40–80 km (25–50 miles) or 2 hours' duration, and are satisfactory for the majority of patients. Despite recent improvements in the design of standard ambulances, however, unmodified multipurpose vehicles are not ideal for transferring critically ill patients. On the other hand, purpose-built mobile ICUs (MICUs) or critical care ambulances are expensive and inflexible.

The advantages of surface ambulances include:

- rapid mobilization,
- door-to-door service;
- no requirement for landing zone or runway;
- little or no restrictions due to weather;
- in an emergency the vehicle can be stopped at the roadside to facilitate performance of procedures;
- can divert to the nearest hospital if the patient deteriorates or supplies are exhausted;
- relative ease of personnel training,
- low cost.

The main disadvantages of surface transport include:

- long journey times, especially when there is traffic congestion, poor road conditions, inclement weather or roadworks;
- the uncomfortable rough ride, 'sway and bounce', vibration, repetitive acceleration/deceleration;
- motion sickness;
- limited accessibility, poor lighting and limited power;
- difficulty gaining access to remote or restricted areas.

AIR TRANSPORT

The main advantage of air transport is the shorter journey time; it is therefore used more frequently in North America and Australia where patients often have to be transported over long distances. Air transport may also be used to achieve rapid delivery of paramedics and doctors to the scene of the incident (see above). Elective movement of patients between hospitals by air may also be preferred because of the reduction in journey times. Generally air transport should be considered for journeys longer than about 80 km (50 miles), although the apparent speed often has to be balanced against organizational delays and the need for transfer between vehicles at the beginning and/or end of the journey.

Secondary transportation of trauma victims by air following stabilization at the receiving hospital can be performed safely and many consider this to be an important aspect of regionalized trauma care. Some authors (Moylan *et al.*, 1988) have demonstrated improved survival of trauma victims transported by air rather than surface ambulance, although the efficacy of air transport may depend on local geography, since in an urban setting the use of a helicopter appeared to offer no advantage compared to a sophisticated paramedic-based system of pre-hospital care (Schiller *et al.*, 1988). Certainly in the immediate vicinity of a trauma centre there appears to be no advantage of a helicopter emergency medical service (HEMS) as compared to ground ambulance. Further, even when the accident is a long distance from the trauma centre, the more aggressive on-site, medically directed approach adopted by HEMS may not be associated with significantly improved survival rates when compared to ground ambulance. On the other hand primary transfer by HEMS to a level 1 trauma centre reduces mortality dramatically when compared to ambulance transfer to a regional hospital, indicating that primary admission to a level 1 trauma centre is perhaps a more important determinant of improved survival than the mode of transport or the composition of the on-site team (Biewener *et al.*, 2004). The evidence regarding the potential benefits associated with HEMS is, however, conflicting and the subject continues to arouse controversy.

Dangers of air transportation

REDUCTION IN ATMOSPHERIC PRESSURE

Helicopter cabins are unpressurized and even in pressurized aircraft the cabin pressure is equivalent to an altitude of 2000–2500 metres (i.e. about 75 kPa). There is therefore a danger of precipitating *hypoxia*, especially in those breathing room air, although critically ill patients will, of course, be receiving supplemental oxygen. Increasing positive end-expiratory pressure seems to be a more effective means of reversing hypoxia than simply increasing inspired oxygen concentrations under these circumstances.

The reduction in atmospheric pressure may also be associated with *expansion of gas in closed cavities*. Pneumothoraces, for example, may enlarge and it is important to ensure that chest drains are patent and correctly positioned; in some cases prophylactic drainage may be indicated. There may also be damage to the middle ear if the eustachian tube is obstructed (e.g. in those with upper respiratory tract infections, sinusitis, ear infections or allergy), while expansion of air trapped in abscesses or behind crowns may cause toothache. Expansion of intracranial air in those with an open head injury may precipitate neurological deterioration. Expansion of gas in the gastrointestinal tract may be associated with discomfort, nausea, vomiting and shortness of breath. In extreme cases, venous return may be compromised and, if pain is severe, the vasovagal response may cause hypotension and syncope. The cuff on the endotracheal tube may also expand and, if the intracuff pressure exceeds about 25 mmHg, it may be wise to remove excess air; during descent the cuff may deflate and a leak can develop around the tube. The air in MASTs may also expand, causing worsening regional compression, while limbs encased in plaster of Paris can swell and may have to be released using plaster shears. Expansion of the air in intravenous fluid containers may increase the rate of transfusion. Finally, decompression sickness can be aggravated.

The effect of air space expansion at altitude (e.g. in those with gut distension, blocked sinuses or intracranial air) can be minimized by administering 100% oxygen to denitrogenate the patient before and during the flight. Patients with bowel obstruction and those who have recently undergone abdominal surgery must have a patent nasogastric tube in place before transport.

EFFECTS OF TURBULENCE

Apart from precipitating *nausea and vomiting* with a risk of aspiration, turbulence may have adverse effects on *unstable spinal fractures* and on an *irritable myocardium*.

TEMPERATURE AND HUMIDITY

Cabin temperature tends to fall at altitude and this may lead to an *increased metabolic rate* and oxygen demand. The reduction in humidity can cause *dehydration* in both the patient and the crew.

NOISE

Noise hampers communication, renders audible alarms useless and makes it difficult or impossible to use a stethoscope. It may also cause discomfort, headache, fatigue, nausea, visual disturbances, vertigo, temporary or permanent ear damage and poor performance of tasks. The use of ear plugs, headsets and helmets ameliorates the effects of noise.

VIBRATION

Vibration causes a slight increase in metabolic rate. Low-frequency vibration may lead to fatigue, shortness of breath, motion sickness, blurred vision and chest or abdominal pain. Vibration may also interfere with thermoregulation by causing vasoconstriction and a reduced ability to perspire.

GRAVITATIONAL FORCES

Gravitational forces occur during ascent and descent as well as during changes in speed or direction (see elsewhere in this chapter).

FLUID LOSSES

As barometric pressure falls, fluid may extravasate from the intravascular to the extravascular space, causing oedema, tachycardia and hypotension, as well as exacerbating the effects of dehydration.

EFFECTS IN THOSE WITH PENETRATING EYE INJURIES

Vomiting, coughing, straining and hypoxia may lead to expulsion of vitreous and other intraocular contents. Expansion of entrapped air may lead to discharge of the globe. Recommended preventive measures have included eye binding, sitting the patient up, the administration of 100% oxygen and antiemetics.

Problems caused by altitude may also be occasionally encountered when transporting by road over mountainous terrain.

Helicopters

When compared to surface transport, helicopters reduce journey times by between one-third and one-half, and, when simultaneously dispatched, provide shorter emergency call to hospital arrival times at distances greater than 16 km (10 miles). Non-simultaneously dispatched helicopter transport is faster than surface vehicles over distances greater than 72 km (45 miles) from the hospital (Diaz *et al.*, 2005). Helicopters also cause less road disruption and can facilitate patient management during a long transfer. They are also able to land close to an incident and gain access to difficult locations. Helicopters have been shown to be a practical means of transporting critically ill patients between hospitals (Kee *et al.*, 1992) but probably offer no advantage for short interhospital transfers (Koppenberg and Taeger, 2002). Although vibration and motion sickness can cause difficulties, transfer by helicopter may be less deleterious to critically ill patients than other forms of transport because:

- acceleration/deceleration can be achieved more smoothly than in a land vehicle;
- a helicopter only accelerates at the beginning of transfer, following which a steady speed can be maintained throughout the flight;
- there is less vibration;
- if patients are flown 'feet first' they will be tilted slightly head-up during acceleration and slightly head-down during deceleration – this may minimize the changes in cardiovascular function and intracranial pressure normally seen during transport (Kee *et al.*, 1992);
- helicopters typically fly at below 600 metres (2000 feet), thereby avoiding the problems associated with depressurization.

The disadvantages of helicopters include the requirement for a helipad or unobstructed landing zone, space and weight limitations, and the noise, which may interfere with monitoring, especially audible warning devices. Communication difficulties are overcome relatively easily by wearing headsets. Finally, helicopters need a minimum visibility to fly, although most other weather conditions are not usually a problem. They are generally more expensive than ground transport and have a poorer safety record.

Fixed-wing aircraft

Fixed-wing aircraft can be used for more rapid transport over longer distances (more than about 240 km (150 miles)). There is usually more space and the patient can often be positioned transversely to minimize the effect of acceleration/deceleration. Fixed-wing aircraft can fly above or around inclement weather. They can, of course, only operate from landing strips, and therefore intermediary transport is normally required.

TRANSPORT BY SEA

It is sometimes necessary to treat severely injured divers in a compression chamber on the surface at the scene of the accident. In some circumstances the patient may subsequently be transferred under pressure. More often the patient is treated and resuscitated before being rapidly evacuated to a specialist facility onshore.

EQUIPMENT FOR TRANSPORT

MICUs consist of a dedicated, purpose-built vehicle and trolley equipped to provide respiratory support and continuous monitoring. Some are large and aim to recreate as closely as possible the intensive care environment, including the provision of advanced ventilatory support, full invasive haemodynamic monitoring and a well-stocked pharmacy (Gebremichael *et al.*, 2000). Alternatively trolleys can be designed to fit into conventional ambulances. Such trolleys should be robust but light, stable and manoeuvrable and fit easily into lifts and through doorways. They must be fully equipped with their own supply of power and gas so that they can provide patient support independently. All equipment must be securely mounted while in transit and should not be placed on the patient. Equipment must be robust, light-weight and battery-powered.

A comprehensive selection of drugs must be available during transfer, including resuscitation drugs, sedatives, analgesics and muscle relaxants, as well as reserve supplies of drugs currently being administered. All battery-operated equipment must be fully charged and capable of functioning for the duration of the transfer, and should be checked before departure.

PROVISION OF RESPIRATORY SUPPORT
Gas supply

The gas supply can be from *cylinders*, which are relatively heavy and cumbersome, require reducing valves and flow gauges, and cannot be refilled on-site, or *portable liquid oxygen containers*, which have a built-in flowmeter, connect directly to the equipment or a facemask and overcome the problem of safety and weight in aircraft. Flexible pipeline extensions can be used to connect to wall supplies in hospitals and to larger cylinders in ambulances. Accurate low-flow oxygen delivery is also required for those breathing spontaneously. Gas-powered ventilators will entrain air, but have a limited selection of inspired oxygen concentrations, whereas minute volume dividers will require a source of diluent gas (either air or nitrous oxide) as well as a supply of oxygen. Compressed air is best provided by a compressor to avoid the difficulties associated with cylinders. An audible alarm must be used to warn of failure of the oxygen supply or the accidental delivery of a hypoxic mixture of gases, bearing in mind the limitations of an audible alarm in a noisy transport vehicle. Vehicles must carry sufficient oxygen to last the journey, with a reserve of 1–2 hours.

Mechanical ventilation

Equipment for establishing and maintaining a secure airway, appropriately sized for the individual patient, must be available during transport. Laryngeal mask airways are not an acceptable means of securing the airway in critically ill patients during transport. Manual ventilation with self-inflating bags may be associated with inadequate ventilation,

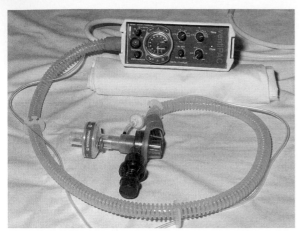

Fig. 21.1 A compact portable ventilator for transporting critically ill patients.

carbon dioxide retention and hypoxaemia. Mechanical ventilation is therefore preferred and it should be possible to apply a positive end-expiratory pressure when necessary. Self-inflating bags for manual ventilation must, however, be available in case the mechanical ventilator fails. Transport ventilators (**Fig. 21.1**) must incorporate disconnect and high-airway-pressure alarms, as well as a back-up battery power supply. Although *capnography* can be unreliable during transport, it is the only continuous method of ensuring that the endotracheal tube has not been displaced. It also provides a visual disconnect alarm and can be helpful in detecting catastrophic reductions in cardiac output. To fulfil these roles, the chosen capnograph must have a continuous graphic display. *Pulse oximeters* are an invaluable means of continuously monitoring oxygenation. Some MICUs designed for the transport of extremely ill patients, such as those with severe ARDS, incorporate facilities for on-board blood gas analysis and fibreoptic bronchoscopy. They also carry conventional intensive care ventilators, rather than smaller transport devices (Gebremichael *et al.*, 2000).

Humidification of inspired gases is best achieved using a heat and moisture exchanger. Electrically operated *suction apparatus* can be used in ambulances and aircraft, but manual or Venturi devices are preferred when transporting patients on trolleys.

PROVISION OF CARDIOVASCULAR MONITORING AND SUPPORT

During transport intravenous fluid is most accurately and reliably administered using an infusion pump. Syringe pumps, which are cheaper, smaller and use less power, may be preferred for administering vasoactive agents and other drugs such as sedatives and analgesics. All intravenous fluids and medications must be stored in plastic, *not glass*, containers. In many helicopters the ceiling is not high enough to guarantee gravitational delivery of fluids/blood for volume replacement. Pressure bags, or additional infusion pumps

are then required. (Beware of air embolism when fluid containers and giving sets are pressurized.)

Clinical assessment of cardiovascular function is extremely difficult during transport and it is therefore essential to establish reliable, accurate continuous monitoring of important haemodynamic variables using a light-weight battery-powered monitor. Devices are now available with excellent screen quality that allow continuous monitoring of two pressures, electrocardiogram (ECG), two temperatures, pulse oximetry, non-invasive blood pressure, capnography and cardiac output. *Continuous ECG monitoring* will detect arrhythmias and alterations in heart rate, and may indicate the development of myocardial ischaemia or biochemical abnormalities such as hyperkalaemia. A monitor capable of storing and retrieving data is preferred. Non-invasive measurement of blood pressure is difficult and unreliable during transport because of artefact and interference. Direct *intra-arterial pressure monitoring* is therefore preferred, and in some cases central venous pressure, intracranial pressure or, very occasionally, pulmonary artery pressures should also be continuously displayed. Because continuous flush systems are relatively bulky, intermittent manual flushing can be used as an alternative. Where possible, alarms should be visible, as well as audible, because of extraneous noise.

A portable external *defibrillator*, which may also display and print the ECG as well as acting as an external pacemaker, should be carried on all transport trolleys and in ambulances. Some trolleys and ambulances are designed to enable intra-aortic balloon counterpulsation to continue during transfer and, in some cases, especially when journey times are long, continuous arteriovenous haemodiafiltration may be necessary.

TRANSPORT WITHIN THE HOSPITAL

Intrahospital transport poses many of the same risks associated with, and may in some instances be more hazardous than, out-of-hospital transfers. Patients may be outside a critical care area (e.g. in the CT scanner) for long periods of time and it is possible to become stranded, for example in a hospital elevator without electricity or in the radiology department with a non-functioning gas supply.

Even for these relatively short journeys, adequate resuscitation and preparation before moving the patient, the provision of comprehensive continuous monitoring and meticulous care by skilled medical and nursing staff during transfer are essential.

Transfer within the hospital may be associated with various complications, including hypotension, hypertension, cardiac arrhythmias, airway obstruction and cardiac arrest (Link *et al.*, 1990). In an analysis of incident reports Beckmann *et al.* (2004) found that 39% of reports identified equipment problems, whilst 61% identified patient/staff management issues. Equipment-related problems commonly involved:

- battery/power supply;
- drug delivery systems;
- intubation equipment;
- transport ventilators;
- oxygen supply;
- monitors;
- access to patient elevators;

Patient/staff/management issues commonly involved:

- communication/liaison;
- airway management (securing, accidental extubation, unplanned reintubation);
- vascular line (dislodgement, disconnection, inadequately secured);
- patient monitoring and positioning;
- equipment set-up.

Significant adverse outcomes, including major physiological derangement and even death, occurred in about a third of these incidents; most seemed to be multifactorial in origin.

Transfer is further complicated if the patient is emerging from anaesthesia on return from the operating theatre. It is important to move at a time and along a route likely to be associated with the least delay, and it is sensible to delegate a team member to commandeer lifts and clear corridors.

TRANSPORT OVER LONG DISTANCES

Transport over long distances poses special problems, especially when international travel is involved. In most cases the patient should not be moved until the acute illness has resolved. Transfer can then be by private aeromedical transport organization, military aircraft, chartered executive jet or commercial airliner, preferably non-stop. Arrangements can be complex, and good liaison is essential. It is important that sufficient staff are employed to allow them to work conventional 8–12-hour shifts. In a commercial jet aircraft up to 15 seats may be required for a complex case – 6–8 for the stretcher, two for the equipment, two for medical gases and one for each team member. A spare ventilator, preferably able to operate using room air, and twice the anticipated gas supplies should be carried. On these long flights waste disposal becomes an important consideration.

REFERENCES

Australian and New Zealand College of Anaesthetists, Joint Faculty of Intensive Care Medicine, Australasian College for Emergency Medicine (2003) Minimum standards for intrahospital transport of critically ill patients. Available online at: www.medeserv.com.au/anzca/publications/profdocs/profstandards/ps39_2003.htm.

Baxt WG, Moody P (1987) The impact of a physician as part of the aeromedical prehospital team in patients with blunt trauma. *Journal of the American Medical Association* 257: 3246–3250.

Beckmann U, Gillies DM, Berenholtz SM, et al. (2004) Incidents relating to the intra-hospital transfer of critically ill patients. *Intensive Care Medicine* 30: 1579–1585.

Bellingan G, Olivier T, Batson S, et al. (2000) Comparison of a specialist retrieval team with current United Kingdom practice for the transport of critically ill patients. *Intensive Care Medicine* 26: 740–744.

Biewener A, Aschenbrenner U, Rammelt S, et al. (2004) Impact of helicopter transport and hospital level on mortality of polytrauma patients. *Journal of Trauma* 56: 94–98.

Bion JF, Edlin SA, Ramsay G, et al. (1985) Validation of a prognostic score in critically ill patients undergoing transport. *British Medical Journal* 291: 432–434.

Bion JF, Wilson IH, Taylor PA (1988) Transporting critically ill patients by ambulance: audit by sickness scoring. *British Medical Journal* 296: 170.

Díaz MA, Hendey GW, Bivins HG (2005) When is the helicopter faster? A comparison of helicopter and ground ambulance transport times. *Journal of Trauma* 58: 148–153.

Gebremichael M, Borg U, Habashi N, et al. (2000) Interhospital transport of the extremely ill patient: the mobile intensive care unit. *Critical Care Medicine* 28: 79–85.

Intensive Care Society (2002) Guidelines for the transport of the critically ill adult. Available online at: www.ics.ac.uk.

Kee SS, Ramage CM, Mendel P, et al. (1992) Interhospital transfers by helicopter: the first 50 patients of the Careflight project. *Journal of the Royal Society of Medicine* 85: 29–31.

Koppenberg J, Taeger K (2002) Interhospital transport: transport of critically ill patients. *Current Opinion in Anaesthesiology* 15: 211–215.

Link J, Krause H, Wagner W, et al. (1990) Intrahospital transport of critically ill patients. *Critical Care Medicine* 18: 1427–1429.

Mackenzie PA, Smith EA, Wallace PG (1997) Transfer of adults between intensive care units in the United Kingdom: postal survey. *British Medical Journal* 314: 1455–1456.

Maguire BJ, Hunting KL, Smith GS, et al. (2002) Occupational fatalities in emergency medical services: a hidden crisis. *Annals of Emergency Medicine* 40: 625–632.

Markakis C, Dalezios M, Chatzicostas C, et al. (2006) Evaluation of a risk score for interhospital transport of critically ill patients. *Emergency Medicine Journal* 23: 313–317.

Moylan JA, Fitzpatrick KT, Beyer AJ III, et al. (1988) Factors improving survival in multisystem trauma patients. *Annals of Surgery* 207: 679–685.

Rossaint R, Pappert D, Gerlach H, et al. (1997) Extracorporeal membrane oxygenation for transport of hypoxaemic patients with severe ARDS. *British Journal of Anaesthesia* 78: 241–246.

Schiller WR, Knox R, Zinnecker H, et al. (1988) Effect of helicopter transport of trauma victims on survival in an urban trauma center. *Journal of Trauma* 28: 1127–1134.

Uusaro A, Parviainen I, Takala J, et al. (2002) Safe long-distance interhospital ground transfer of critically ill patients with acute severe unstable respiratory and circulatory failure. *Intensive Care Medicine* 28: 1122–1125.

Wallace PG, Lawler PG (1997) Bed shortages. Regional intensive care unit transfer teams are needed. *British Medical Journal* 314: 369.

Wallace PG, Ridley SA (1999) Transport of critically ill patients. *British Medical Journal* 319: 368–371.

Wang HE, Callaway CW, Peitzman AB, et al. (2005) Admission hypothermia and outcome after major trauma. *Critical Care Medicine* 33: 1296–1301.

Warren J, Fromm RE, Orr RA, et al. (2004) Guidelines for the inter- and intrahospital transport of critically ill patients. *Critical Care Medicine* 32: 256–262.

Appendices

Normal values

Table A1 Normal haemodynamic values	
Mean arterial pressure (MAP)	70–100 mmHg
Central venous pressure (CVP)	2–8 mmHg
Right ventricular pressures	14–30/0–7 mmHg
Pulmonary artery pressures	16–24/5–12 mmHg
Mean pulmonary artery pressure	9–16 mmHg
Pulmonary artery occlusion pressure (PAOP)	5–12 mmHg
Left ventricular end-diastolic pressure (LVEDP)	4–10 mmHg
Cardiac output (Q_t)	4–6 L/min
Cardiac index (CI)	2.8–3.5 L/min per m^2
Stroke volume (SV)	50–100 mL
Stroke volume index (SVI)	30–50 mL/m^2
Right ventricular stroke work index (RVSWI)	4–12 g/m per m^2
Left ventricular stroke work index (LVSWI)	44–68 g/m per m^2
Systemic vascular resistance (SVR)	900–1200 dyn.s/cm^5
Systemic vascular resistance index (SVRI)	1700–2600 dyn.s/cm^5 per m^2
Pulmonary vascular resistance (PVR)	120–200 dyn.s/cm^5
Pulmonary vascular resistance index (PVRI)	210–360 dyn.s/cm^5 per m^2
Ejection fraction	50–60%

Table A2 Normal oxygen transport values	
Oxygen delivery index ($\dot{D}o_2$)	520–720 mL/min per m^2
Oxygen consumption index ($\dot{V}o_2$)	100–180 mL/min per m^2
Arterial oxygen content (C_ao_2)	18–21 vol%
Mixed venous oxygen content ($C_{\bar{v}}o_2$)	13–16 vol%
Arteriovenous oxygen content difference ($C_{a-\bar{v}}o_2$)	4–5 vol%
Oxygen extraction ratio (OER)	0.22–0.30

Normal values (continued)

Table A3 Normal respiratory values

	Male	Female
Dead-space fraction (V_D/V_T)	< 0.35	
Alveolar–arterial oxygen difference ($P_{A-a}O_2$)		
$F_IO_2 = 0.21$	5–25 mmHg	
$F_IO_2 = 1.0$	< 150 mmHg	
Percentage venous admixture ($\dot{Q}_v/\dot{Q}_t\%$) (shunt fraction)	3–8%	
Static total thoracic compliance	70–100 mL/cm H_2O	
Airflow resistance	< 3 cm H_2O/L per s	
FEV_1 (L)	2.2–4.7	1.3–3.6
FVC (L)	3.2–4.7	1.8–4.5
FEV_1/FVC (%)	66–83	71–81
PEFR (L/min)	460–680	280–400

FEV1, forced expiratory volume in 1 second; FVC, forced vital capacity; PEFR, peak expiratory flow rate.

Table A4 Normal lung volumes in a 60-kg male

Tidal volume (V_T)	400–600 mL
Inspiratory reserve volume (IRV)	3330–3740 mL
Expiratory reserve volume (ERV)	950–1200 mL
Functional residual capacity (FRC)	2300–2600 mL
Residual volume (RV)	1200–1700 mL
Vital capacity (VC)	3800–5000 mL

Index

hypokalaemia 297, 298
hypomagnesaemia 298
invasive respiratory support 169
near-drowning 285
NSTEMI 241
poisoning 509
pulmonary embolism 130
STEMI 241–2, 243
supraventricular *vs* ventricular
    tachycardia 258
during transfer 548
traumatic coma patients 408
electrocution 254
electroencephalography (EEG)
    confirming brain death 426
    continuous monitoring 411
    frequency changes in head injury 411
    hepatic coma 386
    hepatic encephalopathy 383
electrolyte balance/disturbances 291–301
    ALF 384, 386, 391
    brain damage management 419
    cardiorespiratory arrest 251
    fulminant hepatic failure 390
    hyperthermia 535
    management principles 293–4
    near-drowning 285
    tetanus 439
    see also specific disorders
electrolyte measurements 105
electrolyte replacement 478
electromyography 440
electrophysiological testing 447
electrostatic charges at alveolar–capillary
    barrier 42
elemental diets 303
embolic ischaemic colitis 465
emergency back-up equipment 5
emphysema 216, 217
    subcutaneous 164
empyema 199
encephalitis 422
    acute 422
    mortality/survival 422
    viral 341, 343, 422
encephalomyelitis 422
encephalopathy 97–8
    fulminant hepatic failure 390
    hepatic 383, 384
        grading system 385
        pathogenesis 388
end-of-life care 16–21
    comfort care/double effect 19
    consensus 19–21
    decision-making 16–17
        shared decision-making model
        20–1
    withdrawing treatment 19
end-tidal carbon dioxide tension
    ($P_{E}CO_2$) 144
    in cardiopulmonary resuscitation 248

endocardial damage 59
endocarditis 67, 70
endocrine disturbances
    and brain death 425
    calcium metabolism 485–8
    in organ donor 429–30
    pituitary emergencies 491–2
endocrine emergencies 473–93
    adrenal crisis 489–91
    diabetes mellitus 473–81
    phaeochromocytoma 488–9
    thyroid emergencies 481–5
endogenous (autogenous) infection
    331–3
    primary/secondary 331
endoluminal brush sampling 338
endophthalmitis 347
β-endorphin 82
endoscopic oesophageal variceal banding
    459
endoscopic retrograde
        cholangiopancreatography (ERCP)
        469
endoscopic sclerosis 459
endoscopy
    acute pancreatitis 469
    upper gastrointestinal haemorrhage
        454
endothelial injury
    in ARDS/ALI 224, 226
    in sepsis 94
endothelial NOS (eNOS) 90
endothelial permeability 153–4
endothelins
    in ALF 387
    endothelin-1 90
endothelium-derived vasoactive
        mediators 89–90
endotoxins 85
    antibiotic-mediated release 339
    investigation 106
    see also antiendotoxins
endotracheal intubation *see* tracheal
        intubation
endotracheal tubes 266
energy requirements 307
enflurane 316
enkephalins 82
enoxaparin 244
enoximone 116
enteral nutrition 301–3
    administration 302–3
    administration sets 303
    airway protection 303
    benefits 301–2
    choice of feed 303
    elemental diets 303
    prokinetic agents 303
    vs parenteral 302
Enterobacter spp.
    aspiration pneumonia 235

    and malignancy 352
    nosocomial infection 329
Enterococcus spp.
    E. faecalis 339, 342
    vancomycin-resistant (VRE) 329, 333
Entonox
    burn trauma 276
    chest trauma 270
epidermal growth factor (EGF) 368
epidural analgesia/anaesthesia 314–15
    in tetanus 438
    thoracic 271
epiglottitis 221–2
epilepsy 433
    see also status epilepticus
epinephrine *see* adrenaline
epithelial injury 224
epithelial permeability 153–4
Epstein–Barr virus 382
eptifibatide 244
equipment
    emergency back-up 5
    ICU design 5
    required in regional ICU 6
    technical support 7
    transport 543, 547
erythromycin 209
    antibiotic regimens 340, 345
    in enteral nutrition 303
    pneumonia 339
    in tetanus 437
Escherichia coli
    antibiotic regimens 341, 342, 343
    and malignancy 352
    nosocomial infection 329
    toxins 87
esmolol 438
ethanol
    as methanol antidote 513
    poisoning 512–13
ethical issues
    brain death 424–5
    ethics committees/consultants 19
    withholding/withdrawing treatment
        17
etomidate 83, 84
    in brain injury 405, 413, 416
evoked potentials 412
    auditory 312, 412
    somatosensory 412, 414
    in traumatic coma 414
exercise 37
exogenous infection 331, 333–4
    cross-contamination 333
exotoxins 85, 436
expiratory reserve volume (ERV) 45
    normal 553
    in pregnancy 495
expired air gas composition 143–4
expired capnograms 143
expired minute volume ($\dot{V}_{E}$) 38

indications 305–6
liver function tests 309, 310
monitoring 309–10
paediatric feeding tubes 306
perioperative 305
protein/nitrogen 306–7, 308
total thoracic compliance 46–7
normal 553
toxaemia
obstetric deaths 496
pre-eclamptic (PET) 497
TOXBASE 508, 525
toxic megacolon 344
toxic shock syndrome 86
toxins 85
Toxoplasma gondii 353, 422
TPN *see* total parenteral nutrition
tracheal intubation 169–70, 184–6
in brain damage 405–6
in cardiorespiratory arrest 248
complications 184–5
minimization 185
in eclampsia 500
indications 184
in meningitis 422
obstruction 184
prolonged, effects of 184
re-intubation 183–4
in respiratory failure 203
in status epilepticus 433–4
in trauma 266
chest injuries 269, 271
spinal injuries 279, 284
after thermal injury 278
upper-airway obstruction 221
vs nasal 185–6
tracheal rupture 269
tracheal suctioning 203
tracheo-oesophageal fistulae 186
tracheostomy 186–9
benefits 186
in brain injury 416
complications
early 186
intermediate 186–7
late 187
contraindications 186
decannulation 189
indications 186
management 188–9
percutaneous bronchoscopic guidance
188
in respiratory failure 203
in spinal injury 284
techniques
cricothyroidotomy 188
mini-tracheostomy 188
percutaneous 187–8
surgical 187
tracheostomy tubes 188–9
modified 189

in trauma 266, 271, 278–9
upper-airway obstruction 221
tramadol 313
tranexamic acid 456
transcellular fluid 291
tranquillizers 316–17
transcapillary refill 94
transcranial near-infrared spectroscopy
411
transcutaneous measurement 151–2
transfusion, blood 109
blood substitutes 111
complications 109–10
gastrointestinal haemorrhage 454–5
preoperative autologous donation
111
safety 110–11
transfusion-related acute lung injury
(TRALI) 109, 110
transjugular intrahepatic portosystemic
shunting (TIPS) 459–60
translaryngeal tracheostomy technique
187
transoesophageal echocardiography
in aortic trauma 273
in endocarditis 338
transoesophageal echocardiography
(TOE) 66, 68, 71
in shock 104
vs transthoracic 71
transport 541–9
checklist 543
equipment 543, 547
within hospital 548–9
long-distance 549
modes 545–7
air transport 545–7
fixed-wing aircraft 547
helicopters 546–7
long-distance 549
sea transport 547
surface ambulances 545
patient preparation 543
personnel 544
primary 541–3
conduct 542
play and run 542
pre-hospital team composition
541–2
pre-hospital treatment 543
scoop and run 542
stay and play (field stabilization)
542
risk scores 541
risks 541
secondary 541, 543–5
care during transfer 544–5
communication/cooperation 545
patient preparation 543–4
safety principles 543–5
specialist transfer team 544–5

transthoracic echocardiography (TTE)
66, 71
vs transoesophageal 71
transthoracic external pacing 251
transtracheal jet ventilation 221
transtracheal needle aspiration (TTA)
336
trauma 265–90
burns 273–9
causes of death 289
chest injuries 268–73
complications 289
crush injuries 267, 287–8
fat embolism syndrome 267, 288–9
as intensive care admission indication 2
management 289
see also specific conditions
near-drowning 284–7
spinal injuries 279–84
Trauma and Injury Severity Scoring
System (TRISS) 21, 27, 31
trauma centres 289
trauma resuscitation 265–8
ABCDE mnemonic 265, 266
airway/cervical spine control 265–6
life-threatening/hidden injuries
266
breathing 266
circulation 266–7
disability/neurological status 267
exposure/environment control 267
principles 265
radiological assessment 267–8
re-evaluation 267
traumatic brain injury (TBI) 401, 405
immediate care 404
mortality/survival 420
specialist treatment 414
traumatic coma 197
electrocardiography 408
evoked potentials 414
traumatic rhabdomyolysis *see* crush
syndrome
traumatic spinal cord damage 198
treatment plans 8
tricyclic antidepressants 323
in Guillain–Barré syndrome 445
in hyperthermia 533
overdose management 516–17
in respiratory failure 203
triggering receptor expressed on myeloid
cells-1 (TREM-1) 106
trimethoprim 330
antibiotic regimens 342
trismus 436, 438
TRISS *see* Trauma and Injury Severity
Scoring System
troponins
cardiac-specific 242
troponin I 242
troponin T 242